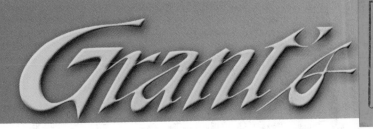

Atlas of Anatomy Twelfth Edition

1   THORAX 1

WEEK DOMEN 95

PELVIS AND PERINEUM 193

4   BACK 285

5   LOWER LIMB 353

6   UPPER LIMB 475

7   HEAD 607

8   NECK 745

9   CRANIAL

INDEX 845

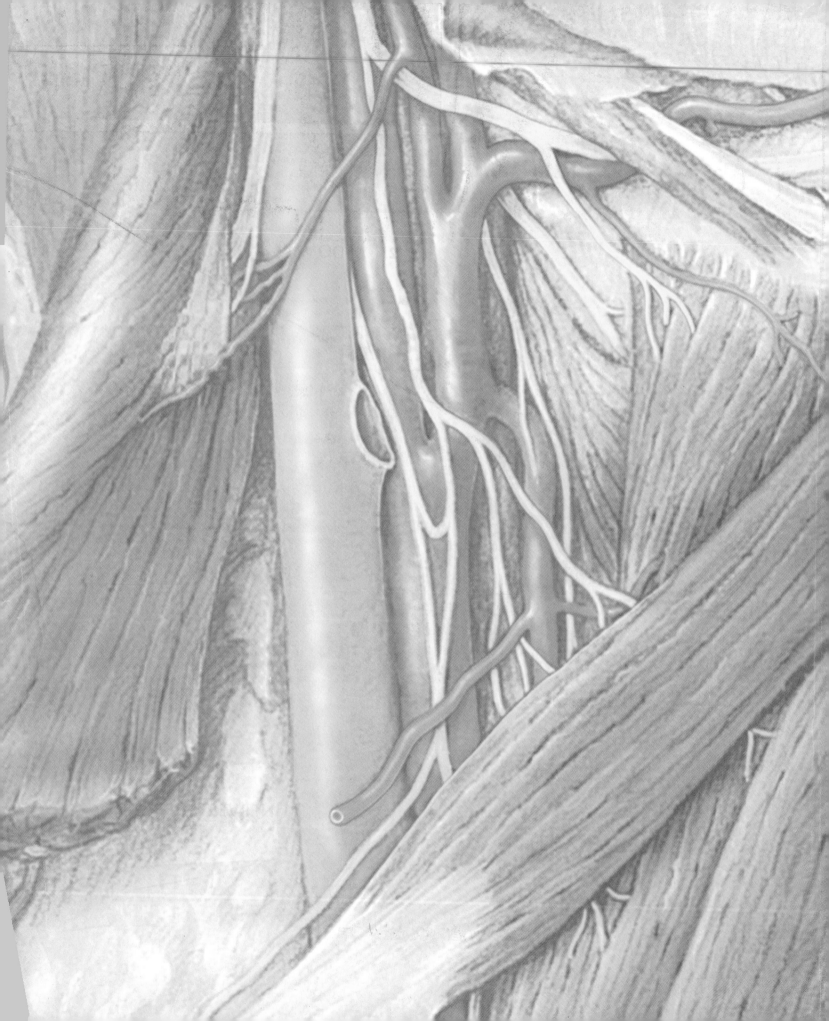

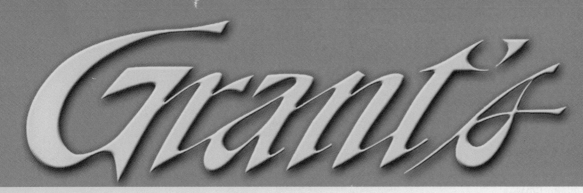

Atlas of Anatomy Twelfth Edition

Anne M.R. Agur, B.Sc. (OT), M.Sc.

Professor, Division of Anatomy, Department of Surgery, Faculty of Medicine
Department of Physical Therapy, Department of Occupational Therapy,
Division of Biomedical Communications, Institute of Medical Science
Graduate Department of Rehabilitation Science, Graduate Department of Dentistry
University of Toronto
Toronto, Ontario, Canada

Arthur F. Dalley II, Ph.D.

Professor, Department of Cell & Developmental Biology
Adjunct Professor, Department of Orthopaedics and Rehabilitation
Vanderbilt University School of Medicine
Adjunct Professor of Anatomy
Belmont University School of Physical Therapy
Nashville, Tennessee, U.S.A.

Wolters Kluwer | Lippincott Williams & Wilkins
Health

Philadelphia · Baltimore · New York · London
Buenos Aires · Hong Kong · Sydney · Tokyo

Acquisitions Editor: Crystal Taylor
Senior Developmental Editor: Kathleen H. Scogna
Marketing Manager: Valerie Sanders
Creative Director: Doug Smock
Managing Editor, Production: Eve Malakoff-Klein
Compositor: Maryland Composition, Inc.
Printer: C&C Offset Printing

Twelfth Edition

By J.C.B. Grant:
First Edition, 1943   Second Edition, 1947
Third Edition, 1951   Fourth Edition, 1956
Fifth Edition, 1962   Sixth Edition, 1972
By J.E. Anderson:
Seventh Edition, 1978   Eighth Edition, 1983
By A.M.R. Agur:
Ninth Edition, 1991   Tenth Edition, 1999
Eleventh Edition, 2005

351 West Camden Street   530 Walnut Street
Baltimore, Maryland 21201-2436 USA   Philadelphia, Pennsylvania 19106-3621 USA

Printed in Hong Kong

9 8 7 6 5 4 3 2 1

Library of Congress Cataloging-in-Publication Data

Agur, A. M. R.
 Grant's atlas of anatomy/Anne M.R. Agur, Arthur F. Dalley II.—12th ed.
   p. ; cm.
 Includes bibliographical references and index.
 ISBN 978-0-7817-9604-0 (hardcover ed.)—ISBN 978-0-7817-7055-2 (softcover ed.) 1. Human anatomy—Atlases. I. Dalley, Arthur F. II. Title. III.
Title: Atlas of anatomy.
 [DNLM: 1. Anatomy, Regional—Atlases. QS 17 A284g 2009]
 QM25.A38 2009
 611.0022'2—dc22

                                        2007043565

DISCLAIMER

Care has been taken to confirm the accuracy of the information presented and to describe generally accepted practices. However, the authors, editors, and publisher are not responsible for errors or omissions or for any consequences from application of the information in this book and make no warranty, expressed or implied, with respect to the currency, completeness, or accuracy of the contents of the publication. Application of this information in a particular situation remains the professional responsibility of the practitioner; the clinical treatments described and recommended may not be considered absolute and universal recommendations.

The authors, editors, and publisher have exerted every effort to ensure that drug selection and dosage set forth in this text are in accordance with the current recommendations and practice at the time of publication. However, in view of ongoing research, changes in government regulations, and the constant flow of information relating to drug therapy and drug reactions, the reader is urged to check the package insert for each drug for any change in indications and dosage and for added warnings and precautions. This is particularly important when the recommended agent is a new or infrequently employed drug.

Some drugs and medical devices presented in this publication have Food and Drug Administration (FDA) clearance for limited use in restricted research settings. It is the responsibility of the health care provider to ascertain the FDA status of each drug or device planned for use in their clinical practice.

To purchase additional copies of this book, call our customer service department at **(800) 638-3030** or fax orders to **(301) 223-2320**. International customers should call (301) 223-2300.

Visit Lippincott Williams & Wilkins on the Internet: http://www.lww.com. Lippincott Williams & Wilkins customer service representatives are available from 8:30 am to 6:00 pm, EST.

To my husband Enno and my children Erik and Kristina
for their support and encouragement
(A.M.R.A.)

To Muriel
My bride, best friend, counselor, and mother of our sons;
To my family
Tristan, Lana, Elijah Grey, and Finley
Denver and Skyler
With great appreciation for their support, humor and patience
(A.F.D.)

DR. JOHN CHARLES BOILEAU GRANT
1886—1973

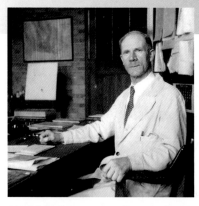

Dr. J.C.B. Grant in his office, McMurrich Building, University of Toronto, 1946. Through his textbooks, Dr. Grant made an indelible impression on the teaching of anatomy throughout the world.

by **Dr. Carlton G. Smith**, M.D., PH.D.
(1905–2003)
Professor Emeritus, Division of
Anatomy, Department of Surgery
Faculty of Medicine
University of Toronto, Canada

The life of J.C. Boileau Grant has been likened to the course of the seventh cranial nerve as it passes out of the skull: complicated, but purposeful.[1] He was born in the parish of Lasswade in Edinburgh, Scotland, on February 6, 1886. Dr. Grant studied medicine at the University of Edinburgh from 1903 to 1908. Here, his skill as a dissector in the laboratory of the renowned anatomist, Dr. Daniel John Cunningham (1850–1909), earned him a number of awards.

Following graduation, Dr. Grant was appointed the resident house officer at the Infirmary in Whitehaven, Cumberland. From 1909 to 1911, Dr. Grant demonstrated anatomy in the University of Edinburgh, followed by two years at the University of Durham, at Newcastle-on-Tyne in England, in the laboratory of Professor Robert Howden, editor of *Gray's Anatomy*.

With the outbreak of World War I in 1914, Dr. Grant joined the Royal Army Medical Corps and served with distinction. He was mentioned in dispatches in September 1916, received the Military Cross in September 1917 for "conspicuous gallantry and devotion to duty during attack," and received a bar to the Military Cross in August 1918.[1]

In October 1919, released from the Royal Army, he accepted the position of Professor of Anatomy at the University of Manitoba in Winnipeg, Canada. With the frontline medical practitioner in mind, he endeavored to "bring up a generation of surgeons who knew exactly what they were doing once an operation had begun."[1] Devoted to research and learning, Dr. Grant took interest in other projects, such as performing anthropometric studies of Indian tribes in northern Manitoba during the 1920s. In Winnipeg, Dr. Grant met Catriona Christie, whom he married in 1922.

Dr. Grant was known for his reliance on logic, analysis, and deduction as opposed to rote memory. While at the University of Manitoba, Dr. Grant began writing *A Method of Anatomy, Descriptive and Deductive*, which was published in 1937.[2]

In 1930, Dr. Grant accepted the position of Chair of Anatomy at the University of Toronto. He stressed the value of a "clean" dissection, with the structures well defined. This required the delicate touch of a sharp scalpel, and students soon learned that a dull tool was anathema. Instructive dissections were made available in the Anatomy Museum, a means of student review on which Dr. Grant placed a high priority. Many of these illustrations have been included in *Grant's Atlas of Anatomy*.

The first edition of the *Atlas*, published in 1943, was the first anatomical atlas to be published in North America.[3] *Grant's Dissector* preceded the *Atlas* in 1940.[4]

Dr. Grant remained at the University of Toronto until his retirement in 1956. At that time, he became Curator of the Anatomy Museum in the University. He also served as Visiting Professor of Anatomy at the University of California at Los Angeles, where he taught for 10 years.

Dr. Grant died in 1973 of cancer. Through his teaching method, still presented in the Grant's textbooks, Dr. Grant's life interest—human anatomy—lives on. In their eulogy, colleagues and friends Ross MacKenzie and J. S. Thompson said: "Dr. Grant's knowledge of anatomical fact was encyclopedic, and he enjoyed nothing better than sharing his knowledge with others, whether they were junior students or senior staff. While somewhat strict as a teacher, his quiet wit and boundless humanity never failed to impress. He was, in the very finest sense, a scholar and a gentleman."[1]

This edition of *Grant's Atlas* has, like its predecessors, required intense research, market input, and creativity. It is not enough to rely on a solid reputation; with each new edition, we have adapted and changed many aspects of the *Atlas* while maintaining the commitment to pedagogical excellence and anatomical realism that has enriched its long history. Medical and health sciences education, and the role of anatomy instruction and application within it, continually evolve to reflect new teaching approaches and educational models. The health care system itself is changing, and the skills and knowledge that future health care practitioners must master are changing along with it. Finally, technologic advances in publishing, particularly in online resources and electronic media, have transformed the way students access content and the methods by which educators teach content. All of these developments have shaped the vision and directed the execution of this twelfth edition of *Grant's Atlas*, as evidenced by the following key features:

Classic "Grant's" images updated for today's students. A unique feature of *Grant's Atlas* is that, rather than providing an idealized view of human anatomy, the classic illustrations represent actual dissections that the student can directly compare with specimens in the lab. Because the original models used for these illustrations were real cadavers, the accuracy of these illustrations is unparalleled, offering students the best introduction to anatomy possible. Over the years we have made many changes to the illustrations to match the shifting expectations of students, adding more vibrant colors and updating the style from the original carbon-dust renderings. In this edition, at the suggestion of reviewers, we have continued this trend by introducing more lifelike skin tones to provide a more realistic—but no less accurate--depiction of anatomy. In addition, almost all of these dissection figures were carefully analyzed to ensure that label placement remained effective and that the illustration's relevance was still clear. Almost every figure in this edition of *Grant's Atlas* was altered, from simple label changes to full-scale revision.

Schematic illustrations to facilitate learning. Full-color schematic illustrations supplement the dissection figures to clarify anatomical concepts, show the relationships of structures, and give an overview of the body region being studied. Many new schematic illustrations have been added to this edition; others have been revised to refine their pedagogical aspects. All conform to Dr. Grant's admonition to "keep it simple": extraneous labels were deleted, and some labels were added to identify key structures and make the illustrations as useful as possible to students. In addition, many new, simple orientation drawings were added for ease of identifying dissected regions.

Legends with easy-to find clinical applications. Admittedly, artwork is the focus of any atlas; however, the *Grant's* legends have long been considered a unique and valuable feature of the *Atlas*.

The observations and comments that accompany the illustrations draw attention to salient points and significant structures that might otherwise escape notice. Their purpose is to interpret the illustrations without providing exhaustive description. Readability, clarity, and practicality were emphasized in the editing of this edition. For the first time, clinical comments, which deliver practical "pearls" that link anatomic features with their significance in health care practice, are highlighted in blue within the figure legends. The clinical comments have also been expanded in this edition, providing even more relevance for students searching for medical application of anatomical concepts.

Enhanced diagnostic and surface anatomy and images. Because medical imaging have taken on increased importance in the diagnosis and treatment of injuries and illnesses, diagnostic images are used liberally throughout the chapters, and a special imaging section appears at the end of each chapter. Over 100 clinically relevant magnetic resonance images (MRIs), computed tomography (CT) scans, ultrasound scans, and corresponding orientation drawings are included in this edition. We have also increased the number of labeled surface anatomy photographs and introduced greater ethnic diversity in the surface anatomy representations.

Tables—updated, expanded, and improved. Another feature unique to *Grant's Atlas* is the use of tables to help students organize complex information in an easy-to-use format ideal for review and study. The eleventh edition saw the introduction of muscle tables. In this edition, we have expanded the tables to include those for nerves, arteries, veins, and other relevant structures. The table format in this edition also received a substantial update; a consistent color code is used to clearly demarcate columns. Many tables are also strategically placed on the same page as the illustrations that demonstrate the structures listed in the tables.

Logical organization and layout. The organization and layout of the *Atlas* has always been determined with ease-of-use as the goal. Although the basic organization by body region was maintained in this edition, the order of plates within every chapter was scrutinized to ensure that it is logical and pedagogically effective. Sections within each chapter further organize the region into discrete subregions; these subregions appear as "titles" on the pages. Readers need only glance at these titles to orient themselves to the region and subregion that the figures on the page belong to. All sections also appear as a "table of contents" on the first page of each chapter.

Helpful learning and teaching tools. For the first time in its history, the twelfth edition of *Grant's Atlas* offers a wide range of electronic ancillaries for both student and teacher on Lippincott Williams & Wilkins' online ancillary site "thePoint" (http://thepoint.lww.com/grantsatlas). Students are given access to an interactive electronic atlas containing all of the atlas images with full search capabilities as well as zoom and compare features, as well as selected video clips from the best-selling *Acland's DVD Atlas of Human Anatomy* collection. Students can test themselves with 300 multiple choice questions, 95 "drag-and-drop" labeling exercises, and a sampling of *Clinical Anatomy Flash Cards*. For instructors, electronic ancillaries include an interactive atlas with slideshow and image-export functions, an image bank, and selected "dissection sequences" of plates.

We hope that you enjoy using this twelfth edition of *Grant's Atlas* and that it becomes a trusted partner in your educational experience. We believe that this new edition safeguards the *Atlas's* historical strengths while enhancing its usefulness to today's students.

Anne M.R. Agur
Arthur F. Dalley II

Starting with the first edition of this *Atlas* published in 1943, many people have given generously of their talents and expertise and we acknowledge their participation with heartfelt gratitude. Most of the original carbon-dust halftones on which this book is based were created by **Dorothy Foster Chubb,** a pupil of Max Brödel and one of Canada's first professionally trained medical illustrators. She was later joined by **Nancy Joy,** who is Professor Emeritus in the Division of Biomedical Communications, University of Toronto. Mrs. Chubb was mainly responsible for the artwork of the first two editions and the sixth edition; Miss Joy for those in between. In subsequent editions, additional line and half-tone illustrations by **Elizabeth Blackstock, Elia Hopper Ross,** and **Marguerite Drummond** were added. In recent editions, the artwork of Valerie Oxorn, Caitlin Duckwall, and Rob Duckwall, and the surface anatomy photography of Anne Rayner of Vanderbilt University Medical Center's Medical Art Group, have augmented the modern look and feel of the atlas.

Much credit is also due to Charles E. Storton for his role in the preparation of the majority of the original dissections and preliminary photographic work. We also wish to acknowledge the work of Dr. James Anderson, a pupil of Dr. Grant, under whose stewardship the seventh and eighth editions were published.

The following individuals also provided invaluable contributions to previous editions of the atlas, and are gratefully acknowledged: C.A. Armstrong, P.G. Ashmore, D. Baker, D.A. Barr, J.V. Basmajian, S. Bensley, D. Bilbey, J. Bottos, W. Boyd, J. Callagan, H.A. Cates, S.A. Crooks, M. Dickie, J.W.A. Duckworth, F.B. Fallis, J.B. Francis, J.S. Fraser, P. George, R.K. George, M.G. Gray, B.L. Guyatt, C.W. Hill, W.J. Horsey, B.S. Jaden, M.J. Lee, G.F. Lewis, I.B. MacDonald, D.L. MacIntosh, R.G. MacKenzie, S. Mader, K.O. McCuaig, D. Mazierski, W.R. Mitchell, K. Nancekivell, A.J.A. Noronha, S. O'Sullivan, W. Pallie, W.M. Paul, D. Rini, C. Sandone, C.H. Sawyer, A.I. Scott, J.S. Simpkins, J.S. Simpson, C.G. Smith, I.M. Thompson, J.S. Thompson, N.A. Watters, R.W. Wilson, B. Vallecoccia, and K. Yu.

Twelfth Edition

We are indebted to our colleagues and former professors for their encouragement—especially Dr. Keith L. Moore for his expert advice and Drs. Daniel O. Graney, Lawrence Ross, Warwick Gorman, and Douglas J. Gould for their invaluable input.

We extend our gratitude to the medical artists who worked on this edition: Valerie Oxorn, and Caitlin and Rob Duckwall of Dragonfly Media Group, who contributed new and modified illustrations. We would also like to acknowledge Wayne Hubbel, former Art Coordinator at Lippincott Williams & Wilkins and now a freelancer, who helped size and label art for this edition.

Special thanks go to everyone at **Lippincott Williams & Wilkins**—especially Crystal Taylor, Acquisitions Editor; Kathleen Scogna, Senior Developmental Editor; and Eve Malakoff-Klein, Managing Editor, Production. All of your efforts and expertise are much appreciated.

We would like to thank the hundreds of instructors and students who have over the years communicated via the publisher and directly with the editor their suggestions for how this *Atlas* might be improved. Finally, we would like to acknowledge the reviewers who reviewed previous editions of the *Atlas* as well as the following reviewers who reviewed the eleventh edition and provided expert advice on the development of this edition in particular:

Faculty Reviewers

Diana Alagna, BS, Branford Hall Career Institute, Southington, Connecticut

Gary Allen, PhD, Dalhousie University, Halifax, Nova Scotia, Canada

Gail Amort-Larson, MS, University of Alberta, Edmonton, Alberta, Canada

Alan W. Budenz, DDS, MS, MBA, Arthur A. Dugoni School of Dentistry, University of the Pacific, San Francisco, California

Anne Burrows, PhD, Duquesne University, Pittsburgh, Pennsylvania

Donald Fletcher, PhD, The Brody School of Medicine, East Carolina University, Greenville, South Carolina

Patricia Jordan, PhD, St. George's University, Grenada, West Indies

Elizabeth Julian, Augusta Technical Institute, Augusta, Georgia

H. Wayne Lambert, PhD, University Of Louisville, Louisville, Kentucky

Hector Lopez, DO, University of North Texas Health Science Center, Texas College of Osteopathic Medicine, Fort Worth, Texas

Brian MacPherson, PhD, University of Kentucky College of Medicine, Lexington, Kentucky

Helen Pearson, PhD, Temple University School of Medicine, Philadelphia, Pennsylvania

Chellapilla Rao, PhD, St. George's University School of Medicine, Grenada, West Indies

Darlene Redenbach, PhD, University of British Columbia, Vancouver, Canada

Heather Roberts, PhD, Sierra College, Rocklin, California

R. Shane Tubbs, PhD, University of Alabama, Birmingham, Alabama

Brad Wright, PhD, University of Vermont College of Medicine, Burlington, Vermont

Student Reviewers

Geoffrey Berbary, Texas A and M University, College Station, Texas

Himanshu Bhatia, University Of Texas Health Sciences, Houston, Texas

Joseph Feuerstein, Boston University School of Medicine, Boston, Massachusetts

David Ficco, Life University, Marietta, Georgia

Eric Gross, Medical College of Wisconsin, Milwaukee, Wisconsin

Kathleen Hong, Boston University School of Medicine, Boston, Massachusetts

Patricia Johnson, Southwest College, Tempe, Arizona

Richy Lee, Medical University of the Americas, Charlestown, Nevis, West Indies

Sharon Phillips, University of Massachusetts Medical School, Worcester, Massachusetts

Karen Weinshelbaum, Mount Sinai School of Medicine, New York, New York

Joshua Weissman, Boston University School of Medicine, Boston, Massachusetts

Heather Willis, The Brody School of Medicine, East Carolina University, Greenville, South Carolina

We hope that readers and reviewers will find many of their suggestions incorporated into the twelfth edition and will continue to provide their valuable input.

Anne M.R. Agur
Arthur F. Dalley II

CONTENTS

Dr. John Charles Boileau Grant **vi**

Preface **vii**

Acknowledgments **ix**

List of Tables **xiii**

Table and Figure Credits **xiv**

References **xvi**

1 THORAX 1
Pectoral Region 2
Breast 4
Bony Thorax and Joints 10
Thoracic Wall 17
Thoracic Contents 25
Pleural Cavities 28
Mediastinum 29
Lungs and Pleura 30
Bronchi and Bronchopulmonary Segments 36
Innervation and Lymphatic Drainage of Lungs 42
External Heart 44
Coronary Vessels 52
Internal Heart and Valves 56
Conducting System of Heart 64
Pericardial Sac 65
Superior Mediastinum and Great Vessels 66
Diaphragm 73
Posterior Thorax 74
Overview of Autonomic Innervation 84
Overview of Lymphatic Drainage of Thorax 86
Sectional Anatomy and Imaging 88

2 ABDOMEN 95
Overview 96
Anterolateral Abdominal Wall 98
Inguinal Region 106
Testis 116
Peritoneum and Peritoneal Cavity 118
Digestive System 128
Stomach 129
Pancreas, Duodenum, and Spleen 131
Intestines 136
Liver and Gallbladder 146
Biliary Ducts 156
Portal Venous System 160
Posterior Abdominal Wall 162

Kidneys 164
Lumbar Plexus 172
Diaphragm 174
Abdominal Aorta and Inferior Vena Cava 175
Autonomic Innervation 176
Lymphatic Drainage 182
Sectional Anatomy and Imaging 186

3 PELVIS AND PERINEUM 193
Pelvic Girdle 194
Ligaments of Pelvic Girdle 200
Floor and Walls of Pelvis 202
Sacral and Coccygeal Plexuses 206
Peritoneal Reflections in Pelvis 208
Rectum and Anal Canal 210
Organs of Male Pelvis 216
Vessels of Male Pelvis 224
Lymphatic Drainage of Male Pelvis and Perineum 228
Innervation of Male Pelvic Organs 230
Organs of Female Pelvis 232
Vessels of Female Pelvis 240
Lymphatic Drainage of Female Pelvis and Perineum 244
Innervation of Female Pelvic Organs 246
Subperitoneal Region of Pelvis 250
Surface Anatomy of Perineum 252
Overview of Male and Female Perineum 254
Male Perineum 261
Female Perineum 269
Imaging of Pelvis and Perineum 276

4 BACK 285
Overview of Vertebral Column 286
Cervical Spine 294
Craniovertebral Joints 298
Thoracic Spine 300
Lumbar Spine 302
Ligaments and Intervertebral Discs 304
Vertebral Venous Plexuses 309
Bones, Joints, and Ligaments of Pelvic Girdle 310
Anomalies of Vertebrae 318
Muscles of Back 320
Suboccipital Region 330
Spinal Cord and Meninges 334
Components of Spinal Nerves 343
Dermatomes and Myotomes 348
Imaging of Vertebral Column 350

5   LOWER LIMB 353
Systemic Overview of Lower Limb 354
Bones 355
Nerves 356
Blood Vessels 362
Lymphatics 366
Musculofascial Compartments 368
Retroinguinal Passage and Femoral Triangle 370
Anterior and Medial Compartments of Thigh 374
Lateral Thigh 383
Gluteal Region and Posterior Compartment of Thigh 384
Hip Joint 394
Knee Region 402
Knee Joint 408
Anterior and Lateral Compartments of Leg, Dorsum of Foot 422
Posterior Compartment of Leg 432
Tibiofibular Joints 442
Sole of Foot 443
Ankle, Subtalar, and Foot Joints 448
Arches of Foot 466
Bony Anomalies 467
Imaging and Sectional Anatomy 468

6   UPPER LIMB 475
Systemic Overview of Upper Limb 476
Bones 476
Nerves 480
Blood Vessels 486
Musculofascial Compartments 492
Pectoral Region 494
Axilla, Axillary Vessels, and Brachial Plexus 501
Scapular Region and Superficial Back 512
Arm and Rotator Cuff 516
Joints of Shoulder Region 530
Elbow Region 538
Elbow Joint 544
Anterior Aspect of Forearm 550
Anterior Aspect of Wrist and Palm of Hand 558
Posterior Aspect of Forearm 574
Posterior Aspect of Wrist and Dorsum of Hand 578
Lateral Aspect of Wrist and Hand 584
Medial Aspect of Wrist and Hand 587
Bones and Joints of Wrist and Hand 588
Function of Hand: Grips, Pinches, and Thumb Movements 596
Imaging and Sectional Anatomy 598

7   HEAD 607
Cranium 608
Face and Scalp 626
Circulation and Innervation of Cranial Cavity 632
Meninges and Meningeal Spaces 636
Cranial Base and Cranial Nerves 640

Blood Supply of Brain 646
Orbit and Eyeball 650
Parotid Region 662
Temporal Region and Infratemporal Fossa 664
Temporomandibular Joint 672
Tongue 676
Palate 682
Teeth 685
Nose, Paranasal Sinuses, and Pterygopalatine Fossa 690
Ear 703
Lymphatic Drainage of Head 716
Autonomic Innervation of Head 717
Imaging of Head 718
Neuroanatomy: Overview and Ventricular System 722
Telencephalon (Cerebrum) and Diencephalon 725
Brainstem and Cerebellum 734
Imaging of Brain 740

8   NECK 745
Subcutaneous Structures and Cervical Fascia 746
Skeleton of Neck 750
Regions of Neck 752
Lateral Region (Posterior Triangle) of Neck 754
Anterior Region (Anterior Triangle) of Neck 758
Neurovascular Structures of Neck 762
Visceral Compartment of Neck 768
Root and Prevertebral Region of Neck 772
Submandibular Region and Floor of Mouth 778
Posterior Cervical Region 783
Pharynx 786
Isthmus of Fauces 792
Larynx 798
Sectional Anatomy and Imaging of Neck 806

9   CRANIAL NERVES 811
Overview of Cranial Nerves 812
Cranial Nerve Nuclei 816
Cranial Nerve I: Olfactory 818
Cranial Nerve II: Optic 819
Cranial Nerves III, IV, and VI: Oculomotor, Trochlear, and Abducent 821
Cranial Nerve V: Trigeminal 824
Cranial Nerve VII: Facial 830
Cranial Nerve VIII: Vestibulocochlear 832
Cranial Nerve IX: Glossopharyngeal 834
Cranial Nerve X: Vagus 836
Cranial Nerve XI: Spinal Accessory 838
Cranial Nerve XII: Hypoglossal 839
Summary of Autonomic Ganglia of Head 840
Summary of Cranial Nerve Lesions 841
Sectional Imaging of Cranial Nerves 842

INDEX 845

LIST OF TABLES

1 THORAX
1.1 Muscles of Thoracic Wall **21**
1.2 Muscles of Respiration **24**
1.3 Surface Markings of Parietal Pleura and Surface Markings of Lungs Covered with Visceral Pleura **31**

2 ABDOMEN
2.1 Principal Muscles of Anterolateral Abdominal Wall **104**
2.2 Structures Forming the Inguinal Canal **108**
2.3 Parts and Relationships of Duodenum **133**
2.4 Schema of Terminology for Subdivisions of the Liver **151**
2.5 Principal Muscles of Posterior Abdominal Wall **172**
2.6 Autonomic Innervation of the Abdominal Viscera (Splanchic Nerves) **179**

3 PELVIS AND PERINEUM
3.1 Differences Between Male and Female Pelves **198**
3.2 Muscles of Pelvic Walls and Floor **203**
3.3 Nerves of Sacral and Coccygeal Plexuses **207**
3.4 Arteries of Male Pelvis **225**
3.5 Lymphatic Drainage of the Male Pelvis and Perineum **229**
3.6 Effect of Sympathetic and Parasympathetic Stimulation on the Urinary Tract, Genital System, and Rectum **230**
3.7 Arteries of Female Pelvis **243**
3.8 Lymphatic Drainage of the Structures of the Female Pelvis and Perineum **245**
3.9 Muscles of Perineum **256**

4 BACK
4.1 Typical Cervical Vertebrae (C3-C7) **294**
4.2 Thoracic Vertebrae **300**
4.3 Lumbar Vertebrae **302**
4.4 Intrinsic Back Muscles **329**
4.5 Muscles of the Atlanto-Occipital and Atlantoaxial Joints **332**

5 LOWER LIMB
5.1 Motor Nerves of Lower Limb **358**
5.2 Muscles of Anterior Thigh **377**
5.3 Muscles of Medial Thigh **378**
5.4 Muscles of Gluteal Region **386**
5.5 Muscles of Posterior Thigh (Hamstring) **387**
5.6 Nerves of Gluteal Region **392**
5.7 Arteries of Gluteal Region and Posterior Thigh **393**
5.8 Bursae Around Knee **415**
5.9 Muscles of the Anterior Compartment of Leg **423**
5.10 Common, Superficial, and Deep Fibular Nerves **424**
5.11 Arterial Supply to Dorsum of Foot **427**
5.12 Muscles of the Lateral Compartment of Leg **429**
5.13 Muscles of the Posterior Compartment of Leg **432**
5.14 Arterial Supply of Leg and Foot **441**
5.15 Muscles in Sole of Foot—First Layer **444**
5.16 Muscles in Sole of Foot—Second Layer **445**
5.17 Muscles in Sole of Foot—Third Layer **446**
5.18 Muscles in Sole of Foot—Fourth Layer **447**
5.19 Joints of Foot **460**

6 UPPER LIMB
6.1 Cutaneous Nerves of Upper Limb **485**
6.2 Anterior Axioappendicular Muscles **499**
6.3 Arteries of Proximal Upper Limb (Shoulder Region and Arm) **505**
6.4 Axilla, Axillary Vessels, and Brachial Plexus **507**
6.5 Superficial Back (Posterior Axioappendicular) and Deltoid Muscles **513**
6.6 Movements of Scapula **515**
6.7 Deep Scapulohumeral/Shoulder Muscles **517**
6.8 Arm Muscles **520**
6.9 Arteries of Forearm **550**
6.10 Muscles of Anterior Surface of the Forearm **553**
6.11 Muscles of Hand **565**
6.12 Arteries of Hand **573**
6.13 Muscles of Posterior Surface of the Forearm **575**

7 HEAD
7.1 Main Muscles of Facial Expression **629**
7.2 Nerves of Face and Scalp **631**
7.3 Arteries of Face and Scalp **632**
7.4 Veins of Face **633**
7.5 Arterial Supply to the Brain **647**
7.6 Arteries of Orbit **657**
7.7 Muscles of Orbit **658**
7.8 Actions of Muscles of the Orbit Starting From Primary Position **659**
7.9 Muscles of Mastication (Acting on Temporomandibular Joint) **672**
7.10 Movements of the Temporomandibular Joint **673**
7.11 Muscles of Tongue **677**
7.12 Muscles of Soft Palate **684**
7.13 Primary and Secondary Dentition **689**

8 NECK
8.1 Platysma **746**
8.2 Cervical Regions and Contents **752**
8.3 Sternocleidomastoid and Trapezius **753**
8.4 Suprahyoid and Infrahyoid Muscles **761**
8.5 Arteries of the Neck **764**
8.6 Anterior Vertebral Muscles **774**
8.7 Lateral Vertebral Muscles **777**
8.8 Muscles of Posterior Cervical Region **783**
8.9 Muscles of Pharynx **788**
8.10 Muscles of Larynx **802**

9 CRANIAL NERVES
9.1 Summary of Cranial Nerves **815**
9.2 Olfactory Nerve (CN I) **818**
9.3 Optic Nerve (CN II) **819**
9.4 Oculomotor (CN III), Trochlear (CN IV), and Abducent (CN VI) Nerves **822**
9.5 Trigeminal Nerve (CN V) **824**
9.6 Branches of Ophthalmic Nerve (CN V^1) **825**
9.7 Branches of Maxillary Nerve (CN V^2) **826**
9.8 Branches of Mandibular Nerve (CN V^3) **828**
9.9 Facial Nerve (CN VII), Including Motor Root and Intermediate Nerve **830**
9.10 Vestibulocochlear Nerve (CN VIII) **832**
9.11 Glossopharyngeal Nerve (CN IX) **834**
9.12 Vagus Nerve (CN X) **837**
9.13 Spinal Accessory Nerve (CN XI) **838**
9.14 Hypoglossal Nerve (CN XII) **839**
9.15 Autonomic Ganglia of the Head **840**
9.16 Summary of Cranial Nerve Lesions **841**

Note: A list of the table and figure sources for this book from previous editions of *Clinically Oriented Anatomy*, *Grant's Atlas*, and *Essential Clinical Anatomy* can be found online at http://thepoint.lww.com/grantsatlas.

CHAPTER 1

1.5AB Courtesy of Dr. K. Bukhanov, University of Toronto, Canada

1.5C Dean D, Herbener TE. Cross-Sectional Human Anatomy, 2000:25 (Plate 2.9).

1.23 Courtesy of Dr. E.L. Lansdown, University of Toronto, Canada

1.33A Courtesy of Dr. D.E. Sanders, University of Toronto, Canada

1.33B Courtesy of Dr. S. Herman, University of Toronto, Canada

1.33C Courtesy of Dr. E.L. Lansdown, University of Toronto, Canada

1.36 Courtesy of I. Verschuur, Joint Department of Medical Imaging, UHN/Mount Sinai Hospital, Toronto, Canada

1.41B&D Courtesy of I. Verschuur, Joint Department of Medical Imaging, UHN/Mount Sinai Hospital, Toronto, Canada

1.46C Courtesy of I. Verschuur, Joint Department of Medical Imaging, UHN/Mount Sinai Hospital, Toronto, Canada

1.47B&D Courtesy of I. Morrow, University of Manitoba, Canada

1.48B Courtesy of Dr. J. Heslin, Toronto, Canada

1.52B Courtesy of I. Verschuur, Joint Department of Medical Imaging, UHN/Mount Sinai Hospital, Toronto, Canada

1.55AB Moore KL, Dalley AF. Clinically Oriented Anatomy. 5th ed, 2006:170 (Fig. 1.55). A is based on Torrent-Guasp F, Buckberg GD, Clemente C et al. The Structure and Function of the Helical Heart and Its Buttress Wrapping. I. The normal macroscopic structure of the heart. Sem. Thor. Cardiovasc Surgery. 13 (4): 301-319, 2001.

1.58B Feigenbaum H, Armstrong WF, Ryan T. Feigenbaum's Echocardiography. 5th ed, 2005:116.

1.66B Courtesy of Dr. E.L. Lansdown, University of Toronto, Canada

1.81A-F MRIs courtesy of Dr. M.A. Haider, University of Toronto, Canada

1.82A-C MRIs courtesy of Dr. M.A. Haider, University of Toronto, Canada

1.83AB MRIs courtesy of Dr. M.A. Haider, University of Toronto, Canada

1.85A-F Courtesy of I. Verschuur, Joint Department of Medical Imaging, UHN/Mount Sinai Hospital, Toronto, Canada

CHAPTER 2

2.22B MRI courtesy of Dr. M.A. Haider, University of Toronto, Canada

2.31 Courtesy of Dr. J. Heslin, Toronto, Canada

2.32A, C, D Courtesy of Dr. E.L. Lansdown, University of Toronto, Canada

2.32B Courtesy of Dr. J. Heslin, Toronto, Canada

2.37A Courtesy of Dr. C.S. Ho, University of Toronto, Canada

2.37B Courtesy of Dr. E.L. Lansdown, University of Toronto, Canada

2.40A Courtesy of Dr. E.L. Lansdown, University of Toronto, Canada

2.40B Courtesy of Dr. J. Heslin, Toronto, Canada

2.42 Courtesy of Dr. K. Sniderman, University of Toronto, Canada

2.48B Courtesy of A. M. Arenson, University of Toronto, Canada

2.54D Courtesy of Dr. G.B. Haber, University of Toronto, Canada

2.56AB Courtesy of Dr. J. Heslin, Toronto, Canada

2.58AB Courtesy of Dr. G.B. Haber, University of Toronto, Canada

2.61B Radiograph courtesy of G.B.Haber, University of Toronto, Canada; photo courtesy of Mission Hospital Regional Center, Mission Viejo, California

2.65B Courtesy of M. Asch, University of Toronto, Canada

2.67B Courtesy of E.L. Lansdown, University of Toronto, Canada

2.68B (right) Courtesy of M. Asch, University of Toronto, Canada

2.85A, C, D Courtesy of Dr. M.A. Haider, University of Toronto, Canada

2.85B The Visible Human Project; National Library of Medicine; Visible Man Image number 1499.

2.86A, B, C Courtesy of Dr. M.A. Haider, University of Toronto, Canada

2.86D The Visible Human Project; National Library of Medicine; Visible Man Image number 1625.

2.87A-D Courtesy of Dr. M.A. Haider, University of Toronto, Canada

2.88A-D Courtesy of Dr. M.A. Haider, University of Toronto, Canada

2.89A-C Ultrasounds courtesy of A.M. Arenson, University of Toronto, Canada.

2.89D, F Courtesy of J. Lai, University of Toronto, Canada

2.86E, G Dean D, Herbener TE. Cross Sectional Human Anatomy, 2000:45,53 (Plates 3.9, 3.13)

CHAPTER 3

3.26A-C Ultrasounds courtesy of Dr. A. Toi, University of Toronto, Canada

3.36D Courtesy of E.L. Lansdown, University of Toronto, Canada

3.36E From Sadler TW. Langman's Medical Embryology. 10th ed, 2006:92 (Fig. 7.5)

3.66A-D Courtesy of Dr. M.A. Haider, University of Toronto, Canada

3.66E Courtesy of The Visible Human Project; National Library of Medicine; Visible Man Image number 1940

3.67 Uflacker R. Atlas of Vascular Anatomy: An Angiographic Approach, 1997:611.

3.68A-C Courtesy of Dr. M.A. Haider, University of Toronto, Canada

3.69 MRIs courtesy of Dr. M.A. Haider, University of Toronto, Canada

3.70A-G MRIs courtesy of Dr. M.A. Haider, University of Toronto, Canada; sectioned specimens from The Visible Human Project; National

Library of Medicine; Visible Woman Image numbers 1870 and 1895

3.71AB Courtesy of Dr. M.A. Haider, University of Toronto, Canada.

3.72A-D Ultrasounds courtesy of A.M. Arenson, University of Toronto, Canada

3.73D Reprinted with permission from Stuart GCE, Reid DF. Diagnostic studies. In Copeland LJ (ed.): Textbook of Gynecology. Philadelphia, WB Saunders, 1993.

CHAPTER 4

4.1B Courtesy of D. Salonen, University of Toronto, Canada

4.7B, D, F, 4.8E Courtesy of Drs. E. Becker and P. Bobechko, University of Toronto, Canada

4.8C&D Courtesy of E. Becker, University of Toronto, Canada

4.11A, B Courtesy of J. Heslin, Unitersity of Toronto, Canada

4.11C, D Courtesy of D. Armstrong, University of Toronto, Canada

4.12C Courtesy of D. Salonen, University of Toronto, Canada

4.40C Clay JH, Pounds DM. Basic Clinical Massage Therapy: Integrating Anatomy and Treatment. 2003:92 (Fig. 3.40)

4.49B Courtesy of D. Salonen, University of Toronto, Canada

4.54AB Courtesy of The Visible Human Project; National Library of Medicine; Visible Man 1168.

4.54C Courtesy of D. Armstrong, University of Toronto, Canada

4.55A, B Courtesy of The Visible Human Project; National Library of Medicine; Visible Man 1715.

4.56A, B Courtesy of The Visible Human Project; National Library of Medicine; Visible Man 1805.

4.57A-D Courtesy of D. Salonen, University of Toronto, Canada

CHAPTER 5

5.7A-D A and B are based on Fender FA. Foerster's scheme of the dermatomes. Arch Neurol Psychiatry 1939; 41:699. C and D are based on Keefan JJ, Garrett FD. The segmental distribution of the cutaneous nerves in the limbs of man. Anat Rec 1948;102:409

5.11B Roche Lexicon Medizin. 4th Ed. Munich: Urban & Schwarzenberg, 1998. (Appeared in Moore KL, Dalley AF. Clincally Oriented Anatomy. 4th Ed., 1999:527.)

5.13B Courtesy of Dr. E.L. Lansdown, University of Toronto, Canada

5.32A Courtesy of E. Becker, University of Toronto, Canada

5.32 C Daffner RH. Clinical Radiology: The Essentials. Baltimore: Williams & Wilkins, 1993:491 (Fig. 11.99)

5.33B Courtesy of Dr. D. Salonen, University of Toronto, Canada

5.46 (inset at page bottom) Roche Lexicon Medizin. 4th Ed. Munich: Urban & Schwarzenberg, 1998.

(Appeared in Moore KL, Dalley AF. and Clincally Oriented Anatomy. 5 Ed., 2006:699.)

5.49A, B Courtesy of Dr. P. Bobechko, University of Toronto, Canada

5.49C Courtesy of Dr. D. Salonen, University of Toronto, Canada

5.50B&C Courtesy of Dr. D. Salonen, University of Toronto, Canada

5.51 Courtesy of Dr. P. Bobechko, University of Toronto, Canada

5.52B, C Courtesy of Dr. D. Salonen, University of Toronto, Canada

5.57C, D Clay JH, Pounds DM. Basic Clinical Massage Therapy: Integrating Anatomy and Treatment. 2002:352,354 (Figs. 10.16 & 10.18)

5.64A Courtesy of Dr. D. K. Sniderman, University of Toronto, Canada

5.71B, 5.76A Courtesy of Dr. E. Becker, University of Toronto, Canada

5.76B Courtesy of Dr. P. Bobechko, University of Toronto, Canada

5.77B Courtesy of E. Becker, University of Toronto, Canada

5.79B Courtesy of Dr. W. Kucharczyk, University of Toronto, Canada

5.80B Courtesy of Dr. W. Kucharczyk, University of Toronto, Canada

5.88C Courtesy of Dr. P. Bobechko, University of Toronto, Canada

5.89B, D Courtesy of P. Babyn, University of Toronto, Canada

5.90C Courtesy of The Visible Human Project; National Library of Medicine; Visible Man 2105.

5.90D, E, F MRIs courtesy of Dr. D. Salonen, University of Toronto, Canada

5.91C Courtesy of The Visible Human Project; National Library of Medicine; Visible Man 2551.

5.91D, E, F MRIs courtesy of Dr. D. Salonen, University of Toronto, Canada

Table 5.2 A-D Modified from Clay JH, Pounds DM. Basic Clinical Massage Therapy: Integrating Anatomy and Treatment. 2002:301 (Plate 9.2).

Table 5.2 E, H Modified from Clay JH, Pounds DM. Basic Clinical Massage Therapy: Integrating Anatomy and Treatment. 2002:280,312 (Figs. 8.10, 9.10)

Table 5.13 Clay JH and Pounds DM. Basic Clinical Massage Therapy: Integrating Anatomy and Treatment. 2002:362,364 (Figs. 10.28, 10.30)

CHAPTER 6

6.5A, B Based on Fender FA. Foerster's scheme of the dermatomes. Arch Neurol Psychiatry 1939;41:688. (Appeared in Moore KL, Dalley AF. Clinically Oriented Anatomy. 4th ed, 1999:682,683.)

6.5C, D Based on Keegan JJ, Garrett FD. The segmental distribution of the cutaneous nerves in the limbs of man. Anat Rec 1948;102:409

6.17A-E Modified from Clay JH, Pounds DM. Basic Clinical Massage Therapy: Integrating Anatomy and Treatment. 2002:120,124,119,149 (Figs. 4.4, 4.9, 4.1, 4.49)

6.22C Courtesy of D. Armstrong, University of Toronto, Canada

6.30B&D Clay JH, Pounds DM. Basic Clinical Massage Therapy: Integrating Anatomy and Treatment. 2002:144,138 (Figs. 4.44, 4.33)

6.44A Courtesy of E. Becker, University of Toronto, Canada

6.44 C, E Courtesy of D. Salonen, University of Toronto, Canada

6.44 D Courtesy of R. Leekam, University of Toronto and West End Diagnostic Imaging, Canada

6.49C Courtesy of E. Becker, University of Toronto, Canada

6.50 Radiographs courtesy of J. Heslin, Toronto, Canada;

6.51B Courtesy of D. Salonen, University of Toronto, Canada

6.52B Courtesy of E. Becker, University of Toronto, Canada

6.55A Courtesy of K. Sniderman, University of Toronto, Canada

6.57A, 6.58A, 6.59A, 6.60A Clay JH, Pounds DM. Basic Clinical Massage Therapy: Integrating Anatomy and Treatment. 2002:170 (Plate 5.3)

6.66ABCD Clay JH, Pounds DM. Basic Clinical Massage Therapy: Integrating Anatomy and Treatment. 2002:174 (Plate 5.55)

6.72A Courtesy of D. Armstrong, University of Toronto, Canada

6.78F Courtesy of E. Becker, University of Toronto, Canada

6.81A, B Courtesy of E. Becker, University of Toronto, Canada

6.82B Courtesy of D. Armstrong, University of Toronto, Canada

6.89L Courtesy of D. Armstrong, University of Toronto, Canada

6.90B-D Courtesy of D. Salonen, University of Toronto, Canada

6.91C-E Courtesy of D. Salonen, University of Toronto, Canada

6.92A-C Courtesy of D. Salonen, University of Toronto, Canada

6.93 B Courtesy of R. Leekam, University of Toronto and West End Diagnostic Imaging, Canada

Table 6.5 Clay JH, Pounds DM. Basic Clinical Massage Therapy: Integrating Anatomy and Treatment. 2002:113,136,132 (Plates 4.4, 4.31, 4.24)

Table 6.8 Clay JH, Pounds DM. Basic Clinical Massage Therapy: Integrating Anatomy and Treatment. 2002:170,171,173,179 (Plates 5.3, 5.4, 5.6, and Fig. 5.1)

Table 6.13 3&4 Clay JH, Pounds DM. Basic Clinical Massage Therapy: Integrating Anatomy and Treatment. 2002:127 (Plate 5.5)

CHAPTER 7

7.1B, E&F Courtesy of Dr. D. Armstrong, University of Toronto, Canada

7.7A, B Courtesy of Dr. E. Becker, University of Toronto, Canada

7.29A-C Courtesy of Dr. D. Armstrong, University of Toronto, Canada

7.30A&B Courtesy of I. Verschuur, Joint Department of Medical Imaging, UHN/Mount Sinai Hospital, Toronto, Canada

7.33C Courtesy of Dr. W. Kucharczyk, University of Toronto, Canada

7.35C Courtesy of Dr. W. Kucharczyk, University of Toronto, Canada

7.38A Courtesy of J.R. Buncic, University of Toronto, Canada

7.46 CTs and MRIs from Langland OE, Langlais RP, Preece JW. Principles of Dental Imaging, 2002:278 (Figs. 11.32A, B; 11.33A, B).

7.53A Langland OE, Langlais RP, Preece JW. Principles of Dental Imaging, 2002:334 (Fig. 14.1).

7.53B Courtesy of M.J. Phatoah, University of Toronto, Canada.

7.54E Courtesy of Dr. B. Libgott, Division of Anatomy/Department of Surgery, University of Toronto, Ontario, Canada

7.55B, C Woelfel JB, Scheid RC. Dental Anatomy: Its Relevance to Dentistry. 6th ed, 2002:86,46 (Figs. 3.5, 1.29).

7.64B Courtesy of D. Armstrong, University of Toronto, Canada

7.64C Courtesy of E. Becker, University of Toronto, Canada

7.65C Courtesy of E. Becker, University of Toronto, Canada

7.67D Courtesy of Dr. E. Becker, University of Toronto, Canada

7.71D Courtesy of Welch Allen, Inc. Skaneateles Falls, NY. (Appeared in Moore KL, Dalley AF. Clinically Oriented Anatomy. 4th ed, 1999:966 (Fig. 8.2)

7.81B Courtesy of W. Kucharczyk, University of Toronto, Canada

7.81C, D Courtesy of W. Kucharczyk, University of Toronto, Canada

7.82B Courtesy of Dr. W. Kucharczyk, University of Toronto, Canada

7.83A-E All photos courtesy of The Visible Human Project; National Library of Medicine; Visible Man 1107 and 1168.

7.86–7.89, 7.91, 7.92B, C, 7.93 Colorized from photographs provided courtesy of Dr. C.G. Smith, which appears in Smith CG. Serial Dissections of the Human Brain. Baltimore: Urban & Schwarzenber, Inc. and Toronto: Gage Publishing Ltd., 1981 (© Carlton G. Smith)

7.90A-F MRIs courtesy of Dr. D. Armstrong, University of Toronto, Canada

7.94A-E MRIs courtesy of Dr. D. Armstrong, University of Toronto, Canada

7.95A-F MRIs courtesy of Dr. D. Armstrong, University of Toronto, Canada

7.96A-C MRIs courtesy of Dr. D. Armstrong, University of Toronto, Canada

Table 7.9 Illustrations from Clay JH, Pounds DM. Basic Clinical Massage Therapy: Integrating Anatomy and Treatment. 2002:76,74,79 (Figs.3.17, 3.15, 3.19).

Table 7.12 (bottom left illustration) Clay JH, Pounds DM. Basic Clinical Massage Therapy: Integrating Anatomy and Treatment, 2002:80 (Fig. 3.22).

CHAPTER 8

8.4B Courtesy of J. Heslin, University of Toronto, Canada

8.18B Modified from Clay JH, Pounds DM. Basic Clinical Massage Therapy: Integrating Anatomy and Treatment. 2003:92 (Fig. 3.40)

8.25B From Liebgott B. The Anatomical Basis of Dentistry. Philadelphia, PA: Mosby, 1982.

8.31A Rohen JW, Yokochi C, Lutjen-DrecollE, Romrell LJ. Color Atlas of Anatomy: A Photographic Study of the Human Body. 5th ed, 2002.

8.31C Courtesy of Dr. D. Salonen, University of Toronto, Canada.

8.34A-C Courtesy of Dr. D. Salonen, University of Toronto, Canada;

8.36B Courtesy of Dr. E. Becker, University of Toronto, Canada

8.37 Photo courtesy of Acuson Corporation, Mt. View, California

Table 8.3 Modified from Clay JH, Pounds DM. Basic Clinical Massage Therapy: Integrating Anatomy and Treatment. 2003:90,91 (Figs. 3.36, 3.48)

Table 8.4 Modified from Clay JH, Pounds DM. Basic Clinical Massage Therapy: Integrating Anatomy and Treatment. 2003:88 (Fig. 3.34)

Table 8.5B Courtesy of Dr. D. Armstrong, University of Toronto, Canada

Table 8.7 Clay JH, Pounds DM. Basic Clinical Massage Therapy: Integrating Anatomy and Treatment. 2003:101,128 (Figs. 3.53, 4.17)

Table 8.8A-D Clay JH, Pounds DM. Basic Clinical Massage Therapy: Integrating Anatomy and Treatment. 2003:96,100,104 (Figs. 3.48, 3.52, 3.56)

CHAPTER 9

9.6A-F Courtesy of Dr. W. Kucharczyk, University of Toronto, Canada

9.7A-C Photos courtesy of Dr. W. Kucharczyk, University of Toronto, Canada

Photograph of Dr. J. C. B. Grant courtesy of Dr. C. G. Smith.

REFERENCES

Tribute to Dr. Grant

1. Robinson C. Canadian Medical Lives: J.C. Boileau Grant: Anatomist Extraordinary. Markham, Ontario, Canada: Associated Medical Services Inc./Fithzenry & Whiteside, 1993.
2. Grant JCB. A Method of Anatomy, Descriptive and Deductive. Baltimore: Williams & Wilkins Co., 1937. (11th edition, J. Basmajian and C. Slonecker, 1989)
3. Grant JCB. Grant's Atlas of Anatomy. Baltimore: Williams & Wilkins Co., 1943 (10th Edition, A. Agur and L. Ming, 1999)
4. Grant JCB, Cates HA. Grant's Dissector (A Handbook for Dissectors). Baltimore: Williams & Wilkins Co., 1940 (12th edition, E.K. Sauerland, 1999)

Chapter 1

(Fig. 1.51) Anson BH. The aortic arch and its branches. *Cardiology*. New York: McGraw-Hill, vol 1: 1963.

Chapter 2

(Fig. 2.49) Couinaud C. Lobes et segments hepatiques: Note sur l'architecture anatomique et chirurgicale du foie. *Presse Med* 1954;62:709.

(Fig. 2.49) Healy JE, Schroy PC. Anatomy of the biliary ducts within the human liver: Analysis of the prevailing pattern of branchings and the major variations of the biliary ducts. *Arch Surg* 1953;66:599.

(Fig. 2.89B) Campbell M. Ureteral reduplication (double ureter). *Urology*. Vol.1. Philadelphia: WB Saunders, 1954:309.

Chapter 3

(Fig. 3.43A) Oelrich TM. The urethral sphincter muscle in the male. *Am J Anat* 1980;158:229.

(Fig. 3.43B) Oelrich TM. The striated urogenital sphincter muscle in the female. *Anat Rec* 1983;205:223.

Chapter 4

(Fig. 4.48A) Jit I, Charnakia VM. The vertebral level of the termination of the spinal cord. *J Anat Soc India* 1959;8:93.

CHAPTER 1

THORAX

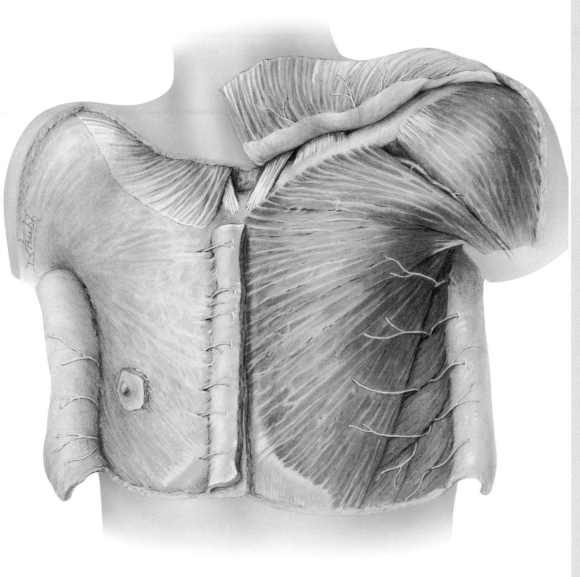

- Pectoral Region 2
- Breast 4
- Bony Thorax and Joints 10
- Thoracic Wall 17
- Thoracic Contents 25
- Pleural Cavities 28
- Mediastinum 29
- Lungs and Pleura 30
- Bronchi and Bronchopulmonary Segments 36
- Innervation and Lymphatic Drainage of Lungs 42
- External Heart 44
- Coronary Vessels 52
- Internal Heart and Valves 56
- Conduction System of Heart 64
- Pericardial Sac 65
- Superior Mediastinum and Great Vessels 66
- Diaphragm 73
- Posterior Thorax 74
- Overview of Autonomic Innervation 84
- Overview of Lymphatic Drainage of Thorax 86
- Sectional Anatomy and Imaging 88

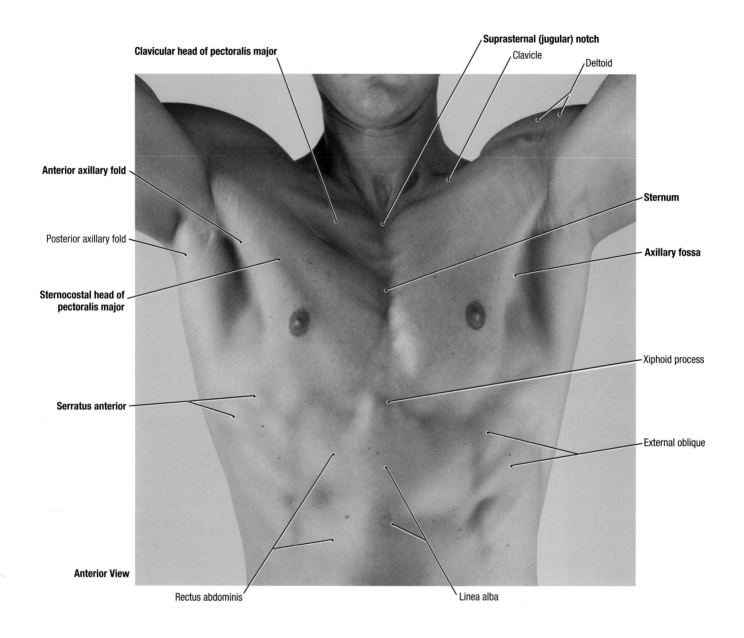

Clavicular head of pectoralis major

Suprasternal (jugular) notch

Clavicle

Deltoid

Anterior axillary fold

Posterior axillary fold

Sternocostal head of pectoralis major

Serratus anterior

Sternum

Axillary fossa

Xiphoid process

External oblique

Anterior View

Rectus abdominis

Linea alba

1.1   **Surface anatomy of male pectoral region**

- The subject is adducting the shoulders against resistance to demonstrate the pectoralis major muscle.
- The pectoralis major muscle has two parts, the sternocostal and clavicular heads.
- The anterior axillary fold is formed by the inferior border of the sternocostal head of the pectoralis major muscle.
- The axillary fossa ("armpit") is a surface feature overlying a fat-filled space, the axilla.

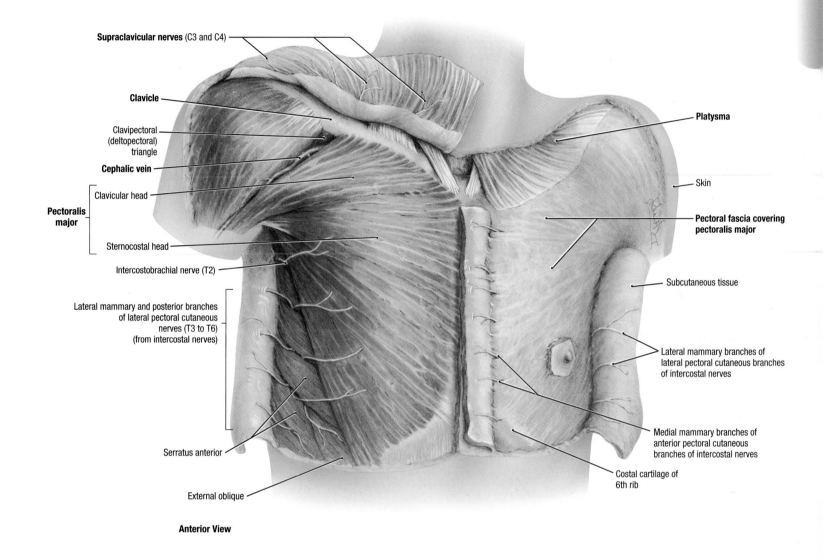

Supraclavicular nerves (C3 and C4)

Clavicle

Clavipectoral
(deltopectoral)
triangle

Cephalic vein

Clavicular head

Pectoralis
major

Sternocostal head

Intercostobrachial nerve (T2)

Lateral mammary and posterior branches
of lateral pectoral cutaneous
nerves (T3 to T6)
(from intercostal nerves)

Serratus anterior

External oblique

Platysma

Skin

Pectoral fascia covering
pectoralis major

Subcutaneous tissue

Lateral mammary branches of
lateral pectoral cutaneous branches
of intercostal nerves

Medial mammary branches of
anterior pectoral cutaneous
branches of intercostal nerves

Costal cartilage of
6th rib

Anterior View

1.2   Superficial dissection, male pectoral region

- The platysma muscle, which descends to the 2nd or 3rd rib, is cut short on the right side of the specimen; together with the supraclavicular nerves, it is reflected on the left side.
- The thin pectoral fascia covers the pectoralis major.
- The clavicle lies deep to the subcutaneous tissue and the platysma muscle.
- The cephalic vein passes deeply in the clavipectoral (deltopectoral) triangle to join the axillary vein.
- Supraclavicular (C3 and C4) and upper thoracic nerves (T2 to T6) supply cutaneous innervation to the pectoral region.
- The clavipectoral (deltopectoral) triangle, bounded by the clavicle superiorly, the deltoid muscle laterally, and the clavicular head of the pectoralis major muscle medially, under-lies a surface depression called the infraclavicular fossa.

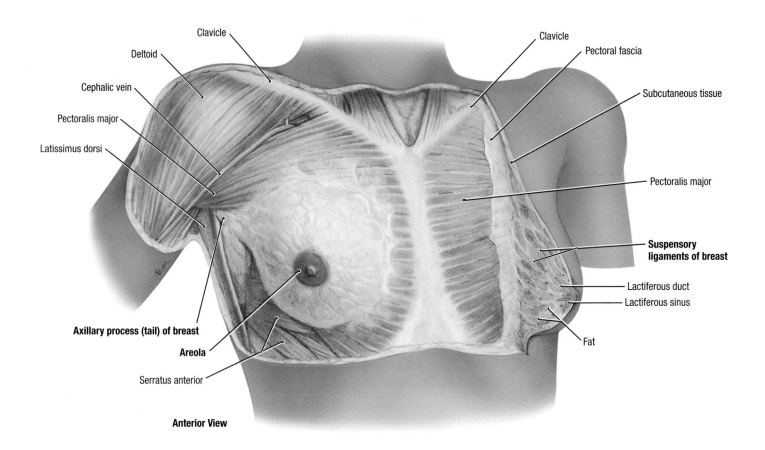

Clavicle

Deltoid

Cephalic vein

Pectoralis major

Latissimus dorsi

Clavicle

Pectoral fascia

Subcutaneous tissue

Pectoralis major

Suspensory ligaments of breast

Lactiferous duct

Lactiferous sinus

Fat

Axillary process (tail) of breast

Areola

Serratus anterior

Anterior View

1.3   Superficial dissection, female pectoral region

- On the specimen's right side, the skin is removed; on the left side, the breast is sagittally sectioned.
- The breast extends from the 2nd to the 6th ribs. The axillary process (tail) of the breast consists of glandular tissue projecting toward the axilla.
- The region of loose connective tissue between the pectoral fascia and the deep surface of the breast, the retromammary bursa, permits the breast to move on the deep fascia.

- Interference with the lymphatic drainage by cancer may cause lymphedema (edema, excess fluid in the subcutaneous tissue), which in turn may result in deviation of the nipple and a leathery, thickened appearance of the breast skin. Prominent (puffy) skin between dimpled pores may develop, which gives the skin an orange-peel appearance (*peau d'orange sign*). Larger dimples may form if pulled by cancerous invasion of the suspensory ligaments of the breast.

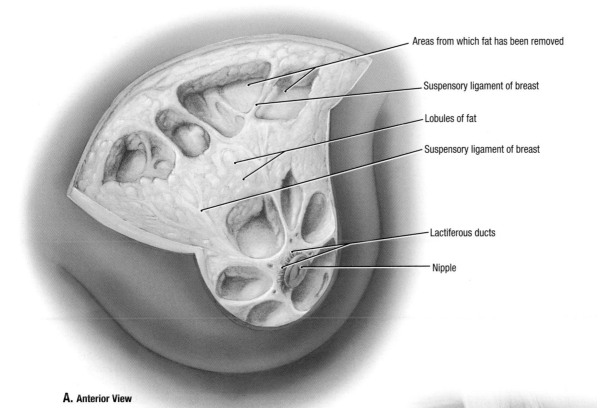

Areas from which fat has been removed

Suspensory ligament of breast

Lobules of fat

Suspensory ligament of breast

Lactiferous ducts

Nipple

A. Anterior View

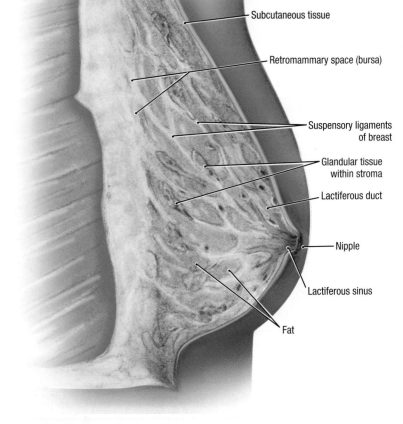

Subcutaneous tissue

Retromammary space (bursa)

Suspensory ligaments of breast

Glandular tissue within stroma

Lactiferous duct

Nipple

Lactiferous sinus

Fat

B. Sagittal Section of Breast

1.4   Female mammary gland

A. The breast consists primarily of fat compartmentalized between connective and glandular tissue septa. The lactiferous ducts (usually 15 to 20 in number) expand to form subareolar lactiferous sinuses and then open on the nipple; the glandular tissue lies within a dense (fibro-) areolar stroma, from which suspensory ligaments extend to the deeper layers of the skin. Areas of superficial fat were scooped out from some compartments between the septa. **B.** Structure of the breast revealed by sagittal section. Cancer can spread by contiguity (invasion of adjacent tissue). When breast cancer cells invade the retromammary space, attach to or invade the pectoral fascia overlaying the pectoralis major muscle, or metastasize to the interpectoral nodes (Fig. 1.8), the breast elevates when the muscle contracts. This movement is a clinical sign of advanced breast cancer.

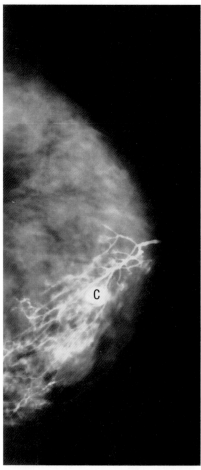

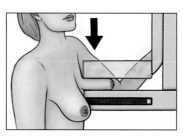

Orientation for Part A

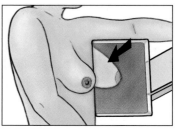

Orientation for Part B

A. Superior View

B. Lateral View

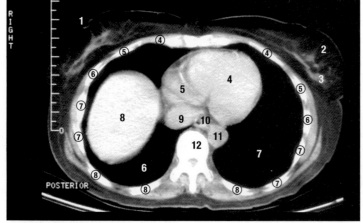

Structures in Part C:

1   Nipple
2   Lactiferous ducts
3   Suspensory ligaments
4   Left ventricle
5   Right atrium
6   Right lung
7   Left lung
8   Liver
9   Inferior vena cava
10   Esophagus
11   Descending aorta
12   T9 vertebra
⑦   Corresponding rib numbers

C. Inferior View

1.5   Imaging of breast

A. Galactogram. Contrast has been injected into a lactiferous duct, outlining the branching pattern of its tributaries. Note the presence of a ductal cyst *(C)*. **B.** Normal mammogram. Observe the connective tissue network of the breast. The stroma is radiopaque and changes with age and during lactation. Pectoralis major muscle *(P)* and an axillary lymph node *(L)* can also be seen. **C.** Axial computed tomographic (CT) scan at the level of the female breasts (T9 level).

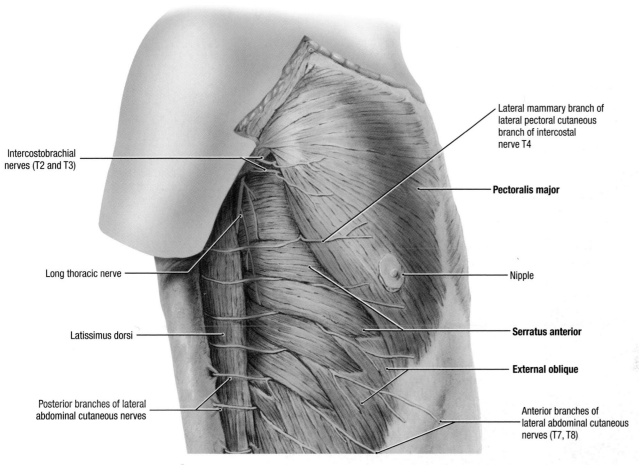

Lateral mammary branch of
lateral pectoral cutaneous
branch of intercostal
nerve T4

Pectoralis major

Intercostobrachial
nerves (T2 and T3)

Long thoracic nerve

Nipple

Latissimus dorsi

Serratus anterior

External oblique

Posterior branches of lateral
abdominal cutaneous nerves

Anterior branches of
lateral abdominal cutaneous
nerves (T7, T8)

A. Anterolateral View

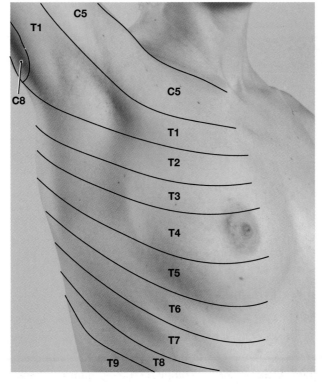

C5

T1

C8

C5

T1

T2

T3

T4

T5

T6

T7

T9   T8

B. Anterolateral View

1.6   Bed of breast

A. Muscles comprising bed of breast and cutaneous nerves. **B.** Dermatomes extending across bed of breast. Local anesthesia of an intercostal space (intercostal nerve block) is produced by injecting a local anesthetic agent around the intercostal nerves between the paravertebral line and the area of required anesthesia. Because any particular area of skin usually receives innervation from two adjacent nerves, considerable overlapping of contiguous dermatomes occurs. Therefore, complete loss of sensation usually does not occur unless two or more intercostal nerves are anesthetized.

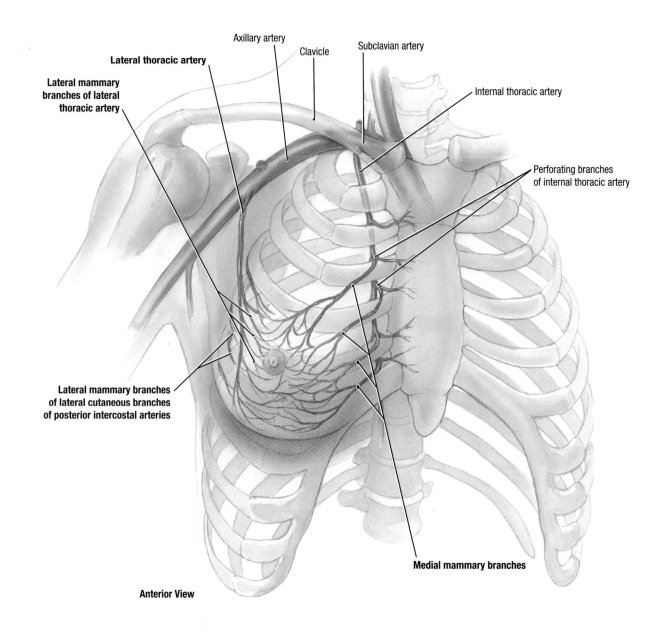

Axillary artery

Clavicle

Subclavian artery

Lateral thoracic artery

Internal thoracic artery

Lateral mammary branches of lateral thoracic artery

Perforating branches of internal thoracic artery

Lateral mammary branches of lateral cutaneous branches of posterior intercostal arteries

Medial mammary branches

Anterior View

1.7   Arterial supply of the breast

Arteries enter the breast from its superomedial and superolateral aspects; vessels also penetrate the deep surface of the breast. The blood supply is from the medial mammary branches of the internal thoracic artery, lateral mammary branches from the lateral thoracic artery, and lateral mammary branches of lateral cutaneous branches of the posterior intercostal arteries. The arteries branch profusely and anastomose with each other.

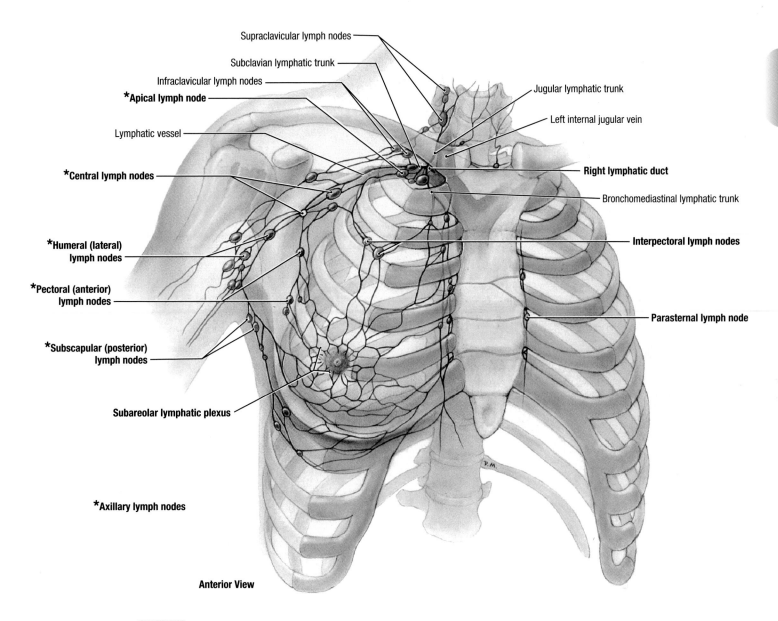

Supraclavicular lymph nodes

Subclavian lymphatic trunk

Infraclavicular lymph nodes

*Apical lymph node

Lymphatic vessel

*Central lymph nodes

*Humeral (lateral) lymph nodes

*Pectoral (anterior) lymph nodes

*Subscapular (posterior) lymph nodes

Subareolar lymphatic plexus

*Axillary lymph nodes

Jugular lymphatic trunk

Left internal jugular vein

Right lymphatic duct

Bronchomediastinal lymphatic trunk

Interpectoral lymph nodes

Parasternal lymph node

Anterior View

1.8 Lymphatic drainage of breast

Lymph drained from the upper limb and breast passes through nodes arranged irregularly in groups of axillary lymph nodes: (a) pectoral, along the inferior border of the pectoralis minor muscle; (b) subscapular, along the subscapular artery and veins; (c) humeral, along the distal part of the axillary vein; (d) central, at the base of the axilla, embedded in axillary fat; and (e) apical, along the axillary vein between the clavicle and the pectoralis minor muscle. Most of the breast drains via the pectoral, central, and apical axillary nodes to the subclavian lymph trunk, which joins the venous system at the junction of the subclavian and internal jugular veins. The medial part of the breast drains to the parasternal nodes, which are located along the internal thoracic vessels.

Breast cancer typically spreads by means of lymphatic vessels (lymphogenic metastasis), which carry cancer cells from the breast to the lymph nodes, chiefly those in the axilla. The cells lodge in the nodes, producing nests of tumor cells (metastases). Abundant communications among lymphatic pathways and among axillary, cervical, and parasternal nodes may also cause metastases from the breast to develop in the supraclavicular lymph nodes, the opposite breast, or the abdomen.

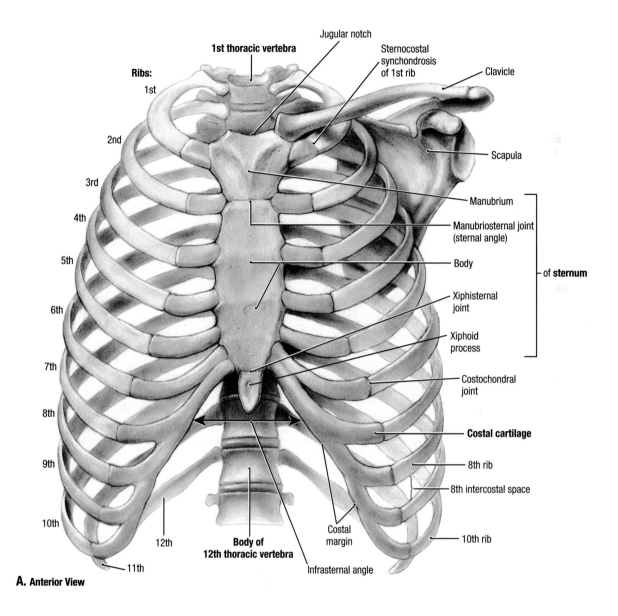

A. Anterior View

1.9   Bony thorax

- The skeleton of the thorax consists of 12 thoracic vertebrae, 12 pairs of ribs and costal cartilages, and the sternum.
- Anteriorly, forming the costal margin, the superior seven costal cartilages articulate with the sternum; the 8th, 9th, and 10th cartilages articulate with the cartilage above; the 11th and 12th are "floating" ribs, i.e., their cartilages do not articulate anteriorly.
- The clavicle lies over the anterosuperior aspect of the 1st rib, making it difficult to palpate.
- The 2nd rib is easy to locate because its costal cartilage articulates with the sternum at the sternal angle, located at the junction of the manubrium and body of the sternum.
- The 3rd to 10th ribs can be palpated in sequence inferolaterally from the 2nd rib; the fused costal cartilages of the 7th to 10th ribs form the costal arch (margin), and the tips of the 11th and 12th ribs can be palpated posterolaterally.

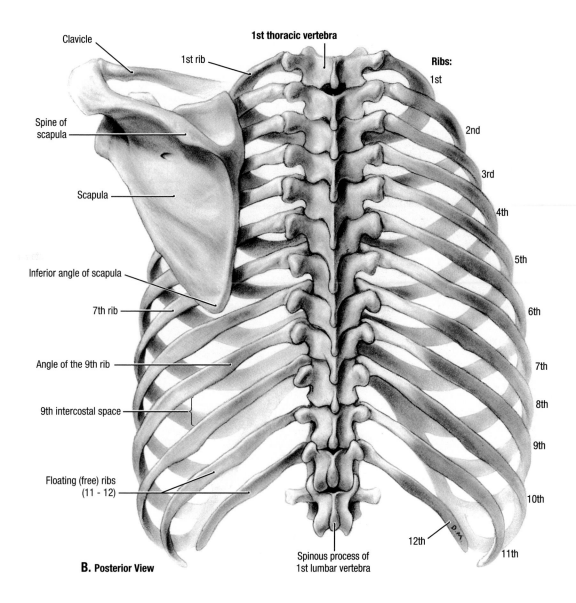

Clavicle

1st thoracic vertebra

1st rib

Ribs:
1st

Spine of scapula

2nd

3rd

Scapula

4th

5th

Inferior angle of scapula

6th

7th rib

Angle of the 9th rib

7th

9th intercostal space

8th

9th

Floating (free) ribs (11 - 12)

10th

12th

11th

Spinous process of 1st lumbar vertebra

B. Posterior View

1.9   Bony thorax (continued)

- The superior thoracic aperture (thoracic inlet) is the doorway between the thoracic cavity and the neck region; it is bounded by the 1st thoracic vertebra, the 1st ribs and their cartilages, and the manubrium of the sternum.
- Each rib articulates posteriorly with the vertebral column.
- Posteriorly, all ribs angle inferiorly; anteriorly, the 3rd to 10th costal cartilages angle superiorly.
- The scapula is suspended from the clavicle and crosses the 2nd to 7th ribs.

- When clinicians refer to the superior thoracic aperture as the thoracic "outlet," they are emphasizing the important nerves and arteries that pass through this aperture into the lower neck and upper limb. Hence, various types of thoracic outlet syndromes exist, such as the costoclavicular syndrome—pallor and coldness of the skin of the upper limb and diminished radial pulse—resulting from compression of the subclavian artery between the clavicle and the 1st rib.

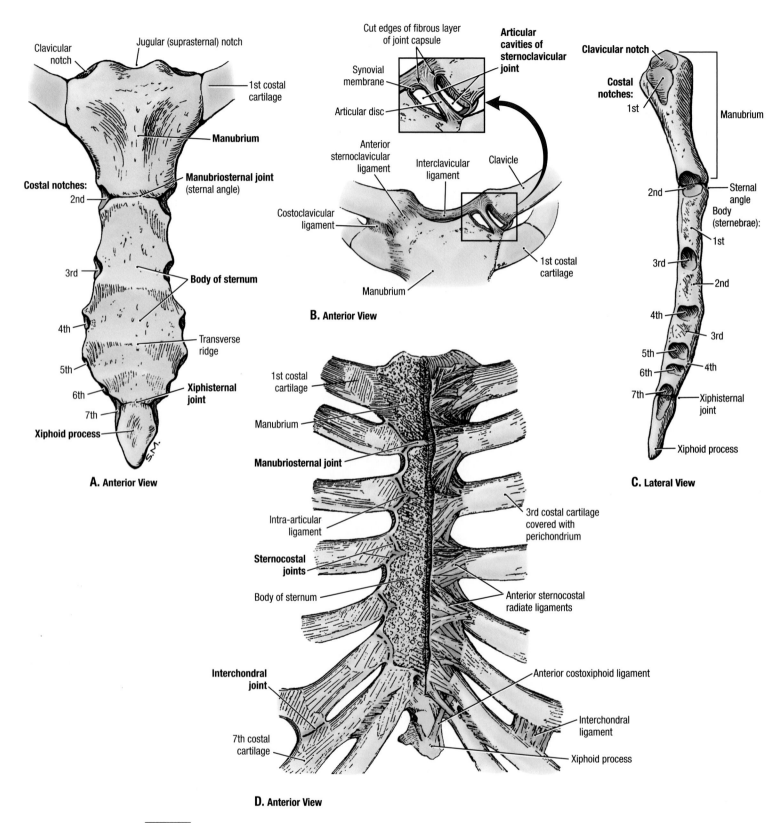

1.10   **Sternum and associated joints**

A. Parts of the anterior aspect of the sternum. **B.** Sternoclavicular joint. **C.** Features of the lateral aspect of the sternum. **D.** Sternocostal, manubriosternal, and interchondral joints. On the right side of the specimen, the cortex of the sternum and the external surface of the costal cartilages have been shaved away.

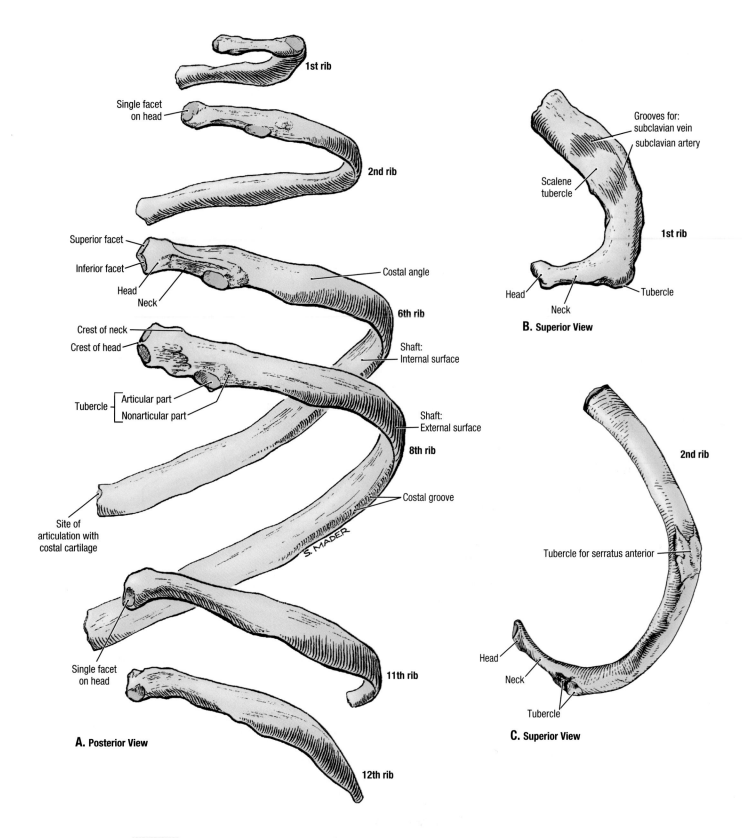

1.11 Ribs

A. "Typical" (6th and 8th) and "atypical" (1st and 2nd, 11th and 12th) ribs. **B.** First rib.
C. Second rib.

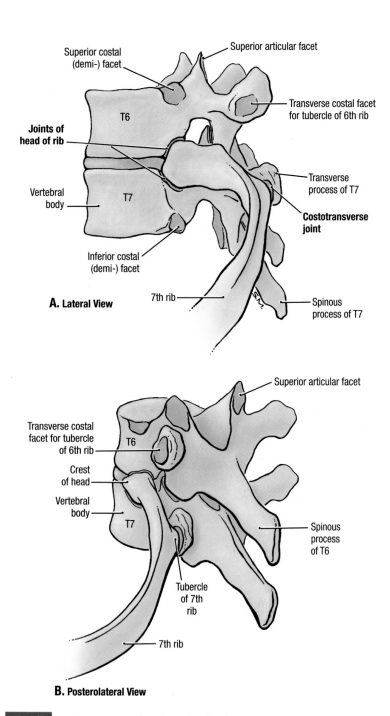

A. Lateral View

B. Posterolateral View

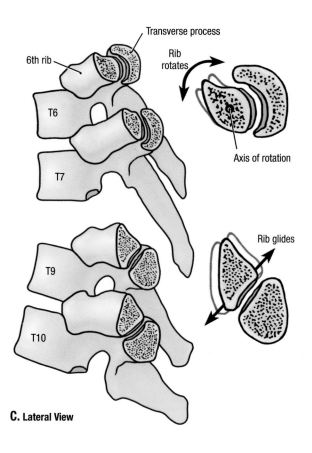

C. Lateral View

1.12   **Costovertebral articulations**

A and B. Articulating structures
- The costovertebral articulations include the joints of the head of the rib with two adjacent vertebral bodies and the tubercle of the rib with the transverse process of a vertebra.
- There are two articular facets on the head of the rib: a larger, inferior costal facet for articulation with the vertebral body of its own number, and a smaller, superior costal facet for articulation with the vertebral body of the vertebra superior to the rib.
- The crest of the head of the rib separates the superior and inferior costal facets.

- The smooth articular part of the tubercle of the rib, the transverse costal facet, articulates with the transverse process of the same numbered vertebra at the costotransverse joint.
C. Movements at the costotransverse joints: At the 1st to 7th costotransverse joints, the ribs rotate, increasing the anteroposterior diameter of the thorax; at the 8th, 9th, and 10th, they glide, increasing the transverse diameter of the upper abdomen.

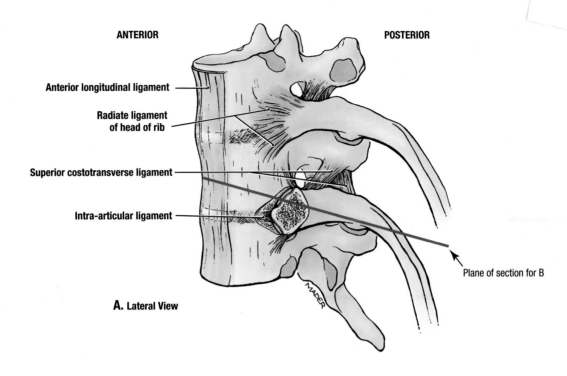

ANTERIOR   POSTERIOR

Anterior longitudinal ligament

Radiate ligament
of head of rib

Superior costotransverse ligament

Intra-articular ligament

Plane of section for B

A. Lateral View

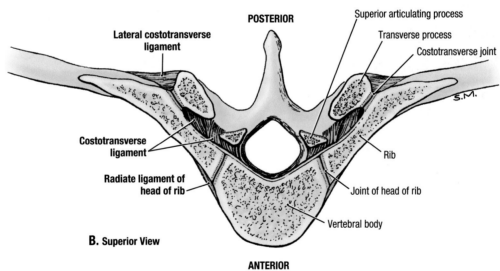

POSTERIOR

Superior articulating process

Transverse process

Costotransverse joint

Lateral costotransverse
ligament

Costotransverse
ligament

Rib

Radiate ligament of
head of rib

Joint of head of rib

Vertebral body

B. Superior View

ANTERIOR

1.13   Ligaments of costovertebral articulations

A.
- The radiate ligament joins the head of the rib to two vertebral bodies and the interposed intervertebral disc.
- The superior costotransverse ligament joins the crest of the neck of the rib to the transverse process above.
- The intra-articular ligament joins the crest of the head of the rib to the intervertebral disc.

B.
- The vertebral body, transverse processes, superior articulating processes, and posterior elements of the articulating ribs have been transversely sectioned to visualize the joint surfaces and ligaments.
- The costotransverse ligament joins the posterior aspect of the neck of the rib to the adjacent transverse process.
- The lateral costotransverse ligament joins the nonarticulating part of the tubercle of the rib to the tip (apex) of the transverse process.
- The articular surfaces of the synovial plane costovertebral joints are colored blue.

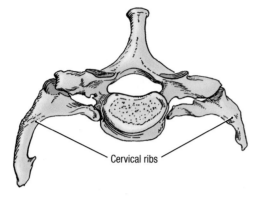

A. Superior View

Cervical ribs

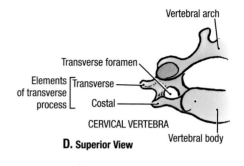

Vertebral arch

Transverse foramen

Elements of transverse process — Transverse

Costal

CERVICAL VERTEBRA

Vertebral body

D. Superior View

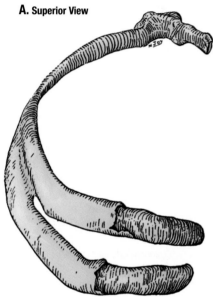

B. Anterior View

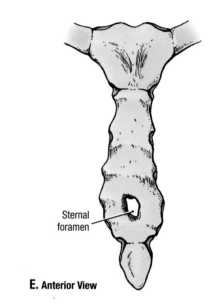

Sternal foramen

E. Anterior View

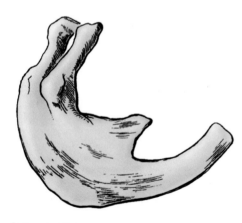

C. Superior View

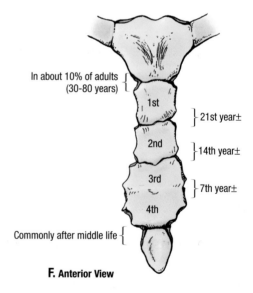

In about 10% of adults (30-80 years)

1st

21st year±

2nd

14th year±

3rd

7th year±

4th

Commonly after middle life

F. Anterior View

1.14   **Rib and sternum anomalies**

A. Cervical ribs. This is an enlarged costal element of the 7th cervical vertebra. (Compare with diagrammatic cervical vertebra in **D.**) Cervical ribs can be unilateral or bilateral, and large and palpable or detectable only radiologically. It can be asymptomatic or, through pressure on the most inferior root of the brachial plexus, can produce sensory and motor changes over the distribution of the ulnar nerve. **B.** Bifid rib. The superior component of this 3rd rib is supernumerary and articulated with the lateral aspect of the 1st sternebra. The inferior component articulated at the junction of the 1st and 2nd sternebrae. **C.** Bicipital rib. In this specimen, there has been partial fusion of the first two thoracic ribs. **E.** Sternal foramen. **F.** Ossification of sternum.

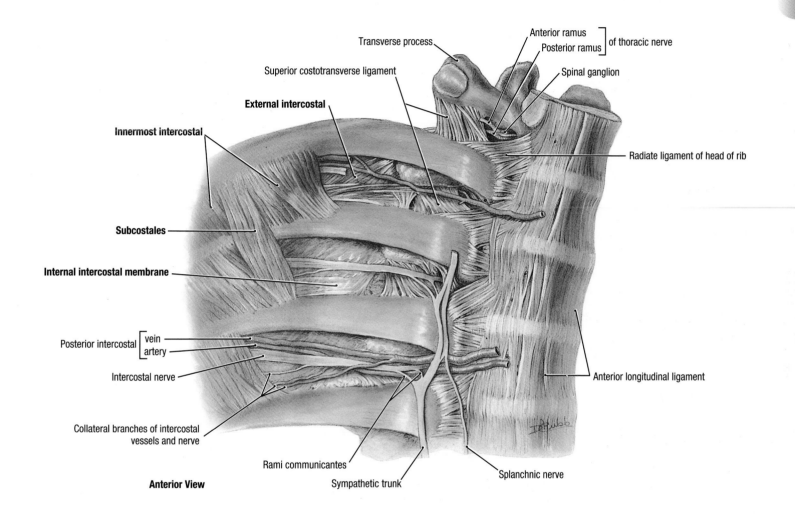

Transverse process
Superior costotransverse ligament
External intercostal
Innermost intercostal
Subcostales
Internal intercostal membrane
Posterior intercostal [vein / artery]
Intercostal nerve
Collateral branches of intercostal vessels and nerve
Rami communicantes
Sympathetic trunk
Anterior View

Anterior ramus] of thoracic nerve
Posterior ramus]
Spinal ganglion
Radiate ligament of head of rib
Anterior longitudinal ligament
Splanchnic nerve

1.15   Vertebral ends of internal aspect of intercostal spaces

- Portions of the innermost intercostal muscle that bridge two intercostal spaces are called subcostales muscles.
- The internal intercostal membrane, in the middle space, is continuous medially with the superior costotransverse ligament.
- Note the order of the structures in the most inferior space: posterior intercostal vein and artery, and intercostal nerve; note also their collateral branches.
- The anterior ramus crosses anterior to the superior costotransverse ligament; the posterior ramus is posterior to it.
- The intercostal nerves attach to the sympathetic trunk by rami communicantes; the splanchnic nerve is a visceral branch of the trunk.

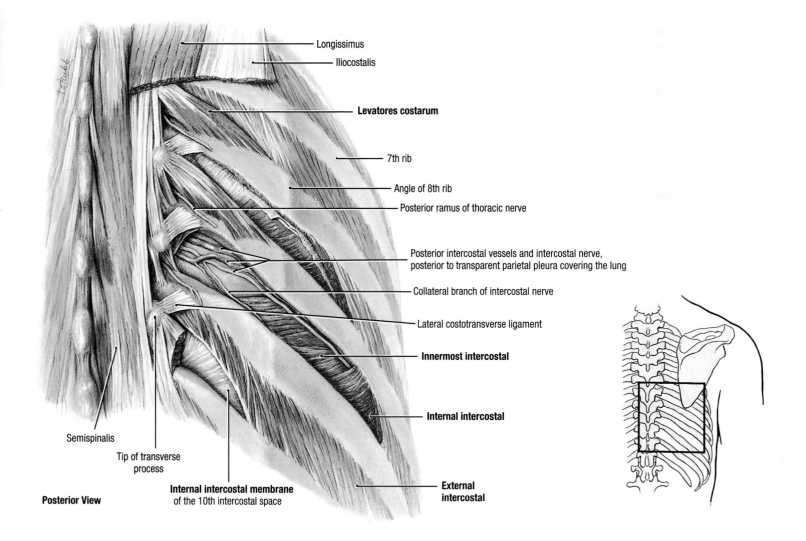

Longissimus

Iliocostalis

Levatores costarum

7th rib

Angle of 8th rib

Posterior ramus of thoracic nerve

Posterior intercostal vessels and intercostal nerve,
posterior to transparent parietal pleura covering the lung

Collateral branch of intercostal nerve

Lateral costotransverse ligament

Innermost intercostal

Internal intercostal

Semispinalis

Tip of transverse
process

Internal intercostal membrane
of the 10th intercostal space

Posterior View

**External
intercostal**

| **1.16** | **Vertebral ends of external aspect of inferior intercostal spaces** |

- The iliocostalis and longissimus muscles have been removed, exposing the levatores costarum muscle. Of the five intercostal spaces shown, the superior two (6th and 7th) are intact. In the 8th and 10th spaces, varying portions of the external intercostal muscle have been removed to reveal the underlying internal intercostal membrane, which is continuous with the internal intercostal muscle. In the 9th space, the levatores costarum muscle has been removed to show the posterior intercostal vessels and intercostal nerve.
- The intercostal vessels and nerve disappear laterally between the internal and innermost intercostal muscles.
- The intercostal nerve is the most inferior of the neurovascular trio (posterior intercostal vein and artery and intercostal nerve) and the least sheltered in the intercostal groove; a collateral branch arises near the angle of the rib.

- Sometimes it is necessary to insert a hypodermic needle through an intercostal space into the pleural cavity (See Fig. 1.24) to obtain a sample of pleural fluid or to remove blood or pus (thoracocentesis). To avoid damage to the intercostal nerve and vessels, the needle is inserted superior to the rib, high enough to avoid the collateral branches.

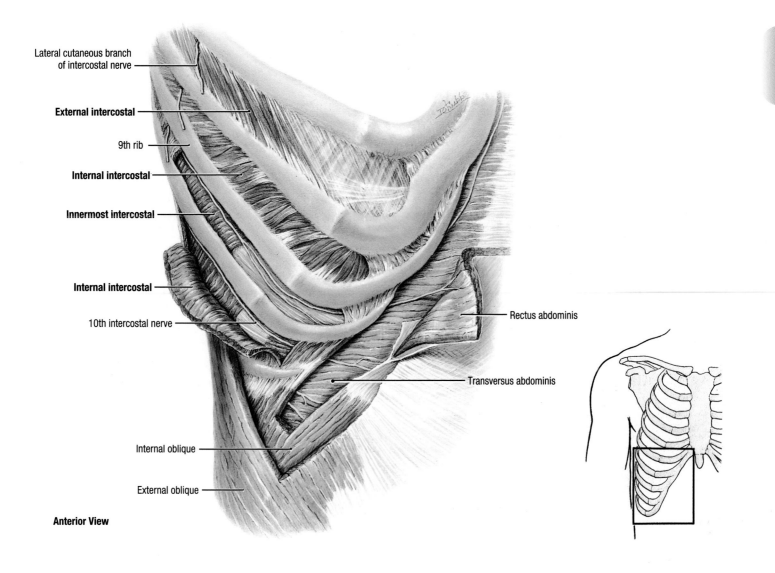

Lateral cutaneous branch
of intercostal nerve

External intercostal

9th rib

Internal intercostal

Innermost intercostal

Internal intercostal

10th intercostal nerve

Internal oblique

External oblique

Anterior View

Rectus abdominis

Transversus abdominis

1.17   Anterior ends of inferior intercostal spaces

- The fibers of the external intercostal and external oblique muscles run inferomedially.
- The internal intercostal and internal oblique muscles are in continuity at the ends of the 9th, 10th, and 11th intercostal spaces.
- The intercostal nerves lie deep to the internal intercostal muscle but superficial to the innermost intercostal muscle; anteriorly, these nerves lie superficial to the transversus thoracis or transversus abdominis muscles.
- Intercostal nerves run parallel to the ribs and costal cartilages; on reaching the abdominal wall, nerves T7 and T8 continue superiorly, T9 continues nearly horizontally, and T10 continues inferomedially toward the umbilicus. These nerves provide cutaneous innervation in overlapping segmental bands.

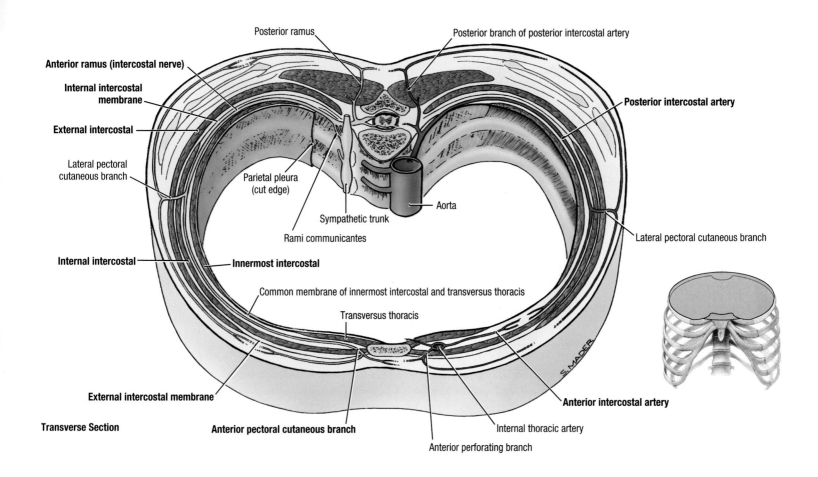

Posterior ramus

Posterior branch of posterior intercostal artery

Anterior ramus (intercostal nerve)

Internal intercostal membrane

Posterior intercostal artery

External intercostal

Lateral pectoral cutaneous branch

Parietal pleura (cut edge)

Aorta

Sympathetic trunk

Lateral pectoral cutaneous branch

Rami communicantes

Internal intercostal   **Innermost intercostal**

Common membrane of innermost intercostal and transversus thoracis

Transversus thoracis

External intercostal membrane

Anterior intercostal artery

Transverse Section

Anterior pectoral cutaneous branch

Internal thoracic artery

Anterior perforating branch

1.18   **Contents of intercostal space, transverse section**

- The diagram is simplified by showing nerves on the right and arteries on the left.
- The three musculomembranous layers are the external intercostal muscle and membrane, internal intercostal muscle and membrane, and the innermost intercostal muscle, transversus thoracis muscle, and the membrane connecting them.
- The intercostal nerves are the anterior rami of spinal nerves T1 to T11; the anterior ramus of T12 is the subcostal nerve.
- Posterior intercostal arteries are branches of the aorta (the superior two spaces are supplied from the superior intercostal branch of the costocervical trunk); the anterior intercostal arteries are branches of the internal thoracic artery or its branch, the musculophrenic artery.
- The posterior rami innervate the deep back muscles and skin adjacent to the vertebral column.

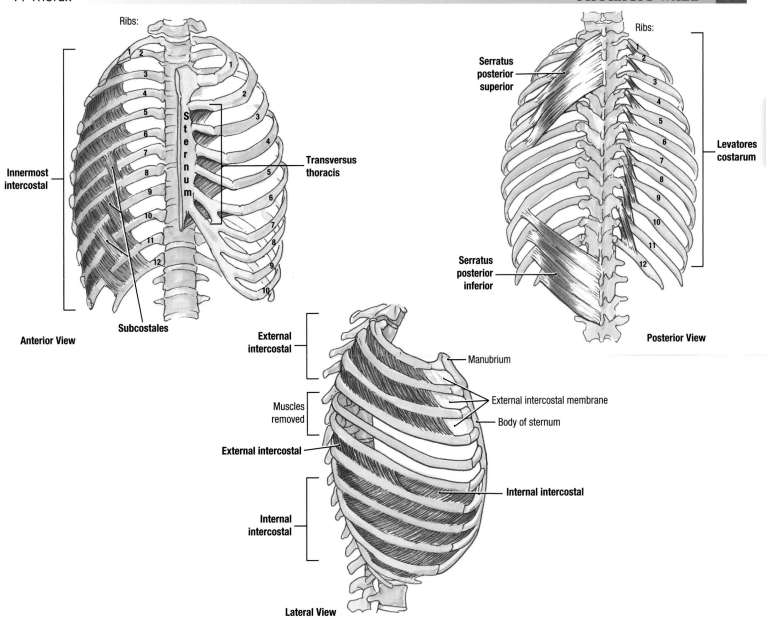

TABLE 1.1 MUSCLES OF THORACIC WALL

Muscle	Superior attachment	Inferior attachment	Innervation	Action[a]
External intercostal				Elevate ribs
Internal intercostal	Inferior border of ribs	Superior border of ribs below		Depress ribs
Innermost intercostal			Intercostal nerve	Probably elevate ribs
Transversus thoracis	Posterior surface of lower sternum	Internal surface of costal cartilages 2–6		Depress ribs
Subcostales	Internal surface of lower ribs near their angles	Superior borders of 2nd or 3rd ribs below		
Levatores costarum	Transverse processes of T7–T11	Subjacent ribs between tubercle and angle	Posterior rami of C8–T11 nerves	Elevate ribs
Serratus posterior superior	Nuchal ligament, spinous processes of C7–T3	Superior borders of 2nd–4th ribs	Second to fifth intercostal nerves	
Serratus posterior inferior	Spinous processes of T11–L2	Inferior borders of 8th–12th ribs near their angles	Anterior rami of T9-T12 nerves	Depress ribs

[a] All intercostal muscles keep intercostal spaces rigid, thereby preventing them from bulging out during expiration and from being drawn in during inspiration. Role of individual intercostal muscles and accessory muscles of respiration in moving the ribs is difficult to interpret despite many electromyographic studies.

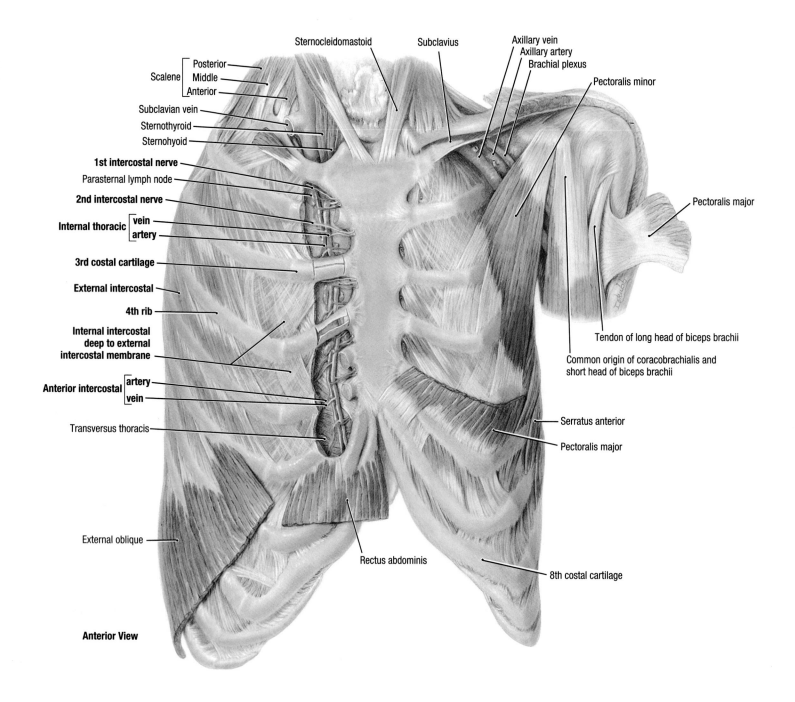

Sternocleidomastoid
Subclavius
Axillary vein
Axillary artery
Brachial plexus
Pectoralis minor

Scalene
Posterior
Middle
Anterior

Subclavian vein
Sternothyroid
Sternohyoid

1st intercostal nerve
Parasternal lymph node
2nd intercostal nerve
Internal thoracic vein / artery
3rd costal cartilage
External intercostal
4th rib
Internal intercostal deep to external intercostal membrane
Anterior intercostal artery / vein
Transversus thoracis

External oblique

Rectus abdominis

Pectoralis major

Tendon of long head of biceps brachii

Common origin of coracobrachialis and short head of biceps brachii

Serratus anterior

Pectoralis major

8th costal cartilage

Anterior View

1.19   **External aspect of thoracic wall**

- H-shaped cuts were made through the perichondrium of the 3rd and 4th costal cartilages to shell out segments of cartilage.
- The internal thoracic (internal mammary) vessels run inferiorly deep to the costal cartilages and just lateral to the edge of the sternum, providing anterior intercostal branches.
- The parasternal lymph nodes (*green*) receive lymphatic vessels from the anterior parts of intercostal spaces, the costal pleura and diaphragm, and the medial part of the breast.
- The subclavian vessels are "sandwiched" between the 1st rib and clavicle and are "padded" by the subclavius.

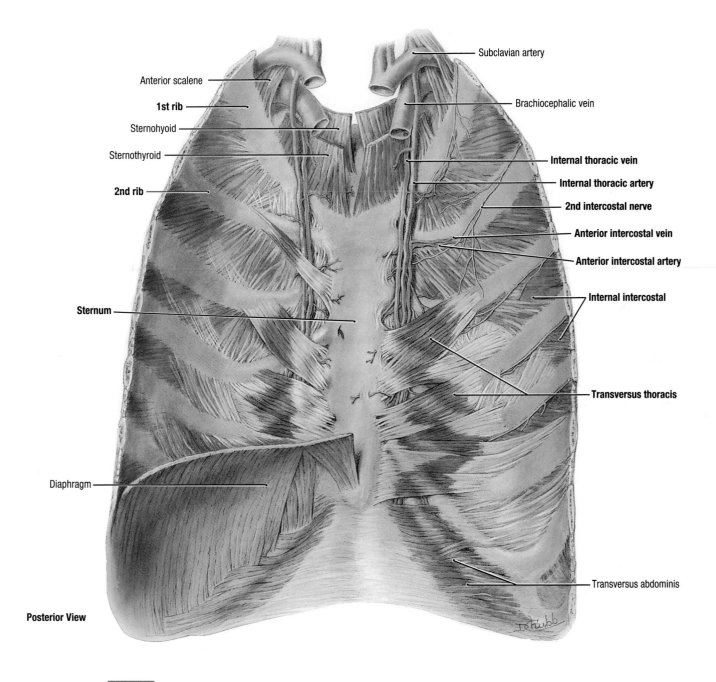

Anterior scalene
1st rib
Sternohyoid
Sternothyroid
2nd rib
Sternum
Diaphragm
Posterior View

Subclavian artery
Brachiocephalic vein
Internal thoracic vein
Internal thoracic artery
2nd intercostal nerve
Anterior intercostal vein
Anterior intercostal artery
Internal intercostal
Transversus thoracis
Transversus abdominis

1.20   **Internal aspect of the anterior thoracic wall**

- The inferior portions of the internal thoracic vessels are covered posteriorly by the transversus thoracis muscle; the superior portions are in contact with the parietal pleura (removed).

- The transversus thoracis muscle is continuous with the transversus abdominis muscle; these form the innermost layer of the three flat muscles of the thoracoabdominal wall.

- The internal thoracic (internal mammary) artery arises from the subclavian artery and is accompanied by two venae comitantes up to the 2nd costal cartilage in this specimen and, superior to this, by the single internal thoracic vein, which drains into the brachiocephalic vein.

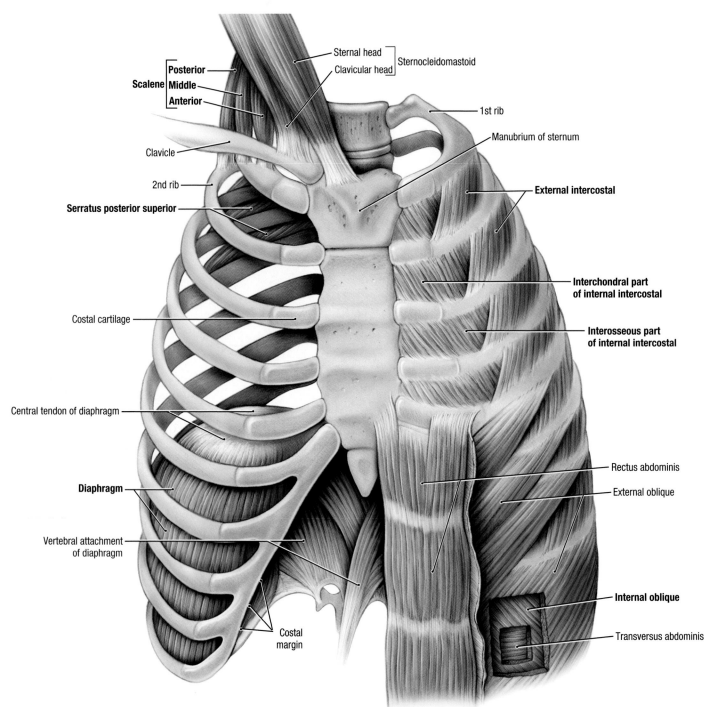

Sternal head
Clavicular head
Sternocleidomastoid
Posterior
Scalene **Middle**
Anterior
Clavicle
2nd rib
Serratus posterior superior
Costal cartilage
Central tendon of diaphragm
Diaphragm
Vertebral attachment of diaphragm
Costal margin
1st rib
Manubrium of sternum
External intercostal
Interchondral part of internal intercostal
Interosseous part of internal intercostal
Rectus abdominis
External oblique
Internal oblique
Transversus abdominis

TABLE 1.2 MUSCLES OF RESPIRATION

Inspiration			Expiration
Normal (Quiet)	Major	Diaphragm (active contraction)	Passive (elastic) recoil of lungs and thoracic cage
	Minor	*Tonic contraction* of external intercostals and interchondral portion of internal intercostals to resist negative pressure	*Tonic contraction* of muscles of anterolateral abdominal walls (rectus abdominis, external and internal obliques, transversus abdominis) to antagonize diaphragm by maintaining intra-abdominal pressure
Active (Forced)		In addition to the above, *active contraction* of	In addition to the above, *active contraction* of
		Sternocleidomastoid, descending (superior) trapezius, pectoralis minor, and scalenes, to elevate and fix upper rib cage	Muscles of anterolateral abdominal wall (antagonizing diaphragm by increasing intra-abdominal pressure and by pulling inferiorly and fixing inferior costal margin): rectus abdominis, external and internal obliques, and transversus abdominis
		External intercostals, interchondral portion of internal intercostals, subcostales, levatores costarum, and serratus posterior superior[a] to elevate ribs	Internal intercostal (interosseous part) and serratus posterior inferior[a] to depress ribs

[a] Recent studies indicate that the serratus posterior superior and inferior muscles may serve primarily as organs of proprioception rather than motion.

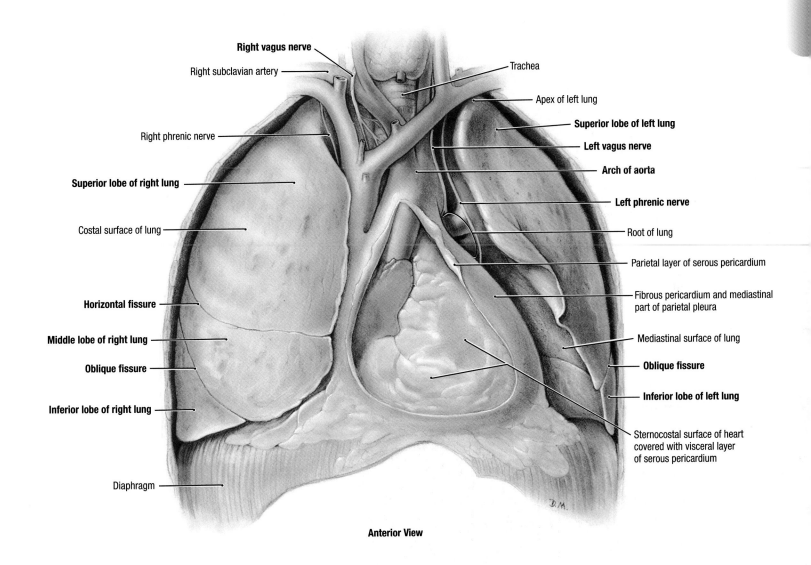

Right vagus nerve

Right subclavian artery

Trachea

Right phrenic nerve

Apex of left lung

Superior lobe of left lung

Left vagus nerve

Arch of aorta

Superior lobe of right lung

Costal surface of lung

Left phrenic nerve

Root of lung

Parietal layer of serous pericardium

Horizontal fissure

Fibrous pericardium and mediastinal part of parietal pleura

Mediastinal surface of lung

Middle lobe of right lung

Oblique fissure

Oblique fissure

Inferior lobe of left lung

Inferior lobe of right lung

Sternocostal surface of heart covered with visceral layer of serous pericardium

Diaphragm

Anterior View

1.21 **Thoracic contents in situ**

- The fibrous pericardium, lined by the parietal layer of serous pericardium, is removed anteriorly to expose the heart and great vessels.
- The right lung has three lobes; the superior lobe is separated from the middle lobe by the horizontal fissure, and the middle lobe is separated from the inferior lobe by the oblique fissure. The left lung has two lobes, superior and inferior, separated by the oblique fissure.
- The anterior border of the left lung is reflected laterally to visualize the phrenic nerve passing anterior to the root of the lung and the vagus nerve lying anterior to the arch of the aorta and then passing posterior to the root of the lung.
- As the right vagus nerve passes anterior to the right subclavian artery, it gives rise to the recurrent branch and then divides to contribute fibers to the esophageal, cardiac, and pulmonary plexuses.

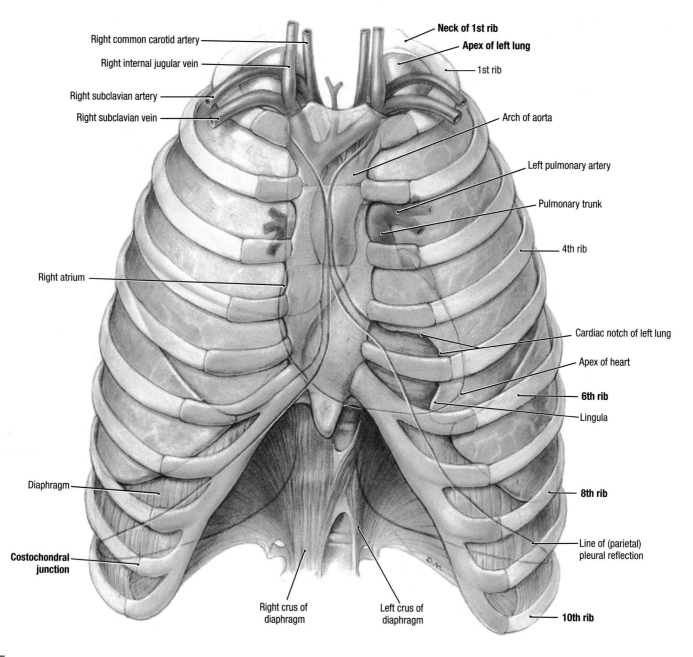

Right common carotid artery

Right internal jugular vein

Right subclavian artery

Right subclavian vein

Right atrium

Diaphragm

Costochondral junction

Right crus of diaphragm

Left crus of diaphragm

Neck of 1st rib

Apex of left lung

1st rib

Arch of aorta

Left pulmonary artery

Pulmonary trunk

4th rib

Cardiac notch of left lung

Apex of heart

6th rib

Lingula

8th rib

Line of (parietal) pleural reflection

10th rib

1.22 **Topography of the lungs and mediastinum**

- The mediastinum is located between the pleural cavities and is occupied by the heart and the tissues anterior, posterior, and superior to the heart.
- The apex of the lungs is at the level of the neck of the 1st rib, and the inferior border of the lungs is at the 6th rib in the left midclavicular line and the 8th rib at the lateral aspect of the bony thorax at the midaxillary line.
- The cardiac notch of the left lung and the deviation of the parietal pleura is away from the median plane toward the left side in the region of the cardiac notch.

- The inferior reflection of parietal pleura is at the 8th costochondral junction in the midclavicular line, at the 10th rib in the midaxillary line.
- The apex of the heart is in the 5th intercostal space at the left midclavicular line.
- The right atrium forms the right border of the heart and extends just beyond the lateral margin of the sternum.
- The branches of the great vessels pass through the superior thoracic aperture.

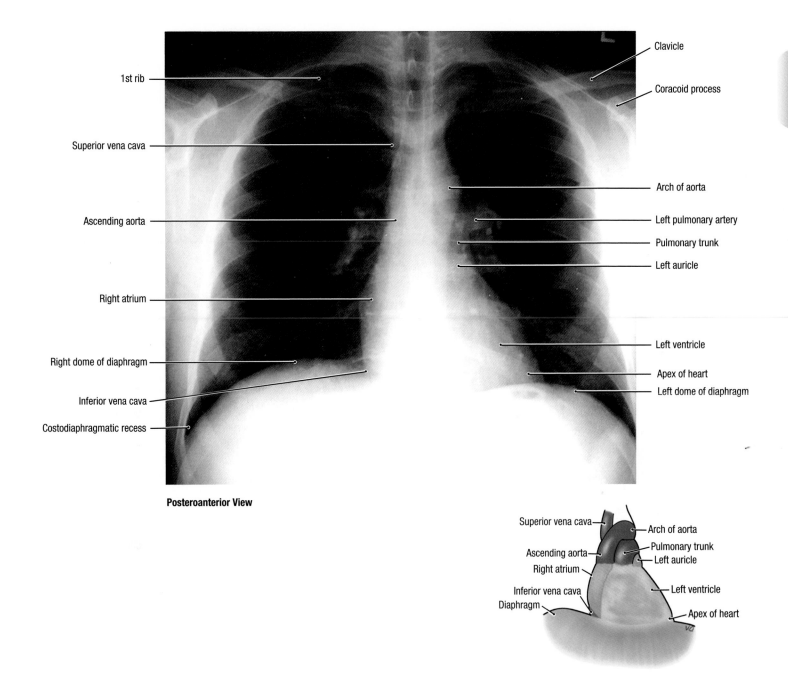

Posteroanterior View

1.23   Radiograph of chest

- The right dome of the diaphragm is higher than the left dome due primarily to the large underlying liver.
- The convex right mediastinal border of the heart is formed by the right atrium; above this, the superior vena cava and ascending aorta produce less convex borders.
- The left border of the mediastinal silhouette is formed by the arch of the aorta, pulmonary trunk, left auricle (normally not prominent), and left ventricle.
- Follow the 1st rib to where it curves laterally and then medially to cross the clavicle.

- Any structure in the mediastinum may contribute to pathological widening of the mediastinal silhouette. It is often observed after trauma resulting from a head-on collision, for example, which produces hemorrhage into the mediastinum from lacerated great vessels such as the aorta or SVC. Frequently, malignant lymphoma (cancer of lymphatic tissue) produces massive enlargement of mediastinal lymph nodes and widening of the mediastinum. Enlargement (hypertrophy) of the heart (occurring with congestive heart failure) is a common cause of widening of the inferior mediastinum.

Nasal cavity
Pharyngeal opening of pharyngotympanic tube
Palate
Tongue
Nasal part
Oral part — **Pharynx**
Laryngeal part
Epiglottis
Larynx
Trachea
Right main bronchus
Left main bronchus
Superior lobe
Superior (upper) lobe
Right lung
Middle lobe
Inferior lobe
Inferior (lower) lobe — **Left lung**
Pleural cavity
Mediastinum
Diaphragm
Costodiaphragmatic recess

A. Anterior View

COLLAPSED LUNG **INFLATED LUNG**
Pleural cavity
*Cervical part
Visceral pleura
*Costal part
Root of lung
*Mediastinal part
*Diaphragmatic part
Parietal pleura
B. Anterior View *Parts of parietal pleura

*Cervical part (cupula)
*Costal part
*Mediastinal part
Left lung
Diaphragm Apex of heart
Right lung
*Diaphragmatic part
Costodiaphragmatic recess
C. Coronal Section *Parts of parietal pleura

1.24 **Respiratory system**

A. Overview. **B.** Pleural cavity and pleura. **C.** Coronal section through heart and lungs.

- The lungs invaginate a continuous membranous pleural sac; the visceral (pulmonary) pleura covers the lungs, and the parietal pleura lines the thoracic cavity; the visceral and parietal pleurae are continuous around the root of the lung.
- The parietal pleura can be divided regionally into the costal, diaphragmatic, mediastinal, and cervical parts; note the costodiaphragmatic recess.

- The pleural cavity is a potential space between the visceral and parietal pleurae that contains a thin layer of fluid. If a sufficient amount of air enters the pleural cavity, the surface tension adhering visceral to parietal pleura (lung to thoracic wall) is broken, and the lung collapses because of its inherent elasticity (elastic recoil). When a lung collapses, the pleural cavity—normally a potential space—becomes a real space (**B**) and may contain air (pneumothorax), blood (hemothorax), etc.

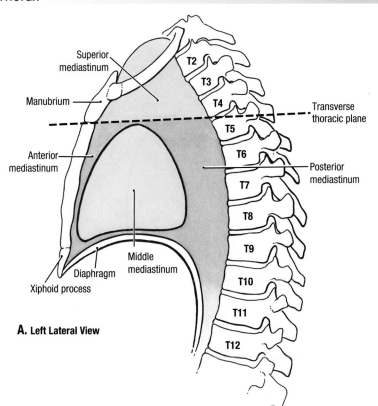

Superior mediastinum

Manubrium

T2

T3

T4

Transverse thoracic plane

T5

Anterior mediastinum

T6

Posterior mediastinum

T7

T8

Middle mediastinum

T9

Diaphragm

T10

Xiphoid process

T11

T12

A. Left Lateral View

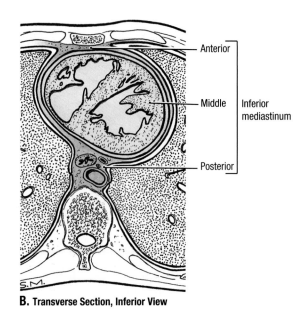

Anterior

Middle — Inferior mediastinum

Posterior

B. Transverse Section, Inferior View

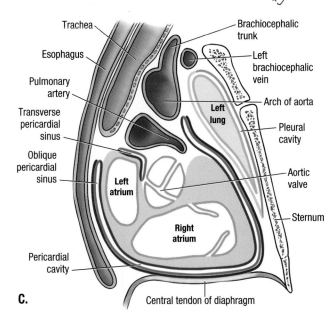

Trachea

Brachiocephalic trunk

Esophagus

Left brachiocephalic vein

Pulmonary artery

Left lung

Transverse pericardial sinus

Arch of aorta

Oblique pericardial sinus

Pleural cavity

Left atrium

Aortic valve

Sternum

Right atrium

Pericardial cavity

Central tendon of diaphragm

C.

Median Section, Right Lateral View

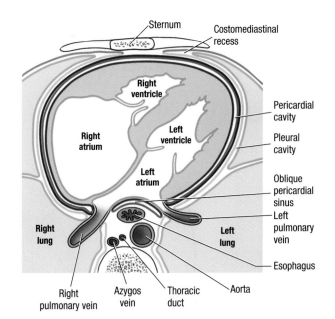

Sternum

Costomediastinal recess

Right ventricle

Right atrium

Left ventricle

Pericardial cavity

Pleural cavity

Left atrium

Oblique pericardial sinus

Right lung

Left pulmonary vein

Left lung

Esophagus

Right pulmonary vein

Azygos vein

Thoracic duct

Aorta

Transverse Section, Inferior View

Key for C.

Pericardium
▬ Fibrous pericardium
Serous pericardium:
▬ Parietal layer of serous pericardium (lines fibrous pericardium)
▬ Visceral layer of serous pericardium (outermost layer of heart wall)

Thin film of fluid in pericardial cavity between visceral and parietal layers allows the heart to move freely within the pericardial sac.

Heart	**Pleurae**
▬ Epicardium (visceral layer of serous pericardium)	▬ Visceral pleura
	Parietal pleura:
▬ Myocardium	▬ Mediastinal
▬ Endocardium	▬ Costal

1.25   **Mediastinum and pericardium**

A and **B.** Subdivisions of mediastinum. **C.** Layers of pericardium and heart.

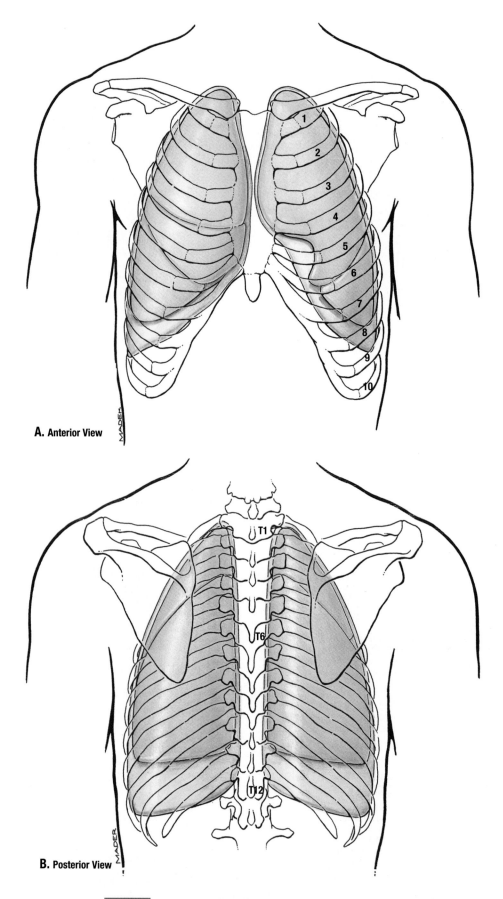

A. Anterior View

B. Posterior View

1.26   Extent of parietal pleura and lungs

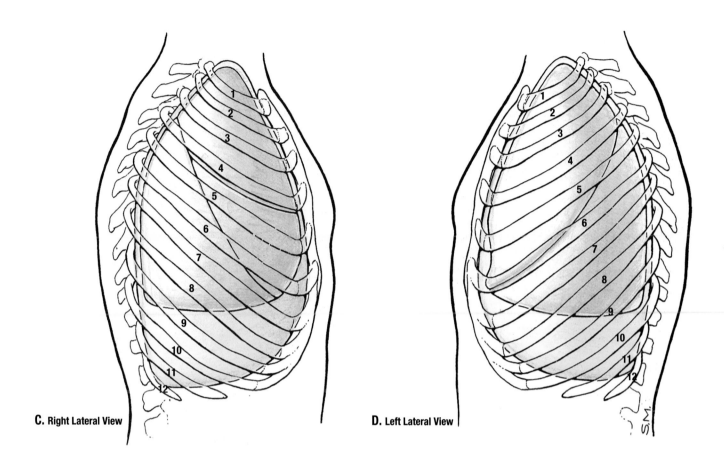

C. Right Lateral View   **D.** Left Lateral View

1.26   **Extent of parietal pleura and lungs** *(continued)*

TABLE 1.3 SURFACE MARKINGS OF PARIETAL PLEURA (BLUE)

Level	Left Pleura	Right Pleura
Apex	About 4 cm superior to middle of clavicle	About 4 cm superior to middle of clavicle
4th costal cartilage	Midline (anteriorly)	Midline (anteriorly)
6th costal cartilage	Lateral margin of sternum	Midline (anteriorly)
8th costal cartilage	Midclavicular line	Midclavicular line
10th rib	Midaxillary line	Midaxillary line
11th rib	Line of inferior angle of scapula	Line of inferior angle of scapula
12th rib	Lateral border of erector spinae to T12 spinous process (slightly lower level than right pleura)	Lateral border of erector spinae to T12 spinous process

SURFACE MARKINGS OF LUNGS COVERED WITH VISCERAL PLEURA (PINK)

Level	Left Lung	Right Lung
Apex	About 4 cm superior to middle of clavicle	About 4 cm superior to middle of clavicle
2nd costal cartilage	Midline (anteriorly)	Midline (anteriorly)
4th costal cartilage	Lateral margin of sternum	Lateral margin of sternum
6th costal cartilage	Follows 4th costal cartilage, turns inferiorly to 6th costal cartilage in the midclavicular line (cardiac notch)	Midclavicular line
8th rib	Midaxillary line	Midaxillary line
10th rib	Line of inferior angle of scapula to T10 spinous process	Line of inferior angle of scapula to T10 spinous process

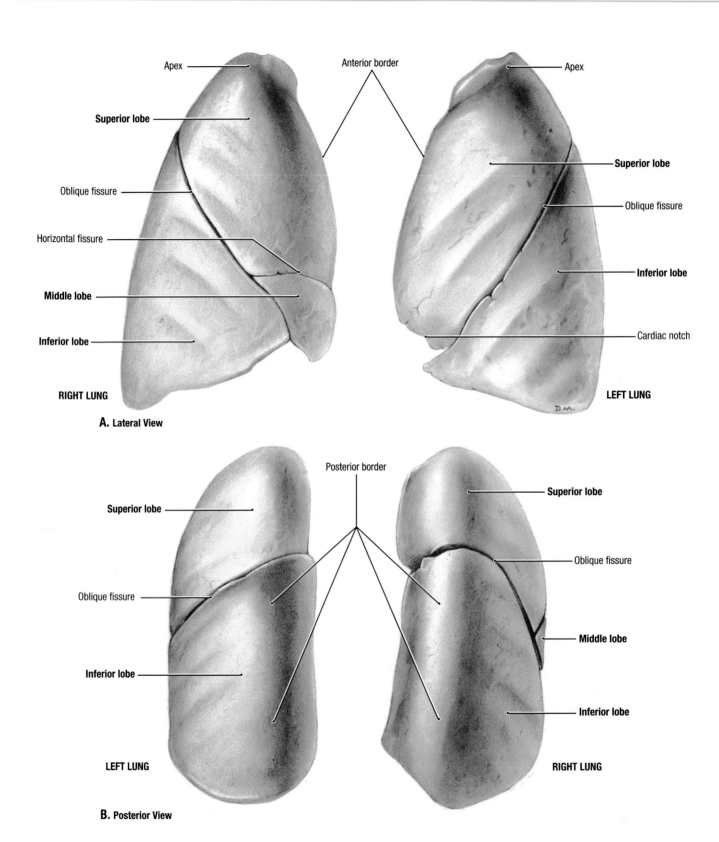

Apex ———— Anterior border ———— Apex

Superior lobe ————

Superior lobe

Oblique fissure ————

———— Oblique fissure

Horizontal fissure ————

Middle lobe ————

———— **Inferior lobe**

Inferior lobe ————

———— Cardiac notch

RIGHT LUNG   **LEFT LUNG**

A. Lateral View

Posterior border

Superior lobe ————

Superior lobe ————

———— Oblique fissure

Oblique fissure ————

———— **Middle lobe**

Inferior lobe ————

———— **Inferior lobe**

LEFT LUNG   **RIGHT LUNG**

B. Posterior View

1.27   Lungs

The right lung usually has three lobes, and the left lung, two lobes. The oblique and horizontal fissures of the right lung and the oblique fissure of the left lung may be incomplete or absent in some specimens.

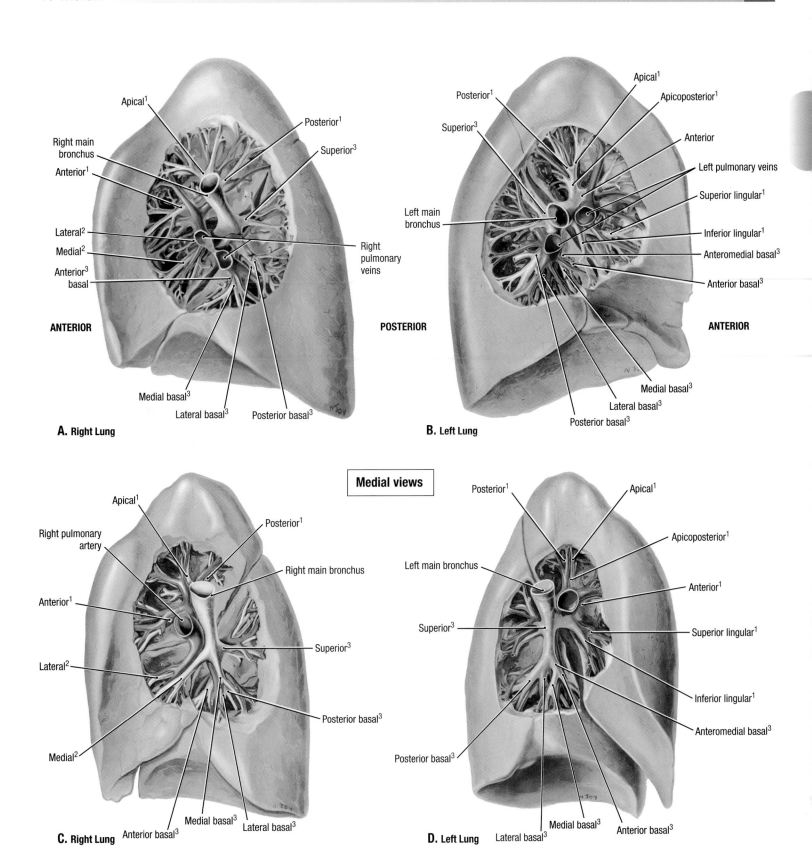

A. Right Lung

- Apical[1]
- Right main bronchus
- Anterior[1]
- Posterior[1]
- Superior[3]
- Lateral[2]
- Medial[2]
- Anterior[3] basal
- Right pulmonary veins
- **ANTERIOR**
- Medial basal[3]
- Lateral basal[3]
- Posterior basal[3]

B. Left Lung

- Posterior[1]
- Superior[3]
- Apical[1]
- Apicoposterior[1]
- Anterior
- Left pulmonary veins
- Superior lingular[1]
- Left main bronchus
- Inferior lingular[1]
- Anteromedial basal[3]
- Anterior basal[3]
- **POSTERIOR**
- **ANTERIOR**
- Medial basal[3]
- Lateral basal[3]
- Posterior basal[3]

Medial views

C. Right Lung

- Apical[1]
- Right pulmonary artery
- Posterior[1]
- Right main bronchus
- Anterior[1]
- Lateral[2]
- Superior[3]
- Medial[2]
- Posterior basal[3]
- Anterior basal[3]
- Medial basal[3]
- Lateral basal[3]

D. Left Lung

- Posterior[1]
- Apical[1]
- Apicoposterior[1]
- Left main bronchus
- Anterior[1]
- Superior[3]
- Superior lingular[1]
- Inferior lingular[1]
- Anteromedial basal[3]
- Posterior basal[3]
- Medial basal[3]
- Anterior basal[3]
- Lateral basal[3]

1.28 **Bronchi, pulmonary veins, and pulmonary arteries**

A and **C.** Right lungs. **B** and **D.** Left lungs. Superscripts indicate segmental bronchi to the [1]superior lobe, [2]middle lobe, and [3]inferior lobe. The pulmonary veins and arteries of fresh lungs were filled with latex, the bronchi were inflated with air. The tissues surrounding the bronchi and vessels were removed.

Obstruction of a pulmonary artery by a blood clot (embolism) results in partial or complete obstruction of blood flow to the lung.

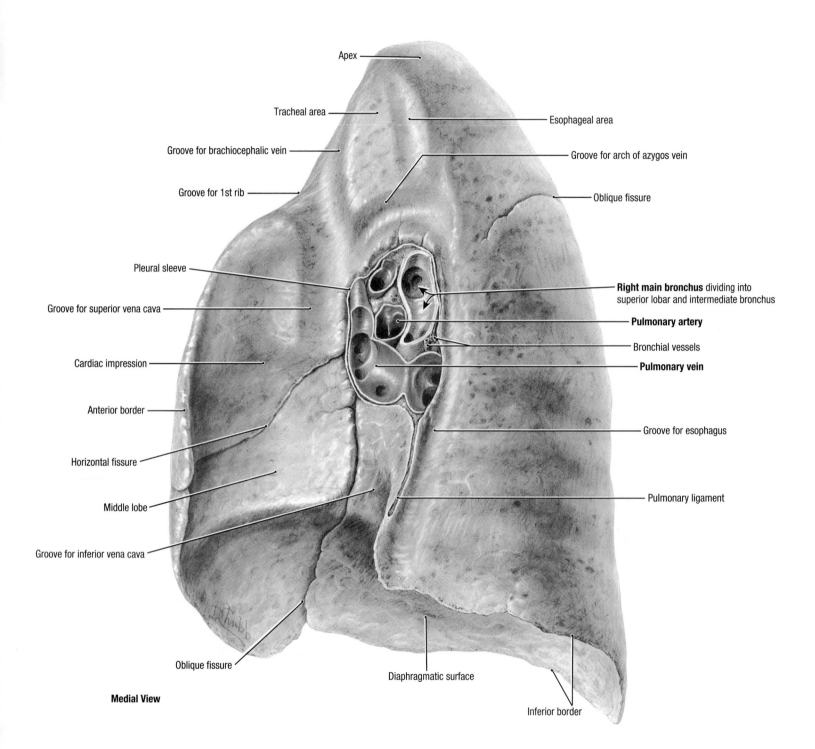

Apex

Tracheal area

Groove for brachiocephalic vein

Groove for 1st rib

Pleural sleeve

Groove for superior vena cava

Cardiac impression

Anterior border

Horizontal fissure

Middle lobe

Groove for inferior vena cava

Oblique fissure

Medial View

Esophageal area

Groove for arch of azygos vein

Oblique fissure

Right main bronchus dividing into superior lobar and intermediate bronchus

Pulmonary artery

Bronchial vessels

Pulmonary vein

Groove for esophagus

Pulmonary ligament

Diaphragmatic surface

Inferior border

1.29   **Mediastinal (medial) surface and hilum of right lung**

The embalmed lung shows impressions of the structures with which it comes into contact, clearly demarcated as surface features; the base is contoured by the domes of the diaphragm; the costal surface bears the impressions of the ribs; distended vessels leave their mark, but nerves do not. The oblique fissure is incomplete here.

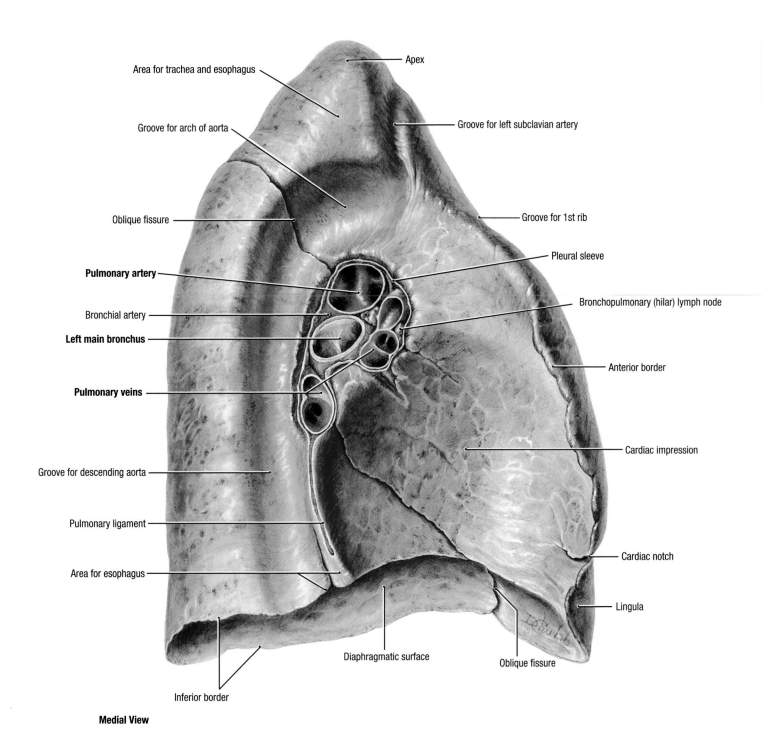

Apex

Area for trachea and esophagus

Groove for left subclavian artery

Groove for arch of aorta

Oblique fissure

Groove for 1st rib

Pleural sleeve

Pulmonary artery

Bronchopulmonary (hilar) lymph node

Bronchial artery

Left main bronchus

Anterior border

Pulmonary veins

Groove for descending aorta

Cardiac impression

Pulmonary ligament

Area for esophagus

Cardiac notch

Lingula

Diaphragmatic surface

Oblique fissure

Inferior border

Medial View

1.30   Mediastinal (medial) surface and hilum of left lung

Note the site of contact with esophagus, between the descending aorta and the inferior end of the pulmonary ligament. In the right and left roots, the artery is superior, the bronchus is posterior, one vein is anterior, and the other is inferior; in the right root, the bronchus to the superior lobe (also called the *eparterial bronchus*) is the most superior structure.

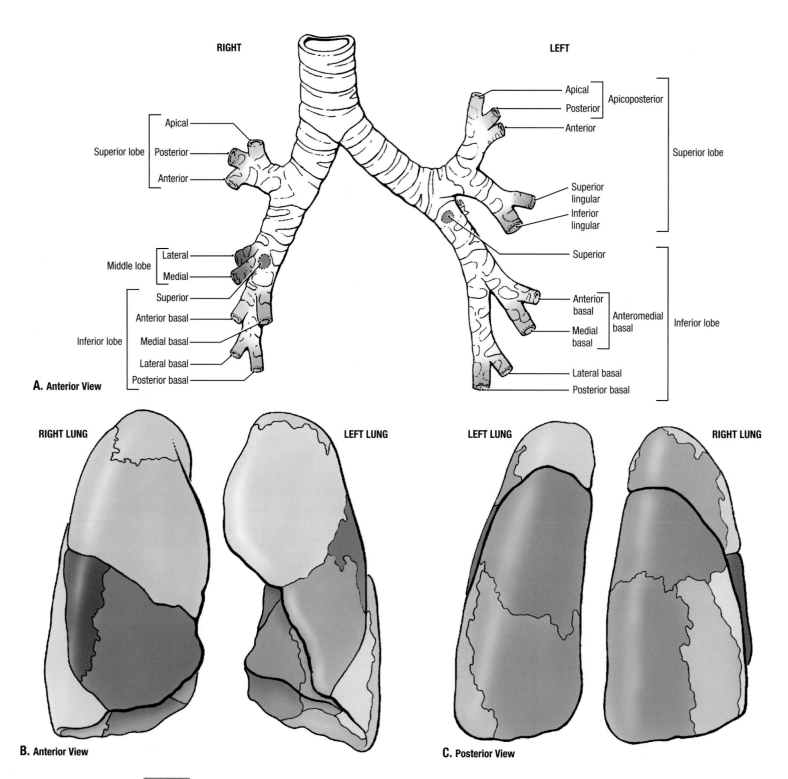

RIGHT

Apical
Posterior — Superior lobe
Anterior

Lateral — Middle lobe
Medial

Superior
Anterior basal
Medial basal — Inferior lobe
Lateral basal
Posterior basal

A. Anterior View

LEFT

Apical
Posterior — Apicoposterior
Anterior

Superior lingular — Superior lobe
Inferior lingular

Superior

Anterior basal
Medial basal — Anteromedial basal — Inferior lobe

Lateral basal
Posterior basal

RIGHT LUNG   **LEFT LUNG**

B. Anterior View

LEFT LUNG   **RIGHT LUNG**

C. Posterior View

1.31   **Segmental bronchi and bronchopulmonary segments**

A. There are 10 tertiary or segmental bronchi on the right, and 8 on the left. Note that on the left, the apical and posterior bronchi arise from a single stem, as do the anterior basal and medial basal. **B** to **F.** A bronchopulmonary segment consists of a tertiary bronchus, pulmonary vein and artery, and the portion of lung they serve. These structures are surgically separable to allow segmental resection of the lung. To prepare these specimens, the tertiary bronchi of fresh lungs were isolated within the hilum and injected with latex of various colors. Minor variations in the branching of the bronchi result in variations in the surface patterns.

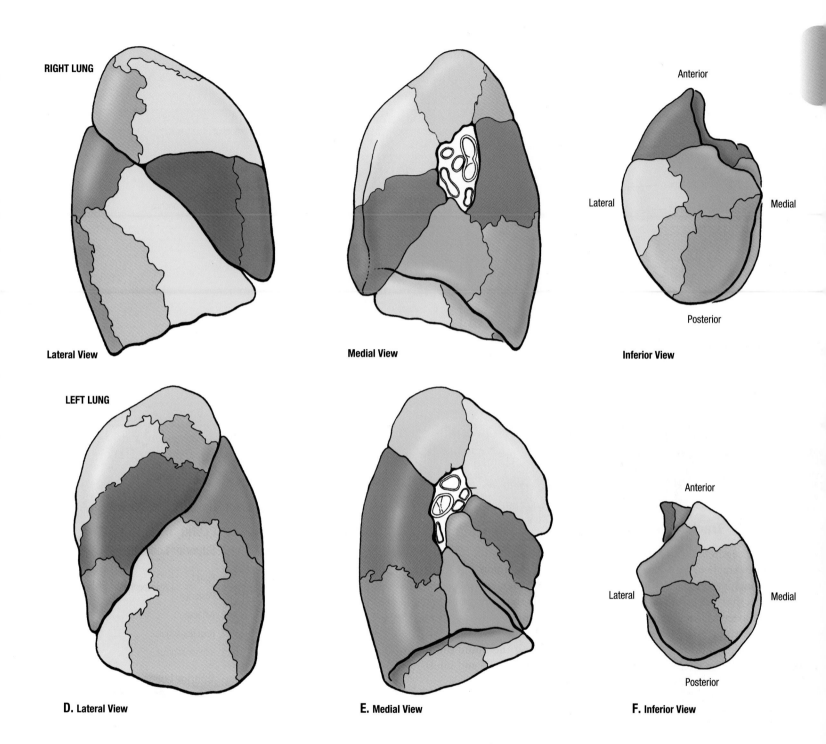

RIGHT LUNG

Lateral View

Medial View

Anterior

Lateral

Medial

Posterior

Inferior View

LEFT LUNG

D. Lateral View

E. Medial View

Anterior

Lateral

Medial

Posterior

F. Inferior View

1.31   **Segmental bronchi and bronchopulmonary segments (*continued*)**

Knowledge of the anatomy of the bronchopulmonary segments is essential for precise interpretations of diagnostic images of the lungs and for surgical resection (removal) of diseased segments. During the treatment of lung cancer, the surgeon may remove a whole lung (*pneumonectomy*), a lobe (*lobectomy*), or one or more bronchopulmonary segments (*segmentectomy*). Knowledge and understanding of the bronchopulmonary segments and their relationship to the bronchial tree are also essential for planning drainage and clearance techniques used in physical therapy for enhancing drainage from specific areas (e.g., in patients with pneumonia or cystic fibrosis).

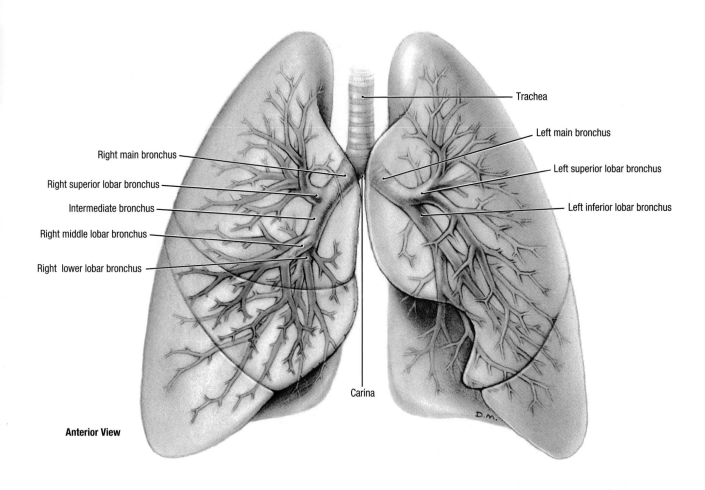

Trachea

Left main bronchus

Left superior lobar bronchus

Right main bronchus

Right superior lobar bronchus

Intermediate bronchus

Left inferior lobar bronchus

Right middle lobar bronchus

Right lower lobar bronchus

Carina

Anterior View

1.32   Trachea and bronchi in situ

- The segmental (tertiary) bronchi are color coded.
- The trachea bifurcates into right and left main (primary) bronchi; the right main bronchus is shorter, wider, and more vertical than the left. Therefore, it is more likely that foreign objects will become lodged in the right main bronchus.
- The right main bronchus gives off the right superior lobe bronchus (eparterial bronchus) before entering the hilum (hilus) of the lung; after entering the hilum, the right middle and inferior lobar bronchi branch off.
- The left main bronchus divides into the left superior and left inferior lobar bronchi; the lobar bronchi further divide into segmental (tertiary) bronchi.

- When examining the bronchi with a *bronchoscope*—an endoscope for inspecting the interior of the tracheobronchial tree for diagnostic purposes—one can observe a ridge, the *carina*, between the orifices of the main bronchi. If the tracheobronchial lymph nodes in the angle between the main bronchi are enlarged because cancer cells have metastasized from a bronchogenic carcinoma, for example, the carina is distorted, widened posteriorly, and immobile.

Segmental bronchi:

RIGHT LUNG	LEFT LUNG
Superior Lobe	**Superior Lobe**
▢ Apical	▢ Apical ⎤ Apicoposterior
▢ Posterior	▢ Posterior ⎦
▢ Anterior	▢ Anterior
	▢ Superior lingular
Middle Lobe	▢ Inferior lingular
▢ Lateral	
▢ Medial	**Inferior Lobe**
	▢ Superior
Inferior Lobe	▢ Anterior basal ⎤ Anteromedial
▢ Superior	▢ Medial basal ⎦ basal
▢ Anterior basal	▢ Lateral basal
▢ Medial basal	▢ Posterior basal
▢ Lateral basal	
▢ Posterior basal	

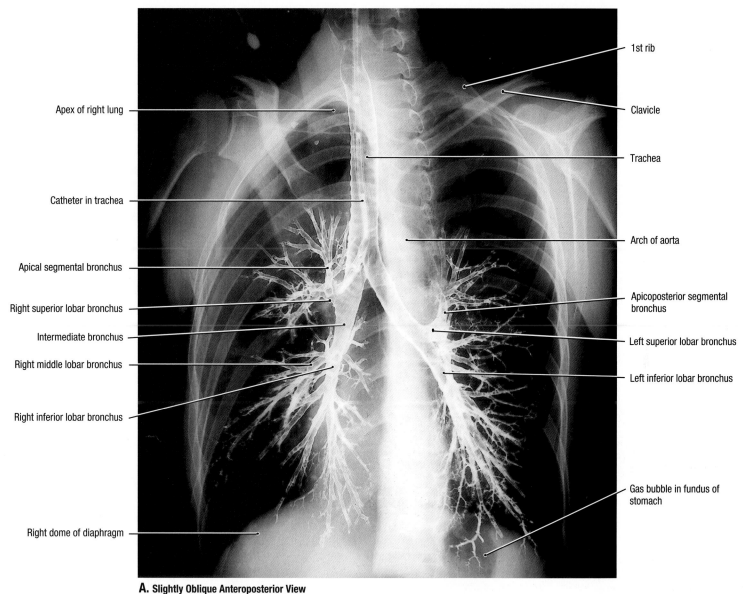

A. Slightly Oblique Anteroposterior View

1.33   **Bronchograms**

A. Bronchogram of tracheobronchial tree.

Because the right bronchus is wider and shorter and runs more vertically than the left bronchus, aspirated foreign bodies are more likely to enter and lodge in it or one of its branches. A potential hazard encountered by dentists is an aspirated foreign body, such as a piece of tooth, filling material, or a small instrument. Such objects are also most likely to enter the right main bronchus.

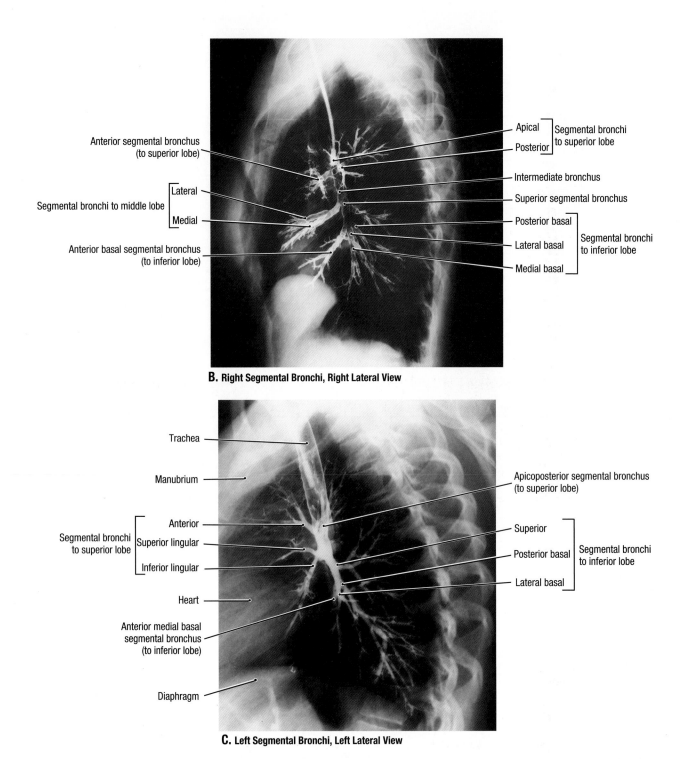

Anterior segmental bronchus (to superior lobe)

Segmental bronchi to middle lobe
Lateral
Medial

Anterior basal segmental bronchus (to inferior lobe)

Apical
Posterior
} Segmental bronchi to superior lobe

Intermediate bronchus

Superior segmental bronchus

Posterior basal
Lateral basal
Medial basal
} Segmental bronchi to inferior lobe

B. Right Segmental Bronchi, Right Lateral View

Trachea

Manubrium

Segmental bronchi to superior lobe
Anterior
Superior lingular
Inferior lingular

Heart

Anterior medial basal segmental bronchus (to inferior lobe)

Diaphragm

Apicoposterior segmental bronchus (to superior lobe)

Superior
Posterior basal
Lateral basal
} Segmental bronchi to inferior lobe

C. Left Segmental Bronchi, Left Lateral View

1.33   **Bronchograms** (*continued*)

B. Right lateral bronchogram, showing segmental bronchi. **C.** Left lateral bronchogram, showing segmental bronchi.

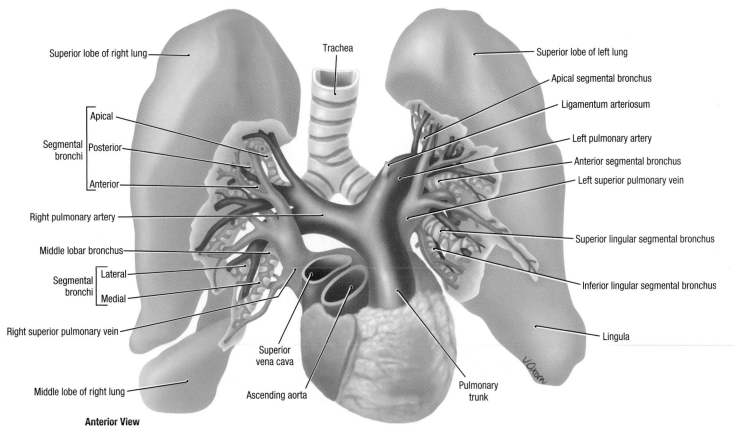

Anterior View

1.34   **Pulmonary artery, lungs retracted (inferior lobes not included)**

The middle lobe of the right lung is drained by the right superior pulmonary vein.

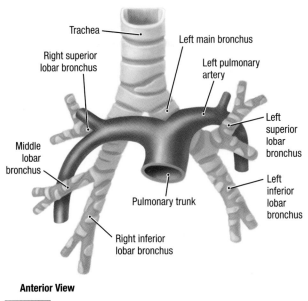

Anterior View

1.35   **Relationship of bronchi and pulmonary arteries**

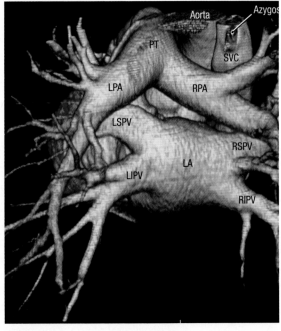

Posterior View

1.36   **3-D volume reconstruction (3DVR) of pulmonary arteries and veins and left atrium**

The pulmonary trunk *(PT)* divides into a longer right pulmonary artery *(RPA)* and shorter left pulmonary artery *(LPA)*; the left superior *(LSPV)* and inferior *(LIPV)* and the right superior *(RSPV)* and inferior *(RIPV)* pulmonary veins drain into the left atrium *(LA)*. Superior vena cava *(SVC)*.

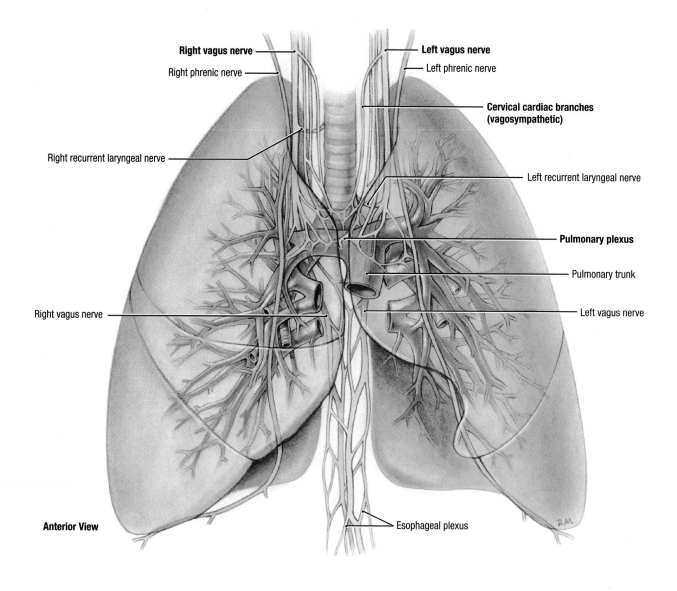

Right vagus nerve

Right phrenic nerve

Right recurrent laryngeal nerve

Right vagus nerve

Anterior View

Left vagus nerve

Left phrenic nerve

Cervical cardiac branches
(vagosympathetic)

Left recurrent laryngeal nerve

Pulmonary plexus

Pulmonary trunk

Left vagus nerve

Esophageal plexus

1.37   Innervation of lungs

- The pulmonary plexuses, located anterior and posterior to the roots of the lungs, receive sympathetic contributions from the right and left sympathetic trunks (2nd to 5th thoracic ganglia, not shown) and parasympathetic contributions from the right and left vagus nerves; cell bodies of postsynaptic parasympathetic neurons are in the pulmonary plexuses and along the branches of the pulmonary tree.
- The right and left vagus nerves continue inferiorly from the posterior pulmonary plexus to contribute fibers to the esophageal plexus.
- The phrenic nerves pass anterior to the root of the lung on their way to the diaphragm.

- The visceral pleura is insensitive to pain because its innervation is autonomic. The autonomic nerves reach the visceral pleura in company with the bronchial vessels. The visceral pleura receives no nerves of general sensation.
- The parietal pleura is sensitive to pain because it is richly supplied by branches of the somatic intercostal and phrenic nerves. Irritation of the parietal pleura produces local pain and referred pain to the areas sharing innervation by the same segments of the spinal cord.

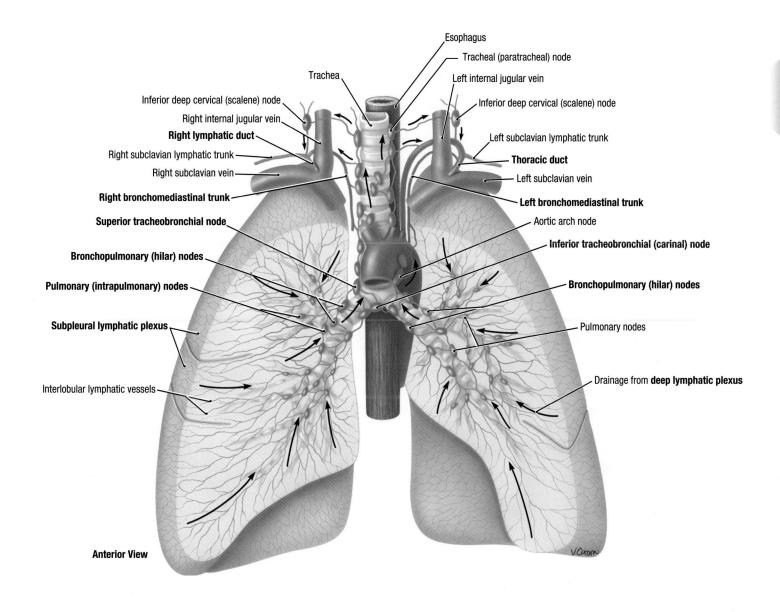

Esophagus

Tracheal (paratracheal) node

Trachea

Left internal jugular vein

Inferior deep cervical (scalene) node

Right internal jugular vein

Inferior deep cervical (scalene) node

Right lymphatic duct

Left subclavian lymphatic trunk

Right subclavian lymphatic trunk

Thoracic duct

Right subclavian vein

Left subclavian vein

Right bronchomediastinal trunk

Left bronchomediastinal trunk

Superior tracheobronchial node

Aortic arch node

Inferior tracheobronchial (carinal) node

Bronchopulmonary (hilar) nodes

Pulmonary (intrapulmonary) nodes

Bronchopulmonary (hilar) nodes

Subpleural lymphatic plexus

Pulmonary nodes

Interlobular lymphatic vessels

Drainage from **deep lymphatic plexus**

Anterior View

V.Oxom

1.38   **Lymphatic drainage of lungs**

- Lymphatic vessels originate in the subpleural (superficial) and deep lymphatic plexuses.
- The subpleural lymphatic plexus is superficial, lying deep to the visceral pleura, and drains lymph from the surface of the lung to the bronchopulmonary (hilar) nodes.
- The deep lymphatic plexus is in the lung and follows the bronchi and pulmonary vessels to the pulmonary, and then bronchopulmonary, nodes located at the root of the lung.
- All lymph from the lungs enters the inferior (carinal) and superior tracheobronchial nodes and then continues to the right and left bronchomediastinal trunks to drain into the venous system via the right lymphatic and thoracic ducts; lymph from the left inferior lobe passes largely to the right side.
- Lymph from the parietal pleura drains into lymph nodes of the thoracic wall (Fig. 1.74).

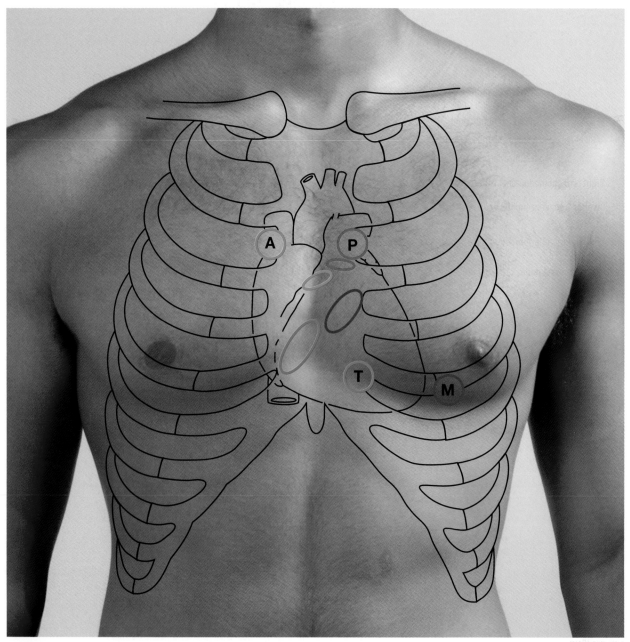

Anterior View

1.39   **Surface markings of the heart, heart valves, and their auscultation areas**

- The location of each heart valve in situ is indicated by a colored oval and the area of auscultation of the valve is indicated as a circle of the same color containing the first letter
of the valve name: the tricuspid valve *(T)* is green, the mitral valve *(M)* is purple, the pulmonary valve *(P)* is pink and the aortic valve *(A)* is blue.
- The auscultation areas are sites where the sounds of each of the heart's valves can be
heard most distinctly through a stethoscope.
- The aortic *(A)* and pulmonary *(P)* auscultation areas are in the 2nd intercostal space to
the right and left of the sternal border; the tricuspid area *(T)* is near the left sternal border in the 5th or 6th intercostal space; the mitral valve *(M)* is heard best near the apex of
the heart in the 5th intercostal space in the midclavicular line.

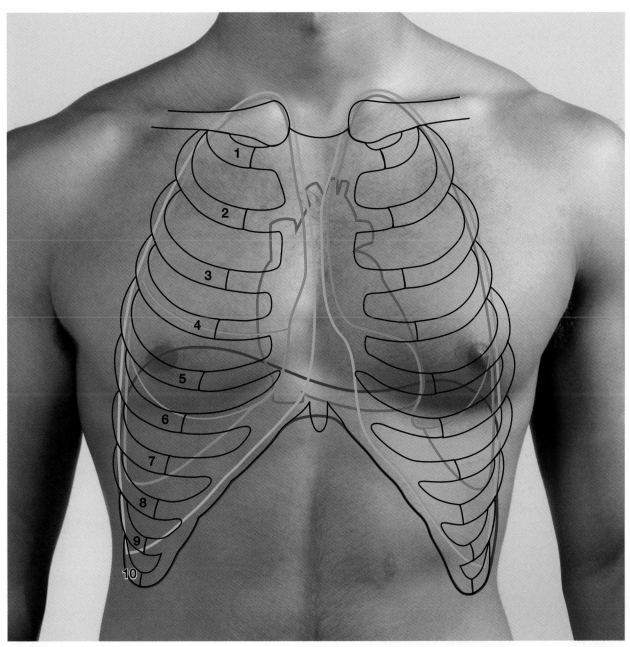

Anterior View

1.40　Surface markings of the heart, lungs, and diaphragm

- Outlined are the heart *(red)*, lungs *(green)*, parietal pleura *(blue)*, and diaphragm *(purple)*.
- The superior border of the heart is represented by a slightly oblique line joining the 3rd costal cartilages; the convex right side of the heart projects lateral to the sternum and inferiorly, lying at the 6th or 7th costochondral junction; the inferior border of the heart lying superior to the central tendon of the diaphragm and sloping slightly inferiorly to the apex at the 5th interspace at the midclavicular line.
- The right dome of the diaphragm is higher than the left because of the large size of the liver inferior to the dome; during expiration the right dome reaches as high as the 5th rib and the left dome ascends to the 5th intercostal space.
- The left pleural cavity is smaller than the right because of the projection of the heart to the left side.

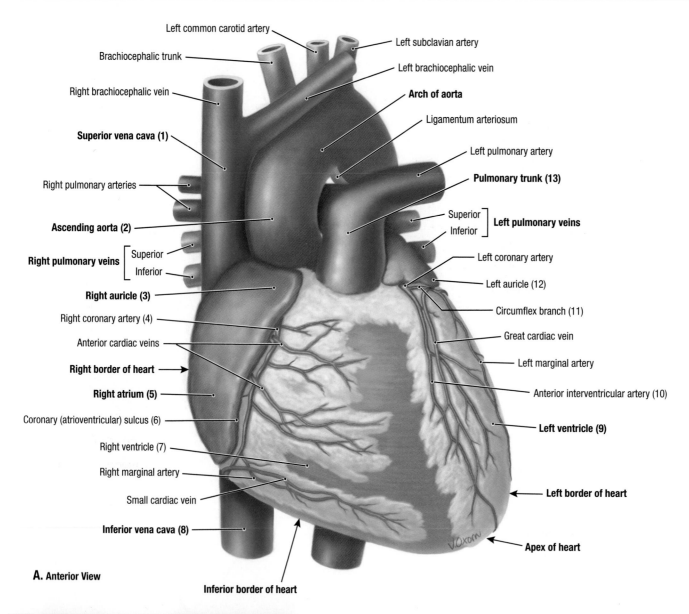

Left common carotid artery

Brachiocephalic trunk

Right brachiocephalic vein

Left subclavian artery

Left brachiocephalic vein

Arch of aorta

Ligamentum arteriosum

Superior vena cava (1)

Right pulmonary arteries

Ascending aorta (2)

Left pulmonary artery

Pulmonary trunk (13)

Superior
Inferior **Left pulmonary veins**

Right pulmonary veins Superior
Inferior

Left coronary artery

Left auricle (12)

Right auricle (3)

Right coronary artery (4)

Anterior cardiac veins

Right border of heart ⟶

Right atrium (5)

Coronary (atrioventricular) sulcus (6)

Right ventricle (7)

Right marginal artery

Small cardiac vein

Inferior vena cava (8) ⟶

Circumflex branch (11)

Great cardiac vein

Left marginal artery

Anterior interventricular artery (10)

Left ventricle (9)

⟵ **Left border of heart**

⟵ **Apex of heart**

A. Anterior View

Inferior border of heart

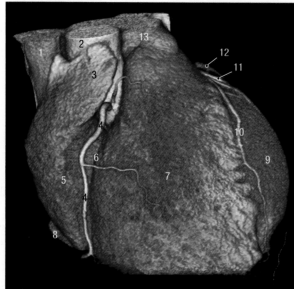

B. Anterior View

1.41   Heart and great vessels

A.

- The right border of the heart, formed by the right atrium, is slightly convex and almost in line with the superior vena cava.
- The inferior border is formed primarily by the right ventricle and part of the left ventricle.
- The left border is formed primarily by the left ventricle and part of the left auricle.

B.

- 3-D volume reconstruction of heart and coronary vessels. Numbers refer to structures in **A.**

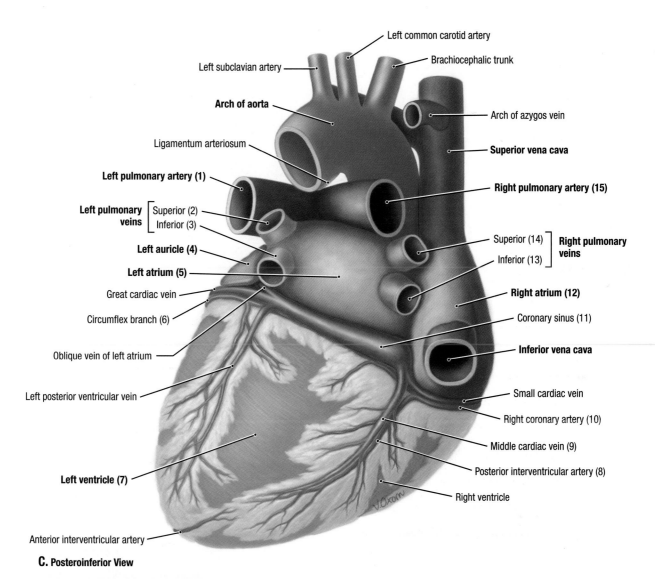

Left common carotid artery

Left subclavian artery

Brachiocephalic trunk

Arch of aorta

Arch of azygos vein

Ligamentum arteriosum

Superior vena cava

Left pulmonary artery (1)

Right pulmonary artery (15)

Left pulmonary veins — Superior (2) / Inferior (3)

Superior (14) / Inferior (13) — **Right pulmonary veins**

Left auricle (4)

Left atrium (5)

Right atrium (12)

Great cardiac vein

Coronary sinus (11)

Circumflex branch (6)

Oblique vein of left atrium

Inferior vena cava

Left posterior ventricular vein

Small cardiac vein

Right coronary artery (10)

Left ventricle (7)

Middle cardiac vein (9)

Posterior interventricular artery (8)

Right ventricle

Anterior interventricular artery

C. Posteroinferior View

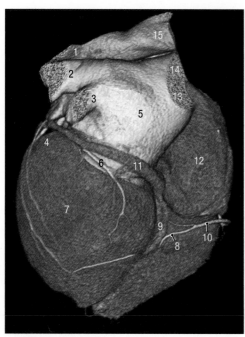

D. Posteroinferior View

1.41   **Heart and great vessels (continued)**

C.

- Most of the left atrium and left ventricle are visible in this posteroinferior view.
- The right and left pulmonary veins open into the left atrium.
- The right and left pulmonary arteries are just superior and parallel to the pulmonary veins.
- The arch of the aorta is arched in two planes: superiorly and to the left.
- The azygos vein arches over the right pulmonary vessels (and bronchus).

D.

- 3-D volume reconstruction of heart and coronary vessels. Numbers refer to structures in C.

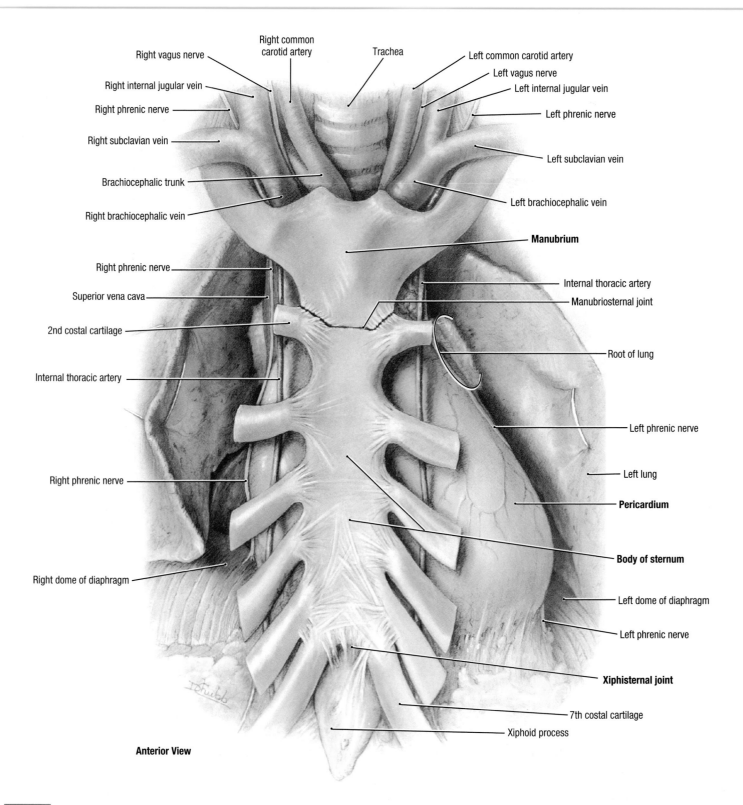

Right common carotid artery
Right vagus nerve
Trachea
Left common carotid artery
Left vagus nerve
Right internal jugular vein
Left internal jugular vein
Right phrenic nerve
Left phrenic nerve
Right subclavian vein
Left subclavian vein
Brachiocephalic trunk
Left brachiocephalic vein
Right brachiocephalic vein
Manubrium
Right phrenic nerve
Internal thoracic artery
Superior vena cava
Manubriosternal joint
2nd costal cartilage
Root of lung
Internal thoracic artery
Left phrenic nerve
Right phrenic nerve
Left lung
Pericardium
Right dome of diaphragm
Body of sternum
Left dome of diaphragm
Left phrenic nerve
Xiphisternal joint
7th costal cartilage
Xiphoid process

Anterior View

1.42   Pericardium in relation to sternum

- The pericardium lies posterior to the body of the sternum, extending from just superior to the sternal angle to the level of the xiphisternal joint; approximately two thirds lies to the left of the median plane.
- The heart lies between the sternum and the anterior mediastinum anteriorly and the vertebral column and the posterior mediastinum posteriorly; in cardiac compression, the sternum is depressed 4 to 5 cm, forcing blood out of the heart and into the great vessels.
- Internal thoracic arteries arise from the subclavian arteries and descend posterior to the costal cartilages, running lateral to the sternum and anterior to the pleura.

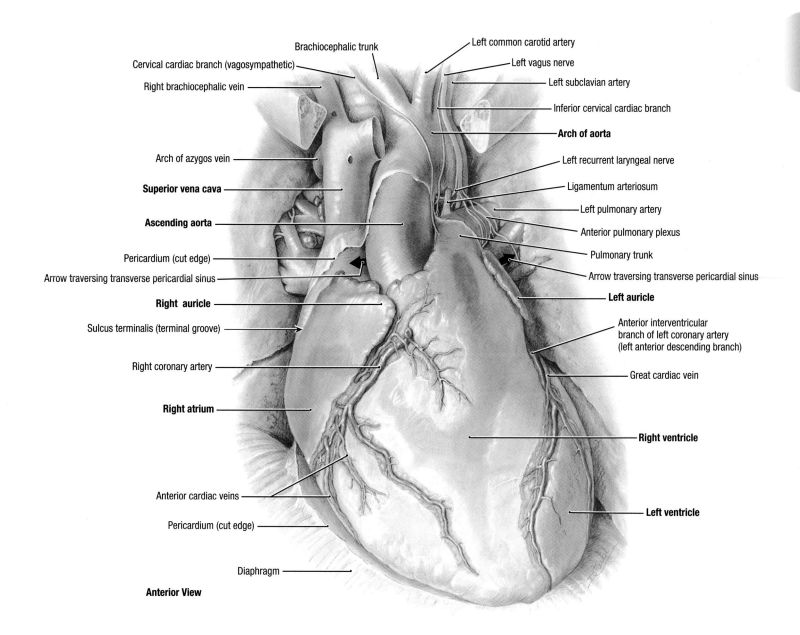

Brachiocephalic trunk

Cervical cardiac branch (vagosympathetic)

Right brachiocephalic vein

Left common carotid artery

Left vagus nerve

Left subclavian artery

Inferior cervical cardiac branch

Arch of aorta

Arch of azygos vein

Superior vena cava

Ascending aorta

Pericardium (cut edge)

Arrow traversing transverse pericardial sinus

Right auricle

Sulcus terminalis (terminal groove)

Right coronary artery

Right atrium

Anterior cardiac veins

Pericardium (cut edge)

Diaphragm

Anterior View

Left recurrent laryngeal nerve

Ligamentum arteriosum

Left pulmonary artery

Anterior pulmonary plexus

Pulmonary trunk

Arrow traversing transverse pericardial sinus

Left auricle

Anterior interventricular
branch of left coronary artery
(left anterior descending branch)

Great cardiac vein

Right ventricle

Left ventricle

1.43 **Sternocostal (anterior) surface of heart and great vessels in situ**

- The right ventricle forms most of the sternocostal surface.
- The entire right auricle and much of the right atrium are visible anteriorly, but only a small portion of the left auricle is visible; the auricles, like a closing claw, grasp the origins of the pulmonary trunk and ascending aorta from a posterior approach.
- The ligamentum arteriosum passes from the origin of the left pulmonary artery to the arch of the aorta.
- The right coronary artery courses in the anterior atrioventricular groove, and the anterior interventricular branch of the left coronary artery (anterior descending branch) courses in the anterior interventricular groove.
- The left vagus nerve passes lateral to the arch of the aorta and then posterior to the root of the lung; the left recurrent laryngeal nerve passes inferior to the arch of the aorta posterior to the ligamentum arteriosum.
- The great cardiac vein ascends beside the anterior interventricular branch of the left coronary artery to drain into the coronary sinus posteriorly.

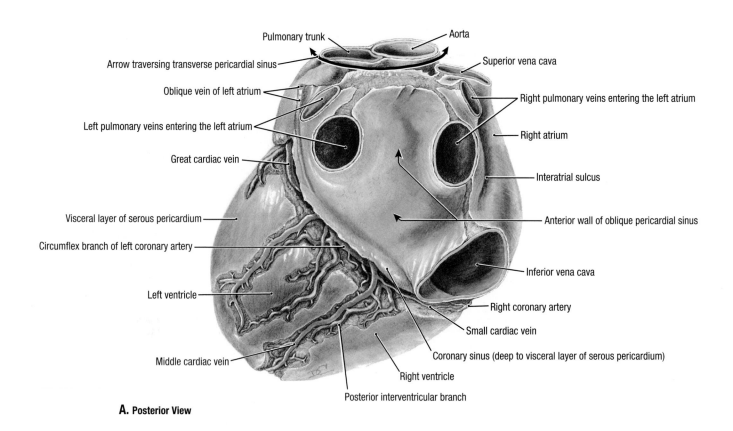

Pulmonary trunk — — Aorta

Arrow traversing transverse pericardial sinus —

Oblique vein of left atrium —

Left pulmonary veins entering the left atrium —

Great cardiac vein —

Visceral layer of serous pericardium —

Circumflex branch of left coronary artery —

Left ventricle —

Middle cardiac vein —

— Superior vena cava

— Right pulmonary veins entering the left atrium

— Right atrium

— Interatrial sulcus

— Anterior wall of oblique pericardial sinus

— Inferior vena cava

— Right coronary artery

Small cardiac vein —

Coronary sinus (deep to visceral layer of serous pericardium) —

Right ventricle —

Posterior interventricular branch —

A. Posterior View

1.44 Heart and pericardium

- This heart **(A)** was removed from the interior of the pericardial sac **(B)**.
- The entire base, or posterior surface, and part of the diaphragmatic or inferior surface of the heart are in view.
- The superior vena cava and larger inferior vena cava join the superior and inferior aspects of the right atrium.
- The left atrium forms the greater part of the base (posterior surface) of the heart.
- The left coronary artery in this specimen is dominant, since it supplies the posterior interventricular branch.
- Most branches of cardiac veins cross branches of the coronary arteries superficially.
- The visceral layer of serous pericardium (epicardium) covers the surface of the heart and reflects onto the great vessels; from around the great vessels, the serous pericardium reflects to line the internal aspect of the fibrous pericardium as the parietal

layer of serous pericardium. The fibrous pericardium and the parietal layer of serous pericardium form the pericardial sac that encases the heart.

- Note the cut edges of the reflections of serous pericardia around the arterial vessels (the pulmonary trunk and aorta) and venous vessels (the superior and inferior venae cavae and the pulmonary veins).

- The transverse pericardial sinus is especially important to cardiac surgeons. After the pericardial sac has been opened anteriorly, a finger can be passed through the transverse pericardial sinus posterior to the aorta and pulmonary trunk. By passing a surgical clamp or placing a ligature around these vessels, inserting the tubes of a coronary bypass machine, and then tightening the ligature, surgeons can stop or divert the circulation of blood in these large arteries while performing cardiac surgery.

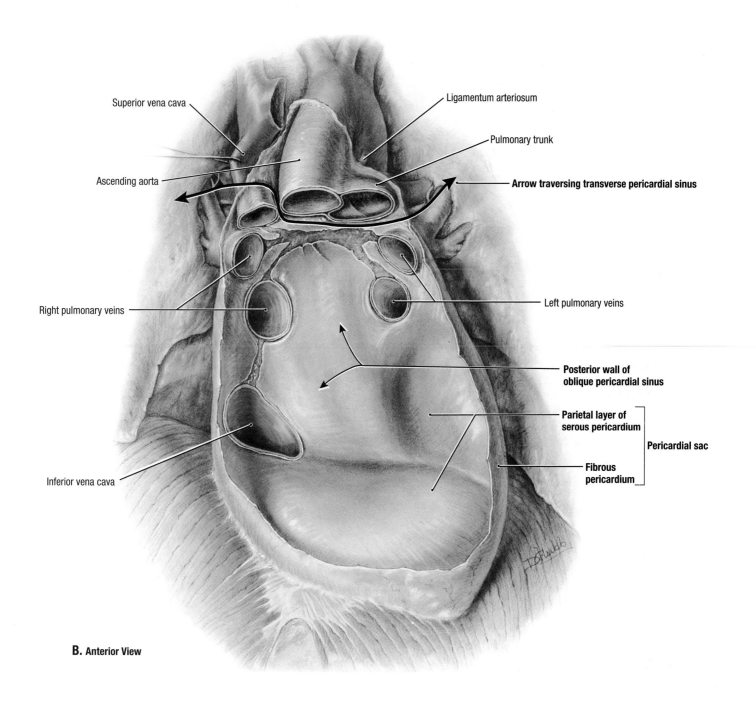

Superior vena cava

Ligamentum arteriosum

Pulmonary trunk

Ascending aorta

Arrow traversing transverse pericardial sinus

Right pulmonary veins

Left pulmonary veins

**Posterior wall of
oblique pericardial sinus**

**Parietal layer of
serous pericardium**

Pericardial sac

Inferior vena cava

**Fibrous
pericardium**

B. Anterior View

1.44   **Heart and pericardium** *(continued)*

- Interior of pericardial sac. Eight vessels were severed to excise the heart: superior and inferior venae cavae, four pulmonary veins, and two pulmonary arteries.
- The oblique sinus is bounded anteriorly by the visceral layer of serous pericardium covering the left atrium (Fig. 1.44A), posteriorly by the parietal layer of serous pericardium lining the fibrous pericardium, and superiorly and laterally by the reflection of serous pericardium around the four pulmonary veins and the superior and inferior venae cavae (Fig. 1.44**B**).

- The transverse sinus is bounded anteriorly by the serous pericardium covering the posterior aspect of the pulmonary trunk and aorta, and posteriorly by the visceral pericardium covering the atria (A).

- Cardiac tamponade (heart compression) is due to critically increased volume of fluid outside the heart but inside the pericardial cavity; e.g., due to stab wounds or from perforation of a weakened area of the heart muscle after heart attack (hemopericardium).

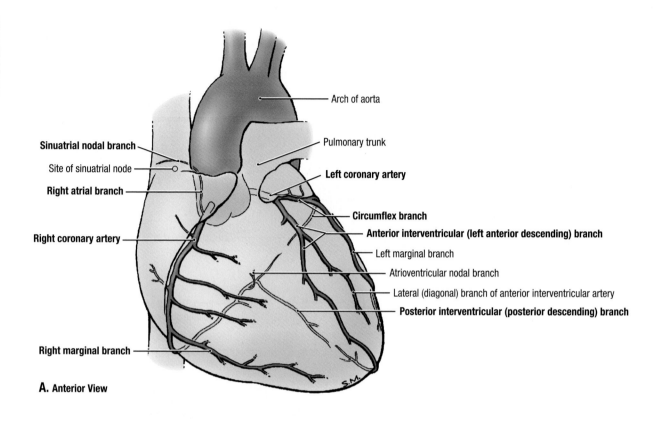

Arch of aorta

Pulmonary trunk

Sinuatrial nodal branch

Site of sinuatrial node

Left coronary artery

Right atrial branch

Circumflex branch

Anterior interventricular (left anterior descending) branch

Right coronary artery

Left marginal branch

Atrioventricular nodal branch

Lateral (diagonal) branch of anterior interventricular artery

Posterior interventricular (posterior descending) branch

Right marginal branch

A. Anterior View

1.45   Coronary arteries

- The right coronary artery travels in the coronary sulcus to reach the posterior surface of the heart, where it anastomoses with the circumflex branch of the left coronary artery. Early in its course, it gives off the right atrial branch, which supplies the sinuatrial (SA) node via the sinuatrial nodal artery; major branches are a marginal branch supplying much of the anterior wall of the right ventricle, an atrioventricular (AV) nodal artery given off near the posterior border of the interventricular septum, and a posterior interventricular artery in the interventricular groove that anastomoses with the anterior interventricular artery, a branch of the left coronary artery.
- The left coronary artery divides into a circumflex branch that passes posteriorly to anastomose with the right coronary on the posterior aspect of the heart and an anterior descending branch in the interventricular groove; the origin of the SA nodal artery is variable and may be a branch of the left coronary artery.
- The interventricular septum receives its blood supply from septal branches of the two interventricular (descending) branches: typically the anterior two thirds from the left coronary, and the posterior one third from the right (see Fig. 1.48A).

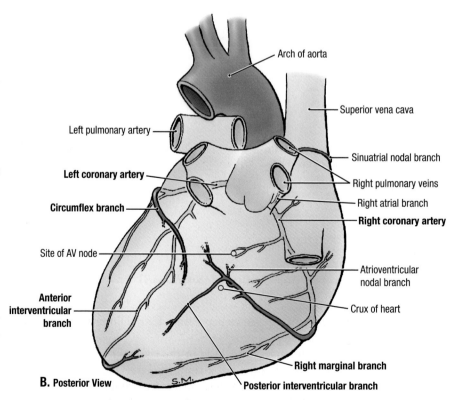

Arch of aorta

Superior vena cava

Left pulmonary artery

Sinuatrial nodal branch

Left coronary artery

Right pulmonary veins

Circumflex branch

Right atrial branch

Right coronary artery

Site of AV node

Atrioventricular nodal branch

Anterior interventricular branch

Crux of heart

Right marginal branch

B. Posterior View

Posterior interventricular branch

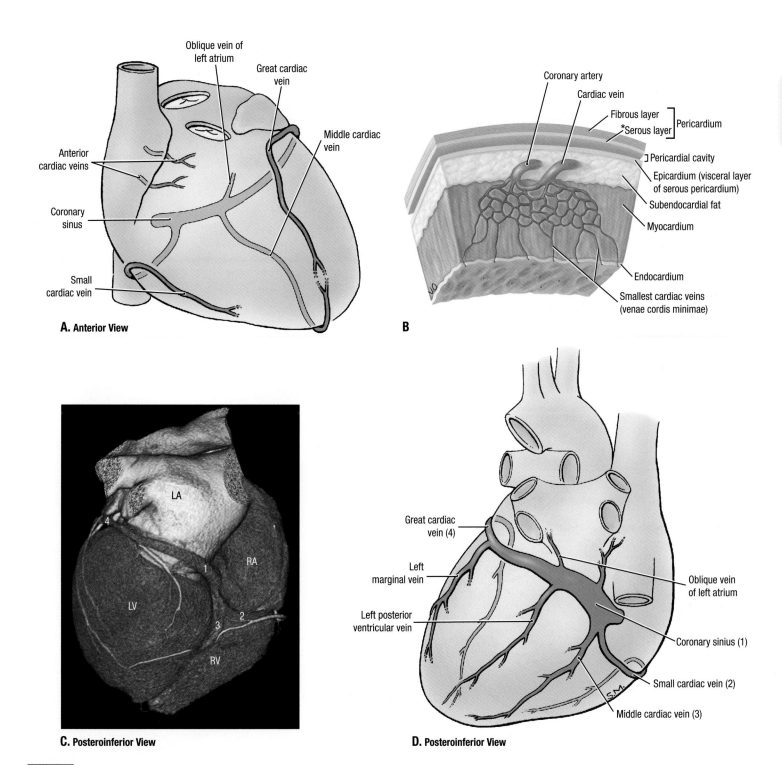

1.46   **Cardiac veins**

A. Anterior aspect. **B.** Smallest cardiac veins. **C.** 3-D volume reconstruction. Numbers refer to veins in **D.** Left atrium *(LA)*. Right atrium *(RA)*. Left ventricle *(LV)*; right ventricle *(RV)*. **D.** Posteroinferior aspect.

The coronary sinus is the major venous drainage vessel of the heart; it is located posteriorly in the atrioventricular (coronary) groove and drains into the right atrium. The great, middle, and small cardiac veins; the oblique vein of the left atrium; and the posterior vein of the left ventricle are the principal vessels draining into the coronary sinus. The anterior cardiac veins drain directly into the right atrium. The smallest cardiac veins (venae cordis minimae) drain the myocardium directly into the atria and ventricles **(B)**. In **B,** the *asterisk* (*) indicates the parietal layer of serous pericardium (epicardium). The cardiac veins accompany the coronary arteries and their branches.

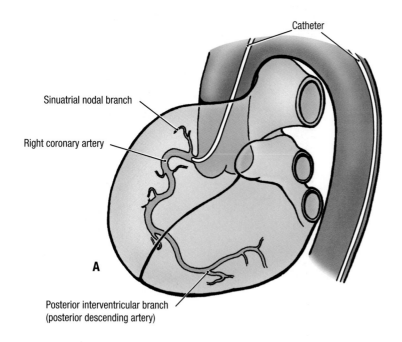

Catheter

Sinuatrial nodal branch

Right coronary artery

A

Posterior interventricular branch
(posterior descending artery)

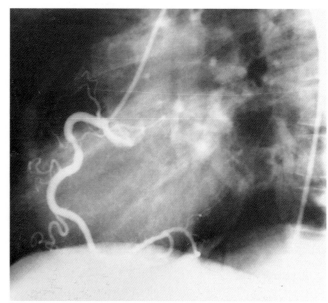

B. *Left Anterior Oblique View*

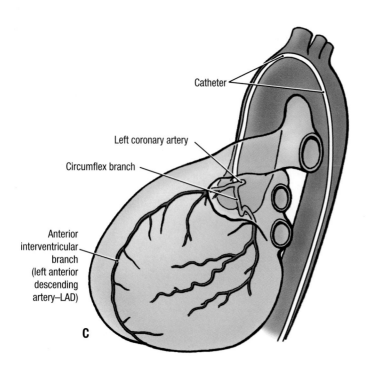

Catheter

Left coronary artery

Circumflex branch

Anterior
interventricular
branch
(left anterior
descending
artery–LAD)

C

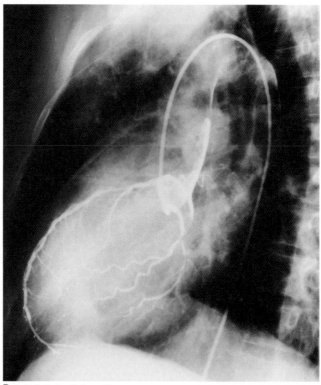

D. *Left Anterior Oblique View*

1.47   **Coronary arteriograms with orientation drawings**

Right (**A** and **B**) and left (**C** and **D**) coronary arteriograms.

Coronary artery disease (CAD) is one of the leading causes of death. CAD has many causes, all of which result in a reduced blood supply to the vital myocardial tissue. The three most common sites of coronary artery occlusion and the percentage of occlusions involving each artery are the (1) Anterior interventricular (clinically referred to as LAD) branch of the left coronary artery (LCA) (40–50%); (2) Right coronary artery (RCA), (30–40%); (3) Circumflex branch of the LCA (15–20%).

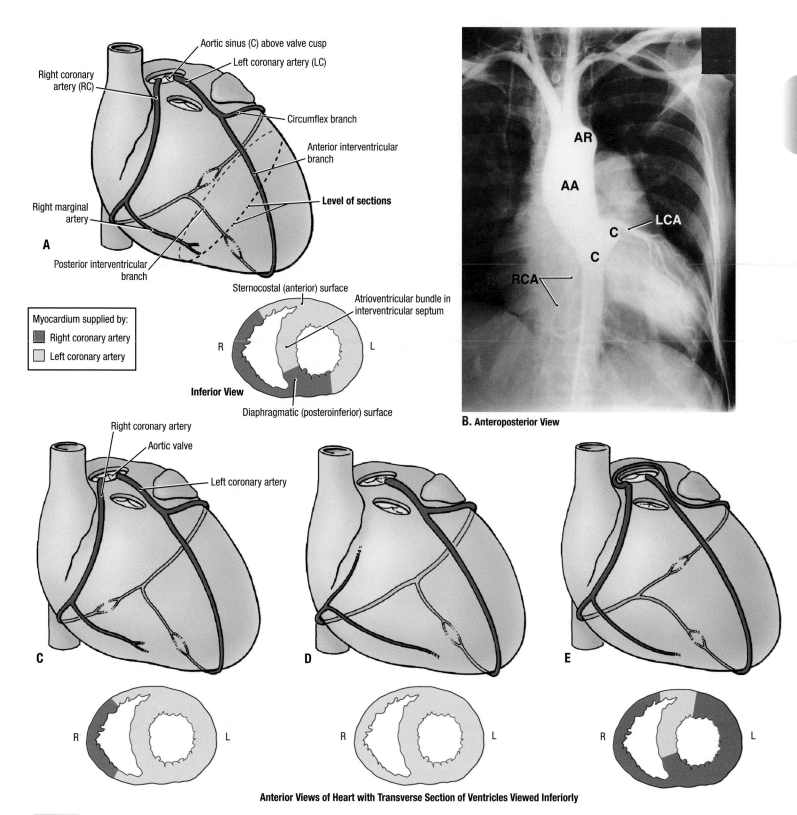

A. Aortic sinus (C) above valve cusp
Left coronary artery (LC)
Right coronary artery (RC)
Circumflex branch
Anterior interventricular branch
Level of sections
Right marginal artery
Posterior interventricular branch

Sternocostal (anterior) surface
Atrioventricular bundle in interventricular septum

Myocardium supplied by:
Right coronary artery
Left coronary artery

R   L

Inferior View
Diaphragmatic (posteroinferior) surface

B. Anteroposterior View

Right coronary artery
Aortic valve
Left coronary artery

R   L

Anterior Views of Heart with Transverse Section of Ventricles Viewed Inferiorly

1.48 Coronary circulation

A. In most cases, the right and left coronary arteries share equally in the blood supply to the heart. The *dotted line* indicates the plane of the cross-section demonstrating the parts of the myocardium supplied by the right and left coronary arteries. **B.** Aortic angiogram. Observe arch of aorta (*AR*), ascending aorta (*AA*), cusp of aortic valve (*C*), left coronary artery (*LCA*), and right coronary artery (*RCA*). **C.** Dominant left coronary artery (about 15% of hearts). The posterior interventicular branch comes off the circumflex branch. **D.** Single coronary artery. **E.** Circumflex branch emerging from the right coronary sinus.

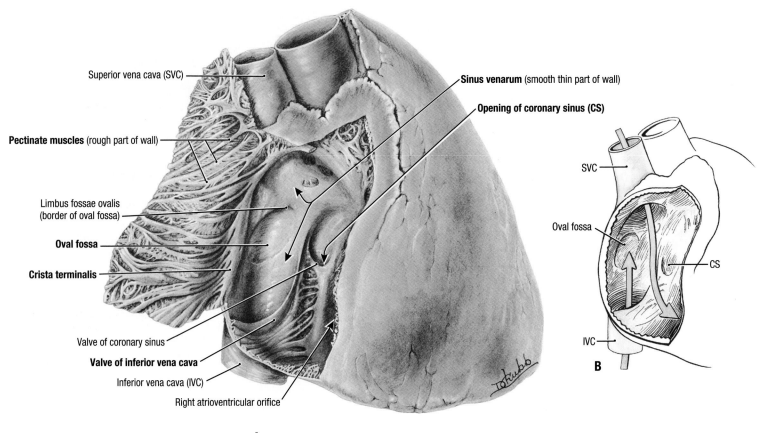

Superior vena cava (SVC)

Pectinate muscles (rough part of wall)

Limbus fossae ovalis
(border of oval fossa)

Oval fossa

Crista terminalis

Valve of coronary sinus

Valve of inferior vena cava

Inferior vena cava (IVC)

Right atrioventricular orifice

Sinus venarum (smooth thin part of wall)

Opening of coronary sinus (CS)

SVC

Oval fossa

CS

IVC

A. Anterior View

B

1.49   Right atrium

A. Interior of right atrium. The anterior wall of the right atrium is reflected. **B.** Blood flow into atrium from the superior and inferior vena cavae.

- The smooth part of the atrial wall is formed by the absorption of the right horn of the sinus venosus, and the rough part is formed from the primitive atrium.
- Crista terminalis, the valve of the inferior vena cava, and the valve of the coronary sinus separate the smooth part from the rough part.
- The pectinate muscle passes anteriorly from the crista terminalis; the crista underlies the sulcus terminalis (not shown), a groove visible externally on the posterolateral surface of the right atrium between the superior and inferior venae cavae.
- The superior and inferior venae cavae and the coronary sinus open onto the smooth part of the right atrium; the anterior cardiac veins and venae cordis minimae (not visible) also open into the atrium.

- The floor of the fossa is the remnant of the fetal septum primum; the crescent-shaped ridge (limbus fossae ovalis) partially surrounding the fossa is the remnant of the septum secundum.
- In **B**, the inflow from the superior vena cava is directed toward the tricuspid orifice, whereas blood from the inferior vena cava is directed toward the fossa ovalis.

- A congenital anomaly of the interatrial septum, usually incomplete closure of the oval foramen, is an atrial septal defect (ASD). A probe-size patency is present in the superior part of the oval fossa in 15–25% of adults (Moore and Persaud, 2003). These small openings, by themselves, cause no hemodynamic abnormalities. Large ASDs allow oxygenated blood from the lungs to be shunted from the left atrium through the ASD into the right atrium, causing enlargement of the right atrium and ventricle and dilation of the pulmonary trunk.

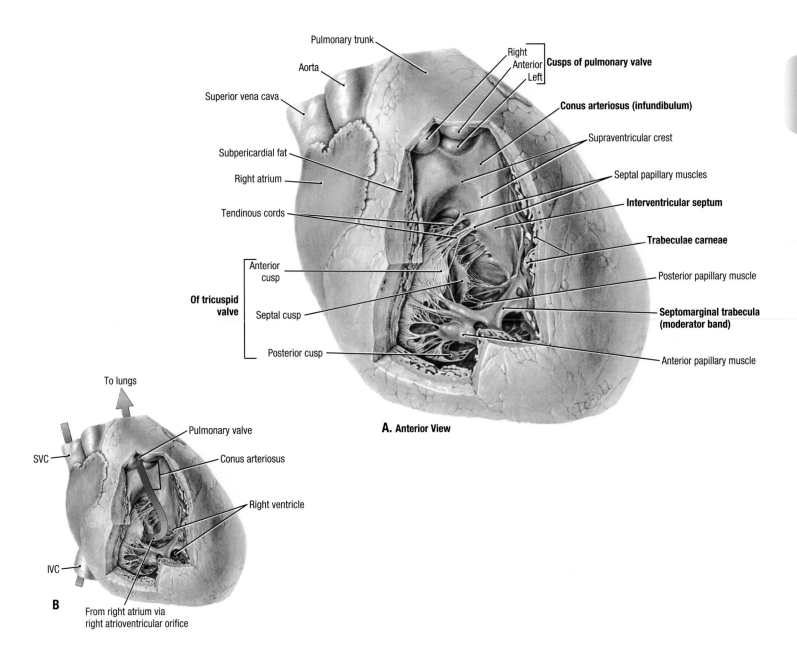

Pulmonary trunk

Aorta

Right ⎤
Anterior ⎬ **Cusps of pulmonary valve**
Left ⎦

Superior vena cava

Conus arteriosus (infundibulum)

Subpericardial fat

Supraventricular crest

Right atrium

Septal papillary muscles

Tendinous cords

Interventricular septum

Trabeculae carneae

Anterior
cusp

Posterior papillary muscle

**Of tricuspid
valve**

Septal cusp

**Septomarginal trabecula
(moderator band)**

Posterior cusp

Anterior papillary muscle

A. Anterior View

To lungs

Pulmonary valve

SVC

Conus arteriosus

Right ventricle

IVC

B

From right atrium via
right atrioventricular orifice

1.50   Right ventricle

A. Interior of right ventricle. **B.** Blood flow through right heart.

- The entrance to this chamber, the right atrioventricular or tricuspid orifice, is situated posteriorly; the exit, the orifice of the pulmonary trunk, is superior.
- The outflow portion of the chamber inferior to the pulmonary orifice (conus arteriosus or infundibulum) has a smooth, funnel-shaped wall; the remainder of the ventricle is rough with fleshy trabeculae.
- There are three types of trabeculae: mere ridges, bridges attached only at each end, and fingerlike projections called papillary muscles. The anterior papillary muscle rises from the anterior wall, the posterior (papillary muscle) from the posterior wall, and a series of small septal papillae from the septal wall.

- The septomarginal trabecula, here thick, extends from the septum to the base of the anterior papillary muscle.

- The membranous part of the interventricular septum develops separately from the muscular part and has a complex embryological origin (Moore and Persaud, 2003). Consequently, this part is the common site of ventricular septal defects (VSDs), although defects also occur in the muscular part, VSDs rank first on all lists of cardiac defects. The size of the defect varies from 1 to 25 mm. A VSD causes a left-to-right shunt of blood through the defect. A large shunt increases pulmonary blood flow, which causes severe pulmonary disease (*hypertension*, or increased blood pressure) and may cause *cardiac failure*.

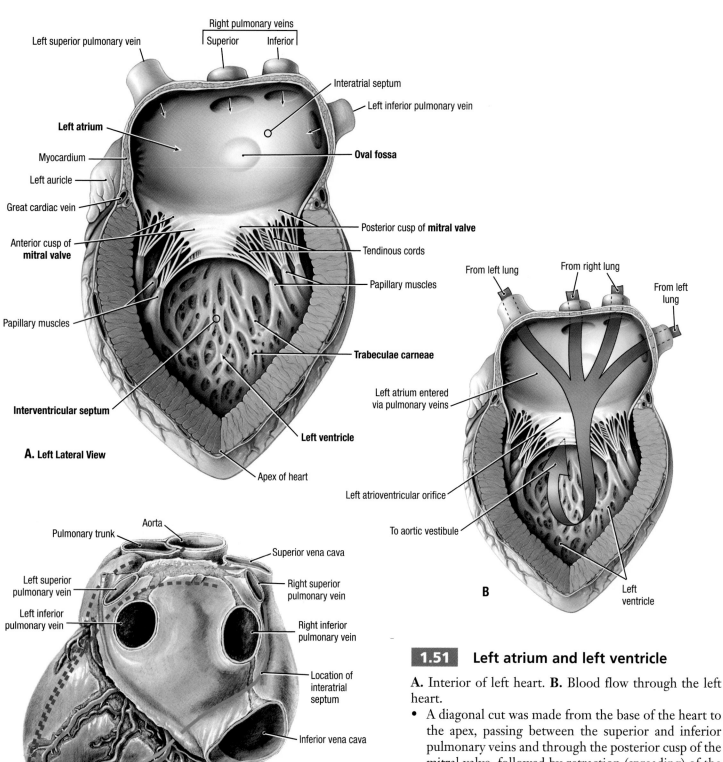

Right pulmonary veins
Superior | Inferior

Left superior pulmonary vein

Interatrial septum

Left inferior pulmonary vein

Left atrium

Myocardium

Oval fossa

Left auricle

Great cardiac vein

Posterior cusp of **mitral valve**

Anterior cusp of **mitral valve**

Tendinous cords

Papillary muscles

Papillary muscles

Trabeculae carneae

Interventricular septum

Left ventricle

A. Left Lateral View

Apex of heart

From left lung   From right lung   From left lung

Left atrium entered via pulmonary veins

Left atrioventricular orifice

To aortic vestibule

Left ventricle

B

Aorta

Pulmonary trunk

Superior vena cava

Left superior pulmonary vein

Right superior pulmonary vein

Left inferior pulmonary vein

Right inferior pulmonary vein

Location of interatrial septum

Inferior vena cava

Location of interventricular septum

Lines of incision:
- - - Figure 1.51 A & B
- - - Figure 1.52 A & B

1.51 Left atrium and left ventricle

A. Interior of left heart. **B.** Blood flow through the left heart.

- A diagonal cut was made from the base of the heart to the apex, passing between the superior and inferior pulmonary veins and through the posterior cusp of the mitral valve, followed by retraction (spreading) of the left heart wall on each side of the incision.
- The entrances (pulmonary veins) to the left atrium are posterior, and the exit (left atrioventricular or mitral orifice) is anterior.
- The left side of the oval fossa is also seen on the left side of the interatrial septum, although the left side is not usually as distinct as the right side is within the right atrium.
- Except for that of the auricle, the atrial wall is smooth.

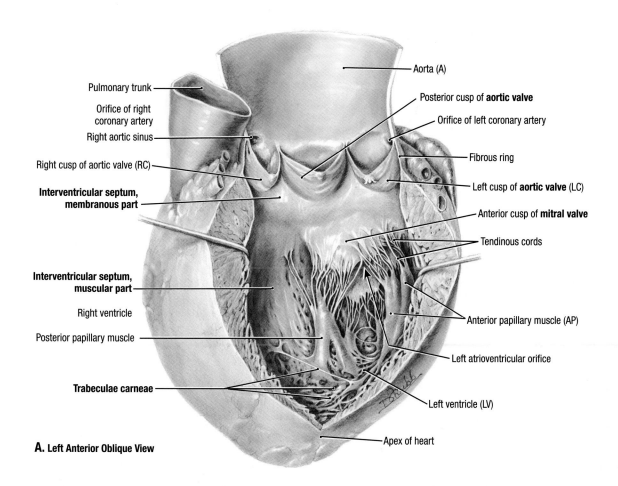

Aorta (A)

Pulmonary trunk

Orifice of right coronary artery

Right aortic sinus

Right cusp of aortic valve (RC)

Interventricular septum, membranous part

Interventricular septum, muscular part

Right ventricle

Posterior papillary muscle

Trabeculae carneae

Posterior cusp of **aortic valve**

Orifice of left coronary artery

Fibrous ring

Left cusp of **aortic valve** (LC)

Anterior cusp of **mitral valve**

Tendinous cords

Anterior papillary muscle (AP)

Left atrioventricular orifice

Left ventricle (LV)

Apex of heart

A. Left Anterior Oblique View

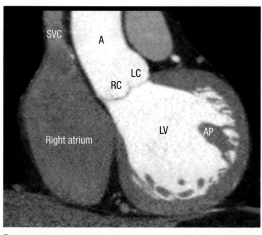

SVC

A

LC

RC

Right atrium

LV

AP

B. Anterior View

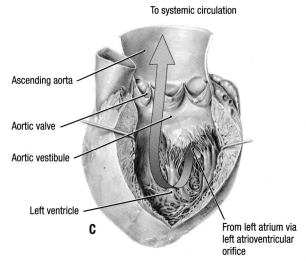

To systemic circulation

Ascending aorta

Aortic valve

Aortic vestibule

Left ventricle

C

From left atrium via left atrioventricular orifice

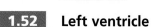

1.52   **Left ventricle**

A cut was made from the apex along the left margin of the heart, passing posterior to the pulmonary trunk, to open the aortic vestibule and ascending aorta.

    A. Interior of left ventricle. **B.** Coronal CT angiogram. Letters refer to structures in **A. C.** Blood flow through the left ventricle.
- The chamber has a conical shape.
- The entrance (left atrioventricular, bicuspid, or mitral orifice) is situated posteriorly, and the exit (aortic orifice) is superior.

- The left ventricular wall is thin and muscular near the apex, thick and muscular superiorly, and thin and fibrous (nonelastic) at the aortic orifice.
- Two large papillary muscles, the anterior from the anterior wall and the posterior from the posterior wall, control the adjacent halves of two cusps of the mitral valve with tendinous cords (chordae tendineae).
- The anterior cusp of the mitral valve lies between the inlet (mitral orifice) and the outlet (aortic orifice).

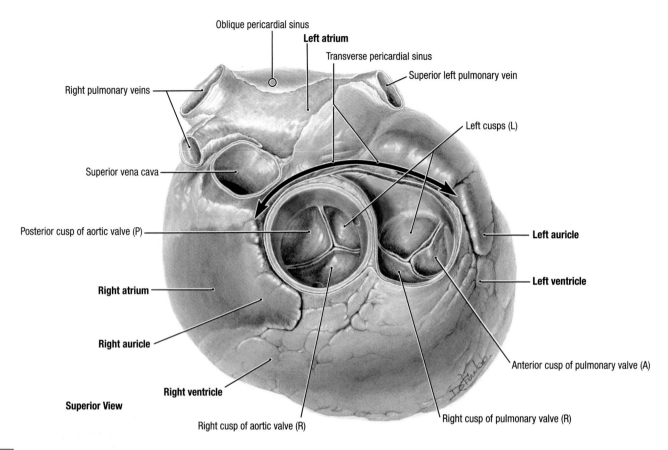

Oblique pericardial sinus

Left atrium

Transverse pericardial sinus

Superior left pulmonary vein

Right pulmonary veins

Left cusps (L)

Superior vena cava

Posterior cusp of aortic valve (P)

Left auricle

Left ventricle

Right atrium

Right auricle

Anterior cusp of pulmonary valve (A)

Right ventricle

Superior View

Right cusp of aortic valve (R)

Right cusp of pulmonary valve (R)

1.53 Excised heart

- The ventricles are positioned anteriorly and to the left, the atria posteriorly and to the right.
- The roots of the aorta and pulmonary artery, which conduct blood from the ventricles, are placed anterior to the atria and their incoming blood vessels (the superior vena cava and pulmonary veins).
- The aorta and pulmonary artery are enclosed within a common tube of serous pericardium and partly embraced by the auricles of the atria.

- The transverse pericardial sinus curves posterior to the enclosed stems of the aorta and pulmonary trunk and anterior to the superior vena cava and upper limits of the atria.
- The three cusps of the aortic and pulmonary valves—and the names of the cusps—have a developmental origin, as explained in Figure 1.54.

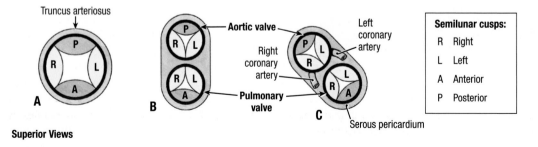

Truncus arteriosus

Aortic valve

Left coronary artery

Right coronary artery

Pulmonary valve

Serous pericardium

Semilunar cusps:
R Right
L Left
A Anterior
P Posterior

Superior Views

1.54 Pulmonary and aortic valve names

The names of these cusps have a developmental origin: the truncus arteriosus with four cusps (**A**) splits to form two valves, each with three cusps (**B**). The heart undergoes partial rotation to the left on its axis, resulting in the arrangement of cusps shown in **C** and in Figure 1.53.

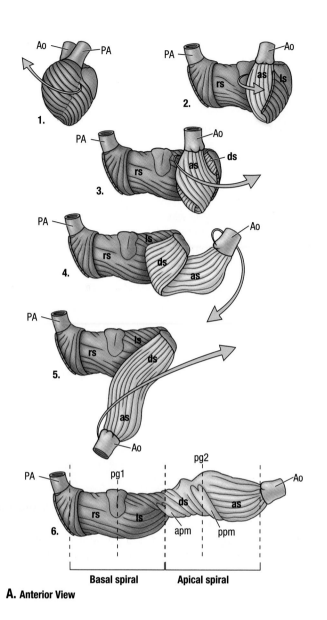

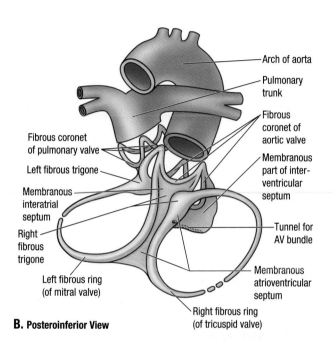

B. Posteroinferior View

A. Anterior View

1.55   **Arrangement of the myocardium and the fibrous skeleton of the heart.**

A. The helical (double spiral) arrangement of the myocardium. (Modified from Torrent-Guasp et al., 2001). *1.* When the superficial myocardium is incised along the anterior interventricular groove *(dashed red line)* and peeled back starting at its origin from the fibrous ring of the pulmonary artery *(PA)*, the thick double spirals of the ventricular myocardial band are revealed *2.* A band of nearly horizontal fibers forms an outer basal spiral *(dark brown)* that comprises the outer wall of the right ventricle (right segment; *rs*) and an external layer of the outer wall of the left ventricle (left segment; *Ls*). *3.* When the left ventricle is rotated to bring the interventricular septum anteriorly, it can be seen that the myocardium then abruptly turns more vertically, descending to the apex (descending segment; *ds*) and then ascends (ascending segment; *as*) to insert onto the fibrous ring of the aorta *(Ao)*. The *ds* and *as* form the deeper apical spiral *(light brown)*, which com-

prises the internal layer of the outer wall of the left ventricle, while the crisscrossing *as* and *ds* fibers make up the interventricular septum. Thus the septum, like the outer wall of the left ventricle, is also double layered. *4* and *5.* The ventricular myocardial band is progressively unwrapped. *6.* The myocardium is completely uncoiled, and its segments are identified. The sequential contraction of the myocardial band enables the ventricles to function as parallel sucking and propelling pumps; on contraction, the ventricles do not merely collapse inward but rather wring themselves out. *apm*, anterior papillary muscles; *pg1* and *pg2*, posterior interventricular groove; *ppm*, posterior papillary muscles. **B.** The isolated fibrous skeleton is composed of four fibrous rings (or two rings and two "coronets"), each encircling a valve; two trigones; and the membranous portions of the interatrial, interventricular, and atrioventricular septa.

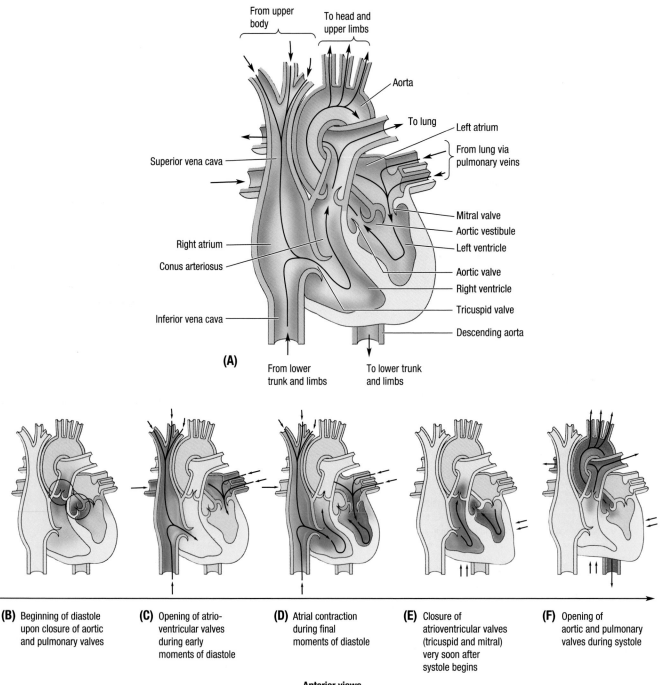

From upper body

To head and upper limbs

Aorta

To lung — Left atrium

From lung via pulmonary veins

Superior vena cava

Mitral valve
Aortic vestibule
Left ventricle

Right atrium

Conus arteriosus

Aortic valve
Right ventricle
Tricuspid valve

Inferior vena cava

Descending aorta

(A)

From lower trunk and limbs

To lower trunk and limbs

(B) Beginning of diastole upon closure of aortic and pulmonary valves

(C) Opening of atrio-ventricular valves during early moments of diastole

(D) Atrial contraction during final moments of diastole

(E) Closure of atrioventricular valves (tricuspid and mitral) very soon after systole begins

(F) Opening of aortic and pulmonary valves during systole

Anterior views

1.56   Cardiac cycle

The cardiac cycle describes the complete movement of the heart or heartbeat and includes the period from the beginning of one heartbeat to the beginning of the next one. The cycle consists of diastole (ventricular relaxation and filling) and systole (ventricular contraction and emptying). The right heart *(blue side)* is the pump for the pulmonary circuit; the left heart *(red side)* is the pump for the systemic circuit.

Disorders involving the valves of the heart disturb the pumping efficiency of the heart. Valvular heart disease produces either stenosis (narrowing) or insufficiency. Valvular stenosis is the failure of a valve to open fully, slowing blood flow from a chamber. Valvular insufficiency, or regurgitation, on the other hand, is failure of the valve to close completely, usually owing to nodule formation on (or scarring and contraction of) the cusps so that the edges do not meet or align. This allows a variable amount of blood (depending on the severity) to flow back into the chamber it was just ejected from. Both stenosis and insufficiency result in an increased workload for the heart. Because valvular diseases are mechanical problems, damaged or defective cardiac valves are often replaced surgically in a procedure called valvuloplasty. Most commonly, artificial valve prostheses made of synthetic materials are used in these valve replacement procedures, but xenografted valves (valves transplanted from other species, such as pigs) are also used.

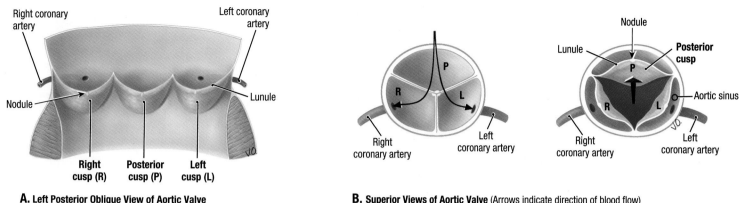

A. Left Posterior Oblique View of Aortic Valve

B. Superior Views of Aortic Valve (Arrows indicate direction of blood flow)

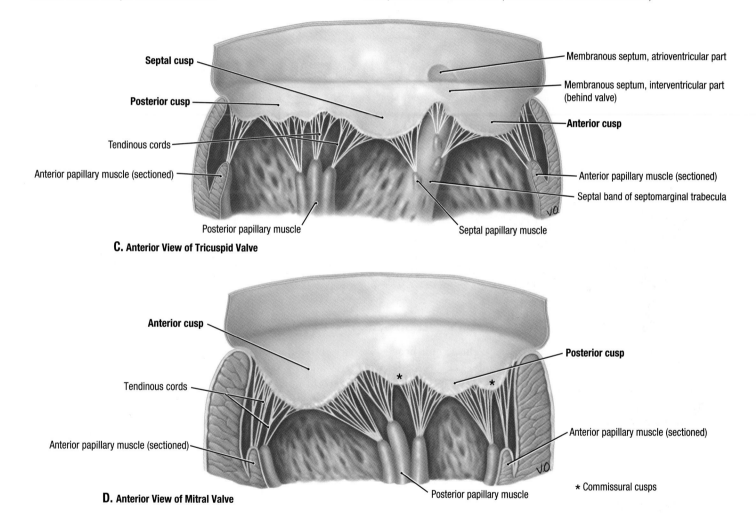

C. Anterior View of Tricuspid Valve

D. Anterior View of Mitral Valve

★ Commissural cusps

1.57   **Valves of the heart**

A and **B.** Semilunar valves. **C** and **D.** Atrioventricular valves.

In **(A),** as in Figure 1.52A, the anulus of the aortic valve has been incised between the right and left cusps and spread open. Each cusp of the semilunar valves bears a nodule in the midpoint of its free edge, flanked by thin connective tissue areas (lunules). When the ventricles relax to fill (diastole), backflow of blood from aortic recoil or pulmonary resistance fills the sinus (space between cusp and dilated part of the aortic or pulmonary wall), causing the nod-

ules and lunules to meet centrally, closing the valve **(B).** Filling of the coronary arteries occurs during diastole (when ventricular walls are relaxed) as backflow "inflates" the cusps to close the valve. Tendinous cords pass from the tips of the papillary muscles to the free margins and ventricular surfaces of the cusps of the tricuspid **(C)** and mitral **(D)** valves. Each papillary muscle or muscle group controls the adjacent sides of two cusps, resisting valve prolapse during systole.

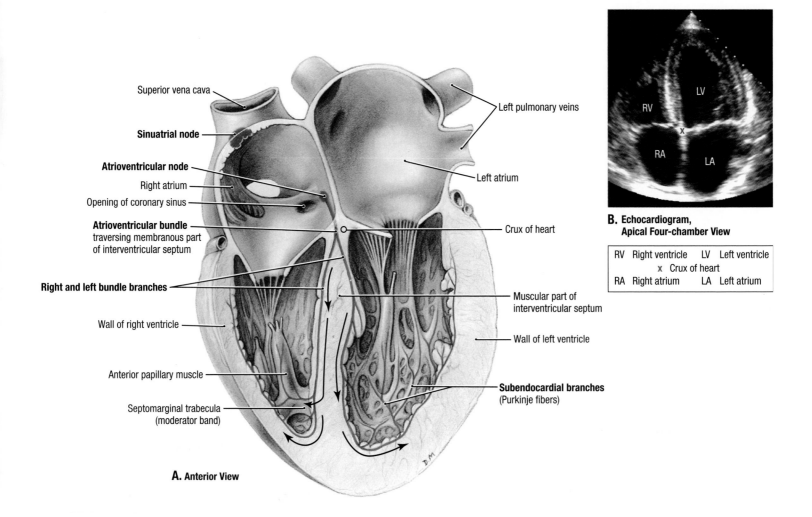

Superior vena cava

Sinuatrial node

Atrioventricular node

Right atrium

Opening of coronary sinus

Atrioventricular bundle
traversing membranous part
of interventricular septum

Right and left bundle branches

Wall of right ventricle

Anterior papillary muscle

Septomarginal trabecula
(moderator band)

Left pulmonary veins

Left atrium

Crux of heart

Muscular part of
interventricular septum

Wall of left ventricle

Subendocardial branches
(Purkinje fibers)

A. Anterior View

**B. Echocardiogram,
Apical Four-chamber View**

LV

RV

x

RA

LA

RV	Right ventricle	LV	Left ventricle
	x	Crux of heart	
RA	Right atrium	LA	Left atrium

1.58 Conduction system of heart, coronal section

- The sinuatrial (SA) node in the wall of the right atrium near the superior end of the sulcus terminalis extends over the opening of the superior vena cava. The SA node is the "pacemaker" of the heart because it initiates muscle contraction and determines the heart rate. It is supplied by the sinuatrial nodal artery, usually a branch of the right atrial branch of the right coronary artery (see Fig. 1.45A–B), but it may arise from the left coronary artery.

- Contraction spreads through the atrial wall (myogenic induction) until it reaches the atrioventricular (AV) node in the interatrial septum superomedial to the opening of the coronary sinus. The AV node is supplied by the atrioventricular nodal artery, usually arising from the right coronary artery posteriorly at the inferior margin of the interatrial septum.

- The AV bundle, usually supplied by the right coronary artery, passes from the AV node in the membranous part of the interventricular septum, dividing into right and left bundle branches on either side of the muscular part of the interventricular septum.

- The right bundle branch travels inferiorly in the interventricular septum to the anterior wall of the ventricle, with part passing via the septomarginal trabecula to the anterior papil-

lary muscle; excitation spreads throughout the right ventricular wall through a network of subendocardial branches from the right bundle (Purkinje fibers).

- The left bundle branch lies beneath the endocardium on the left side of the interventricular septum and branches to enter the anterior and posterior papillary muscles and the wall of the left ventricle; further branching into a plexus of subendocardial branches (Purkinje fibers) allows the impulses to be conveyed throughout the left ventricular wall. The bundle branches are mostly supplied by the left coronary, except the posterior limb of the left bundle branch, which is supplied by both coronary arteries.

- Damage to the cardiac conduction system (often by compromised blood supply as in coronary artery disease) leads to disturbances of muscle contraction. Damage to the AV node results in "heart block" because the atrial excitation wave does not reach the ventricles, which begin to contract independently at their own slower rate. Damage to one of the branches results in "bundle branch block," in which excitation goes down the unaffected branch to cause systole of that ventricle; the impulse then spreads to the other ventricle, producing later, asynchronous contraction.

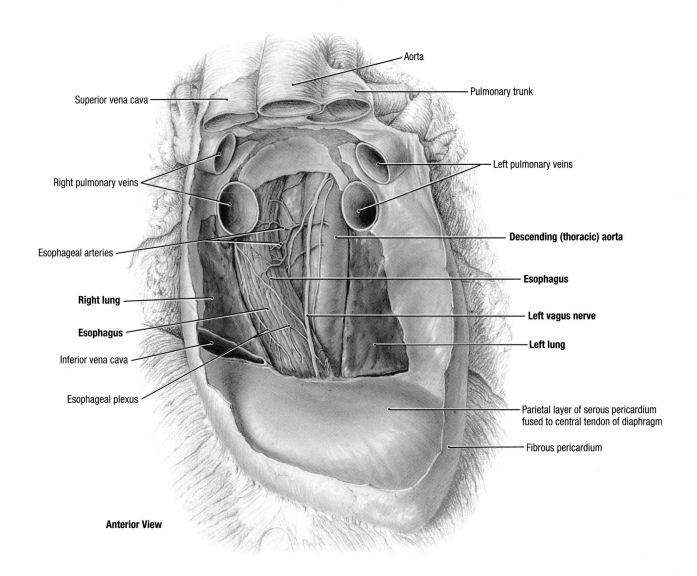

Aorta

Pulmonary trunk

Superior vena cava

Right pulmonary veins

Left pulmonary veins

Esophageal arteries

Descending (thoracic) aorta

Esophagus

Right lung

Left vagus nerve

Esophagus

Left lung

Inferior vena cava

Esophageal plexus

Parietal layer of serous pericardium
fused to central tendon of diaphragm

Fibrous pericardium

Anterior View

1.59   **Posterior relationships of heart and pericardium**

Posterior relationships. The fibrous and parietal layers of serous pericardium have been removed from posterior and lateral to the oblique sinus. The esophagus in this specimen is deflected to the right; it usually lies in contact with the aorta. Compare with Figure 1.44.

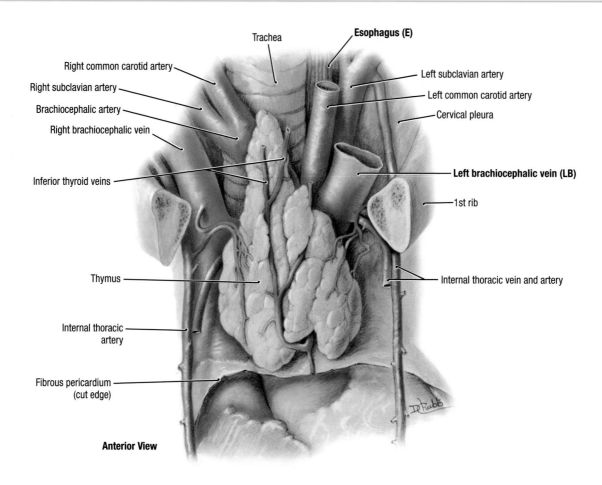

Trachea

Esophagus (E)

Right common carotid artery

Right subclavian artery

Brachiocephalic artery

Right brachiocephalic vein

Inferior thyroid veins

Thymus

Internal thoracic artery

Fibrous pericardium (cut edge)

Left subclavian artery

Left common carotid artery

Cervical pleura

Left brachiocephalic vein (LB)

1st rib

Internal thoracic vein and artery

Anterior View

1.60 **Superior mediastinum I: superficial dissection**

The sternum and ribs have been excised and the pleurae removed. It is unusual in an adult to see such a discrete thymus, which is impressive during puberty but subsequently regresses and is largely replaced by fat and fibrous tissue.

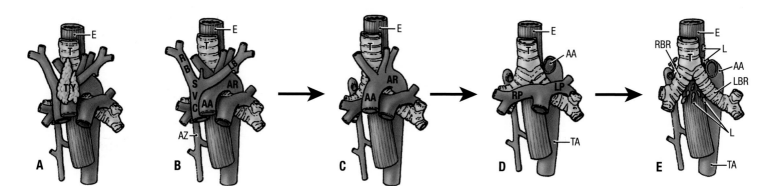

A   B   C   D   E

1.61 **Relations of great vessels and trachea**

Observe, from superficial to deep: (A) Thymus (TY); (B) the right (RB) and left (LB) brachiocephalic veins form the superior vena cava (SVC) and receive the arch of the azygos vein (AZ) posteriorly; (C) the ascending aorta (AA) and arch of the aorta (AR) arch over the right pulmonary artery and left main bronchus; (D) the pulmonary arteries (RP and LP); and (E) the tracheobronchial lymph nodes (L) at the tracheal bifurcation (T).

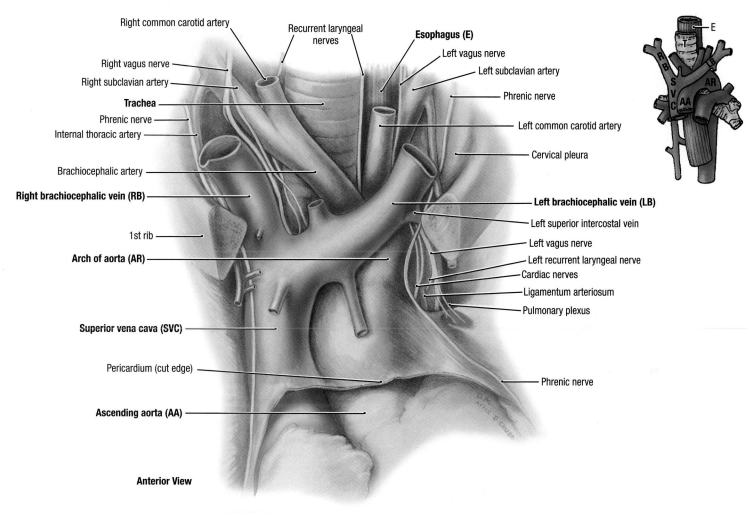

Right common carotid artery

Recurrent laryngeal nerves

Esophagus (E)

Right vagus nerve

Left vagus nerve

Right subclavian artery

Left subclavian artery

Trachea

Phrenic nerve

Phrenic nerve

Left common carotid artery

Internal thoracic artery

Brachiocephalic artery

Cervical pleura

Right brachiocephalic vein (RB)

Left brachiocephalic vein (LB)

Left superior intercostal vein

1st rib

Left vagus nerve

Arch of aorta (AR)

Left recurrent laryngeal nerve

Cardiac nerves

Ligamentum arteriosum

Pulmonary plexus

Superior vena cava (SVC)

Pericardium (cut edge)

Phrenic nerve

Ascending aorta (AA)

Anterior View

1.62   **Superior mediastinum II: root of neck**

The thymus gland has been removed.

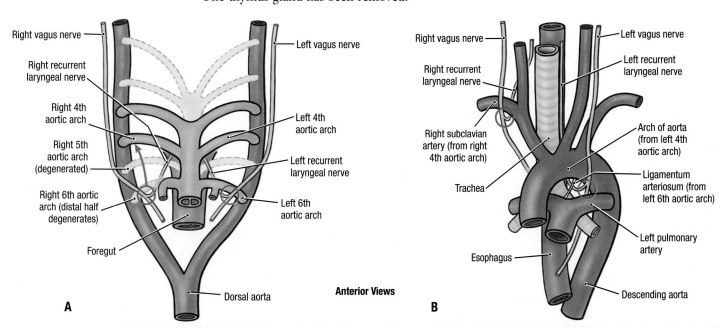

Right vagus nerve

Left vagus nerve

Right recurrent laryngeal nerve

Right 4th aortic arch

Left 4th aortic arch

Right 5th aortic arch (degenerated)

Left recurrent laryngeal nerve

Right 6th aortic arch (distal half degenerates)

Left 6th aortic arch

Foregut

Dorsal aorta

A

Right vagus nerve

Left vagus nerve

Right recurrent laryngeal nerve

Left recurrent laryngeal nerve

Right subclavian artery (from right 4th aortic arch)

Arch of aorta (from left 4th aortic arch)

Ligamentum arteriosum (from left 6th aortic arch)

Trachea

Esophagus

Left pulmonary artery

Descending aorta

B

Anterior Views

1.63   **Relationship of recurrent laryngeal nerve to the aortic arches**

A. Six weeks. **B.** Child.

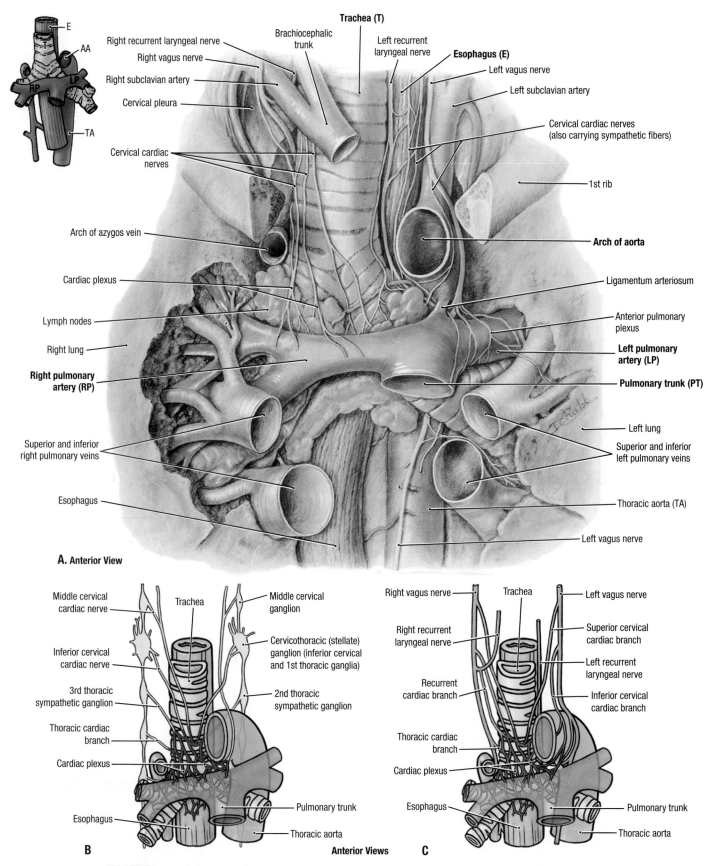

A. Anterior View

Labels, clockwise from top:

Trachea (T)

Right recurrent laryngeal nerve

Brachiocephalic trunk

Left recurrent laryngeal nerve

Right vagus nerve

Esophagus (E)

Right subclavian artery

Left vagus nerve

Cervical pleura

Left subclavian artery

Cervical cardiac nerves

Cervical cardiac nerves (also carrying sympathetic fibers)

1st rib

Arch of azygos vein

Arch of aorta

Cardiac plexus

Ligamentum arteriosum

Lymph nodes

Anterior pulmonary plexus

Right lung

Left pulmonary artery (LP)

Right pulmonary artery (RP)

Pulmonary trunk (PT)

Left lung

Superior and inferior right pulmonary veins

Superior and inferior left pulmonary veins

Esophagus

Thoracic aorta (TA)

Left vagus nerve

B (Sympathetic contribution)

Middle cervical cardiac nerve

Trachea

Middle cervical ganglion

Inferior cervical cardiac nerve

Cervicothoracic (stellate) ganglion (inferior cervical and 1st thoracic ganglia)

3rd thoracic sympathetic ganglion

2nd thoracic sympathetic ganglion

Thoracic cardiac branch

Cardiac plexus

Esophagus

Pulmonary trunk

Thoracic aorta

C (Parasympathetic contribution)

Right vagus nerve

Trachea

Left vagus nerve

Right recurrent laryngeal nerve

Superior cervical cardiac branch

Recurrent cardiac branch

Left recurrent laryngeal nerve

Inferior cervical cardiac branch

Thoracic cardiac branch

Cardiac plexus

Esophagus

Pulmonary trunk

Thoracic aorta

Anterior Views

1.64   Superior mediastinum III: cardiac plexus and pulmonary arteries

A. Dissection. **B.** Sympathetic and **(C)** parasympathetic contribution to the cardiac plexus. *Yellow*, sympathetic; *blue*, parasympathetic; *green*, mixed sympathetic and parasympathetic nerves.

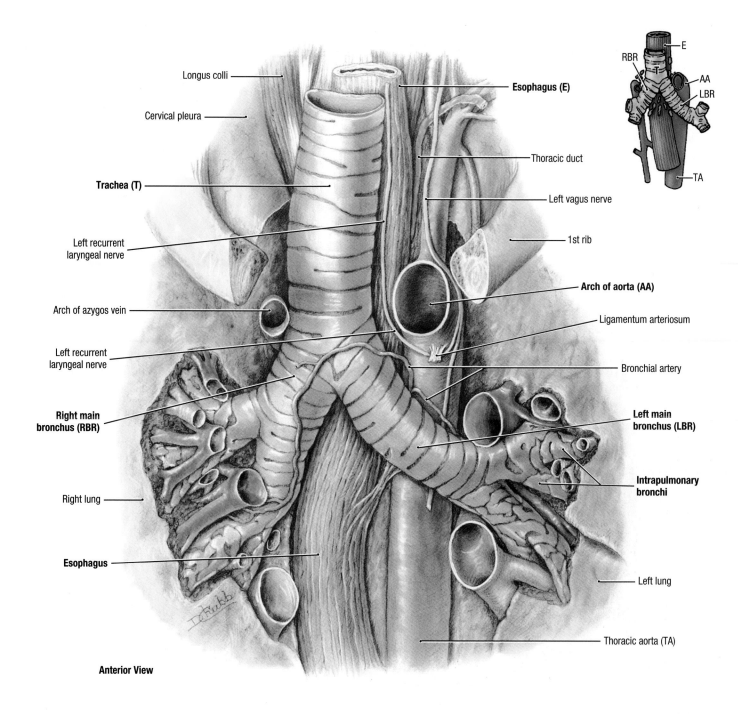

Longus colli

Cervical pleura

Trachea (T)

Left recurrent
laryngeal nerve

Arch of azygos vein

Left recurrent
laryngeal nerve

**Right main
bronchus (RBR)**

Right lung

Esophagus

Anterior View

Esophagus (E)

Thoracic duct

Left vagus nerve

1st rib

Arch of aorta (AA)

Ligamentum arteriosum

Bronchial artery

**Left main
bronchus (LBR)**

**Intrapulmonary
bronchi**

Left lung

Thoracic aorta (TA)

E
RBR
T
AA
LBR
TA

1.65   **Superior mediastinum IV: tracheal bifurcation and bronchi**

- Note the four parallel structures: the trachea, esophagus, left recurrent laryngeal nerve, and thoracic duct. The esophagus bulges to the left of the trachea, the recurrent nerve lies in the angle between the trachea and esophagus, and the duct is at the left side of the esophagus. The trachea bifurcates at the level of the sternal angle.
- The arch of the aorta passes posterior to the left of these four structures as it arches over the left main bronchus; the arch of the azygos vein passes anterior to their right as it arches over the right main bronchus.
- The right main bronchus is (1) more vertical, (2) of greater caliber, and (3) shorter than the left main bronchus.

- The recurrent laryngeal nerves supply all the intrinsic muscles of the larynx, except one. Consequently, any investigative procedure or disease process in the superior mediastinum may involve these nerves and affect the voice. Because the left recurrent laryngeal nerve hooks around the arch of the aorta and ascends between the trachea and the esophagus, it may be involved when there is a bronchial or esophageal carcinoma, enlargement of mediastinal lymph nodes, or an aneurysm of the arch of the aorta.

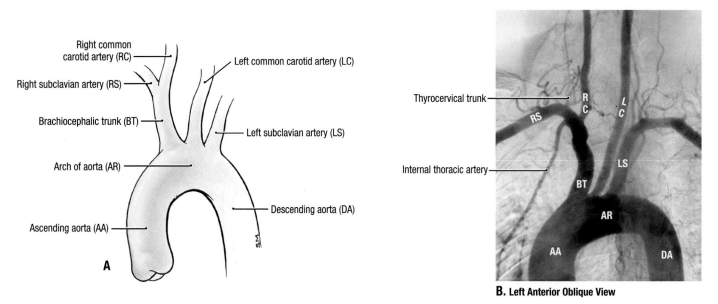

B. Left Anterior Oblique View

1.66   **Branches of aortic arch**

A. Aortic arch. **B.** Aortic angiogram. Observe the ascending aorta *(AA)*, the arch of the aorta *(AR)*, the descending aorta *(DA)*, the brachiocephalic *(BT)* trunk (artery) branching into the right subclavian *(RS)* and right common carotid *(RC)* arteries, and the left subclavian *(LS)* and left common carotid *(LC)* arteries arising directly from the aorta.

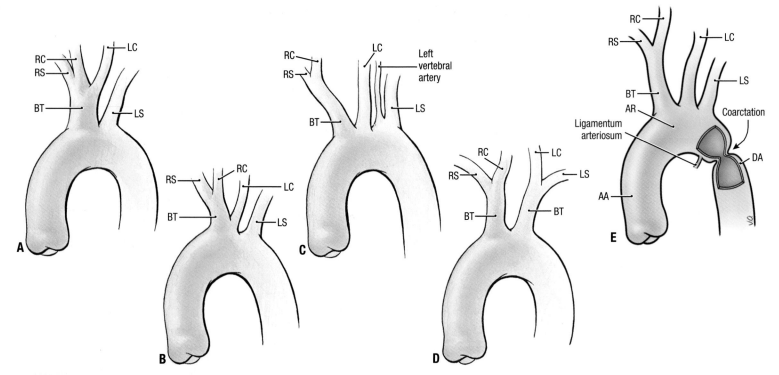

1.67   **Variations in origins of branches of aortic arch**

The most common pattern (65%) is shown in Figure 1.66. Less common variations include (**A** and **B**) left common carotid artery originating from the brachiocephalic trunk (27%); (**C**) each of the four arteries originating independently from the arch of the aorta (2.5%); (**D**) right and left brachiocephalic trunks originating from the arch of the aorta (1.2%); (**E**) Coarctation of aorta. In coarctation of the aorta, the arch or descending aorta has an abnormal narrowing (stenosis) that diminishes the caliber of the aortic lumen, producing an obstruction to blood flow. The most common site is near the ligamentum arteriosum. When the coarctation is inferior to this site (postductal coarctation), a good collateral circulation usually develops between the proximal and distal parts of the aorta through the intercostal and internal thoracic arteries.

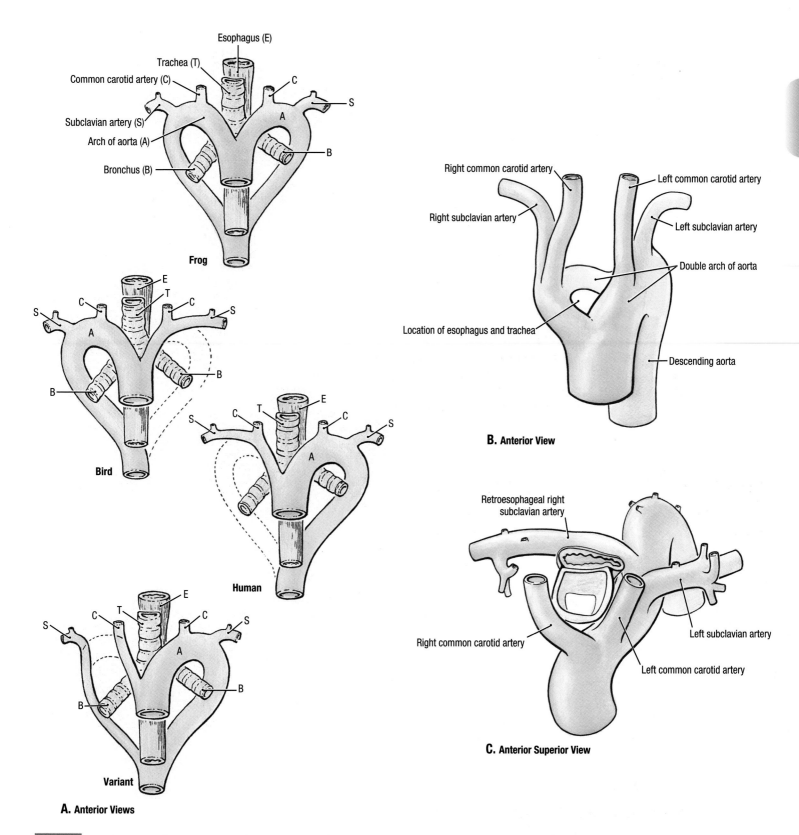

1.68   Scheme of varieties of aortic arches

A. Comparative anatomy. The double aortic arch of the frog; the right aortic arch of the bird; the left aortic arch of the mammal, including man, and a variant. **B.** Double aortic arch. The right and left aortic arches persist completely, as in the frog. In this rare condition, the esophagus and trachea pass through the so-formed "aortic ring." **C.** Retroesophageal right subclavian artery. The artery arises as the last branch of the arch of the aorta, passing posterior to the esophagus and trachea.

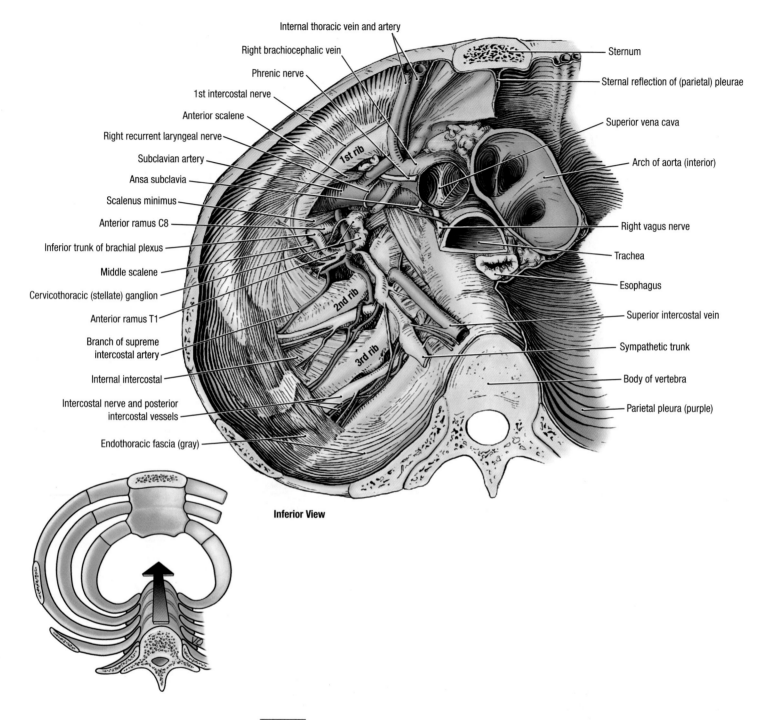

Internal thoracic vein and artery

Right brachiocephalic vein

Phrenic nerve

1st intercostal nerve

Anterior scalene

Right recurrent laryngeal nerve

Subclavian artery

Ansa subclavia

Scalenus minimus

Anterior ramus C8

Inferior trunk of brachial plexus

Middle scalene

Cervicothoracic (stellate) ganglion

Anterior ramus T1

Branch of supreme intercostal artery

Internal intercostal

Intercostal nerve and posterior intercostal vessels

Endothoracic fascia (gray)

Sternum

Sternal reflection of (parietal) pleurae

Superior vena cava

Arch of aorta (interior)

Right vagus nerve

Trachea

Esophagus

Superior intercostal vein

Sympathetic trunk

Body of vertebra

Parietal pleura (purple)

1st rib

2nd rib

3rd rib

Inferior View

1.69   **Superior mediastinum and roof of pleural cavity**

- The cervical, costal, and mediastinal parietal pleura *(purple)* and portions of the endothoracic fascia *(gray)* have been removed from the right side of the specimen to demonstrate structures traversing the superior thoracic aperture.
- The first part of the subclavian artery disappears as it crosses the first rib anterior to the anterior scalene muscle.
- The ansa subclavian from the sympathetic trunk and right recurrent laryngeal nerve from the vagus are seen looping inferior to the subclavian artery.
- The anterior rami of C8 and T1 merge to form the inferior trunk of the brachial plexus, which crosses the first rib posterior to the anterior scalene muscle.

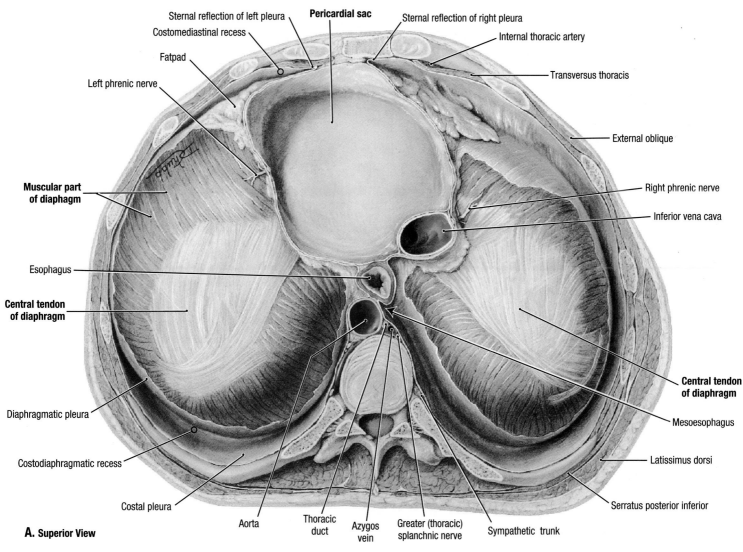

Sternal reflection of left pleura
Costomediastinal recess
Fatpad
Left phrenic nerve

Pericardial sac

Sternal reflection of right pleura
Internal thoracic artery
Transversus thoracis

External oblique

**Muscular part
of diaphagm**

Right phrenic nerve
Inferior vena cava

Esophagus

**Central tendon
of diaphragm**

**Central tendon
of diaphragm**

Mesoesophagus

Diaphragmatic pleura

Costodiaphragmatic recess

Latissimus dorsi

Serratus posterior inferior

Costal pleura

Aorta

Thoracic
duct

Azygos
vein

Greater (thoracic)
splanchnic nerve

Sympathetic trunk

A. Superior View

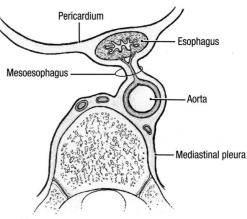

Pericardium

Esophagus

Mesoesophagus

Aorta

Mediastinal pleura

B. Inferior View

1.70   Diaphragm and pericardial sac

A. The diaphragmatic pleura is mostly removed. The pericardial sac is situated on the anterior half of the diaphragm; one third is to the right of the median plane, and two thirds to the left. Note also that anterior to the pericardium, the sternal reflection of the left pleural sac approaches but fails to meet that of the right sac in the median plane; and on reaching the vertebral column, the costal pleura becomes the mediastinal pleura. Irritation of the parietal pleura produces local pain and referred pain to the areas sharing innervation by the same segments of the spinal cord. Irritation of the costal and peripheral parts of the diaphragmatic pleura results in local pain and referred pain along the intercostal nerves to the thoracic and abdominal walls. Irritation of the mediastinal and central diaphragmatic areas of the parietal pleura results in pain that is referred to the root of the neck and over the shoulder (C3–C5 dermatomes). **B.** Between the inferior part of the esophagus and the aorta, the right and left layers of mediastinal pleura form a dorsal mesoesophagus.

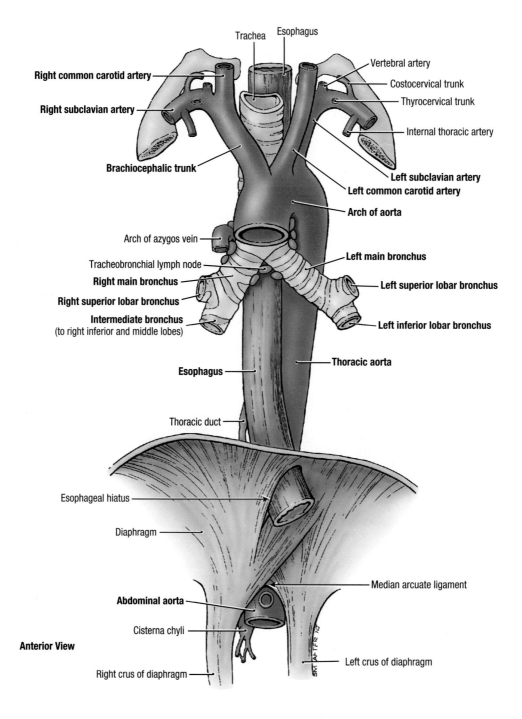

Trachea   Esophagus

Right common carotid artery

Right subclavian artery

Brachiocephalic trunk

Vertebral artery

Costocervical trunk

Thyrocervical trunk

Internal thoracic artery

Left subclavian artery

Left common carotid artery

Arch of aorta

Arch of azygos vein

Tracheobronchial lymph node

Right main bronchus

Right superior lobar bronchus

Intermediate bronchus
(to right inferior and middle lobes)

Left main bronchus

Left superior lobar bronchus

Left inferior lobar bronchus

Thoracic aorta

Esophagus

Thoracic duct

Esophageal hiatus

Diaphragm

Median arcuate ligament

Abdominal aorta

Cisterna chyli

Anterior View

Left crus of diaphragm

Right crus of diaphragm

1.71 Esophagus, trachea, and aorta

- The anterior relations of the thoracic part of the esophagus from superior to inferior are the trachea (from origin at cricoid cartilage to bifurcation), right and left bronchi, inferior tracheobronchial lymph nodes, pericardium (not shown) and, finally, the diaphragm.
- The arch of the aorta passes posterior to the left of these four structures as it arches over the left main bronchus; the arch of the azygos vein passes anterior to their right as it arches over the right main bronchus.

- The impressions produced in the esophagus by adjacent structures (aorta, left main bronchus) are of clinical interest because of the slower passage of substances at these sites. The impressions indicate where swallowed foreign objects are most likely to lodge and where a stricture may develop after the accidental drinking of a caustic liquid such as lye.

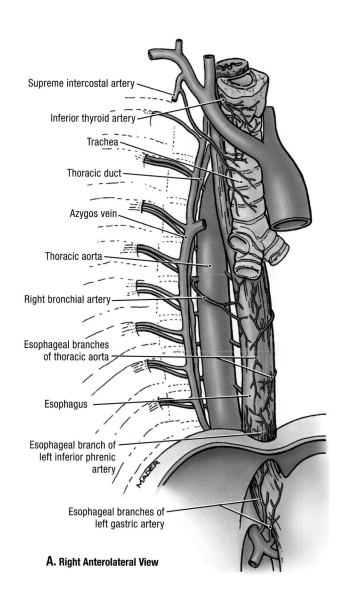

Supreme intercostal artery

Inferior thyroid artery

Trachea

Thoracic duct

Azygos vein

Thoracic aorta

Right bronchial artery

Esophageal branches of thoracic aorta

Esophagus

Esophageal branch of left inferior phrenic artery

Esophageal branches of left gastric artery

A. Right Anterolateral View

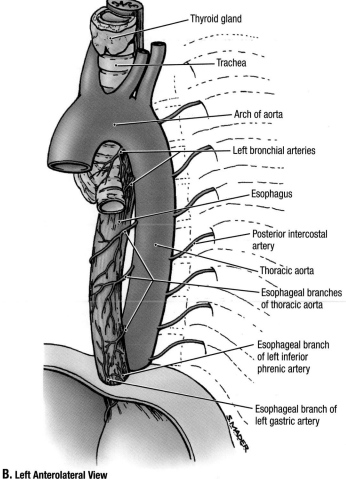

Thyroid gland

Trachea

Arch of aorta

Left bronchial arteries

Esophagus

Posterior intercostal artery

Thoracic aorta

Esophageal branches of thoracic aorta

Esophageal branch of left inferior phrenic artery

Esophageal branch of left gastric artery

B. Left Anterolateral View

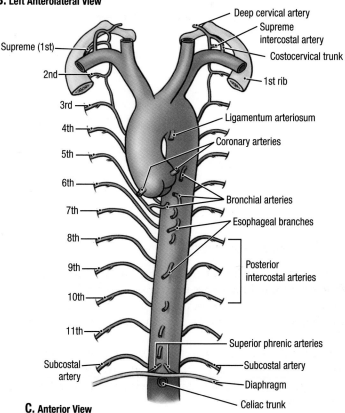

Deep cervical artery

Supreme intercostal artery

Costocervical trunk

Supreme (1st)

1st rib

2nd

3rd

Ligamentum arteriosum

4th

Coronary arteries

5th

6th

Bronchial arteries

7th

Esophageal branches

8th

Posterior intercostal arteries

9th

10th

11th

Superior phrenic arteries

Subcostal artery

Subcostal artery

Diaphragm

Celiac trunk

C. Anterior View

1.72   Arterial supply to trachea and esophagus

A and **B.** The continuous anastomotic chain of arteries on the esophagus is formed (a) by branches of the right and left inferior thyroid and right supreme intercostal arteries superiorly, (b) by the unpaired median aortic (bronchial and esophageal) branches, and (c) by branches of the left gastric and left inferior phrenic arteries inferiorly. The right bronchial artery usually arises from the superior left bronchial or 3rd right posterior intercostal artery (here the 5th) or from the aorta directly. The unpaired median aortic branches also supply the trachea and bronchi. **C.** Branches of the thoracic aorta.

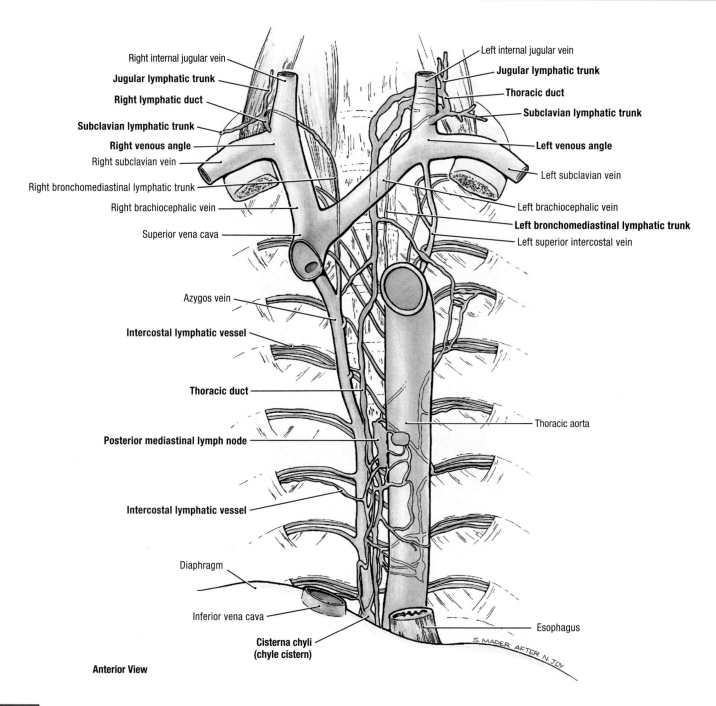

Right internal jugular vein
Jugular lymphatic trunk
Right lymphatic duct
Subclavian lymphatic trunk
Right venous angle
Right subclavian vein
Right bronchomediastinal lymphatic trunk
Right brachiocephalic vein
Superior vena cava

Left internal jugular vein
Jugular lymphatic trunk
Thoracic duct
Subclavian lymphatic trunk
Left venous angle
Left subclavian vein
Left brachiocephalic vein
Left bronchomediastinal lymphatic trunk
Left superior intercostal vein

Azygos vein
Intercostal lymphatic vessel

Thoracic duct

Thoracic aorta

Posterior mediastinal lymph node

Intercostal lymphatic vessel

Diaphragm

Inferior vena cava
Cisterna chyli (chyle cistern)

Esophagus

S. MADER AFTER N. JOY

Anterior View

1.73   Thoracic duct

- The descending aorta is located to the left, and the azygos vein slightly to the right of the midline.
- The thoracic duct (a) originates from the cisterna chyli at the T12 vertebral level, (b) ascends on the vertebral column between the azygos vein and the descending aorta, (c) passes to the left at the junction of the posterior and superior mediastina, and continues its ascent to the neck, where (d) it arches laterally to enter the venous system near or at the angle of union of the left internal jugular and subclavian veins (left venous angle).
- The thoracic duct is commonly plexiform (resembling a network) in the posterior mediastinum.

- The termination of the thoracic duct typically receives the jugular, subclavian, and bronchomediastinal trunks.
- The right lymph duct is short and formed by the union of the right jugular, subclavian, and bronchomediastinal trunks.

- Because the thoracic duct is thin walled and may be colorless, it may not be easily identified. Consequently, it is vulnerable to inadvertent injury during investigative and/or surgical procedures in the posterior mediastinum. Laceration of the thoracic duct results in chyle escaping into the thoracic cavity. Chyle may also enter the pleural cavity, producing chylothorax.

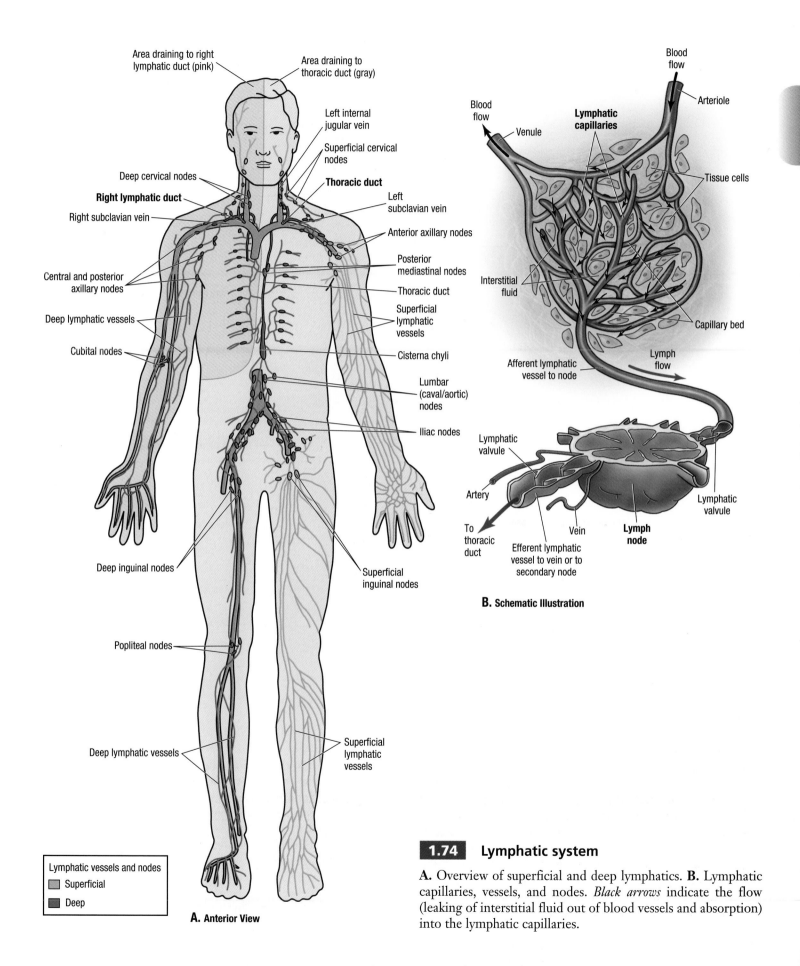

Area draining to right lymphatic duct (pink)
Area draining to thoracic duct (gray)
Left internal jugular vein
Superficial cervical nodes
Thoracic duct
Deep cervical nodes
Right lymphatic duct
Left subclavian vein
Right subclavian vein
Anterior axillary nodes
Posterior mediastinal nodes
Central and posterior axillary nodes
Thoracic duct
Superficial lymphatic vessels
Deep lymphatic vessels
Cisterna chyli
Cubital nodes
Lumbar (caval/aortic) nodes
Iliac nodes
Deep inguinal nodes
Superficial inguinal nodes
Popliteal nodes
Deep lymphatic vessels
Superficial lymphatic vessels

Lymphatic vessels and nodes
☐ Superficial
■ Deep

A. Anterior View

Blood flow
Arteriole
Blood flow
Lymphatic capillaries
Venule
Tissue cells
Interstitial fluid
Capillary bed
Afferent lymphatic vessel to node
Lymph flow
Lymphatic valvule
Artery
Lymphatic valvule
To thoracic duct
Vein
Lymph node
Efferent lymphatic vessel to vein or to secondary node

B. Schematic Illustration

1.74   **Lymphatic system**

A. Overview of superficial and deep lymphatics. **B.** Lymphatic capillaries, vessels, and nodes. *Black arrows* indicate the flow (leaking of interstitial fluid out of blood vessels and absorption) into the lymphatic capillaries.

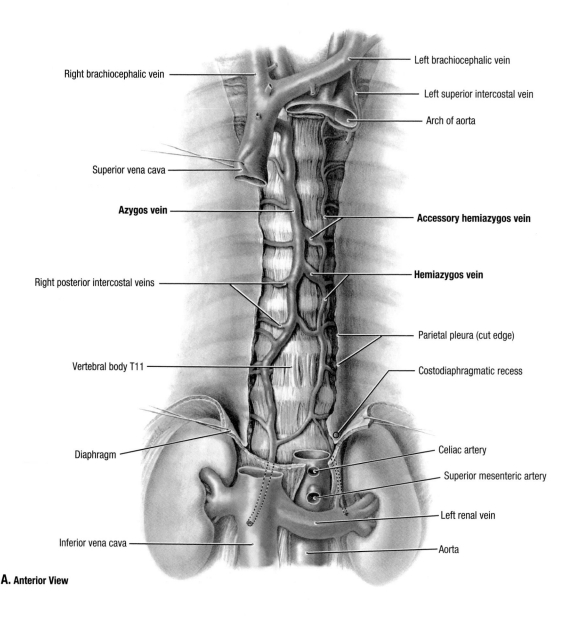

Right brachiocephalic vein

Superior vena cava

Azygos vein

Right posterior intercostal veins

Vertebral body T11

Diaphragm

Inferior vena cava

Left brachiocephalic vein

Left superior intercostal vein

Arch of aorta

Accessory hemiazygos vein

Hemiazygos vein

Parietal pleura (cut edge)

Costodiaphragmatic recess

Celiac artery

Superior mesenteric artery

Left renal vein

Aorta

A. Anterior View

1.75   Azygos system of veins

The ascending lumbar veins connect the common iliac veins to the lumbar veins and join the subcostal veins to become the lateral roots of the azygos and hemiazygos veins; the medial roots of the azygos and hemiazygos veins are usually from the inferior vena cava and left renal vein, if present. Typically the upper four left posterior intercostal veins drain into the left brachiocephalic vein, directly and via the left superior intercostal veins.

In **A,** the hemiazygos, accessory hemiazygos, and left superior intercostals veins are continuous, but commonly they are discontinuous. The hemiazygos vein crosses the vertebral column at approximately T9, and the accessory hemiazygos vein crosses at T8, to enter the azygos vein. In **A,** there are four cross-connecting channels between the azygos and hemiazygos systems. The azygos vein arches superior to the root of the right lung at T4 to drain into the superior vena cava.

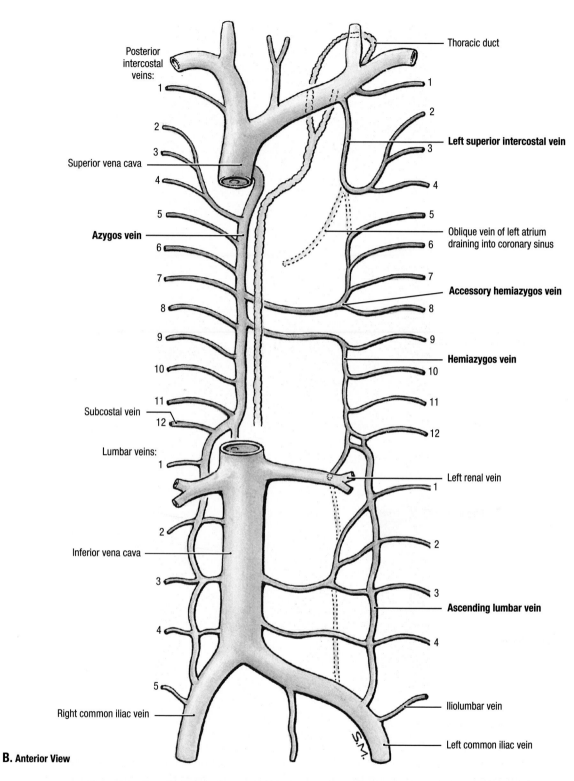

Posterior intercostal veins:

Thoracic duct

1

1

2

2

3

Left superior intercostal vein

Superior vena cava

3

4

4

5

5

Azygos vein

Oblique vein of left atrium draining into coronary sinus

6

6

7

7

Accessory hemiazygos vein

8

8

9

9

Hemiazygos vein

10

10

11

11

Subcostal vein

12

12

Lumbar veins:

1

Left renal vein

1

2

Inferior vena cava

2

3

3

Ascending lumbar vein

4

4

5

Iliolumbar vein

Right common iliac vein

S.M.

Left common iliac vein

B. Anterior View

1.75   Azygos system of veins (continued)

The azygos, hemiazygos, and accessory hemiazygos veins offer alternate means of venous drainage from the thoracic, abdominal, and back regions when *obstruction of the IVC* occurs. In some people, an accessory azygos vein parallels the main azygos vein on the right side. Other people have no hemiazygos system of veins. A clinically important variation, although uncommon, is when the azygos system receives all the blood from the IVC, except that from the liver. In these people, the azygos system drains nearly all the blood inferior to the diaphragm, except that from the digestive tract. When *obstruction of the SVC* occurs superior to the entrance of the azygos vein, blood can drain inferiorly into the veins of the abdominal wall and return to the right atrium through the IVC and azygos system of veins.

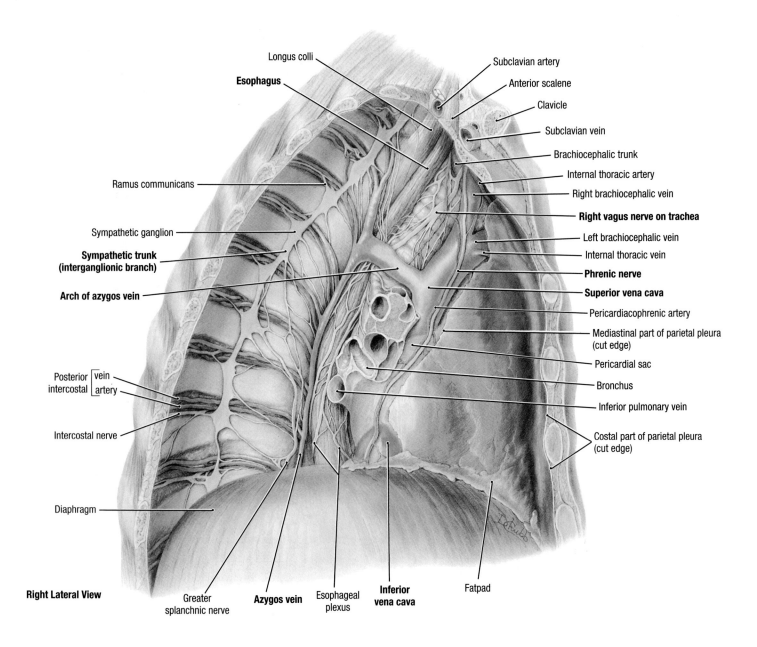

Longus colli

Esophagus

Ramus communicans

Sympathetic ganglion

Sympathetic trunk (interganglionic branch)

Arch of azygos vein

Posterior intercostal ⌈ vein ⌊ artery

Intercostal nerve

Diaphragm

Right Lateral View

Greater splanchnic nerve

Azygos vein

Esophageal plexus

Inferior vena cava

Fatpad

Subclavian artery

Anterior scalene

Clavicle

Subclavian vein

Brachiocephalic trunk

Internal thoracic artery

Right brachiocephalic vein

Right vagus nerve on trachea

Left brachiocephalic vein

Internal thoracic vein

Phrenic nerve

Superior vena cava

Pericardiacophrenic artery

Mediastinal part of parietal pleura (cut edge)

Pericardial sac

Bronchus

Inferior pulmonary vein

Costal part of parietal pleura (cut edge)

1.76   **Mediastinum, right side**

- The costal and mediastinal pleurae have mostly been removed, exposing the underlying structures. Compare with the mediastinal surface of the right lung in Figure 1.29.
- The right side of the mediastinum is the "blue side," dominated by the arch of the azygos vein and the superior vena cava.
- Both the trachea and the esophagus are visible from the right side.
- The right vagus nerve descends on the medial surface of the trachea, passes medial to the arch of the azygos vein, posterior to the root of the lung, and then enters the esophageal plexus.
- The right phrenic nerve passes anterior to the root of the lung lateral to both venae cavae.

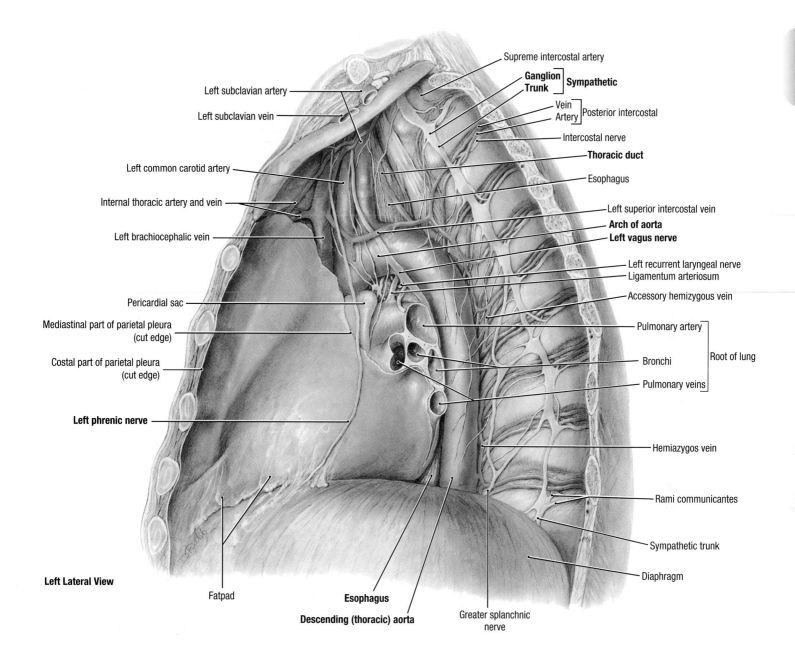

Supreme intercostal artery

Ganglion Trunk ⎱ **Sympathetic**

Left subclavian artery

Left subclavian vein

Vein ⎱ Posterior intercostal
Artery ⎰

Intercostal nerve

Thoracic duct

Left common carotid artery

Esophagus

Internal thoracic artery and vein

Left superior intercostal vein

Arch of aorta
Left vagus nerve

Left brachiocephalic vein

Left recurrent laryngeal nerve
Ligamentum arteriosum

Accessory hemizygous vein

Pericardial sac

Pulmonary artery

Mediastinal part of parietal pleura
(cut edge)

Bronchi ⎱ Root of lung

Costal part of parietal pleura
(cut edge)

Pulmonary veins ⎰

Left phrenic nerve

Hemiazygos vein

Rami communicantes

Sympathetic trunk

Diaphragm

Left Lateral View

Fatpad

Esophagus

Greater splanchnic
nerve

Descending (thoracic) aorta

1.77　Mediastinum, left side

- Compare with the mediastinal surface of the left lung in Figure 1.30.
- The left side of the mediastinum is the "red side," dominated by the arch and descending portion of the aorta, the left common carotid and subclavian arteries; the latter obscure the trachea from view.
- The thoracic duct can be seen on the left side of the esophagus.
- The left vagus nerve passes posterior to the root of the lung, sending its recurrent laryngeal branch around the ligamentum arteriosum inferior, then medial to the aortic arch.
- The phrenic nerve passes anterior to the root of the lung and penetrates the diaphragm more anteriorly than on the right side.

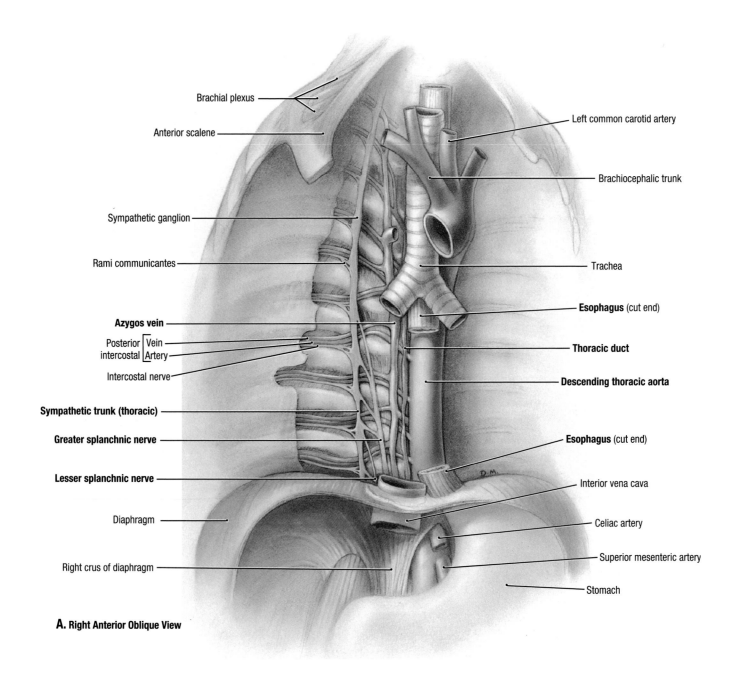

Brachial plexus

Anterior scalene

Left common carotid artery

Brachiocephalic trunk

Sympathetic ganglion

Rami communicantes

Trachea

Esophagus (cut end)

Azygos vein

Posterior [Vein
intercostal [Artery

Thoracic duct

Intercostal nerve

Descending thoracic aorta

Sympathetic trunk (thoracic)

Greater splanchnic nerve

Esophagus (cut end)

Lesser splanchnic nerve

Interior vena cava

Diaphragm

Celiac artery

Superior mesenteric artery

Right crus of diaphragm

Stomach

A. Right Anterior Oblique View

1.78   Structures of posterior mediastinum

- In this specimen, the parietal pleura is intact on the left side and partially removed on the right side. A portion of the esophagus, between the bifurcation of the trachea and the diaphragm, is also removed.
- The thoracic sympathetic trunk is connected to each intercostal nerve by rami communicantes.
- The greater splanchnic nerve is formed by fibers from the 5th to 10th thoracic ganglia, and the lesser splanchnic nerve receives fibers from the 10th and 11th thoracic ganglia. Both nerves contain presynaptic and visceral afferent fibers.
- The azygos vein ascends anterior to the intercostal vessels and to the right of the thoracic duct and aorta.

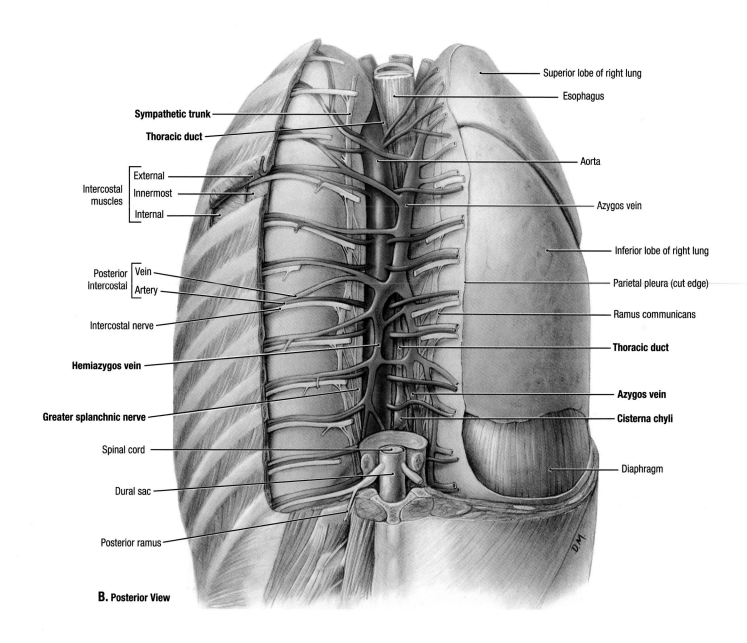

Sympathetic trunk

Thoracic duct

Intercostal muscles
- External
- Innermost
- Internal

Posterior Intercostal
- Vein
- Artery

Intercostal nerve

Hemiazygos vein

Greater splanchnic nerve

Spinal cord

Dural sac

Posterior ramus

Superior lobe of right lung

Esophagus

Aorta

Azygos vein

Inferior lobe of right lung

Parietal pleura (cut edge)

Ramus communicans

Thoracic duct

Azygos vein

Cisterna chyli

Diaphragm

B. Posterior View

1.78   Structures of posterior mediastinum *(continued)*

- The thoracic vertebral column and thoracic cage are removed on the right. On the left, the ribs and intercostal musculature are removed posteriorly as far laterally as the angles of the ribs. The parietal pleura is intact on the left side but partially removed on the right to reveal the visceral pleura covering the right lung.
- The azygos vein is on the right side, and the hemiazygos vein is on the left, crossing the midline (usually at T9, but higher in this specimen) to join the azygos vein. The accessory hemiazygos vein is absent in this specimen; instead, three most superior posterior intercostal veins drain directly into the azygos vein.

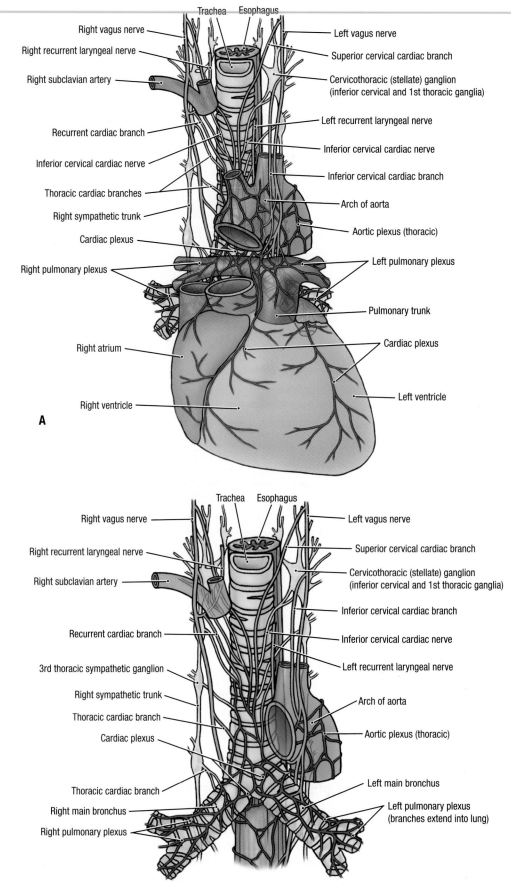

Trachea Esophagus

Right vagus nerve

Right recurrent laryngeal nerve

Right subclavian artery

Recurrent cardiac branch

Inferior cervical cardiac nerve

Thoracic cardiac branches

Right sympathetic trunk

Cardiac plexus

Right pulmonary plexus

Right atrium

Right ventricle

Left vagus nerve

Superior cervical cardiac branch

Cervicothoracic (stellate) ganglion
(inferior cervical and 1st thoracic ganglia)

Left recurrent laryngeal nerve

Inferior cervical cardiac nerve

Inferior cervical cardiac branch

Arch of aorta

Aortic plexus (thoracic)

Left pulmonary plexus

Pulmonary trunk

Cardiac plexus

Left ventricle

A

Trachea Esophagus

Right vagus nerve

Right recurrent laryngeal nerve

Right subclavian artery

Recurrent cardiac branch

3rd thoracic sympathetic ganglion

Right sympathetic trunk

Thoracic cardiac branch

Cardiac plexus

Thoracic cardiac branch

Right main bronchus

Right pulmonary plexus

Left vagus nerve

Superior cervical cardiac branch

Cervicothoracic (stellate) ganglion
(inferior cervical and 1st thoracic ganglia)

Inferior cervical cardiac branch

Inferior cervical cardiac nerve

Left recurrent laryngeal nerve

Arch of aorta

Aortic plexus (thoracic)

Left main bronchus

Left pulmonary plexus
(branches extend into lung)

B

Anterior Views

1.79 **Overview of autonomic innervation of thorax**

A. Innervation of heart. **B.** Innervation of trachea and bronchial tree.

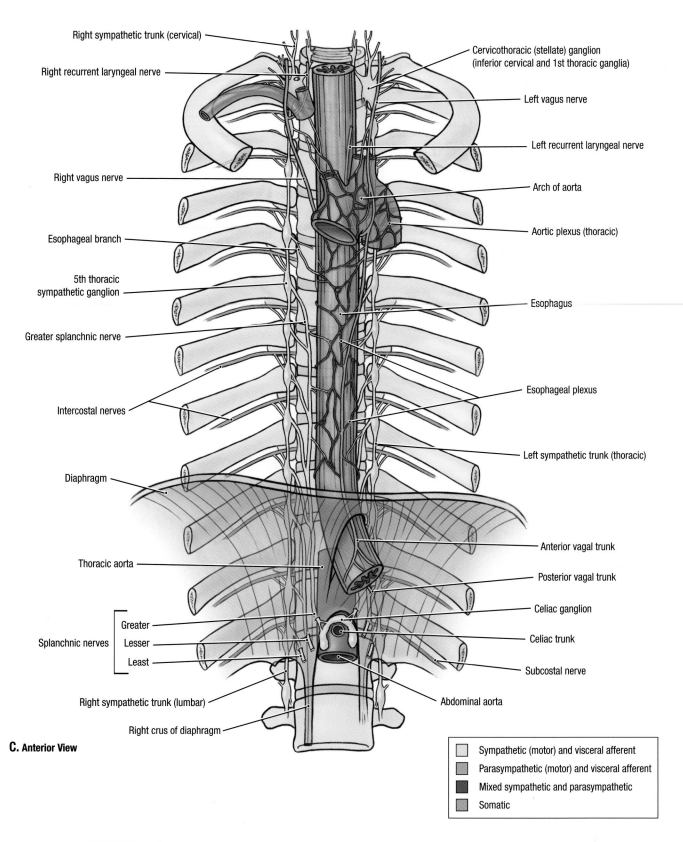

Right sympathetic trunk (cervical)

Right recurrent laryngeal nerve

Right vagus nerve

Esophageal branch

5th thoracic sympathetic ganglion

Greater splanchnic nerve

Intercostal nerves

Diaphragm

Thoracic aorta

Splanchnic nerves — Greater / Lesser / Least

Right sympathetic trunk (lumbar)

Right crus of diaphragm

Cervicothoracic (stellate) ganglion (inferior cervical and 1st thoracic ganglia)

Left vagus nerve

Left recurrent laryngeal nerve

Arch of aorta

Aortic plexus (thoracic)

Esophagus

Esophageal plexus

Left sympathetic trunk (thoracic)

Anterior vagal trunk

Posterior vagal trunk

Celiac ganglion

Celiac trunk

Subcostal nerve

Abdominal aorta

C. Anterior View

Legend:
- Sympathetic (motor) and visceral afferent
- Parasympathetic (motor) and visceral afferent
- Mixed sympathetic and parasympathetic
- Somatic

1.79   **Overview of autonomic innervation of thorax (continued)**

C. Innervation of posterior and superior mediastina.

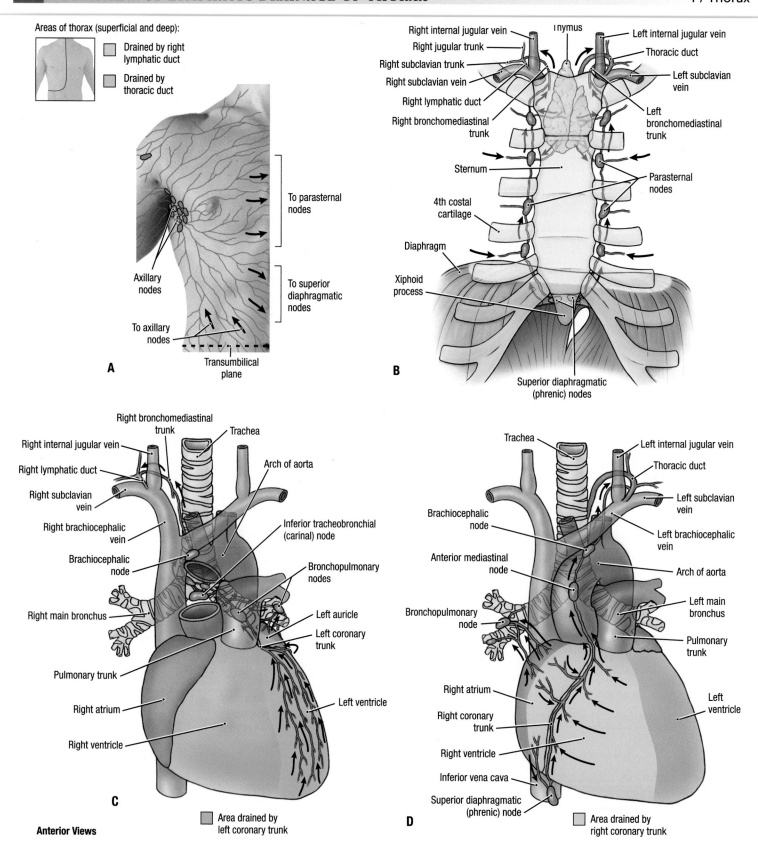

Areas of thorax (superficial and deep):

☐ Drained by right lymphatic duct

☐ Drained by thoracic duct

To parasternal nodes

Axillary nodes

To superior diaphragmatic nodes

To axillary nodes

Transumbilical plane

A

Right internal jugular vein

Thymus

Left internal jugular vein

Right jugular trunk

Thoracic duct

Right subclavian trunk

Left subclavian vein

Right subclavian vein

Right lymphatic duct

Left bronchomediastinal trunk

Right bronchomediastinal trunk

Sternum

Parasternal nodes

4th costal cartilage

Diaphragm

Xiphoid process

Superior diaphragmatic (phrenic) nodes

B

Right bronchomediastinal trunk

Trachea

Right internal jugular vein

Arch of aorta

Right lymphatic duct

Right subclavian vein

Inferior tracheobronchial (carinal) node

Right brachiocephalic vein

Brachiocephalic node

Bronchopulmonary nodes

Right main bronchus

Left auricle

Left coronary trunk

Pulmonary trunk

Right atrium

Left ventricle

Right ventricle

☐ Area drained by left coronary trunk

C

Anterior Views

Trachea

Left internal jugular vein

Thoracic duct

Brachiocephalic node

Left subclavian vein

Anterior mediastinal node

Left brachiocephalic vein

Arch of aorta

Bronchopulmonary node

Left main bronchus

Pulmonary trunk

Right atrium

Right coronary trunk

Left ventricle

Right ventricle

Inferior vena cava

Superior diaphragmatic (phrenic) node

☐ Area drained by right coronary trunk

D

1.80 **Overview of lymphatic drainage of thorax**

A. Superficial lymphatic drainage. **B.** Lymphatic drainage of parasternal nodes. **C.** Lymphatic drainage of left side of heart. **D.** Lymphatic drainage of right side of heart.

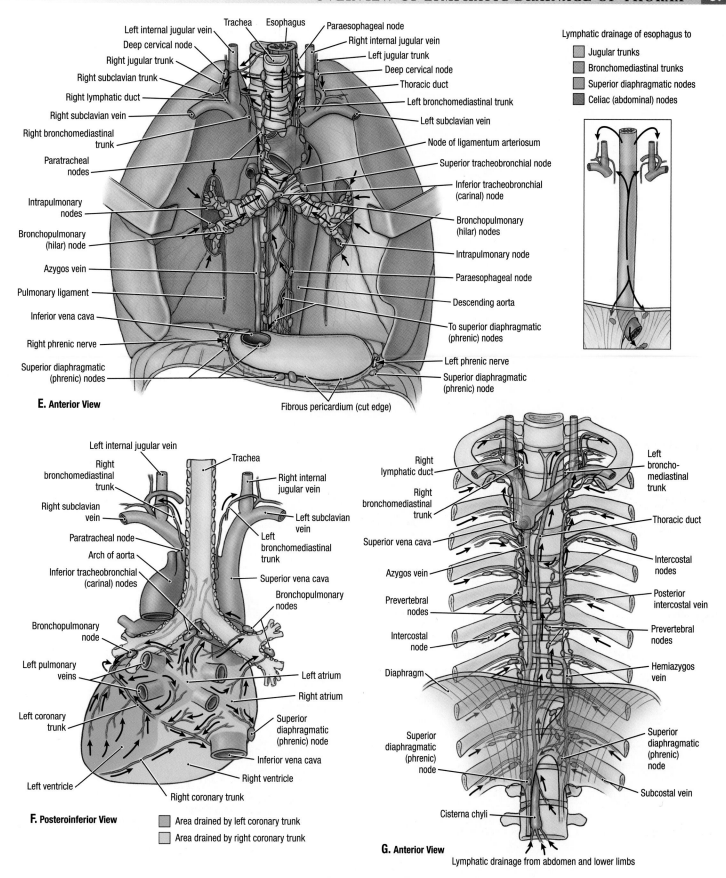

Lymphatic drainage of esophagus to
- Jugular trunks
- Bronchomediastinal trunks
- Superior diaphragmatic nodes
- Celiac (abdominal) nodes

E. Anterior View

F. Posteroinferior View

- Area drained by left coronary trunk
- Area drained by right coronary trunk

G. Anterior View

Lymphatic drainage from abdomen and lower limbs

1.80   **Overview of lymphatic drainage of thorax (continued)**

E. Lymphatic drainage of lungs, esophagus, and superior surface of diaphragm. **F.** Lymphatic drainage of posterior and inferior surfaces of heart. **G.** Lymphatic drainage of posterior mediastinum.

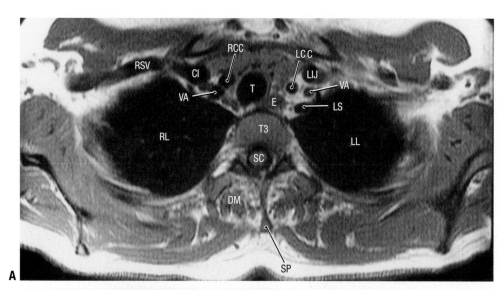

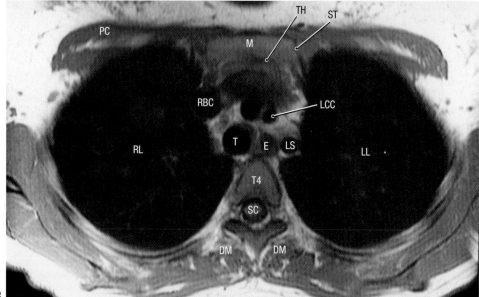

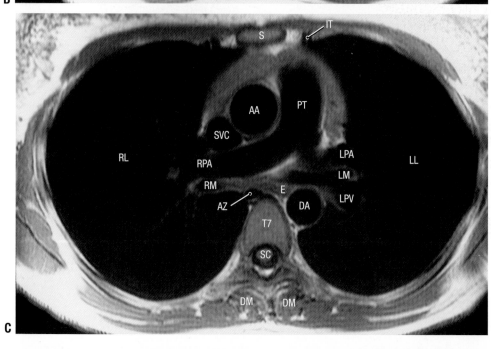

AA	Ascending aorta
AI	Anterior interventricular artery
AZ	Azygos vein
CA	Cusp of aortic valve
CI	Confluence of internal jugular vein
DA	Descending aorta
DM	Deep back muscles
E	Esophagus
HR	Head of rib
HZ	Hemiazygos vein
IT	Internal thoracic vessels
IVS	Interventricular septum
LA	Left atrium
LC	Left coronary artery
LCC	Left common carotid artery
LIJ	Left internal jugular vein
LL	Left lung
LM	Left main bronchus
LPA	Left pulmonary artery
LPV	Left pulmonary vein
LS	Left subclavian artery
LV	Left vertebral artery
M	Manubrium
P	Pericardium
PC	Pectoralis major
PI	Pulmonary infundibulum
PM	Papillary muscle
PT	Pulmonary trunk
RA	Right atrium
RBC	Right brachiocephalic vein
RCC	Right common carotid artery
RL	Right lung
RM	Right middle lobar bronchus
RPA	Right pulmonary artery
RPV	Right pulmonary vein
RSV	Right subclavian vein
RV	Right vertebral artery
S	Sternum
SC	Spinal cord
SP	Spinous process
ST	Sternoclavicular joint
SVC	Superior vena cava
T3-T10	Vertebral body
T	Trachea
TH	Thymus
VA	Vertebral artery

1.81 **Transverse (axial) MRIs of the thorax (A–F)**

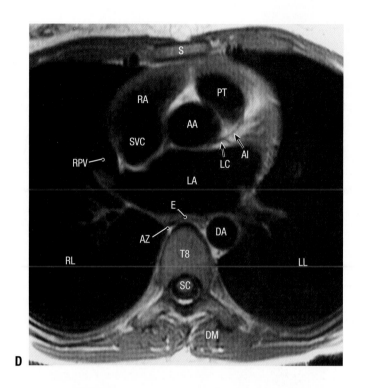

D

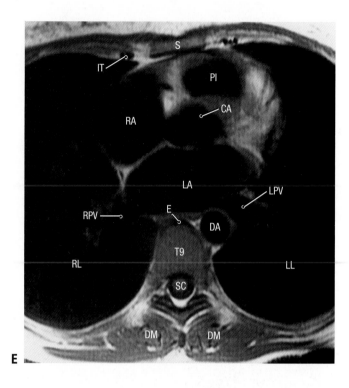

E

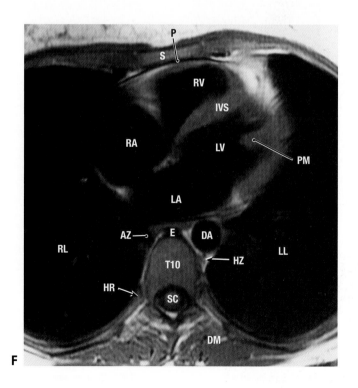

F

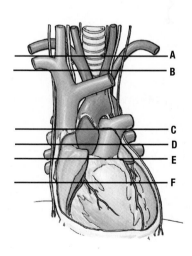

1.81   Transverse (axial) MRIs of the thorax *(continued)*

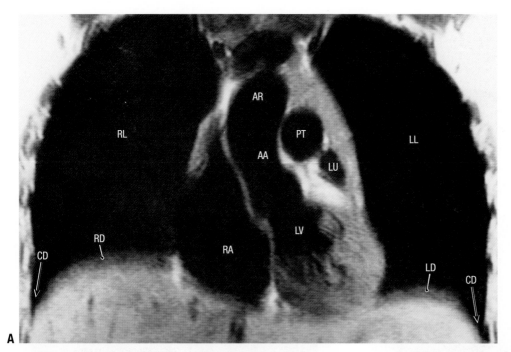

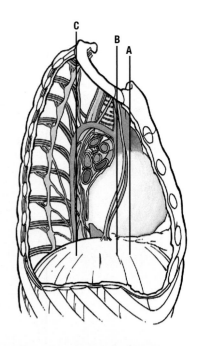

A

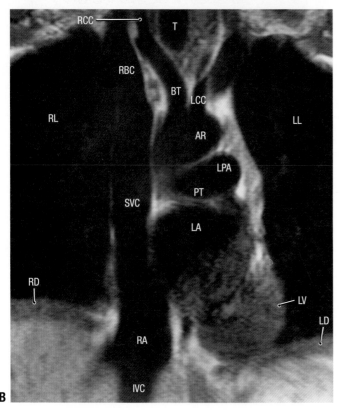

B

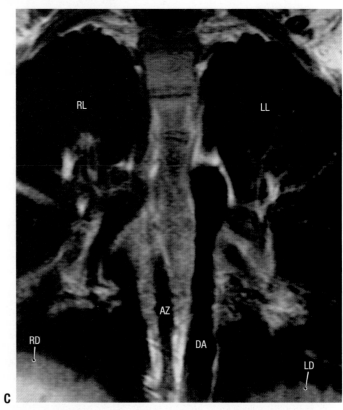

C

AA	Ascending aorta	IVC	Inferior vena cava	LU	Left auricle	RD	Right dome of diaphragm
AR	Arch of aorta	LA	Left atrium	LV	Left ventricle	RL	Right lung
AZ	Azygos vein	LCC	Left common carotid artery	PT	Pulmonary trunk	RV	Right ventricle
BT	Brachiocephalic trunk	LD	Left dome of diaphragm	RA	Right atrium	SVC	Superior vena cava
CD	Costodiaphragmatic recess	LL	Left lung	RBC	Right brachiocephalic vein	T	Trachea
DA	Descending aorta	LPA	Left pulmonary artery	RCC	Right common carotid artery	V	Vertebral body

1.82   **Coronal MRIs of the thorax**

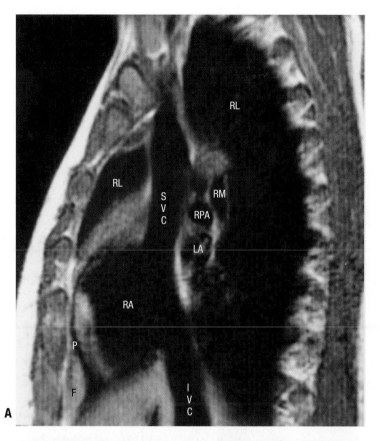

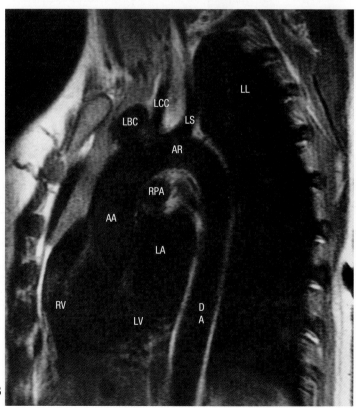

AR	Arch of aorta
AA	Ascending aorta
DA	Descending aorta
F	Fat
IVC	Inferior vena cava
LA	Left atrium
LBC	Left brachiocephalic vein
LCC	Left common carotid artery
LL	Left lung
LS	Left subclavian artery
LV	Left ventricle
P	Pericardium
RA	Right atrium
RL	Right lung
RM	Right main bronchus
RPA	Right pulmonary artery
RV	Right ventricle
SVC	Superior vena cava

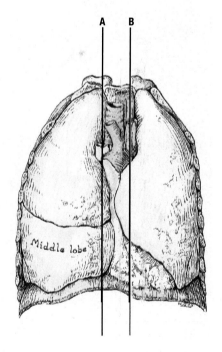

1.83   **Sagittal MRIs of the thorax**

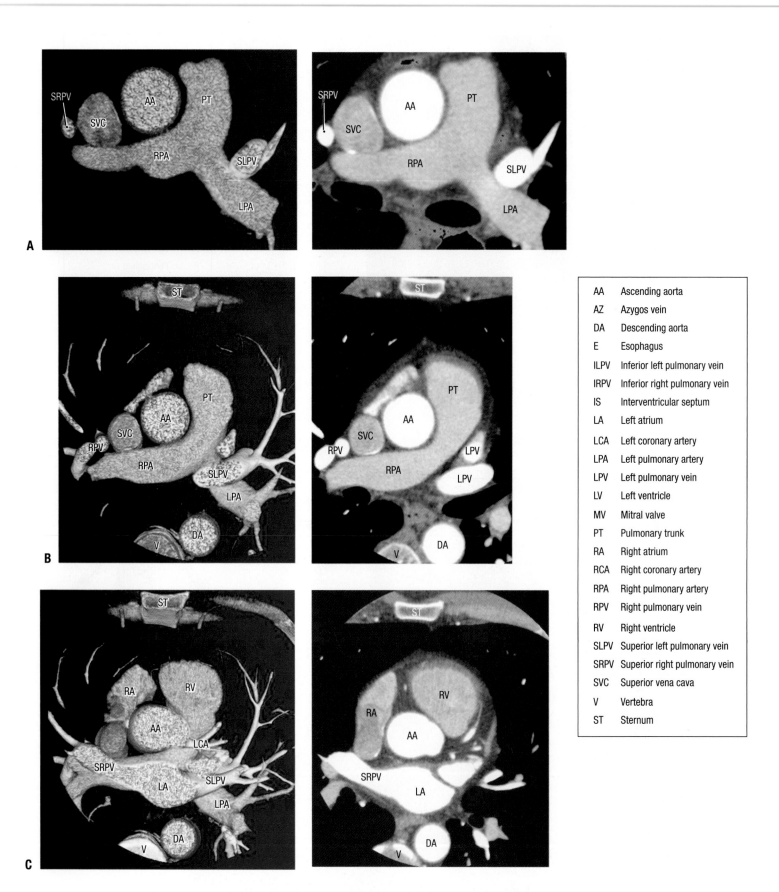

AA	Ascending aorta
AZ	Azygos vein
DA	Descending aorta
E	Esophagus
ILPV	Inferior left pulmonary vein
IRPV	Inferior right pulmonary vein
IS	Interventricular septum
LA	Left atrium
LCA	Left coronary artery
LPA	Left pulmonary artery
LPV	Left pulmonary vein
LV	Left ventricle
MV	Mitral valve
PT	Pulmonary trunk
RA	Right atrium
RCA	Right coronary artery
RPA	Right pulmonary artery
RPV	Right pulmonary vein
RV	Right ventricle
SLPV	Superior left pulmonary vein
SRPV	Superior right pulmonary vein
SVC	Superior vena cava
V	Vertebra
ST	Sternum

1.84   Transverse or horizontal (axial) 3-D volume reconstructions (on left side of page) and CT angiograms of the thorax (A–F) *(continued)*

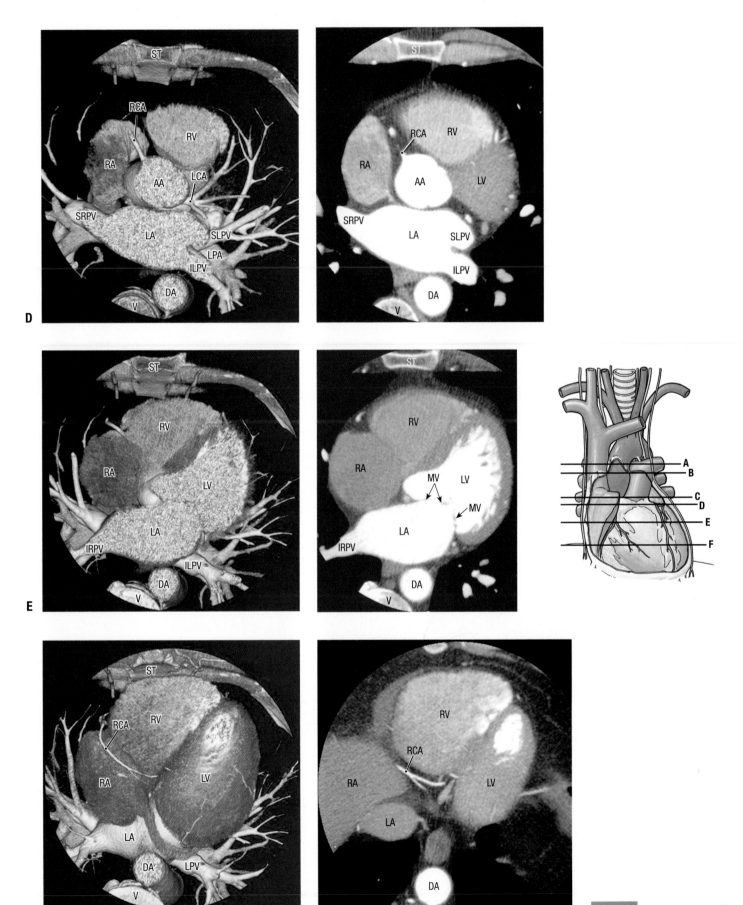

CHAPTER 2

ABDOMEN

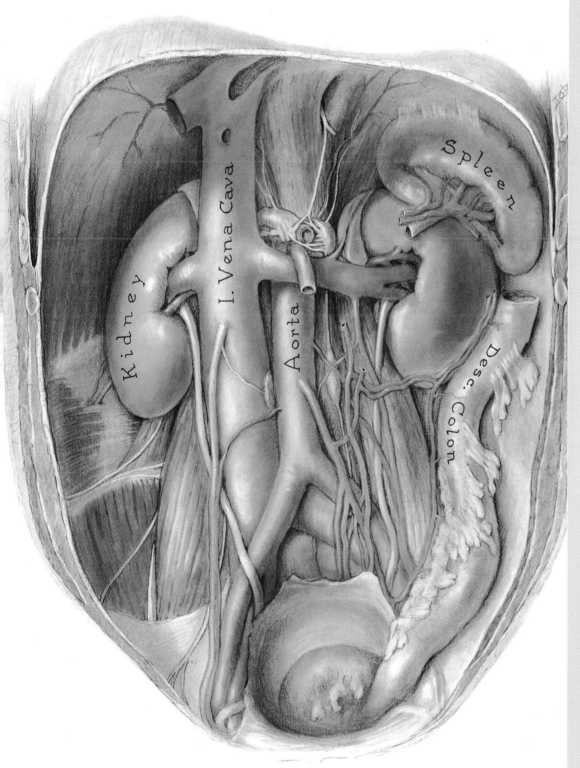

- Overview **96**
- Anterolateral Abdominal Wall **98**
- Inguinal Region **106**
- Testis **116**
- Peritoneum and Peritoneal Cavity **118**
- Digestive System **128**
- Stomach **129**
- Pancreas, Duodenum, and Spleen **131**
- Intestines **136**
- Liver and Gallbladder **146**
- Biliary Ducts **156**
- Portal Venous System **160**
- Posterior Abdominal Wall **162**
- Kidneys **164**
- Lumbar Plexus **172**
- Diaphragm **174**
- Abdominal Aorta and Inferior Vena Cava **175**
- Autonomic Innervation **176**
- Lymphatic Drainage **182**
- Sectional Anatomy and Imaging **186**

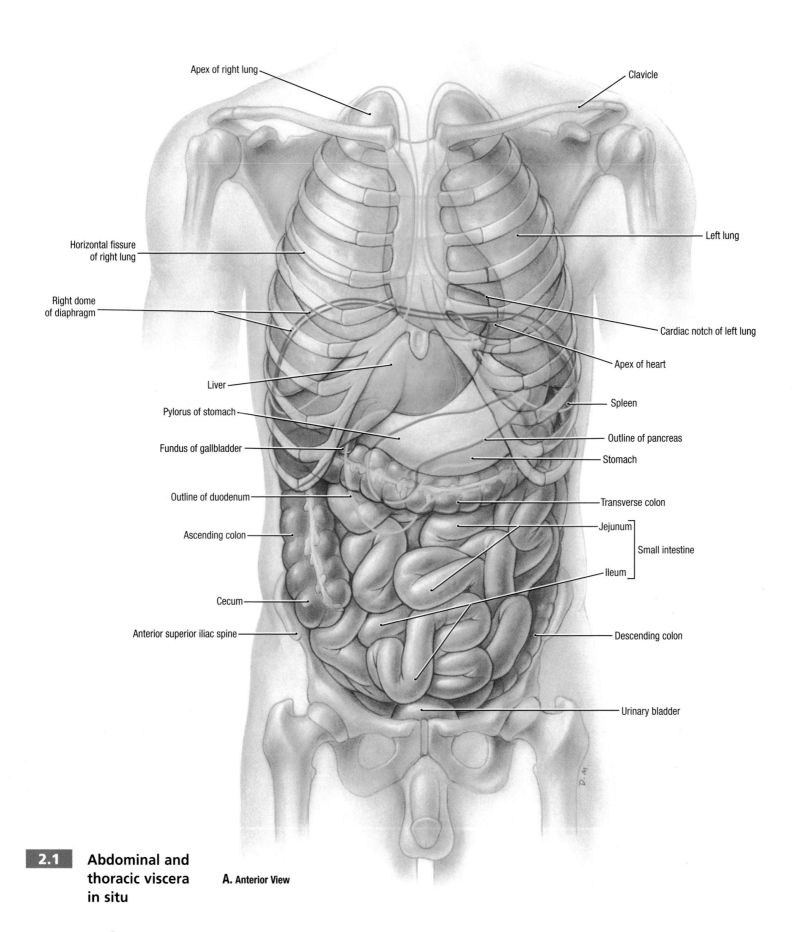

Apex of right lung

Clavicle

Horizontal fissure
of right lung

Left lung

Right dome
of diaphragm

Cardiac notch of left lung

Apex of heart

Liver

Spleen

Pylorus of stomach

Outline of pancreas

Fundus of gallbladder

Stomach

Outline of duodenum

Transverse colon

Ascending colon

Jejunum

Small intestine

Ileum

Cecum

Anterior superior iliac spine

Descending colon

Urinary bladder

2.1   **Abdominal and
thoracic viscera
in situ**   **A. Anterior View**

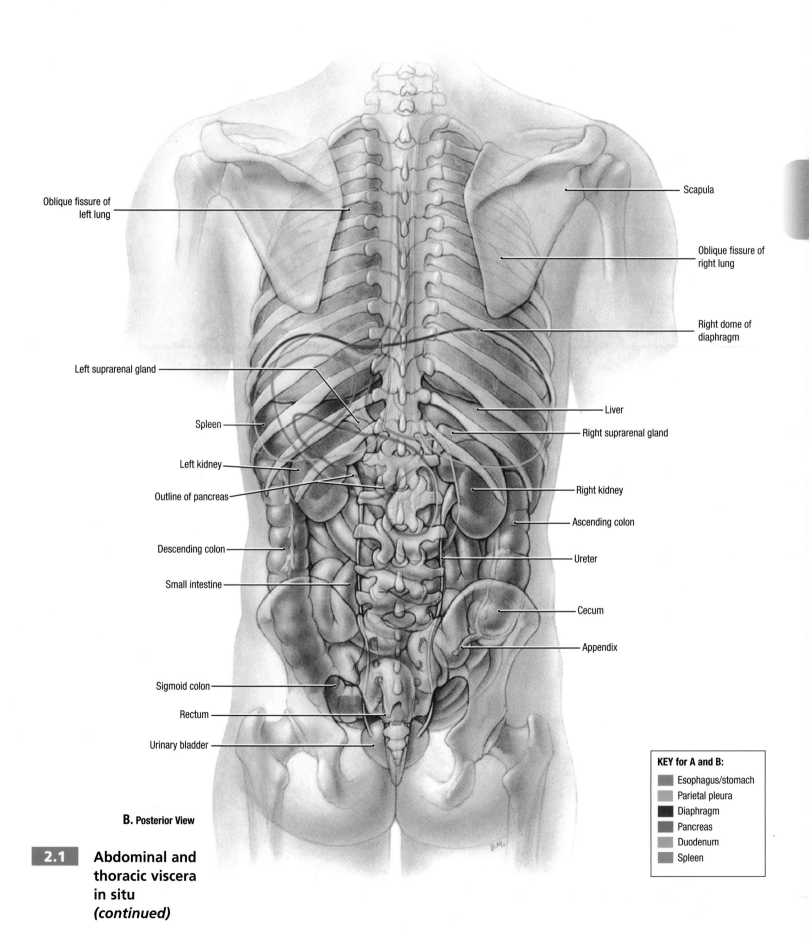

Oblique fissure of
left lung

Scapula

Oblique fissure of
right lung

Right dome of
diaphragm

Left suprarenal gland

Spleen

Liver

Right suprarenal gland

Left kidney

Outline of pancreas

Right kidney

Ascending colon

Descending colon

Ureter

Small intestine

Cecum

Appendix

Sigmoid colon

Rectum

Urinary bladder

B. Posterior View

KEY for A and B:

Esophagus/stomach
Parietal pleura
Diaphragm
Pancreas
Duodenum
Spleen

2.1   **Abdominal and
thoracic viscera
in situ**
(continued)

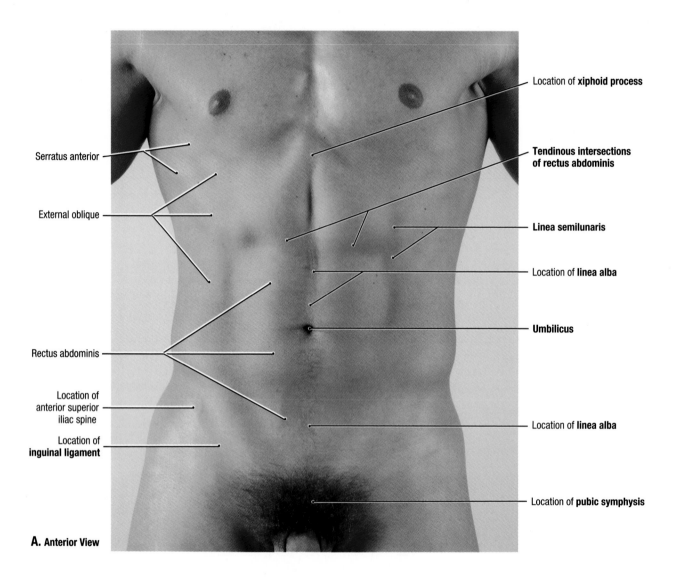

Serratus anterior

External oblique

Rectus abdominis

Location of anterior superior iliac spine

Location of inguinal ligament

A. Anterior View

Location of **xiphoid process**

Tendinous intersections of rectus abdominis

Linea semilunaris

Location of **linea alba**

Umbilicus

Location of **linea alba**

Location of **pubic symphysis**

2.2   Surface anatomy

A. Surface features.

- The umbilicus is where the umbilical cord entered into the fetus and indicates the level of the T10 dermatome, typically at the level of the IV disc between the L3 and L4 vertebrae.
- The linea alba is a subcutaneous fibrous band extending from the xiphoid process to the pubic symphysis that is demarcated by a midline vertical skin groove as far inferiorly as the umbilicus.

- Curved skin grooves, the linea semilunaris, demarcate the lateral borders of the rectus abdominis muscle and rectus sheath.
- Three transverse skin grooves overlie the tendinous intersections of the rectus abdominis muscle.
- The site of the inguinal ligament is indicated by a skin crease, the inguinal groove, just inferior and parallel to the ligament, marking the division between the anterolateral abdominal wall and the thigh.

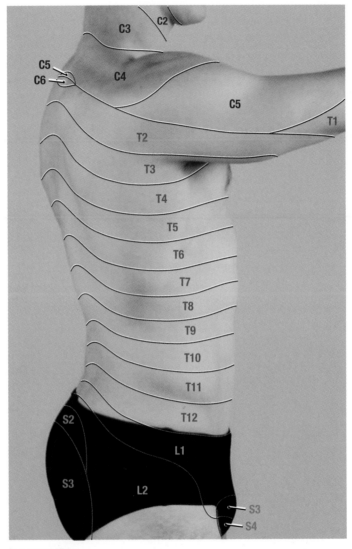

B. Lateral View

2.2   Surface anatomy *(continued)*

B. Dermatomes. The thoracoabdominal (T7–T11) nerves run between the external and internal oblique muscles to supply sensory innervation to the overlying skin. The T10 nerve supplies the region of the umbilicus. The subcostal nerve (T12) runs along the inferior border of the 12th rib to supply the skin over the anterior superior iliac spine and hip. The iliohypogastric nerve (L1) innervates the skin over the iliac crest and hypogastric region and the ilioinguinal nerve (L1), the skin of the medial aspect of the thigh, the scrotum or labium majus and mons pubis.

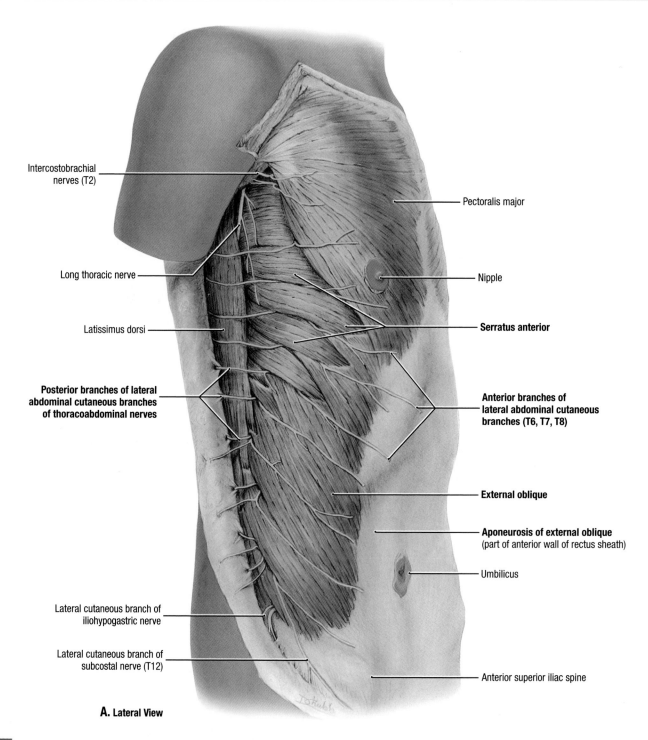

Intercostobrachial nerves (T2)

Long thoracic nerve

Latissimus dorsi

Posterior branches of lateral abdominal cutaneous branches of thoracoabdominal nerves

Lateral cutaneous branch of iliohypogastric nerve

Lateral cutaneous branch of subcostal nerve (T12)

Pectoralis major

Nipple

Serratus anterior

Anterior branches of lateral abdominal cutaneous branches (T6, T7, T8)

External oblique

Aponeurosis of external oblique (part of anterior wall of rectus sheath)

Umbilicus

Anterior superior iliac spine

A. Lateral View

2.3 Anterolateral abdominal wall, superficial dissection

The muscular portion of the external oblique muscle interdigitates with slips of the serratus anterior muscle, and the aponeurotic portion contributes to the anterior wall of the rectus sheath. The anterior and posterior branches of the lateral abdominal cutaneous branches of the thoracoabdominal nerves course superficially in the subcutaneous tissue.

- Umbilical hernias are usually small protrusions of extraperitoneal fat and/or peritoneum abdomen omentum and sometimes bowel. They result from increased intraabdominal pressure in the presence of weakness or incomplete closure of the anterior abdominal wall after ligation of the umbilical cord at birth, or may be acquired later, most commonly in women and obese people.

- The lines along which the fibers of the abdominal aponeurosis interlace (see Fig. 2.6**A**, **B** & **D**) are also potential sites of herniation. These gaps may be congenital, the result of the stresses of obesity and aging, or the consequence of surgical or traumatic wounds.

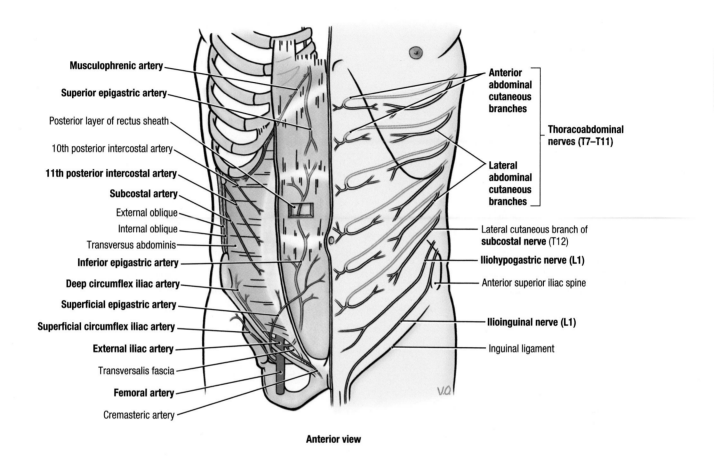

Anterior view

2.4   Arteries and nerves of anterolateral abdominal wall

The skin and muscles of the anterolateral abdominal wall are supplied mainly by the:
- Thoracoabdominal nerves: distal, abdominal parts of the anterior rami of the inferior six thoracic spinal nerves (T7–T11), which have muscular branches and anterior and lateral abdominal cutaneous branches. The anterior abdominal cutaneous branches pierce the rectus sheath a short distance from the median plane, after the rectus abdominis muscle has been supplied. Spinal nerves T7–T9 supply the skin superior to the umbilicus; T10 innervates the skin around the umbilicus.
- Subcostal nerve: large anterior ramus of spinal nerve T12.
- Iliohypogastric and ilioinguinal nerves: terminal branches of the anterior ramus of spinal nerve L1.

- Spinal nerve T11, plus the cutaneous branches of the subcostal (T12), iliohypogastric, and ilioinguinal (L1) nerves: supply the skin inferior to the umbilicus.

The blood vessels of the anterolateral abdominal wall are the:
- Superior epigastric vessels and branches of the musculophrenic vessels from the internal thoracic vessels.
- Inferior epigastric and deep circumflex iliac vessels from the external iliac vessels.
- Superficial circumflex iliac and superficial epigastric vessels from the femoral artery and great saphenous vein.
- Posterior intercostal vessels in the 11th intercostal space and anterior branches of subcostal vessels.

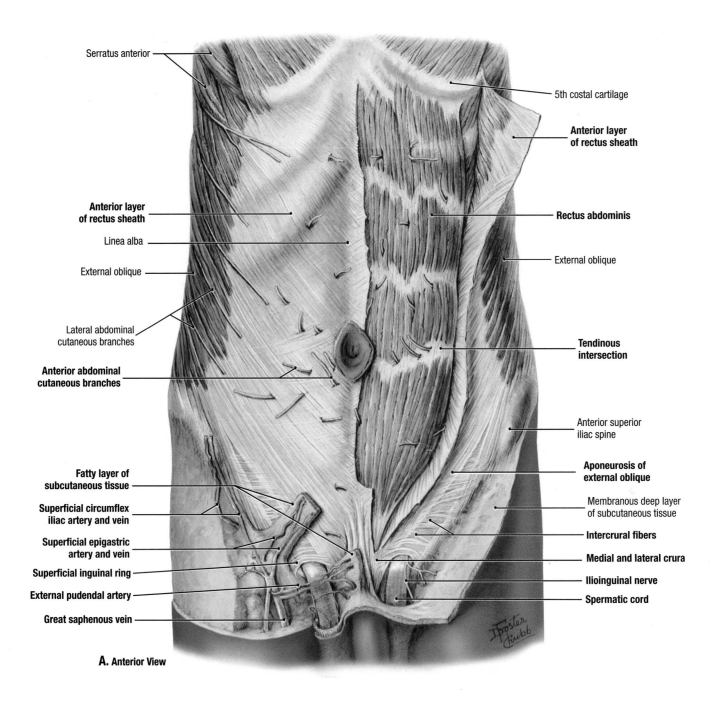

Serratus anterior

5th costal cartilage

Anterior layer of rectus sheath

Anterior layer of rectus sheath

Linea alba

External oblique

Lateral abdominal cutaneous branches

Anterior abdominal cutaneous branches

Rectus abdominis

External oblique

Tendinous intersection

Anterior superior iliac spine

Aponeurosis of external oblique

Fatty layer of subcutaneous tissue

Superficial circumflex iliac artery and vein

Superficial epigastric artery and vein

Superficial inguinal ring

External pudendal artery

Great saphenous vein

Membranous deep layer of subcutaneous tissue

Intercrural fibers

Medial and lateral crura

Ilioinguinal nerve

Spermatic cord

A. Anterior View

2.5   Anterior abdominal wall

A. Superficial dissection demonstrating the relationship of the cutaneous nerves and superficial vessels to the musculoaponeurotic structures. The anterior wall of the left rectus sheath is reflected, revealing the rectus abdominis muscle, segmented by tendinous intersections.

- After the T7 to T12 spinal nerves supply the muscles, their anterior abdominal cutaneous branches emerge from the rectus abdominis muscle and pierce the anterior wall of its sheath.
- The three superficial inguinal branches of the femoral artery (superficial circumflex iliac artery, superficial epigastric artery,

and external pudendal artery) and the great saphenous vein lie in the fatty layer of subcutaneous tissue.

- The fibers of the external oblique aponeurosis separate into medial and lateral crura which, with the intercrural fibers that unite them, form the superficial inguinal ring. The spermatic cord of the male (shown here), or round ligament of the female, exit the inguinal canal through the superficial inguinal ring along with the ilioinguinal nerve.

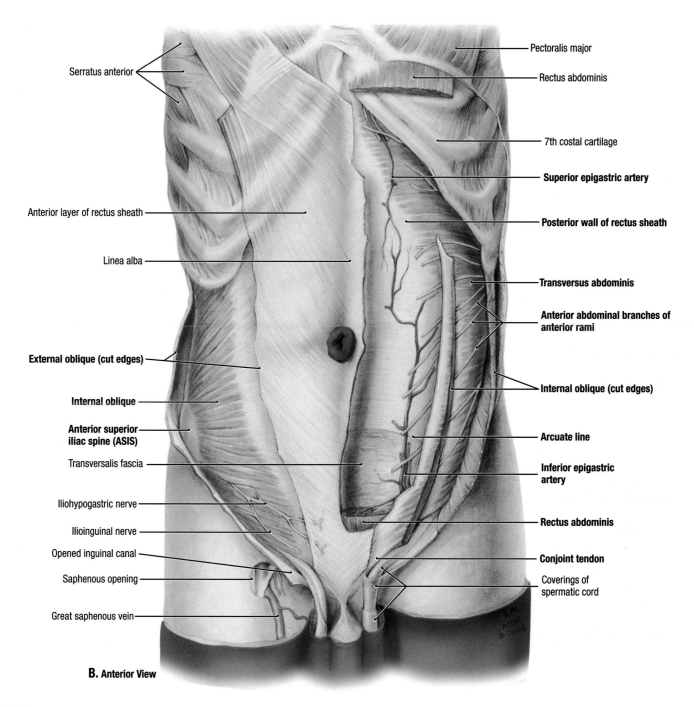

Serratus anterior

Anterior layer of rectus sheath

Linea alba

External oblique (cut edges)

Internal oblique

Anterior superior iliac spine (ASIS)

Transversalis fascia

Iliohypogastric nerve

Ilioinguinal nerve

Opened inguinal canal

Saphenous opening

Great saphenous vein

Pectoralis major

Rectus abdominis

7th costal cartilage

Superior epigastric artery

Posterior wall of rectus sheath

Transversus abdominis

Anterior abdominal branches of anterior rami

Internal oblique (cut edges)

Arcuate line

Inferior epigastric artery

Rectus abdominis

Conjoint tendon

Coverings of spermatic cord

B. Anterior View

| 2.5 | **Anterior abdominal wall (continued)** |

B. Deep dissection. On the right side of the specimen, most of the external oblique muscle is excised. On the left, the internal oblique muscle is divided and the rectus abdominis muscle is excised, revealing the posterior wall of the rectus sheath.

- The fibers of the internal oblique muscle run horizontally at the level of the anterior superior iliac spine (ASIS), obliquely upward superior to the ASIS, and obliquely downward inferior to the ASIS.
- The arcuate line is at the level of the ASIS; inferior to the line, only transversalis fascia lies posterior to the rectus abdominis muscle.

- Initially, the anterior abdominal branches of the anterior rami course between the internal oblique and transversus abdominis muscles.
- The anastomosis between the superior and inferior epigastric arteries indirectly unites the subclavian artery of the upper limb to the external iliac arteries of the lower limb. The anastomosis can become functionally patent in response to slowly developing occlusion of the aorta.

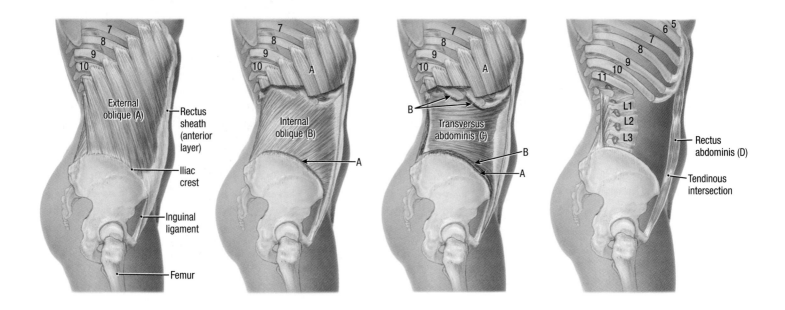

TABLE 2.1 PRINCIPAL MUSCLES OF ANTEROLATERAL ABDOMINAL WALL

Muscles[a]	Origin	Insertion	Innervation	Action(s)
External oblique (A)	External surfaces of 5th–12th ribs	Linea alba, pubic tubercle, and anterior half of iliac crest	Thoracoabdominal nerves (T7–T11) and subcostal nerve	Compresses and supports abdominal viscera[b]; flexes and rotates trunk
Internal oblique (B)	Thoracolumbar fascia, anterior two thirds of iliac crest	Inferior borders of 10th–12th ribs, linea alba, and pubis via conjoint tendon		
Transversus abdominis (C)	Internal surfaces of 7th–12th costal cartilages, thoracolumbar fascia, iliac crest, and lateral third of inguinal ligament	Linea alba with aponeurosis of internal oblique, pubic crest, and pecten pubis via conjoint tendon	Thoracoabdominal (T7–T11), subcostal and first lumbar nerves	Compresses and supports abdominal viscera[b]
Rectus abdominis (D)	Pubic symphysis and pubic crest	Xiphoid process and 5th–7th costal cartilages	Thoracoabdominal nerves and anterior rami of inferior thoracic nerves	Flexes trunk (lumbar vertebrae) and compresses abdominal viscera[b]; stabilizes and controls tilt of pelvis (antilordosis)

[a]Approximately 80% of people have a pyramidal muscle, which is located in the rectus sheath anterior to the most inferior part of the rectus abdominis. It extends from the pubic crest of the hip bone to the linea alba. This small muscle draws down on the linea alba.

[b]In so doing, these muscles act as antagonists of the diaphragm to produce expiration.

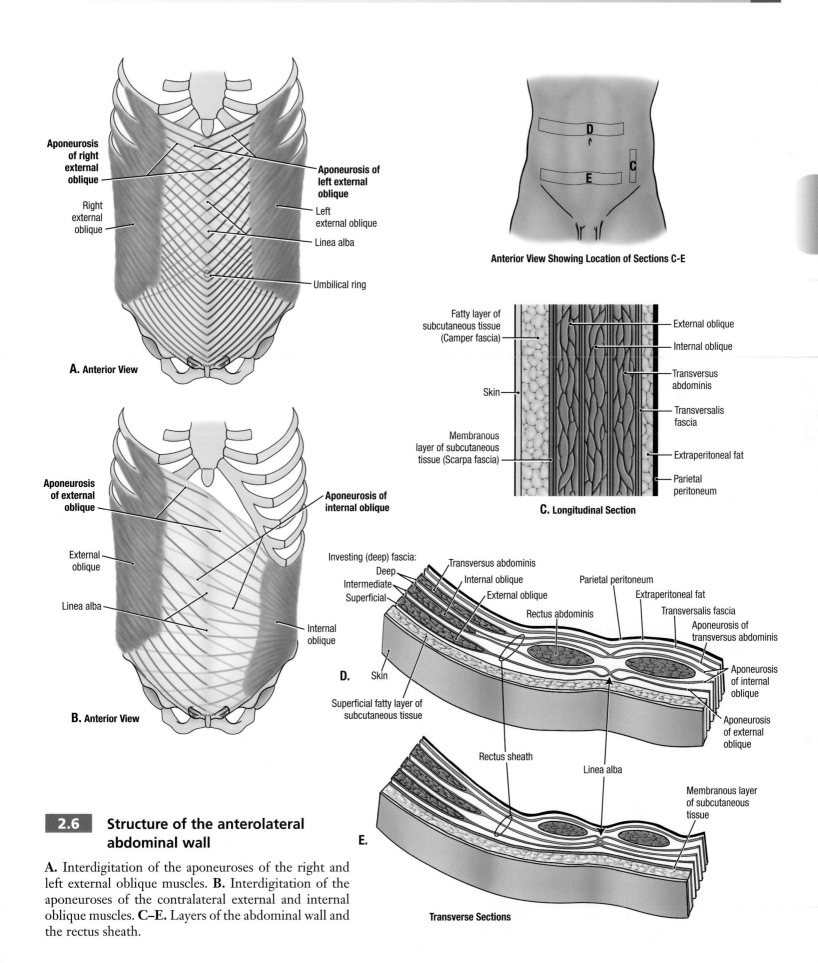

Aponeurosis of right external oblique

Right external oblique

Aponeurosis of left external oblique

Left external oblique

Linea alba

Umbilical ring

A. Anterior View

Aponeurosis of external oblique

External oblique

Linea alba

Aponeurosis of internal oblique

Internal oblique

B. Anterior View

Anterior View Showing Location of Sections C-E

Fatty layer of subcutaneous tissue (Camper fascia)

Skin

Membranous layer of subcutaneous tissue (Scarpa fascia)

External oblique

Internal oblique

Transversus abdominis

Transversalis fascia

Extraperitoneal fat

Parietal peritoneum

C. Longitudinal Section

Investing (deep) fascia:
Deep
Intermediate
Superficial

Transversus abdominis
Internal oblique
External oblique
Rectus abdominis

Parietal peritoneum
Extraperitoneal fat
Transversalis fascia
Aponeurosis of transversus abdominis

Aponeurosis of internal oblique

Aponeurosis of external oblique

D. Skin

Superficial fatty layer of subcutaneous tissue

Rectus sheath

Linea alba

Membranous layer of subcutaneous tissue

E.

Transverse Sections

2.6 Structure of the anterolateral abdominal wall

A. Interdigitation of the aponeuroses of the right and left external oblique muscles. **B.** Interdigitation of the aponeuroses of the contralateral external and internal oblique muscles. **C–E.** Layers of the abdominal wall and the rectus sheath.

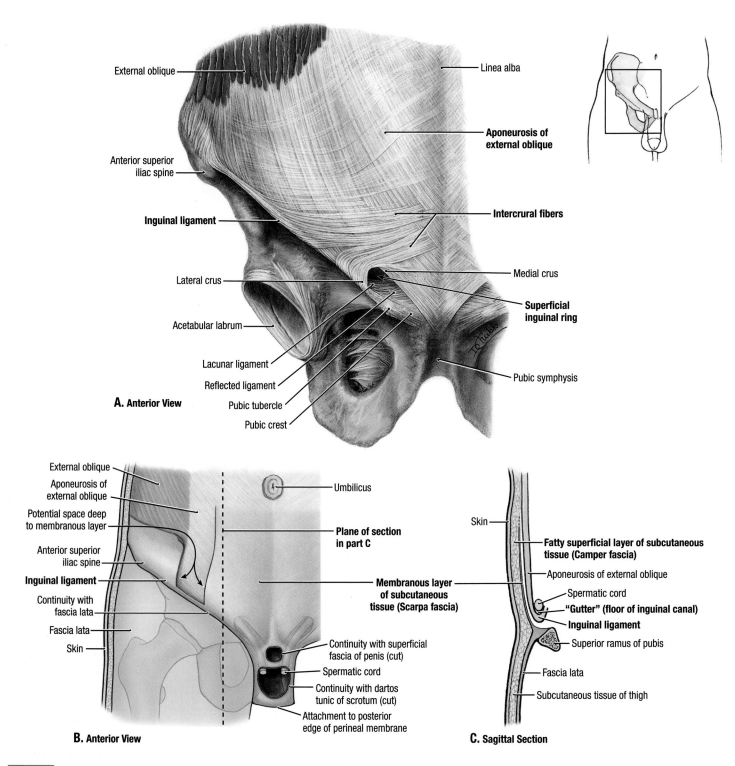

External oblique

Linea alba

**Aponeurosis of
external oblique**

Anterior superior
iliac spine

Inguinal ligament

Intercrural fibers

Lateral crus

Medial crus

**Superficial
inguinal ring**

Acetabular labrum

Lacunar ligament

Reflected ligament

Pubic symphysis

A. Anterior View

Pubic tubercle

Pubic crest

External oblique

Aponeurosis of
external oblique

Umbilicus

Potential space deep
to membranous layer

**Plane of section
in part C**

Skin

**Fatty superficial layer of subcutaneous
tissue (Camper fascia)**

Anterior superior
iliac spine

Aponeurosis of external oblique

Inguinal ligament

Spermatic cord

Continuity with
fascia lata

**Membranous layer
of subcutaneous
tissue (Scarpa fascia)**

"Gutter" (floor of inguinal canal)

Inguinal ligament

Fascia lata

Superior ramus of pubis

Skin

Continuity with superficial
fascia of penis (cut)

Fascia lata

Spermatic cord

Subcutaneous tissue of thigh

Continuity with dartos
tunic of scrotum (cut)

Attachment to posterior
edge of perineal membrane

B. Anterior View

C. Sagittal Section

2.7   Inguinal region of male-I

A. Formations of the aponeurosis of the external oblique muscle. **B** and **C.** Membranous (deep) layer of subcutaneous tissue. Inferior to the umbilicus, the subcutaneous tissue is composed of two layers: a superficial fatty layer and a deep membranous layer. Laterally, the membranous layer fuses with the fascia lata of the thigh about a finger's breadth inferior to the inguinal ligament. Medially, it fuses with the linea alba and pubic symphysis in the midline, and inferiorly, it continues as the membranous layer of the subcutaneous tissue of the perineum and penis and the dartos fascia of the scrotum. The inferior margin of the external oblique aponeurosis is thickened and turned internally forming the inguinal ligament. The superior surface of the in-turning inguinal ligament forms a shallow trough or "gutter" that is the floor of the inguinal canal.

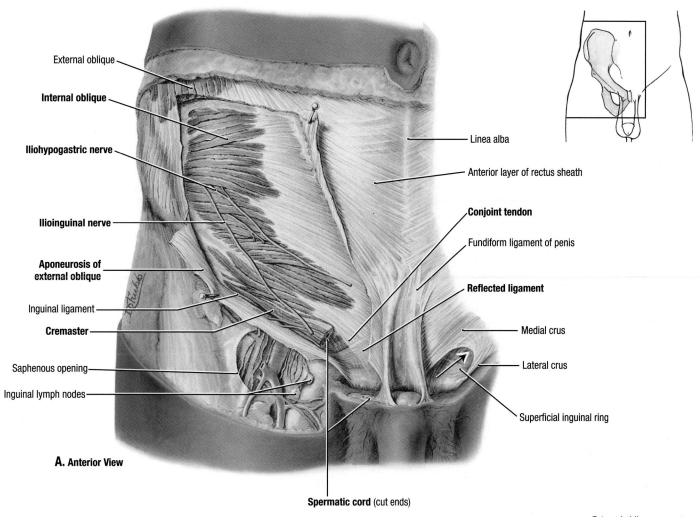

Internal oblique and cremaster muscle, with labels:

External oblique

Internal oblique

Iliohypogastric nerve

Ilioinguinal nerve

Aponeurosis of external oblique

Inguinal ligament

Cremaster

Saphenous opening

Inguinal lymph nodes

Linea alba

Anterior layer of rectus sheath

Conjoint tendon

Fundiform ligament of penis

Reflected ligament

Medial crus

Lateral crus

Superficial inguinal ring

A. Anterior View

Spermatic cord (cut ends)

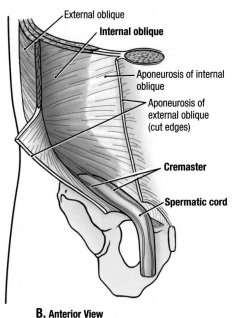

External oblique

Internal oblique

Aponeurosis of internal oblique

Aponeurosis of external oblique (cut edges)

Cremaster

Spermatic cord

B. Anterior View

2.8   **Inguinal region of male—II**

A. Internal oblique and cremaster muscle. Part of the aponeurosis of the external oblique muscle is cut away, and the spermatic cord is cut short. **B.** Schematic illustration.

• The cremaster muscle covers the spermatic cord.

• The reflected ligament is formed by aponeurotic fibers of the external oblique muscle and lies anterior to the conjoint tendon. The conjoint tendon is formed by the fusion of the aponeurosis of the internal oblique and transversus abdominis muscles.

• The cutaneous branches of the iliohypogastric and ilioinguinal nerves (L1) course between the internal and external oblique muscles and must be avoided when an appendectomy incision is made in this region.

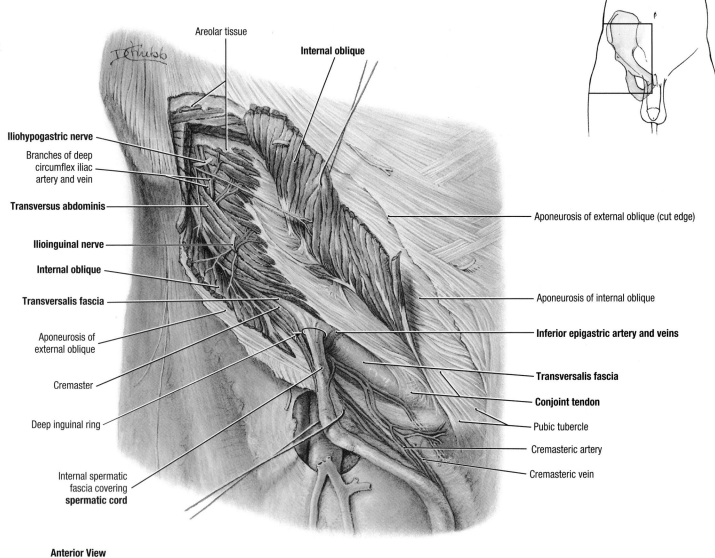

Areolar tissue

Internal oblique

Iliohypogastric nerve

Branches of deep
circumflex iliac
artery and vein

Transversus abdominis

Ilioinguinal nerve

Internal oblique

Transversalis fascia

Aponeurosis of
external oblique

Cremaster

Deep inguinal ring

Internal spermatic
fascia covering
spermatic cord

Aponeurosis of external oblique (cut edge)

Aponeurosis of internal oblique

Inferior epigastric artery and veins

Transversalis fascia

Conjoint tendon

Pubic tubercle

Cremasteric artery

Cremasteric vein

Anterior View

2.9 Inguinal region of male—III

The internal oblique muscle is reflected, and the spermatic cord is retracted.

- The internal oblique muscle portion of the conjoint tendon is attached to the pubic crest, and the transversus abdominis portion to the pectineal line.
- The iliohypogastric and ilioinguinal nerves (L1) supply the internal oblique and transversus abdominis muscles.
- The transversalis fascia is evaginated to form the tubular internal spermatic fascia. The mouth of the tube, called the deep inguinal ring, is situated lateral to the inferior epigastric vessels.

TABLE 2.2 STRUCTURES FORMING THE INGUINAL CANAL

Boundaries	Lateral Third	Middle Third	Medial Third
Posterior wall	Transversalis fascia including deep inguinal ring	Transversalis fascia	Transversalis fascia Conjoint tendon
Anterior wall	Aponeurosis of external oblique Internal oblique	Aponeurosis of external oblique	Aponeurosis of external oblique Superficial inguinal ring
Roof	Arching fibers of internal oblique and transversus abdominis		
Floor	Inguinal ligament	Inguinal ligament	Inguinal ligament Lacunar ligament

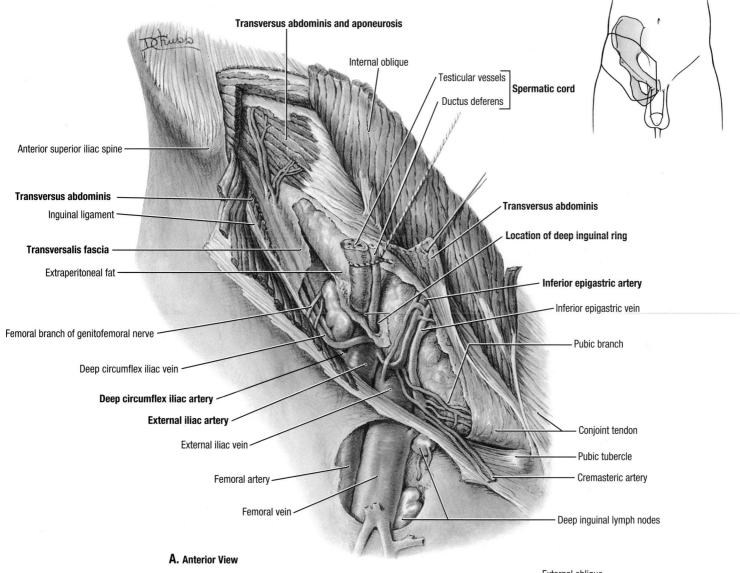

A. Anterior View

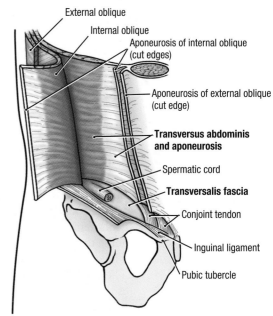

B. Anterior View

2.10   Inguinal region of male—IV

A. The inguinal part of the transversus abdominis muscle and transversalis fascia is partially cut away, the spermatic cord is excised, and the ductus deferens is retracted. **B.** Schematic illustration.

- The deep inguinal ring is located superior to the inguinal ligament at the midpoint between the anterior superior iliac spine and pubic tubercle.
- The external iliac artery has two branches, the deep circumflex iliac and inferior epigastric arteries. Note also the cremasteric artery and pubic branch arising from the latter.

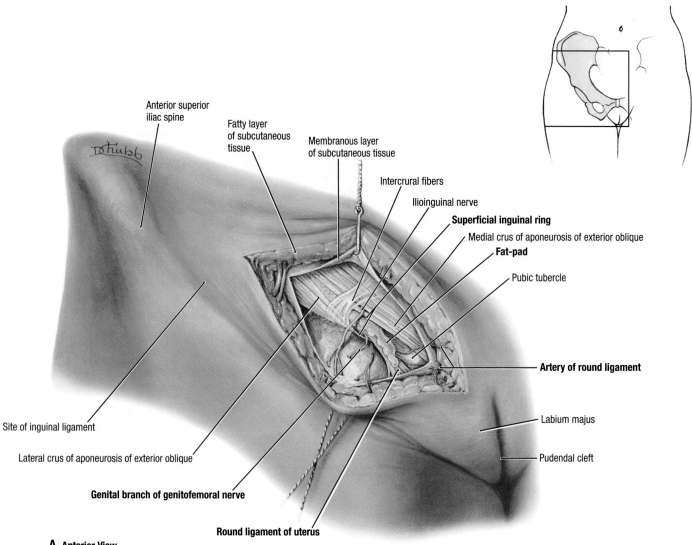

Anterior superior iliac spine

Fatty layer of subcutaneous tissue

Membranous layer of subcutaneous tissue

Intercrural fibers

Ilioinguinal nerve

Superficial inguinal ring

Medial crus of aponeurosis of exterior oblique

Fat-pad

Pubic tubercle

Artery of round ligament

Labium majus

Pudendal cleft

Site of inguinal ligament

Lateral crus of aponeurosis of exterior oblique

Genital branch of genitofemoral nerve

Round ligament of uterus

A. Anterior View

2.11   Inguinal canal of female

Progressive dissections of the female inguinal canal **(A–D).**

- In **A,** the superficial inguinal ring is small. Passing through the superficial inguinal ring are the round ligament of the uterus, a closely applied fat-pad, the genital branch of the genitofemoral nerve, and the artery of the round ligament of the uterus. The ilioinguinal nerve may also pass through the ring.
- The cremaster muscle does not extend beyond the superficial inguinal ring **(B).**
- The round ligament breaks up into strands as it leaves the inguinal canal and approaches the labium majus **(C).**
- The external iliac artery and vein are exposed deep to the inguinal canal by excising the transversalis fascia **(D).**

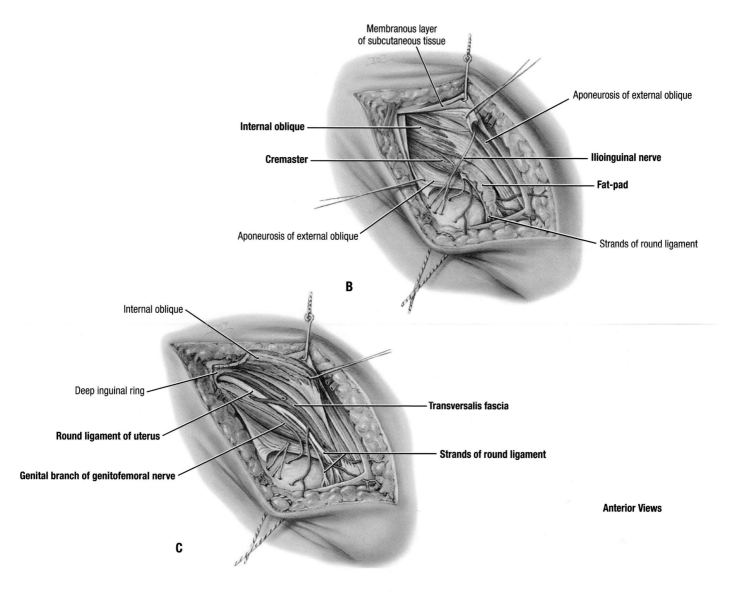

Membranous layer
of subcutaneous tissue

Aponeurosis of external oblique

Internal oblique

Cremaster

Ilioinguinal nerve

Fat-pad

Aponeurosis of external oblique

Strands of round ligament

B

Internal oblique

Deep inguinal ring

Transversalis fascia

Round ligament of uterus

Strands of round ligament

Genital branch of genitofemoral nerve

Anterior Views

C

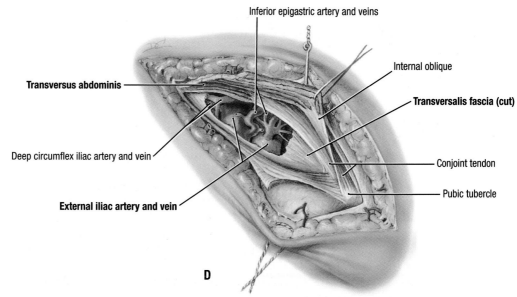

Inferior epigastric artery and veins

Internal oblique

Transversus abdominis

Transversalis fascia (cut)

Deep circumflex iliac artery and vein

Conjoint tendon

Pubic tubercle

External iliac artery and vein

D

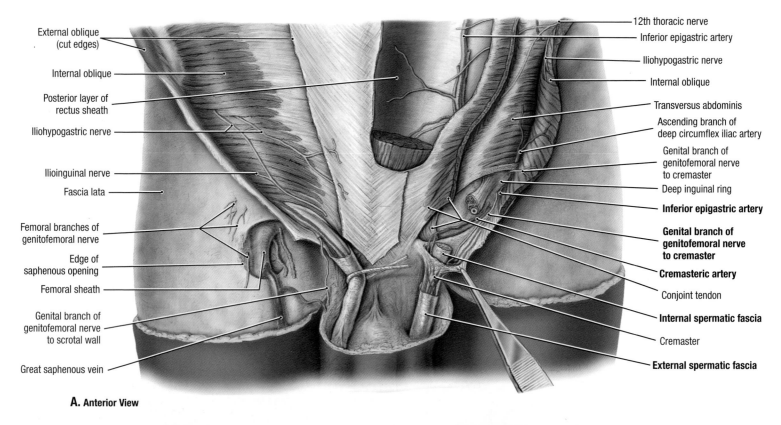

External oblique (cut edges)

Internal oblique

Posterior layer of rectus sheath

Iliohypogastric nerve

Ilioinguinal nerve

Fascia lata

Femoral branches of genitofemoral nerve

Edge of saphenous opening

Femoral sheath

Genital branch of genitofemoral nerve to scrotal wall

Great saphenous vein

12th thoracic nerve

Inferior epigastric artery

Iliohypogastric nerve

Internal oblique

Transversus abdominis

Ascending branch of deep circumflex iliac artery

Genital branch of genitofemoral nerve to cremaster

Deep inguinal ring

Inferior epigastric artery

Genital branch of genitofemoral nerve to cremaster

Cremasteric artery

Conjoint tendon

Internal spermatic fascia

Cremaster

External spermatic fascia

A. Anterior View

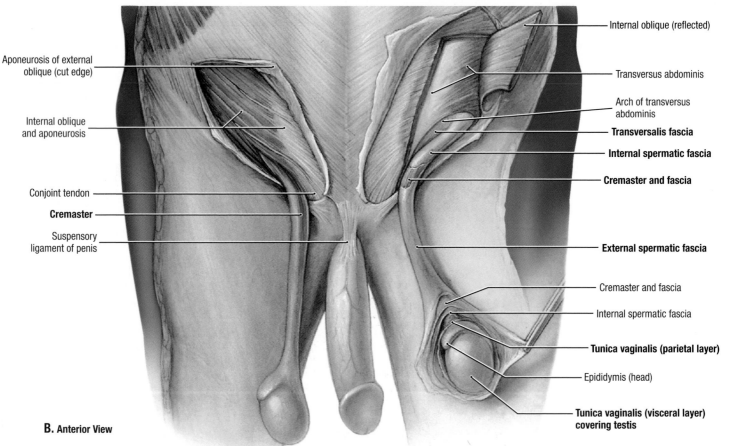

Aponeurosis of external oblique (cut edge)

Internal oblique and aponeurosis

Conjoint tendon

Cremaster

Suspensory ligament of penis

Internal oblique (reflected)

Transversus abdominis

Arch of transversus abdominis

Transversalis fascia

Internal spermatic fascia

Cremaster and fascia

External spermatic fascia

Cremaster and fascia

Internal spermatic fascia

Tunica vaginalis (parietal layer)

Epididymis (head)

Tunica vaginalis (visceral layer) covering testis

B. Anterior View

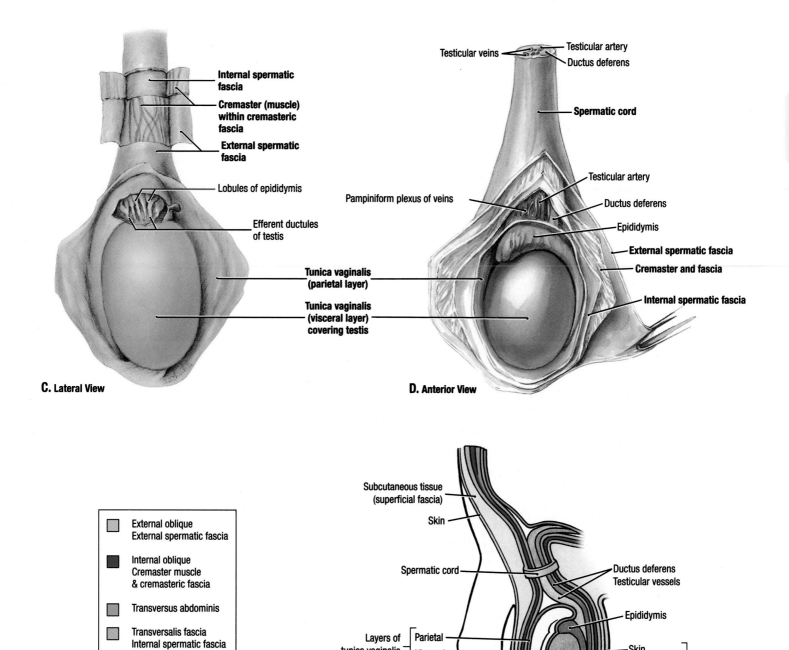

C. Lateral View

Internal spermatic fascia
Cremaster (muscle) within cremasteric fascia
External spermatic fascia
Lobules of epididymis
Efferent ductules of testis
Tunica vaginalis (parietal layer)
Tunica vaginalis (visceral layer) covering testis

D. Anterior View

Testicular veins
Testicular artery
Ductus deferens
Spermatic cord
Testicular artery
Pampiniform plexus of veins
Ductus deferens
Epididymis
External spermatic fascia
Cremaster and fascia
Internal spermatic fascia

External oblique
External spermatic fascia

Internal oblique
Cremaster muscle
& cremasteric fascia

Transversus abdominis

Transversalis fascia
Internal spermatic fascia

Parietal peritoneum
Tunica vaginalis (parietal and visceral layers)

E. Schematic Illustration

Subcutaneous tissue (superficial fascia)
Skin
Spermatic cord
Ductus deferens
Testicular vessels
Epididymis
Layers of tunica vaginalis — Parietal / Visceral
Skin
Dartos muscle and fascia — Scrotum
Cavity of tunica vaginalis
Testis

2.12   Inguinal canal, spermatic cord, and testis

A. Dissection of inguinal canal. **B.** Dissection of inguinal region and coverings of the spermatic cord and testis. **C–E.** Coverings of spermatic cord and testis.

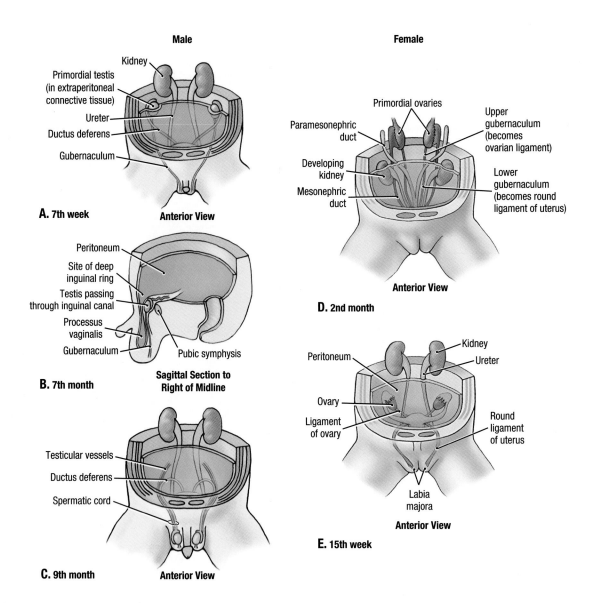

Male

Kidney
Primordial testis (in extraperitoneal connective tissue)
Ureter
Ductus deferens
Gubernaculum

A. 7th week **Anterior View**

Peritoneum
Site of deep inguinal ring
Testis passing through inguinal canal
Processus vaginalis
Gubernaculum
Pubic symphysis

B. 7th month **Sagittal Section to Right of Midline**

Testicular vessels
Ductus deferens
Spermatic cord

C. 9th month **Anterior View**

Female

Primordial ovaries
Paramesonephric duct
Upper gubernaculum (becomes ovarian ligament)
Developing kidney
Mesonephric duct
Lower gubernaculum (becomes round ligament of uterus)

Anterior View

D. 2nd month

Peritoneum
Kidney
Ureter
Ovary
Ligament of ovary
Round ligament of uterus
Labia majora

Anterior View

E. 15th week

2.13   Descent of gonads

The inguinal canals in females are narrower than those in males, and the canals in infants of both sexes are shorter and much less oblique than in adults. For a complete description of the embryology of the inguinal region, see Moore and Persaud (2003).

The fetal testes descend from the dorsal abdominal wall in the superior lumbar region to the deep inguinal rings during the 9th–12th fetal weeks. This movement probably results from growth of the vertebral column and pelvis. The male gubernaculum, attached to the caudal pole of the testis and accompanied by an outpouching of peritoneum, the processus vaginalis, projects into the scrotum. The testis descends posterior to the processus vaginalis. The inferior remnant of the processus vaginalis forms the tunica vaginalis covering the testis. The ductus deferens, tes-

ticular vessels, nerves, and lymphatics accompany the testis. The final descent of the testis usually occurs before or shortly after birth.

The fetal ovaries also descend from the dorsal abdominal wall in the superior lumbar region during the 12th week but pass into the lesser pelvis. The female gubernaculum attaches to the caudal pole of the ovary and projects into the labia majora, attaching en route to the uterus; the part passing from the uterus to the ovary forms the ovarian ligament, and the remainder of it becomes the round ligament of the uterus. Because of the attachment of the ovarian ligaments to the uterus, the ovaries do not descend to the inguinal region; however, the round ligament passes through the inguinal canal and attaches to the subcutaneous tissue of the labium majus.

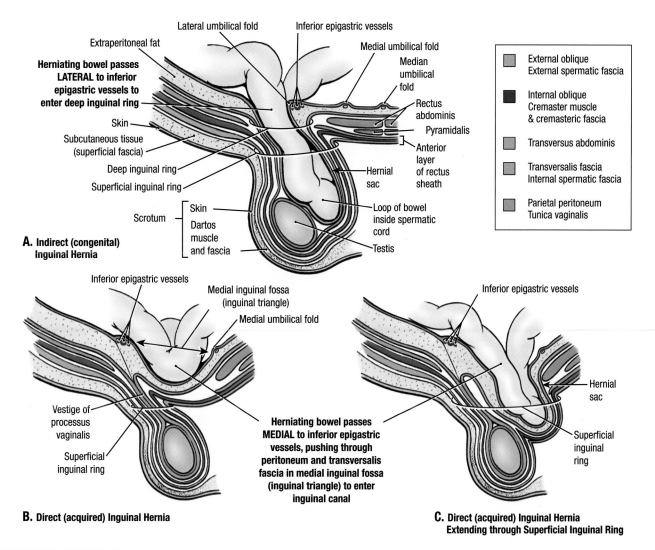

A. Indirect (congenital) Inguinal Hernia

B. Direct (acquired) Inguinal Hernia

C. Direct (acquired) Inguinal Hernia Extending through Superficial Inguinal Ring

Legend:
- External oblique / External spermatic fascia
- Internal oblique / Cremaster muscle & cremasteric fascia
- Transversus abdominis
- Transversalis fascia / Internal spermatic fascia
- Parietal peritoneum / Tunica vaginalis

2.14 Inguinal hernias

An inguinal hernia is a protrusion of parietal peritoneum and viscera, such as the small intestine, through the abdominal wall in the inguinal region. There are two major categories of inguinal hernia: indirect and direct. More than two-thirds are indirect hernias, most commonly occurring in males.

Characteristics[a]	Direct (Acquired)	Indirect (Congenital)
Predisposing factors	Weakness of anterior abdominal wall in inguinal triangle (e.g., owing to distended superficial ring, narrow conjoint tendon, or attenuation of aponeurosis in males > 40 years of age)	Patency of processus vaginalis (complete or at least of superior part) in younger persons, the great majority of whom are males
Frequency	Less common (1/3 to 1/4 of inguinal hernias)	More common (2/3 to 3/4 of inguinal hernias)
Coverings at exit from abdominal cavity (**A** and **B**)	Peritoneum plus transversalis fascia (lies outside inner one or two fascial coverings of cord)	Peritoneum of persistent processus vaginalis plus all three fascial coverings of cord/round ligament
Course (**C**)	Usually traverses only medial third of inguinal canal, external and parallel to vestige of processus vaginalis	Traverses inguinal canal (entire canal if it is sufficient size) within processus vaginalis
Exit from anterior abdominal wall	Via superficial ring, lateral to cord; rarely enters scrotum	Via superficial ring inside cord, commonly passing into scrotum/labium majus

[a]Letters in parentheses refer to the figure parts.

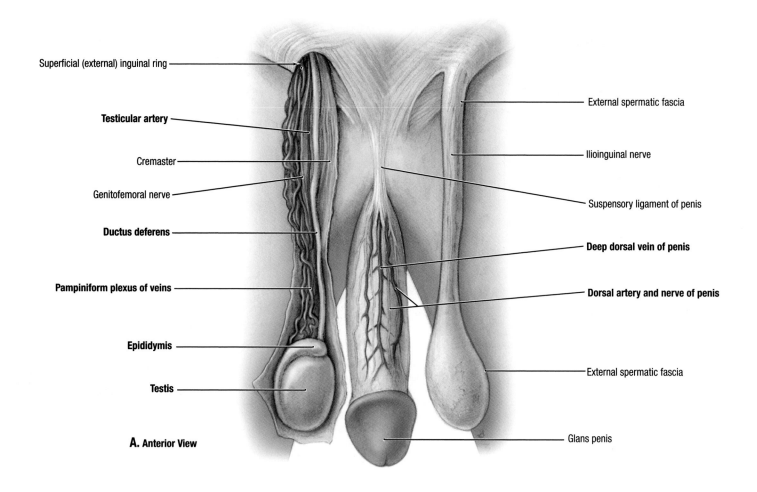

Superficial (external) inguinal ring

Testicular artery

Cremaster

Genitofemoral nerve

Ductus deferens

Pampiniform plexus of veins

Epididymis

Testis

A. Anterior View

External spermatic fascia

Ilioinguinal nerve

Suspensory ligament of penis

Deep dorsal vein of penis

Dorsal artery and nerve of penis

External spermatic fascia

Glans penis

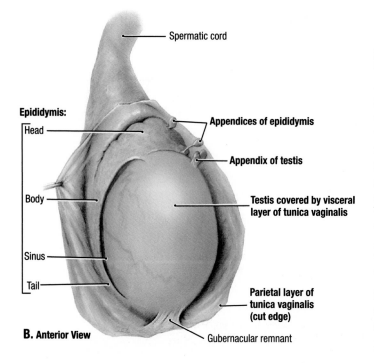

Spermatic cord

Epididymis:
Head
Body
Sinus
Tail

Appendices of epididymis

Appendix of testis

Testis covered by visceral layer of tunica vaginalis

Parietal layer of tunica vaginalis (cut edge)

B. Anterior View

Gubernacular remnant

2.15 Spermatic cord, testis, and epididymis

A. Dissection of spermatic cord. The subcutaneous tissue (dartos fascia) covering the penis has been removed and the deep fascia rendered transparent to demonstrate the median deep dorsal vein and the bilateral dorsal arteries and nerves of the penis. On the specimen's right, the coverings of the spermatic cord and testis are reflected, and the contents of the cord are separated. The testicular artery has been separated from the pampiniform plexus of veins that surrounds it as it courses parallel to the ductus deferens. Lymphatic vessels and autonomic nerve fibers (not shown) are also present. **B.** The tunica vaginalis has been incised longitudinally to expose its cavity, surrounding the testis anteriorly and laterally, and extending between the testis and epididymis at the sinus of the epididymis. The epididymis is located posterolateral to the left testis, i.e., on the right side of the right testis and on the left side of the left testis. The appendices of the testis and epididymis may be observed in some specimens. These structures are small remnants of the embryonic genital (paramesonephric) duct.

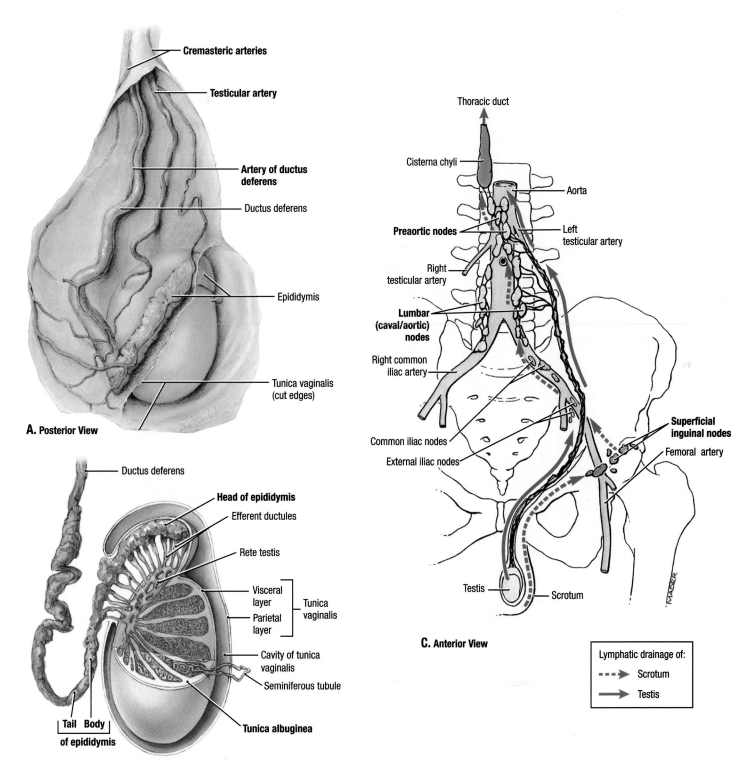

A. Posterior View

- Cremasteric arteries
- Testicular artery
- Artery of ductus deferens
- Ductus deferens
- Epididymis
- Tunica vaginalis (cut edges)

**B. Longitinal Section of Tunica Vaginalis;
Testis Sectioned in Sagittal and Transverse Planes**

- Ductus deferens
- Head of epididymis
- Efferent ductules
- Rete testis
- Visceral layer
- Parietal layer } Tunica vaginalis
- Cavity of tunica vaginalis
- Seminiferous tubule
- Tail Body of epididymis
- Tunica albuginea

C. Anterior View

- Thoracic duct
- Cisterna chyli
- Aorta
- Preaortic nodes
- Left testicular artery
- Right testicular artery
- Lumbar (caval/aortic) nodes
- Right common iliac artery
- Common iliac nodes
- External iliac nodes
- Superficial inguinal nodes
- Femoral artery
- Testis
- Scrotum

Lymphatic drainage of:
----▶ Scrotum
——▶ Testis

2.16   Blood supply and lymphatic drainage of testis

A. Blood supply. **B.** Internal structure. **C.** Lymphatic drainage. Because the testes descend from the posterior abdominal wall into the scrotum during fetal development, their lymphatic drainage differs from that of the scrotum, which is an outpouching of the abdominal skin. Consequently, cancer of the testis metastasizes initially to the lumbar lymph nodes and cancer of the scrotum metastasizes initially to the superficial inguinal lymph nodes.

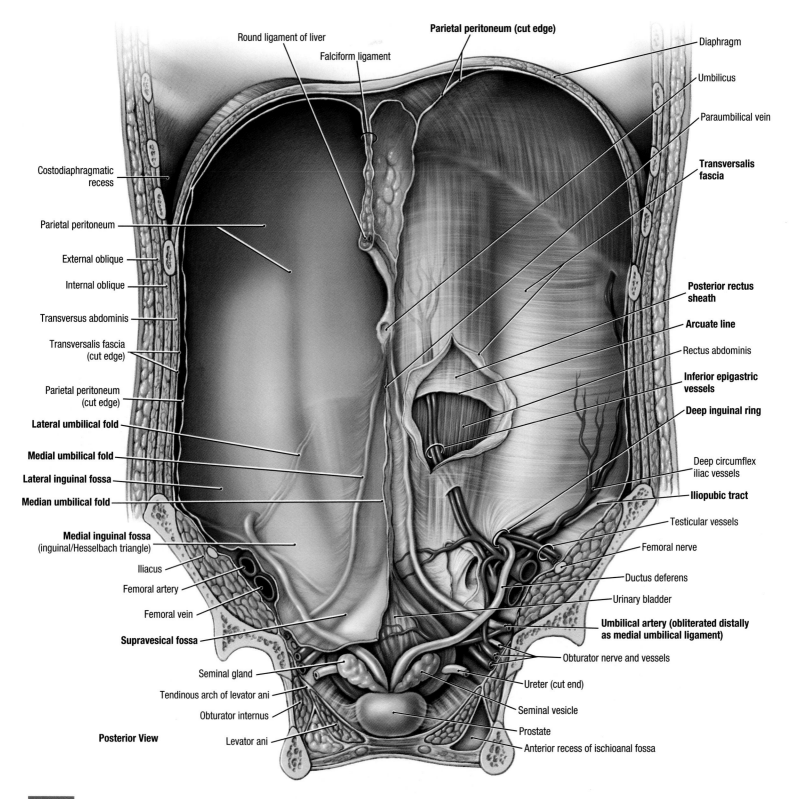

Round ligament of liver
Falciform ligament
Parietal peritoneum (cut edge)
Diaphragm
Umbilicus
Paraumbilical vein
Transversalis fascia
Costodiaphragmatic recess
Parietal peritoneum
External oblique
Internal oblique
Transversus abdominis
Transversalis fascia (cut edge)
Parietal peritoneum (cut edge)
Lateral umbilical fold
Medial umbilical fold
Lateral inguinal fossa
Median umbilical fold
Medial inguinal fossa (inguinal/Hesselbach triangle)
Iliacus
Femoral artery
Femoral vein
Supravesical fossa
Seminal gland
Tendinous arch of levator ani
Obturator internus
Posterior View   Levator ani
Posterior rectus sheath
Arcuate line
Rectus abdominis
Inferior epigastric vessels
Deep inguinal ring
Deep circumflex iliac vessels
Iliopubic tract
Testicular vessels
Femoral nerve
Ductus deferens
Urinary bladder
Umbilical artery (obliterated distally as medial umbilical ligament)
Obturator nerve and vessels
Ureter (cut end)
Seminal vesicle
Prostate
Anterior recess of ischioanal fossa

2.17   **Posterior aspect of the anterolateral abdominal wall**

Umbilical folds (median, medial, and lateral) are reflections of the parietal peritoneum that are raised from the body wall by underlying structures. The median umbilical fold extends from the urinary bladder to the umbilicus and covers the median umbilical ligament (the remnant of the urachus). The two medial umbilical folds cover the medial umbilical ligaments (occluded remnants of the fetal umbilical arteries). Two lateral umbilical folds cover the inferior epigastric vessels. The supravesical fossae are between the median and medial umbilical folds, the medial inguinal fossae (inguinal triangles) are between the medial and lateral umbilical folds, and the lateral inguinal fossae and deep inguinal rings are lateral to the lateral umbilical folds.

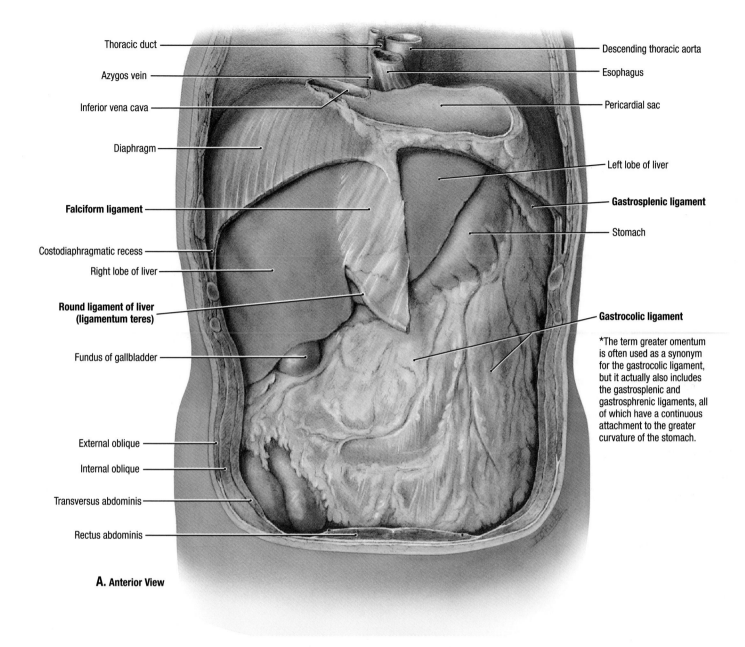

Thoracic duct

Azygos vein

Inferior vena cava

Diaphragm

Falciform ligament

Costodiaphragmatic recess

Right lobe of liver

Round ligament of liver (ligamentum teres)

Fundus of gallbladder

External oblique

Internal oblique

Transversus abdominis

Rectus abdominis

Descending thoracic aorta

Esophagus

Pericardial sac

Left lobe of liver

Gastrosplenic ligament

Stomach

Gastrocolic ligament

*The term greater omentum is often used as a synonym for the gastrocolic ligament, but it actually also includes the gastrosplenic and gastrophrenic ligaments, all of which have a continuous attachment to the greater curvature of the stomach.

A. Anterior View

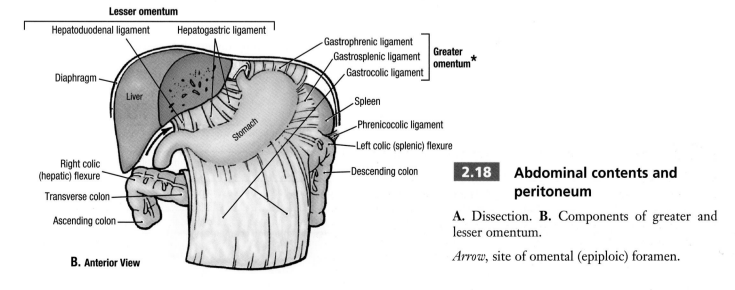

Lesser omentum

Hepatoduodenal ligament   Hepatogastric ligament

Diaphragm

Liver

Right colic (hepatic) flexure

Transverse colon

Ascending colon

Stomach

Gastrophrenic ligament

Gastrosplenic ligament

Gastrocolic ligament

} **Greater omentum** *

Spleen

Phrenicocolic ligament

Left colic (splenic) flexure

Descending colon

B. Anterior View

2.18   **Abdominal contents and peritoneum**

A. Dissection. **B.** Components of greater and lesser omentum.

Arrow, site of omental (epiploic) foramen.

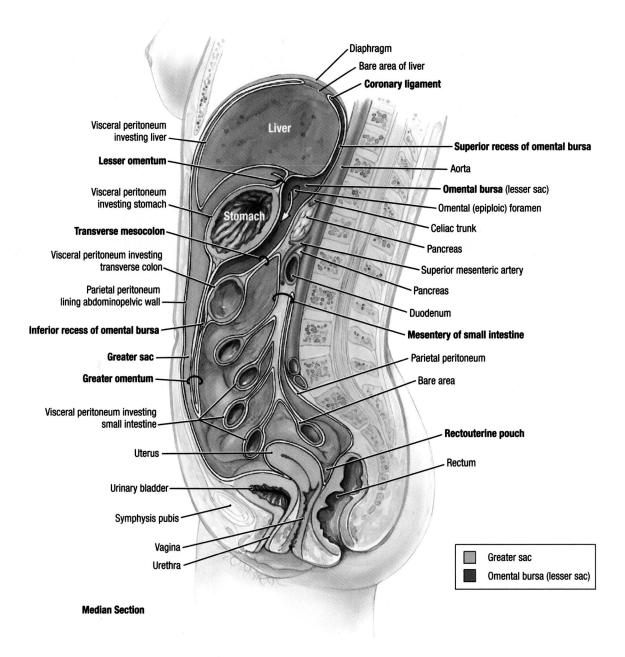

Diaphragm
Bare area of liver
Coronary ligament
Visceral peritoneum investing liver
Liver
Superior recess of omental bursa
Aorta
Lesser omentum
Omental bursa (lesser sac)
Visceral peritoneum investing stomach
Omental (epiploic) foramen
Stomach
Celiac trunk
Transverse mesocolon
Pancreas
Visceral peritoneum investing transverse colon
Superior mesenteric artery
Pancreas
Parietal peritoneum lining abdominopelvic wall
Duodenum
Mesentery of small intestine
Inferior recess of omental bursa
Parietal peritoneum
Greater sac
Bare area
Greater omentum
Visceral peritoneum investing small intestine
Rectouterine pouch
Uterus
Rectum
Urinary bladder
Symphysis pubis
Vagina
Urethra

Greater sac
Omental bursa (lesser sac)

Median Section

2.19   Peritoneal formations and bare areas

Various terms are used to describe the parts of the peritoneum that connect organs with other organs or to the abdominal wall, and to describe the compartments and recesses that are formed as a consequence. The *arrow* passes through the omental (epiploic) foramen.

Term	Definition
Peritoneal ligament	Double layer of peritoneum that connects an organ with another organ or to the abdominal wall.
Mesentery	Double layer of peritoneum that occurs as a result of the invagination of the peritoneum by an organ and constitutes a continuity of the visceral and parietal peritoneum.
Omentum	Double-layered extension of peritoneum passing from the stomach and proximal part of the duodenum to adjacent organs. The greater omentum extends from the greater curvature of the stomach and the proximal duodenum; the lesser omentum from the lesser curvature.
Bare area	Every organ must have an area, the bare area, that is not covered with visceral peritoneum, to allow the entrance and exit of neurovascular structures. Bare areas are formed in relation to the attachments of mesenteries, omenta, and ligaments.

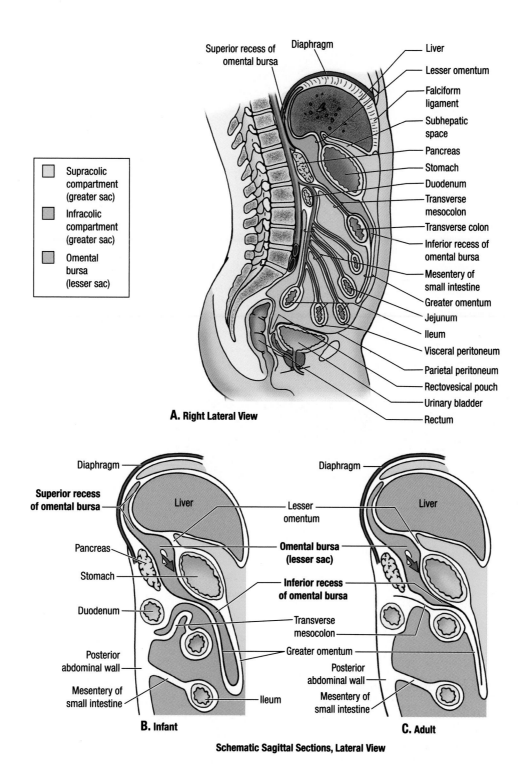

Superior recess of omental bursa

Diaphragm

Liver

Lesser omentum

Falciform ligament

Subhepatic space

Pancreas

Stomach

Duodenum

Transverse mesocolon

Transverse colon

Inferior recess of omental bursa

Mesentery of small intestine

Greater omentum

Jejunum

Ileum

Visceral peritoneum

Parietal peritoneum

Rectovesical pouch

Urinary bladder

Rectum

A. Right Lateral View

Supracolic compartment (greater sac)

Infracolic compartment (greater sac)

Omental bursa (lesser sac)

Diaphragm

Superior recess of omental bursa

Liver

Lesser omentum

Pancreas

Stomach

Duodenum

Posterior abdominal wall

Mesentery of small intestine

Ileum

B. Infant

Diaphragm

Liver

Omental bursa (lesser sac)

Inferior recess of omental bursa

Transverse mesocolon

Greater omentum

Posterior abdominal wall

Mesentery of small intestine

C. Adult

Schematic Sagittal Sections, Lateral View

2.20   Subdivisions of peritoneal cavity

A. Sagittal section. **B.** In an infant, the omental bursa (lesser sac) is an isolated part of the peritoneal cavity, lying dorsal to the stomach and extending superiorly to the liver and diaphragm (superior recess of the omental bursa) and inferiorly between the layers of the greater omentum (inferior recess of the omental bursa). **C.** In an adult, after fusion of the layers of the greater omentum, the inferior recess of the omental bursa now extends inferiorly only as far as the transverse colon. The *red arrows* pass from the greater sac through the omental (epiploic) foramen into the omental bursa.

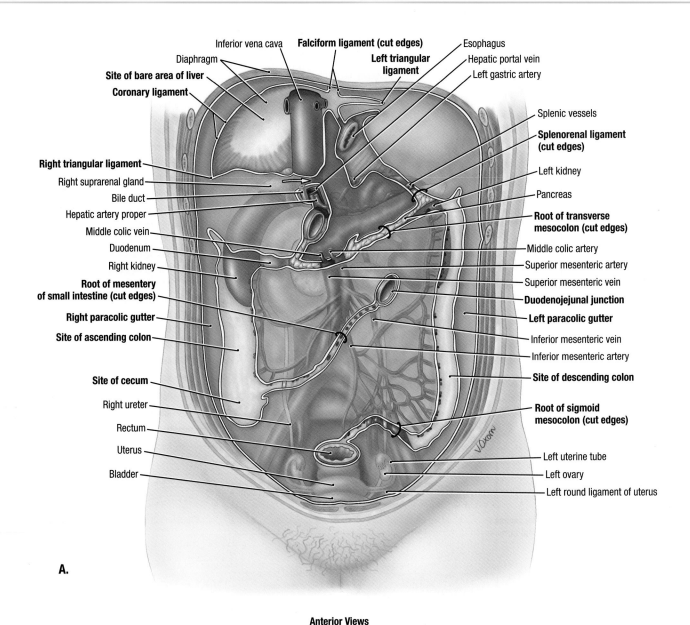

Inferior vena cava
Diaphragm
Site of bare area of liver
Coronary ligament
Right triangular ligament
Right suprarenal gland
Bile duct
Hepatic artery proper
Middle colic vein
Duodenum
Right kidney
**Root of mesentery
of small intestine (cut edges)**
Right paracolic gutter
Site of ascending colon
Site of cecum
Right ureter
Rectum
Uterus
Bladder

Falciform ligament (cut edges)
**Left triangular
ligament**
Esophagus
Hepatic portal vein
Left gastric artery
Splenic vessels
**Splenorenal ligament
(cut edges)**
Left kidney
Pancreas
**Root of transverse
mesocolon (cut edges)**
Middle colic artery
Superior mesenteric artery
Superior mesenteric vein
Duodenojejunal junction
Left paracolic gutter
Inferior mesenteric vein
Inferior mesenteric artery
Site of descending colon
**Root of sigmoid
mesocolon (cut edges)**
Left uterine tube
Left ovary
Left round ligament of uterus

A.

Anterior Views

2.21 Posterior wall of peritoneal cavity

A. Roots of the peritoneal reflections. The peritoneal reflections from the posterior abdominal wall (mesenteries and reflections surrounding bare areas of liver and secondarily retroperitoneal organs) have been cut at their roots, and the intraperitoneal and secondarily retroperitoneal viscera have been removed. The *white arrow* passes through the omental (epiploic) foramen. **B.** Supracolic and infracolic compartments of the greater sac. The infracolic spaces and paracolic gutters are of clinical importance because they determine the paths (*black arrows*) for the flow of ascetic fluid with changes in position, and the spread of intraperitoneal reflections.

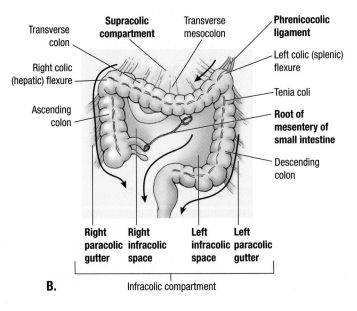

Transverse colon
Supracolic compartment
Right colic (hepatic) flexure
Ascending colon
Transverse mesocolon
Phrenicocolic ligament
Left colic (splenic) flexure
Tenia coli
Root of mesentery of small intestine
Descending colon

Right paracolic gutter **Right infracolic space** **Left infracolic space** **Left paracolic gutter**

Infracolic compartment

B.

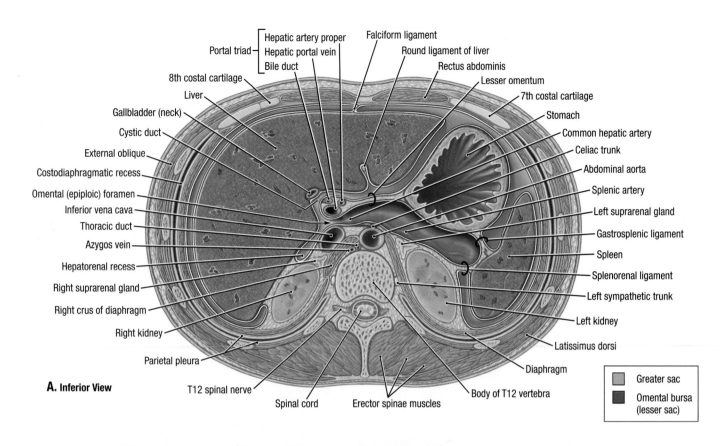

Portal triad— { Hepatic artery proper
Hepatic portal vein
Bile duct }

Falciform ligament

Round ligament of liver

8th costal cartilage

Rectus abdominis

Liver

Lesser omentum

Gallbladder (neck)

7th costal cartilage

Cystic duct

Stomach

External oblique

Common hepatic artery

Costodiaphragmatic recess

Celiac trunk

Omental (epiploic) foramen

Abdominal aorta

Inferior vena cava

Splenic artery

Thoracic duct

Left suprarenal gland

Azygos vein

Gastrosplenic ligament

Hepatorenal recess

Spleen

Right suprarenal gland

Splenorenal ligament

Right crus of diaphragm

Left sympathetic trunk

Right kidney

Left kidney

Parietal pleura

Latissimus dorsi

A. Inferior View

Diaphragm

T12 spinal nerve

Spinal cord   Erector spinae muscles

Body of T12 vertebra

| | Greater sac |
| | Omental bursa (lesser sac) |

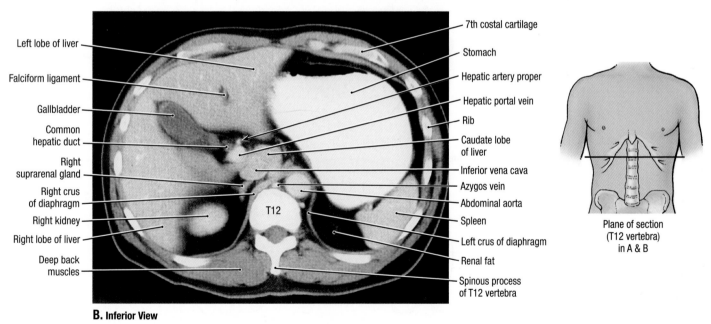

Left lobe of liver

7th costal cartilage

Falciform ligament

Stomach

Gallbladder

Hepatic artery proper

Common hepatic duct

Hepatic portal vein

Right suprarenal gland

Rib

Right crus of diaphragm

Caudate lobe of liver

Right kidney

Inferior vena cava

Right lobe of liver

Azygos vein

Deep back muscles

Abdominal aorta

Spleen

Left crus of diaphragm

Renal fat

Spinous process of T12 vertebra

T12

Plane of section (T12 vertebra) in A & B

B. Inferior View

2.22   **Transverse sections through greater sac and omental bursa.**

- When bacterial contamination occurs or when the gut is traumatically penetrated or ruptured as the result of infection and inflammation, gas, fecal matter, and bacteria enter the peritoneal cavity. The result is infection and inflammation of the peritoneum, called peritonitis.
- Under certain pathological conditions such as peritonitis, the peritoneal cavity may be distended with abnormal fluid (ascites). Widespread metastases (spread) of cancer cells to the abdominal viscera cause exudation (escape) of fluid that is often blood stained. Thus the peritoneal cavity may be distended with several liters of abnormal fluid. Surgical puncture of the peritoneal cavity for the aspiration of drainage of fluid is called paracentesis.

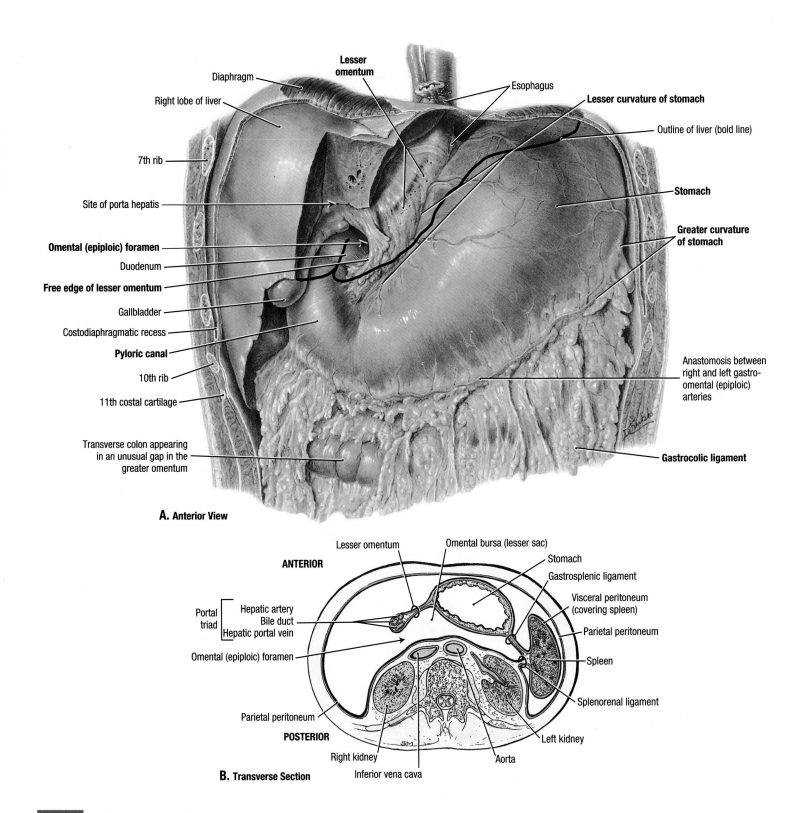

A. Anterior View

B. Transverse Section

2.23 **Stomach and omenta**

A. Lesser and greater omenta. The stomach is inflated with air, and the left part of the liver is cut away. The gallbladder, followed superiorly, leads to the free margin of the lesser omentum and serves as a guide to the omental epiploic foramen, which lies posterior to that free margin. **B.** Omental bursa (lesser sac), schematic transverse section.

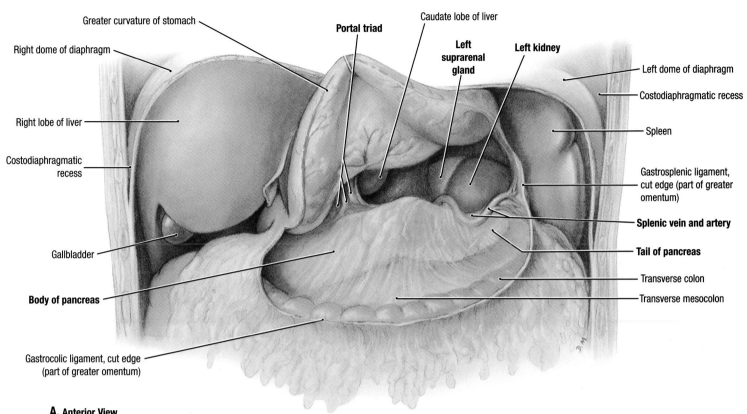

Greater curvature of stomach

Right dome of diaphragm

Right lobe of liver

Costodiaphragmatic recess

Gallbladder

Body of pancreas

Gastrocolic ligament, cut edge (part of greater omentum)

Portal triad

Caudate lobe of liver

Left suprarenal gland

Left kidney

Left dome of diaphragm

Costodiaphragmatic recess

Spleen

Gastrosplenic ligament, cut edge (part of greater omentum)

Splenic vein and artery

Tail of pancreas

Transverse colon

Transverse mesocolon

A. Anterior View

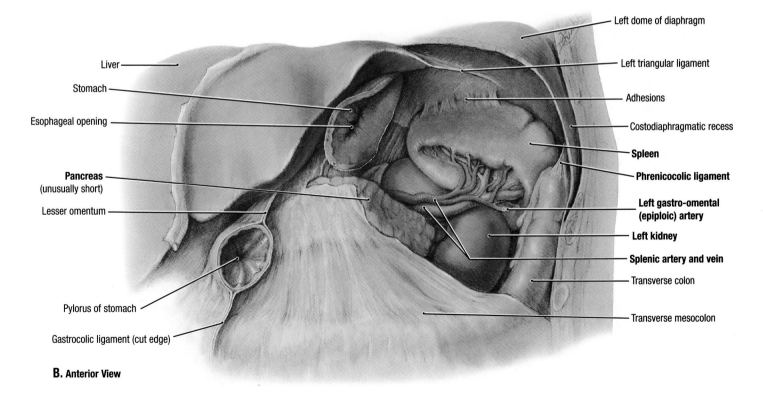

Liver

Stomach

Esophageal opening

Pancreas (unusually short)

Lesser omentum

Pylorus of stomach

Gastrocolic ligament (cut edge)

Left dome of diaphragm

Left triangular ligament

Adhesions

Costodiaphragmatic recess

Spleen

Phrenicocolic ligament

Left gastro-omental (epiploic) artery

Left kidney

Splenic artery and vein

Transverse colon

Transverse mesocolon

B. Anterior View

2.24   **Posterior relationships of omental bursa (lesser sac)**

A. Opened omental bursa. The greater omentum has been cut along the greater curvature of the stomach; the stomach is reflected superiorly. Peritoneum of the stomach bed is partially removed. **B.** Stomach bed. The stomach is excised. Peritoneum covering the stomach bed and inferior part of the kidney and pancreas is largely removed. Adhesions binding the spleen to the diaphragm are pathological, but not unusual.

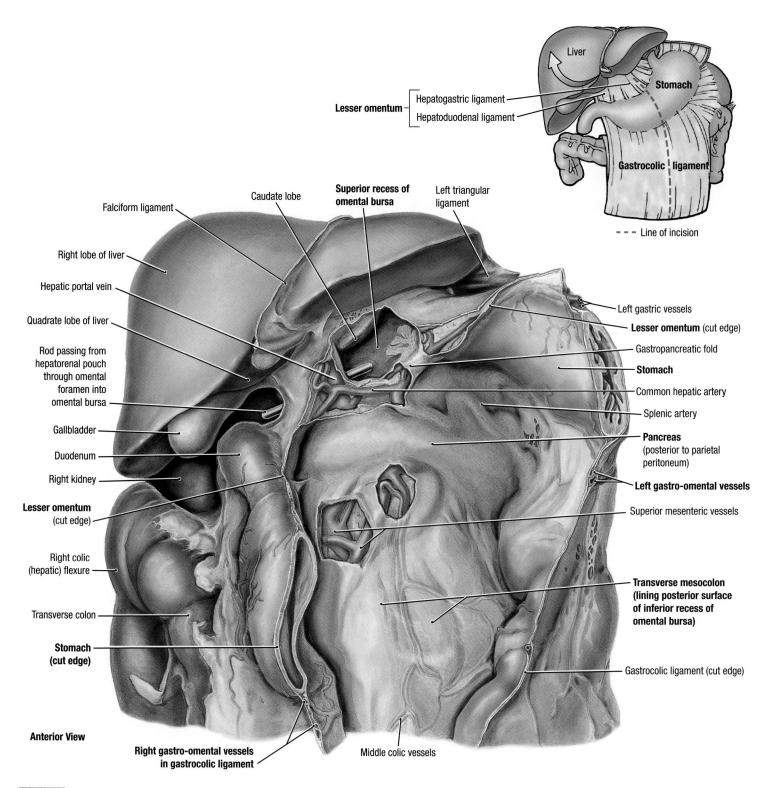

Anterior View

2.25 Omental bursa (lesser sac), opened

The anterior wall of the omental bursa, consisting of the stomach, lesser omentum, anterior layer of the greater omentum, and vessels along the curvatures of the stomach, has been sectioned sagittally. The two halves have been retracted to the left and right: the body of the stomach on the left side, and the pyloric part of the stomach and first part of the duodenum on the right. The right kidney forms the posterior wall of the hepatorenal pouch (part of

greater sac), and the pancreas lies horizontally on the posterior wall of the main compartment of the omental bursa (lesser sac). The gastrocolic ligament forms the anterior wall and the lower part of the posterior wall of the inferior recess of the omental bursa. The transverse mesocolon forms the upper part of the posterior wall of the inferior recess of the omental bursa.

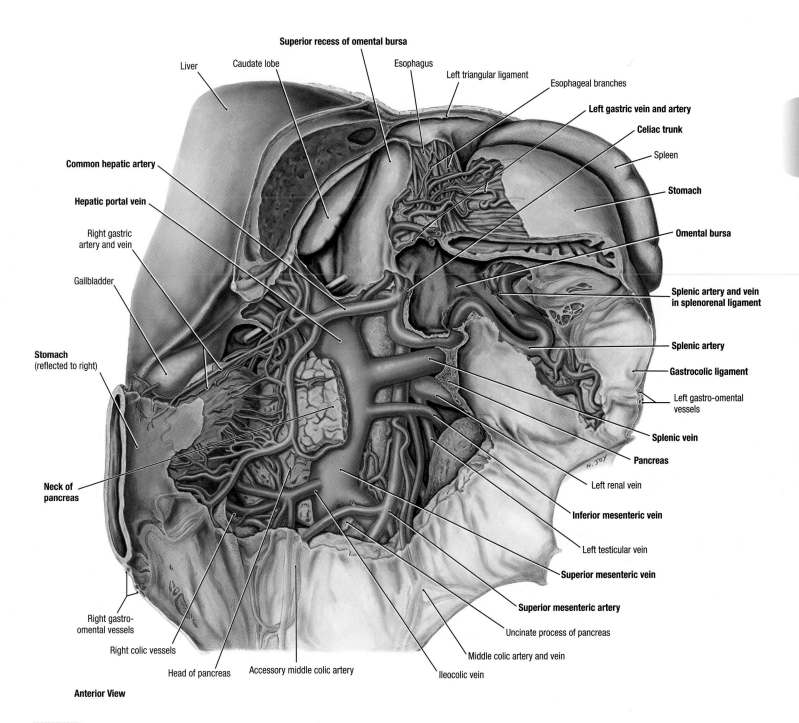

Superior recess of omental bursa

Liver   Caudate lobe   Esophagus

Left triangular ligament

Esophageal branches

Left gastric vein and artery

Celiac trunk

Spleen

Common hepatic artery

Stomach

Hepatic portal vein

Omental bursa

Right gastric
artery and vein

Gallbladder

**Splenic artery and vein
in splenorenal ligament**

Splenic artery

Gastrocolic ligament

Left gastro-omental
vessels

Stomach
(reflected to right)

Splenic vein

Pancreas

Left renal vein

**Neck of
pancreas**

Inferior mesenteric vein

Left testicular vein

Superior mesenteric vein

Right gastro-
omental vessels

Superior mesenteric artery

Right colic vessels

Uncinate process of pancreas

Head of pancreas   Accessory middle colic artery

Middle colic artery and vein

Ileocolic vein

Anterior View

2.26   Posterior wall of omental bursa

The parietal peritoneum of the posterior wall of the omental bursa has been mostly removed, and a section of the pancreas has been excised. The rod passes through the omental foramen.

- The celiac trunk gives rise to the left gastric artery, the splenic artery that runs tortuously to the left, and the common hepatic artery that runs to the right, passing anterior to the hepatic portal vein.

- The hepatic portal vein is formed posterior to the neck of the pancreas by the union of the superior mesenteric and splenic veins, with the inferior mesenteric vein joining at or near the angle of union.

- The left testicular vein usually drains into the left renal vein. Both are systemic veins.

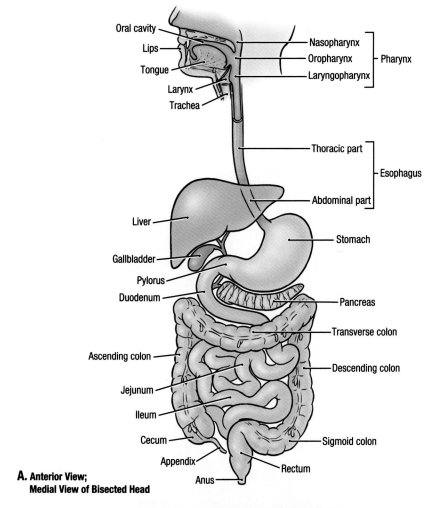

A. Anterior View;
Medial View of Bisected Head

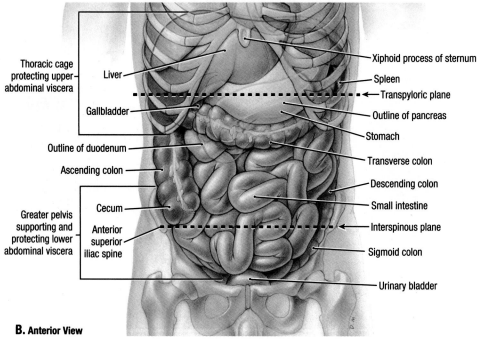

B. Anterior View

2.27 **Digestive system**

A. Schematic illustration. **B.** Abdominal portion. The digestive system extends from the lips to the anus. Associated organs include the liver, gallbladder, and pancreas.

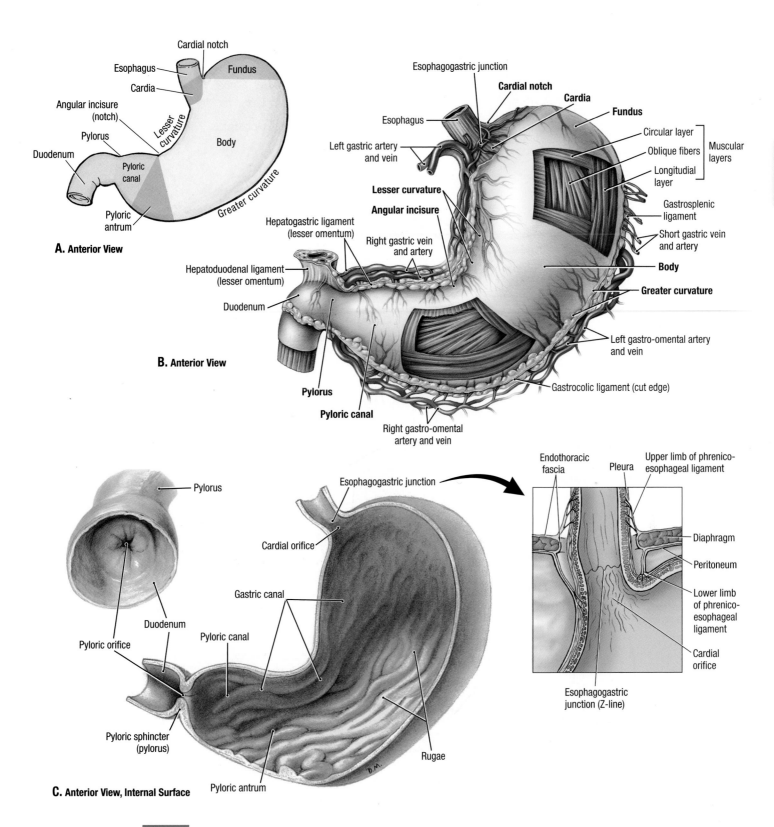

Cardial notch
Esophagus
Cardia
Fundus
Angular incisure (notch)
Pylorus
Duodenum
Pyloric canal
Lesser curvature
Body
Pyloric antrum
Greater curvature

A. Anterior View

Esophagogastric junction
Cardial notch
Cardia
Fundus
Esophagus
Circular layer
Oblique fibers — Muscular layers
Longitudial layer
Left gastric artery and vein
Lesser curvature
Angular incisure
Gastrosplenic ligament
Short gastric vein and artery
Hepatogastric ligament (lesser omentum)
Right gastric vein and artery
Body
Hepatoduodenal ligament (lesser omentum)
Duodenum
Greater curvature
Left gastro-omental artery and vein
Gastrocolic ligament (cut edge)
Pylorus
Pyloric canal
Right gastro-omental artery and vein

B. Anterior View

Pylorus
Esophagogastric junction
Endothoracic fascia
Pleura
Upper limb of phrenico-esophageal ligament
Cardial orifice
Diaphragm
Gastric canal
Peritoneum
Duodenum
Pyloric canal
Lower limb of phrenico-esophageal ligament
Pyloric orifice
Cardial orifice
Pyloric sphincter (pylorus)
Esophagogastric junction (Z-line)
Rugae
Pyloric antrum

C. Anterior View, Internal Surface

2.28 **Stomach**

A. Parts. **B.** External surface. **C.** Internal surface (mucous membrane), anterior wall removed. Insets: Left side of page—pylorus, viewed from the duodenum. Right side of page—details of the esophagogastric junction.

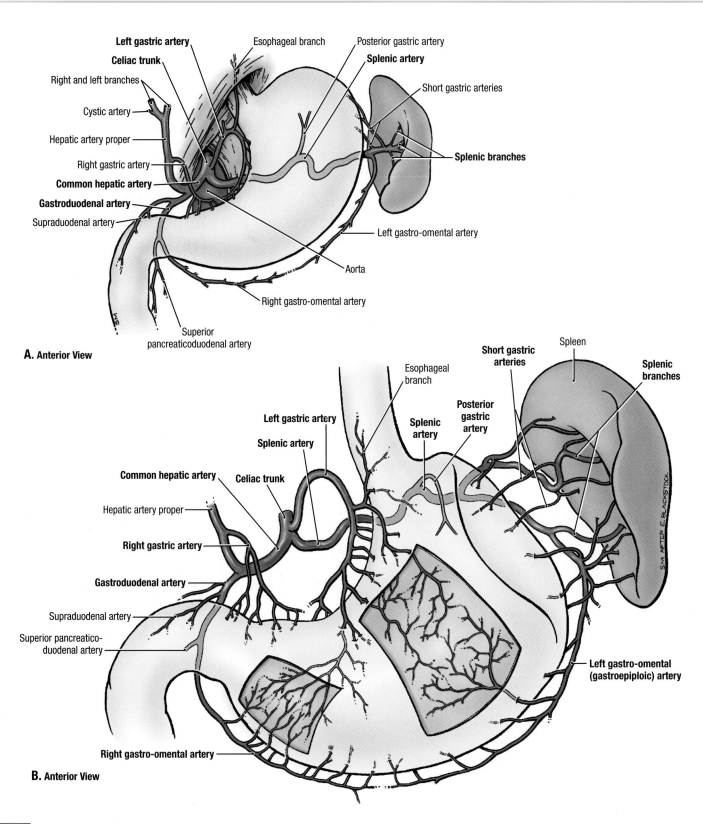

Left gastric artery
Celiac trunk
Right and left branches
Cystic artery
Hepatic artery proper
Right gastric artery
Common hepatic artery
Gastroduodenal artery
Supraduodenal artery

Esophageal branch
Posterior gastric artery
Splenic artery
Short gastric arteries
Splenic branches
Left gastro-omental artery
Aorta
Right gastro-omental artery
Superior pancreaticoduodenal artery

A. Anterior View

Esophageal branch
Short gastric arteries
Spleen
Splenic branches
Left gastric artery
Splenic artery
Posterior gastric artery
Common hepatic artery
Celiac trunk
Hepatic artery proper
Right gastric artery
Gastroduodenal artery
Supraduodenal artery
Superior pancreatico-duodenal artery
Left gastro-omental (gastroepiploic) artery
Right gastro-omental artery

B. Anterior View

2.29 Celiac artery

A. Branches of celiac trunk. The celiac trunk is a branch of the abdominal aorta, arising immediately inferior to the aortic hiatus of the diaphragm (T12 vertebral level). The vessel is usually 1 to 2 cm long and divides into the left gastric, common hepatic, and splenic arteries. The celiac trunk supplies the liver, gall bladder, inferior esophagus, stomach, pancreas, spleen, and duodenum. **B.** Arteries of stomach and spleen. The serous and muscular coats are removed from two areas of the stomach, revealing anastomotic networks in the submucous coat.

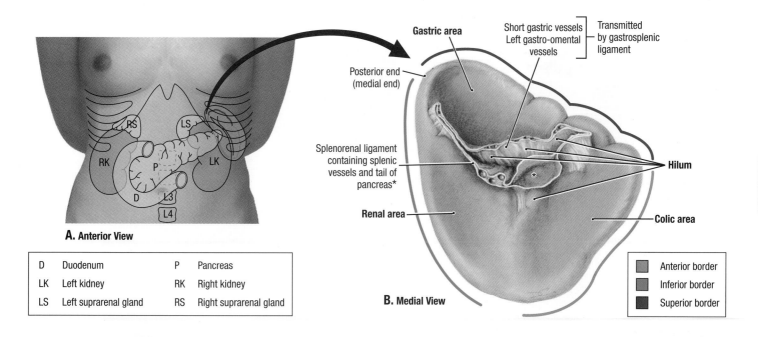

A. Anterior View

D	Duodenum	P	Pancreas
LK	Left kidney	RK	Right kidney
LS	Left suprarenal gland	RS	Right suprarenal gland

B. Medial View

- Anterior border
- Inferior border
- Superior border

2.30 **Spleen**

A. The surface anatomy of the spleen. The spleen lies superficially in the left upper abdominal quadrant between the 9th and 11th ribs. **B.** Note the impressions (colic, renal and gastric areas) made by structures in contact with its visceral surface. The superior border is notched.

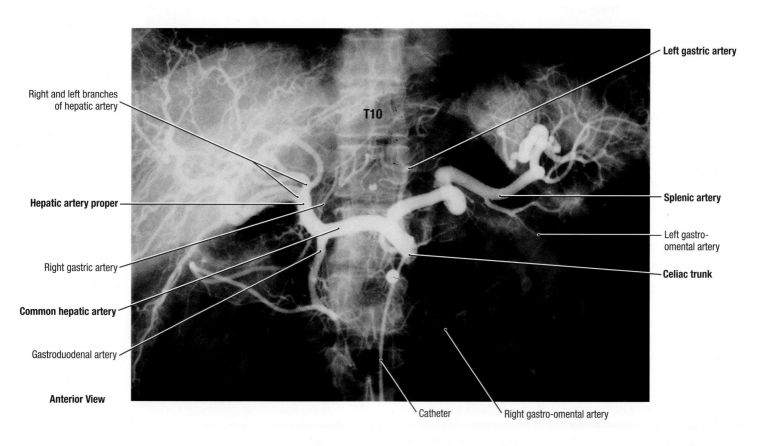

2.31 **Celiac arteriogram**

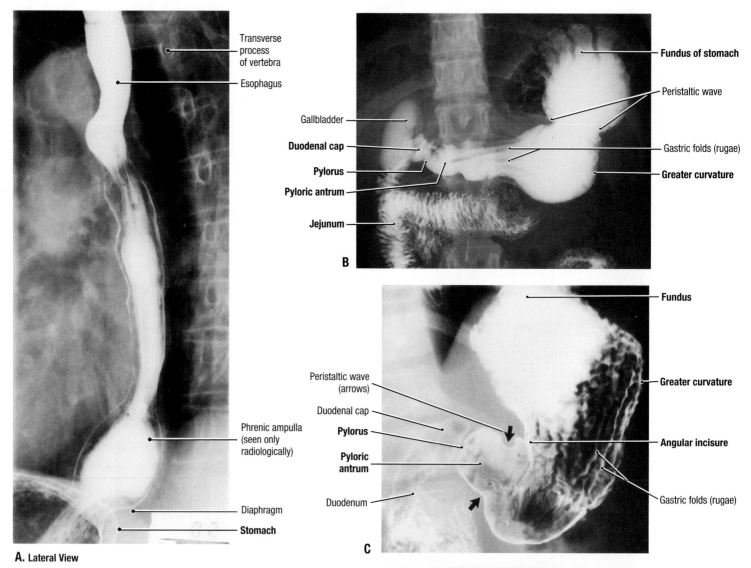

Transverse process of vertebra

Esophagus

Fundus of stomach

Peristaltic wave

Gallbladder

Duodenal cap

Gastric folds (rugae)

Pylorus

Greater curvature

Pyloric antrum

Jejunum

B

Phrenic ampulla (seen only radiologically)

Diaphragm

Stomach

A. Lateral View

Fundus

Peristaltic wave (arrows)

Duodenal cap

Pylorus

Greater curvature

Pyloric antrum

Angular incisure

Duodenum

Gastric folds (rugae)

C

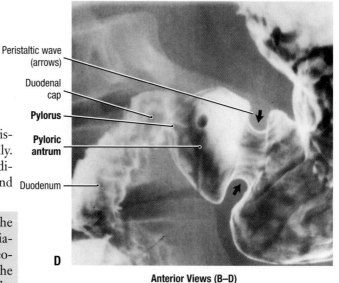

Peristaltic wave (arrows)

Duodenal cap

Pylorus

Pyloric antrum

Duodenum

D

Anterior Views (B–D)

2.32 **Radiographs of esophagus, stomach, duodenum (barium swallow)**

A. Esophagus. The esophageal (phrenic) ampulla is the distensible portion of the esophagus seen only radiologically. **B.** Stomach, small intestine, and gallbladder. Note additional contrast medium in gallbladder. **C.** Stomach and duodenum. **D.** Pyloric antrum and duodenal cap.

A hiatal—or hiatus—hernia is a protrusion of a part of the stomach into the mediastinum through the esophageal hiatus of the diaphragm. The hernias occur most often in people after middle age, possibly because of weakening of the muscular part of the diaphragm and widening of the esophageal hiatus.

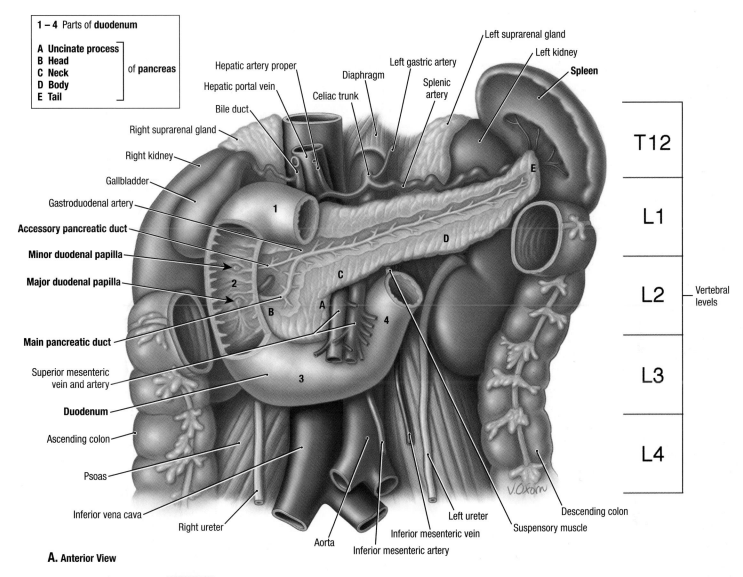

1 – 4 Parts of **duodenum**

A **Uncinate process**
B **Head**
C **Neck**   of **pancreas**
D **Body**
E **Tail**

2.33 **Parts and relationships of pancreas and duodenum**

A. Pancreas and duodenum in situ.

TABLE 2.3 PARTS AND RELATIONSHIPS OF DUODENUM

Part of Duodenum	Anterior	Posterior	Medial	Superior	Inferior	Vertebral Level
Superior (**1**st part)	Peritoneum Gallbladder Quadrate lobe of liver	Bile duct Gastroduodenal artery Hepatic portal vein Inferior vena cava		Neck of gallbladder	Neck of pancreas	Anterolateral to L1 vertebra
Descending (**2**nd part)	Transverse colon Transverse mesocolon Coils of small intestine	Hilum of right kidney Renal vessels Ureter Psoas major	Head of pancreas Pancreatic duct Bile duct			Right of L2–L3 vertebrae
Inferior (horizontal or **3**rd part)	Superior mesenteric artery Superior mesenteric vein Coils of small intestine	Right psoas major Inferior vena cava Aorta Right ureter		Head and uncinate process of pancreas Superior mesenteric artery and vein		Anterior to L3 vertebra
Ascending (**4**th part)	Beginning of root of mesentery Coils of jejunum	Left psoas major Left margin of aorta	Superior mesenteric artery and vein	Body of pancreas		Left of L3 vertebra

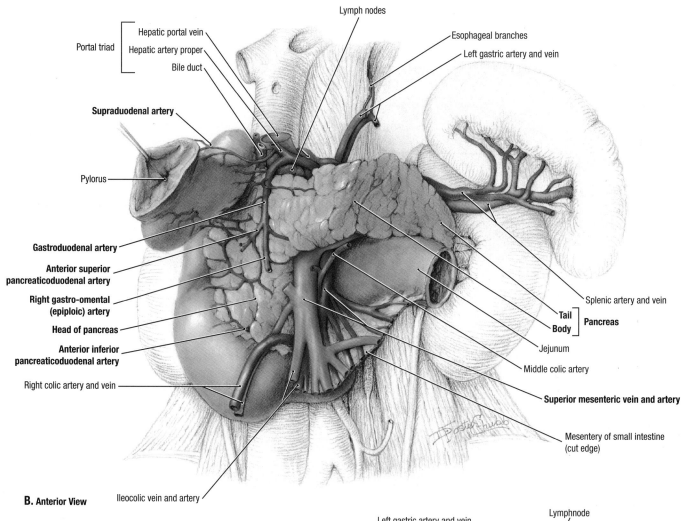

B. Anterior View

2.33 **Parts and relationships of the duodenum and pancreas (continued)**

B. Anterior relationships. The gastroduodenal artery descends anterior to the neck of the pancreas. **C. Posterior relationships.** The splenic artery and vein course on the posterior aspect of the pancreatic tail, which usually extends to the spleen. The pancreas "loops" around the right side of the superior mesenteric vessels so that its neck is anterior, its head is to the right, and its uncinate process is posterior to the vessels. The splenic and superior mesenteric veins unite posterior to the neck to form the hepatic portal vein. The bile duct descends in a fissure (opened up) in the posterior part of the head of the pancreas. Most inflammatory erosions of the duodenal wall, duodenal (peptic) ulcers, are in the posterior wall of the superior (1st) part of the duodenum within 3 cm of the pylorus.

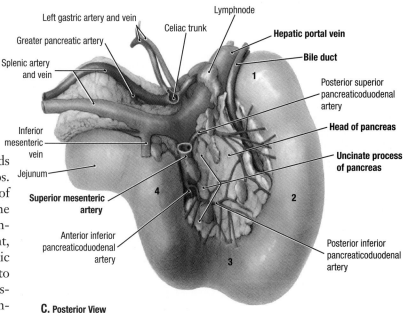

C. Posterior View

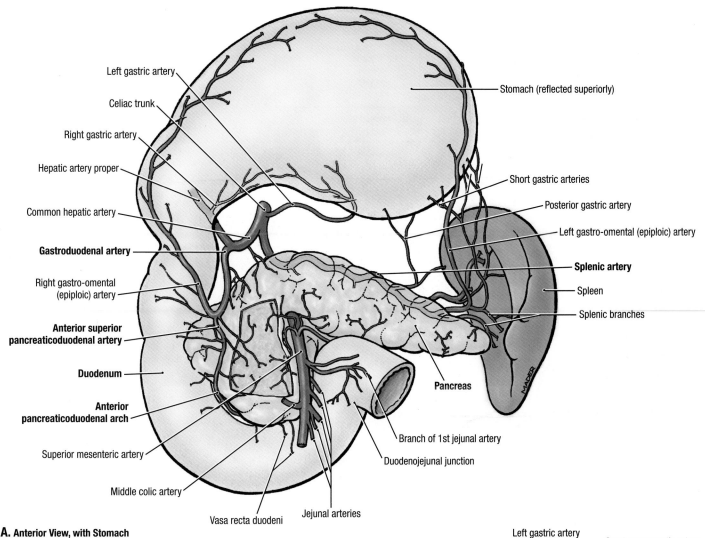

Left gastric artery

Celiac trunk

Right gastric artery

Hepatic artery proper

Common hepatic artery

Gastroduodenal artery

Right gastro-omental
(epiploic) artery

**Anterior superior
pancreaticoduodenal artery**

Duodenum

**Anterior
pancreaticoduodenal arch**

Superior mesenteric artery

Middle colic artery

Vasa recta duodeni

Jejunal arteries

Stomach (reflected superiorly)

Short gastric arteries

Posterior gastric artery

Left gastro-omental (epiploic) artery

Splenic artery

Spleen

Splenic branches

Pancreas

Branch of 1st jejunal artery

Duodenojejunal junction

**A. Anterior View, with Stomach
Reflected Superiorly**

**2.34   Blood supply to the pancreas,
duodenum, and spleen**

A. Celiac trunk and superior mesenteric artery. **B.** Pancreatic
and pancreaticoduodenal arteries.

- The anterior superior pancreaticoduodenal artery from
  the gastroduodenal artery and the anterior inferior pancreaticoduodenal artery of the superior mesenteric artery
  form the anterior pancreaticoduodenal arch anterior to
  the head of the pancreas. The posterior superior and posterior inferior branches of the same two arteries form the
  posterior pancreaticoduodenal arch posterior to the pancreas. The anterior and posterior inferior arteries often
  arise from a common stem.
- Arteries supplying the pancreas are derived from the
  common hepatic artery, gastroduodenal artery, pancreaticoduodenal arches, splenic artery, and superior mesenteric artery.

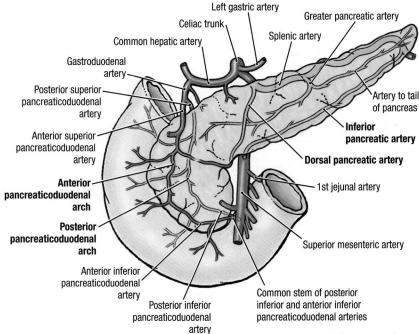

Left gastric artery

Celiac trunk

Common hepatic artery

Gastroduodenal
artery

Posterior superior
pancreaticoduodenal
artery

Anterior superior
pancreaticoduodenal
artery

**Anterior
pancreaticoduodenal
arch**

**Posterior
pancreaticoduodenal
arch**

Anterior inferior
pancreaticoduodenal
artery

Posterior inferior
pancreaticoduodenal
artery

Splenic artery

Greater pancreatic artery

Artery to tail
of pancreas

**Inferior
pancreatic artery**

Dorsal pancreatic artery

1st jejunal artery

Superior mesenteric artery

Common stem of posterior
inferior and anterior inferior
pancreaticoduodenal arteries

B. Anterior View

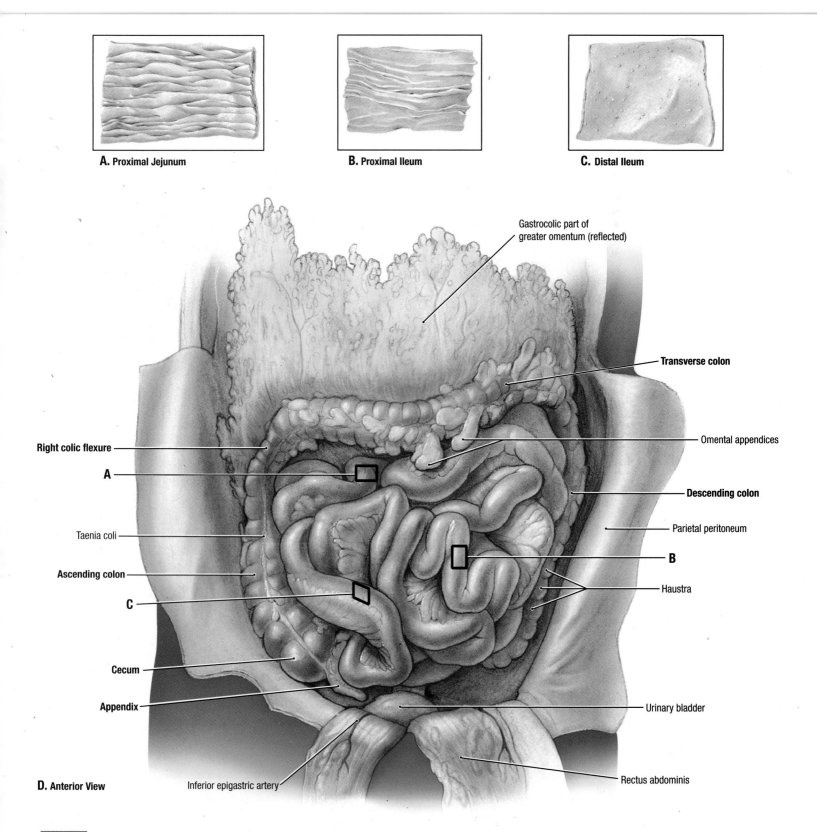

A. Proximal Jejunum

B. Proximal Ileum

C. Distal Ileum

Gastrocolic part of
greater omentum (reflected)

Transverse colon

Right colic flexure

A

Omental appendices

Descending colon

Parietal peritoneum

Taenia coli

B

Ascending colon

Haustra

C

Cecum

Appendix

Urinary bladder

Rectus abdominis

D. Anterior View　　Inferior epigastric artery

2.35　　**Intestines in situ, interior of small intestine**

A. Proximal jejunum. The circular folds are tall, closely packed, and commonly branched. **B.** Proximal ileum. The circular folds are low and becoming sparse. The caliber of the gut is reduced, and the wall is thinner. **C.** Distal ileum. Circular folds are absent, and solitary lymph nodules stud the wall. **D.** Intestines in situ, greater omentum reflected. The ileum is reflected to expose the appendix. The appendix usually lies posterior to the cecum (retrocecal) or, as in this case, projects over the pelvic brim. The features of the large intestines are the taeniae coli; haustra; and omental appendices.

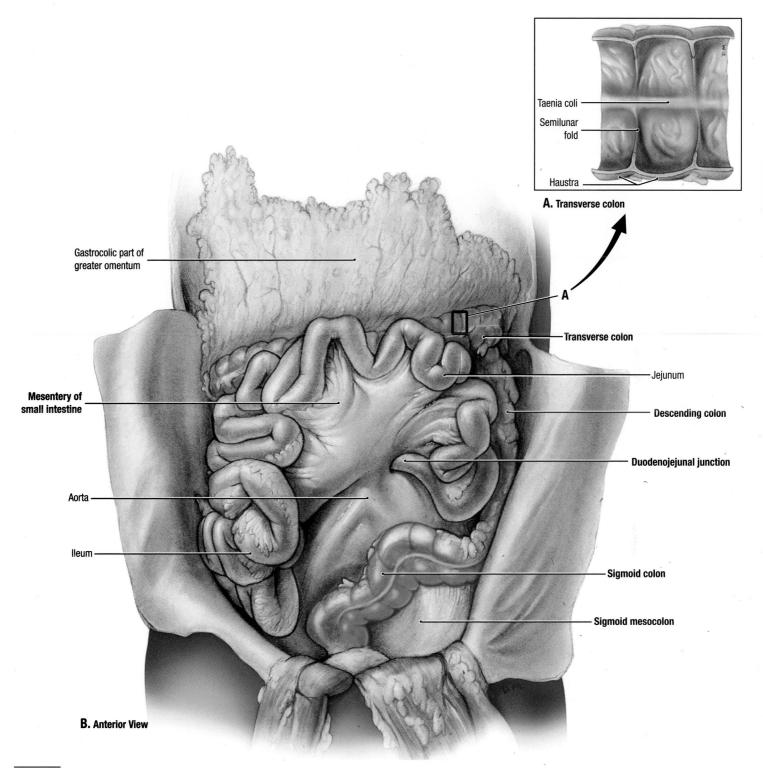

Taenia coli

Semilunar fold

Haustra

A. Transverse colon

A

Gastrocolic part of greater omentum

A

Transverse colon

Jejunum

Mesentery of small intestine

Descending colon

Duodenojejunal junction

Aorta

Ileum

Sigmoid colon

Sigmoid mesocolon

B. Anterior View

2.36 Sigmoid mesocolon and mesentry of small intestine, interior of transverse colon

A. Transverse colon. The semilunar folds and taeniae coli form prominent features on the smooth-surfaced wall. **B.** Sigmoid mesocolon and mesentry of the small intestine.

- The duodenojejunal junction is situated to the left of the median plane.
- The mesentery of the small intestine fans out extensively from its short root to accommodate the length of jejunum and ileum (approximately 6m).

- The descending colon is the narrowest part of the large intestine and is retroperitoneal. The sigmoid colon has a mesentery, the sigmoid mesocolon; the sigmoid colon is continuous with the rectum at the point at which the sigmoid mesocolon ends.

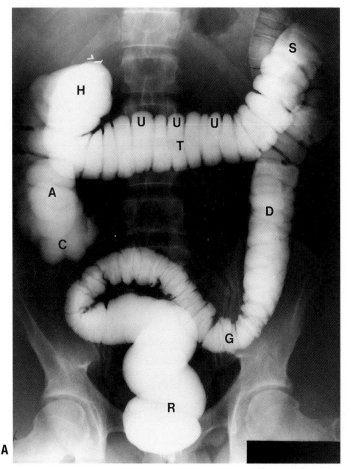

A

Posteroanterior Radiographs

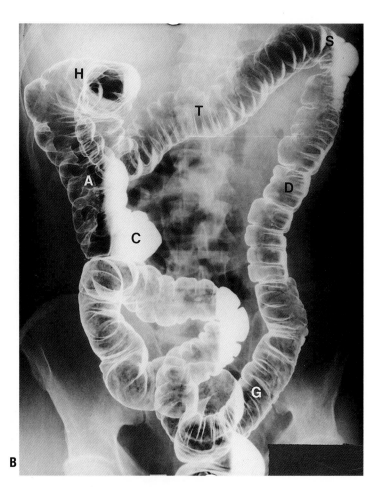

B

A	Ascending colon	G	Sigmoid colon	S	Splenic flexure
C	Cecum	H	Hepatic flexure	T	Transverse colon
D	Descending colon	R	Rectum	U	Haustra

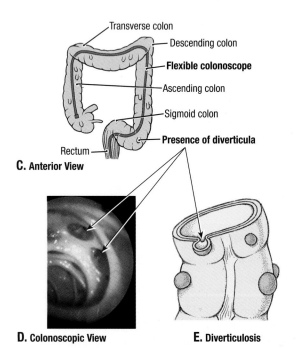

C. Anterior View

D. Colonoscopic View

E. Diverticulosis

(labels in figure C:) Transverse colon · Descending colon · **Flexible colonoscope** · Ascending colon · Sigmoid colon · **Presence of diverticula** · Rectum

2.37   Barium enema and colonoscopy of colon

A. Single-contrast study. A barium enema has filled the colon. **B.** Double-contrast study. Barium can be seen coating the walls of the colon, which is distended with air, providing a vivid view of the mucosal relief and haustra. **C.** The interior of the colon can be observed with an elongated endoscope, usually a fiberoptic flexible colonoscope. The endoscope is a tube that inserts into the colon through the anus and rectum. **D.** Diverticulosis of the colon can be photographed through a colonoscope.

E. Diverticulosis is a disorder in which multiple false diverticula (external evaginations or out-pocketings of the mucosa of the colon) develop along the intestine. It primarily affects middle-aged and elderly people. Diverticulosis is commonly (60%) found in the sigmoid colon. Diverticula are subject to infection and rupture, leading to diverticulitis, and they can distort and erode the nutrient arteries, leading to hemorrhage.

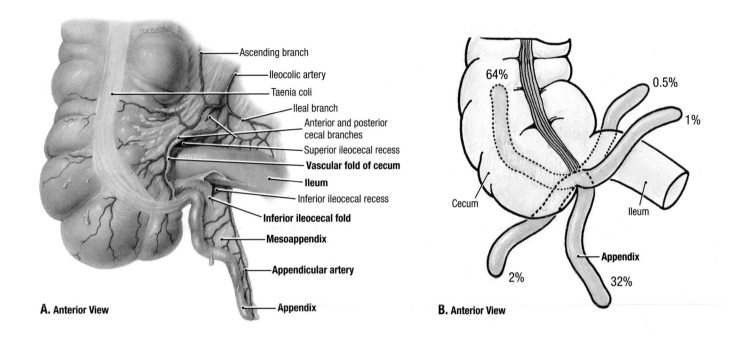

A. Anterior View

- Ascending branch
- Ileocolic artery
- Taenia coli
- Ileal branch
- Anterior and posterior cecal branches
- Superior ileocecal recess
- **Vascular fold of cecum**
- **Ileum**
- Inferior ileocecal recess
- **Inferior ileocecal fold**
- **Mesoappendix**
- **Appendicular artery**
- **Appendix**

B. Anterior View

- 64%
- 0.5%
- 1%
- Cecum
- Ileum
- Appendix
- 2%
- 32%

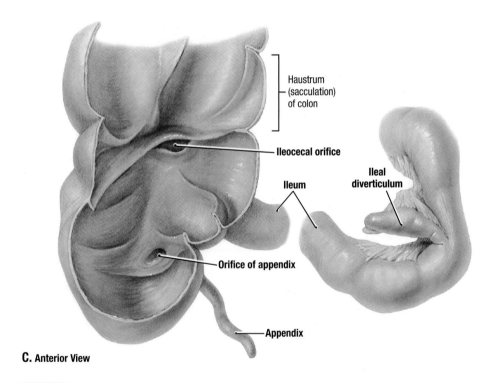

C. Anterior View

- Haustrum (sacculation) of colon
- **Ileocecal orifice**
- **Ileum**
- **Ileal diverticulum**
- **Orifice of appendix**
- **Appendix**

2.38   Ileocecal region and appendix

A. Blood supply. The appendicular artery is located in the free edge of the mesoappendix. The inferior ileocecal fold is bloodless, whereas the superior ileocecal fold is called the vascular fold of the cecum. **B.** The approximate incidence of various locations of the appendix. **C.** Interior of a dried cecum and ileal diverticulum (of Meckel). This cecum was filled with air until dry, opened, and varnished. Ileal diverticulum is a congenital anomaly that occurs in 1 to 2% of persons. It is a pouchlike remnant (3–6 cm long) of the proximal part of the yolk stalk, typically within 50 cm of the ileocecal junction. It sometimes becomes inflamed and produces pain that may mimic that produced by appendicitis.

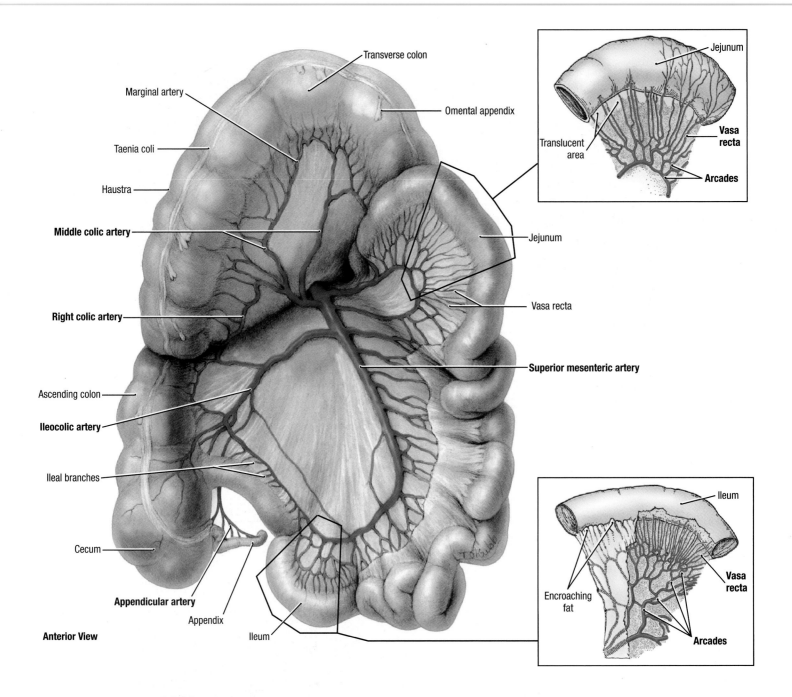

2.39   **Superior mesenteric artery and arterial arcades**

The peritoneum is partially stripped off.
- The superior mesenteric artery ends by anastomosing with one of its own branches, the ileal branch of the ileocolic artery.
- On the inset drawings of jejunum and ileum compare the diameter, thickness of wall, number of arterial arcades, long or short vasa recta, presence of translucent (fat free) areas at the mesenteric border, and fat encroaching on the wall of the gut between the jejunum and ileum.

- Acute inflammation of the appendix is a common cause of an acute abdomen (severe abdominal pain arising suddenly). The pain of appendicitis usually commences as a vague pain in the periumbilical region because afferent pain fibers enter the spinal cord at the T10 level. Later, severe pain in the right lower quadrant results from irritation of the parietal peritoneum lining the posterior abdominal wall.

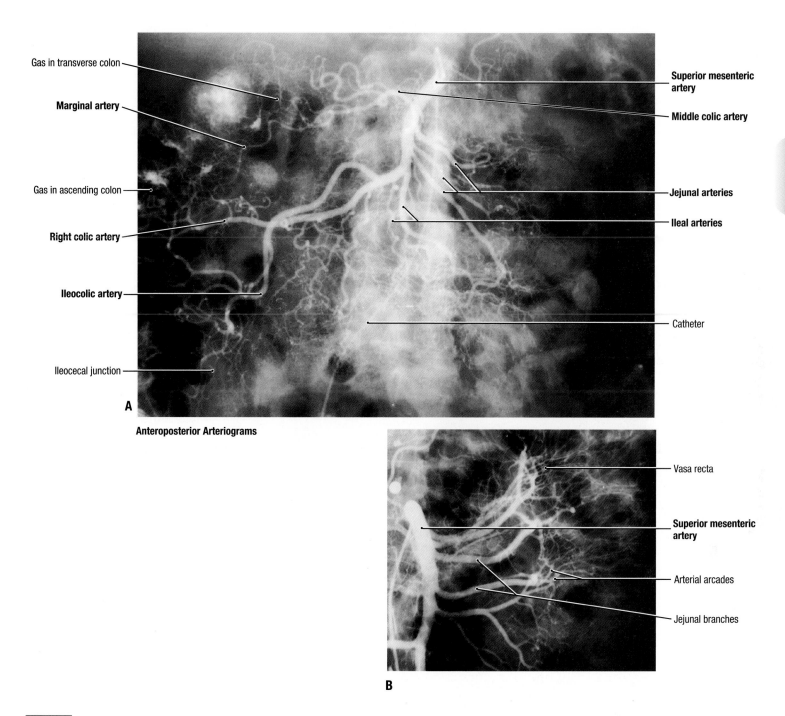

Gas in transverse colon

Marginal artery

Gas in ascending colon

Right colic artery

Ileocolic artery

Ileocecal junction

A

Superior mesenteric artery

Middle colic artery

Jejunal arteries

Ileal arteries

Catheter

Anteroposterior Arteriograms

Vasa recta

Superior mesenteric artery

Arterial arcades

Jejunal branches

B

| 2.40 | **Superior mesenteric arteriograms** |

A. Branches of superior mesenteric artery. Consult Figure 2.39 to identify the branches. **B.** Enlargement to show the jejunal branches, arterial arcades, and vasa recta.

• The branches of the superior mesenteric artery include, from its left side, 12 or more jejunal and ileal branches that anastomose to form arcades from which vasa recta pass to the small intestine and, from its right side, the middle colic, ileocolic, and commonly (but not here) an independent right colic artery that anastomose to form a marginal artery that parallels the mesenteric border at the colon and from which vasa recta pass to the large intestine. Occlusion of the vasa recta by emboli results in ischemia of the part of the intestine concerned. If the ischemia is severe, necrosis of the involved segment results and ileus (obstruction of the intestine) of the paralytic type occurs. Ileus is accompanied by a severe colicky pain, along with abdominal distension, vomiting, and often fever and dehydration. If the condition is diagnosed early (e.g., using a superior mesenteric arteriogram), the obstructed part of the vessel may be cleared surgically

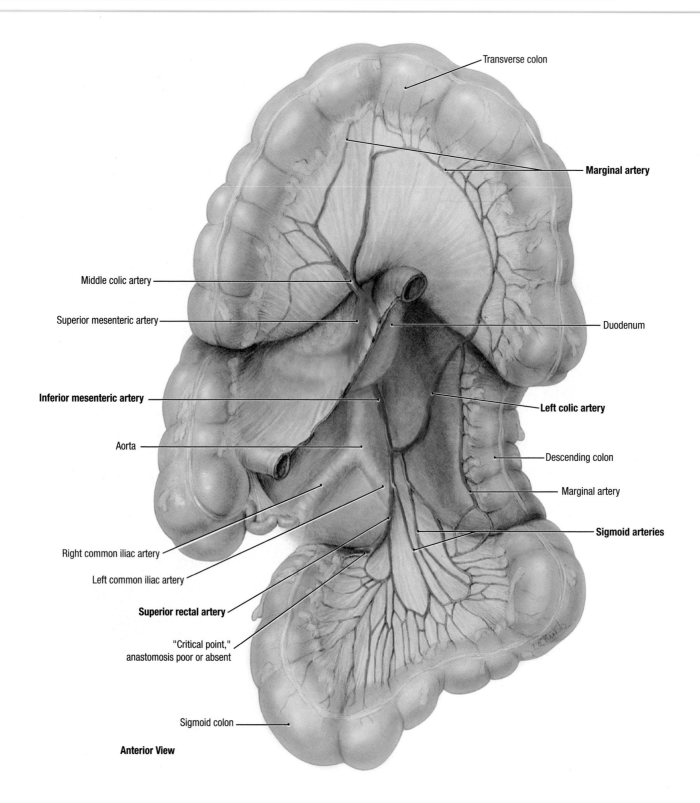

Transverse colon

Marginal artery

Middle colic artery

Superior mesenteric artery

Duodenum

Inferior mesenteric artery

Left colic artery

Aorta

Descending colon

Marginal artery

Sigmoid arteries

Right common iliac artery

Left common iliac artery

Superior rectal artery

"Critical point,"
anastomosis poor or absent

Sigmoid colon

Anterior View

2.41   **Inferior mesenteric artery**

The mesentery of the small intestine has been cut at its root.

- The inferior mesenteric artery arises posterior to the ascending part of the duodenum, about 4 cm superior to the bifurcation of the aorta; on crossing the left common iliac artery, it becomes the superior rectal artery.
- The branches of the inferior mesenteric artery include the left colic artery and several sigmoid arteries; the inferior two sigmoid arteries branch from the superior rectal artery.

- The point at which the last artery to the colon branches from the superior rectal artery is known as the "critical point"; this branch has poor or no anastomotic connections with the superior rectal artery.

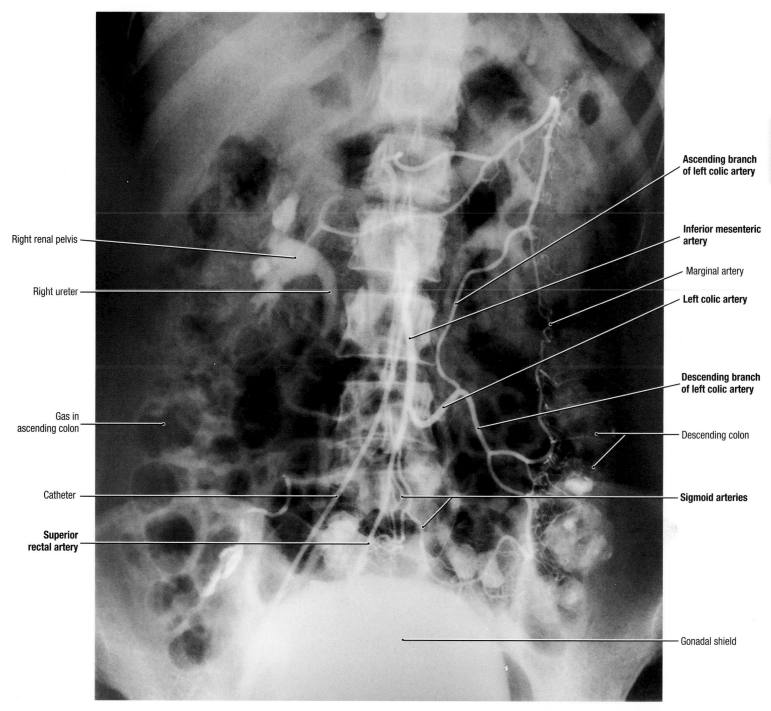

Right renal pelvis

Right ureter

Gas in
ascending colon

Catheter

**Superior
rectal artery**

**Ascending branch
of left colic artery**

**Inferior mesenteric
artery**

Marginal artery

Left colic artery

**Descending branch
of left colic artery**

Descending colon

Sigmoid arteries

Gonadal shield

Posteroanterior Arteriogram

2.42   Inferior mesenteric arteriogram

- The left colic artery courses to the left toward the descending colon and splits into ascending and descending branches.
- The sigmoid arteries, two to four in number, supply the sigmoid colon.
- The superior rectal artery, which is the continuation of the inferior mesenteric artery, supplies the rectum; the superior rectal anastomoses is formed by branches of the middle and inferior rectal arteries (from the internal iliac artery).

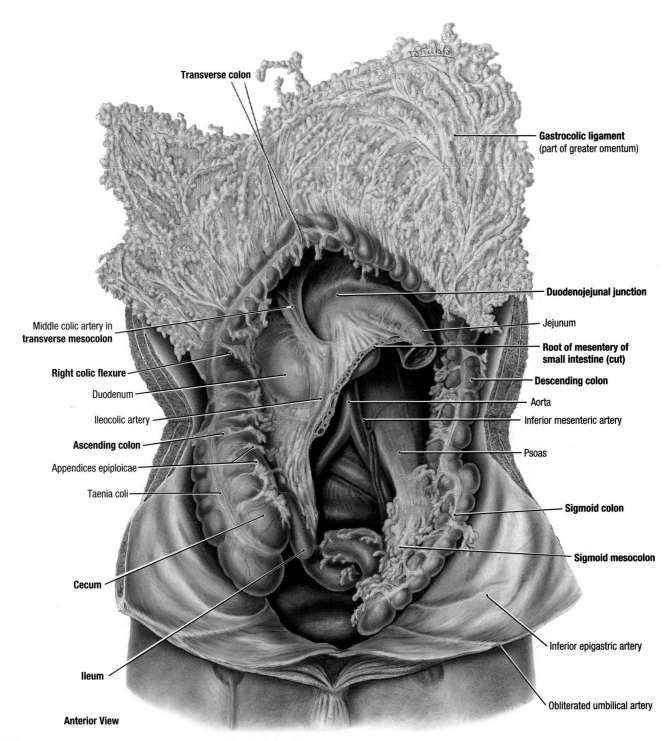

Anterior View

Transverse colon
Gastrocolic ligament
(part of greater omentum)
Duodenojejunal junction
Jejunum
Middle colic artery in
transverse mesocolon
**Root of mesentery of
small intestine (cut)**
Right colic flexure
Descending colon
Duodenum
Aorta
Ileocolic artery
Inferior mesenteric artery
Ascending colon
Psoas
Appendices epiploicae
Taenia coli
Sigmoid colon
Sigmoid mesocolon
Cecum
Inferior epigastric artery
Ileum
Obliterated umbilical artery

2.43 **Peritoneum of posterior abdominal cavity**

The gastrocolic ligament is retracted superiorly, along with the transverse colon and transverse mesocolon. The appendix had been surgically removed. This dissection is continued in Figure 2.44.

- The root of the mesentery of the small intestine, approximately 15 to 20 cm in length, extends between the duodenojejunal junction and ileocecal junction.
- The large intestine forms 3½ sides of a square around the jejunum and ileum. On the right are the cecum and ascending colon,

superior is the transverse colon, on the left is the descending and sigmoid colon, inferiorly is the sigmoid colon.

- Chronic inflammation of the colon (ulcerative colitis, Crohn disease) is characterized by severe inflammation and ulceration of the colon and rectum. In some patients, a colectomy is performed, during which the terminal ileum and colon as well as the rectum and anal canal are removed. An ileostomy is then constructed to establish an artificial cutaneous opening between the ileum and the skin of the anterolateral abdominal wall.

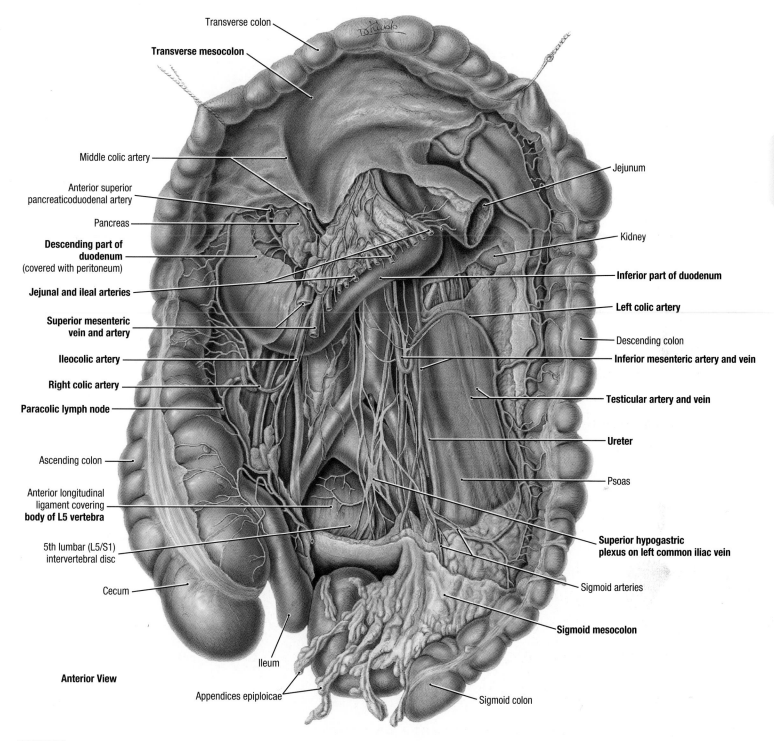

Transverse colon, Transverse mesocolon, Middle colic artery, Anterior superior pancreaticoduodenal artery, Pancreas, Descending part of duodenum (covered with peritoneum), Jejunal and ileal arteries, Superior mesenteric vein and artery, Ileocolic artery, Right colic artery, Paracolic lymph node, Ascending colon, Anterior longitudinal ligament covering body of L5 vertebra, 5th lumbar (L5/S1) intervertebral disc, Cecum, Anterior View, Ileum, Appendices epiploicae, Jejunum, Kidney, Inferior part of duodenum, Left colic artery, Descending colon, Inferior mesenteric artery and vein, Testicular artery and vein, Ureter, Psoas, Superior hypogastric plexus on left common iliac vein, Sigmoid arteries, Sigmoid mesocolon, Sigmoid colon

2.44 Posterior abdominal cavity with peritoneum removed

The jejunal and ileal branches (cut) pass from the left side of the superior mesenteric artery. The right colic artery here is a branch of the ileocolic artery. This is the same specimen as in Figure 2.43.
- The duodenum is large in diameter before crossing the superior mesenteric vessels and narrow afterward.
- On the right side, there are lymph nodes on the colon, paracolic nodes beside the colon, and nodes along the ileocolic artery, which drain into nodes anterior to the pancreas.
- The intestines and intestinal vessels lie on a resectable plane anterior to that of the testicular vessels; these in turn lie anterior to the plane of the kidney, its vessels, and the ureter.
- The superior hypogastric plexus lies within the bifurcation of the aorta and anterior to the left common iliac vein, the body of the 5th lumbar vertebra, and the 5th intervertebral disc.

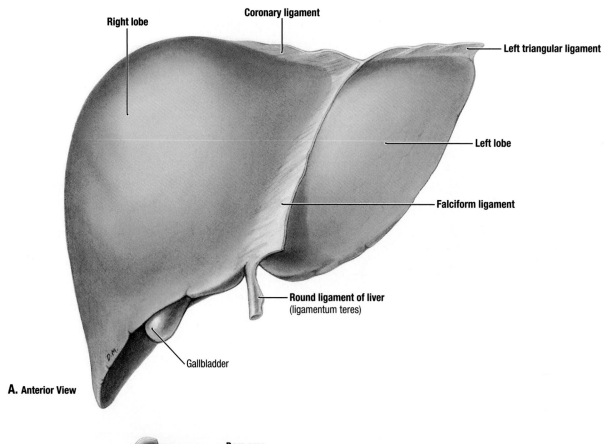

Right lobe
Coronary ligament
Left triangular ligament
Left lobe
Falciform ligament
Round ligament of liver (ligamentum teres)
Gallbladder

A. Anterior View

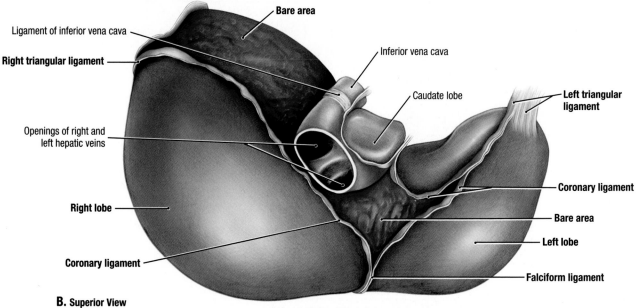

Bare area
Ligament of inferior vena cava
Inferior vena cava
Right triangular ligament
Caudate lobe
Left triangular ligament
Openings of right and left hepatic veins
Coronary ligament
Right lobe
Bare area
Left lobe
Coronary ligament
Falciform ligament

B. Superior View

2.45 **Diaphragmatic (anterior and superior) surface of liver**

A. The falciform ligament has been severed close to its attachment to the diaphragm and anterior abdominal wall and demarcates the right and left lobes of the liver. The round ligament of the liver (ligamentum teres) lies within the free edge of the falciform ligament.
B. The two layers of peritoneum that form the falciform ligament separate over the superior aspect (surrounding the bare area) of the liver to form the superior layer of the coronary ligament and the right and left triangular ligaments.

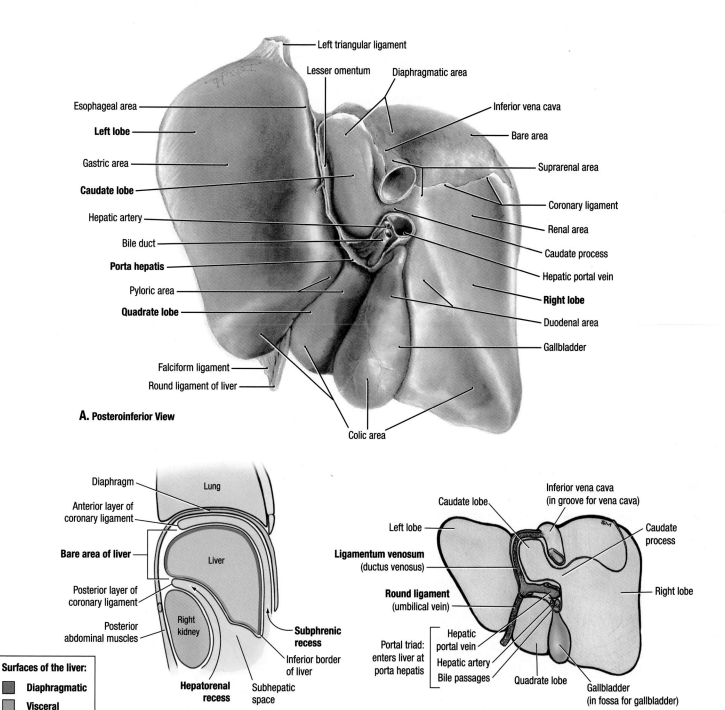

A. Posteroinferior View

B. Sagittal Section

Surfaces of the liver:
Diaphragmatic
Visceral

C. Posteroinferior View

2.46 **Visceral (posteroinferior) surface of liver**

A. Isolated specimen demonstrating lobes, and impressions of adjacent viscera. **B.** Hepatic surfaces and peritoneal recesses. **C.** Round ligament of liver and ligamentum venosum. The round ligament of liver includes the obliterated remains of the umbilical vein that carried well-oxygenated blood from the placenta to the fetus. The ligamentum venosum is the fibrous remnant of the fetal ductus venosus that shunted blood from the umbilical vein to the inferior vena cava, short circuiting the liver. Hepatic tissue may be obtained for diagnostic purposes by liver biopsy. The needle puncture is commonly made through the right 10th intercostal space in the midaxillary line. Before the physician takes the biopsy, the person is asked to hold his or her breath in full expiration to reduce the costodiaphragmatic recess and to lessen the possibility of damaging the lung and contaminating the pleural cavity.

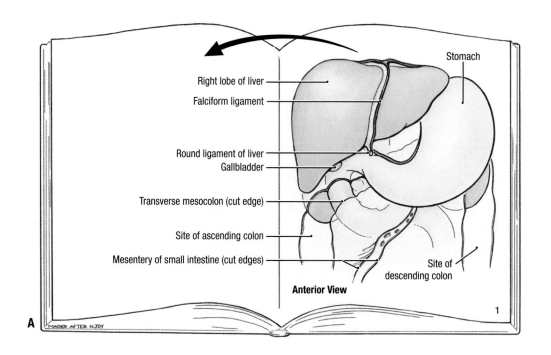

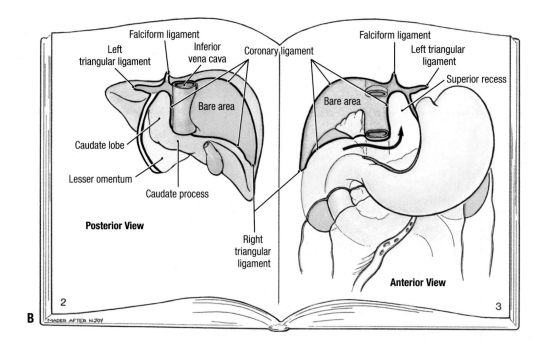

2.47 **Liver and its posterior relations, schematic illustration**

A. Liver in situ. The jejunum, ileum, and the ascending, transverse, and descending colon have been removed. **B.** The liver is drawn schematically on a page in a book, so that as the page is turned (*arrow in A*), the liver is reflected to the right to reveal its posterior surface, and on the facing page, the posterior relations that compose the bed of the liver are viewed. The *arrow in B* traverses the site of the omental (epiploic) foramen. The bare area is triangular, hence the coronary ligament that surrounds it is three-sided; its left side, or base, is between the inferior vena cava and caudate lobe, and its apex is at the right triangular ligament, where the superior and inferior layers of the coronary ligament meet.

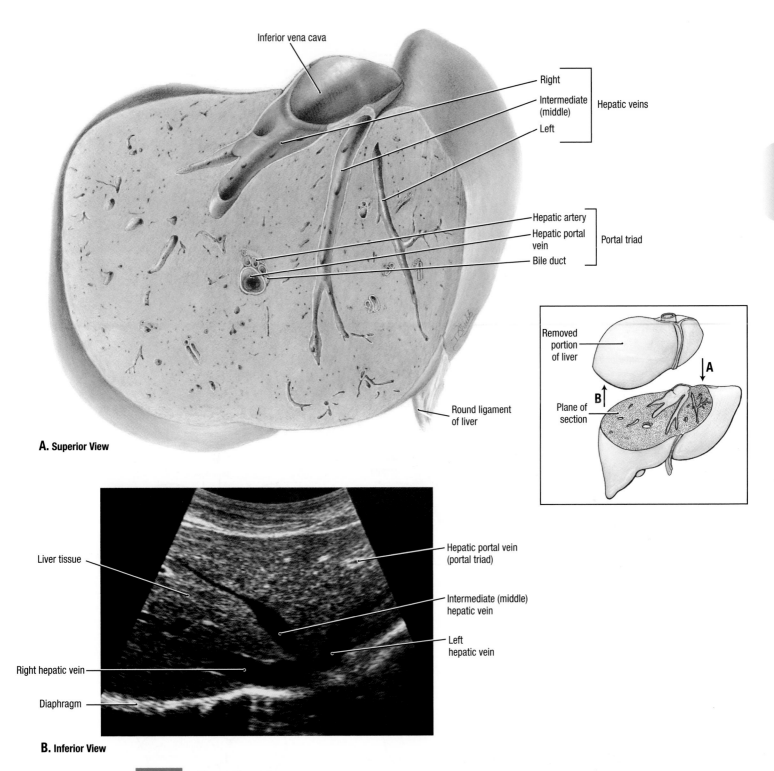

Inferior vena cava

Right ⎤
Intermediate (middle) ⎬ Hepatic veins
Left ⎦

Hepatic artery ⎤
Hepatic portal vein ⎬ Portal triad
Bile duct ⎦

Round ligament of liver

A. Superior View

Removed portion of liver

Plane of section

A

B

Liver tissue

Hepatic portal vein (portal triad)

Intermediate (middle) hepatic vein

Left hepatic vein

Right hepatic vein

Diaphragm

B. Inferior View

2.48   Hepatic veins

A. Approximately horizontal section of liver with the posterior aspect at top of page. Note the multiple perivascular fibrous capsules sectioned throughout the cut surface, each containing a portal triad (the hepatic portal vein, hepatic artery, bile ductules) plus lymph vessels. Interdigitating with these are branches of the three main hepatic veins (right, intermediate, and left), which, unaccompanied and lacking capsules, converge on the inferior vena cava. **B.** Ultrasound scan. The transducer was placed under the costal margin, and directed posteriorly producing an inverted image corresponding to **A.**

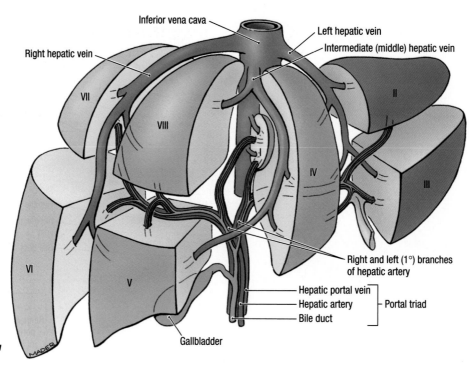

Inferior vena cava

Right hepatic vein

Left hepatic vein

Intermediate (middle) hepatic vein

VII

VIII

II

IV

III

VI

V

Right and left (1°) branches of hepatic artery

Hepatic portal vein ⎤
Hepatic artery   ⎥ Portal triad
Bile duct   ⎦

Gallbladder

A. Anterior View

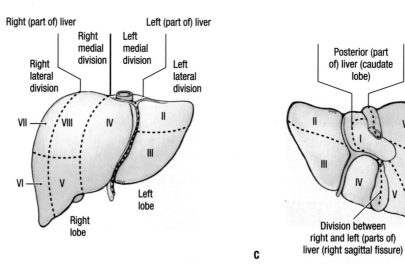

Right (part of) liver

Left (part of) liver

Right medial division

Left medial division

Right lateral division

Left lateral division

VII — VIII   IV   II

III

VI — V

Left lobe

Right lobe

B

Posterior (part of) liver (caudate lobe)

II   VII

I

III

IV   V   VI

Division between right and left (parts of) liver (right sagittal fissure)

C

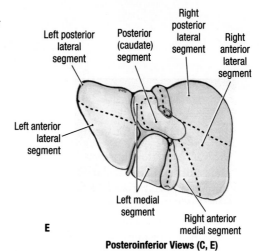

Right posterior medial segment

Left medial segment

Left posterior lateral segment

Right posterior lateral segment

Right anterior lateral segment

Left anterior lateral segment

Right anterior medial segment

D

Anterior Views (B, D)

Left posterior lateral segment

Posterior (caudate) segment

Right posterior lateral segment

Right anterior lateral segment

Left anterior lateral segment

Left medial segment

Right anterior medial segment

E

Posteroinferior Views (C, E)

2.49   Hepatic segmentation

Each segment is supplied by a secondary or tertiary branch of the hepatic artery, bile duct, and portal vein. The hepatic veins interdigitate between the structures of the portal triad and are intersegmental in that they drain adjacent segments. Since the right and left hepatic arteries and ducts and branches of the right and left portal veins do not communicate, it is possible to perform hepatic lobectomies (removal of the right or left part of the liver) and segmentectomies. Each segment can be identified numerically or by name (Table 2.4).

TABLE 2.4   SCHEMA OF TERMINOLOGY FOR SUBDIVISIONS OF THE LIVER

Anatomical Term	Right Lobe		Left Lobe		Caudate Lobe	
Functional/ surgical term**	Right (part of) liver [Right portal lobe*]		Left (part of) liver [Left portal lobe+]		Posterior (part of) liver	
	Right lateral division	Right medial division	Left medial division	Left lateral division	[Right caudate lobe*]	[Left caudate lobe+]
	Posterior lateral segment **Segment VII** [Posterior superior area]	Posterior medial segment **Segment VIII** [Anterior superior area]	[Medial superior area] Left medial segment **Segment IV**	Lateral segment **Segment II** [Lateral superior area]	Posterior segment **Segment I**	
	Right anterior lateral segment **Segment VI** [Posterior inferior area]	Anterior medial segment **Segment V** [Anterior inferior area]	[Medial inferior area = quadrate lobe]	Left anterior lateral segment **Segment III** [Lateral inferior area]		

** The labels in the table and figure above reflect the new Terminologia Anatomica: International Anatomical Terminology Previous terminology is in brackets.

*+ Under the schema of the previous terminology, the caudate lobe was divided into right and left halves, and *the right half of the caudate lobe was considered a subdivision of the right portal lobe; + the left half of the caudate lobe was considered a subdivision of the left portal lobe.

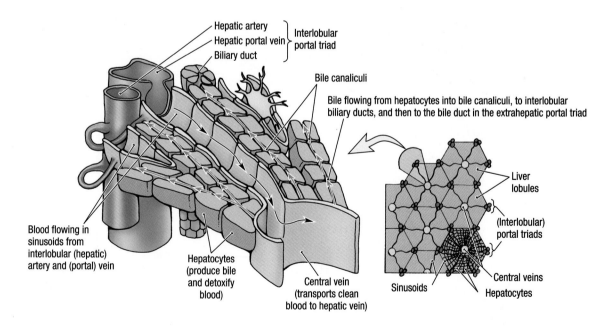

2.50   Flow of blood and bile in the liver

This small part of a liver lobule shows the components of the interlobular portal triad and the positioning of the sinusoids and bile canaliculi. Right: The cut surface of the liver shows the hexagonal pattern of the lobules.

- With the exception of lipids, every substance absorbed by the alimentary tract is received first by the liver, via the hepatic portal vein. In addition to its many metabolic activities, the liver stores glycogen and secretes bile.

- There is progressive destruction of hepatocytes in cirrhosis of the liver and replacement of them by fibrous tissue. This tissue surrounds the intrahepatic blood vessels and biliary ducts, making the liver firm and impeding circulation of blood through it.

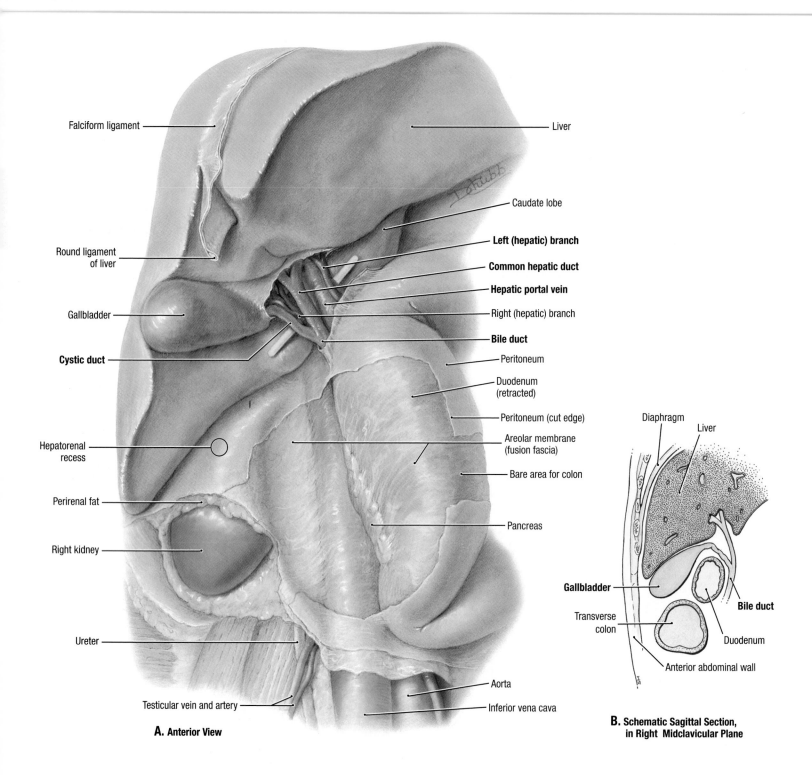

Falciform ligament

Liver

Caudate lobe

Left (hepatic) branch

Round ligament of liver

Common hepatic duct

Hepatic portal vein

Gallbladder

Right (hepatic) branch

Cystic duct

Bile duct

Peritoneum

Duodenum (retracted)

Peritoneum (cut edge)

Hepatorenal recess

Areolar membrane (fusion fascia)

Bare area for colon

Perirenal fat

Pancreas

Right kidney

Ureter

Aorta

Testicular vein and artery

Inferior vena cava

A. Anterior View

Diaphragm

Liver

Gallbladder

Bile duct

Transverse colon

Duodenum

Anterior abdominal wall

B. Schematic Sagittal Section, in Right Midclavicular Plane

2.51 **Exposure of the portal triad**

A. The portal triad typically consists of the hepatic portal vein (posteriorly), the hepatic artery proper (ascending from the left), and the bile passages (descending to the right). Here, the hepatic artery proper is replaced by a left hepatic branch, arising directly from the common hepatic artery, and a right hepatic branch, arising from the superior mesenteric artery (a common variation). A rod traverses the omental (epiploic) foramen. The lesser omen-tum and transverse colon are removed, and the peritoneum is cut along the right border of the duodenum; this part of the duodenum is retracted anteriorly. The space opened up reveals two smooth areolar membranes (fusion fascia) normally applied to each other that are vestiges of the embryonic peritoneum originally covering these surfaces **B.** Typical relations of gallbladder, cystic duct, and bile duct to the duodenum.

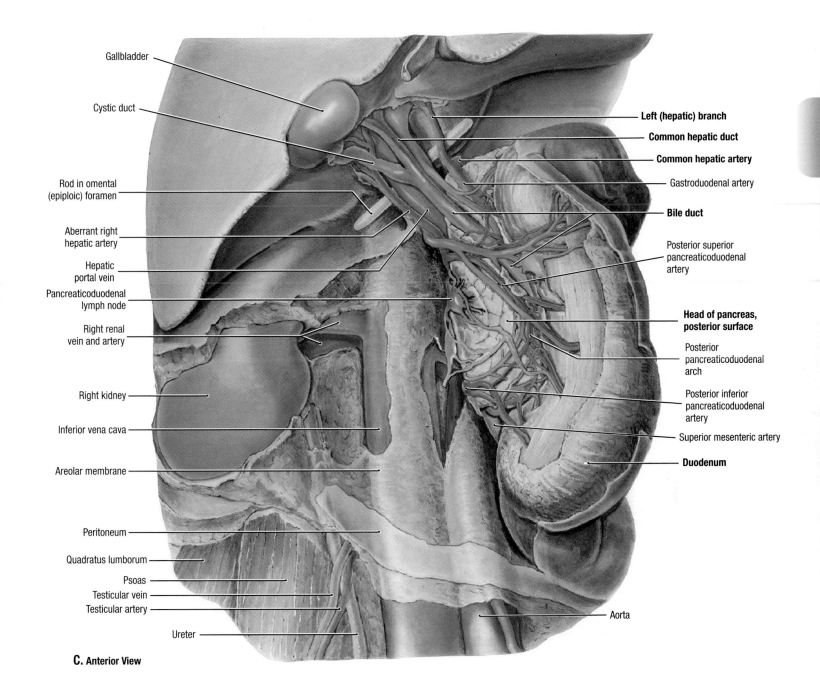

Gallbladder

Cystic duct

Rod in omental (epiploic) foramen

Aberrant right hepatic artery

Hepatic portal vein

Pancreaticoduodenal lymph node

Right renal vein and artery

Right kidney

Inferior vena cava

Areolar membrane

Peritoneum

Quadratus lumborum

Psoas

Testicular vein

Testicular artery

Ureter

Left (hepatic) branch

Common hepatic duct

Common hepatic artery

Gastroduodenal artery

Bile duct

Posterior superior pancreaticoduodenal artery

Head of pancreas, posterior surface

Posterior pancreaticoduodenal arch

Posterior inferior pancreaticoduodenal artery

Superior mesenteric artery

Duodenum

Aorta

C. Anterior View

2.51 **Exposure of the portal triad** *(continued)*

C. Continuing the dissection in **A,** the secondarily retroperitoneal viscera (duodenum and head of the pancreas) are retracted anteriorly and to the left. The areolar membrane (fusion fascia) covering the posterior aspect of the pancreas and duodenum is largely removed, and that covering the anterior aspect of the great vessels is partly removed. A common method for reducing portal hypertension is to divert blood from the portal venous system to the systemic venous system by creating a communication between the portal vein and the IVC. This portacaval anastomosis of portosystemic shunt may be created where these vessels lie close to each other posterior to the liver.

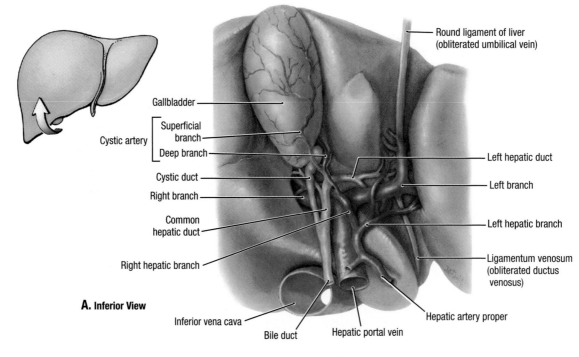

A. Inferior View

Round ligament of liver
(obliterated umbilical vein)

Gallbladder

Cystic artery
— Superficial branch
— Deep branch

Cystic duct

Right branch

Common hepatic duct

Right hepatic branch

Left hepatic duct

Left branch

Left hepatic branch

Ligamentum venosum
(obliterated ductus venosus)

Inferior vena cava

Bile duct

Hepatic portal vein

Hepatic artery proper

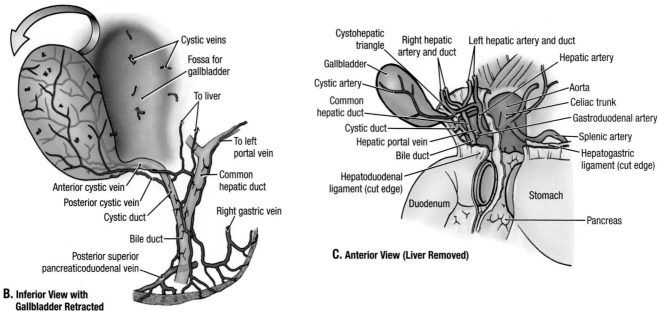

B. Inferior View with Gallbladder Retracted

Cystic veins

Fossa for gallbladder

To liver

To left portal vein

Common hepatic duct

Right gastric vein

Anterior cystic vein
Posterior cystic vein
Cystic duct

Bile duct

Posterior superior pancreaticoduodenal vein

C. Anterior View (Liver Removed)

Cystohepatic triangle
Right hepatic artery and duct
Left hepatic artery and duct
Hepatic artery

Gallbladder

Cystic artery

Common hepatic duct

Cystic duct

Hepatic portal vein

Bile duct

Hepatoduodenal ligament (cut edge)

Duodenum

Aorta

Celiac trunk

Gastroduodenal artery

Splenic artery

Hepatogastric ligament (cut edge)

Stomach

Pancreas

2.52 **Gallbladder and structures of porta hepatis**

A. Gallbladder, cystic artery and extrahepatic bile ducts. The inferior border of the liver is elevated to demonstrate its visceral surface (as in orientation figure). **B.** Venous drainage of the gall bladder and extrahepatic ducts. Most veins are tributaries of the hepatic portal vein, but some drain directly to the liver. **C.** Portal triad within the hepatoduodenal ligament (free edge of lesser omentum).

Gallstones are concretions, pebble(s), in the gallbladder or extrahepatic biliary ducts. The cystohepatic triangle (Calot), between the common hepatic duct, cystic duct, and liver is an important endoscopic landmark for locating the cystic artery.

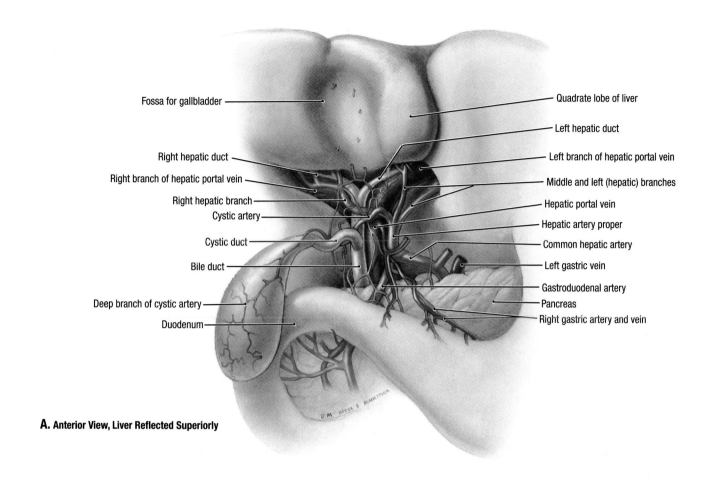

Fossa for gallbladder

Right hepatic duct

Right branch of hepatic portal vein

Right hepatic branch

Cystic artery

Cystic duct

Bile duct

Deep branch of cystic artery

Duodenum

Quadrate lobe of liver

Left hepatic duct

Left branch of hepatic portal vein

Middle and left (hepatic) branches

Hepatic portal vein

Hepatic artery proper

Common hepatic artery

Left gastric vein

Gastroduodenal artery

Pancreas

Right gastric artery and vein

A. Anterior View, Liver Reflected Superiorly

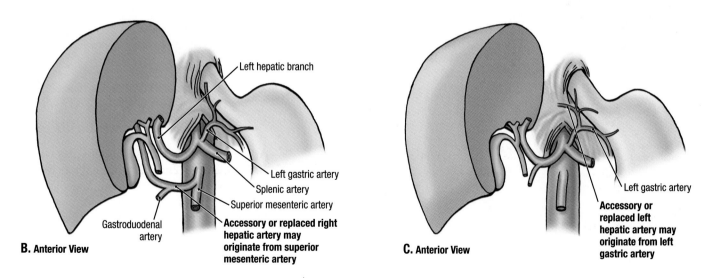

Left hepatic branch

Left gastric artery

Splenic artery

Superior mesenteric artery

Accessory or replaced right hepatic artery may originate from superior mesenteric artery

Gastroduodenal artery

B. Anterior View

Left gastric artery

Accessory or replaced left hepatic artery may originate from left gastric artery

C. Anterior View

2.53   Vessels in porta hepatis

A. Hepatic and cystic vessels. The liver is reflected superiorly. The gallbladder, freed from its bed, or fossa, has remained nearly in its anatomical position, pulled slightly to the right. The deep branch of the cystic artery on the deep, or attached, surface of the gallbladder anastomoses with branches of the superficial branch of the cystic artery and sends twigs into the bed of the gallbladder. Veins (not all shown) accompany most arteries. **B.** Aberrant (accessory or replaced) right hepatic artery. **C.** Aberrant left hepatic artery.

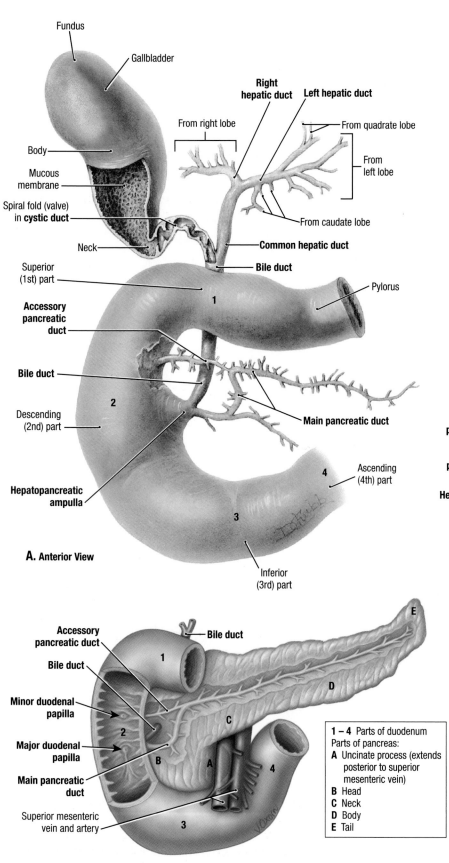

Fundus

Gallblader

Right hepatic duct

Left hepatic duct

From right lobe

From quadrate lobe

Body

From left lobe

Mucous membrane

Spiral fold (valve) in **cystic duct**

From caudate lobe

Neck

Common hepatic duct

Bile duct

Superior (1st) part

Pylorus

1

Accessory pancreatic duct

Bile duct

2

Descending (2nd) part

Main pancreatic duct

4

Ascending (4th) part

Hepatopancreatic ampulla

3

A. Anterior View

Inferior (3rd) part

Accessory pancreatic duct

Bile duct

E

Bile duct

1

Bile duct

D

Minor duodenal papilla

2

C

Major duodenal papilla

B

A

4

Main pancreatic duct

Superior mesenteric vein and artery

3

1 – 4 Parts of duodenum
Parts of pancreas:
A Uncinate process (extends posterior to superior mesenteric vein)
B Head
C Neck
D Body
E Tail

B. Anterior View

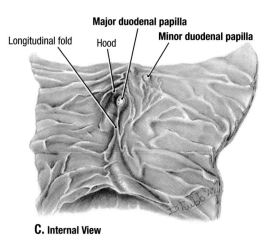

Longitudinal fold

Major duodenal papilla

Hood

Minor duodenal papilla

C. Internal View

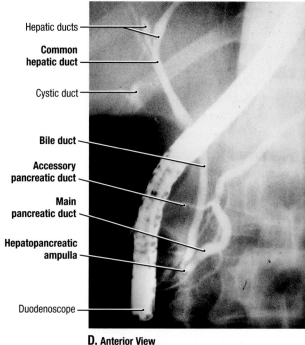

Hepatic ducts

Common hepatic duct

Cystic duct

Bile duct

Accessory pancreatic duct

Main pancreatic duct

Hepatopancreatic ampulla

Duodenoscope

D. Anterior View

2.54 Bile and pancreatic ducts

A. Extrahepatic bile passages and pancreatic ducts. **B.** Descending (2nd) part of the duodenum (interior). **C.** Endoscopic retrograde cholangiography and pancreatography (ERCP) demonstrating the bile and pancreatic ducts. The right and left hepatic ducts collect bile from the liver; the common hepatic duct unites with the cystic duct superior to the duodenum to form the bile duct which descends posterior to the superior (1st) part of the duodenum. The bile duct joins the main pancreatic duct, forming the hepatopancreatic ampulla, which opens on the major duodenal papilla. This opening is the narrowest part of the biliary passages and is the common site for impaction of a gallstone. Gallstones may produce biliary colic (pain in the epigastric region). The accessory pancreatic duct opens on the minor duodenal papilla.

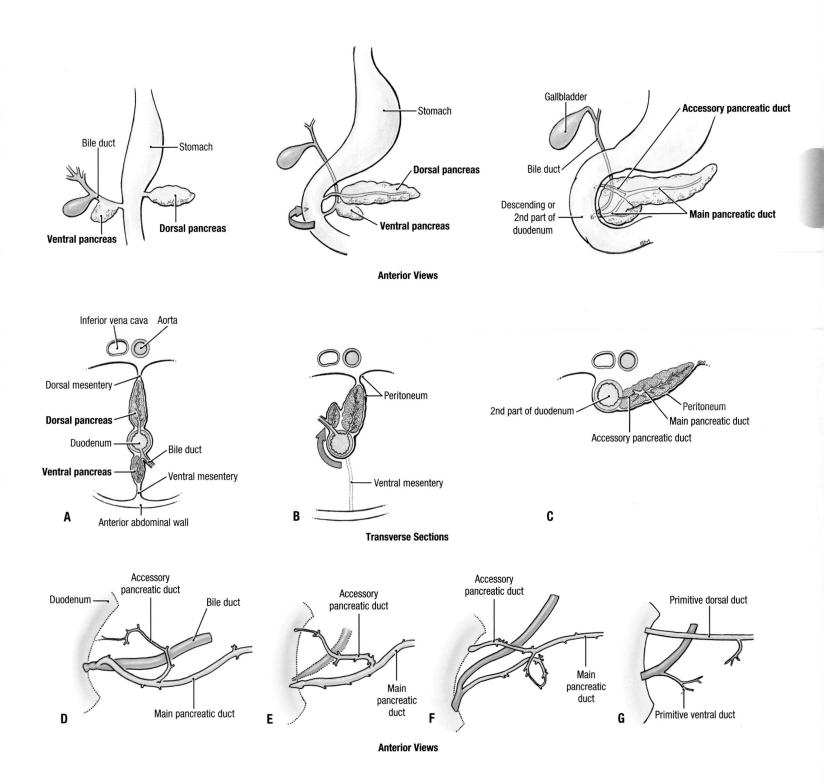

Anterior Views

Transverse Sections

Anterior Views

2.55 Development and variability of the pancreatic ducts

A–C. Anterior views (top) and transverse sections (bottom) of the stages in the development of the pancreas. **A.** The small, primitive ventral bud arises in common with the bile duct, and a larger, primitive dorsal bud arises independently from the duodenum. **B.** The 2nd, or descending, part of the duodenum rotates on its long axis, which brings the ventral bud and bile duct posterior to the dorsal bud. **C.** A connecting segment unites the dorsal duct to the ventral duct, whereupon the duodenal end of the dorsal duct atrophies, and the direction of flow within it is reversed. **D–G.** Common variations of the pancreatic duct. **D.** An accessory duct that has lost its connection with the duodenum. **E.** An accessory duct that is large enough to relieve an obstructed main duct. **F.** An accessory duct that could probably substitute for the main duct. **G.** A persisting primitive dorsal duct unconnected to the primitive ventral duct.

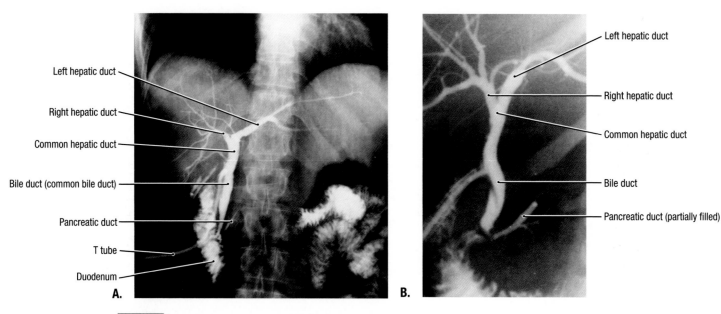

2.56   **Radiographs of biliary passages**

After a cholecystectomy (removal of the gallbladder), contrast medium was injected with a T tube inserted into the bile passages. The biliary passages are visualized in the superior abdomen in **A** and are more localized in **B.**

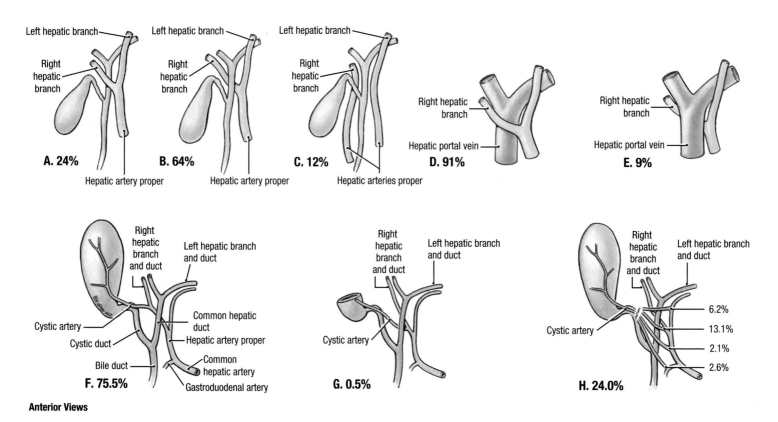

Anterior Views

2.57   **Variations in hepatic and cystic arteries**

In a study of 165 cadavers, five patterns were observed. **A.** Right hepatic artery crossing anterior to bile passages, 24%. **B.** Right hepatic artery crossing posterior to bile passages, 64%. **C.** Aberrant artery arising from the superior mesenteric artery, 12%. The artery crossed anterior (**D**) to the portal vein in 91%, and posterior (**E**) in 9%. The cystic artery usually arises from the right hepatic artery in the angle between the common hepatic duct and cystic duct, without crossing the common hepatic duct (**F** and **G**). However, when it arises on the left of the bile passages, it almost always crosses anterior to the passages (**H**).

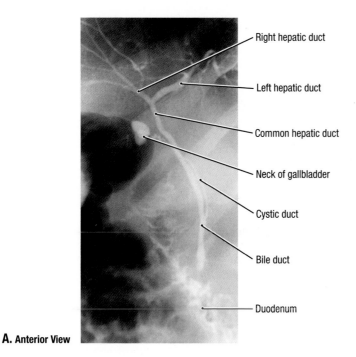

- Right hepatic duct
- Left hepatic duct
- Common hepatic duct
- Neck of gallbladder
- Cystic duct
- Bile duct
- Duodenum

A. Anterior View

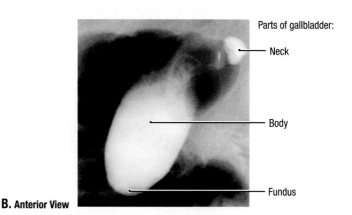

Parts of gallbladder:
- Neck
- Body
- Fundus

B. Anterior View

2.58   Endoscopic retrograde cholangiography of gallbladder and biliary passages

A. Cystic duct. **B.** Parts of gallbladder.

Endoscopic retrograde cholangiography (ERCP) is done by first passing a fiberoptic endoscope through the mouth, esophagus, and stomach. Then the duodenum is entered and a cannula is inserted into the major duodenal papilla and advanced under fluoroscopic control into the duct of choice (bile duct or pancreatic duct) for injection of radiographic contrast medium.

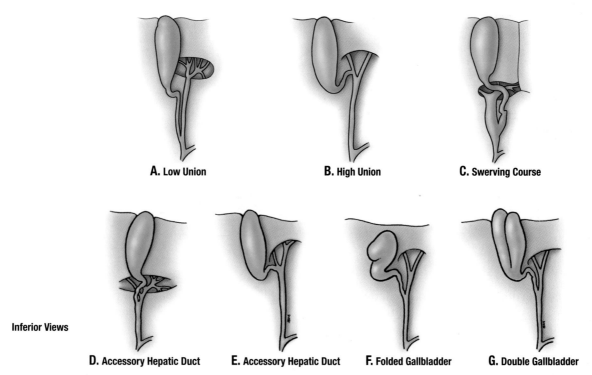

A. Low Union   **B. High Union**   **C. Swerving Course**

Inferior Views

D. Accessory Hepatic Duct   **E. Accessory Hepatic Duct**   **F. Folded Gallbladder**   **G. Double Gallbladder**

2.59   Variations of cystic and hepatic ducts and gallbladder

The cystic duct usually lies on the right side of the common hepatic duct, joining it just above the superior (1st) part of the duodenum, but this varies as in **A–C**. Of 95 gallbladders and bile passages studied, 7 had accessory ducts. Of these, 4 joined the common hepatic duct near the cystic duct **(D)**, 2 joined the cystic duct **(E)**, and 1 was an anastomosing duct connecting the cystic with the common hepatic duct. **F.** Folded gallbladder. **G.** Double gallbladder.

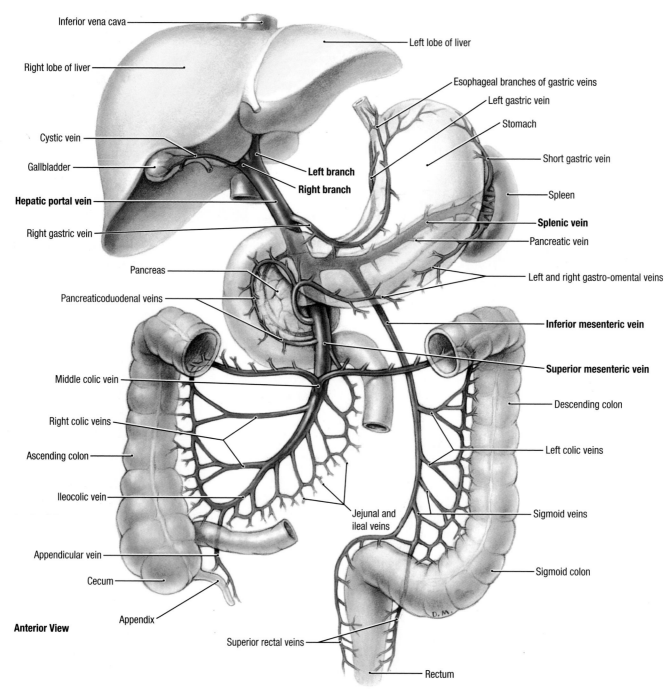

Inferior vena cava

Left lobe of liver

Right lobe of liver

Esophageal branches of gastric veins

Left gastric vein

Stomach

Cystic vein

Gallbladder

Short gastric vein

Left branch

Right branch

Spleen

Hepatic portal vein

Splenic vein

Right gastric vein

Pancreatic vein

Pancreas

Left and right gastro-omental veins

Pancreaticoduodenal veins

Inferior mesenteric vein

Superior mesenteric vein

Middle colic vein

Descending colon

Right colic veins

Ascending colon

Left colic veins

Ileocolic vein

Jejunal and ileal veins

Sigmoid veins

Appendicular vein

Cecum

Sigmoid colon

Anterior View

Appendix

Superior rectal veins

Rectum

2.60 Portal venous system

- The hepatic portal vein drains venous blood from the gastrointestinal tract, spleen, pancreas, and gallbladder to the sinusoids of the liver; from here, the blood is conveyed to the systemic venous system by the hepatic veins that drain directly to the inferior vena cava.
- The hepatic portal vein forms posterior to the neck of the pancreas by the union of the superior mesenteric and splenic veins, with the inferior mesenteric vein joining at or near the angle of union.
- The splenic vein drains blood from the inferior mesenteric, left gastro-omental (epiploic), short gastric, and pancreatic veins.

- The right gastro-omental, pancreaticoduodenal, jejunal, ileal, right, and middle colic veins drain into the superior mesenteric vein.
- The inferior mesenteric vein commences in the rectal plexus as the superior rectal vein and, after crossing the common iliac vessels, becomes the inferior mesenteric vein; branches include the sigmoid and left colic veins.
- The hepatic portal vein divides into right and left branches at the porta hepatis. The left branch carries mainly, but not exclusively, blood from the inferior mesenteric, gastric, and splenic veins, and the right branch carries blood mainly from the superior mesenteric vein.

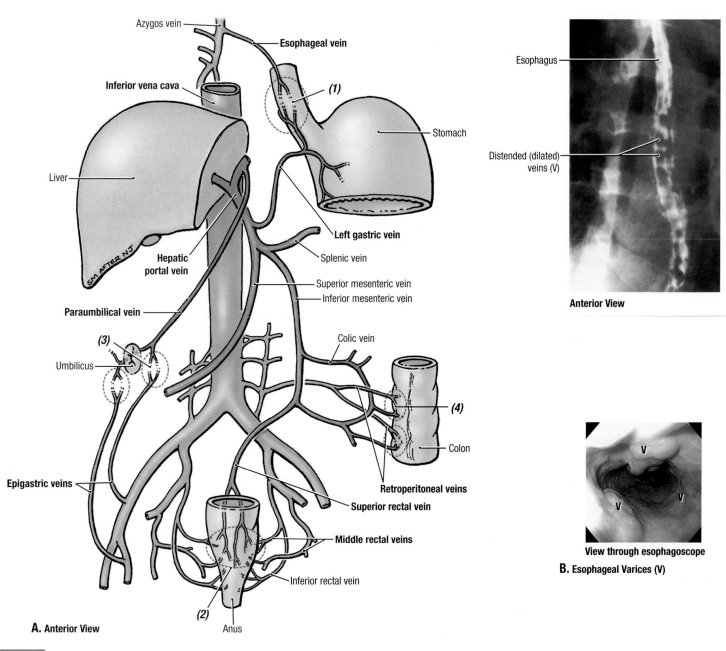

A. Anterior View

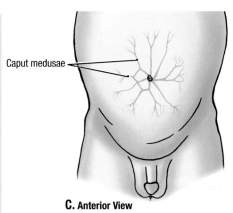

C. Anterior View

2.61   **Portacaval system**

A. Portacaval system. In this diagram, portal tributaries are dark blue, and systemic tributaries and communicating veins are light blue. In portal hypertension (as in hepatic cirrhosis), the portal blood cannot pass freely through the liver, and the portocaval anastomoses become engorged, dilated, or even varicose; as a consequence, these veins may rupture. The sites of the portocaval anastomosis shown are between *(1)* esophageal veins draining into the azygos vein (systemic) and left gastric vein (portal), which when dilated are esophageal varices, also shown in **B**; *(2)* the inferior and middle rectal veins, draining into the inferior vena cava (systemic) and the superior rectal vein continuing as the inferior mesenteric vein (portal) (hemorrhoids result if the vessels are dilated); *(3)* paraumbilical veins (portal) and small epigastric veins of the anterior abdominal wall (systemic), which when varicose form "caput medusae" (so named because of the resemblance of the radiating veins to the serpents on the head of Medusa, a character in Greek mythology); and *(4)* twigs of colic veins (portal) anastomosing with systemic retroperitoneal veins. **B.** Esophageal varices. **C.** Caput medusae.

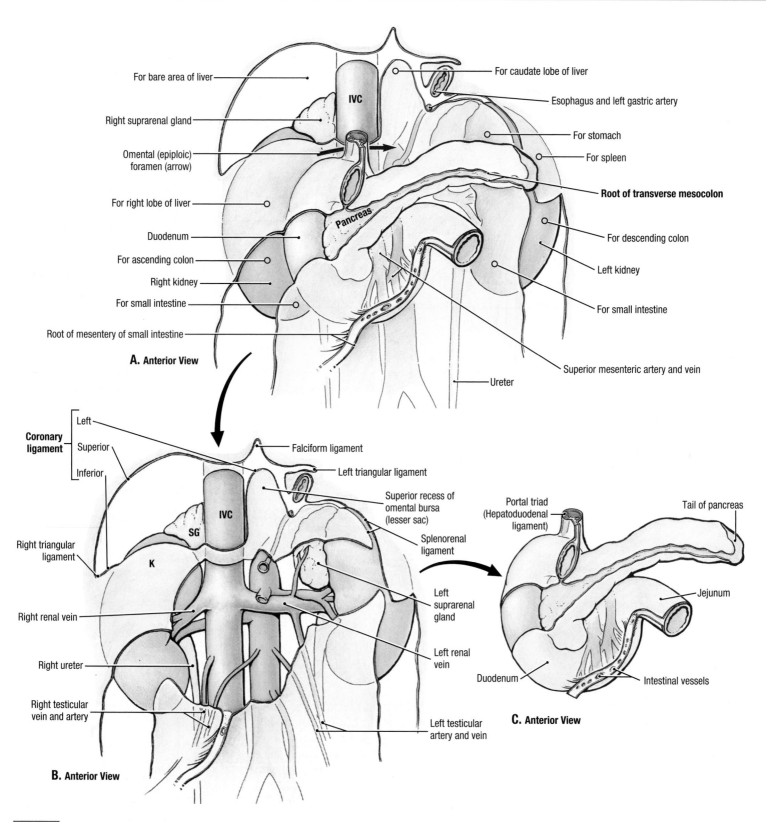

2.62   Posterior abdominal viscera and their anterior relations

The peritoneal coverings are yellow. **A.** Duodenum and pancreas in situ. Note the line of attachment of the root of the transverse mesocolon is to the body and tail of the pancreas. The viscera contacting specific regions are indicated by the term "for." The omental (epiploic) foramen is traversed by an arrow. **B.** After removal of duodenum and pancreas. The three parts of the coronary ligament are attached to the diaphragm, except where the inferior vena cava (IVC), suprarenal gland (SG), and kidney (K) intervene. **C.** Pancreas and duodenum removed from **A.**

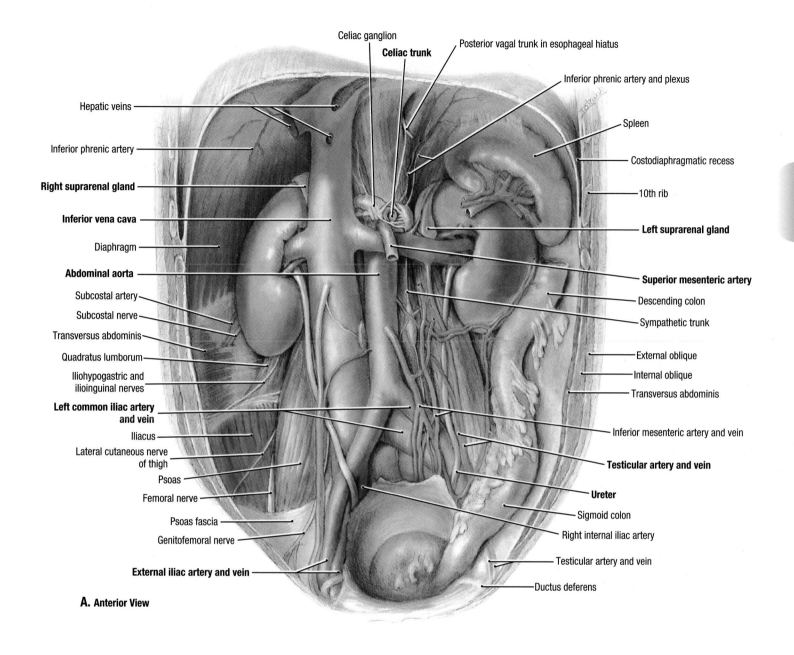

Celiac ganglion

Celiac trunk

Posterior vagal trunk in esophageal hiatus

Inferior phrenic artery and plexus

Hepatic veins

Inferior phrenic artery

Right suprarenal gland

Inferior vena cava

Diaphragm

Abdominal aorta

Subcostal artery

Subcostal nerve

Transversus abdominis

Quadratus lumborum

Iliohypogastric and ilioinguinal nerves

Left common iliac artery and vein

Iliacus

Lateral cutaneous nerve of thigh

Psoas

Femoral nerve

Psoas fascia

Genitofemoral nerve

External iliac artery and vein

A. Anterior View

Spleen

Costodiaphragmatic recess

10th rib

Left suprarenal gland

Superior mesenteric artery

Descending colon

Sympathetic trunk

External oblique

Internal oblique

Transversus abdominis

Inferior mesenteric artery and vein

Testicular artery and vein

Ureter

Sigmoid colon

Right internal iliac artery

Testicular artery and vein

Ductus deferens

2.63   **Viscera and vessels of posterior abdominal wall**

A. Great vessels, kidneys, and suprarenal glands. **B.** Relationships of left renal vein and inferior (3rd) part of duodenum to aorta and superior mesenteric artery.

- The abdominal aorta is shorter and smaller in caliber than the inferior vena cava.
- The inferior mesenteric artery arises about 4 cm superior to the aortic bifurcation and crosses the left common iliac vessels to become the superior rectal artery.
- The left renal vein drains the left testis, left suprarenal gland, and left kidney; the renal arteries are posterior to the renal veins.
- The ureter crosses the external iliac artery just beyond the common iliac bifurcation.
- The testicular vessels cross anterior to the ureter and join the ductus deferens at the deep inguinal ring.
- In **B**, the left renal vein and duodenum (and uncinate process of pancreas—not shown) pass between the aorta posteriorly and the superior mesenteric artery, anteriorly; they may be compressed like nuts in a nutcracker.

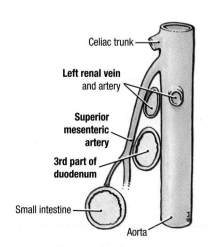

Celiac trunk

Left renal vein and artery

Superior mesenteric artery

3rd part of duodenum

Small intestine

Aorta

B. Lateral View (from left)

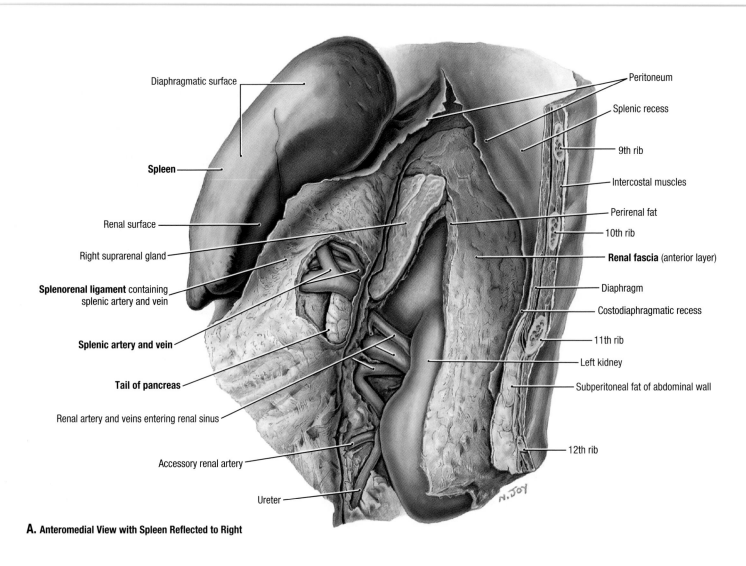

Diaphragmatic surface

Spleen

Renal surface

Right suprarenal gland

Splenorenal ligament containing splenic artery and vein

Splenic artery and vein

Tail of pancreas

Renal artery and veins entering renal sinus

Accessory renal artery

Ureter

Peritoneum

Splenic recess

9th rib

Intercostal muscles

Perirenal fat

10th rib

Renal fascia (anterior layer)

Diaphragm

Costodiaphragmatic recess

11th rib

Left kidney

Subperitoneal fat of abdominal wall

12th rib

N. Joy

A. Anteromedial View with Spleen Reflected to Right

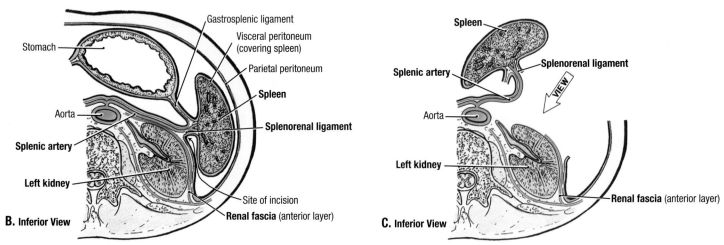

Stomach

Aorta

Splenic artery

Left kidney

Gastrosplenic ligament

Visceral peritoneum (covering spleen)

Parietal peritoneum

Spleen

Splenorenal ligament

Site of incision

Renal fascia (anterior layer)

B. Inferior View

Spleen

Splenic artery

Aorta

Left kidney

Splenorenal ligament

VIEW

Renal fascia (anterior layer)

C. Inferior View

2.64   **Exposure of the left kidney and suprarenal gland**

A. Dissection. **B.** Schematic section with spleen and splenorenal ligament intact. **C.** Procedure used in **A** to expose the kidney. The spleen and splenorenal ligament are reflected anteriorly, with the splenic vessels and tail of the pancreas. Part of the renal fascia of the kidney is removed. Note the proximity of the splenic vein and left renal vein, enabling a splenorenal shunt to be established surgically to relieve portal hypertension.

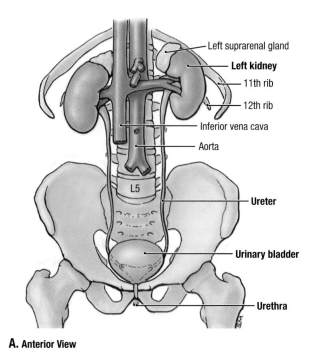

A. Anterior View

Left suprarenal gland
Left kidney
11th rib
12th rib
Inferior vena cava
Aorta
L5
Ureter
Urinary bladder
Urethra

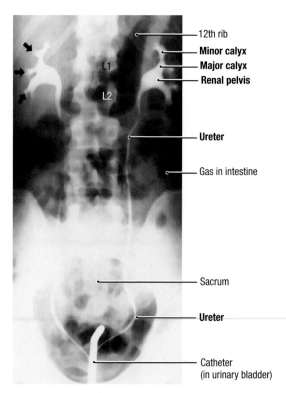

B. Anteroposterior Pyelogram

12th rib
Minor calyx
Major calyx
Renal pelvis
L1
L2
Ureter
Gas in intestine
Sacrum
Ureter
Catheter
(in urinary bladder)

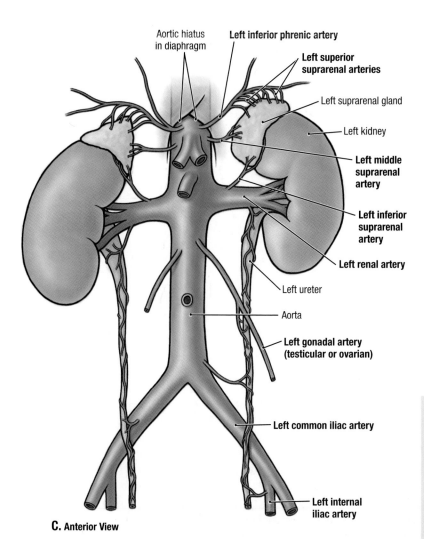

C. Anterior View

Aortic hiatus
in diaphragm
Left inferior phrenic artery
**Left superior
suprarenal arteries**
Left suprarenal gland
Left kidney
**Left middle
suprarenal
artery**
**Left inferior
suprarenal
artery**
Left renal artery
Left ureter
Aorta
**Left gonadal artery
(testicular or ovarian)**
Left common iliac artery
**Left internal
iliac artery**

2.65 Kidneys and suprarenal glands

A. Overview of urinary system. **B.** Pyelogram. Radiopaque material occupies the cavities that normally conduct urine. Note the papillae (indicated with arrows) bulging into the minor calices, which empty into a major calyx that opens, in turn, into the renal pelvis drained by the ureter. **C.** Arterial supply of the suprarenal glands, kidneys and ureters.

Renal transplantation is now an established operation for the treatment of selected cases of chronic renal failure. The kidney can be removed from the donor without damaging the suprarenal gland because of the weak septum of renal fascia that separates the kidney from this gland. The site for transplanting a kidney is in the iliac fossa of the greater pelvis. The renal artery and vein are joined to the external iliac artery and vein, respectively, and the ureter is sutured into the urinary bladder.

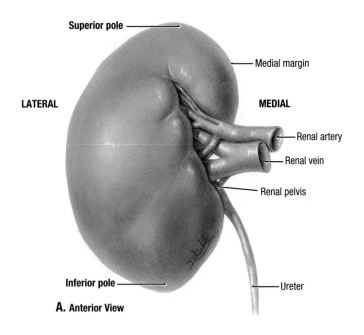

A. Anterior View

Superior pole

Medial margin

LATERAL

MEDIAL

Renal artery

Renal vein

Renal pelvis

Inferior pole

Ureter

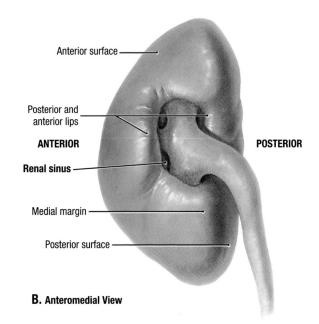

B. Anteromedial View

Anterior surface

Posterior and anterior lips

ANTERIOR

POSTERIOR

Renal sinus

Medial margin

Posterior surface

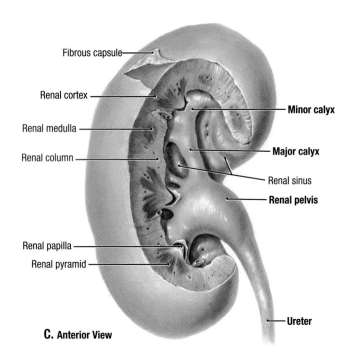

C. Anterior View

Fibrous capsule

Renal cortex

Renal medulla

Renal column

Minor calyx

Major calyx

Renal sinus

Renal pelvis

Renal papilla

Renal pyramid

Ureter

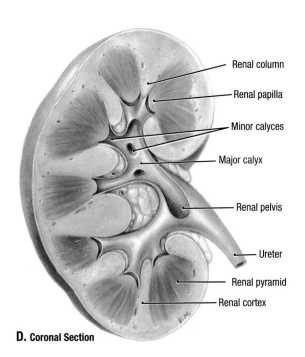

D. Coronal Section

Renal column

Renal papilla

Minor calyces

Major calyx

Renal pelvis

Ureter

Renal pyramid

Renal cortex

2.66 Structure of kidney

A. External features. The superior pole of the kidney is closer to the median plane than the inferior pole. Approximately 25% of kidneys may have a 2nd, 3rd, and even 4th accessory renal artery branching from the aorta. These multiple vessels enter through the renal sinus or at the superior or inferior pole. **B.** Renal sinus. The renal sinus is a vertical "pocket" opening on the medial side of the kidney. Tucked into the pocket are the renal pelvis and renal vessels in a matrix of perirenal fat. **C.** Renal calices. The anterior wall of the renal sinus has been cut away to expose the renal pelvis and the calices. **D.** Internal features. Cysts in the kidney, multiple or solitary, are common and usually benign findings during ultrasound examinations and dissection of cadavers. Adult polycystic disease of the kidneys, however, is an important cause of renal failure.

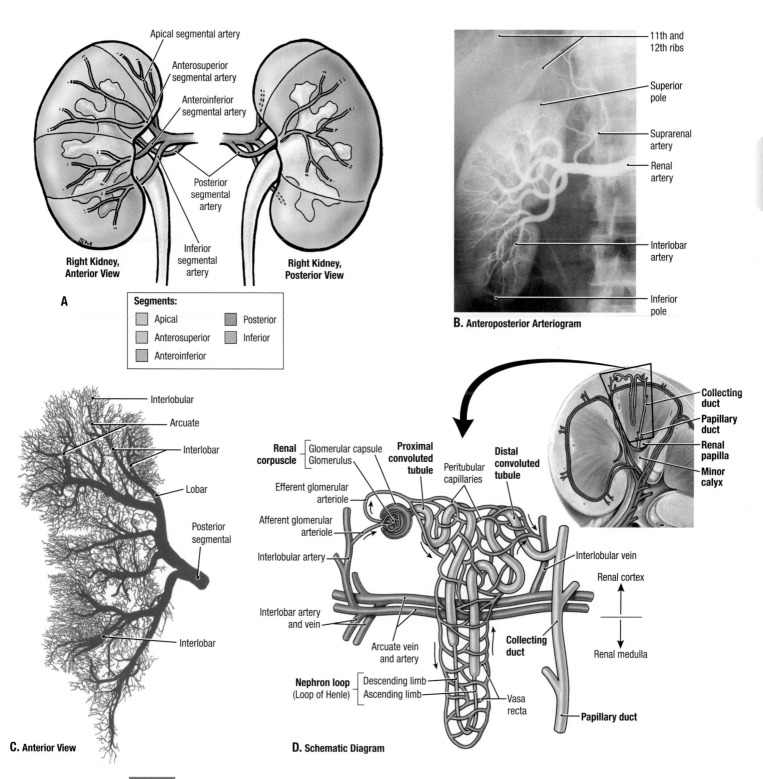

2.67 **Segments of the kidneys**

A. Segmental arteries. Segmental arteries do not anastomose significantly with other segmental arteries; they are end arteries. The area supplied by each segmented artery is an independent, surgically respectable unit or renal segment. **B.** Renal arteriogram. **C.** Corrosion cast of posterior segmental artery of kidney. **D.** The nephron is the functional unit of the kidney consisting of a renal corpuscle, proximal tubule, nephron loop and distal tubule. Papillary ducts open onto renal papillae, emptying into minor calices.

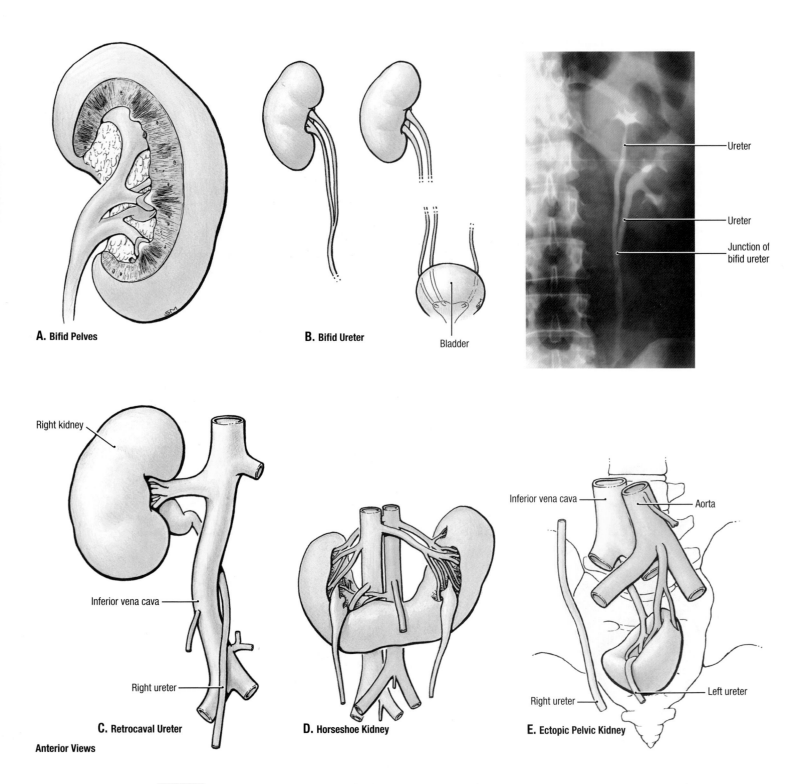

A. Bifid Pelves

B. Bifid Ureter

Bladder

Ureter

Ureter

Junction of
bifid ureter

Right kidney

Inferior vena cava

Right ureter

C. Retrocaval Ureter

Anterior Views

D. Horseshoe Kidney

Inferior vena cava

Aorta

Right ureter

Left ureter

E. Ectopic Pelvic Kidney

2.68 **Anomalies of kidney and ureter**

A. Bifid pelves. The pelves are almost replaced by two long major calices, which extend out-side the sinus. **B.** Duplicated, or bifid, ureters. These can be unilateral or bilateral, and com-plete or incomplete. **C.** Retrocaval ureter. The ureter courses posterior and then anterior to the inferior vena cava. **D.** Horseshoe kidney. The right and left kidneys are fused in the midline. **E.** Ectopic pelvic kidney. Pelvic kidneys have no fatty capsule and can be unilater-al or bilateral. During childbirth, they may cause obstruction and suffer injury.

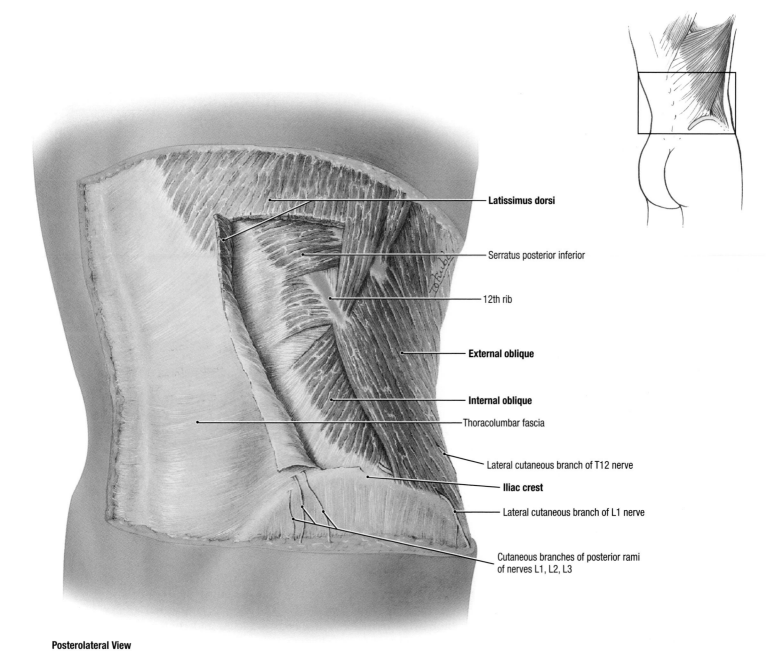

Latissimus dorsi

Serratus posterior inferior

12th rib

External oblique

Internal oblique

Thoracolumbar fascia

Lateral cutaneous branch of T12 nerve

Iliac crest

Lateral cutaneous branch of L1 nerve

Cutaneous branches of posterior rami
of nerves L1, L2, L3

Posterolateral View

2.69 Exposure of kidney

The latissimus dorsi is partially reflected.

- The external oblique muscle has an oblique, free posterior border that extends from the tip of the 12th rib to the midpoint of the iliac crest.
- The internal oblique muscle extends posteriorly beyond the border of the external oblique muscle.

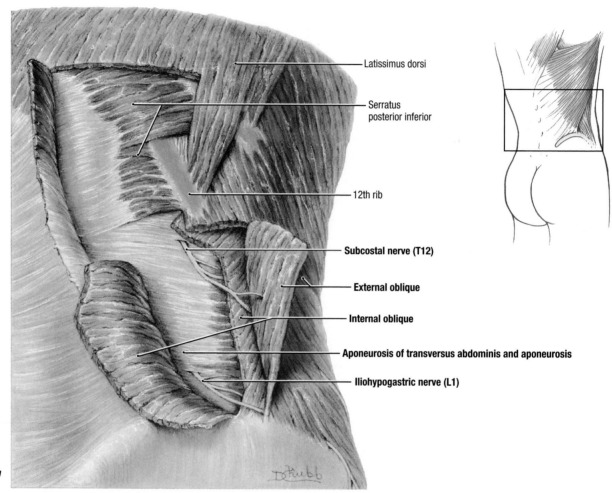

Latissimus dorsi

Serratus
posterior inferior

12th rib

Subcostal nerve (T12)

External oblique

Internal oblique

Aponeurosis of transversus abdominis and aponeurosis

Iliohypogastric nerve (L1)

Posterolateral View

2.70 Exposure of kidney—II

The external oblique muscle is incised and reflected laterally, and the internal oblique muscle is incised and reflected medially; the transversus abdominis muscle and its posterior aponeurosis are exposed where pierced by the subcostal (T12) and iliohypogastric (L1) nerves. These nerves give off motor twigs and lateral cutaneous branches and continue anteriorly between the internal oblique and transversus abdominis muscles.

2.71 Exposure of kidney—III and renal fascia

A. Dissection. The posterior aponeurosis of the transversus abdominis muscle is divided between the subcostal and iliohypogastric nerves and lateral to the oblique lateral border of the quadratus lumborum muscle; the retroperitoneal fat surrounding the kidney is exposed. **B.** Renal fascia and retroperitoneal fat, schematic transverse section. The renal fascia is within this fat; the portion of fat internal to the renal fascia is termed perinephric fat (perirenal fat capsule), and the fat immediately external is paranephric fat (pararenal fat body).

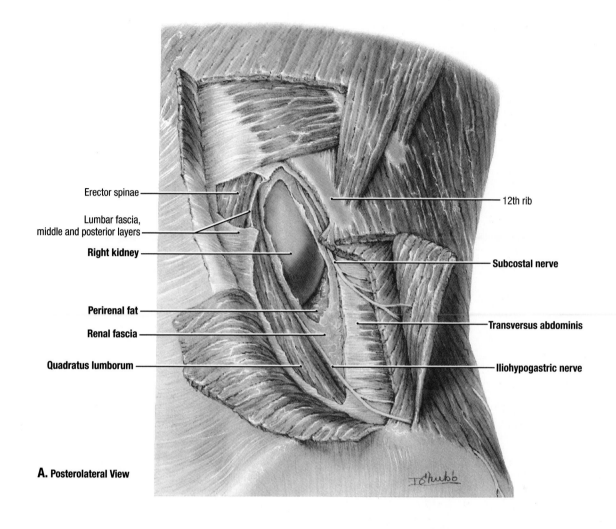

Erector spinae

Lumbar fascia,
middle and posterior layers

Right kidney

Perirenal fat

Renal fascia

Quadratus lumborum

12th rib

Subcostal nerve

Transversus abdominis

Iliohypogastric nerve

A. Posterolateral View

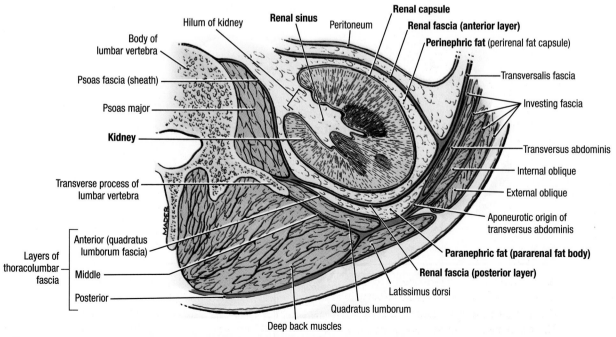

Hilum of kidney

Body of
lumbar vertebra

Psoas fascia (sheath)

Psoas major

Kidney

Transverse process of
lumbar vertebra

Layers of
thoracolumbar
fascia

Anterior (quadratus
lumborum fascia)

Middle

Posterior

Renal sinus

Peritoneum

Renal capsule

Renal fascia (anterior layer)

Perinephric fat (perirenal fat capsule)

Transversalis fascia

Investing fascia

Transversus abdominis

Internal oblique

External oblique

Aponeurotic origin of
transversus abdominis

Paranephric fat (pararenal fat body)

Renal fascia (posterior layer)

Latissimus dorsi

Quadratus lumborum

Deep back muscles

B. Transverse Section

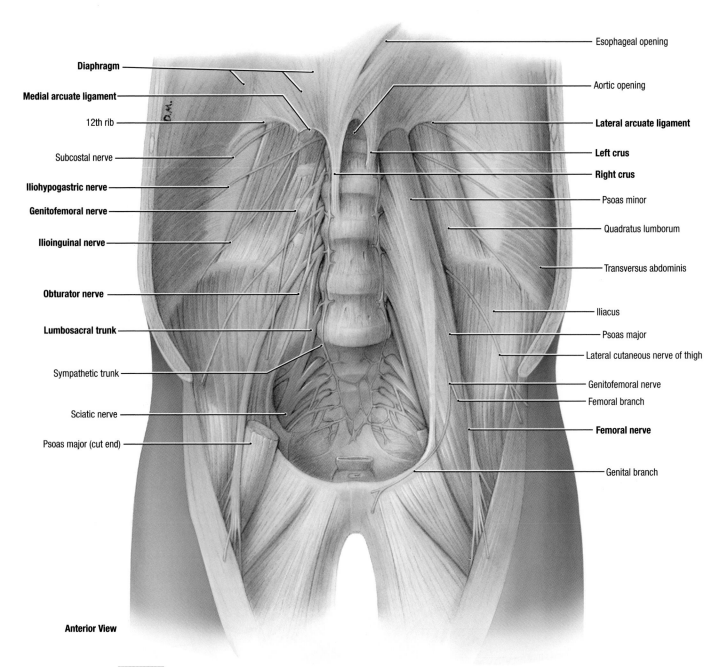

Esophageal opening

Diaphragm

Aortic opening

Medial arcuate ligament

12th rib

Lateral arcuate ligament

Subcostal nerve

Left crus

Iliohypogastric nerve

Right crus

Genitofemoral nerve

Psoas minor

Ilioinguinal nerve

Quadratus lumborum

Transversus abdominis

Obturator nerve

Iliacus

Lumbosacral trunk

Psoas major

Lateral cutaneous nerve of thigh

Sympathetic trunk

Genitofemoral nerve

Femoral branch

Sciatic nerve

Femoral nerve

Psoas major (cut end)

Genital branch

Anterior View

2.72   Lumbar plexus and vertebral attachment of diaphragm

TABLE 2.5   PRINCIPAL MUSCLES OF POSTERIOR ABDOMINAL WALL

Muscle	Superior Attachments	Inferior Attachments	Innervation	Actions
Psoas major,[a][b]	Transverse processes of lumbar vertebrae; sides of bodies of T12–L5 vertebrae and intervening invertebral discs	By a strong tendon to lesser trochanter of femur	Anterior rami of lumbar nerves (**L1, L2,** L3)	Acting inferiorly with iliacus, it flexes thigh at hip; acting superiorly, it flexes vertebral column laterally; it is used to balance the trunk; during sitting it acts inferiorly with iliacus to flex trunk
Iliacus[a]	Superior two thirds of iliac fossa, ala of sacrum; and anterior sacroiliac ligaments	Lesser trochanter of femur and shaft inferior to it, and to psoas major tendon	Femoral nerve (**L2,** L3)	Flexes thigh and stabilizes hip joint; acts with psoas major
Quadratus lumborum	Medial half of inferior border of 12th rib and tips of lumbar transverse processes	Iliolumbar ligament and internal lip of iliac crest	Anterior rami of T12 and L1-L4 nerves	Extends and laterally flexes vertebral column; fixes 12th rib during inspiration

[a]Psoas major and iliacus muscles are often described together as the iliopsoas muscle when flexion of the thigh is discussed.

[b]Psoas minor attaches proximally to the sides of bodies of T12–L1 vertebrae and intervertebral disc and distally to the pectineal line and iliopectineal eminence via the iliopectineal arch; it does not cross the hip joint. It is used to balance the trunk, in conjunction with psoas major. Innervation is from the anterior rami of lumbar nerves (L1, L2).

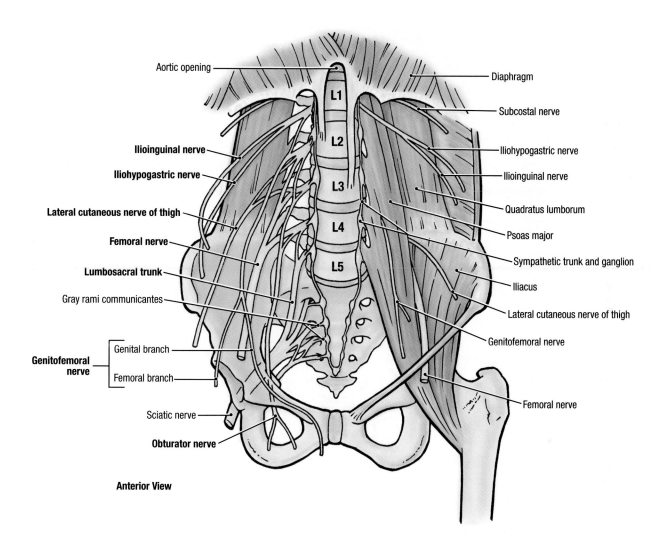

Aortic opening

Diaphragm

L1

Subcostal nerve

L2

Ilioinguinal nerve

Iliohypogastric nerve

Iliohypogastric nerve

Ilioinguinal nerve

L3

Lateral cutaneous nerve of thigh

Quadratus lumborum

L4

Femoral nerve

Psoas major

L5

Lumbosacral trunk

Sympathetic trunk and ganglion

Gray rami communicantes

Iliacus

Lateral cutaneous nerve of thigh

Genital branch

Genitofemoral nerve

Genitofemoral nerve

Femoral branch

Femoral nerve

Sciatic nerve

Obturator nerve

Anterior View

2.73   Nerves of the lumbar plexus

The lumbar plexus of nerves is in the posterior part of the psoas major, anterior to the lumbar transverse processes. This nerve network is composed of the anterior rami of L1-L4 nerves. All rami receive gray rami communicates from the sympathetic trunks. The following nerves are branches of the lumbar plexus:

- Ilioinguinal and iliohypogastric nerves (L1) arise from the anterior ramus of L1 and enter the abdomen posterior to the medial arcuate ligaments and pass inferolaterally, anterior to the quadratus lumborum muscle; they pierce the transversus abdominis muscle near the anterior superior iliac spine and pass through the internal and external oblique muscles to supply the skin of the suprapubic and inguinal regions.
- Lateral cutaneous nerve of thigh (L2, L3) runs inferolaterally on the iliacus muscle and enters the thigh posterior to the inguinal ligament, just medial to the anterior superior iliac

spine; it supplies the skin on the anterolateral surface of the thigh.
- Femoral nerve (L2-L4) emerges from the lateral border of the psoas and innervates the iliacus muscle and the extensor muscles of the knee.
- Genitofemoral nerve (L1, L2) pierces the anterior surface of the psoas major muscle and runs inferiorly on it deep to the psoas fascia; it divides lateral to the common and external iliac arteries into femoral and genital branches.
- Obturator nerve (L2-L4) emerges from the medial border of the psoas to supply the adductor muscles of the thigh.
- Lumbosacral trunk (L4, L5) passes over the ala (wing) of the sacrum and descends into the pelvis to take part in the formation of the sacral plexus along with the anterior rami of S1-S4 nerves.

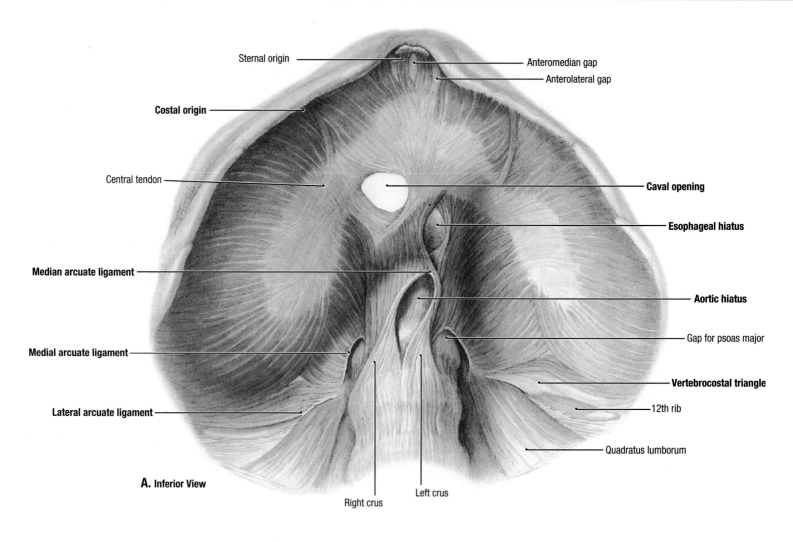

Sternal origin — Anteromedian gap
Anterolateral gap
Costal origin —
Central tendon — **Caval opening**
Esophageal hiatus
Median arcuate ligament — **Aortic hiatus**
Gap for psoas major
Medial arcuate ligament — **Vertebrocostal triangle**
12th rib
Lateral arcuate ligament — Quadratus lumborum
A. Inferior View
Right crus   Left crus

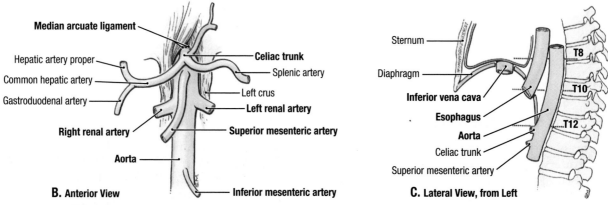

Median arcuate ligament —
Hepatic artery proper — **Celiac trunk**
— Splenic artery
Common hepatic artery — — Left crus
Gastroduodenal artery — **Left renal artery**
Right renal artery — **Superior mesenteric artery**
Aorta —
B. Anterior View   **Inferior mesenteric artery**

Sternum — T8
Diaphragm —
Inferior vena cava — T10
Esophagus —
Aorta — T12
Celiac trunk —
Superior mesenteric artery —
C. Lateral View, from Left

2.74   **Diaphragm**

A. Dissection. The clover-shaped central tendon is the aponeurotic insertion of the muscle.
The diaphragm in this specimen fails to arise from the left lateral arcuate ligament, leaving
a potential opening, the vertebrocostal triangle, through which abdominal contents may be
herniated into the thoracic cavity. **B.** Median arcuate ligament and branches of the aorta.
C. Openings of the diaphragm. There are three major openings through which major structures pass from the thorax into the abdomen: the caval opening for the inferior vena cava,
most anterior, at the T8 vertebral level to the right of the midline; the esophageal hiatus,
intermediate, at T10 level and to the left; and the aortic hiatus, which allows the aorta to
pass posterior to the vertebral attachment of the diaphragm in the midline at T12.

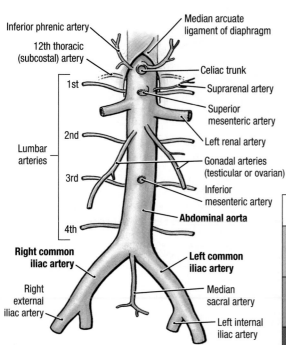

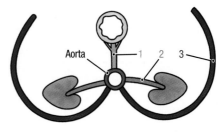

Three Vascular Planes

	Vascular plane	Class	Distribution	Abdominal Branches (Arteries)	Vertebral Level
1	Anterior midline	Unpaired visceral	Alimentary tract	Celiac	T12
				Superior mesenteric (SMA)	L1
				Inferior mesenteric (IMA)	L3
2	Lateral	Paired visceral	Urogenital and endocrine organs	Suprarenal	L1
				Renal	L1
				Gonadal (testicular or ovarian)	L2
3	Postero-lateral	Paired parietal (segmental)	Diaphragm Body Wall	Subcostal	T12
				Inferior phrenic	T12
				Lumbar	L1–L4

A. Anterior View

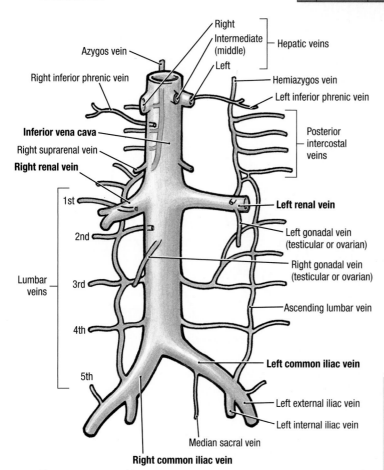

B. Anterior View

2.75 **Abdominal aorta and inferior vena cava and their branches**

A. Branches of abdominal aorta. **B.** Tributaries of the inferior vena cava (IVC). The asymmetry in the renal and common iliac veins reflects the placement of the IVC to the right of the midline.

Rupture of an aneurysm (localized enlargement) of the abdominal aorta causes severe pain in the abdomen or back. If unrecognized, a ruptured aneurysm has a mortality of nearly 90% because of heavy blood loss. Surgeons can repair an aneurysm by opening it, inserting a prosthetic graft (such as one made of Dacron), and sewing the wall of the aneurysmal aorta over the graft to protect it. Aneurysms may also be treated by endovascular catheterization procedures.

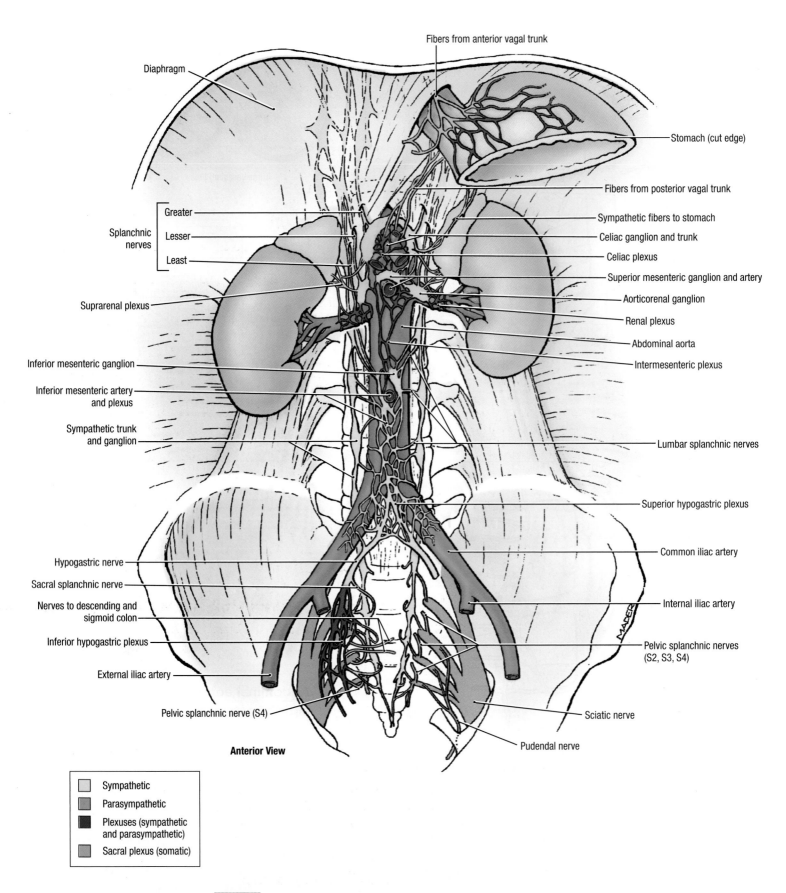

Fibers from anterior vagal trunk

Diaphragm

Stomach (cut edge)

Fibers from posterior vagal trunk

Sympathetic fibers to stomach

Splanchnic nerves
- Greater
- Lesser
- Least

Celiac ganglion and trunk

Celiac plexus

Superior mesenteric ganglion and artery

Aorticorenal ganglion

Suprarenal plexus

Renal plexus

Abdominal aorta

Inferior mesenteric ganglion

Intermesenteric plexus

Inferior mesenteric artery and plexus

Sympathetic trunk and ganglion

Lumbar splanchnic nerves

Superior hypogastric plexus

Common iliac artery

Hypogastric nerve

Internal iliac artery

Sacral splanchnic nerve

Nerves to descending and sigmoid colon

Pelvic splanchnic nerves (S2, S3, S4)

Inferior hypogastric plexus

External iliac artery

Pelvic splanchnic nerve (S4)

Sciatic nerve

Pudendal nerve

Anterior View

Legend:
- Sympathetic
- Parasympathetic
- Plexuses (sympathetic and parasympathetic)
- Sacral plexus (somatic)

2.76 **Abdominopelvic nerve plexuses and ganglia**

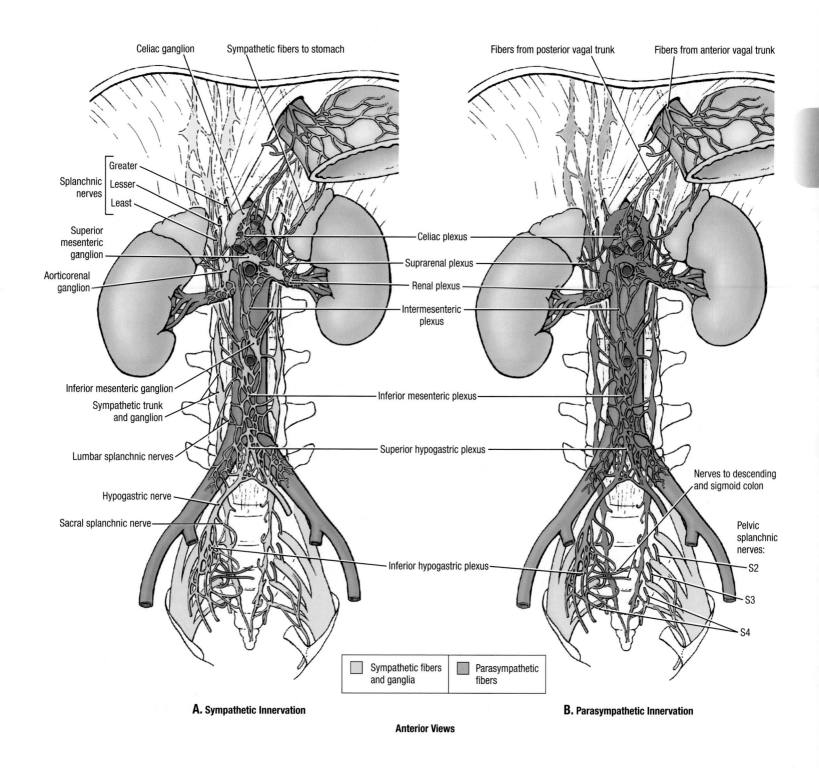

Celiac ganglion

Sympathetic fibers to stomach

Fibers from posterior vagal trunk

Fibers from anterior vagal trunk

Splanchnic nerves
- Greater
- Lesser
- Least

Superior mesenteric ganglion

Aorticorenal ganglion

Celiac plexus

Suprarenal plexus

Renal plexus

Intermesenteric plexus

Inferior mesenteric ganglion

Sympathetic trunk and ganglion

Lumbar splanchnic nerves

Inferior mesenteric plexus

Hypogastric nerve

Sacral splanchnic nerve

Superior hypogastric plexus

Nerves to descending and sigmoid colon

Pelvic splanchnic nerves:
- S2
- S3
- S4

Inferior hypogastric plexus

| Sympathetic fibers and ganglia | Parasympathetic fibers |

A. Sympathetic Innervation

B. Parasympathetic Innervation

Anterior Views

2.77   Overview of autonomic nervous system

A. Sympathetic. **B.** Parasympathetic.

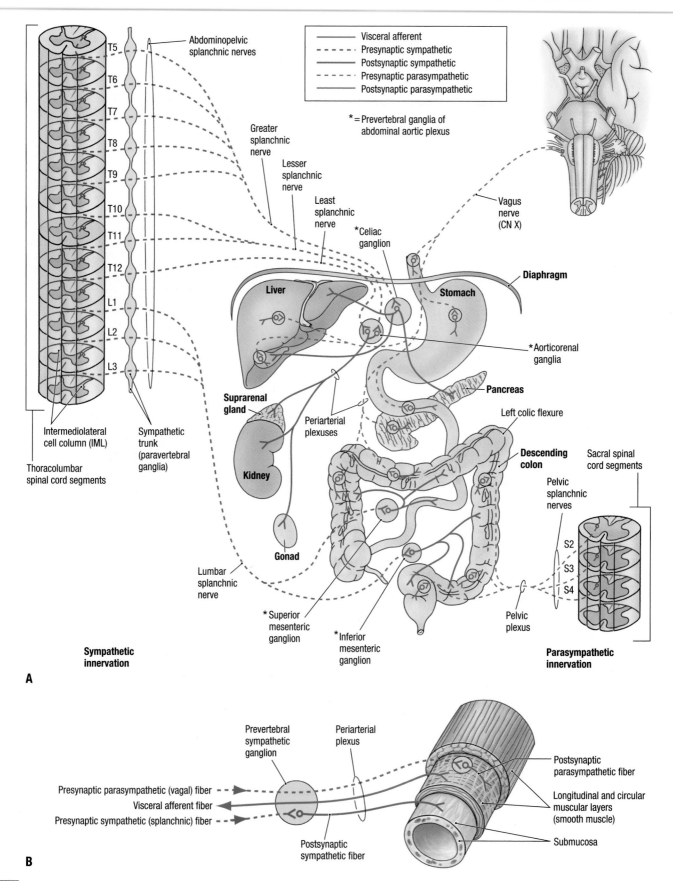

A. Overview. B. Fibers supplying the intrinsic plexuses of abdominal viscera.

2.78 Origin and distribution of presynaptic and postsynaptic sympathetic and parasympathetic fibers, and the ganglia involved in supplying abdominal viscera

TABLE 2.6   AUTONOMIC INNERVATION OF THE ABDOMINAL VISCERA (SPLANCHNIC NERVES)

Splanchnic Nerves	Autonomic Fiber Type[a]	System	Origin	Destination
A. **Cardiopulmonary** (Cervical and upper thoracic)	Postsynaptic		Cervical and upper thoracic sympathetic trunk	Thoracic cavity (viscera superior to level of diaphragm)
B. **Abdominopelvic**			Lower thoracic and abdomino-pelvic sympathetic trunk:	Abdominopelvic cavity (prevertebral ganglia serving viscera and suprarenal glands inferior to level of diaphragm)

1. Lower thoracic
  a. Greater
  b. Lesser
  c. Least
2. Lumbar
 	
3. Sacral
	Presynaptic	Sympathetic	1. Thoracic sympathetic trunk:
			  a. T5–T9 or T10 level
			  b. T10–T11 level
			  c. T12 level
			2. Abdominal sympathetic trunk
			
			3. Pelvic (sacral) sympathetic trunk
				1. Abdominal prevertebral ganglia:
				  a. Celiac ganglia
				  b. Aorticorenal ganglia
				  c. & 2. Other abdominal prevertebral ganglia (superior and inferior mesenteric, and of inter-mesenteric/hypogastric plexuses
				3. Pelvic prevertebral ganglia

C. **Pelvic**	Presynaptic	Parasympathetic	Anterior rami of S2–S4 spinal nerves	Intrinsic ganglia of descending and sigmoid colon, rectum, and pelvic viscera

[a]Splanchnic nerves also convey visceral afferent fibers, which are not part of the autonomic nervous system.

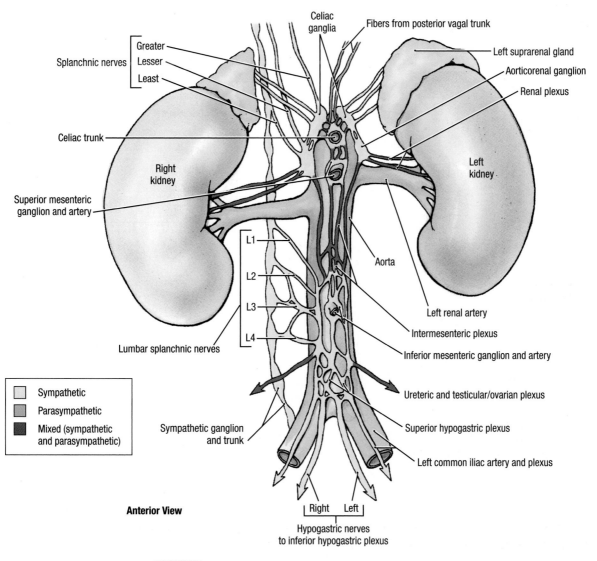

2.79   **Abdominal nerve plexuses and ganglia**

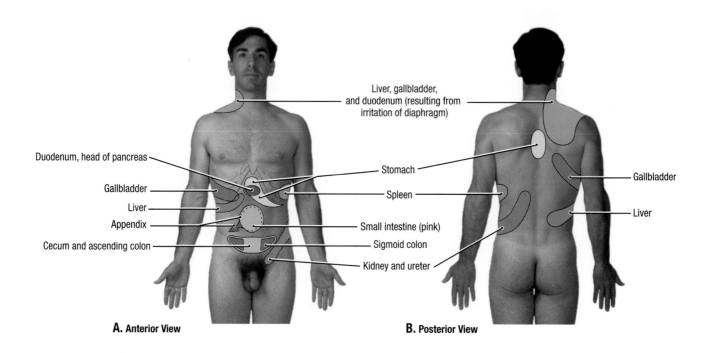

Liver, gallbladder, and duodenum (resulting from irritation of diaphragm)

Duodenum, head of pancreas

Gallbladder

Liver

Appendix

Cecum and ascending colon

Stomach

Spleen

Small intestine (pink)

Sigmoid colon

Kidney and ureter

Gallbladder

Liver

A. Anterior View

B. Posterior View

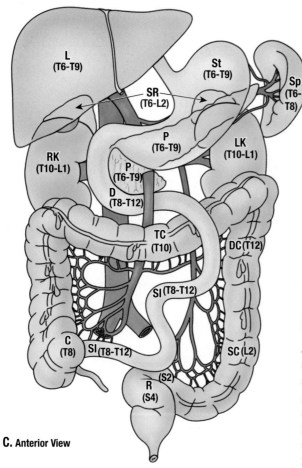

C. Anterior View

C	Cecum	RK	Right kidney
D	Duodenum	SC	Sigmoid colon
DC	Descending colon	SI	Small intestine
L	Liver	Sp	Spleen
LK	Left kidney	SR	Suprarenal glands
P	Pancreas	St	Stomach
R	Rectum	TC	Transverse colon

2.80 **Surface projections of visceral pain**

A. and **B.** Pain arising from a viscus (organ) varies from dull to severe but is poorly localized. It radiates to the part of the body supplied by somatic sensory fibers associated with the same spinal ganglion and segment of the spinal cord that receive visceral sensory (autonomic) fibers from the viscus concerned. The pain is interpreted by the brain as though the irritation occurred in the area of skin supplied by the posterior roots of the affected segments. This is called visceral referred pain. **C.** Approximate spinal cord segments and spinal sensory ganglia involved in sympathetic and visceral afferent (pain) innervation of abdominal viscera.

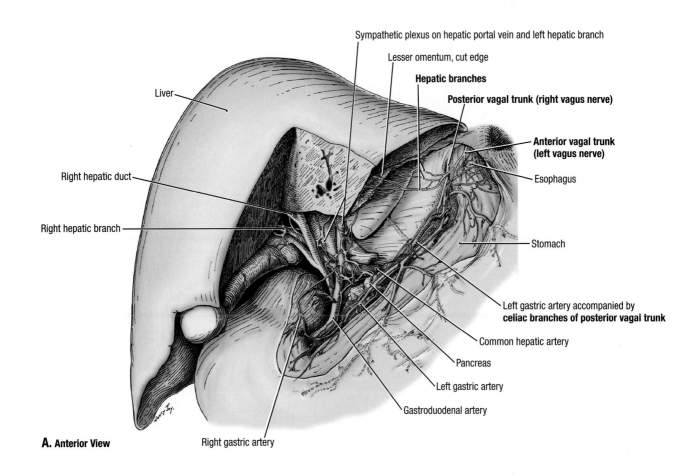

Sympathetic plexus on hepatic portal vein and left hepatic branch

Lesser omentum, cut edge

Hepatic branches

Posterior vagal trunk (right vagus nerve)

Anterior vagal trunk (left vagus nerve)

Esophagus

Liver

Right hepatic duct

Right hepatic branch

Stomach

Left gastric artery accompanied by **celiac branches of posterior vagal trunk**

Common hepatic artery

Pancreas

Left gastric artery

Gastroduodenal artery

Right gastric artery

A. Anterior View

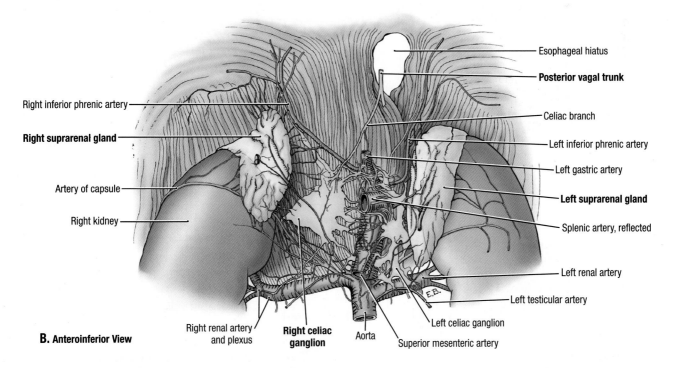

Esophageal hiatus

Posterior vagal trunk

Right inferior phrenic artery

Right suprarenal gland

Celiac branch

Left inferior phrenic artery

Left gastric artery

Left suprarenal gland

Splenic artery, reflected

Artery of capsule

Right kidney

Left renal artery

Left testicular artery

Right renal artery and plexus

Right celiac ganglion

Aorta

Superior mesenteric artery

Left celiac ganglion

B. Anteroinferior View

2.81   Vagus nerves in abdomen

A. Anterior and posterior vagal trunks. **B.** Celiac plexus and ganglia and suprarenal glands.

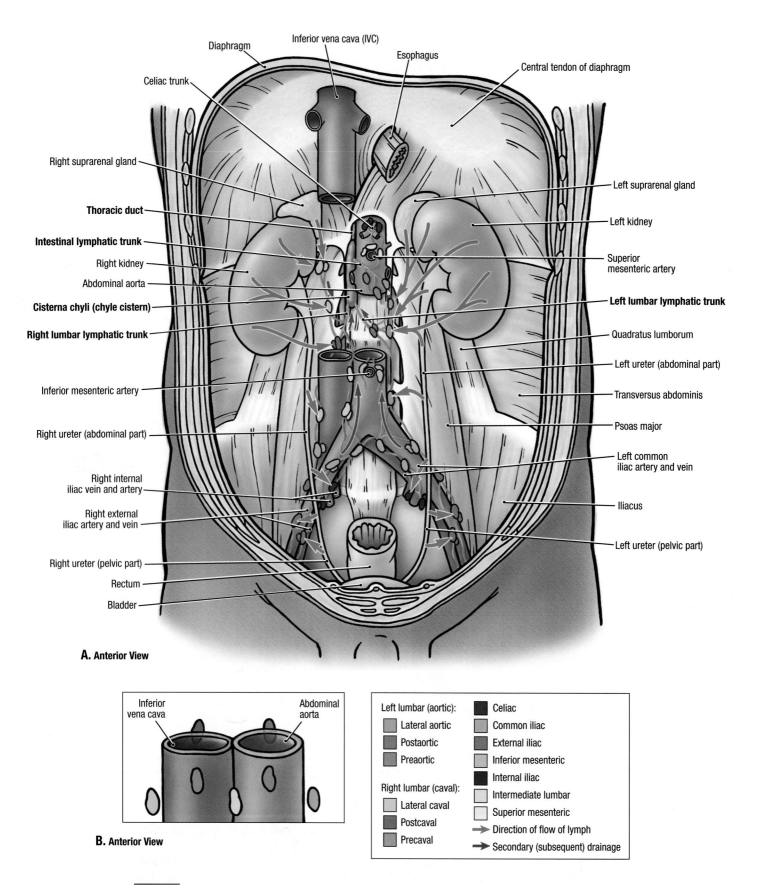

Diaphragm

Inferior vena cava (IVC)

Esophagus

Central tendon of diaphragm

Celiac trunk

Right suprarenal gland

Thoracic duct

Intestinal lymphatic trunk

Right kidney

Abdominal aorta

Cisterna chyli (chyle cistern)

Right lumbar lymphatic trunk

Inferior mesenteric artery

Right ureter (abdominal part)

Right internal
iliac vein and artery

Right external
iliac artery and vein

Right ureter (pelvic part)

Rectum

Bladder

Left suprarenal gland

Left kidney

Superior
mesenteric artery

Left lumbar lymphatic trunk

Quadratus lumborum

Left ureter (abdominal part)

Transversus abdominis

Psoas major

Left common
iliac artery and vein

Iliacus

Left ureter (pelvic part)

A. Anterior View

Inferior
vena cava

Abdominal
aorta

B. Anterior View

Left lumbar (aortic):
- Lateral aortic
- Postaortic
- Preaortic

Right lumbar (caval):
- Lateral caval
- Postcaval
- Precaval

- Celiac
- Common iliac
- External iliac
- Inferior mesenteric
- Internal iliac
- Intermediate lumbar
- Superior mesenteric
→ Direction of flow of lymph
→ Secondary (subsequent) drainage

2.82 Lymphatic drainage of suprarenal glands, kidneys, and ureters

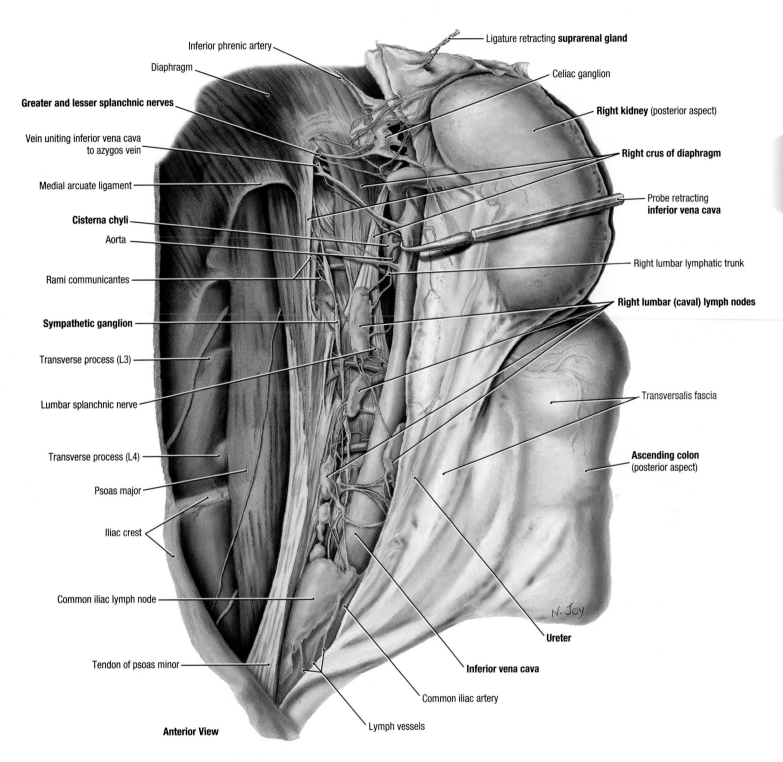

Inferior phrenic artery

Diaphragm

Greater and lesser splanchnic nerves

Vein uniting inferior vena cava
to azygos vein

Medial arcuate ligament

Cisterna chyli

Aorta

Rami communicantes

Sympathetic ganglion

Transverse process (L3)

Lumbar splanchnic nerve

Transverse process (L4)

Psoas major

Iliac crest

Common iliac lymph node

Tendon of psoas minor

Anterior View

Ligature retracting **suprarenal gland**

Celiac ganglion

Right kidney (posterior aspect)

Right crus of diaphragm

Probe retracting
inferior vena cava

Right lumbar lymphatic trunk

Right lumbar (caval) lymph nodes

Transversalis fascia

Ascending colon
(posterior aspect)

Ureter

Inferior vena cava

Common iliac artery

Lymph vessels

N. Joy

2.83   **Lumbar lymph nodes, sympathetic trunk, nerves, and ganglia**

The right suprarenal gland, kidney, ureter, and colon are reflected to the left; the inferior vena cava is pulled medially, and the third and fourth lumbar veins are removed. In this specimen, the greater and lesser splanchnic nerves, the sympathetic trunk, and a communicating vein pass through an unusually wide cleft in the right crus. The splanchnic nerves convey preganglionic fibers arising from the cell bodies in the (thoracolumbar) sympathetic trunk. The greater splanchnic nerve is from thoracic ganglia 5 to 9, and the lesser from thoracic ganglia 10 to 11.

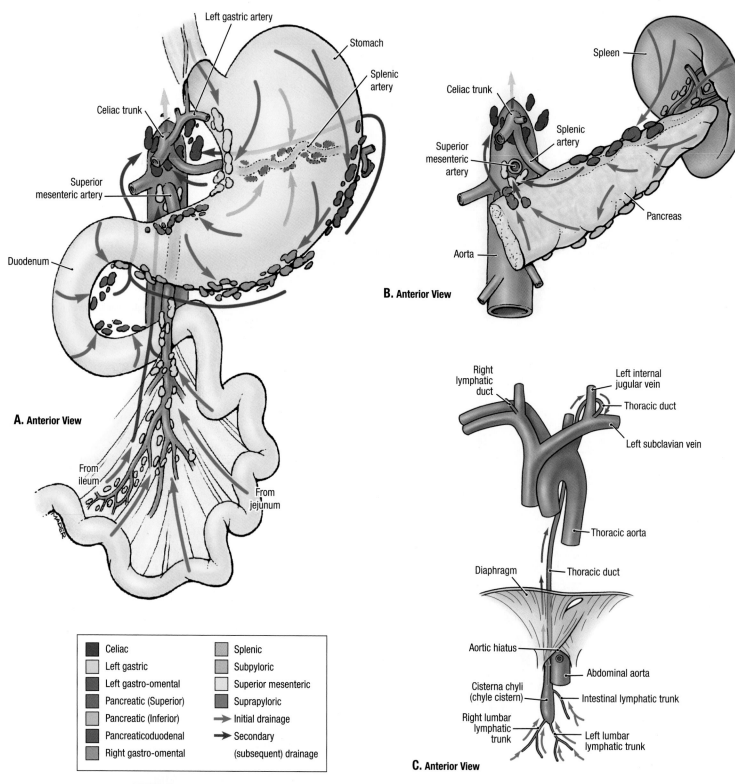

Left gastric artery

Stomach

Splenic artery

Celiac trunk

Superior mesenteric artery

Duodenum

A. Anterior View

From ileum

From jejunum

KAGER

Spleen

Celiac trunk

Splenic artery

Superior mesenteric artery

Pancreas

Aorta

B. Anterior View

Right lymphatic duct

Left internal jugular vein

Thoracic duct

Left subclavian vein

Thoracic aorta

Thoracic duct

Diaphragm

Aortic hiatus

Abdominal aorta

Cisterna chyli (chyle cistern)

Intestinal lymphatic trunk

Right lumbar lymphatic trunk

Left lumbar lymphatic trunk

C. Anterior View

Celiac	Splenic
Left gastric	Subpyloric
Left gastro-omental	Superior mesenteric
Pancreatic (Superior)	Suprapyloric
Pancreatic (Inferior)	→ Initial drainage
Pancreaticoduodenal	→ Secondary
Right gastro-omental	(subsequent) drainage

2.84 **Lymphatic drainage**

A. Stomach and small intestine. **B.** Spleen and pancreas. **C.** Drainage from lumbar and intestinal lymphatic trunks. The *arrows* indicate the direction of lymph flow; each group of lymph nodes is color coded. Lymph from the abdominal nodes drains into the cisterna chyli, origin of the inferior end of the thoracic duct. The thoracic duct receives all lymph that forms inferior to the diaphragm and left upper quadrant (thorax and left upper limb) and empties into the junction of the left subclavian and left internal jugular veins.

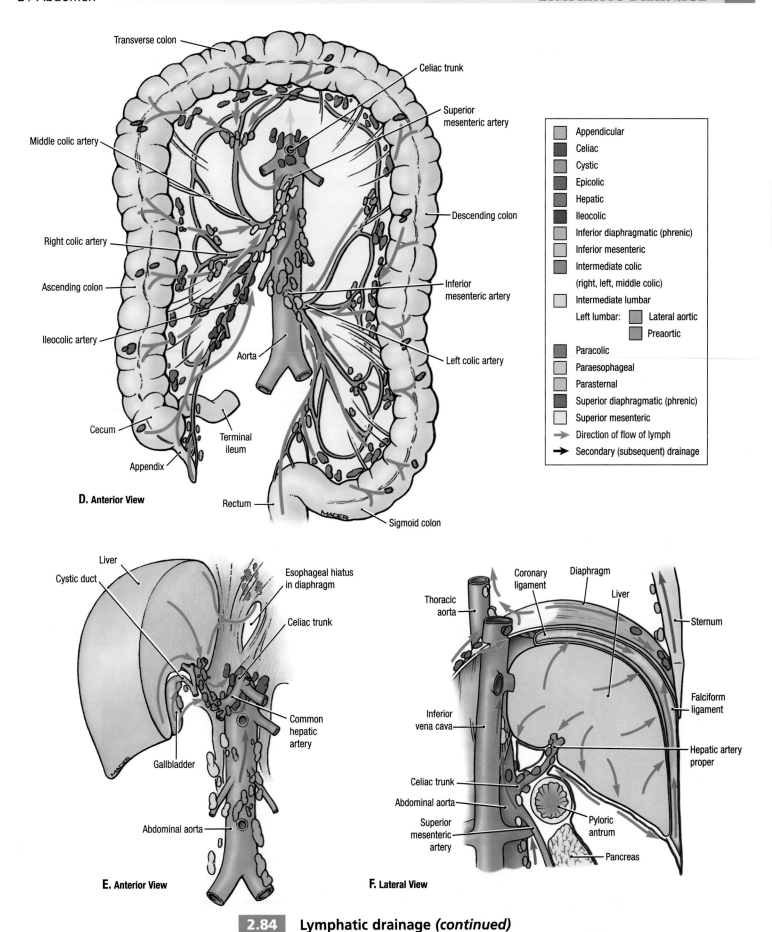

D. Anterior View

E. Anterior View

F. Lateral View

2.84   **Lymphatic drainage (continued)**

D. Large intestine. **E.** Liver and gallbladder. **F.** Liver.

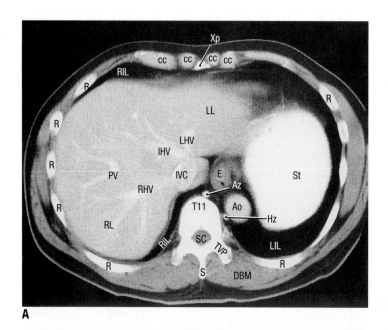

A

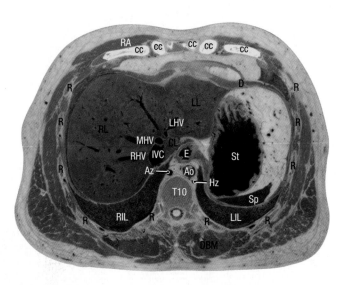

B

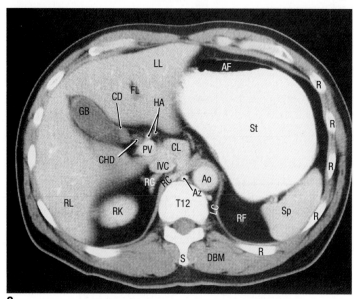

C

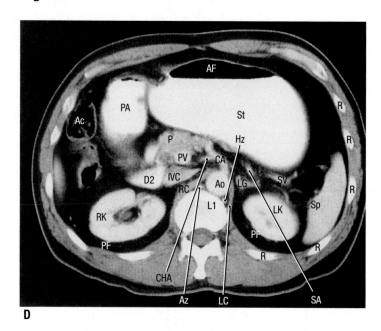

D

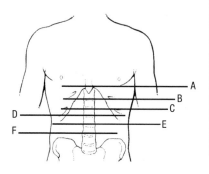

Ac	Ascending colon	DBM	Deep back muscles	LC	Left crus of diaphragm
AF	Air-fluid level of stomach	Dc	Descending colon	LG	Left suprarenal gland
Ao	Aorta	D2	Descending part of duodenum	LHV	Left hepatic vein
Az	Azygos vein	D3	Inferior part of duodenum	LIL	Left inferior lobe of lung
CA	Celiac artery	E	Esophagus	LK	Left kidney
cc	Costal cartilage	FL	Falciform ligament	LL	Left lobe of liver
CD	Cystic duct	GB	Gallbladder	LRV	Left renal vein
CHA	Common hepatic artery	HA	Hepatic artery	LU	Left ureter
CHD	Common hepatic duct	Hz	Hemiazygos vein	IHV	Intermediate hepatic vein
CL	Caudate lobe of liver	IMV	Inferior mesenteric vein	P	Pancreas
D	Diaphragm	IVC	Inferior vena cava	PA	Pyloric antrum of stomach

2.85   Transverse or horizontal (axial) MRIs of the abdomen

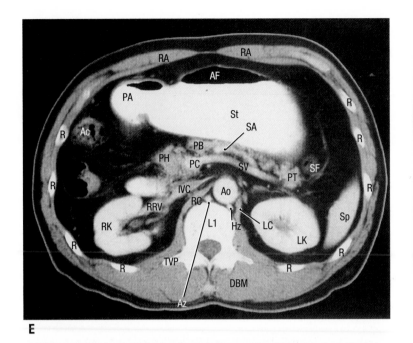

E

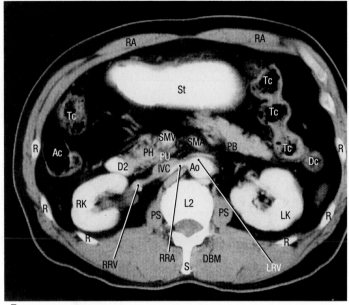

F

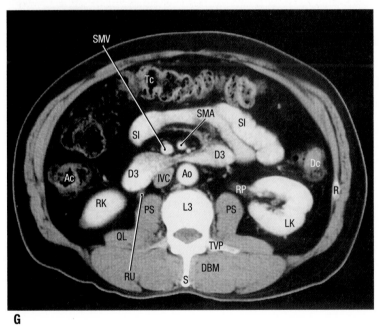

G

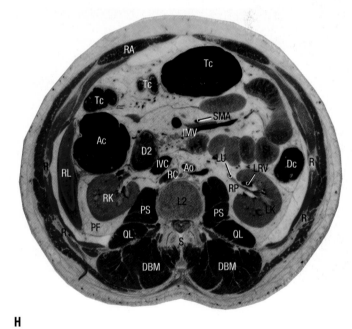

H

PB	Body of pancreas	R	Rib	RP	Renal pelvis	SMA	Superior mesenteric artery
PC	Portal confluence	RA	Rectus abdominis	RRA	Right renal artery	SMV	Superior mesenteric vein
PF	Perinephric fat	RC	Right crus of diaphragm	RRV	Right renal vein	Sp	Spleen
PH	Head of pancreas	RF	Retroperitoneal fat	RU	Right ureter	St	Stomach
PS	Psoas muscle	RG	Right suprarenal gland	S	Spinous process	SV	Splenic vein
PT	Tail of pancreas	RHV	Right hepatic vein	SA	Splenic artery	Tc	Transverse colon
PU	Uncinate process of pancreas	RIL	Right inferior lobe of lung	SC	Spinal cord	TVP	Transverse process
PV	Hepatic portal vein	RK	Right kidney	SF	Splenic flexure	Xp	Xiphoid process
QL	Quadratus lumborum	RL	Right lobe of liver	SI	Small intestine		

2.85 **Transverse or horizontal (axial) MRIs of the abdomen (*continued*)**

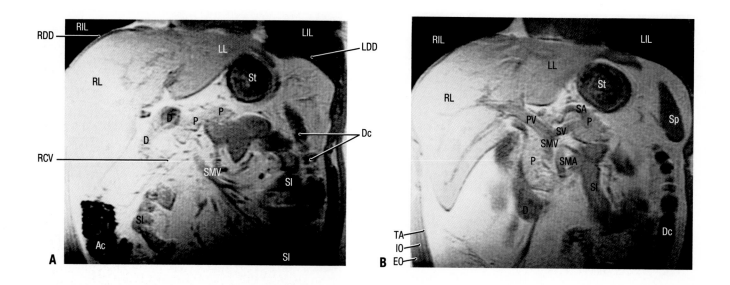

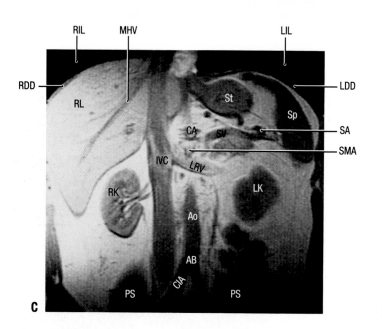

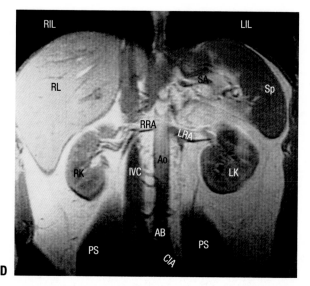

AB	Aortic bifurcation	LIL	Left lung (inferior lobe)	RK	Right kidney
Ac	Ascending colon	LK	Left kidney	RL	Right lobe of liver
Ao	Aorta	LL	Left lobe of liver	RRA	Right renal artery
CA	Celiac artery	LRA	Left renal artery	SA	Splenic artery
CIA	Common iliac artery	LRV	Left renal vein	SI	Small intestine
D	Duodenum	MHV	Middle hepatic vein	SMA	Superior mesenteric artery
Dc	Descending colon	P	Pancreas	SMV	Superior mesenteric vein
E	Esophagus	PV	Portal vein	Sp	Spleen
EO	External oblique	PS	Psoas	St	Stomach
IO	Internal oblique	RCV	Right colic vein	SV	Splenic vein
IVC	Inferior vena cava	RDD	Right dome of diaphragm	TA	Transversus abdominis
LDD	Left dome of diaphragm	RIL	Right lung (inferior lobe)		

2.86   Coronal MRIs of the abdomen

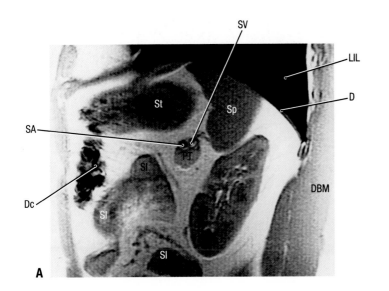

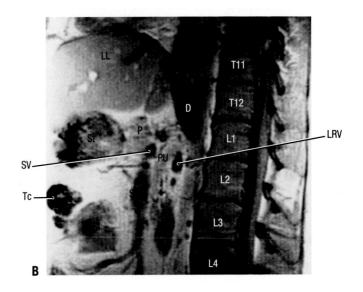

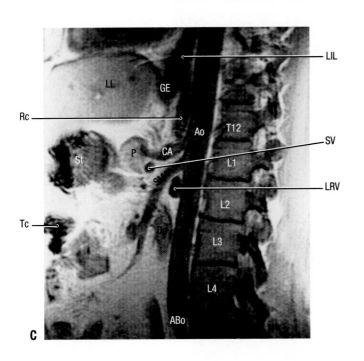

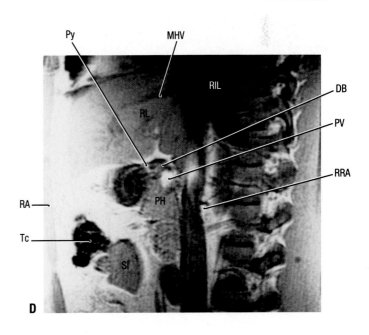

Ao	Aorta	LL	Left lobe of liver	RC	Right crus
ABo	Bifurcation of aorta	LRV	Left renal vein	RIL	Inferior lobe of right lung
CA	Celiac artery	MHV	Middle hepatic vein	RL	Right lobe of right liver
D	Diaphragm	P	Pancreas	RRA	Right renal artery
DB	Bulb of duodenum	Pa	Pyloric antrum	SA	Splenic artery
Dc	Descending colon	PC	Portal confluence	SI	Small intestine
Do	Duodenum	PH	Head of pancreas	SMA	Superior mesenteric artery
DBM	Deep back muscles	PT	Tail of pancreas	SMV	Superior mesenteric vein
GE	Gastroesophageal junction	PV	Portal vein	Sp	Spleen
IVC	Inferior vena cava	PU	Uncinate process of pancreas	St	Stomach
LIL	Inferior lobe of left lung	Py	Pylorus of stomach	SV	Splenic vein
LK	Left kidney	RA	Rectus abdominus	Tc	Transverse colon

2.87   **Sagittal MRIs of the abdomen**

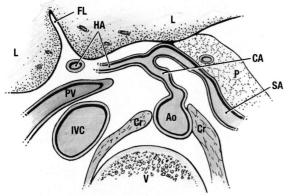

A. Transverse Section, Inferior View

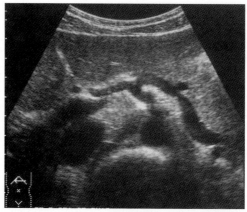

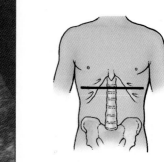

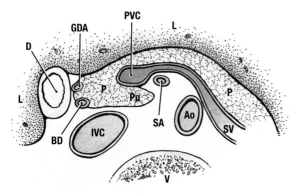

B. Transverse Section, Inferior View

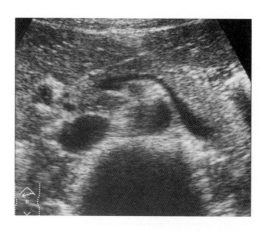

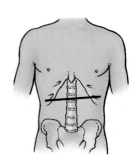

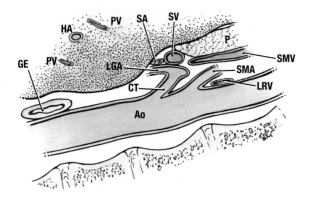

C. Median Section, Right Lateral View

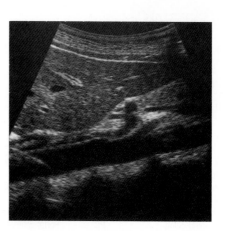

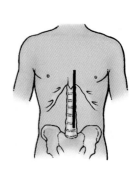

2.88 **Ultrasound scans and MR angiogram of the abdomen**

A. Transverse ultrasound scan through celiac trunk. **B.** Transverse ultrasound scan through pancreas. **C** and **D.** Sagittal ultrasound scans through the aorta, celiac trunk, and superior mesenteric artery. (**D.** With Doppler.) **E.** MR angiogram of abdominal aorta and branches. **F.** Transverse ultrasound scan at hilum of left kidney with the left renal artery and vein (with Doppler). **G.** Sagittal ultrasound scan of the right kidney.

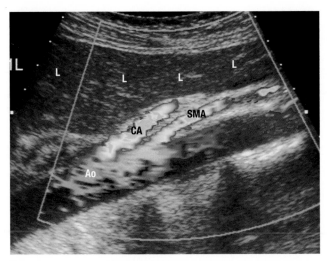

D. Median Section, Right Lateral View

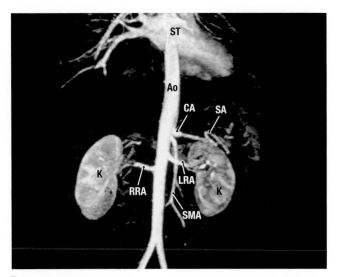

E. Anterior View

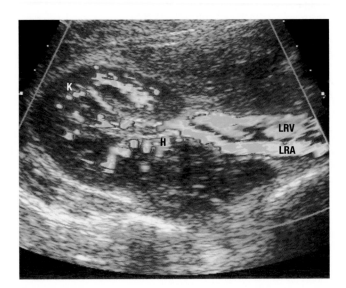

F. Transverse Section

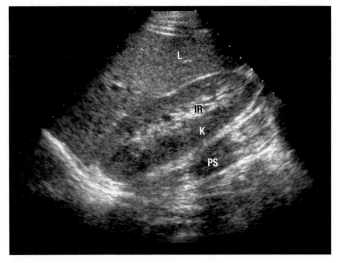

G. Sagittal Section, Right Lateral View

A major advantage of ultrasonography is its ability to produce real-time images, demonstrating motion of structures and flow within blood vessels. In Doppler ultrasonography (**D** and **F**) the shifts in frequency between emitted ultrasonic waves and their echoes are used to measure the velocities of moving objects. This technique is based on the principle of the Doppler effect. Blood flow through vessels is displayed in color, superimposed on the two-dimensional cross-sectional image. (slow flow: blue, fast flow: orange)

Ao	Aorta	IR	Intrarenal fat	PV	Portal vein		
BD	Bile duct	IVC	Inferior vena cava	PVC	Portal venous confluence		
CA	Celiac artery	K	Cortex of kidney	RRA	Right renal artery		
Cr	Crus of diaphragm	L	Liver	SA	Splenic artery		
D	Duodenum	LGA	Left gastric artery	SMA	Superior mesenteric artery		
FL	Falciform ligament	LRA	Left renal artery	SMV	Superior mesenteric vein		
GDA	Gastroduodenal artery	LRV	Left renal vein	ST	Stomach		
GE	Gastroesophageal junction	P	Pancreas	SV	Splenic vein		
H	Hilum of kidney	PS	Psoas	V	Vertebra		
HA	Hepatic artery	Pu	Uncinate process of pancreas				

2.88   **Ultrasound scans and MR angiogram of the abdomen *(continued)***

CHAPTER 3

PELVIS AND PERINEUM

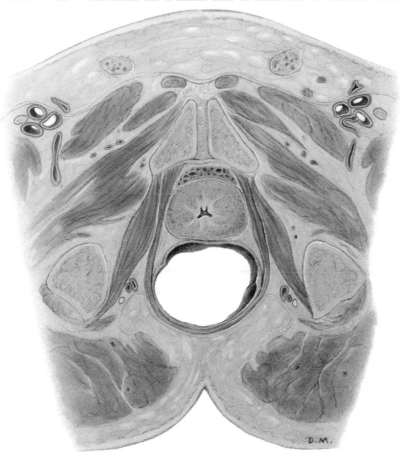

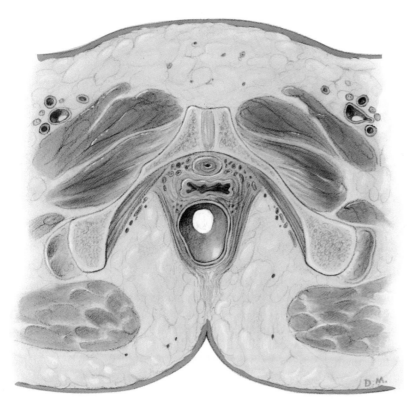

- Pelvic Girdle **194**
- Ligaments of Pelvic Girdle **200**
- Floor and Walls of Pelvis **202**
- Sacral and Coccygeal Plexuses **206**
- Peritoneal Reflections in Pelvis **208**
- Rectum and Anal Canal **210**
- Organs of Male Pelvis **216**
- Vessels of Male Pelvis **224**
- Lymphatic Drainage of Male Pelvis and Perineum **228**
- Innervation of Male Pelvic Organs **230**
- Organs of Female Pelvis **232**
- Vessels of Female Pelvis **240**
- Lymphatic Drainage of Female Pelvis and Perineum **244**
- Innervation of Female Pelvic Organs **246**
- Subperitoneal Region of Pelvis **250**
- Surface Anatomy of Perineum **252**
- Overview of Male and Female Perineum **254**
- Male Perineum **261**
- Female Perineum **269**
- Imaging of Pelvis and Perineum **276**

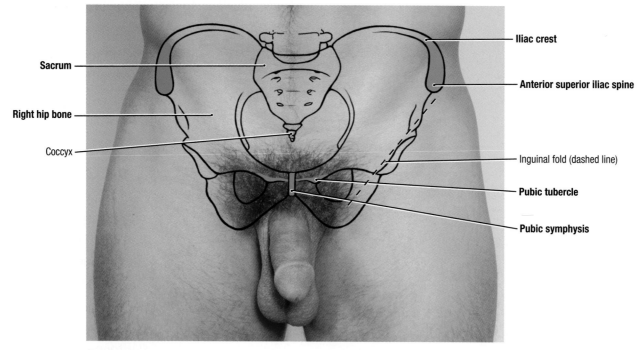

Sacrum

Right hip bone

Coccyx

Iliac crest

Anterior superior iliac spine

Inguinal fold (dashed line)

Pubic tubercle

Pubic symphysis

A. Anterior View

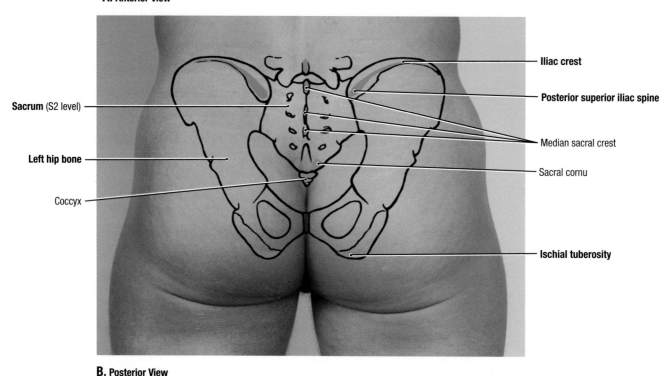

Sacrum (S2 level)

Left hip bone

Coccyx

Iliac crest

Posterior superior iliac spine

Median sacral crest

Sacral cornu

Ischial tuberosity

B. Posterior View

3.1   **Surface anatomy of the male pelvic girdle**

The pelvic girdle (bony pelvis) is a basin-shaped ring of three bones (right and left hip bones and sacrum) that connects the vertebral column to the femora. Palpable features (*green*) should be symmetrical across the midline. **A.** The anterior third of the iliac crests are subcutaneous and usually easily palpable. The remainder of the crests may also be palpable, depending on the thickness of the overlying subcutaneous tissue (fat). The inguinal ligament spans between the palpable anterior superior iliac spine (ASIS) and pubic tubercle, located superior to the lateral and medial ends of the inguinal fold. **B.** The posterior superior iliac spine is usually palpable and often lies deep to a visible dimple, indicating the S-2 vertebral level. The ischial tuberosities may be palpated when the thigh is flexed at the hip joint.

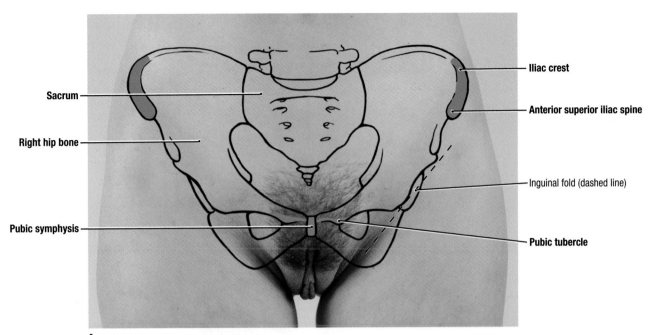

Sacrum

Right hip bone

Pubic symphysis

Iliac crest

Anterior superior iliac spine

Inguinal fold (dashed line)

Pubic tubercle

A. Anterior View

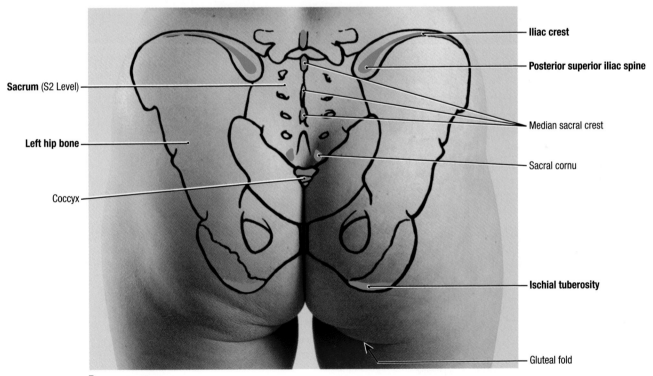

Sacrum (S2 Level)

Left hip bone

Coccyx

Iliac crest

Posterior superior iliac spine

Median sacral crest

Sacral cornu

Ischial tuberosity

Gluteal fold

B. Posterior View

3.2   **Surface anatomy of the female pelvic girdle**

The female pelvic girdle is relatively wider and shallower than that of the male, related to its additional roles of bearing the weight of the gravid uterus in late pregnancy, and allowing passage of the fetus through the pelvic outlet during childbirth (parturition). (*Green:* palpable features) **A.** The hip bones are joined anteriorly at the pubic symphysis. The presence of a thick overlying pubic fat-pad forming the mons pubis may interfere with palpation of the pubic tubercles and symphysis. **B.** Posteriorly the hip bones are joined to the sacrum at the sacroiliac joints.

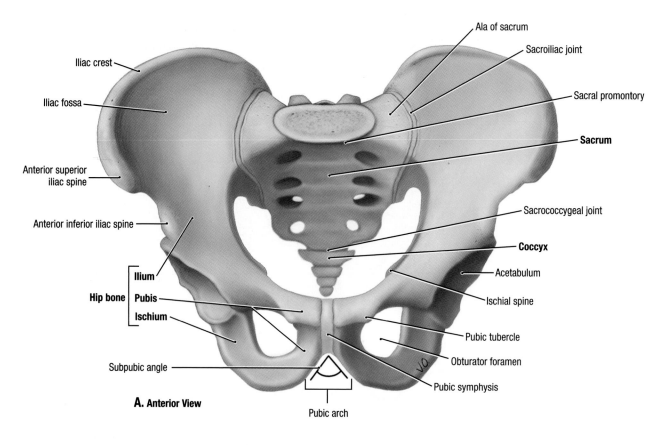

Iliac crest

Iliac fossa

Anterior superior
iliac spine

Anterior inferior iliac spine

Ilium

Hip bone Pubis

Ischium

Subpubic angle

A. Anterior View

Ala of sacrum

Sacroiliac joint

Sacral promontory

Sacrum

Sacrococcygeal joint

Coccyx

Acetabulum

Ischial spine

Pubic tubercle

Obturator foramen

Pubic symphysis

Pubic arch

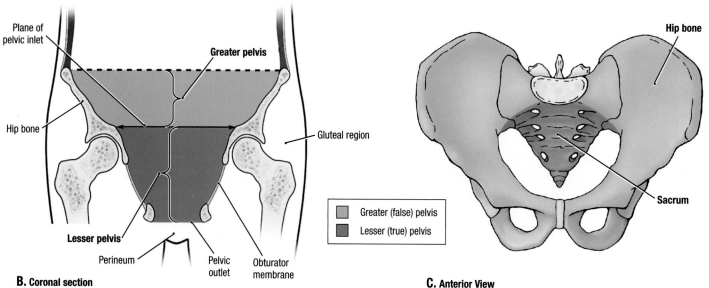

Plane of
pelvic inlet

Greater pelvis

Hip bone

Gluteal region

Lesser pelvis

Perineum   Pelvic
            outlet   Obturator
                      membrane

B. Coronal section

| | Greater (false) pelvis |
| | Lesser (true) pelvis |

Hip bone

Sacrum

C. Anterior View

3.3   Bones and divisions of pelvis

A. Bones of pelvis. The three bones composing the pelvis are the pubis, ischium, and ilium. **B** and **C.** Lesser and greater pelvis, schematic illustrations. The plane of the pelvic inlet (*double-headed arrow* in **B**) separates the greater pelvis (part of the abdominal cavity) from the lesser pelvis (pelvic cavity).

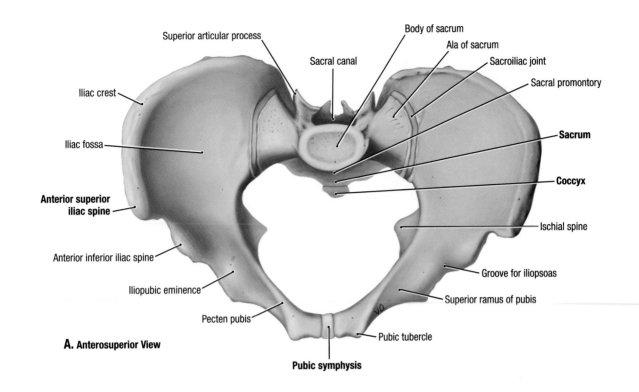

Superior articular process
Body of sacrum
Sacral canal
Ala of sacrum
Sacroiliac joint
Sacral promontory
Iliac crest
Iliac fossa
Sacrum
Anterior superior iliac spine
Coccyx
Ischial spine
Anterior inferior iliac spine
Groove for iliopsoas
Iliopubic eminence
Superior ramus of pubis
Pecten pubis
Pubic tubercle
A. Anterosuperior View
Pubic symphysis

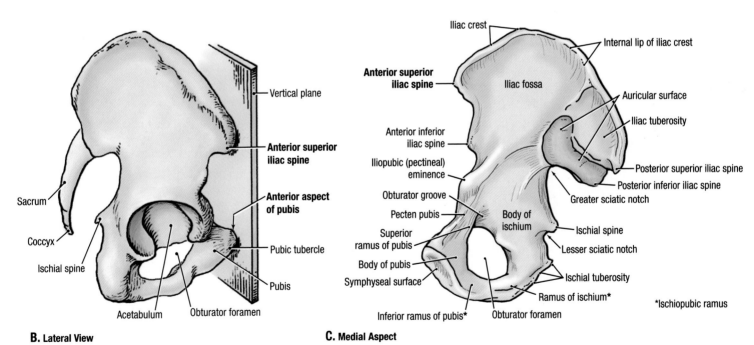

Vertical plane
Anterior superior iliac spine
Anterior aspect of pubis
Sacrum
Pubic tubercle
Coccyx
Ischial spine
Pubis
Acetabulum
Obturator foramen
B. Lateral View

Iliac crest
Internal lip of iliac crest
Anterior superior iliac spine
Iliac fossa
Auricular surface
Iliac tuberosity
Anterior inferior iliac spine
Iliopubic (pectineal) eminence
Posterior superior iliac spine
Posterior inferior iliac spine
Obturator groove
Greater sciatic notch
Pecten pubis
Body of ischium
Superior ramus of pubis
Ischial spine
Lesser sciatic notch
Body of pubis
Symphyseal surface
Ischial tuberosity
Inferior ramus of pubis*
Ramus of ischium*
Obturator foramen
*Ischiopubic ramus
C. Medial Aspect

3.4　**Pelvis, anatomical position**

A. Pelvic girdle. **B.** Placement of hip bone in anatomical position. In the anatomical position: (1) the anterior superior iliac spine and the anterior aspect of the pubis lie in the same vertical plane; (2) the sacrum is located superiorly, the coccyx posteriorly and the pubic symphysis anteroinferiorly. **C.** Features of hip bone.

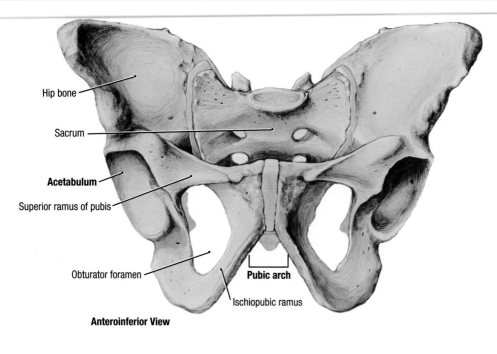

Hip bone

Sacrum

Acetabulum

Superior ramus of pubis

Obturator foramen

Pubic arch

Ischiopubic ramus

Anteroinferior View

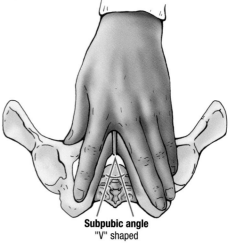

Subpubic angle
"V" shaped

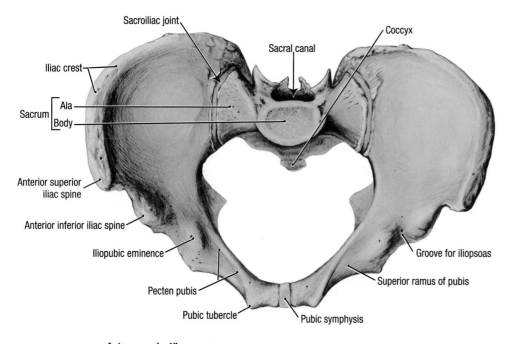

Sacroiliac joint

Coccyx

Sacral canal

Iliac crest

Sacrum { Ala
         Body

Anterior superior
iliac spine

Anterior inferior iliac spine

Iliopubic eminence

Groove for iliopsoas

Superior ramus of pubis

Pecten pubis

Pubic tubercle

Pubic symphysis

Anterosuperior View

3.5   **Male pelvic girdle**

TABLE 3.1 DIFFERENCES BETWEEN MALE AND FEMALE PELVES (continued on next page)

Bony pelvis	Male	Female
General structure	Thick and heavy	Thin and light
Greater pelvis (pelvis major)	Deep	Shallow
Lesser pelvis (pelvis minor)	Narrow and deep, tapering	Wide and shallow, cylindrical
Pelvic inlet (superior pelvic aperture)	Heart shaped, narrow	Oval or rounded, wide

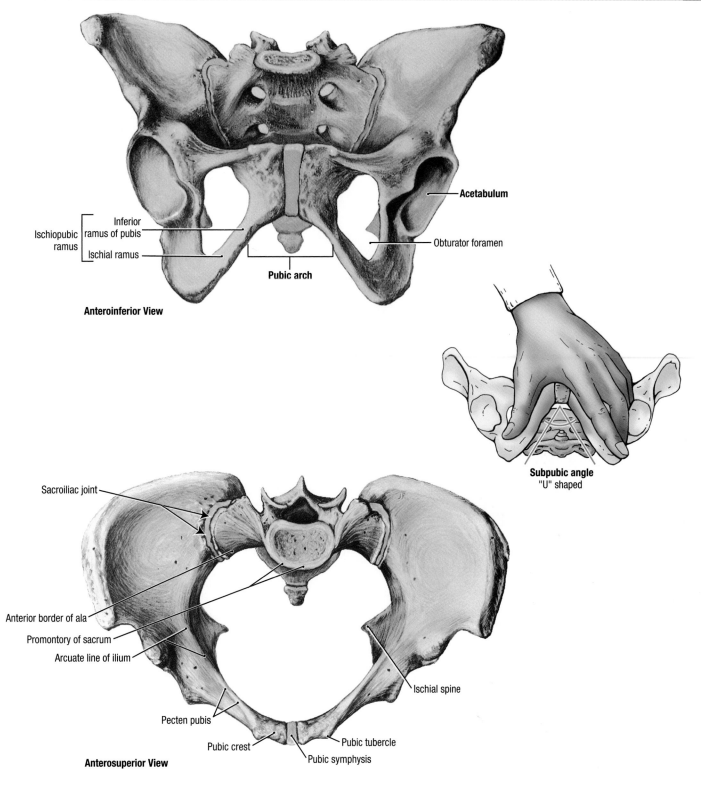

Acetabulum

Ischiopubic
ramus

Inferior
ramus of pubis

Ischial ramus

Obturator foramen

Pubic arch

Anteroinferior View

Subpubic angle
"U" shaped

Sacroiliac joint

Anterior border of ala

Promontory of sacrum

Arcuate line of ilium

Ischial spine

Pecten pubis

Pubic crest

Pubic tubercle

Pubic symphysis

Anterosuperior View

3.6 Female pelvic girdle

TABLE 3.1 DIFFERENCES BETWEEN MALE AND FEMALE PELVES *(continued)*

Bony pelvis	Male	Female
Pelvic outlet (inferior pelvic aperture)	Comparatively small	Comparatively large
Pubic arch and subpubic angle	Narrow	Wide
Obturator foramen	Round	Oval
Acetabulum	Large	Small

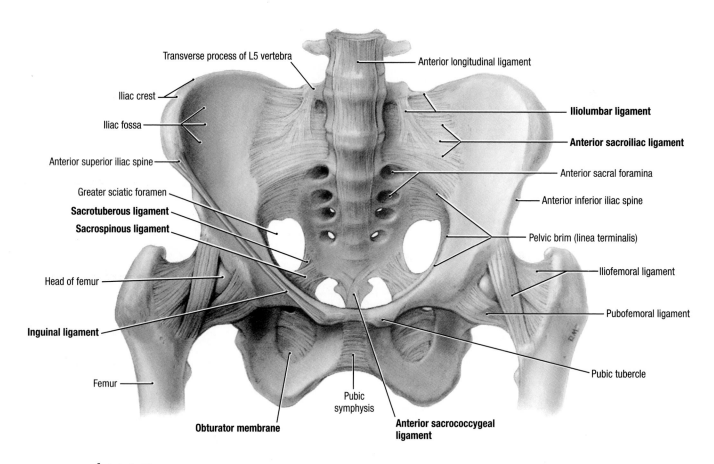

Transverse process of L5 vertebra

Anterior longitudinal ligament

Iliac crest

Iliolumbar ligament

Iliac fossa

Anterior sacroiliac ligament

Anterior superior iliac spine

Anterior sacral foramina

Anterior inferior iliac spine

Greater sciatic foramen

Pelvic brim (linea terminalis)

Sacrotuberous ligament

Sacrospinous ligament

Iliofemoral ligament

Head of femur

Pubofemoral ligament

Inguinal ligament

Pubic tubercle

Femur

Pubic symphysis

Obturator membrane

Anterior sacrococcygeal ligament

A. Anterior View

3.7 **Pelvis and pelvic ligaments**

A. Ligaments of pelvis, anterior aspect of pelvis.

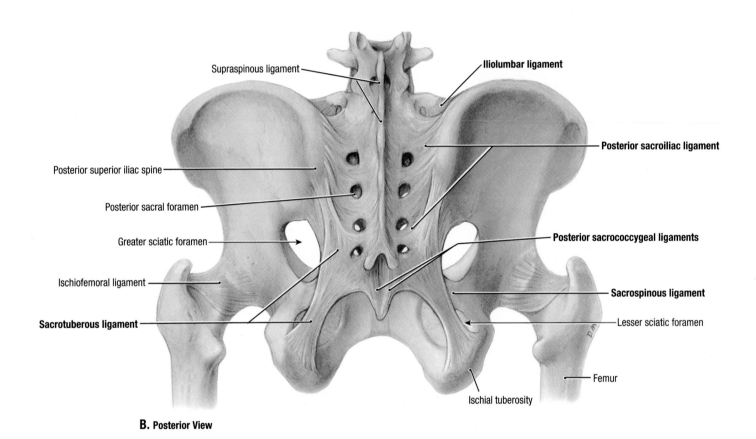

Supraspinous ligament

Iliolumbar ligament

Posterior superior iliac spine

Posterior sacroiliac ligament

Posterior sacral foramen

Greater sciatic foramen

Posterior sacrococcygeal ligaments

Ischiofemoral ligament

Sacrospinous ligament

Sacrotuberous ligament

Lesser sciatic foramen

Femur

Ischial tuberosity

B. Posterior View

3.7   **Pelvis and pelvic ligaments** *(continued)*

B. Ligaments of pelvis, posterior aspect of pelvis.

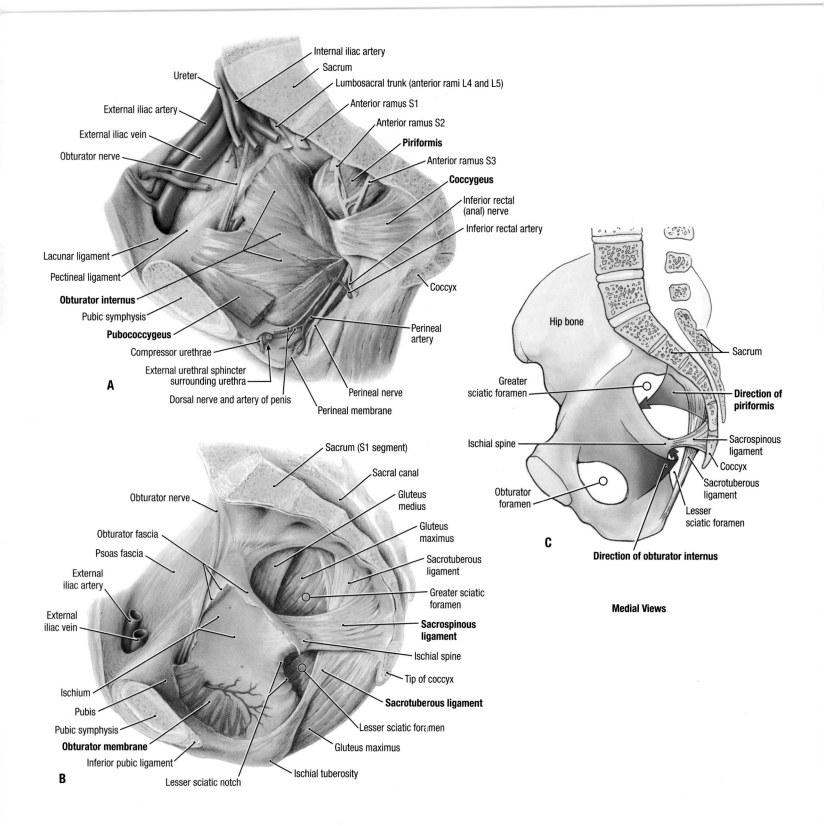

A

Internal iliac artery
Sacrum
Ureter
Lumbosacral trunk (anterior rami L4 and L5)
External iliac artery
Anterior ramus S1
External iliac vein
Anterior ramus S2
Obturator nerve
Piriformis
Anterior ramus S3
Coccygeus
Inferior rectal (anal) nerve
Inferior rectal artery
Lacunar ligament
Pectineal ligament
Coccyx
Obturator internus
Pubic symphysis
Perineal artery
Pubococcygeus
Compressor urethrae
External urethral sphincter surrounding urethra
Perineal nerve
Dorsal nerve and artery of penis
Perineal membrane

B

Sacrum (S1 segment)
Sacral canal
Obturator nerve
Gluteus medius
Obturator fascia
Gluteus maximus
Psoas fascia
Sacrotuberous ligament
External iliac artery
Greater sciatic foramen
External iliac vein
Sacrospinous ligament
Ischial spine
Tip of coccyx
Ischium
Pubis
Sacrotuberous ligament
Pubic symphysis
Lesser sciatic foramen
Obturator membrane
Gluteus maximus
Inferior pubic ligament
Ischial tuberosity
Lesser sciatic notch

C

Hip bone
Sacrum
Greater sciatic foramen
Direction of piriformis
Ischial spine
Sacrospinous ligament
Coccyx
Obturator foramen
Sacrotuberous ligament
Lesser sciatic foramen
Direction of obturator internus

Medial Views

3.8   Obturator internus and piriformis

- On the lateral pelvic wall the obturator foramen is closed by the obturator membrane; the obturator internus muscle attaches mainly to the obturator membrane and exits the lesser pelvis through the lesser sciatic foramen; obturator fascia lies on the medial surface of the muscle.

- Piriformis lies on the posterolateral pelvic wall and leaves the lesser pelvis through the greater sciatic foramen.

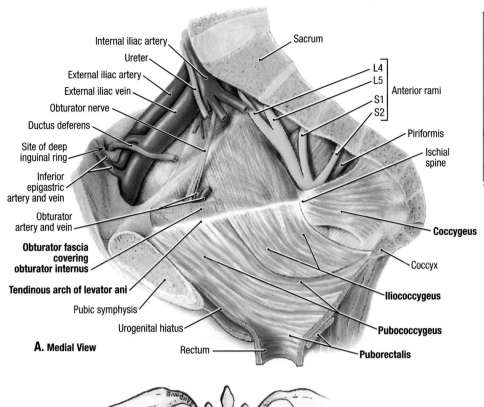

A. Medial View

Labels (clockwise from upper left):
Internal iliac artery
Ureter
External iliac artery
External iliac vein
Obturator nerve
Ductus deferens
Site of deep inguinal ring
Inferior epigastric artery and vein
Obturator artery and vein
Obturator fascia covering obturator internus
Tendinous arch of levator ani
Pubic symphysis
Urogenital hiatus
Rectum
Sacrum
L4
L5
S1
S2
Anterior rami
Piriformis
Ischial spine
Coccygeus
Coccyx
Iliococcygeus
Pubococcygeus
Puborectalis

> **Muscles of floor of pelvis*:**
>
> Pelvic diaphragm (PD) = Levator ani (LA) + Coccygeus (C)
> (PD = LA + C)
>
> Levator ani (LA) = Pubococcygeus (PC) + Iliococcygeus (IC)
> (LA = PC + IC)
>
> Pubococcygeus (PC ♀) = Puborectalis (PR) + Pubovaginalis (PV)
> (PC = PR + PV ♀)
>
> Pubococcygeus (PC ♂) = Puborectalis (PR) + Puboprostaticus
> (PC = PR + LP ♂) (Levator prostatae [LP])

*Formulas: Dr. Larry M. Ross.
The Univesity of Texas Medical School at Houston

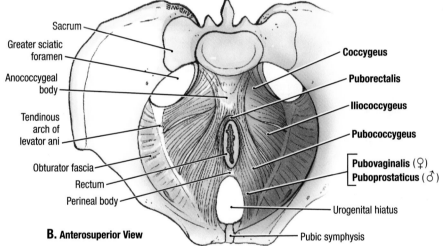

B. Anterosuperior View

Labels:
Sacrum
Greater sciatic foramen
Anococcygeal body
Tendinous arch of levator ani
Obturator fascia
Rectum
Perineal body
Coccygeus
Puborectalis
Iliococcygeus
Pubococcygeus
Pubovaginalis (♀)
Puboprostaticus (♂)
Urogenital hiatus
Pubic symphysis

3.9 **Muscles of the pelvic diaphragm**

A. The pelvic floor is formed by the funnel- or bowl-shaped pelvic diaphragm. The funnel shape can be seen in a medial view of a median section. **B.** The bowl shape from a superior view.

TABLE 3.2 MUSCLES OF PELVIC WALLS AND FLOOR

Boundary	Muscle	Proximal attachment	Distal attachment	Innervation	Main Action
Lateral wall	Obturator internus	Pelvic surfaces of ilium and ischium, obturator membrane	Greater trochanter of femur	Nerve to obturator internus (L5, S1, S2)	Rotates thigh laterally; assists in holding head of femur in acetabulum
Posterolateral wall	Piriformis	Pelvic surface of S2–S4 segments, superior margin of greater sciatic notch, sacrotuberous ligament		Anterior rami of S1 and S2	Rotates thigh laterally; abducts thigh; assists in holding head of femur in acetabulum
Floor	Levator ani (pubococcygeus, puborectalis, and iliococcygeus)	Body of pubis, tendinous arch of obturator fascia, ischial spine	Perineal body, coccyx, anococcygeal ligament, walls of prostate or vagina, rectum, and anal canal	Nerve to levator ani (branches of S4), inferior anal (rectal) nerve, and coccygeal plexus	Forms most of pelvic diaphragm that helps support pelvic viscera and resists increases in intra-abdominal pressure
	Coccygeus (ischiococcygeus)	Ischial spine	Inferior end of sacrum and coccyx	Branches of S4 and S5 spinal nerves	Forms small part of pelvic diaphragm that supports pelvic viscera; flexes coccyx

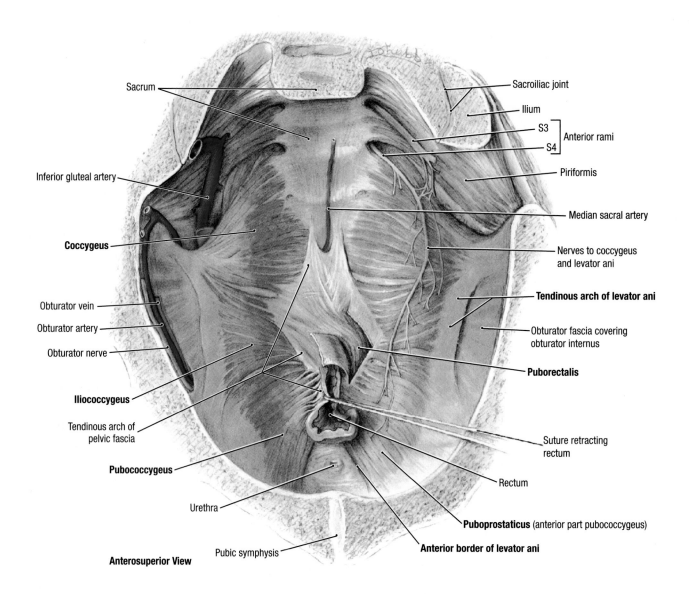

Sacrum

Sacroiliac joint

Ilium

S3 ⎫
S4 ⎬ Anterior rami

Piriformis

Inferior gluteal artery

Median sacral artery

Coccygeus

Nerves to coccygeus and levator ani

Tendinous arch of levator ani

Obturator vein

Obturator artery

Obturator fascia covering obturator internus

Obturator nerve

Puborectalis

Iliococcygeus

Tendinous arch of pelvic fascia

Suture retracting rectum

Pubococcygeus

Rectum

Urethra

Puboprostaticus (anterior part pubococcygeus)

Pubic symphysis

Anterior border of levator ani

Anterosuperior View

3.10   Floor and walls of male pelvis, pelvic diaphragm

The pelvic viscera are removed, and the bony pelvis has been cut to show the levator ani and coccygeus muscles.

- The pubococcygeus muscle arises mainly from the pubic bone, the iliococcygeus muscle from the tendinous arch, and the coccygeus muscle from the ischial spine.
- In the male, the anterior part of the pubococcygeus muscle that lies adjacent to the prostate is the puboprostaticus.
- Although not part of the pelvic diaphragm, the piriformis assists in closure of the pelvic outlet, largely occluding the greater sciatic foramen.

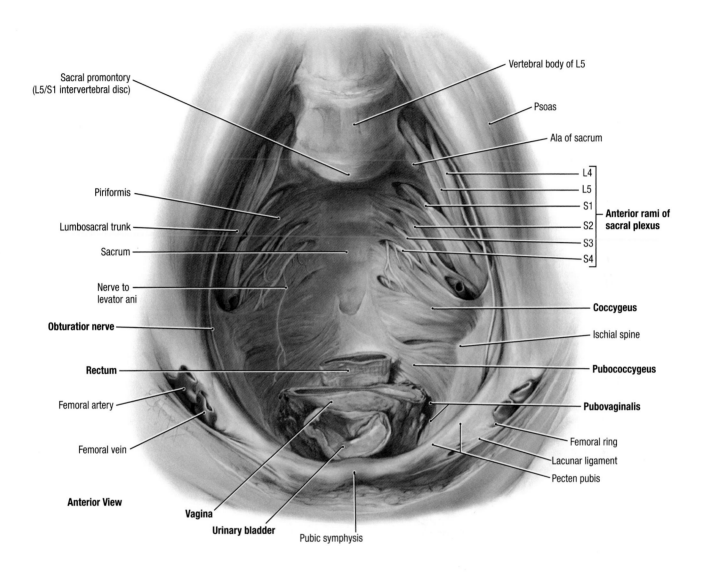

Sacral promontory
(L5/S1 intervertebral disc)

Piriformis

Lumbosacral trunk

Sacrum

Nerve to
levator ani

Obturatior nerve

Rectum

Femoral artery

Femoral vein

Anterior View

Vagina

Urinary bladder   Pubic symphysis

Vertebral body of L5

Psoas

Ala of sacrum

L4
L5
S1
S2   **Anterior rami of**
S3   **sacral plexus**
S4

Coccygeus

Ischial spine

Pubococcygeus

Pubovaginalis

Femoral ring

Lacunar ligament

Pecten pubis

3.11   **Floor and walls of female pelvis**

The pelvic viscera are removed to reveal the levator ani and coccygeus muscles.

- Note the relative positions of the bladder, vagina, and rectum as they penetrate the pelvic floor.
- Branches of S3 and S4 nerves supply the levator ani and coccygeus muscles; the pudendal nerve, through its perineal branch, also supplies the levator ani muscle (see Table 3.2).
- The obturator nerve runs along the lateral wall of the pelvis and enters the thigh by passing through the obturator canal.
- The anterior rami of L4–S4 are part of the sacral plexus, almost all of which exits the pelvis via the greater sciatic foramen with the piriformis.

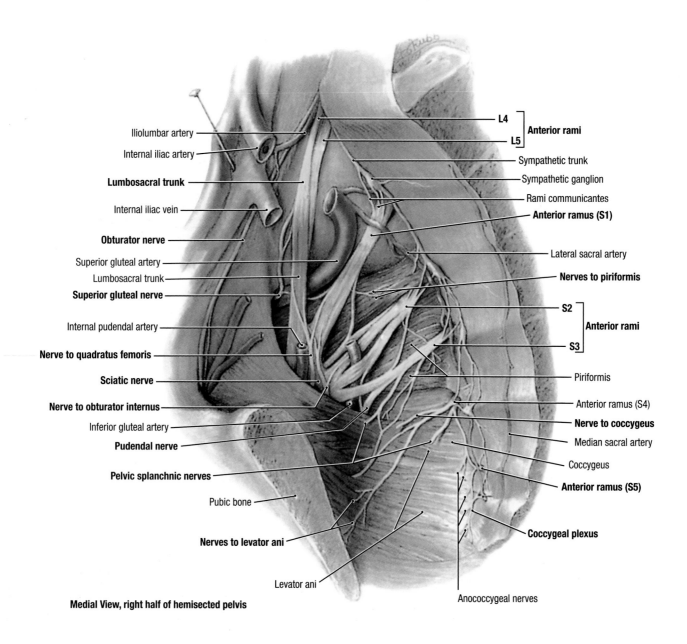

Iliolumbar artery

Internal iliac artery

Lumbosacral trunk

Internal iliac vein

Obturator nerve

Superior gluteal artery

Lumbosacral trunk

Superior gluteal nerve

Internal pudendal artery

Nerve to quadratus femoris

Sciatic nerve

Nerve to obturator internus

Inferior gluteal artery

Pudendal nerve

Pelvic splanchnic nerves

Pubic bone

Nerves to levator ani

Levator ani

L4 ⎤
L5 ⎦ **Anterior rami**

Sympathetic trunk

Sympathetic ganglion

Rami communicantes

Anterior ramus (S1)

Lateral sacral artery

Nerves to piriformis

S2 ⎤
     Anterior rami
S3 ⎦

Piriformis

Anterior ramus (S4)

Nerve to coccygeus

Median sacral artery

Coccygeus

Anterior ramus (S5)

Coccygeal plexus

Anococcygeal nerves

Medial View, right half of hemisected pelvis

3.12   Sacral and coccygeal nerve plexuses

- The sympathetic trunk or its ganglia send rami communicantes to each sacral and coccygeal nerve.
- The anterior ramus from L4 joins that of L5 to form the lumbosacral trunk.
- The anterior rami of S1 and S2 supply the piriformis muscle; S3 and S4 supply the coccygeus and levator ani muscles.
- The sciatic nerve arises from anterior rami of L4, L5, S1, S2, and S3; the pudendal nerve from S2, S3, and S4; and the coccygeal plexus from S4, S5, and coccygeal segments.

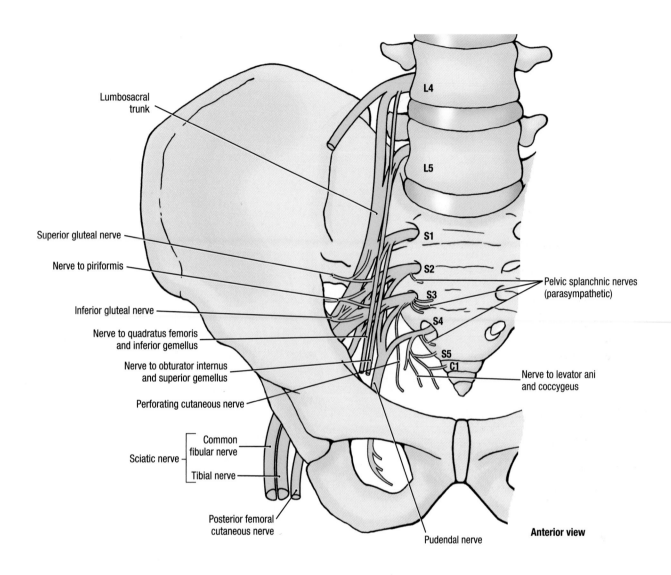

Lumbosacral trunk

Superior gluteal nerve

Nerve to piriformis

Inferior gluteal nerve

Nerve to quadratus femoris and inferior gemellus

Nerve to obturator internus and superior gemellus

Perforating cutaneous nerve

Sciatic nerve — Common fibular nerve / Tibial nerve

Posterior femoral cutaneous nerve

L4

L5

S1

S2

S3

S4

S5

C1

Pelvic splanchnic nerves (parasympathetic)

Nerve to levator ani and coccygeus

Pudendal nerve

Anterior view

TABLE 3.3 NERVES OF SACRAL AND COCCYGEAL PLEXUSES

Nerve	Origin	Distribution
Sciatic	L4, L5, S1, S2, S3	Articular branches to hip joint and muscular branches to flexors of knee in thigh and all muscles in leg and foot
Superior gluteal	L4, L5, S1	Gluteus medius and gluteus minimus muscles
Nerve to quadratus femoris and inferior gemellus	L4, L5, S1	Quadratus femoris and inferior gemellus muscles
Inferior gluteal	L5, S1, S2	Gluteus maximus muscle
Nerve to obturator internus and superior gemellus	L5, S1, S2	Obturator internus and superior gemellus muscles
Nerve to piriformis	S1, S2	Piriformis muscle
Posterior femoral cutaneous	S2, S3	Cutaneous branches to buttock and uppermost medial and posterior surfaces of thigh
Perforating cutaneous	S2, S3	Cutaneous branches to medial part of buttock
Pudendal	S2, S3, S4	Structures in perineum, sensory to genitalia, muscular branches to perineal muscles, external urethral sphincter, and external anal sphincter
Pelvic splanchnic	S2, S3, S4	Pelvic viscera via inferior hypogastric and pelvic plexuses
Nerves to levator ani and coccygeus	S3, S4	Levator ani and coccygeus muscles

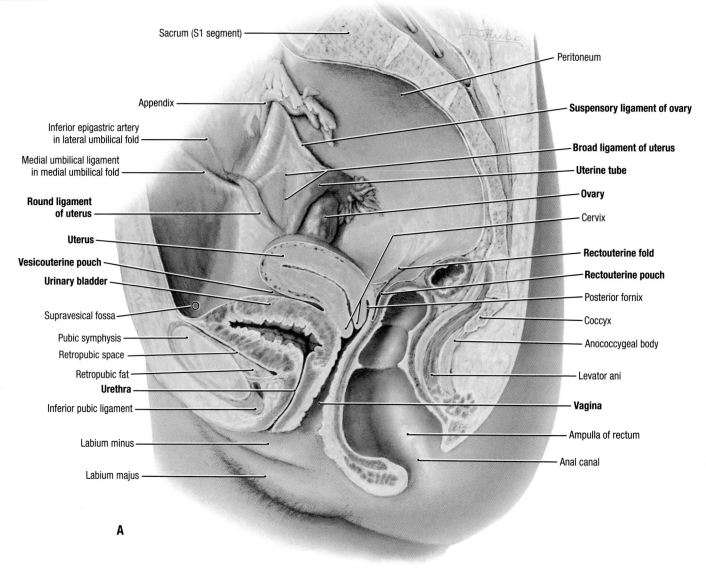

Sacrum (S1 segment)

Appendix

Inferior epigastric artery in lateral umbilical fold

Medial umbilical ligament in medial umbilical fold

Round ligament of uterus

Uterus

Vesicouterine pouch

Urinary bladder

Supravesical fossa

Pubic symphysis

Retropubic space

Retropubic fat

Urethra

Inferior pubic ligament

Labium minus

Labium majus

Peritoneum

Suspensory ligament of ovary

Broad ligament of uterus

Uterine tube

Ovary

Cervix

Rectouterine fold

Rectouterine pouch

Posterior fornix

Coccyx

Anococcygeal body

Levator ani

Vagina

Ampulla of rectum

Anal canal

A

Medial Views

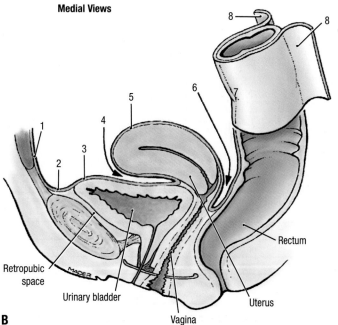

Retropubic space

Urinary bladder

Vagina

Uterus

Rectum

B

Female:
Peritoneum passes:
- From the anterior abdominal wall (1)
- Superior to the pubic bone (2)
- On the superior surface of the urinary bladder (3)
- From the bladder to the uterus, forming the vesicouterine pouch (4)
- On the fundus and body of the uterus, posterior formix. and all of the vagina (5)
- Between the rectum and uterus, forming the rectouterine pouch (6)
- On the anterior and lateral sides of the rectum (7)
- Posteriorly to become the sigmoid mesocolon (8)

3.13 **Right half of hemisected female pelvis**

A. Organs in situ.
- The urethra, the vagina, and the rectum are parallel to one another; the uterus is nearly at right angles to these structures when the bladder is empty.

B. Peritoneum covering female pelvic organs.

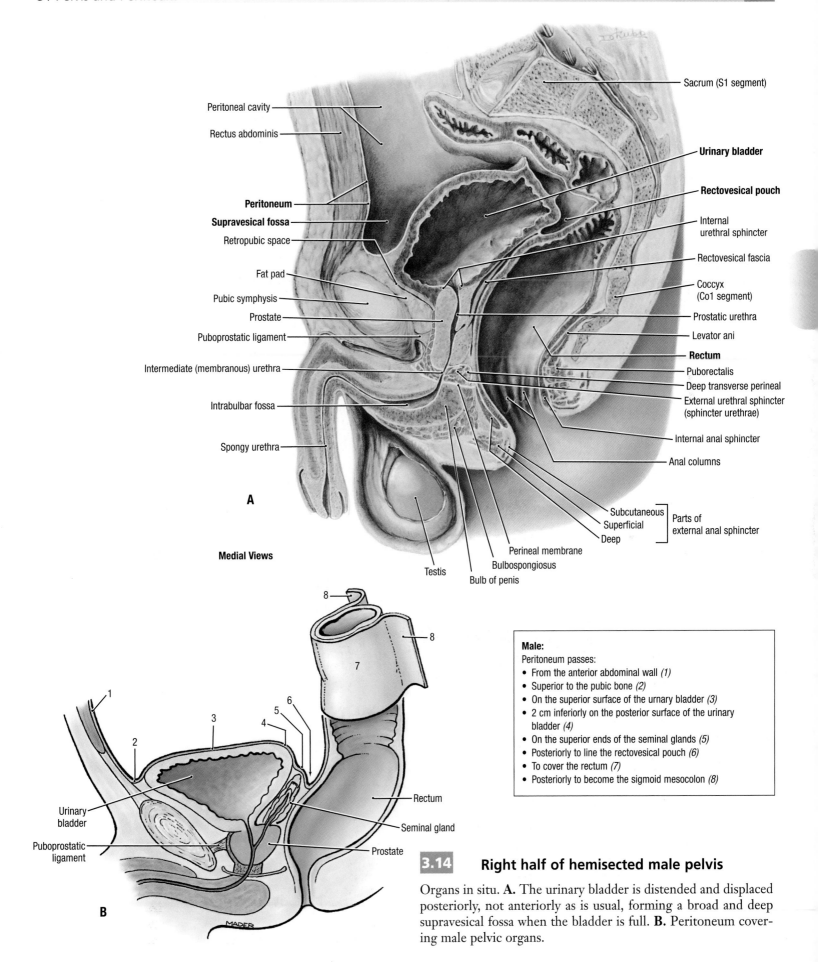

A

Medial Views

Peritoneal cavity
Rectus abdominis
Peritoneum
Supravesical fossa
Retropubic space
Fat pad
Pubic symphysis
Prostate
Puboprostatic ligament
Intermediate (membranous) urethra
Intrabulbar fossa
Spongy urethra
Testis

Sacrum (S1 segment)
Urinary bladder
Rectovesical pouch
Internal urethral sphincter
Rectovesical fascia
Coccyx (Co1 segment)
Prostatic urethra
Levator ani
Rectum
Puborectalis
Deep transverse perineal
External urethral sphincter (sphincter urethrae)
Internal anal sphincter
Anal columns
Subcutaneous / Superficial / Deep — Parts of external anal sphincter
Perineal membrane
Bulbospongiosus
Bulb of penis

B

Urinary bladder
Puboprostatic ligament
Rectum
Seminal gland
Prostate

MADER

Male:
Peritoneum passes:
- From the anterior abdominal wall *(1)*
- Superior to the pubic bone *(2)*
- On the superior surface of the urinary bladder *(3)*
- 2 cm inferiorly on the posterior surface of the urinary bladder *(4)*
- On the superior ends of the seminal glands *(5)*
- Posteriorly to line the rectovesical pouch *(6)*
- To cover the rectum *(7)*
- Posteriorly to become the sigmoid mesocolon *(8)*

3.14 **Right half of hemisected male pelvis**

Organs in situ. **A.** The urinary bladder is distended and displaced posteriorly, not anteriorly as is usual, forming a broad and deep supravesical fossa when the bladder is full. **B.** Peritoneum covering male pelvic organs.

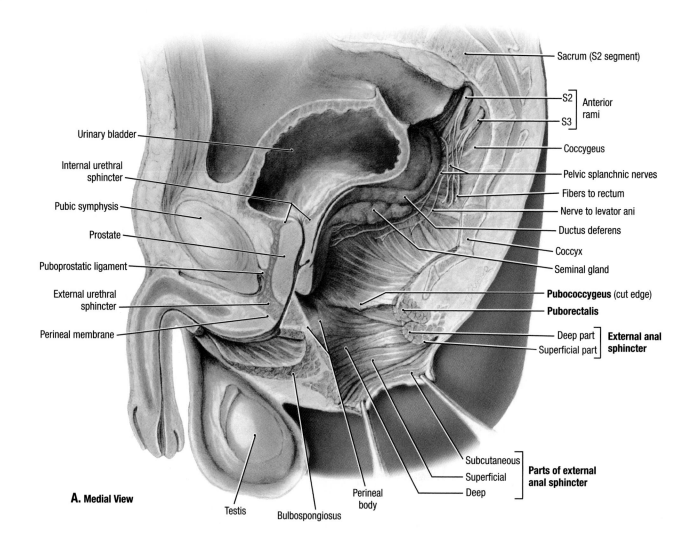

Urinary bladder

Internal urethral
sphincter

Pubic symphysis

Prostate

Puboprostatic ligament

External urethral
sphincter

Perineal membrane

Sacrum (S2 segment)

S2
S3 } Anterior
rami

Coccygeus

Pelvic splanchnic nerves

Fibers to rectum

Nerve to levator ani

Ductus deferens

Coccyx

Seminal gland

Pubococcygeus (cut edge)

Puborectalis

Deep part
Superficial part } **External anal
sphincter**

Subcutaneous
Superficial
Deep } **Parts of external
anal sphincter**

Perineal
body

Testis   Bulbospongiosus

A. Medial View

3.15   Anal sphincters and anal canal

A. Levator ani, in right half of hemisected pelvis.

- The subcutaneous fibers of the external anal sphincter are reflected with forceps. The pubococcygeus muscle is cut to reveal
  the anal canal, to which it is, in part, attached.

B. Puborectalis.

- The innermost part of the pubococcygeus muscle, the puborectalis, forms a U-shaped muscular "sling" around the anorectal
  junction, which maintains the anorectal (perineal) flexure.

C. External and internal anal sphincters.

- The internal anal sphincter is a thickening of the inner, circular
  muscular coat of the anal canal.

- The external anal sphincter has three continuous zones: deep, superficial, and subcutaneous; the deep part intermingles with the
  puborectalis muscle posteriorly.

- The longitudinal muscle layer of the rectum separates the internal and external anal sphincters and terminates in the subcutaneous tissue and skin around the anus.

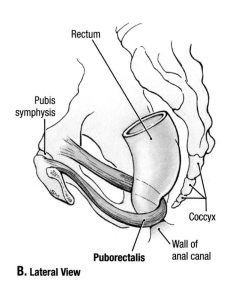

Rectum

Pubis
symphysis

Coccyx

Wall of
anal canal

Puborectalis

B. Lateral View

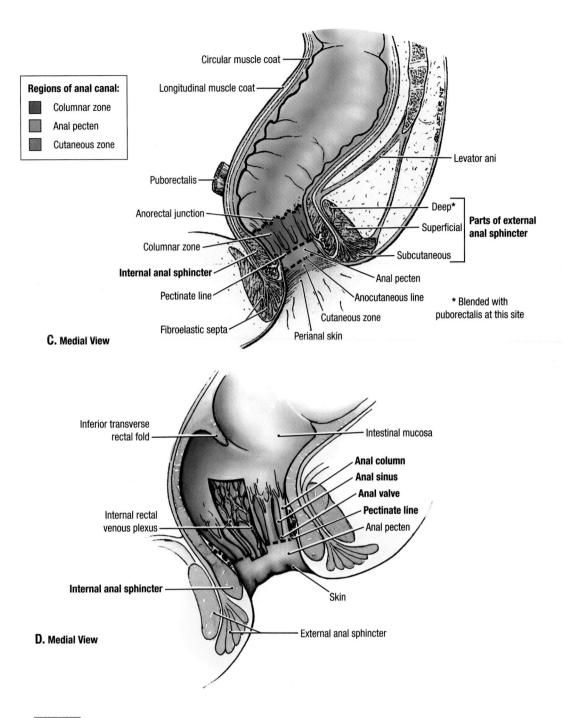

Regions of anal canal:
- Columnar zone
- Anal pecten
- Cutaneous zone

Circular muscle coat

Longitudinal muscle coat

Puborectalis

Anorectal junction

Columnar zone

Internal anal sphincter

Pectinate line

Fibroelastic septa

C. Medial View

Levator ani

Deep* ⎫
Superficial ⎬ **Parts of external anal sphincter**
Subcutaneous ⎭

Anal pecten

Anocutaneous line

Cutaneous zone

Perianal skin

* Blended with puborectalis at this site

Inferior transverse rectal fold

Internal rectal venous plexus

Internal anal sphincter

D. Medial View

Intestinal mucosa

Anal column

Anal sinus

Anal valve

Pectinate line

Anal pecten

Skin

External anal sphincter

3.15   **Anal sphincters and anal canal *(continued)***

D. Features of the anal canal.
- The anal columns are 5 to 10 vertical folds of mucosa separated by anal valves; they contain portions of the rectal venous plexus.
- The pecten is a smooth area of hairless stratified epithelium that lies between the anal valves superiorly and the inferior border of the internal anal sphincter inferiorly.
- The pectinate line is an irregular line at the base of the anal valves where the intestinal mucosa is continuous with the pecten; this indicates the junction of the *superior part of the anal canal (derived from embryonic hindgut)* and the inferior part of the *anal canal (derived from the anal pit [proctodeum])*. Innervation is visceral proximal to the line and somatic distally; lymphatic drainage is to the pararectal nodes proximally and to the superficial inguinal nodes distally.

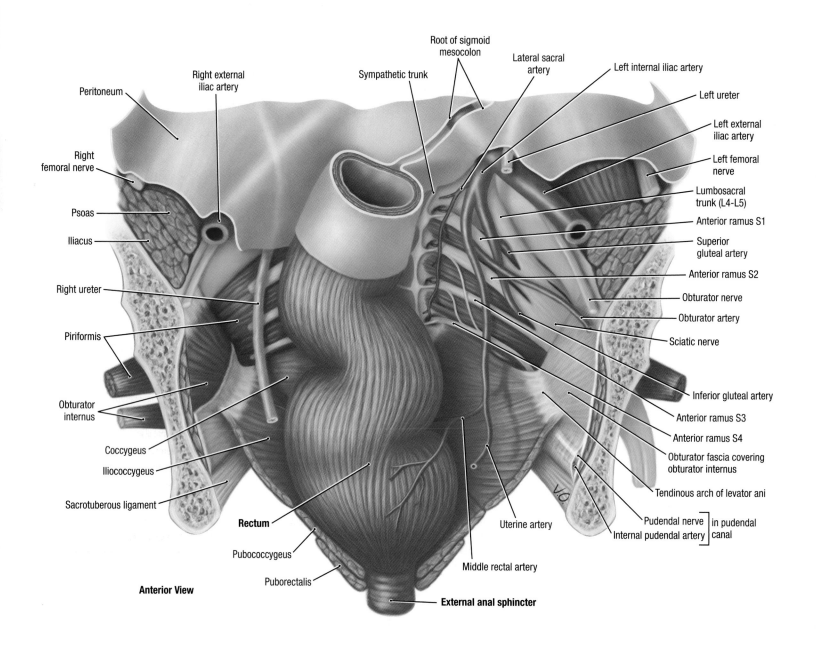

Peritoneum

Right external
iliac artery

Root of sigmoid
mesocolon

Sympathetic trunk

Lateral sacral
artery

Left internal iliac artery

Left ureter

Left external
iliac artery

Right
femoral nerve

Left femoral
nerve

Psoas

Lumbosacral
trunk (L4-L5)

Iliacus

Anterior ramus S1

Superior
gluteal artery

Right ureter

Anterior ramus S2

Obturator nerve

Piriformis

Obturator artery

Sciatic nerve

Obturator
internus

Inferior gluteal artery

Anterior ramus S3

Coccygeus

Anterior ramus S4

Iliococcygeus

Obturator fascia covering
obturator internus

Sacrotuberous ligament

Tendinous arch of levator ani

Rectum

Pudendal nerve ⎫ in pudendal
Internal pudendal artery ⎭ canal

Pubococcygeus

Uterine artery

Puborectalis

Middle rectal artery

Anterior View

External anal sphincter

3.16 **Rectum, anal canal, and neurovascular structures of the
posterior pelvis**

The pelvis is coronally bisected anterior to the rectum and anal canal. The superior gluteal
artery often passes posteriorly between the anterior rami of L5 and S1, and the inferior
gluteal artery between S2 and S3.

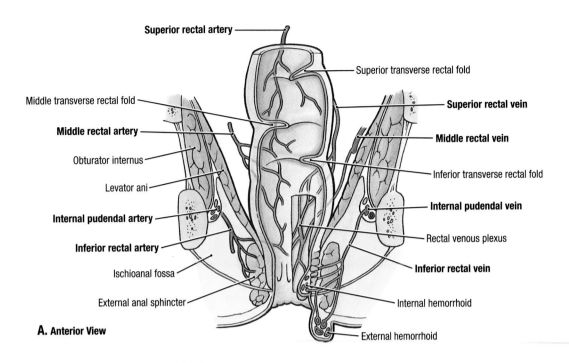

A. Anterior View

Superior rectal artery

Middle transverse rectal fold

Middle rectal artery

Obturator internus

Levator ani

Internal pudendal artery

Inferior rectal artery

Ischioanal fossa

External anal sphincter

Superior transverse rectal fold

Superior rectal vein

Middle rectal vein

Inferior transverse rectal fold

Internal pudendal vein

Rectal venous plexus

Inferior rectal vein

Internal hemorrhoid

External hemorrhoid

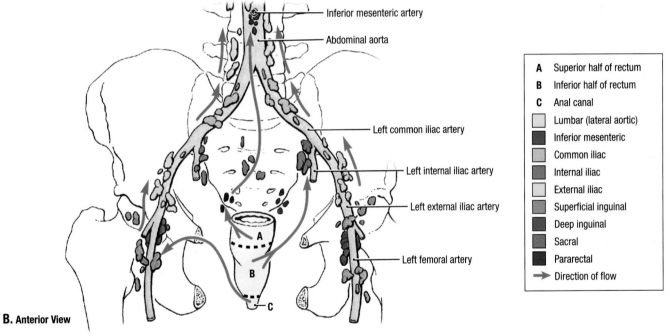

B. Anterior View

Inferior mesenteric artery

Abdominal aorta

Left common iliac artery

Left internal iliac artery

Left external iliac artery

Left femoral artery

A	Superior half of rectum
B	Inferior half of rectum
C	Anal canal
	Lumbar (lateral aortic)
	Inferior mesenteric
	Common iliac
	Internal iliac
	External iliac
	Superficial inguinal
	Deep inguinal
	Sacral
	Pararectal
→	Direction of flow

3.17   Vasculature of rectum

A. Arterial and venous drainage.
- The continuation of the inferior mesenteric artery, the superior rectal artery, supplies the proximal part of rectum.
- Right and left middle rectal arteries, usually arising from the inferior vesical (male) or uterine (female) arteries, supply the middle and inferior parts of the rectum.
- Inferior rectal arteries, arising from the internal pudendal arteries, supply the anorectal junction and the anal canal.

B. Lymphatic drainage.
- The superior, middle, and inferior rectal veins drain the rectum and anal canal; there are anastomoses between the plexuses formed by all three veins.

- The rectal venous plexus surrounds the distal rectum and anal canal and consists of an internal rectal plexus deep to the epithelium of the anal canal and an external rectal plexus external to the muscular coats of the wall of the anal canal.
- The superior rectal vein drains into the portal system, and the middle and inferior veins drain into the systemic system; thus, this is an important area of portacaval anastomosis.

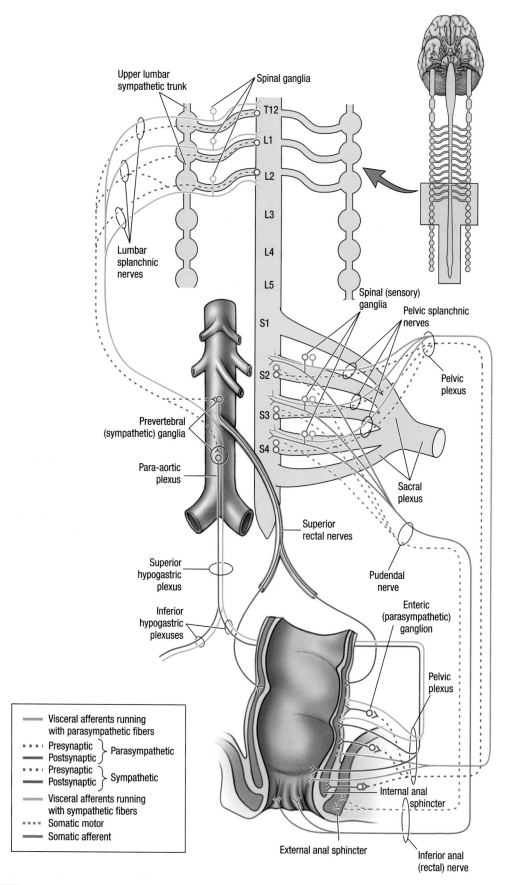

Upper lumbar
sympathetic trunk

Spinal ganglia

T12

L1

L2

L3

L4

L5

S1

S2

S3

S4

Lumbar
splanchnic
nerves

Spinal (sensory)
ganglia

Pelvic splanchnic
nerves

Pelvic
plexus

Prevertebral
(sympathetic) ganglia

Para-aortic
plexus

Sacral
plexus

Superior
rectal nerves

Superior
hypogastric
plexus

Pudendal
nerve

Enteric
(parasympathetic)
ganglion

Inferior
hypogastric
plexuses

Pelvic
plexus

Internal anal
sphincter

External anal sphincter

Inferior anal
(rectal) nerve

Visceral afferents running
with parasympathetic fibers

Presynaptic } Parasympathetic
Postsynaptic

Presynaptic } Sympathetic
Postsynaptic

Visceral afferents running
with sympathetic fibers

Somatic motor

Somatic afferent

3.18 **Innervation of rectum and anal canal**

The lumbar and pelvic spinal nerves and hypogastric plexuses have been retracted laterally for clarity.

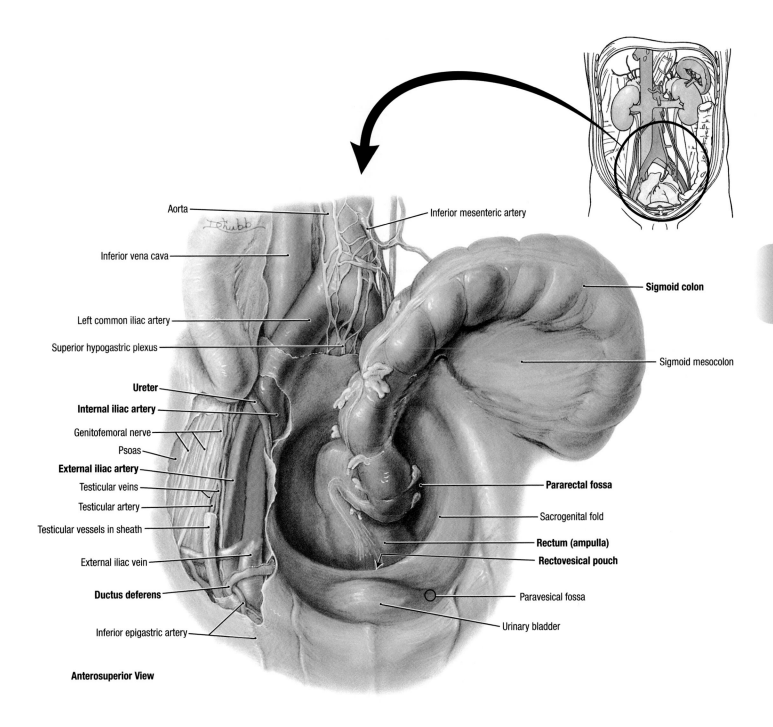

Aorta

Inferior mesenteric artery

Inferior vena cava

Sigmoid colon

Left common iliac artery

Sigmoid mesocolon

Superior hypogastric plexus

Ureter

Internal iliac artery

Genitofemoral nerve

Psoas

Pararectal fossa

External iliac artery

Sacrogenital fold

Testicular veins

Testicular artery

Rectum (ampulla)

Testicular vessels in sheath

Rectovesical pouch

External iliac vein

Paravesical fossa

Ductus deferens

Urinary bladder

Inferior epigastric artery

Anterosuperior View

3.19   **Rectum in situ**

- The sigmoid colon begins at the left pelvic brim and becomes the rectum anterior to the third sacral segment in the midline.
- The superior hypogastric plexus lies inferior to the bifurcation of the aorta and anterior to the left common iliac vein.
- The ureter adheres to the external aspect of the peritoneum, crosses the external iliac vessels, and descends anterior to the internal iliac artery. The ductus deferens and its artery also adhere to the peritoneum, cross the external iliac vessels, and then hook around the inferior epigastric artery to join the other components of the spermatic cord.
- The genitofemoral nerve lies on the psoas.

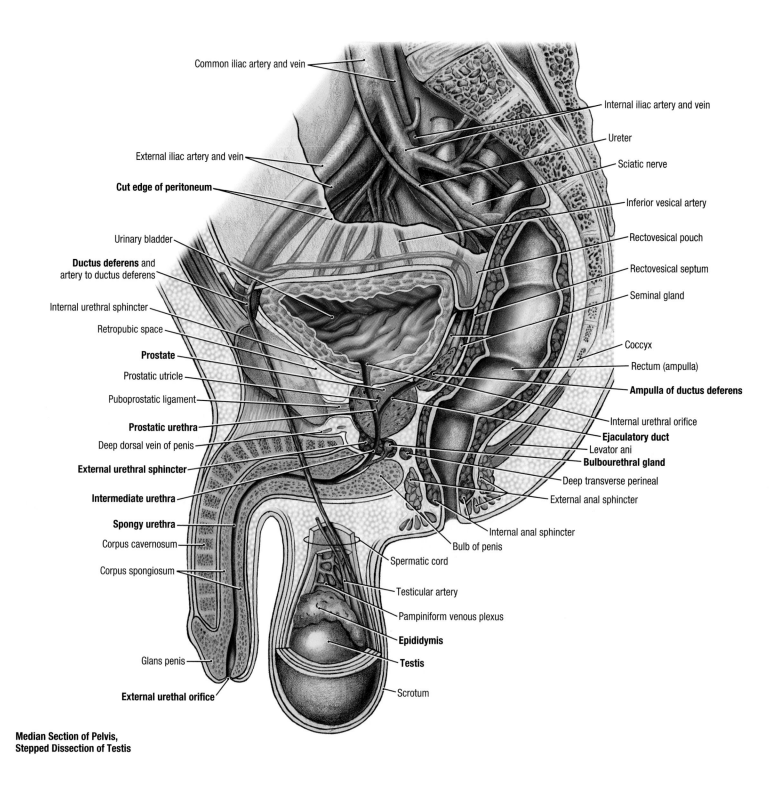

Common iliac artery and vein

External iliac artery and vein

Cut edge of peritoneum

Urinary bladder

Ductus deferens and artery to ductus deferens

Internal urethral sphincter

Retropubic space

Prostate

Prostatic utricle

Puboprostatic ligament

Prostatic urethra

Deep dorsal vein of penis

External urethral sphincter

Intermediate urethra

Spongy urethra

Corpus cavernosum

Corpus spongiosum

Glans penis

External urethal orifice

Internal iliac artery and vein

Ureter

Sciatic nerve

Inferior vesical artery

Rectovesical pouch

Rectovesical septum

Seminal gland

Coccyx

Rectum (ampulla)

Ampulla of ductus deferens

Internal urethral orifice

Ejaculatory duct

Levator ani

Bulbourethral gland

Deep transverse perineal

External anal sphincter

Internal anal sphincter

Bulb of penis

Spermatic cord

Testicular artery

Pampiniform venous plexus

Epididymis

Testis

Scrotum

Median Section of Pelvis, Stepped Dissection of Testis

3.20 Male pelvic organs and external genitalia

- Most of the pelvic viscera are subperitoneal, embedded in a matrix of fatty endopelvic fascia.
- The genital tract is demonstrated in its entirety; it merges with the urinary tract in the prostatic urethra.

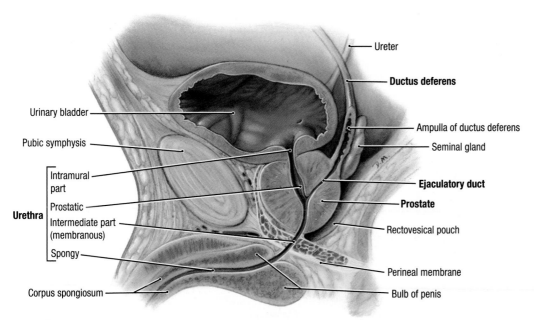

A. Median Section

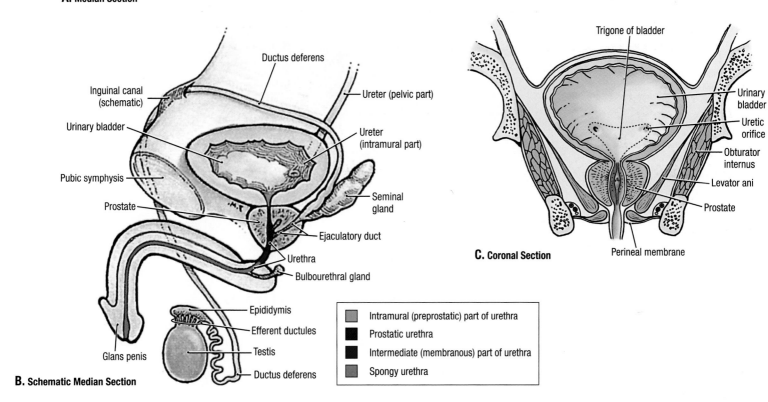

B. Schematic Median Section

C. Coronal Section

	Intramural (preprostatic) part of urethra
	Prostatic urethra
	Intermediate (membranous) part of urethra
	Spongy urethra

3.21   **Urinary bladder, prostate, and ductus deferens**

A. Dissection. The ejaculatory duct (approximately 2 cm in length) is formed by the union of the ductus deferens and duct of the seminal gland; it passes anteriorly and inferiorly through the substance of the prostate to enter the prostatic urethra on the seminal colliculus. **B.** Overview of urogenital system, schematic illustration. **C.** Coronal section through urinary bladder and prostate.

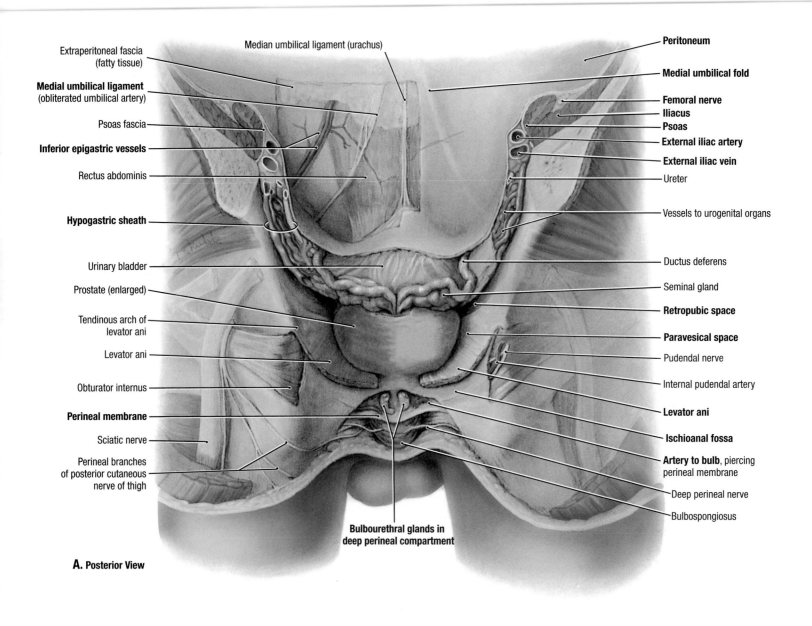

Extraperitoneal fascia (fatty tissue)

Median umbilical ligament (urachus)

Peritoneum

Medial umbilical fold

Medial umbilical ligament (obliterated umbilical artery)

Femoral nerve

Iliacus

Psoas fascia

Psoas

Inferior epigastric vessels

External iliac artery

External iliac vein

Rectus abdominis

Ureter

Hypogastric sheath

Vessels to urogenital organs

Urinary bladder

Ductus deferens

Prostate (enlarged)

Seminal gland

Retropubic space

Tendinous arch of levator ani

Paravesical space

Levator ani

Pudendal nerve

Obturator internus

Internal pudendal artery

Perineal membrane

Levator ani

Sciatic nerve

Ischioanal fossa

Perineal branches of posterior cutaneous nerve of thigh

Artery to bulb, piercing perineal membrane

Deep perineal nerve

Bulbospongiosus

Bulbourethral glands in deep perineal compartment

A. Posterior View

3.22   **Posterior approach to anterior pelvic and perineal structures and spaces**

A. Dissection. The rectovesical septum and all pelvic and perineal structures posterior to it have been removed. **B.** Posterior surface of inferior part of anterior abdominal wall with umbilical folds and ligaments and anterior pelvic viscera. **C.** Schematic coronal section through the anterior pelvis (plane of urinary bladder and prostate) demonstrating pelvic fascia.

- In **A** and **B**, the inferior epigastric artery and accompanying veins enter the rectus sheath, covered posteriorly with peritoneum to form the lateral umbilical fold. The medial umbilical fold is formed by peritoneum overlying the medial umbilical ligament (obliterated umbilical artery), and the median umbilical fold is formed by the median umbilical ligament (urachus).

- In **A**, the femoral nerve lies between the psoas and iliacus muscles, covered on their internal aspects with psoas (membranous parietal) fascia; the external iliac artery and vein lie within the areolar extraperitoneal fascia.

- The pelvic genitourinary organs are subperitoneal. Near the bladder, the ureter accompanies a "leash" of internal iliac vessels and derivatives within the fibroareolar hypogastric sheath.

- The levator ani and its fascial coverings separate the retropubic and paravesical spaces of the pelvis from the ischioanal fossae of the perineum. The fat that occupies these spaces has been removed.

- The bulbourethral glands and the initial part of the artery to the bulb lie superior to the perineal membrane in the deep perineal compartment.

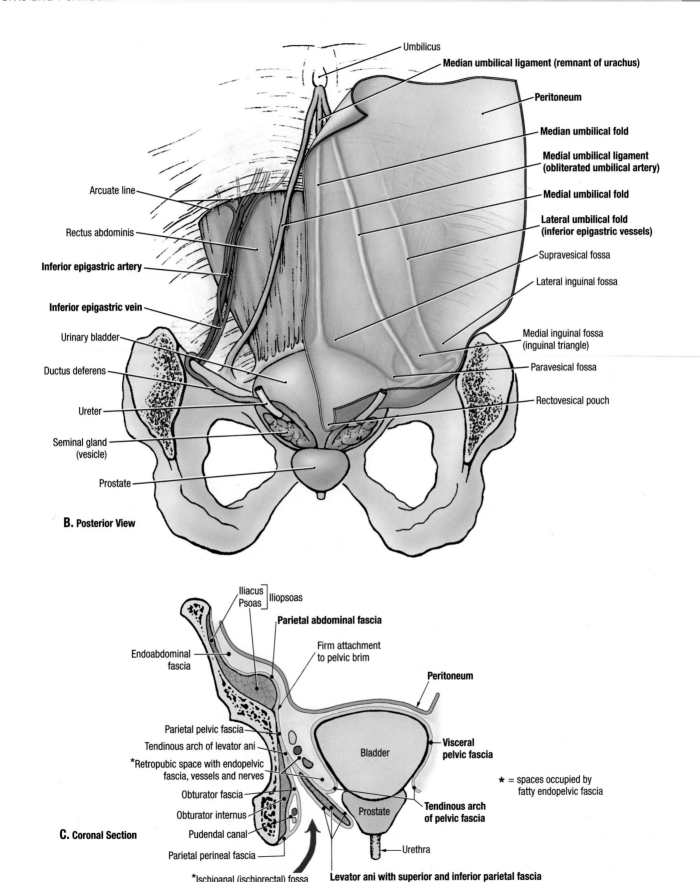

Umbilicus

Median umbilical ligament (remnant of urachus)

Peritoneum

Median umbilical fold

Medial umbilical ligament (obliterated umbilical artery)

Medial umbilical fold

Lateral umbilical fold (inferior epigastric vessels)

Supravesical fossa

Lateral inguinal fossa

Medial inguinal fossa (inguinal triangle)

Paravesical fossa

Rectovesical pouch

Arcuate line

Rectus abdominis

Inferior epigastric artery

Inferior epigastric vein

Urinary bladder

Ductus deferens

Ureter

Seminal gland (vesicle)

Prostate

B. Posterior View

Iliacus | Psoas | Iliopsoas

Parietal abdominal fascia

Firm attachment to pelvic brim

Peritoneum

Endoabdominal fascia

Parietal pelvic fascia

Tendinous arch of levator ani

*Retropubic space with endopelvic fascia, vessels and nerves

Obturator fascia

Obturator internus

Pudendal canal

Parietal perineal fascia

Visceral pelvic fascia

Bladder

Prostate

Tendinous arch of pelvic fascia

Urethra

★ = spaces occupied by fatty endopelvic fascia

C. Coronal Section

*Ischioanal (ischiorectal) fossa

Levator ani with superior and inferior parietal fascia

3.22 **Posterior approach to anterior pelvic and perineal structures and spaces (continued)**

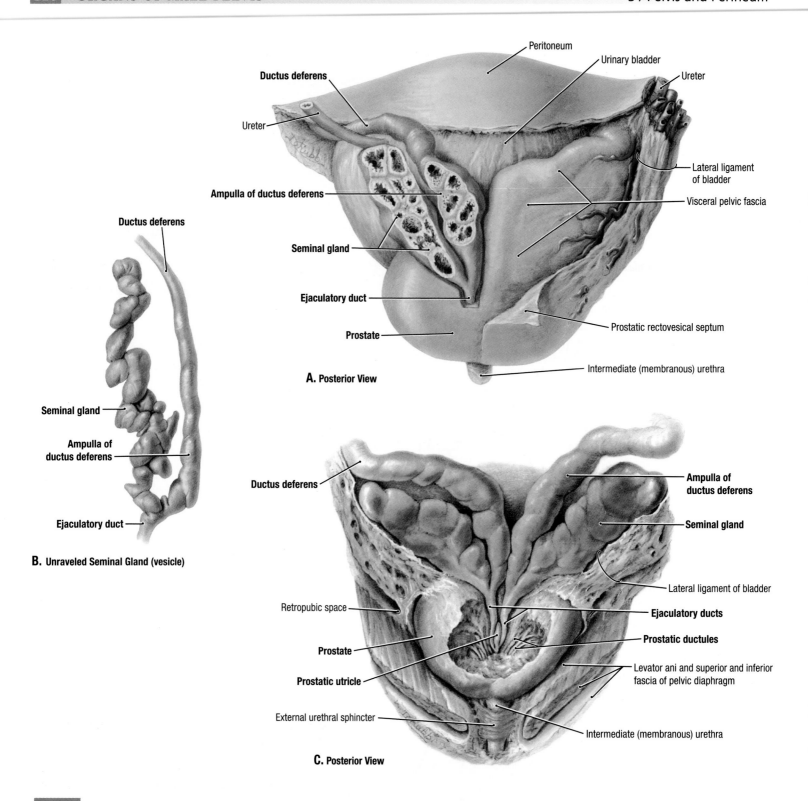

Peritoneum

Ductus deferens

Urinary bladder

Ureter

Ureter

Lateral ligament of bladder

Ampulla of ductus deferens

Visceral pelvic fascia

Seminal gland

Ejaculatory duct

Prostatic rectovesical septum

Prostate

Intermediate (membranous) urethra

A. Posterior View

Ductus deferens

Seminal gland

Ampulla of ductus deferens

Ejaculatory duct

B. Unraveled Seminal Gland (vesicle)

Ductus deferens

Ampulla of ductus deferens

Seminal gland

Lateral ligament of bladder

Retropubic space

Ejaculatory ducts

Prostatic ductules

Prostate

Prostatic utricle

Levator ani and superior and inferior fascia of pelvic diaphragm

External urethral sphincter

Intermediate (membranous) urethra

C. Posterior View

3.23 Seminal glands and prostate

A. Bladder, ductus deferens, seminal glands (vesicles), and prostate. The left seminal gland and ampulla of the ductus deferens are dissected and opened; part of the prostate is cut away to expose the ejaculatory duct. **B.** Seminal vesicle, unraveled. The vesicle is a tortuous tube with numerous dilatations. The ampulla of the ductus deferens has similar dilatations. **C.** Prostate, dissected posteriorly. The ejaculatory duct (approximately 2 cm in length) is formed by the union of the ductus deferens and the duct of the seminal gland; it passes anteriorly and inferiorly through the substance of the prostate to enter the prostatic urethra on the seminal colliculus. The prostatic utricle lies between the ends of the two ejaculatory ducts. The prostatic ductules mostly open onto the prostatic sinus.

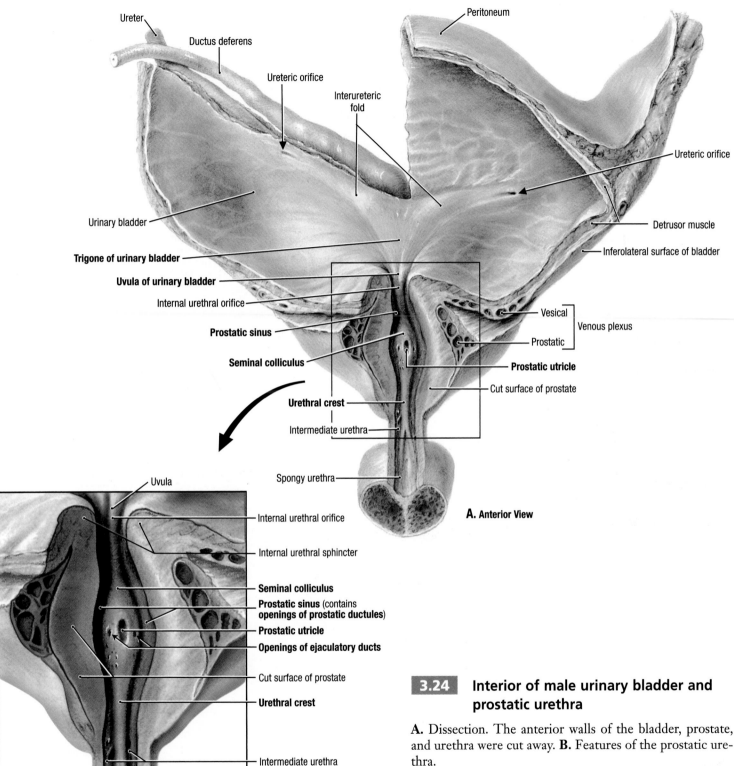

3.24 Interior of male urinary bladder and prostatic urethra

A. Dissection. The anterior walls of the bladder, prostate, and urethra were cut away. **B.** Features of the prostatic urethra.

- The mucous membrane is smooth over the trigone of the urinary bladder (triangular region demarcated by ureteric and internal urethral orifices) but folded elsewhere, especially when the bladder is empty.
- The opening of the prostatic utricle is in the seminal colliculus on the urethral crest; there is an orifice of an ejaculatory duct on each side of the prostatic utricle. The prostatic fascia encloses a venous plexus..

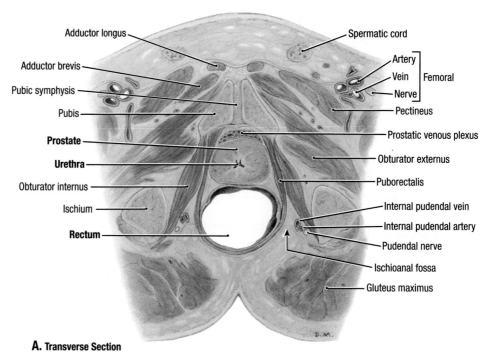

Adductor longus — Spermatic cord
Adductor brevis — Artery — Vein — Nerve } Femoral
Pubic symphysis
Pubis — Pectineus
Prostate — Prostatic venous plexus
Urethra — Obturator externus
Obturator internus — Puborectalis
Ischium — Internal pudendal vein
Rectum — Internal pudendal artery
— Pudendal nerve
— Ischioanal fossa
— Gluteus maximus

A. Transverse Section

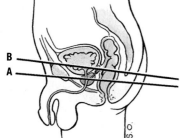

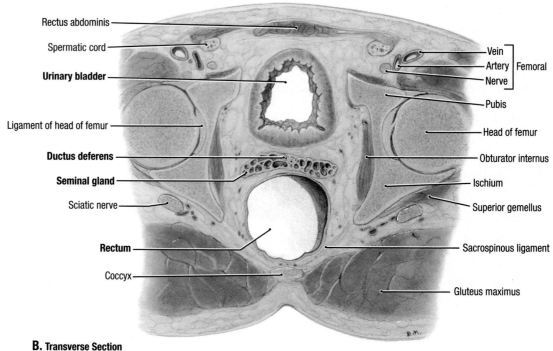

Rectus abdominis
Spermatic cord — Vein — Artery — Nerve } Femoral
Urinary bladder — Pubis
Ligament of head of femur — Head of femur
Ductus deferens — Obturator internus
Seminal gland — Ischium
Sciatic nerve — Superior gemellus
Rectum — Sacrospinous ligament
Coccyx — Gluteus maximus

B. Transverse Section

3.25   **Male pelvis, transverse sections**

A. Section through prostate and puborectalis. **B.** Section through urinary bladder and seminal gland.

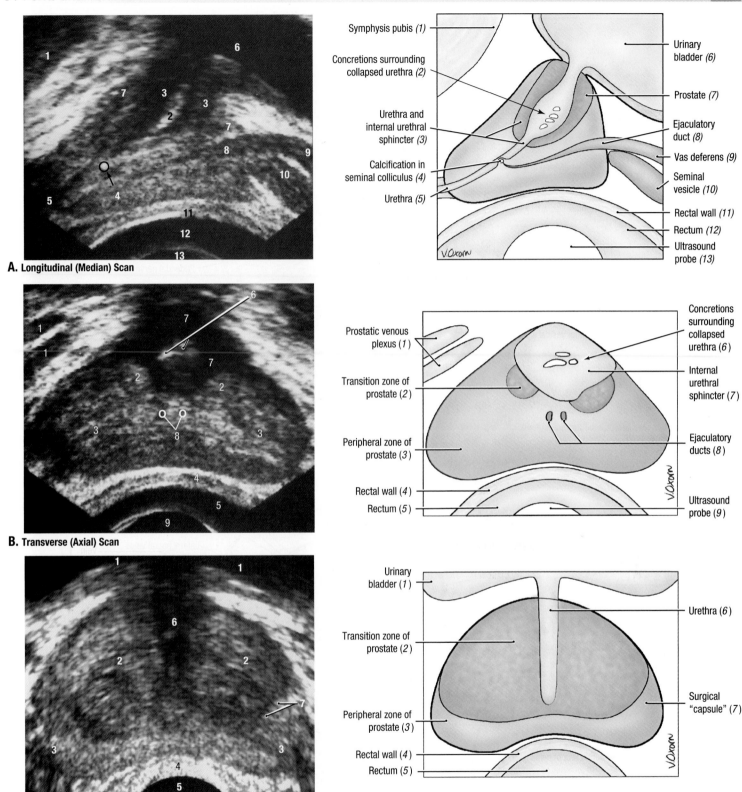

A. Longitudinal (Median) Scan

Symphysis pubis *(1)*
Concretions surrounding collapsed urethra *(2)*
Urethra and internal urethral sphincter *(3)*
Calcification in seminal colliculus *(4)*
Urethra *(5)*
Urinary bladder *(6)*
Prostate *(7)*
Ejaculatory duct *(8)*
Vas deferens *(9)*
Seminal vesicle *(10)*
Rectal wall *(11)*
Rectum *(12)*
Ultrasound probe *(13)*

V.Oxorn

B. Transverse (Axial) Scan

Prostatic venous plexus *(1)*
Transition zone of prostate *(2)*
Peripheral zone of prostate *(3)*
Rectal wall *(4)*
Rectum *(5)*
Concretions surrounding collapsed urethra *(6)*
Internal urethral sphincter *(7)*
Ejaculatory ducts *(8)*
Ultrasound probe *(9)*

V.Oxorn

C. Transverse (Axial) Scan

Urinary bladder *(1)*
Transition zone of prostate *(2)*
Peripheral zone of prostate *(3)*
Rectal wall *(4)*
Rectum *(5)*
Urethra *(6)*
Surgical "capsule" *(7)*

V.Oxorn

3.26   Transrectal ultrasound scans of male pelvis

A. In this longitudinal ultrasound scan, the probe was inserted into the rectum to scan the anteriorly located prostate. The ducts of the glands in the peripheral zone open into the prostatic sinuses, whereas the ducts of the glands in the central (internal) zone open into the prostatic sinuses and onto the seminal colliculus. The large peripheral zone (3) is the common site for carcinomas.

B. Normal prostate of young male. **C.** Benign prostatic hyperplasia. Note the enlarged transition zone (2). The transition zone of the prostate normally starts becoming hyperplastic after age 30. The numbers in parentheses correspond to labels on the ultrasound scan.

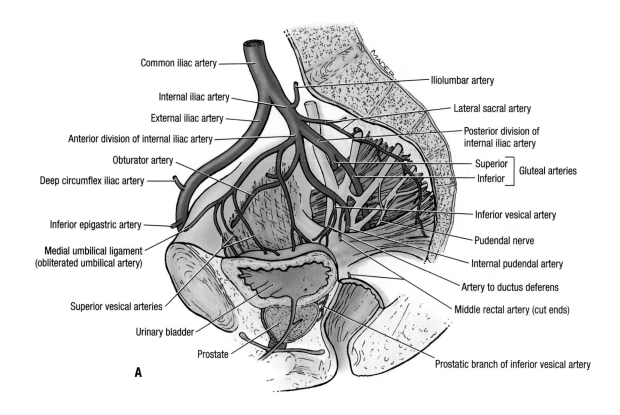

Common iliac artery

Internal iliac artery

External iliac artery

Anterior division of internal iliac artery

Obturator artery

Deep circumflex iliac artery

Inferior epigastric artery

Medial umbilical ligament
(obliterated umbilical artery)

Superior vesical arteries

Urinary bladder

Prostate

A

Iliolumbar artery

Lateral sacral artery

Posterior division of
internal iliac artery

Superior ⎤
            ⎥ Gluteal arteries
Inferior ⎦

Inferior vesical artery

Pudendal nerve

Internal pudendal artery

Artery to ductus deferens

Middle rectal artery (cut ends)

Prostatic branch of inferior vesical artery

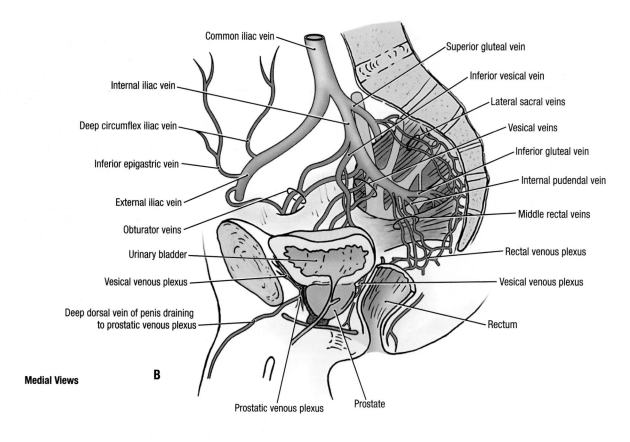

Common iliac vein

Internal iliac vein

Deep circumflex iliac vein

Inferior epigastric vein

External iliac vein

Obturator veins

Urinary bladder

Vesical venous plexus

Deep dorsal vein of penis draining
to prostatic venous plexus

Medial Views

B

Superior gluteal vein

Inferior vesical vein

Lateral sacral veins

Vesical veins

Inferior gluteal vein

Internal pudendal vein

Middle rectal veins

Rectal venous plexus

Vesical venous plexus

Rectum

Prostatic venous plexus

Prostate

3.27   Arteries and veins of male pelvis

A. Arteries. **B.** Pelvic veins and venous plexuses.

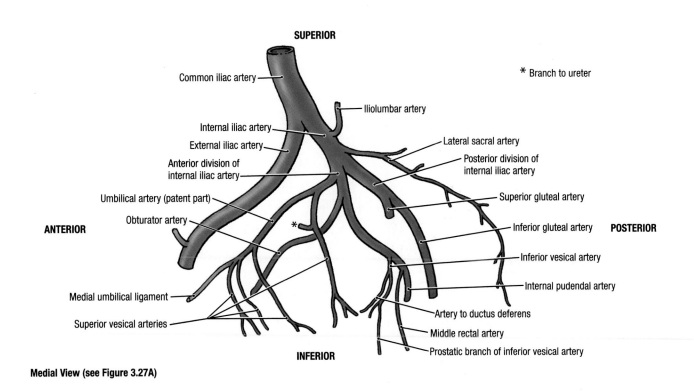

Medial View (see Figure 3.27A)

TABLE 3.4 ARTERIES OF MALE PELVIS

Artery	Origin	Course	Distribution
Internal iliac	Common iliac artery	Passes medially over pelvic brim and descends into pelvic cavity; often forms anterior and posterior divisions	Main blood supply to pelvic organs, gluteal muscles, and perineum
Anterior division of internal iliac	Internal iliac artery	Passes laterally along lateral wall of pelvis, dividing into visceral, obturator, and internal pudendal arteries	Pelvic viscera, perineum, and muscles of superior medial thigh
Umbilical	Anterior division of internal iliac artery	Short pelvic course; gives off superior vesical arteries, then obliterates, becoming medial umbilical ligament	Urinary bladder and, in some males, ductus deferens
Superior vesical	Patent part of umbilical artery	Usually multiple; pass to superior aspect of urinary bladder	Superior aspect of urinary bladder and distal ureter
Artery to ductus deferens	Superior or inferior vesical artery	Runs subperitoneally to ductus deferens	Ductus deferens
Obturator	Anterior division of internal iliac artery	Runs anteroinferiorly on lateral pelvic wall	Pelvic muscles, nutrient artery to ilium, head of femur and medial compartment of thigh
Inferior vesical		Passes subperitoneally giving rise to prostatic artery and occasionally the artery to the ductus deferens	Inferior aspect of urinary bladder, pelvic ureter, seminal glands, and prostate
Middle rectal		Descends in pelvis to rectum	Seminal glands, prostate, and inferior part of rectum
Internal pudendal		Exits pelvis through greater sciatic foramen and enters perineum via lesser sciatic foramen	Main artery to perineum, including muscles and skin of anal and urogenital triangles; erectile bodies
Posterior division of internal iliac artery	Internal iliac artery	Passes posteriorly and gives rise to parietal branches	Pelvic wall and gluteal region
Iliolumbar	Posterior division of internal iliac artery	Ascends anterior to sacroiliac joint and posterior to common iliac vessels and psoas major	Iliacus, psoas major, quadratus lumborum muscles, and cauda equina in vertebral canal
Lateral sacral (superior and inferior)		Run on anteromedial aspect of piriformis to send branches into pelvic sacral foramina	Piriformis muscle, structures in sacral canal and erector spinae muscles
Testicular (gonadal) [see Fig. 3.28A]	Abdominal aorta	Descends retroperitoneally; traverses inguinal canal and enters scrotum	Abdominal ureter, testis and epididymis

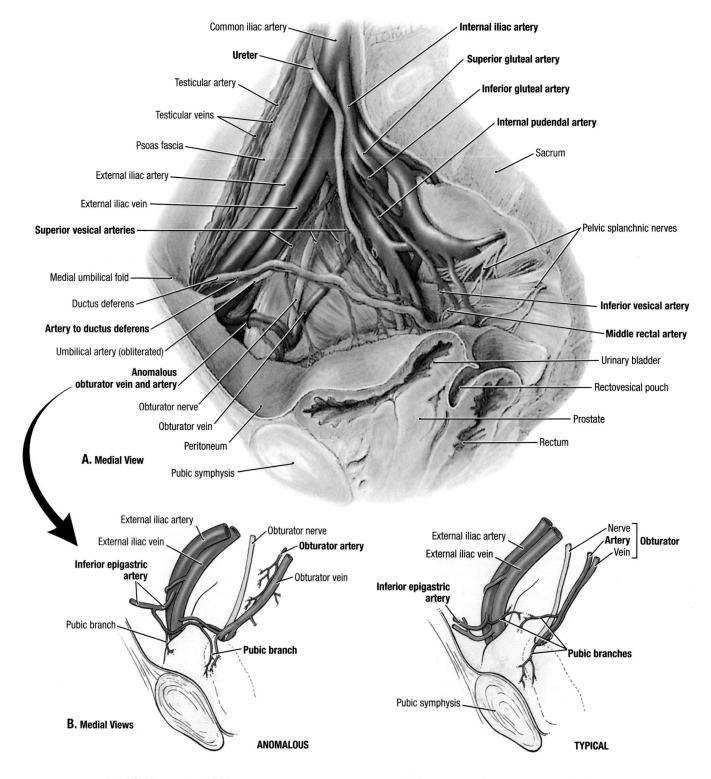

A. Medial View

B. Medial Views

ANOMALOUS

TYPICAL

3.28   Pelvic vessels in situ; lateral pelvic wall

A. Dissection. B. Usual and anomalous obturator arteries.

• The ureter crosses the external iliac artery at its origin (common iliac bifurcation), and the ductus deferens crosses the external iliac artery at its termination (deep inguinal ring).

• In this specimen, an anomalous (replaced) obturator artery branches from the inferior epigastric artery (**B**).

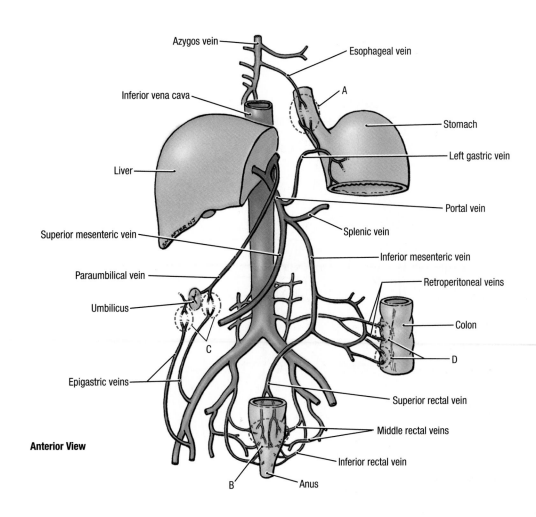

Anterior View

3.29 Portal–systemic anastomoses

The portal tributaries are *purple*, and systemic tributaries are *blue*. *A–D* indicate sites of portal systemic anastomoses. *A*, between portal and systemic esophageal veins; *B*, between portal and systemic rectal veins; *C*, paraumbilical veins (portal) anastomosing with small epigastric veins of the anterior abdominal wall (systemic); *D*, twigs of colic veins (portal) anastomosing with retroperitoneal veins (systemic).

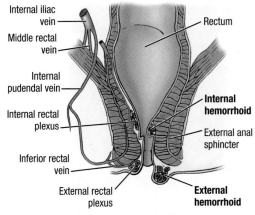

Anterior view of coronal section

Internal hemorrhoids (piles) are prolapses of rectal mucosa containing the normally dilated veins of the *internal rectal venous plexus*. Internal hemorrhoids are thought to result from a breakdown of the muscularis mucosae, a smooth muscle layer deep to the mucosa (see figure at right). Internal hemorrhoids that prolapse through the anal canal are often compressed by the contracted sphincters, impeding blood flow. As a result, they tend to strangulate, ulcerate, and bleed.

External hemorrhoids are thromboses (blood clots) in the veins of the *external rectal venous plexus* and are covered by skin. Predisposing factors for hemorrhoids include pregnancy, chronic constipation, and any disorder that impedes venous return. The superior rectal vein drains into the inferior mesenteric vein, whereas the middle and inferior rectal veins drain through the systemic system into the inferior vena cava. Any abnormal in- crease in pressure in the valveless portal system or veins of the trunk may cause enlargement of the superior rectal veins, resulting in an increase in blood flow or stasis in the internal rectal venous plexus. In *portal hypertension* that occurs in relation to *hepatic cirrhosis*, the portocaval anastomosis (e.g., esophageal) may become varicose and rupture.

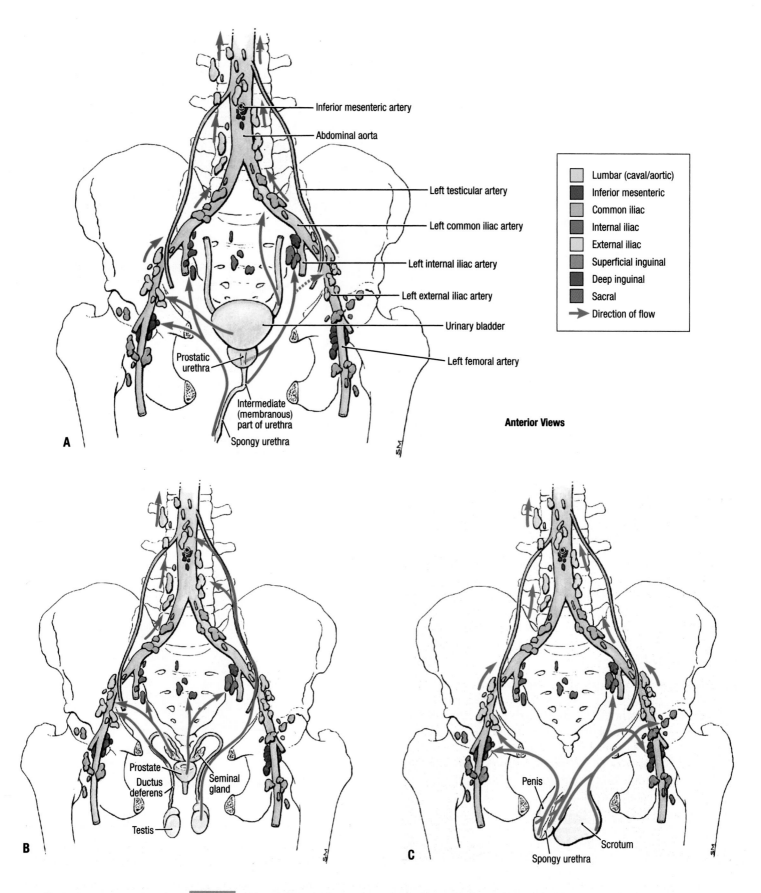

Inferior mesenteric artery

Abdominal aorta

Left testicular artery

Left common iliac artery

Left internal iliac artery

Left external iliac artery

Urinary bladder

Left femoral artery

Prostatic urethra

Intermediate (membranous) part of urethra

Spongy urethra

Anterior Views

Lumbar (caval/aortic)
Inferior mesenteric
Common iliac
Internal iliac
External iliac
Superficial inguinal
Deep inguinal
Sacral
Direction of flow

A

Prostate
Ductus deferens
Seminal gland
Testis

B

Penis
Scrotum
Spongy urethra

C

3.30   **Lymphatic drainage of male pelvis and perineum**

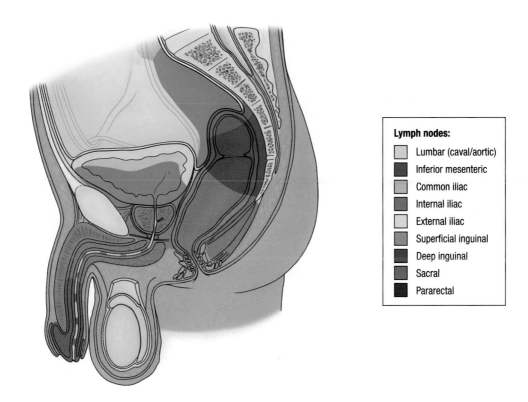

Lymph nodes:

- Lumbar (caval/aortic)
- Inferior mesenteric
- Common iliac
- Internal iliac
- External iliac
- Superficial inguinal
- Deep inguinal
- Sacral
- Pararectal

TABLE 3.5 LYMPHATIC DRAINAGE OF THE MALE PELVIS AND PERINEUM

Lymph Node Group	Structures Typically Draining to Lymph Node Group
Lumbar	Gonads and associated structures (including testicular vessels), urethra, testis, epididymis, common iliac nodes
Inferior mesenteric nodes	Superiormost rectum, sigmoid colon, descending colon, pararectal nodes
Common iliac nodes	External and internal iliac lymph nodes
Internal iliac nodes	Inferior pelvic structures, deep perineal structures, sacral nodes, prostatic urethra, prostate, base of bladder, inferior part of pelvic ureter, inferior part of seminal glands, cavernous bodies, anal canal (above pectinate line), inferior rectum
External iliac nodes	Anterosuperior pelvic structures, deep inguinal nodes, superior aspect of bladder, superior part of pelvic ureter, upper part of seminal gland, pelvic part of ductus deferens, intermediate and spongy urethra
Superficial inguinal nodes	Lower limb, superficial drainage of inferolateral quadrant of trunk, including anterior abdominal wall inferior to umbilicus, gluteal region, superficial perineal structures, skin of perineum including skin and prepuce of penis, scrotum, perianal skin, anal canal inferior to pectinate line
Deep inguinal nodes	Glans of penis, distal spongy urethra, superficial inguinal nodes
Sacral nodes	Posteroinferior pelvic structures, inferior rectum
Pararectal nodes	Superior rectum

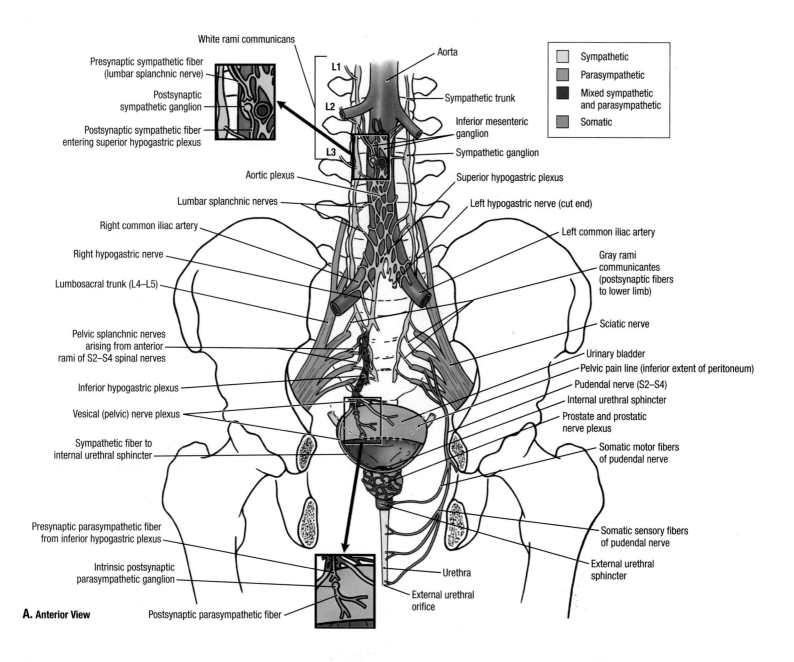

White rami communicans

Presynaptic sympathetic fiber
(lumbar splanchnic nerve)

Postsynaptic
sympathetic ganglion

Postsynaptic sympathetic fiber
entering superior hypogastric plexus

Aorta

Sympathetic trunk

Inferior mesenteric
ganglion

Sympathetic ganglion

Aortic plexus

Lumbar splanchnic nerves

Right common iliac artery

Right hypogastric nerve

Lumbosacral trunk (L4–L5)

Pelvic splanchnic nerves
arising from anterior
rami of S2–S4 spinal nerves

Inferior hypogastric plexus

Vesical (pelvic) nerve plexus

Sympathetic fiber to
internal urethral sphincter

Presynaptic parasympathetic fiber
from inferior hypogastric plexus

Intrinsic postsynaptic
parasympathetic ganglion

Superior hypogastric plexus

Left hypogastric nerve (cut end)

Left common iliac artery

Gray rami
communicantes
(postsynaptic fibers
to lower limb)

Sciatic nerve

Urinary bladder

Pelvic pain line (inferior extent of peritoneum)

Pudendal nerve (S2–S4)

Internal urethral sphincter

Prostate and prostatic
nerve plexus

Somatic motor fibers
of pudendal nerve

Somatic sensory fibers
of pudendal nerve

External urethral
sphincter

Urethra

External urethral
orifice

Symbols:
- Sympathetic
- Parasympathetic
- Mixed sympathetic and parasympathetic
- Somatic

A. Anterior View

Postsynaptic parasympathetic fiber

TABLE 3.6 EFFECT OF SYMPATHETIC AND PARASYMPATHETIC STIMULATION ON THE URINARY TRACT, GENITAL SYSTEM, AND RECTUM

Organ, Tract, or System	Effect of Sympathetic Stimulation	Effect of Parasympathetic Stimulation
Urinary tract	Vasoconstriction of renal vessels slows urine formation; internal sphincter of male bladder contracted to prevent retrograde ejaculation and maintain urinary continence	Inhibits contraction of internal sphincter of bladder in males; contracts detrusor muscle of the bladder wall causing urination
Genital system	Causes ejaculation and vasoconstriction resulting in remission of erection	Produces engorgement (erection) of erectile tissues of the external genitals
Rectum	Maintains tonus of internal anal sphincter; inhibits peristalsis of rectum	Rectal contraction (peristalsis) for defecation; inhibition of contraction of internal anal sphincter

The parasympathetic system is restricted in its distribution to the head, neck, and body cavities (except for erectile tissues of genitalia); otherwise, parasympathetic fibers are never found in the body wall and limbs. Sympathetic fibers, by comparison, are distributed to all vascularized portions of the body.

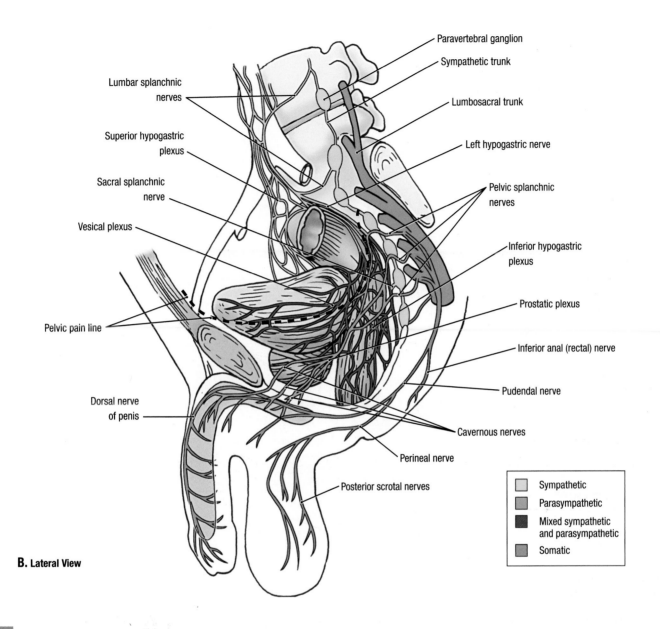

B. Lateral View

Labels (top to bottom, left):
- Lumbar splanchnic nerves
- Superior hypogastric plexus
- Sacral splanchnic nerve
- Vesical plexus
- Pelvic pain line
- Dorsal nerve of penis

Labels (right):
- Paravertebral ganglion
- Sympathetic trunk
- Lumbosacral trunk
- Left hypogastric nerve
- Pelvic splanchnic nerves
- Inferior hypogastric plexus
- Prostatic plexus
- Inferior anal (rectal) nerve
- Pudendal nerve
- Cavernous nerves
- Perineal nerve
- Posterior scrotal nerves

Legend:
- Sympathetic
- Parasympathetic
- Mixed sympathetic and parasympathetic
- Somatic

3.31   Innervation of male pelvis and perineum

A. Overview. B. Innervation of prostate and external genitalia.
- The primary function of the sacral sympathetic trunks is to provide postsynaptic fibers to the sacral plexus for sympathetic innervation of the lower limb.
- The periarterial plexuses of the ovarian, superior rectal, and internal iliac arteries are minor routes by which sympathetic fibers enter the pelvis. Their primary function is vasomotion of the arteries they accompany.
- The hypogastric plexuses (superior and inferior) are networks of sympathetic and visceral afferent nerve fibers.
- The superior hypogastric plexus carries fibers conveyed to and from the aortic (intermesenteric) plexus by the L3 and L4 splanchnic nerves. The superior hypogastric plexus divides into right and left hypogastric nerves that merge with the parasympathetic pelvic splanchnic nerves to form the inferior hypogastric plexuses.

- The fibers of the inferior hypogastric plexuses continue to the pelvic viscera upon which they form pelvic plexuses, e.g., prostatic nerve plexus.
- The pelvic splanchnic nerves convey presynaptic parasympathetic fibers from the S2–S4 spinal cord segments, which make up the sacral outflow of the parasympathetic system.
- Visceral afferents conveying unconscious reflex sensation follow the course of the parasympathetic fibers retrogradely to the spinal sensory ganglia of S2–S4, as do those transmitting pain sensations from the viscera inferior to the pelvic pain line (structures that do not contact the peritoneum plus the distal sigmoid colon and rectum). Visceral afferent fibers conducting pain from structures superior to the pelvic pain line (structures in contact with the peritoneum, except for the distal sigmoid colon and rectum) follow the sympathetic fibers retrogradely to inferior thoracic and superior lumbar spinal ganglia.

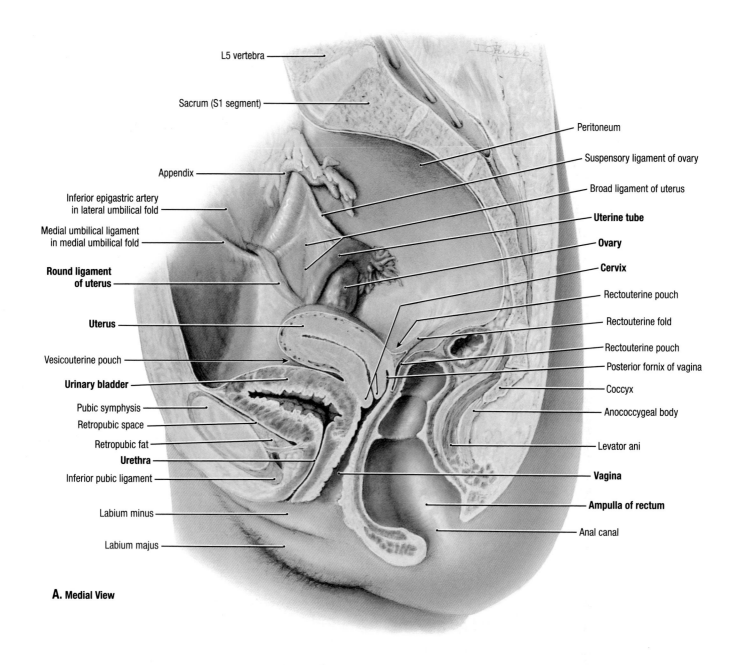

L5 vertebra

Sacrum (S1 segment)

Peritoneum

Suspensory ligament of ovary

Appendix

Broad ligament of uterus

Inferior epigastric artery
in lateral umbilical fold

Uterine tube

Medial umbilical ligament
in medial umbilical fold

Ovary

**Round ligament
of uterus**

Cervix

Rectouterine pouch

Uterus

Rectouterine fold

Vesicouterine pouch

Rectouterine pouch

Urinary bladder

Posterior fornix of vagina

Pubic symphysis

Coccyx

Retropubic space

Anococcygeal body

Retropubic fat

Levator ani

Urethra

Vagina

Inferior pubic ligament

Ampulla of rectum

Labium minus

Anal canal

Labium majus

A. Medial View

3.32   Female pelvic organs in situ

A. Median section. The uterus is bent on itself (anteflexed) at the
junction of its body and the cervix; the cervix, opening on the
anterior wall of the vagina, has a short, round, anterior lip and a
long, thin, posterior lip. **B.** Hysterectomy (excision of the uterus) is
performed through the lower anterior abdominal wall or through
the vagina. Because the uterine artery crosses superior to the ureter
near the lateral fornix of the vagina, the ureter is in danger of being
inadvertently clamped or severed when the uterine artery is tied off
during a hysterectomy.

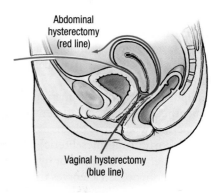

Abdominal
hysterectomy
(red line)

Vaginal hysterectomy
(blue line)

B. Medial View

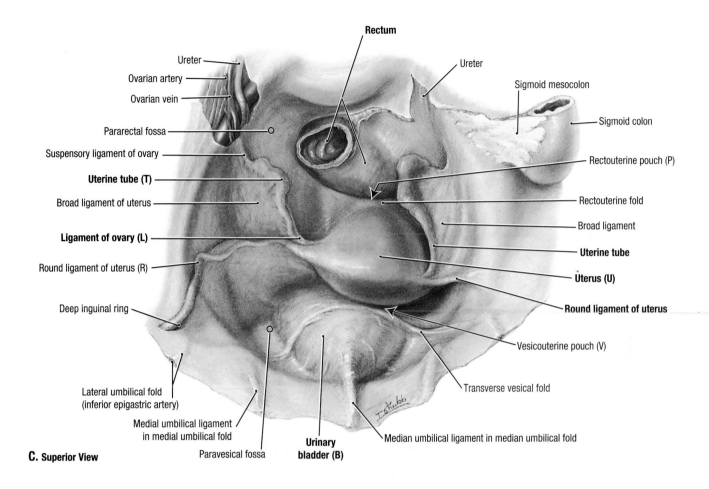

C. Superior View

D. Laparoscopic View of Normal Pelvis

3.32   **Female pelvic organs in situ** *(continued)*

C. True pelvis with peritoneum intact, viewed from above. The uterus is usually asymmetrically placed. The round ligament of the female takes the same subperitoneal course as the ductus deferens of the male.

D. Laparoscopy involves inserting a laparoscope into the peritoneal cavity through a small incision below the umbilicus. Insufflation of inert gas creates a pneumoperitoneum to provide space to visualize the pelvic organs. Additional openings (ports) can be made to introduce other instruments for manipulation or to enable therapeutic procedures (e.g., ligation of the uterine tubes).

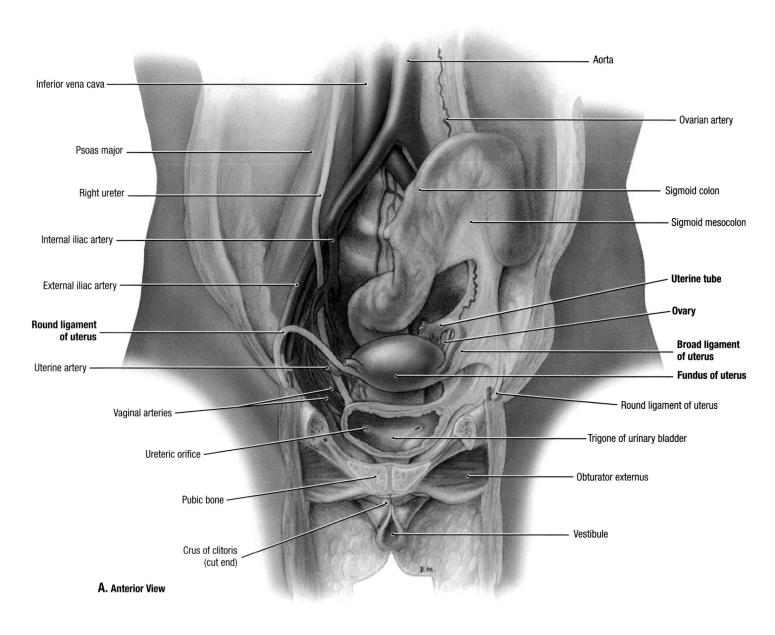

Aorta

Inferior vena cava

Ovarian artery

Psoas major

Right ureter

Sigmoid colon

Sigmoid mesocolon

Internal iliac artery

External iliac artery

Uterine tube

Ovary

Round ligament of uterus

Broad ligament of uterus

Uterine artery

Fundus of uterus

Vaginal arteries

Round ligament of uterus

Trigone of urinary bladder

Ureteric orifice

Obturator externus

Pubic bone

Vestibule

Crus of clitoris (cut end)

A. Anterior View

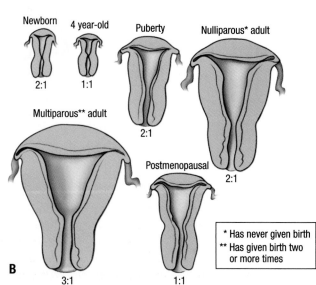

Newborn   4 year-old   Puberty   Nulliparous* adult

2:1   1:1

Multiparous** adult

2:1

Postmenopausal

3:1   1:1

2:1

* Has never given birth
** Has given birth two or more times

B

3.33   **Female genital organs**

A. Dissection. Part of the pubic bones, the anterior aspect of the bladder, and—on the specimen's right side—the uterine tube, ovary, broad ligament, and peritoneum covering the lateral wall of the pelvis have been removed. **B.** Lifetime changes in uterine size and proportion (body to cervical ratio, e.g., 2:1). All these stages represent normal anatomy for the particular age and reproductive status of the woman.

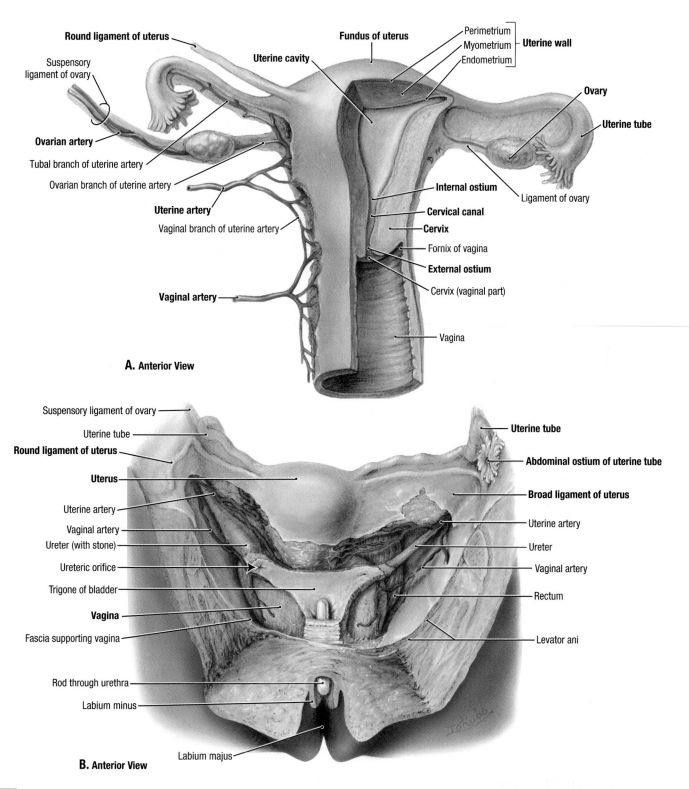

A. Anterior View

B. Anterior View

3.34   Uterus and its adnexa

A. Blood supply. On the specimen's left side, part of the uterine wall with the round ligament and the vaginal wall have been cut away to expose the cervix, uterine cavity, and thick muscular wall of the uterus, the myometrium. On the specimen's right side, the ovarian artery (from the aorta) and uterine artery (from the internal iliac) supply the ovary, uterine tube, and uterus and anasto-

mose in the broad ligament along the lateral aspect of the uterus. The uterine artery sends a uterine branch to supply the uterine body and fundus and a vaginal branch to supply the cervix and vagina. **B.** Uterus and broad ligament. The pubic bones and bladder, trigone excepted, are removed, as a continued dissection from Figure 3.33.

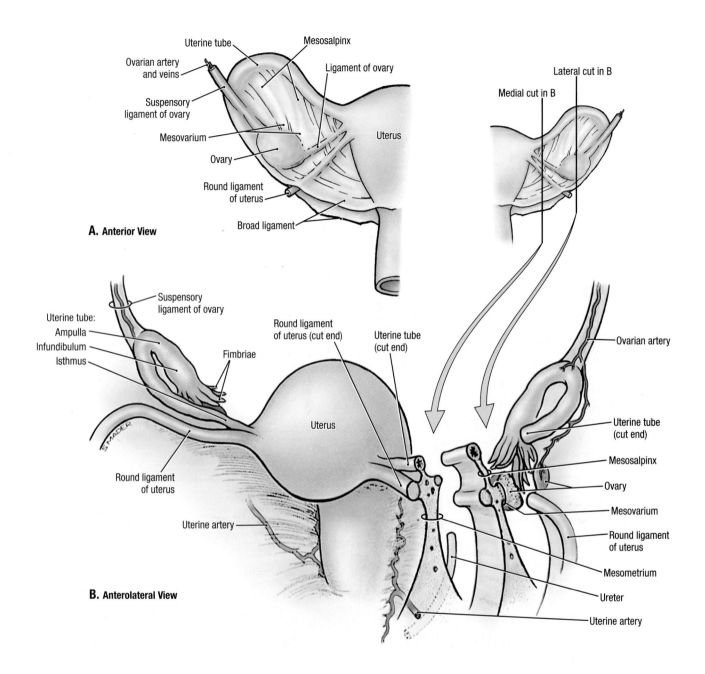

3.35 Uterus and broad ligament

A and **B.** Two paramedian sections show "mesenteries" with the prefix meso-. "Salpinx" is the Greek word for trumpet or tube, "metro" for uterus. The mesentery of the uterus and uterine tube is called the broad ligament. The major part of the broad ligament, the *mesometrium*, is attached to the uterus. The ovary is attached: to the broad ligament by a mesentery of its own, called the *mesovarium*; to the uterus by the ligament of the ovary; and near the pelvic brim, by the suspensory ligament of the ovary containing the ovarian vessels. The part of the broad ligament superior to the level of the mesovarium is called the *mesosalpinx*. **C.** Uterus in situ. **D.** Uterus and adnexa, removed from cadaver.

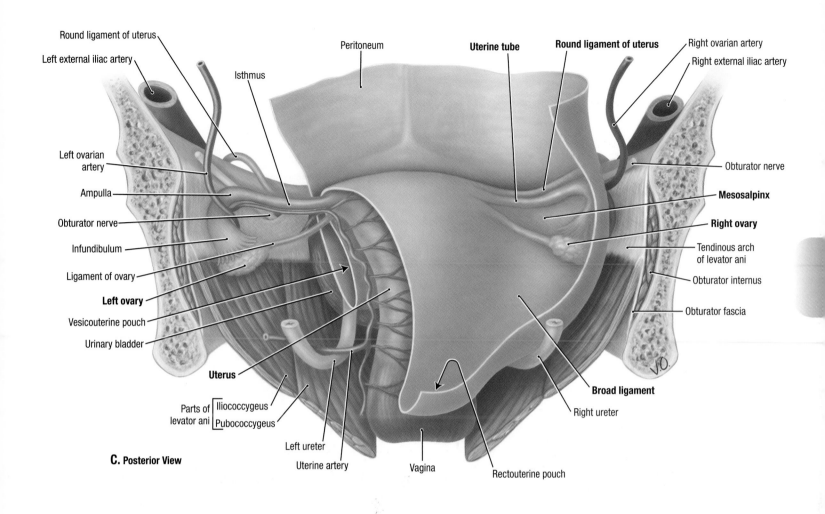

Round ligament of uterus

Left external iliac artery

Isthmus

Peritoneum

Uterine tube

Round ligament of uterus

Right ovarian artery

Right external iliac artery

Left ovarian artery

Ampulla

Obturator nerve

Infundibulum

Ligament of ovary

Left ovary

Vesicouterine pouch

Urinary bladder

Uterus

Parts of levator ani [Iliococcygeus / Pubococcygeus]

Left ureter

Uterine artery

Vagina

Obturator nerve

Mesosalpinx

Right ovary

Tendinous arch of levator ani

Obturator internus

Obturator fascia

Broad ligament

Right ureter

Rectouterine pouch

C. Posterior View

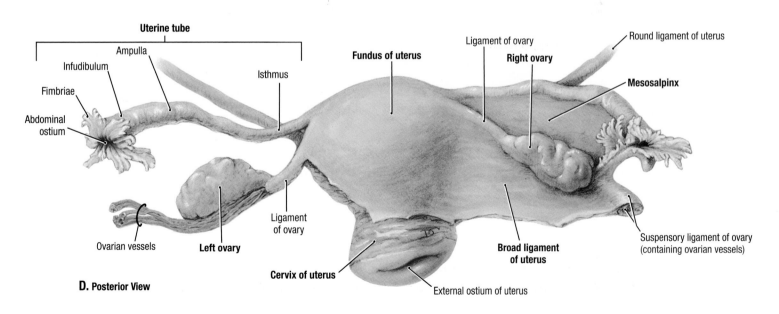

Uterine tube

Ampulla

Infudibulum

Fimbriae

Abdominal ostium

Isthmus

Fundus of uterus

Ligament of ovary

Right ovary

Round ligament of uterus

Mesosalpinx

Ligament of ovary

Ovarian vessels

Left ovary

Cervix of uterus

External ostium of uterus

Broad ligament of uterus

Suspensory ligament of ovary (containing ovarian vessels)

D. Posterior View

3.35   **Uterus and broad ligament** *(continued)*

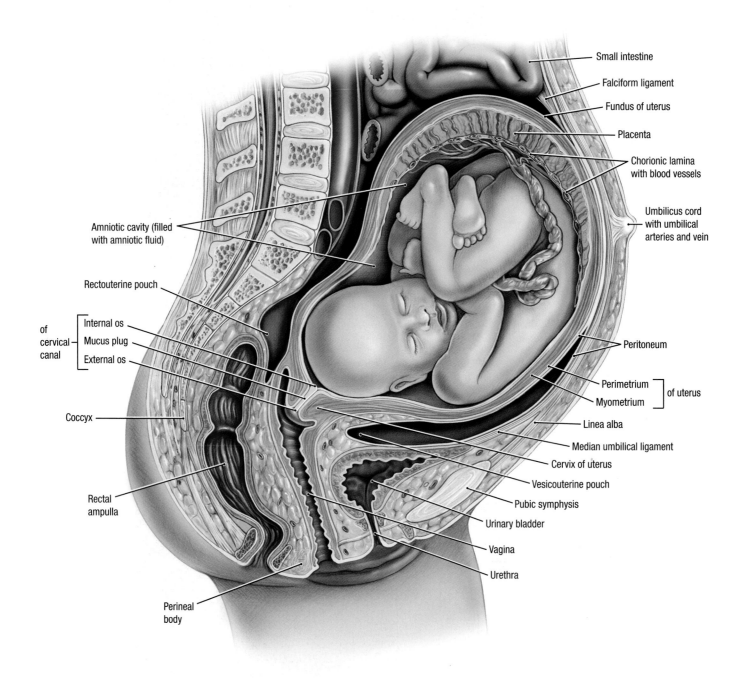

Small intestine

Falciform ligament

Fundus of uterus

Placenta

Chorionic lamina
with blood vessels

Umbilicus cord
with umbilical
arteries and vein

Amniotic cavity (filled
with amniotic fluid)

Rectouterine pouch

of cervical canal
Internal os
Mucus plug
External os

Peritoneum

Perimetrium
Myometrium
of uterus

Linea alba

Median umbilical ligament

Cervix of uterus

Vesicouterine pouch

Pubic symphysis

Urinary bladder

Vagina

Urethra

Coccyx

Rectal
ampulla

Perineal
body

3.36   Pregnant uterus

A. Median section; fetus is intact.

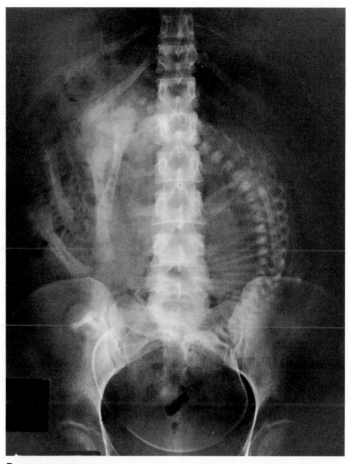

B. Anteroposterior View

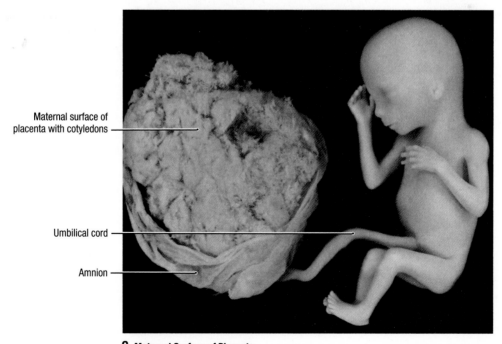

Maternal surface of
placenta with cotyledons

Umbilical cord

Amnion

C. Maternal Surface of Placenta

3.36   **Pregnant uterus** *(continued)*

B. Radiograph of fetus. **C.** Photograph of an 18-week-old fetus connected to the placenta
by the umbilical cord.

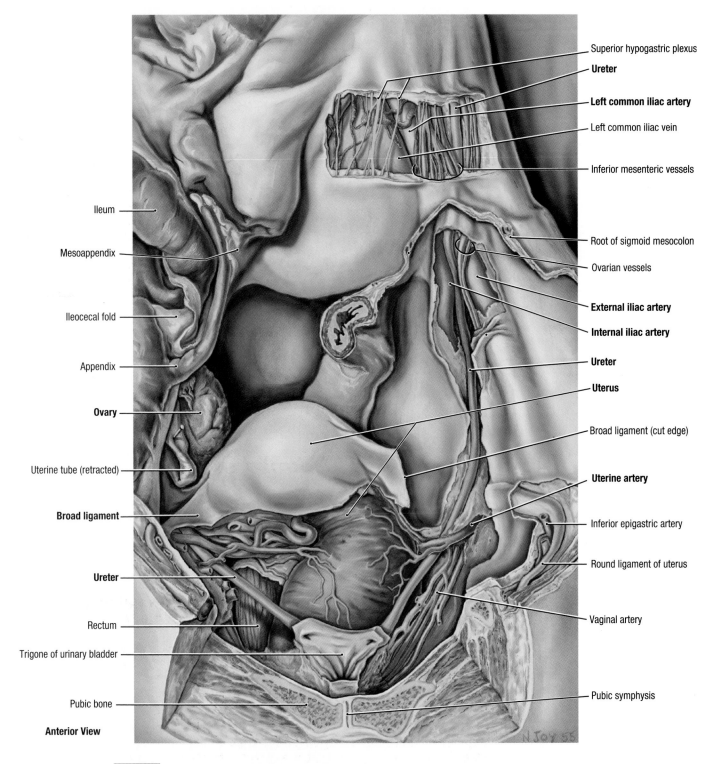

Ileum

Mesoappendix

Ileocecal fold

Appendix

Ovary

Uterine tube (retracted)

Broad ligament

Ureter

Rectum

Trigone of urinary bladder

Pubic bone

Anterior View

Superior hypogastric plexus

Ureter

Left common iliac artery

Left common iliac vein

Inferior mesenteric vessels

Root of sigmoid mesocolon

Ovarian vessels

External iliac artery

Internal iliac artery

Ureter

Uterus

Broad ligament (cut edge)

Uterine artery

Inferior epigastric artery

Round ligament of uterus

Vaginal artery

Pubic symphysis

3.37   **Ureter and relationship to uterine artery**

- Most of the pubic symphysis and most of the bladder (except the trigone) have been removed as in Figure 3.34B.
- The left ureter is crossed by the ovarian vessels and nerves; the apex of the inverted V-shaped root of the sigmoid mesocolon is situated anterior to the left ureter.
- The left ureter crosses the external iliac artery at the bifurcation of the common iliac artery and then descends anterior to the internal iliac artery; its course is subperitoneal from where it enters the pelvis to where it passes deep to the broad ligament and is crossed by the uterine artery.

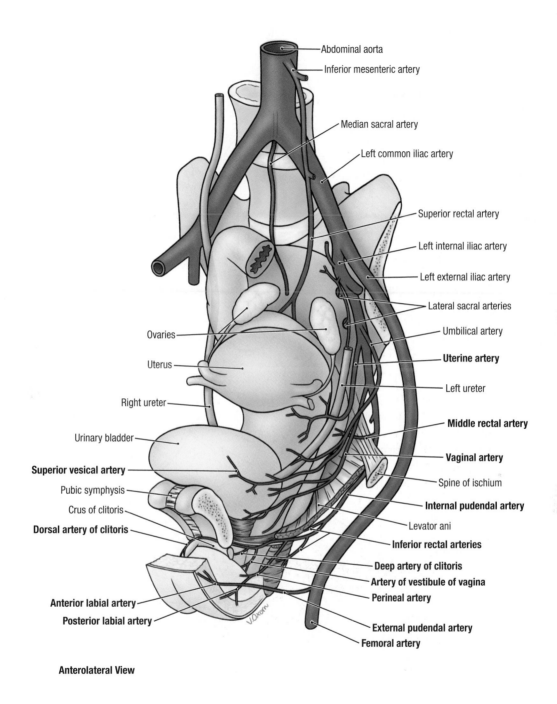

Abdominal aorta

Inferior mesenteric artery

Median sacral artery

Left common iliac artery

Superior rectal artery

Left internal iliac artery

Left external iliac artery

Lateral sacral arteries

Umbilical artery

Uterine artery

Left ureter

Middle rectal artery

Vaginal artery

Spine of ischium

Internal pudendal artery

Levator ani

Deep artery of clitoris

Inferior rectal arteries

Artery of vestibule of vagina

Perineal artery

External pudendal artery

Femoral artery

Ovaries

Uterus

Right ureter

Urinary bladder

Superior vesical artery

Pubic symphysis

Crus of clitoris

Dorsal artery of clitoris

Anterior labial artery

Posterior labial artery

Anterolateral View

3.38   **Arterial supply of female pelvis and perineum**

- The blood supply of the uterus is mainly from the *uterine arteries*, with potential collateral supply from the ovarian arteries.
- The arteries supplying the superior part of the vagina derive from the *uterine arteries*; the arteries supplying the middle and inferior parts of the vagina derive from the *vaginal* and *internal pudendal arteries*.
- The superior vesical arteries supply the anterosuperior parts of the bladder; the vaginal arteries supply the posteroinferior parts of the bladder.

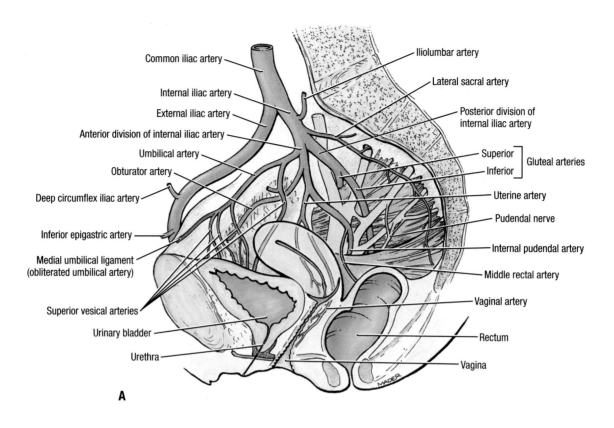

Common iliac artery

Internal iliac artery

External iliac artery

Anterior division of internal iliac artery

Umbilical artery

Obturator artery

Deep circumflex iliac artery

Inferior epigastric artery

Medial umbilical ligament (obliterated umbilical artery)

Superior vesical arteries

Urinary bladder

Urethra

Iliolumbar artery

Lateral sacral artery

Posterior division of internal iliac artery

Superior ⎤
          ⎥ Gluteal arteries
Inferior ⎦

Uterine artery

Pudendal nerve

Internal pudendal artery

Middle rectal artery

Vaginal artery

Rectum

Vagina

A

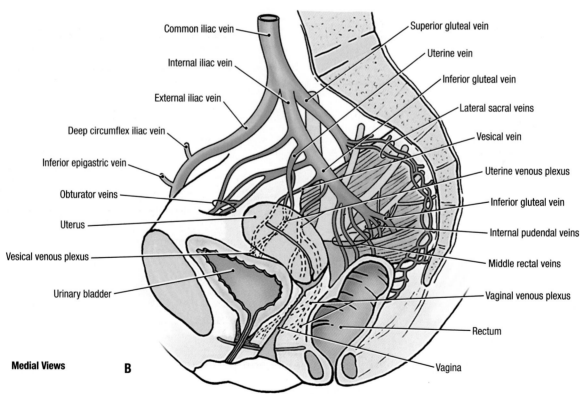

Common iliac vein

Internal iliac vein

External iliac vein

Deep circumflex iliac vein

Inferior epigastric vein

Obturator veins

Uterus

Vesical venous plexus

Urinary bladder

Superior gluteal vein

Uterine vein

Inferior gluteal vein

Lateral sacral veins

Vesical vein

Uterine venous plexus

Inferior gluteal vein

Internal pudendal veins

Middle rectal veins

Vaginal venous plexus

Rectum

Vagina

Medial Views   **B**

3.39 **Arteries and veins of female pelvis**

A. Arteries. **B.** Pelvic veins and venous plexuses.

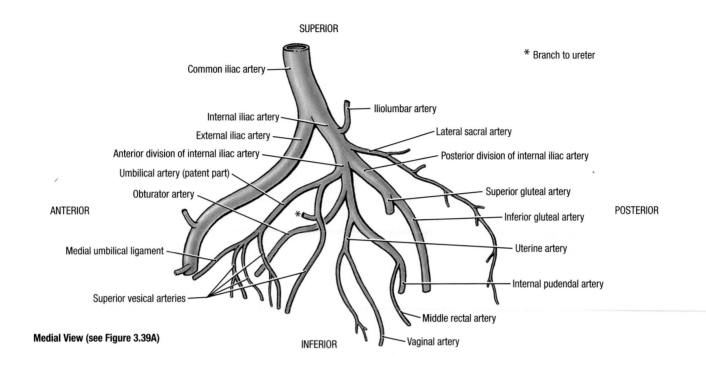

SUPERIOR

* Branch to ureter

Medial View (see Figure 3.39A)

ANTERIOR   POSTERIOR

INFERIOR

TABLE 3.7 ARTERIES OF FEMALE PELVIS

Artery	Origin	Course	Distribution
Internal iliac	Common iliac artery	Passes over pelvic brim and descends into pelvic cavity	Main blood supply to pelvic organs, gluteal muscles, and perineum
Anterior division of internal iliac artery	Internal iliac artery	Passes anteriorly along lateral wall of pelvis, dividing into visceral, obturator, and internal pudendal arteries	Pelvic viscera and muscles of superior medial thigh, and perineum
Umbilical	Anterior division of internal iliac artery	Short pelvic course, gives off superior vesical arteries	Superior aspect of urinary bladder
Superior vesical artery	Patent proximal part of umbilical artery	Usually multiple, pass to superior aspect of urinary bladder	Superior aspect of urinary bladder
Obturator	Anterior division of internal iliac artery	Runs anteroinferiorly on lateral pelvic wall	Pelvic muscles, nutrient artery to ilium, head of femur, and muscles of medial compartment of thigh
Uterine		Runs anteromedially in base of broad ligament/ superior cardinal ligament; gives rise to vaginal branch, then crosses ureter superiorly to reach lateral aspect of uterine cervix	Uterus, ligaments of uterus, medial parts of uterine tube and ovary, and superior vagina
Vaginal		Divides into vaginal and inferior vesical branches	Vaginal branch: lower vagina, vestibular bulb, and adjacent rectum; inferior vesical branch: fundus of urinary bladder
Middle rectal		Descends in pelvis to inferior part of rectum	Inferior part of rectum
Internal pudendal		Exits pelvis via greater sciatic foramen and enters perineum (ischioanal fossa) via lesser sciatic foramen	Main artery to perineum including muscles of anal canal and perineum, skin and urogenital triangle, and erectile bodies
Posterior division of internal iliac artery	Internal iliac artery	Passes posteriorly and gives rise to parietal branches	Pelvic wall and gluteal region
Iliolumbar	Posterior division of internal iliac artery	Ascends anterior to sacroiliac joint and posterior to common iliac vessels and psoas major	Iliacus, psoas major, quadratus lumborum muscles, and cauda equina in vertebral canal
Lateral sacral (superior and inferior)		Run on anteromedial aspect of piriformis	Piriformis muscle, structures in sacral canal and erector spinae muscles
Ovarian	Abdominal aorta	Crosses pelvic brim and descends in suspensory ligament to ovary	Abdominal and/or pelvic ureter, ovary, and ampullary end of uterine tube

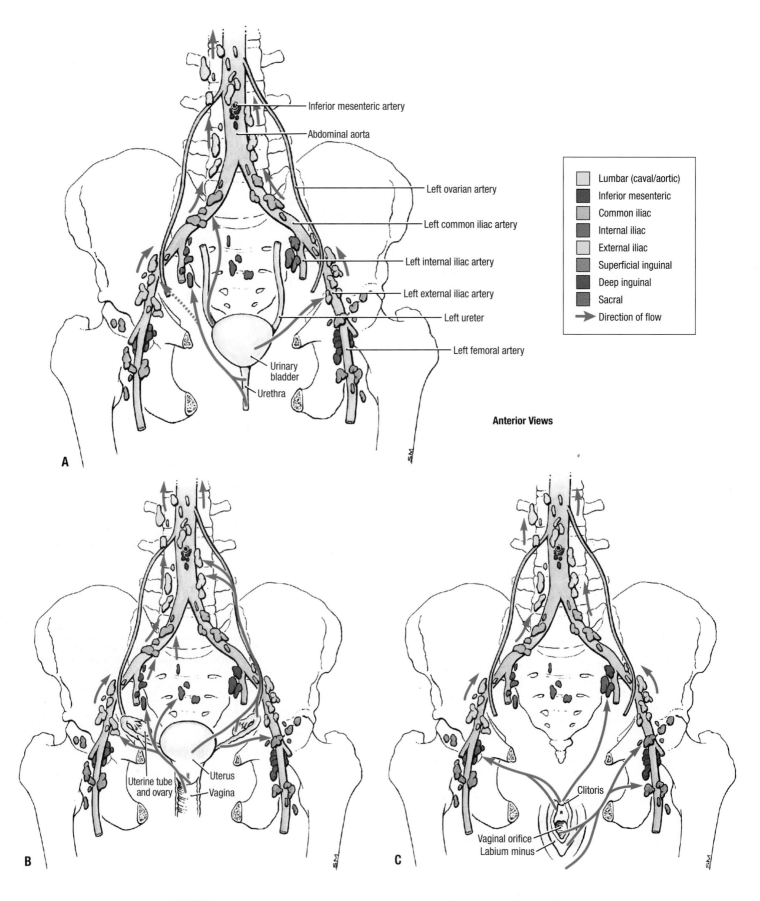

Inferior mesenteric artery

Abdominal aorta

Left ovarian artery

Left common iliac artery

Left internal iliac artery

Left external iliac artery

Left ureter

Left femoral artery

Urinary bladder

Urethra

Lumbar (caval/aortic)
Inferior mesenteric
Common iliac
Internal iliac
External iliac
Superficial inguinal
Deep inguinal
Sacral
Direction of flow

Anterior Views

A

Uterine tube and ovary
Uterus
Vagina

B

Clitoris

Vaginal orifice
Labium minus

C

3.40   Lymphatic drainage of female pelvis and perineum

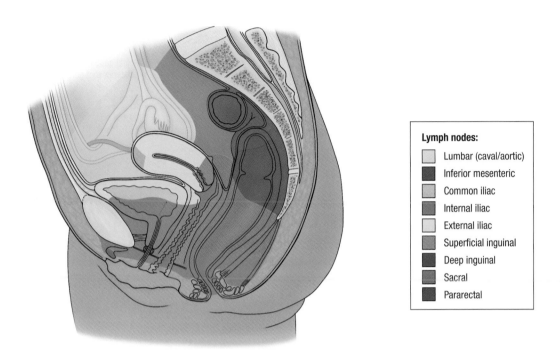

Lymph nodes:

- Lumbar (caval/aortic)
- Inferior mesenteric
- Common iliac
- Internal iliac
- External iliac
- Superficial inguinal
- Deep inguinal
- Sacral
- Pararectal

TABLE 3.8 LYMPHATIC DRAINAGE OF THE STRUCTURES OF THE FEMALE PELVIS AND PERINEUM

Lymph Node Group	Structures Typically Draining to Lymph Node Group
Lumbar	Gonads and associated structures (along ovarian vessels), ovary, uterine tube (except isthmus and intrauterine parts), fundus of uterus, common iliac nodes
Inferior mesenteric	Superiormost rectum, sigmoid colon, descending colon, pararectal nodes
Common iliac	External and internal iliac lymph nodes
Internal iliac	Inferior pelvic structures, deep perineal structures, sacral nodes, base of bladder, inferior pelvic ureter, anal canal (above pectinate line), inferior rectum, middle and upper vagina, cervix, body of uterus , sacral nodes
External iliac	Anterosuperior pelvic structures, deep inguinal nodes, superior bladder, superior pelvic ureter, upper vagina, cervix, lower body of uterus
Superficial inguinal	Lower limb, superficial drainage of inferolateral quadrant of trunk, including anterior abdominal wall inferior to umbilicus, gluteal region, superolateral uterus (near attachment of round ligament), skin of perineum including vulva, ostium of vagina (inferior to hymen), prepuce of clitoris, perianal skin, anal canal inferior to pectinate line
Deep inguinal	Glans of clitoris, superficial inguinal nodes
Sacral	Posteroinferior pelvic structures, inferior rectum, inferior vagina
Pararectal	Superior rectum

3.41 Innervation of female pelvic viscera

- Pelvic splanchnic nerves (S2–S4) supply parasympathetic motor fibers to the uterus and vagina (and vasodilator fibers to the erectile tissue of the clitoris and bulb of the vestibule; not shown).
- Presynaptic sympathetic fibers pass through the lumbar splanchnic nerves to synapse in prevertebral ganglia; the postsynaptic fibers travel through the superior and inferior hypogastric plexuses to reach the pelvic viscera.
- Visceral afferent fibers conducting pain from intraperitoneal viscera travel with the sympathetic fibers to the T12–L2 spinal ganglia. Visceral afferent fibers conducting pain from subperitoneal viscera travel with parasympathetic fibers to the S2–S4 spinal ganglia.
- Somatic sensation from the opening of the vagina also passes to the S2–S4 spinal ganglia via the pudendal nerve.
- Muscular contractions of the uterus are hormonally induced.

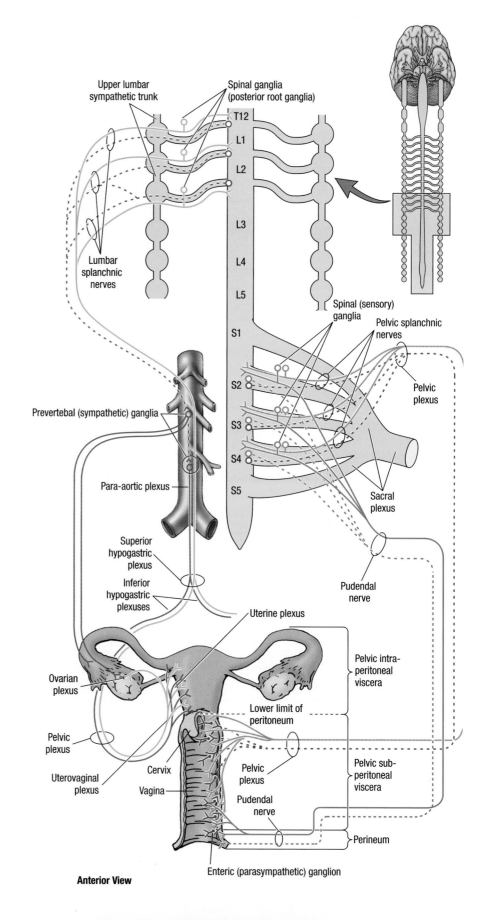

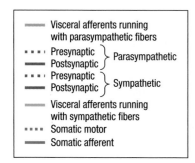

Visceral afferents running with parasympathetic fibers

····· Presynaptic } Parasympathetic
───── Postsynaptic

····· Presynaptic } Sympathetic
───── Postsynaptic

Visceral afferents running with sympathetic fibers

····· Somatic motor

───── Somatic afferent

Anterior View

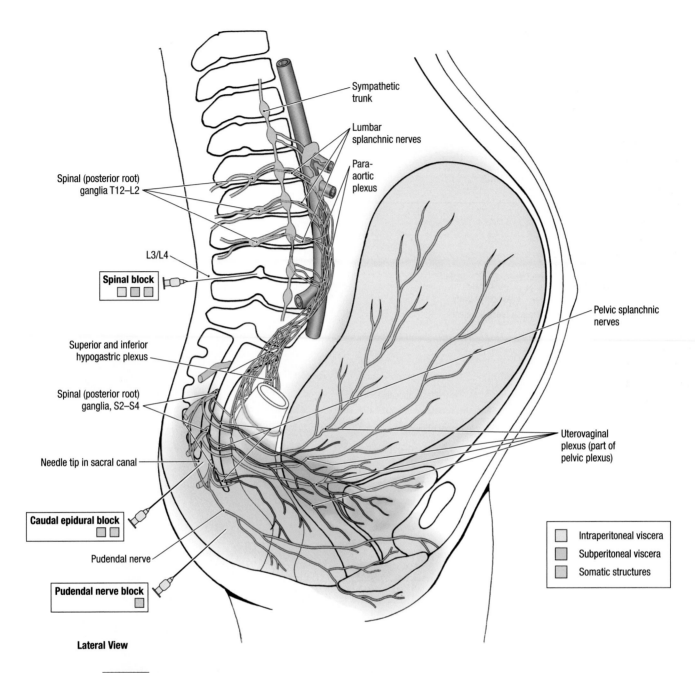

Lateral View

Sympathetic trunk

Lumbar splanchnic nerves

Para-aortic plexus

Spinal (posterior root) ganglia T12–L2

L3/L4

Spinal block

Superior and inferior hypogastric plexus

Spinal (posterior root) ganglia, S2–S4

Needle tip in sacral canal

Caudal epidural block

Pudendal nerve

Pudendal nerve block

Pelvic splanchnic nerves

Uterovaginal plexus (part of pelvic plexus)

Intraperitoneal viscera
Subperitoneal viscera
Somatic structures

3.42 Innervation of pelvic viscera during pregnancy; nerve blocks

- A spinal block, in which the anesthetic agent is introduced with a needle into the spinal subarachnoid space at the L3–L4 vertebral level produces complete anesthesia inferior to approximately the waist level. The perineum, pelvic floor, and birth canal are anesthetized, and motor and sensory functions of the entire lower limbs, as well as sensation of uterine contractions, are temporarily eliminated.
- With the caudal epidural block, the anesthetic agent is administered using an in-dwelling catheter in the sacral canal. The entire birth canal, pelvic floor, and most of the perineum are anesthetized, but the lower limbs are not usually affected. The mother is aware of her uterine contractions.
- A pudendal nerve block is a peripheral nerve block that provides local anesthesia over the S2–S4 dermatomes (most of the perineum) and the inferior quarter of the vagina. It does not block pain from the superior birth canal (uterine cervix and superior vagina, so the mother is able to feel uterine contractions.

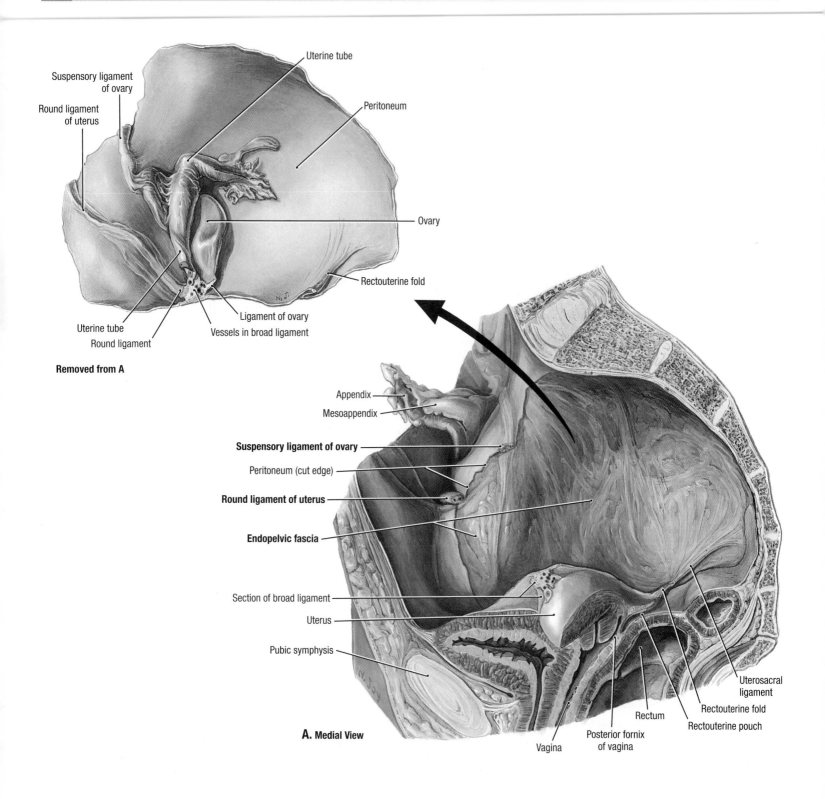

Suspensory ligament
of ovary

Round ligament
of uterus

Uterine tube

Peritoneum

Ovary

Rectouterine fold

Uterine tube

Round ligament

Ligament of ovary

Vessels in broad ligament

Removed from A

Appendix

Mesoappendix

Suspensory ligament of ovary

Peritoneum (cut edge)

Round ligament of uterus

Endopelvic fascia

Section of broad ligament

Uterus

Pubic symphysis

A. Medial View

Vagina

Posterior fornix
of vagina

Rectum

Rectouterine pouch

Rectouterine fold

Uterosacral
ligament

3.43   **Serial dissection of autonomic nerves of female pelvis**

A. Broad ligament and peritoneum of the lateral wall of the pelvic cavity have been removed
to expose the endopelvic fascia.

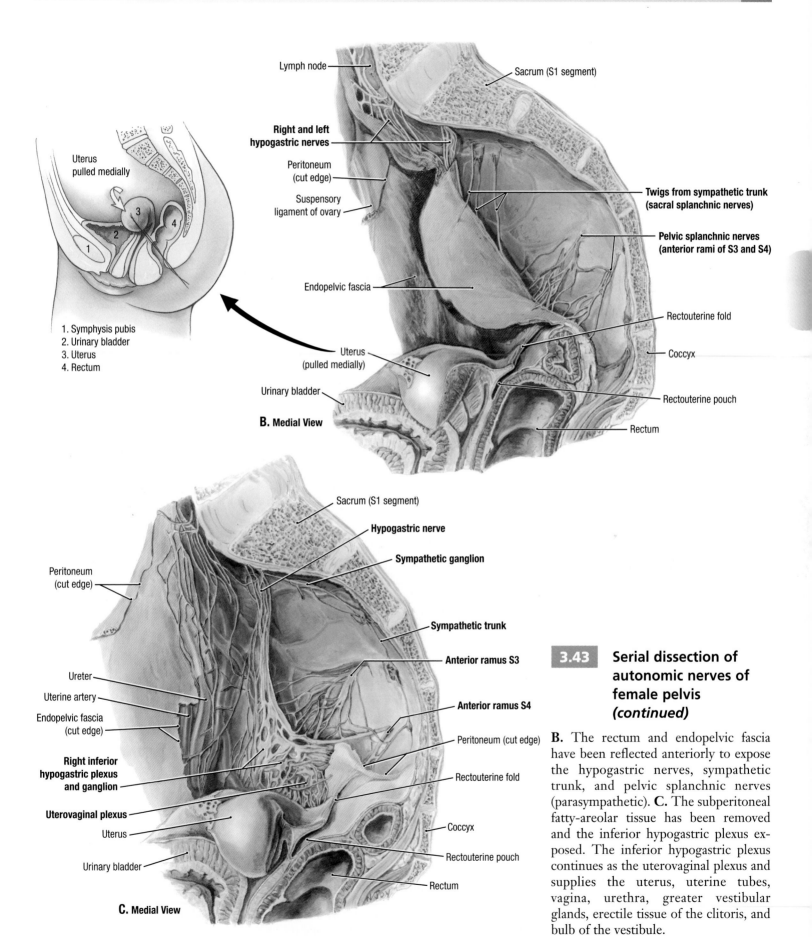

Uterus
pulled medially

1. Symphysis pubis
2. Urinary bladder
3. Uterus
4. Rectum

Lymph node
Sacrum (S1 segment)

**Right and left
hypogastric nerves**

Peritoneum
(cut edge)

Suspensory
ligament of ovary

Endopelvic fascia

**Twigs from sympathetic trunk
(sacral splanchnic nerves)**

**Pelvic splanchnic nerves
(anterior rami of S3 and S4)**

Rectouterine fold

Coccyx

Uterus
(pulled medially)

Urinary bladder

Rectouterine pouch

B. Medial View

Rectum

Sacrum (S1 segment)

Hypogastric nerve

Sympathetic ganglion

Sympathetic trunk

Anterior ramus S3

Anterior ramus S4

Peritoneum
(cut edge)

Ureter

Uterine artery

Endopelvic fascia
(cut edge)

**Right inferior
hypogastric plexus
and ganglion**

Uterovaginal plexus

Uterus

Urinary bladder

Peritoneum (cut edge)

Rectouterine fold

Coccyx

Rectouterine pouch

Rectum

C. Medial View

3.43   **Serial dissection of autonomic nerves of female pelvis** *(continued)*

B. The rectum and endopelvic fascia have been reflected anteriorly to expose the hypogastric nerves, sympathetic trunk, and pelvic splanchnic nerves (parasympathetic). **C.** The subperitoneal fatty-areolar tissue has been removed and the inferior hypogastric plexus exposed. The inferior hypogastric plexus continues as the uterovaginal plexus and supplies the uterus, uterine tubes, vagina, urethra, greater vestibular glands, erectile tissue of the clitoris, and bulb of the vestibule.

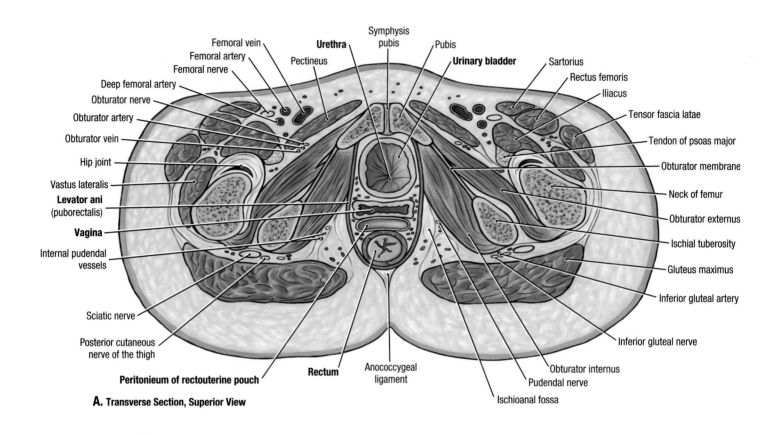

Femoral vein
Femoral artery
Femoral nerve
Deep femoral artery
Obturator nerve
Obturator artery
Obturator vein
Hip joint
Vastus lateralis
Levator ani
(puborectalis)
Vagina
Internal pudendal
vessels
Sciatic nerve
Posterior cutaneous
nerve of the thigh
Peritonieum of rectouterine pouch

Pectineus
Symphysis
pubis
Urethra
Pubis
Urinary bladder

Sartorius
Rectus femoris
Iliacus
Tensor fascia latae
Tendon of psoas major
Obturator membrane
Neck of femur
Obturator externus
Ischial tuberosity
Gluteus maximus
Inferior gluteal artery
Inferior gluteal nerve
Obturator internus
Pudendal nerve

Rectum
Anococcygeal
ligament
Ischioanal fossa

A. Transverse Section, Superior View

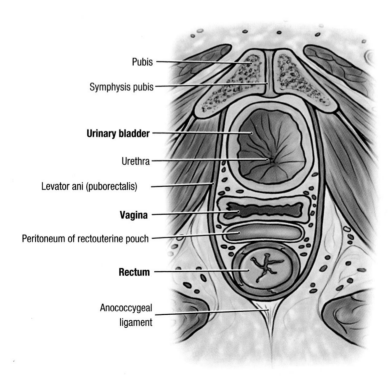

Pubis
Symphysis pubis
Urinary bladder
Urethra
Levator ani (puborectalis)
Vagina
Peritoneum of rectouterine pouch
Rectum
Anococcygeal
ligament

B. Transverse Section

3.44   Transverse section through female pelvis

A. Transverse section through the ischial tuberosities. **B.** Enlargement of central part of
section including the bladder, vagina, rectum, and rectouterine pouch.

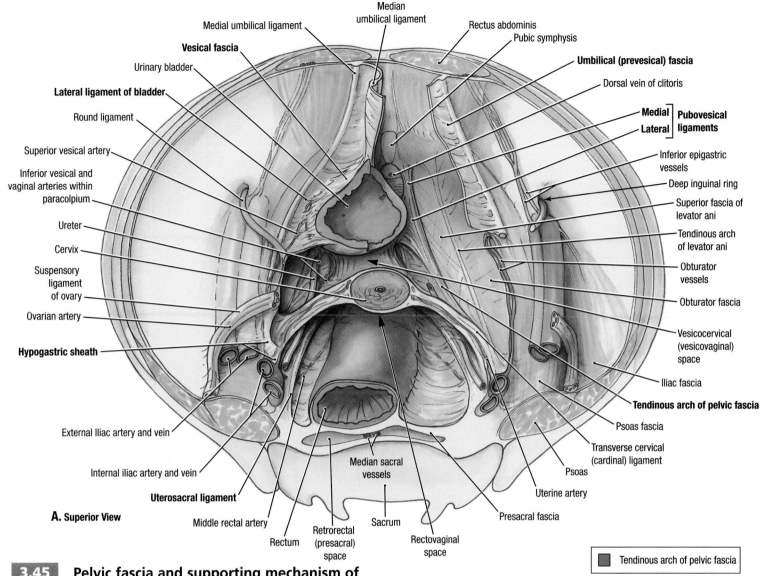

Median umbilical ligament
Medial umbilical ligament
Vesical fascia
Urinary bladder
Lateral ligament of bladder
Round ligament
Superior vesical artery
Inferior vesical and vaginal arteries within paracolpium
Ureter
Cervix
Suspensory ligament of ovary
Ovarian artery
Hypogastric sheath
External Iliac artery and vein
Internal iliac artery and vein
Uterosacral ligament
Middle rectal artery
Rectum
Retrorectal (presacral) space
Sacrum
Median sacral vessels
Rectovaginal space
Presacral fascia
Uterine artery
Psoas
Transverse cervical (cardinal) ligament
Psoas fascia
Tendinous arch of pelvic fascia
Iliac fascia
Vesicocervical (vesicovaginal) space
Obturator fascia
Obturator vessels
Tendinous arch of levator ani
Superior fascia of levator ani
Deep inguinal ring
Inferior epigastric vessels
Medial **Lateral** **Pubovesical ligaments**
Dorsal vein of clitoris
Umbilical (prevesical) fascia
Pubic symphysis
Rectus abdominis

A. Superior View

3.45 **Pelvic fascia and supporting mechanism of cervix and upper vagina**

A. Greater and lesser pelvis demonstrating pelvic viscera and endopelvic fascia. **B.** Schematic illustration of fascial ligaments and areolar spaces at level of tendinous arch of pelvic fascia.

- Note the parietal pelvic fascia covering the obturator internus and levator ani muscles and the visceral pelvic fascia surrounding the pelvic organs. These membranous fasciae are continuous where the organs penetrate the pelvic floor, forming a tendinous arch of pelvic fascia bilaterally.
- The endopelvic fascia lies between, and is continuous with, both visceral and parietal layers of pelvic fascia. The loose, areolar portions of the endopelvic fascia have been removed; the fibrous, condensed portions remain. Note the condensation of this fascia into the hypogastric sheath, containing the vessels to the pelvic viscera, the ureters, and (in the male) the ductus deferens.
- Observe the ligamentous extensions of the hypogastric sheath: the lateral ligament of the urinary bladder, the transverse cervical ligament at the base of the broad ligament, and a less prominent lamina posteriorly containing the middle rectal vessels.

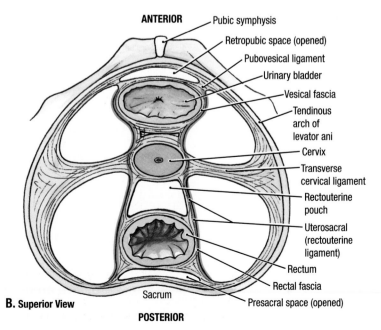

Tendinous arch of pelvic fascia

ANTERIOR
Pubic symphysis
Retropubic space (opened)
Pubovesical ligament
Urinary bladder
Vesical fascia
Tendinous arch of levator ani
Cervix
Transverse cervical ligament
Rectouterine pouch
Uterosacral (rectouterine ligament)
Rectum
Rectal fascia
Presacral space (opened)
Sacrum
B. Superior View
POSTERIOR

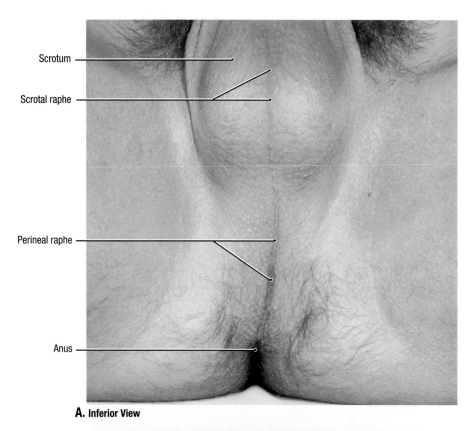

Scrotum

Scrotal raphe

Perineal raphe

Anus

A. Inferior View

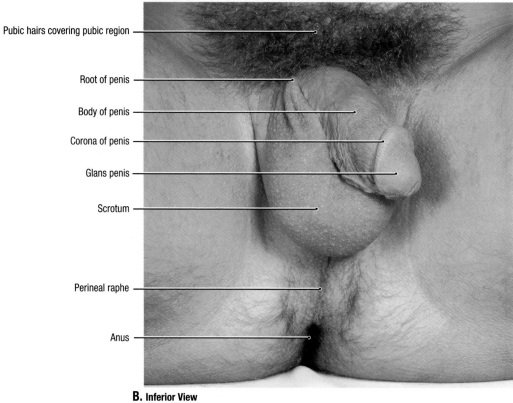

Pubic hairs covering pubic region

Root of penis

Body of penis

Corona of penis

Glans penis

Scrotum

Perineal raphe

Anus

B. Inferior View

3.46   **Surface anatomy of male perineum**

A. Scrotum and anal region. **B.** Penis, scrotum, and anal region.

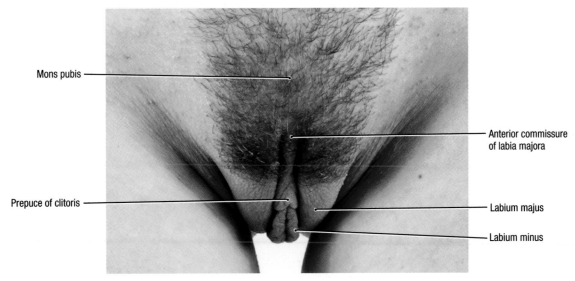

Mons pubis

Anterior commissure
of labia majora

Prepuce of clitoris

Labium majus

Labium minus

A. Anterior View

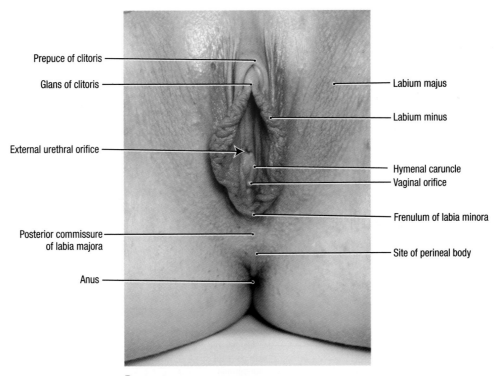

Prepuce of clitoris

Glans of clitoris

Labium majus

Labium minus

External urethral orifice

Hymenal caruncle

Vaginal orifice

Frenulum of labia minora

Posterior commissure
of labia majora

Site of perineal body

Anus

B. Antero-inferior View (Lithotomy Position)

3.47   Surface anatomy of the female perineum

A. External genitalia (pudendum; vulva), standing position. **B.** Vestibule of vagina and the
external urethral and vaginal orifices opening into it (recumbent position).

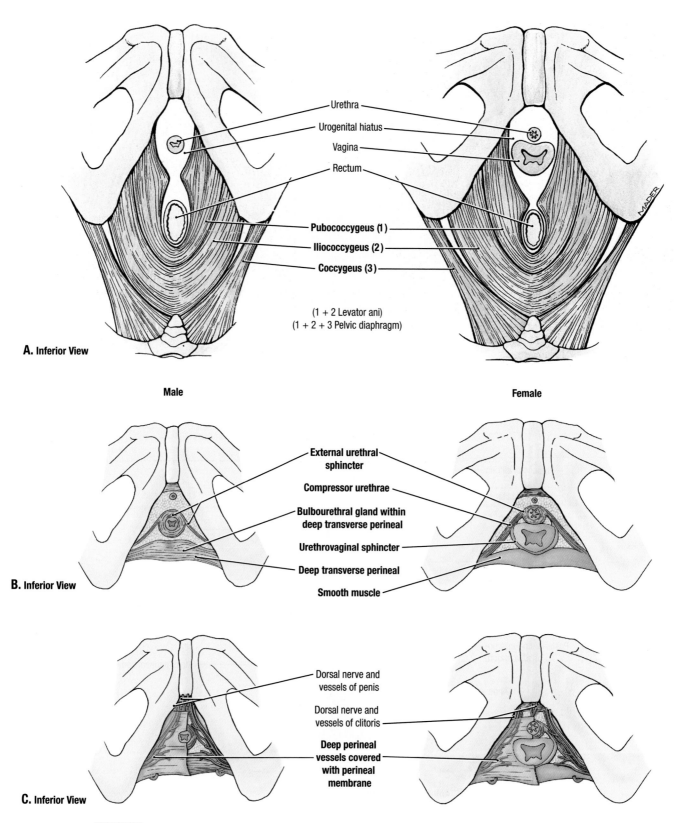

A. Inferior View

Urethra
Urogenital hiatus
Vagina
Rectum
Pubococcygeus (1)
Iliococcygeus (2)
Coccygeus (3)

(1 + 2 Levator ani)
(1 + 2 + 3 Pelvic diaphragm)

Male   Female

B. Inferior View

External urethral sphincter
Compressor urethrae
Bulbourethral gland within deep transverse perineal
Urethrovaginal sphincter
Deep transverse perineal
Smooth muscle

C. Inferior View

Dorsal nerve and vessels of penis
Dorsal nerve and vessels of clitoris
Deep perineal vessels covered with perineal membrane

3.48   Male and female perineal compartments

A–F. Sequential demonstration of structures of the perineal compartments, from deep to superficial. **A–C.** Deep perineal compartment (superior to perineal membrane). **A.** Pelvic diaphragm. **B.** Muscles of deep perineal compartment. **C.** Deep perineal vessels and nerves, covered by perineal membrane on right side.

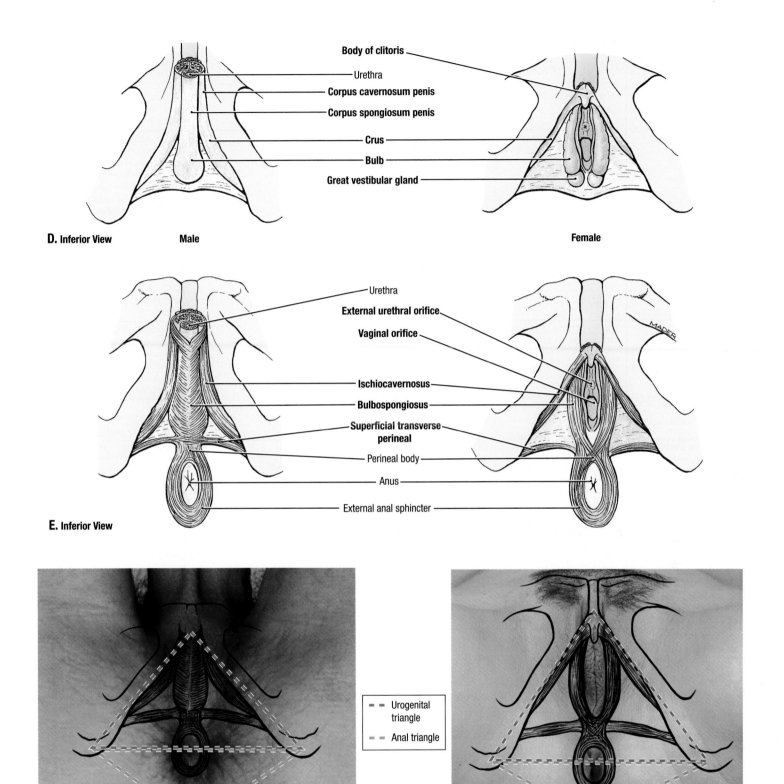

D. Inferior View   Male   Female

Body of clitoris
Urethra
Corpus cavernosum penis
Corpus spongiosum penis
Crus
Bulb
Great vestibular gland

Urethra
External urethral orifice
Vaginal orifice
Ischiocavernosus
Bulbospongiosus
Superficial transverse perineal
Perineal body
Anus
External anal sphincter

E. Inferior View

F. Inferior View

- - Urogenital triangle
- - Anal triangle

3.48   **Male and female perineal compartments (continued)**

D–F. Superficial perineal compartment (inferior to perineal membrane). **D.** Erectile bodies. **E.** Muscles of superficial perineal compartment. **F.** Superficial muscles imposed on surface anatomy of perineum.

TABLE 3.9 MUSCLES OF PERINEUM

Muscle	Origin	Course and Insertion	Innervation	Main Action
External anal sphincter	Skin and fascia surrounding anus; coccyx via anococcygeal ligament	Passes around lateral aspects of anal canal; insertion into perineal body	Inferior anal (rectal) nerve, a branch of pudendal nerve (S2–S4)	Constricts anal canal during peristalsis, resisting defecation; supports and fixes perineal body and pelvic floor
Bulbospongiosus	*Male:* median raphe on ventral surface of bulb of penis; perineal body	*Male:* surrounds lateral aspects of bulb of penis and most proximal part of body of penis, inserting into perineal membrane, dorsal aspect of corpora spongiosum and cavernosa, and fascia of bulb of penis		*Male:* supports and fixes perineal body/pelvic floor; compresses bulb of penis to expel last drops of urine/semen; assists erection by compressing outflow via deep perineal vein and by pushing blood from bulb into body of penis
	Female: perineal body	*Female:* passes on each side of lower vagina, enclosing bulb and greater vestibular gland; inserts onto pubic arch and fascia of corpora cavernosa of clitoris	Muscular (deep) branch of perineal nerve, a branch of the pudendal nerve (S2–S4)	*Female:* supports and fixes perineal body/pelvic floor; "sphincter" of vagina; assists in erection of clitoris (and perhaps bulb of vestibule); compresses greater vestibular gland
Ischiocavernosus	Internal surface of ischiopubic ramus and ischial tuberosity	Embraces crus of penis or clitoris, inserting onto the inferior and medial aspects of the crus and to the perineal membrane medial to the crus		Maintains erection of penis or clitoris by compressing outflow veins and pushing blood from the root of penis or clitoris into the body of penis or clitoris
Superficial transverse perineal	Internal surface of ischiopubic ramus and ischial tuberosity	Passes along inferior aspect of posterior border of perineal membrane to perineal body		Supports and fixes perineal body (pelvic floor) to support abdominopelvic viscera and resist increased intraabdominal pressure
Deep transverse perineal (male only)		Passes along superior aspect of posterior border of perineal membrane to perineal body, and external anal sphincter	Muscular (deep) branch of perineal nerve	
Smooth muscle (female only)	Ischiopubic rami	Passes to lateral wall of urethra and vagina	Autonomic nerves	Quantity of smooth muscle increases with age; function uncertain
External urethral sphincter		Surrounds urethra superior to perineal membrane; in males, also ascends anterior aspect of prostate		Compresses urethra to maintain urinary continence
Compressor urethrae (females only)	Internal surface of ischiopubic ramus	Continuous with external urethral sphincter	Dorsal nerve of penis or clitoris, the terminal branch of the pudendal nerve (S2–S4)	Compresses urethra; with pelvic diaphragm; assists in elongation of urethra
Urethrovaginal sphincter (females only)	Anterior side of urethra	Continuous with compressor urethrae; extends posteriorly on lateral wall of urethra and vagina to interdigitate with fibers from opposite side of perineal body		Compresses urethra and vagina

Oelrich TM. The urethral sphincter muscle in the male. Am J Anat 1980;158:229–246.
Oelrich TM. The striated urogenital sphincter muscle in the female. Anat Rec 1983;205:223–232.
Mirilas P, Skandalakis JE. Urogenital diaphragm: an erroneous concept casting its shadow over the sphincter urethrae and deep perineal space. J Am Coll Surg 2004;198:279–290.
DeLancey JO. Correlative study of paraurethral anatomy. Obstet Gynecol 1986;68:91–97.

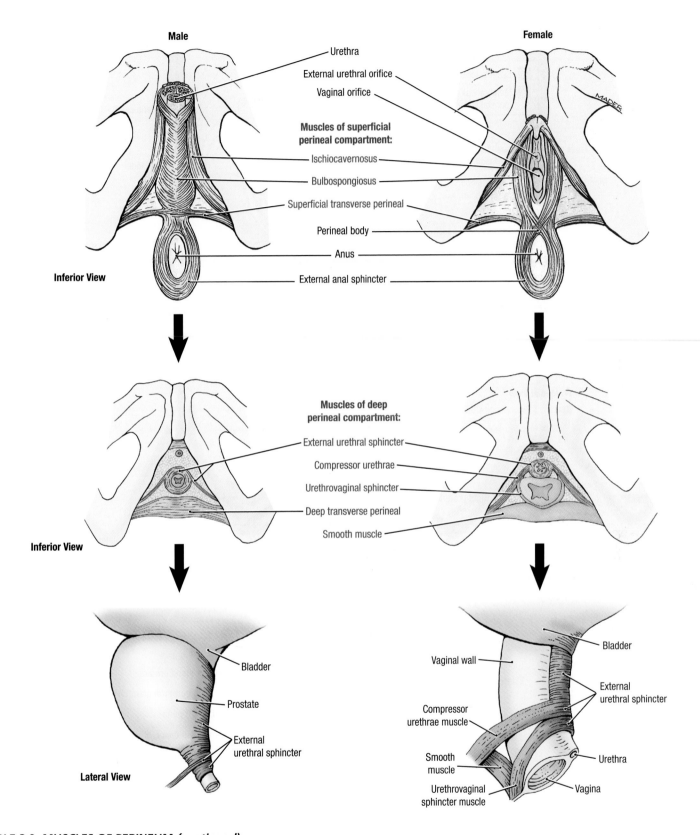

TABLE 3.9 MUSCLES OF PERINEUM *(continued)*

A potential subcutaneous perineal space (pouch) lies between the membranous layer of the subcutaneous tissue of the perineum and the perineal fascia (investing fascia of the superficial perineal muscles). The superficial perineal compartment (pouch) is an enclosed compartment bounded inferiorly by the perineal fascia and superiorly by the perineal membrane. The deep compartment is bounded inferiorly by the perineal membrane and continues superiorly to the (inferior investing fascia of the) pelvic diaphragm. (Oelich, 1980, 1983; DeLancy 1986; Mirilus, 2004).

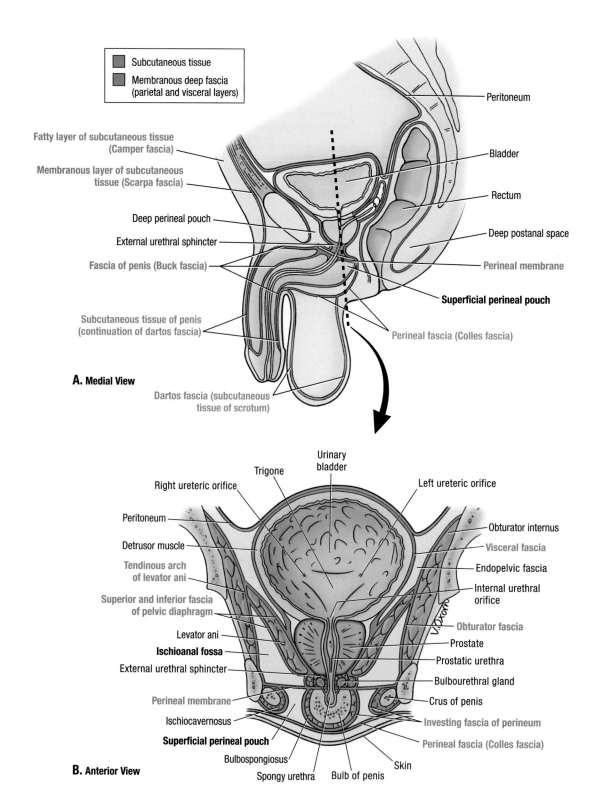

Subcutaneous tissue

Membranous deep fascia
(parietal and visceral layers)

A. Medial View

Fatty layer of subcutaneous tissue
(Camper fascia)

Membranous layer of subcutaneous
tissue (Scarpa fascia)

Deep perineal pouch

External urethral sphincter

Fascia of penis (Buck fascia)

Subcutaneous tissue of penis
(continuation of dartos fascia)

Dartos fascia (subcutaneous
tissue of scrotum)

Peritoneum

Bladder

Rectum

Deep postanal space

Perineal membrane

Superficial perineal pouch

Perineal fascia (Colles fascia)

B. Anterior View

Urinary
bladder

Trigone

Right ureteric orifice

Peritoneum

Detrusor muscle

Tendinous arch
of levator ani

Superior and inferior fascia
of pelvic diaphragm

Levator ani

Ischioanal fossa

External urethral sphincter

Perineal membrane

Ischiocavernosus

Superficial perineal pouch

Bulbospongiosus

Spongy urethra

Left ureteric orifice

Obturator internus

Visceral fascia

Endopelvic fascia

Internal urethral
orifice

Obturator fascia

Prostate

Prostatic urethra

Bulbourethral gland

Crus of penis

Investing fascia of perineum

Perineal fascia (Colles fascia)

Skin

Bulb of penis

3.49   **Perineal fascia and perineal compartments**

A. Fascia of male perineum, median section. **B.** Compartments of male perineum, coronal section.

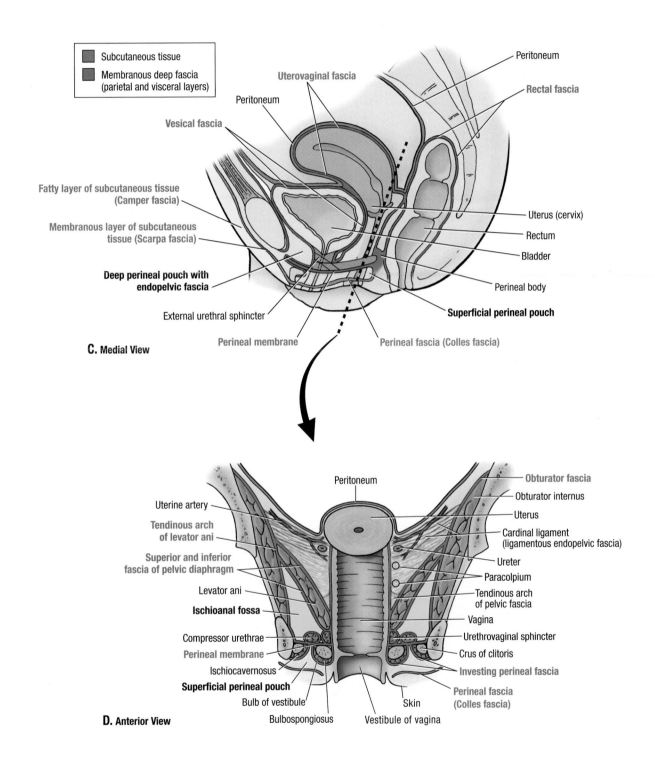

3.49   **Perineal fascia and perineal compartments (*continued*)**

C. Fascia of female perineum, median section. **D.** Compartments of female perineum, coronal section.

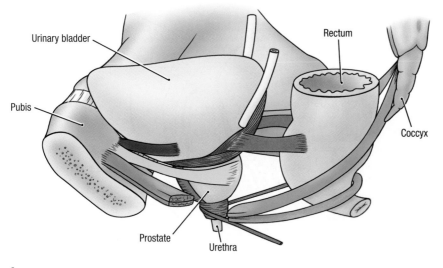

Urinary bladder

Rectum

Pubis

Coccyx

Prostate

Urethra

A. Left Lateral View, Male

MALE:

Puboprostaticus

Pubococcygeus

Puborectalis

Muscle of uvula

Rectovesicalis

Muscles compressing urethra:

Internal urethral sphincter

Pubovesicalis

External urethral sphincter

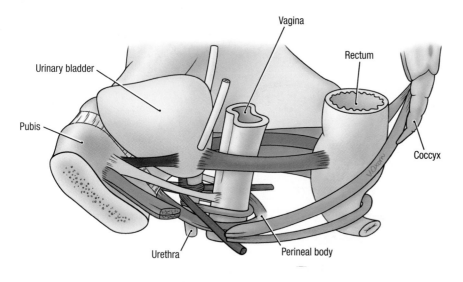

Vagina

Rectum

Urinary bladder

Pubis

Coccyx

Urethra

Perineal body

B. Left Lateral View, Female

FEMALE:

Pubovesicalis

Pubococcygeus

Puborectalis

Rectovesicalis

Muscles compressing urethra:

Compressor urethrae

External urethral sphincter

Muscles compressing vagina:

Pubovaginalis

Urethrovaginal sphincter
(part of external urethral
sphincter)

Bulbospongiosus

3.50   Supporting and compressor/sphincteric muscles of pelvis

A. Male. **B.** Female.

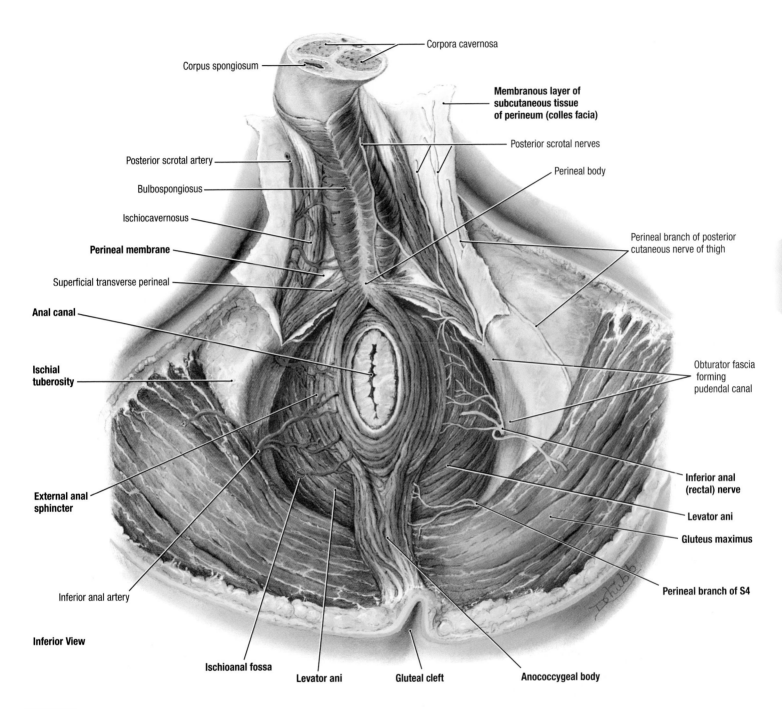

3.51 **Dissection of male perineum—I**

Superficial dissection.

- The membranous layer of subcutaneous tissue of the perineum was incised and reflected, opening the subcutaneous perineal compartment (pouch) in which the cutaneous nerves course.
- The perineal membrane is exposed between the three paired muscles of the superficial compartment; although not evident here, the muscles are individually ensheathed with investing fascia.
- The anal canal is surrounded by the external anal sphincter. The superficial fibers of the sphincter anchor the anal canal anteriorly to the perineal body and posteriorly, via the anococcygeal body (ligament), to the coccyx and skin of the gluteal cleft.

- Ischioanal (ischiorectal) fossae, from which fat bodies have been removed, lie on each side of the external anal sphincter. The fossae are also bound medially and superiorly by the levator ani; laterally by the ischial tuberosities and obturator internus fascia; and posteriorly by the gluteus maximus overlying the sacrotuberous ligaments. An anterior recess of each ischioanal fossa extends superior to the perineal membrane.
- In the lateral wall of the fossa, the inferior anal (rectal) nerve emerges from the pudendal canal and, with the perineal branch of S4, supplies the voluntary external anal sphincter and perianal skin; most cutaneous twigs have been removed.

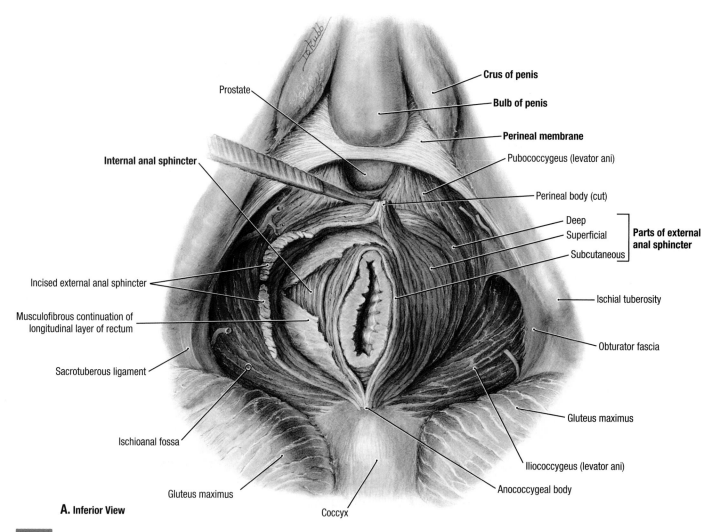

A. Inferior View

3.52   **Dissection of the male perineum—II**

A. The superficial perineal muscles have been removed, revealing the roots of the erectile bodies (crura and bulb) of the penis, attached to the ischiopubic rami and perineal membrane. On the left side the superficial and deep parts of the external anal sphincter were incised and reflected; the underlying musculofibrous continuation of the outer longitudinal layer of the muscular layer of the rectum is cut to reveal thickening of the inner circular layer that comprises the internal anal sphincter. **B.** Rupture of the spongy urethra in the bulb of the penis results in urine passing (extravasating) into the subcutaneous perineal compartment. The attachments of the membranous layer of subcutaneous tissue determine the direction and restrictions of flow of the extravasated urine. Urine and blood may pass deep to the continuations of the membranous layer in the scrotum, penis, and inferior abdominal wall. The urine cannot pass laterally and inferiorly into the thighs because the membranous layer fuses with the fascia lata (deep fascia of the thigh), nor posteriorly into the anal triangle due to continuity with the perineal membrane and perineal body.

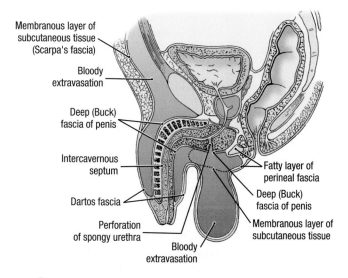

B. Medial view (from left)

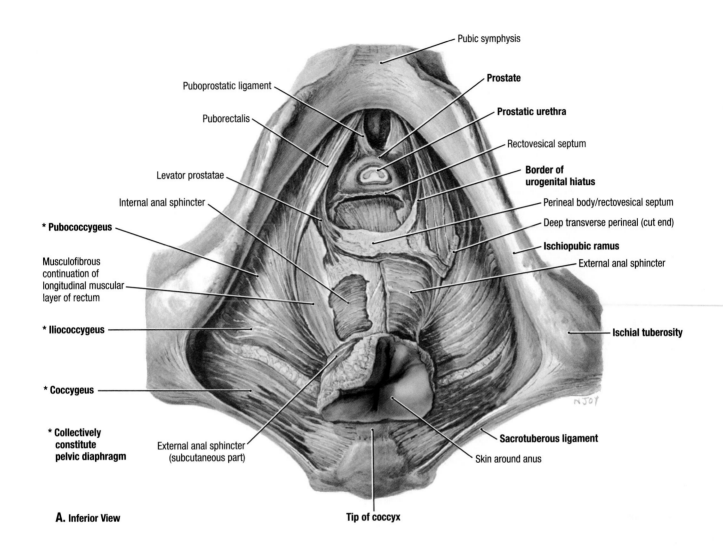

Pubic symphysis

Puboprostatic ligament

Prostate

Puborectalis

Prostatic urethra

Levator prostatae

Rectovesical septum

Internal anal sphincter

Border of urogenital hiatus

* **Pubococcygeus**

Perineal body/rectovesical septum

Musculofibrous continuation of longitudinal muscular layer of rectum

Deep transverse perineal (cut end)

Ischiopubic ramus

External anal sphincter

* **Iliococcygeus**

Ischial tuberosity

* **Coccygeus**

* **Collectively constitute pelvic diaphragm**

External anal sphincter (subcutaneous part)

Sacrotuberous ligament

Skin around anus

Tip of coccyx

A. Inferior View

3.53   Dissection of the male perineum—III

A. The perineal membrane and structures superficial to it have been removed. The prostatic urethra, base of the prostate, and rectum are visible through the urogenital hiatus of the pelvic diaphragm. The osseofibrous boundaries are demonstrated. **B.** Rupture of the intermediate part of the urethra results in extravasation of urine and blood into the deep perineal compartment. The fluid may pass superiorly through the urogenital hiatus and distribute extraperitoneally around the prostate and bladder.

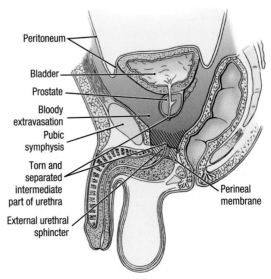

Peritoneum

Bladder

Prostate

Bloody extravasation

Pubic symphysis

Torn and separated intermediate part of urethra

External urethral sphincter

Perineal membrane

B. Medial View (from left)

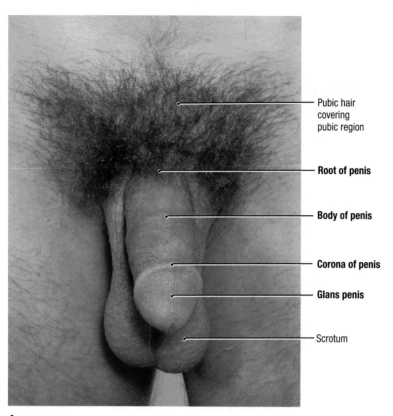

Pubic hair
covering
pubic region

Root of penis

Body of penis

Corona of penis

Glans penis

Scrotum

A. Anterior View

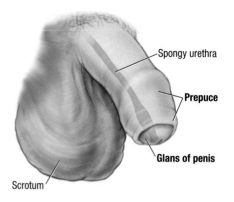

Spongy urethra

Prepuce

Glans of penis

Scrotum

B. Right Anterolateral View

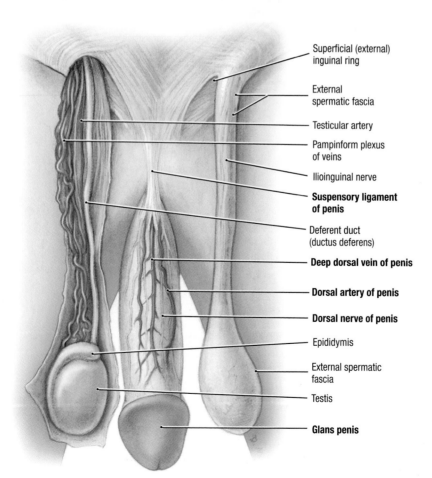

Superficial (external)
inguinal ring

External
spermatic fascia

Testicular artery

Pampiniform plexus
of veins

Ilioinguinal nerve

**Suspensory ligament
of penis**

Deferent duct
(ductus deferens)

Deep dorsal vein of penis

Dorsal artery of penis

Dorsal nerve of penis

Epididymis

External spermatic
fascia

Testis

Glans penis

C. Anterior View

<table>
<tr><td>3.54</td><td>**Glans, prepuce, and
neurovascular bundle of penis**</td></tr>
</table>

A. Surface anatomy, penis circumcised. **B.**
Uncircumcised penis. **C.** Vessels and nerves of penis
and contents of spermatic cord.

In **C:**

- The superficial and deep fasciae covering the
  penis are removed to expose the midline deep
  dorsal vein and the bilateral dorsal arteries and
  nerves of the penis. The triangular suspensory
  ligament of the penis attaches to the region of the
  pubic symphysis and blends with the deep fascia
  of the penis.
- On the specimen's left, the spermatic cord passes
  through the external inguinal ring and picks up a
  covering of external spermatic fascia from the
  margins of the superficial inguinal ring.
- On the specimen's right, the coverings of the spermatic cord and testis are incised and reflected, and
  the contents of the cord are separated.

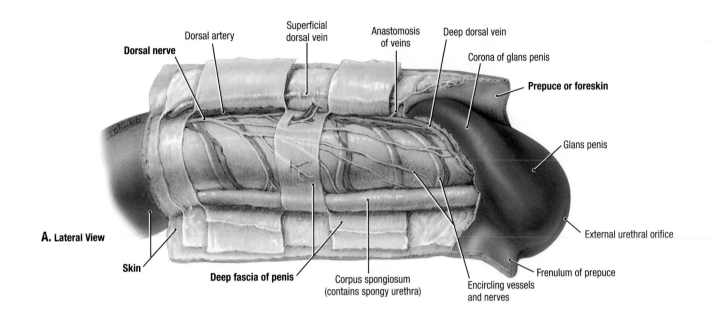

A. Lateral View

- Dorsal nerve
- Dorsal artery
- Superficial dorsal vein
- Anastomosis of veins
- Deep dorsal vein
- Corona of glans penis
- Prepuce or foreskin
- Glans penis
- External urethral orifice
- Frenulum of prepuce
- Encircling vessels and nerves
- Corpus spongiosum (contains spongy urethra)
- Deep fascia of penis
- Skin

Regions traversed by pudendal nerve and its branches:

- Pelvis
- Gluteal region
- Pudendal canal
- Deep perineal pouch
- Dorsum of penis
- Superficial perineum (superficial compartment, ischioanal fossae)

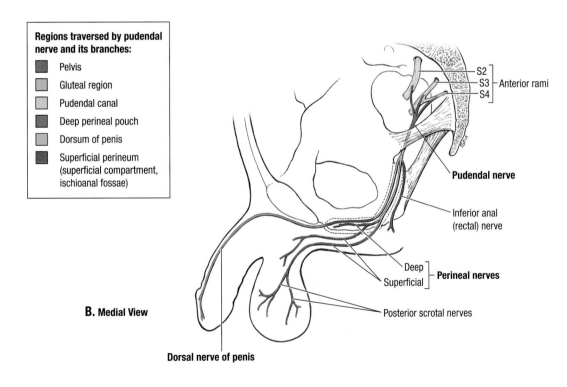

B. Medial View

- S2
- S3 — Anterior rami
- S4
- **Pudendal nerve**
- Inferior anal (rectal) nerve
- Deep
- Superficial — **Perineal nerves**
- Posterior scrotal nerves
- **Dorsal nerve of penis**

3.55   Layers and nerves of penis

A. Dissection. The skin, subcutaneous tissue, and deep fascia of the penis and prepuce are reflected separately. **B.** Distribution of pudendal nerve, right hemipelvis. Five regions traversed by the nerve are demonstrated.

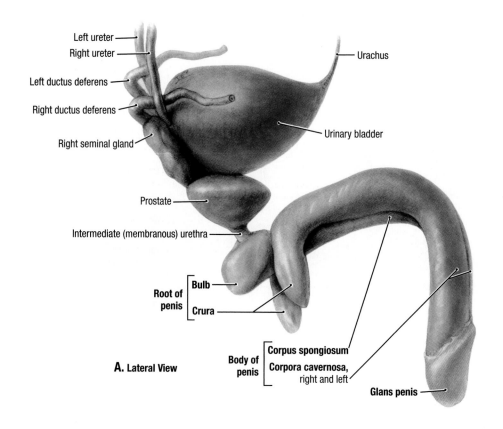

Left ureter

Right ureter

Left ductus deferens

Right ductus deferens

Right seminal gland

Urachus

Urinary bladder

Prostate

Intermediate (membranous) urethra

Root of penis
- Bulb
- Crura

Body of penis
- Corpus spongiosum
- Corpora cavernosa, right and left

Glans penis

A. Lateral View

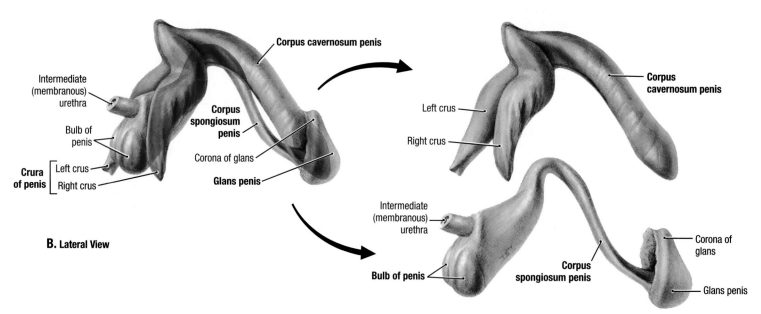

Corpus cavernosum penis

Intermediate (membranous) urethra

Bulb of penis

Crura of penis
- Left crus
- Right crus

Corpus spongiosum penis

Corona of glans

Glans penis

B. Lateral View

Corpus cavernosum penis

Left crus

Right crus

Intermediate (membranous) urethra

Bulb of penis

Corpus spongiosum penis

Corona of glans

Glans penis

C. Lateral View

3.56   Male urogenital system, erectile bodies

A. Pelvic components of genital and urinary tracts and erectile bodies of perineum. **B.** Dissection of male erectile bodies (corpora cavernosa and corpus spongiosum). **C.** Corpus spongiosum and corpora cavernosa, separated. The corpora cavernosa is bent where the penis is suspended by the suspensory ligament of the penis from the pubic symphysis. The corpus spongiosum extends posteriorly as the bulb of the penis and terminates anteriorly as the glans.

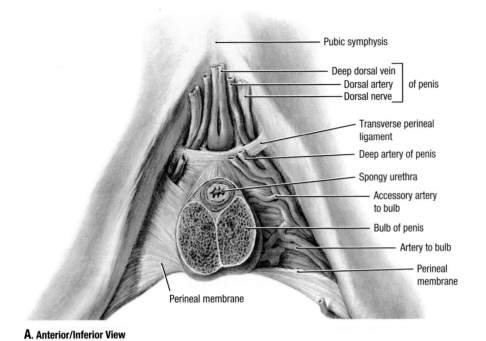

A. Anterior/Inferior View

Pubic symphysis
Deep dorsal vein
Dorsal artery } of penis
Dorsal nerve
Transverse perineal ligament
Deep artery of penis
Spongy urethra
Accessory artery to bulb
Bulb of penis
Artery to bulb
Perineal membrane
Perineal membrane

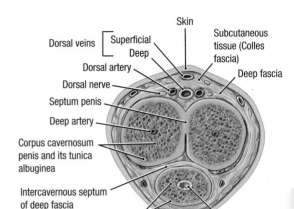

C. Transverse Section

DORSUM
Skin
Dorsal veins { Superficial / Deep }
Subcutaneous tissue (Colles fascia)
Dorsal artery
Deep fascia
Dorsal nerve
Septum penis
Deep artery
Corpus cavernosum penis and its tunica albuginea
Intercavernous septum of deep fascia
Corpus spongiosum penis and its tunica albuginea
Spongy urethra
URETHRAL SURFACE

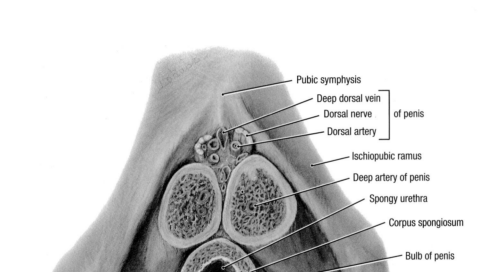

B. Anterior View

Pubic symphysis
Deep dorsal vein
Dorsal nerve } of penis
Dorsal artery
Ischiopubic ramus
Deep artery of penis
Spongy urethra
Corpus spongiosum
Bulb of penis
Crus of penis

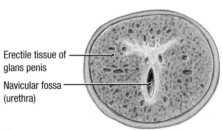

D. Transverse Section

Erectile tissue of glans penis
Navicular fossa (urethra)

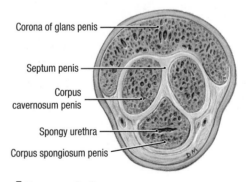

E. Transverse Section

Corona of glans penis
Septum penis
Corpus cavernosum penis
Spongy urethra
Corpus spongiosum penis

3.57   Cross sections of penis

A. Transverse section through bulb of penis with crura removed. The bulb is cut posterior to the entry of the intermediate urethra. On the left side, the perineal membrane is partially removed, opening the deep perineal compartment. **B.** The crura and bulb of penis have been sectioned obliquely. The spongy urethra is dilated within the bulb of the penis. **C.** Transverse section through body of penis. **D.** Transverse section through the proximal part of the glans penis. **E.** Transverse section through the distal part of the glans penis.

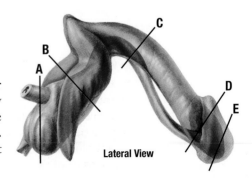

Lateral View

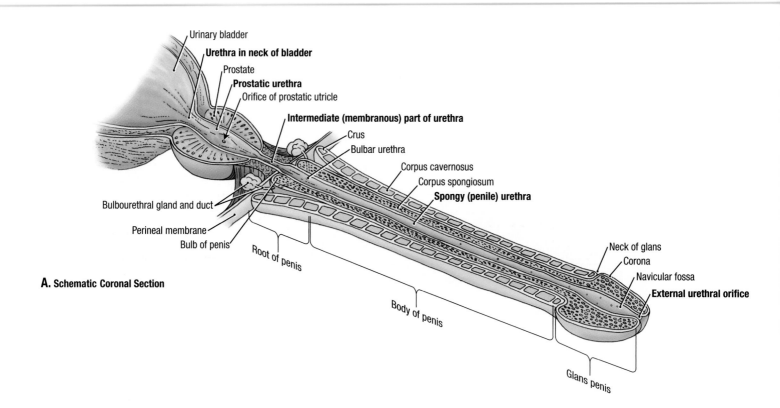

A. Schematic Coronal Section

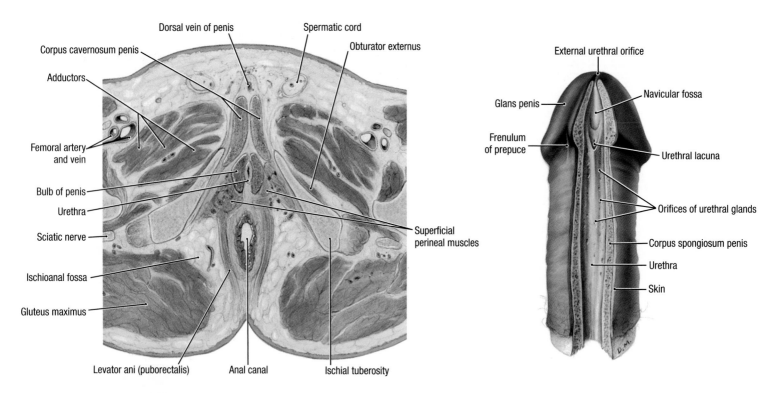

B. Transverse Section, Inferior View

C. Urethal Aspect of Distal Penis

3.58   Urethra

A. Urethra and related structures. **B.** Transverse section of body passing through the bulb of the penis. **C.** Spongy urethra, interior. A longitudinal incision was made on the urethral surface of the penis and carried through the floor of the urethra, allowing a view of the dorsal surface of the interior of the urethra.

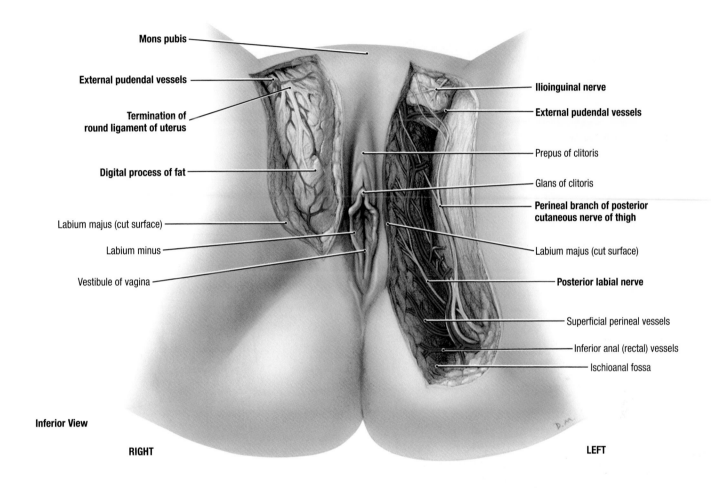

Mons pubis

External pudendal vessels

Termination of
round ligament of uterus

Digital process of fat

Labium majus (cut surface)

Labium minus

Vestibule of vagina

Ilioinguinal nerve

External pudendal vessels

Prepus of clitoris

Glans of clitoris

Perineal branch of posterior
cutaneous nerve of thigh

Labium majus (cut surface)

Posterior labial nerve

Superficial perineal vessels

Inferior anal (rectal) vessels

Ischioanal fossa

Inferior View

RIGHT

LEFT

3.59   Female perineum—I

Superficial dissection. On the right side of the specimen:
- A long digital process of fat lies deep to the subcutaneous fatty tissue and descends into the labium majus.
- The round ligament of the uterus ends as a branching band of fascia that spreads out superficial to the fatty digital process.

On the left side of the specimen:
- Most of the fatty digital process is removed.
- The mons pubis is the rounded fatty prominence anterior to the pubic symphysis and bodies of the pubic bones.
- The posterior labial vessels and nerves (S2, S3) are joined by the perineal branch of the posterior cutaneous nerve of thigh (S1, S2, S3) and run anteriorly to the mons pubis. At the mons pubis the vessels anastomose with the external pudendal vessels, and the nerves overlap in supply with the ilioinguinal nerve (L1).

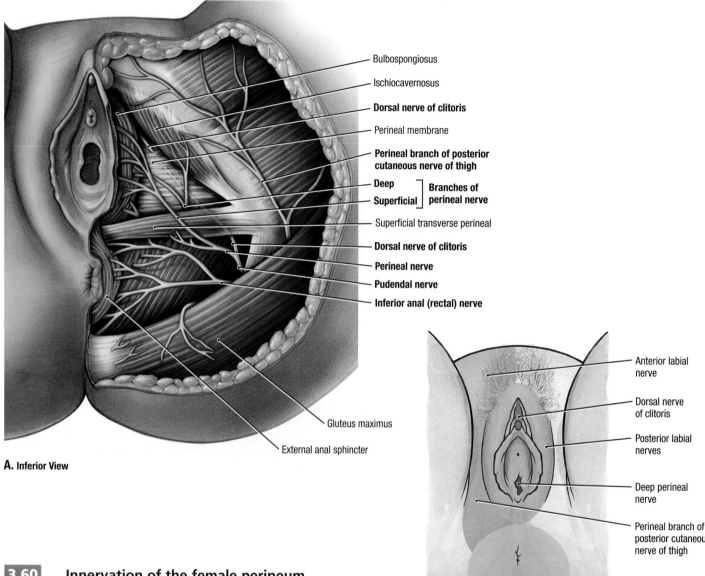

Bulbospongiosus

Ischiocavernosus

Dorsal nerve of clitoris

Perineal membrane

Perineal branch of posterior cutaneous nerve of thigh

Deep ⎤ **Branches of**
Superficial ⎦ **perineal nerve**

Superficial transverse perineal

Dorsal nerve of clitoris

Perineal nerve

Pudendal nerve

Inferior anal (rectal) nerve

Gluteus maximus

External anal sphincter

A. Inferior View

3.60   Innervation of the female perineum

A and **B.** The anterior aspect of the perineum is supplied by anterior labial nerves, derived from the ilioinguinal nerve and genital branch of the genitofemoral nerve. The pudendal nerve is the main nerve of the perineum. Posterior labial nerves, derived from the superficial perineal nerve, supply most of the vulva. The deep perineal nerve supplies the orifice of the vagina and superficial perineal muscles; and the dorsal nerve of the clitoris supplies deep perineal muscles and sensations to the clitoris. The inferior anal (rectal) nerve, also from the pudendal nerve, innervates the external anal sphincter and the perianal skin. The lateral perineum is supplied by the perineal branch of the posterior cutaneous nerve of the thigh. **C.** To relieve the pain experienced during childbirth, pudendal nerve block anesthesia may be performed by injecting a local anesthetic agent into the tissue surrounding the pudendal nerve, near the ischial spine. A pudendal nerve block does not abolish sensations from the anterior and lateral parts of the perineum. Therefore, a block of the ilioinguinal and/or perineal branch of the posterior cutaneous nerve of the thigh may also need to be performed.

Anterior labial nerve

Dorsal nerve of clitoris

Posterior labial nerves

Deep perineal nerve

Perineal branch of posterior cutaneous nerve of thigh

Inferior rectal (anal) nerve

Inferior clunial nerves

B. Inferior View

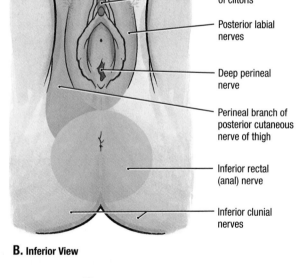

Ilioinguinal nerve block site

Perineal branch of posterior cutaneous nerve of thigh

Ischial spine (pudendal nerve block site)

Sacrospinous ligament

Pudendal nerve

C. Inferior View

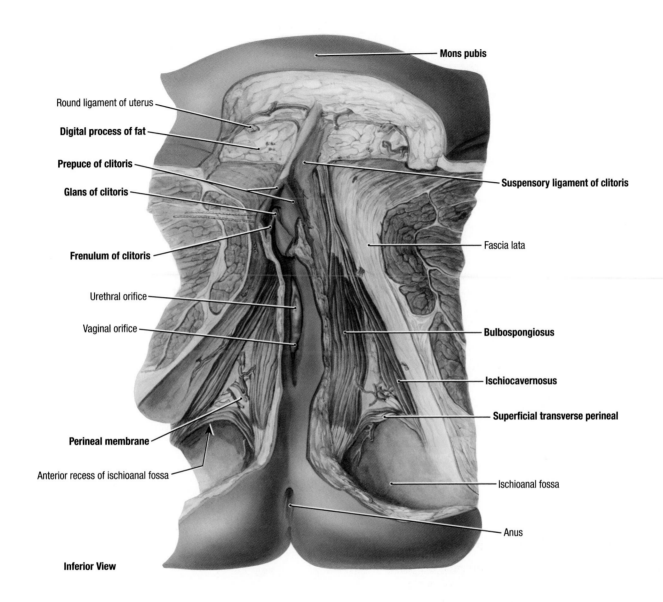

Mons pubis

Round ligament of uterus

Digital process of fat

Prepuce of clitoris

Glans of clitoris

Frenulum of clitoris

Urethral orifice

Vaginal orifice

Perineal membrane

Anterior recess of ischioanal fossa

Suspensory ligament of clitoris

Fascia lata

Bulbospongiosus

Ischiocavernosus

Superficial transverse perineal

Ischioanal fossa

Anus

Inferior View

3.61 **Female perineum—II**

- Note the thickness of the subcutaneous fatty tissue of the mons pubis and the encapsulated digital process of fat deep to this. The suspensory ligament of the clitoris descends from the linea alba.
- Anteriorly, each labium minus forms two laminae or folds: the lateral laminae of the labia pass on each side of the glans clitoris and unite, forming a hood that partially or completely covers the glans, the prepuce (foreskin) of the clitoris. The medial laminae of the labia merge posterior to the glans, forming the frenulum of the clitoris.
- There are three muscles on each side: bulbospongiosus, ischiocavernosus, and superficial transverse perineal; the perineal membrane is visible between them.
- The bulbospongiosus muscle overlies the bulb of the vestibule and the great vestibular gland. In the male, the muscles of the two sides are united by a median raphe; in the female, the orifice of the vagina separates the right from the left.

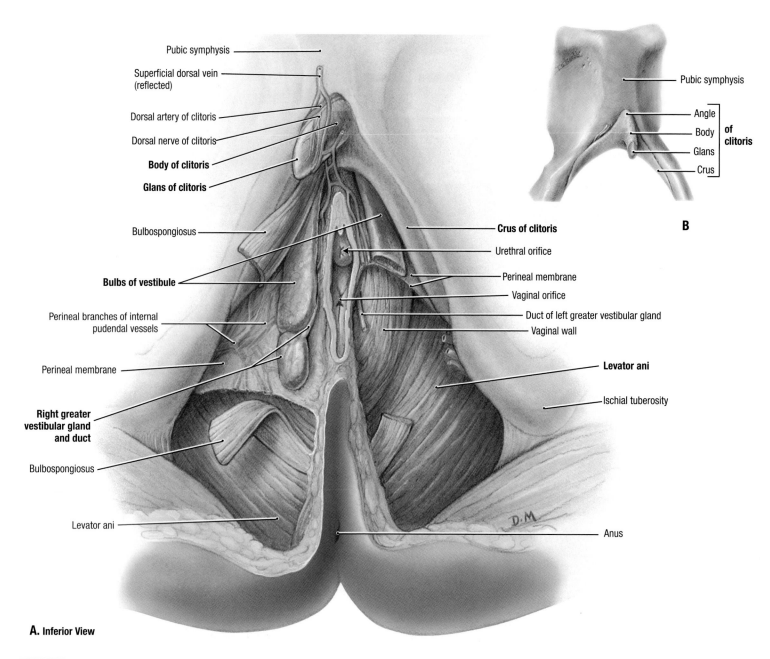

Pubic symphysis

Superficial dorsal vein (reflected)

Dorsal artery of clitoris

Dorsal nerve of clitoris

Body of clitoris

Glans of clitoris

Bulbospongiosus

Bulbs of vestibule

Perineal branches of internal pudendal vessels

Perineal membrane

Right greater vestibular gland and duct

Bulbospongiosus

Levator ani

Crus of clitoris

Urethral orifice

Perineal membrane

Vaginal orifice

Duct of left greater vestibular gland

Vaginal wall

Levator ani

Ischial tuberosity

Anus

Pubic symphysis

Angle
Body **of clitoris**
Glans
Crus

B

A. Inferior View

3.62   **Female perineum—III**

A. Deeper dissection. **B.** Clitoris.
  In **A:**
- The bulbospongiosus muscle is reflected on the right side and mostly removed on the left side; the posterior portion of the bulb of the vestibule and the greater vestibular gland have been removed on the left side.
- The glans and body of the clitoris is displaced to the right so that the distribution of the dorsal vessels and nerve of the clitoris can be seen.
- Homologues of the bulb of the penis, the bulbs of the vestibule exist as two masses of elongated erectile tissue that lie along the sides of the vaginal orifice; veins connect the bulbs of the vestibule to the glans of the clitoris.

- On the specimen's right side, the greater vestibular gland is situated at the posterior end of the bulb; both structures are covered by bulbospongiosus muscle.
- On the specimen's left side, the bulb, gland, and perineal membrane are cut away, thereby revealing the external aspect of the vaginal wall.
In **B:**
- The body of the clitoris, composed of two crura (corpora cavernosa), is capped by the glans.

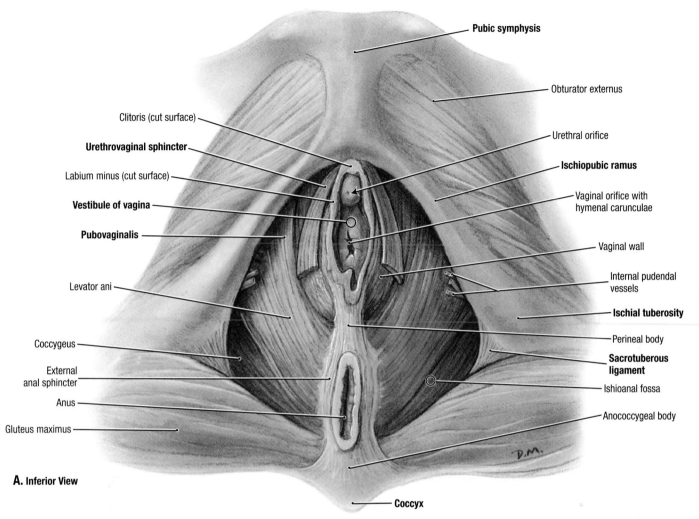

A. Inferior View

- Pubic symphysis
- Clitoris (cut surface)
- **Urethrovaginal sphincter**
- Labium minus (cut surface)
- **Vestibule of vagina**
- **Pubovaginalis**
- Levator ani
- Coccygeus
- External anal sphincter
- Anus
- Gluteus maximus
- Obturator externus
- Urethral orifice
- **Ischiopubic ramus**
- Vaginal orifice with hymenal carunculae
- Vaginal wall
- Internal pudendal vessels
- **Ischial tuberosity**
- Perineal body
- **Sacrotuberous ligament**
- Ishioanal fossa
- Anococcygeal body
- **Coccyx**

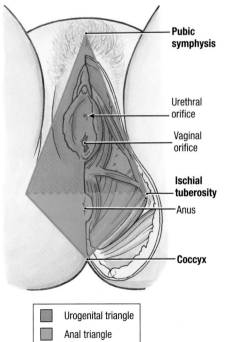

B. Inferior View

- Pubic symphysis
- Urethral orifice
- Vaginal orifice
- **Ischial tuberosity**
- Anus
- **Coccyx**

Urogenital triangle
Anal triangle

3.63   Female perineum—IV

A. Deep perineal compartment. The perineal membrane and smooth muscle corresponding in position to the deep transverse perineal muscle in the male have been removed.

- The most anterior and medial part of the levator ani muscle, the pubo-vaginalis, passes posterior to the vaginal orifice.
- The urethrovaginal sphincter, part of the external urethral sphincter of the female, rests on the urethra and straddles the vagina.
- The labia minora (cut short here) bound the vestibule of the vagina.

A and **B.** The osseoligamentous boundaries of the diamond-shaped perineum are the pubic symphysis, ischiopubic rami, ischial tuberosities, sacrotuberous ligaments, and coccyx. For descriptive purposes, a transverse line connecting the ischial tuberosities subdivides the diamond into urogenital and anal triangles.

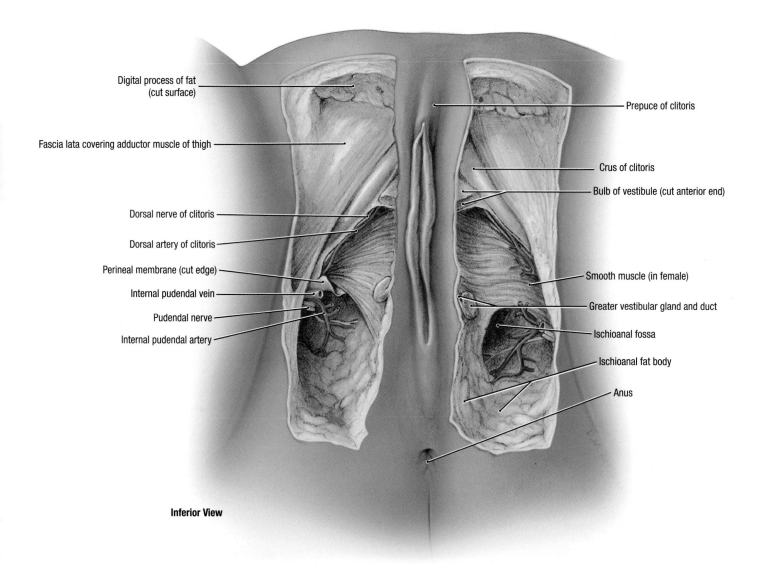

Digital process of fat
(cut surface)

Fascia lata covering adductor muscle of thigh

Dorsal nerve of clitoris

Dorsal artery of clitoris

Perineal membrane (cut edge)

Internal pudendal vein

Pudendal nerve

Internal pudendal artery

Prepuce of clitoris

Crus of clitoris

Bulb of vestibule (cut anterior end)

Smooth muscle (in female)

Greater vestibular gland and duct

Ischioanal fossa

Ischioanal fat body

Anus

Inferior View

3.64   Female perineum—V

This is a different dissection than the previous series, with the vulva undissected centrally
but the perineum dissected deeply on each side. Although most of the perineal membrane
and bulbs of the vestibule have been removed, the greater vestibular glands (structures of
the superficial perineal compartment) have been left in place. The development and extent
of the smooth muscle layer corresponding in position to the voluntary deep transverse perineal muscles of the male is highly variable, being relatively extensive in this case, blending
centrally with voluntary fibers of the external urethral sphincter and the perineal body.

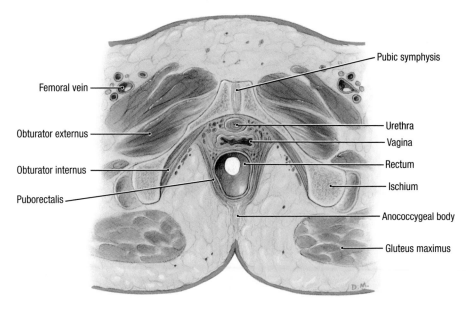

Femoral vein

Obturator externus

Obturator internus

Puborectalis

Pubic symphysis

Urethra

Vagina

Rectum

Ischium

Anococcygeal body

Gluteus maximus

A. Transverse Section

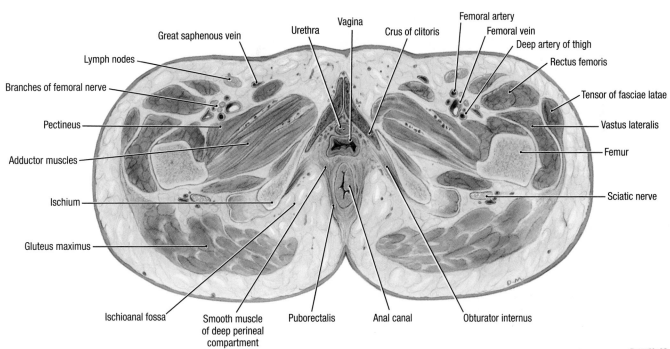

Great saphenous vein

Lymph nodes

Branches of femoral nerve

Pectineus

Adductor muscles

Ischium

Gluteus maximus

Ischioanal fossa

Smooth muscle of deep perineal compartment

Puborectalis

Urethra

Vagina

Crus of clitoris

Anal canal

Femoral artery

Femoral vein

Deep artery of thigh

Rectus femoris

Tensor of fasciae latae

Vastus lateralis

Femur

Sciatic nerve

Obturator internus

B. Transverse Section

3.65   Female perineum—V

A. Section through vagina and urethra at base of urinary bladder. **B.** Section through vagina, urethra, and crura of clitoris.

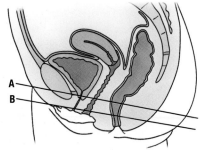

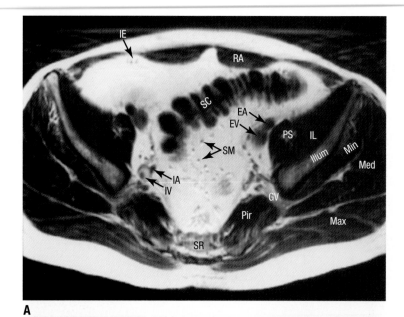

A

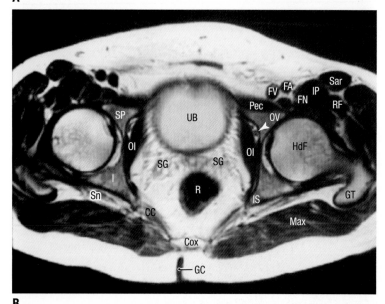

B

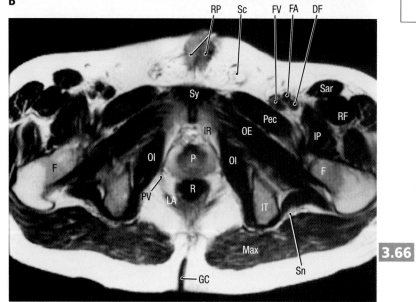

C

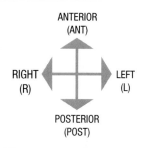

ANTERIOR
(ANT)

RIGHT
(R)

LEFT
(L)

POSTERIOR
(POST)

A	**Anus**	IV	Internal iliac vein
Ad	Adductor muscles	**LA**	**Levator ani**
Bi	Biceps femoris tendon	Max	Gluteus maximus
Bu	**Bulb of penis**	Med	Gluteus medius
Cav	**Corpus cavernosum penis**	Min	Gluteus minimus
CC	Coccygeus	OE	Obturator externus
Cox	Coccyx	OI	Obturator internus
Cr	**Crus of penis**	OV	Obturator vessels and nerve
DD	Ductus deferens		
DF	Deep femoral artery	**P**	**Prostate**
DVP	Dorsal vein of penis	**PB**	**Perineal body**
EA	External iliac artery	Pec	Pectineus
EAS	External anal sphincter	Pir	Piriformis
EV	External iliac vein	**PR**	**Puborectalis**
F	Femur	PS	Psoas
FA	Femoral artery	PV	Pudenal vessels and nerves
FN	Femoral nerve	QF	Quadratus femoris
FV	Femoral vein	**R**	**Rectum**
GC	Gluteal cleft	RA	Rectus abdominis
GSV	Great saphenous vein	RF	Rectus femoris
GT	Greater trochanter	**RP**	**Root of penis**
GV	Superior gluteal vein	Sar	Sartorius
HdF	Head of femur	Sc	Spermatic cord
I	Body of ischium	SC	Sigmoid colon
IA	Internal iliac artery	**SG**	**Seminal gland**
IAF	**Ischioanal fossa (pararectal fat)**	SM	Sigmoidal vessels in mesentery of sigmoid colon
IC	**Ischiocavernosus**	Sn	Sciatic nerve
IE	Inferior epigastric vessels	SP	Superior ramus of pubis
IL	Iliacus	SR	Sacrum
IP	Iliopsoas	Sy	Pubic symphysis
IPR	Ischiopubic ramus	**U**	**Urethra**
IR	Inferior pubic ramus	**UB**	**Urinary bladder**
IS	Ischial spine	VI	Vastus intermedius
IT	Ischial tuberosity		

(Organs/structures of male pelvis and perineum are in boldface)

3.66 Transverse (axial) MRIs and sectional specimen of the male pelvis and perineum, inferior views

A–D. MRIs. **E.** Anatomical section.

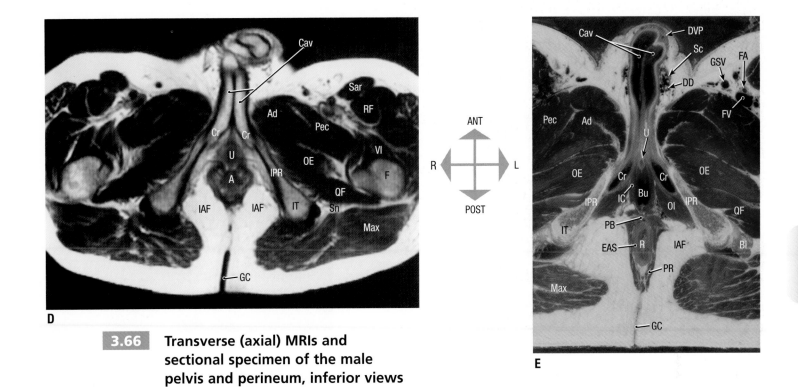

3.66 Transverse (axial) MRIs and sectional specimen of the male pelvis and perineum, inferior views *(continued)*

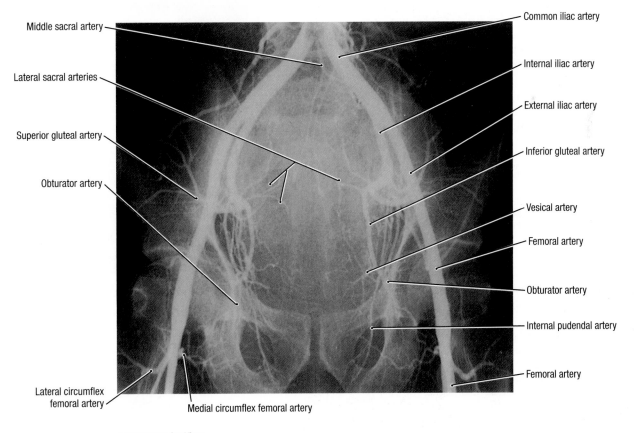

Anteroposterior View

3.67 Pelvic angiography

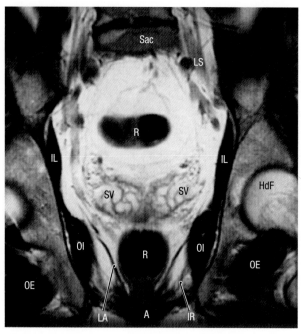

A

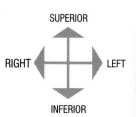

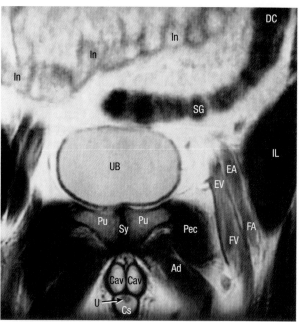

B

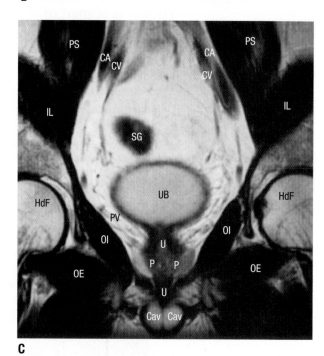

C

A	Anus
Ad	Adductors
CA	Common iliac artery
Cav	**Corpus cavernosum penis**
Cs	**Corpus spongiosum penis**
CV	Common iliac vein
DC	Descending colon
EA	External iliac artery
EV	External iliac vein
FA	Femoral artery
FV	Femoral vein
HdF	Head of femur
IL	Iliacus
In	Small intestine
IR	**Inferior rectal nerve and vessels**
LA	**Levator ani**
LS	Lumbosacral trunk
OE	Obturator externus
OI	**Obturator internus**
P	**Prostate**
Pec	Pectineus
PS	Psoas
Pu	Pubic bone
PV	**Pelvic vessels and nerves**
R	**Rectum**
Sac	Sacrum
SC	Sigmoid colon
SG	**Seminal vesicle**
Sy	**Pubic symphysis**
U	**Urethra**
UB	**Urinary bladder**

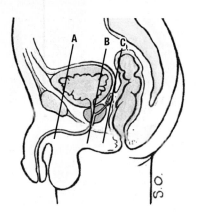

3.68   Coronal MRIs of the male pelvis and perineum, anterior views

MALE

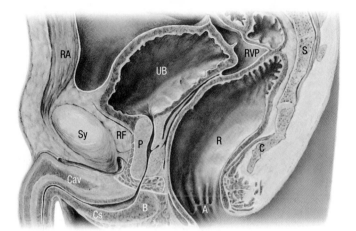

FEMALE

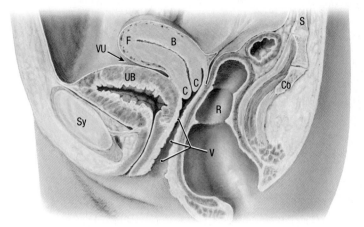

Median Section   **Median Section**

A	Anus
B	Bulb of penis
Co	Coccyx
Cav	Corpus cavernosum penis
Cs	Corpus spongiosum penis
P	Prostate
PP	Prostatic venous plexus
R	Rectum
RA	Rectus abdominis
RF	Retropubic fat
RVP	Rectovesical pouch
S	Sacrum
SG	Seminal gland
SN	Sacral nerves
Sy	Pubic symphysis
UB	Urinary bladder

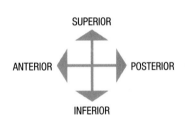

SUPERIOR

ANTERIOR — POSTERIOR

INFERIOR

B	Body of uterus
C	Cervix of uterus
Co	Coccyx
E	Endometrium
EF	Endopelvic fascia
F	Fundus of uterus
M	Myometrium
R	Rectum
RA	Rectus abdominis
S	Sacrum
Sy	Pubis symphysis
UB	Urinary bladder
V	Vagina
VU	Vesicouterine pouch

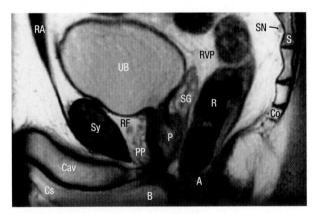

Median MRI Scan

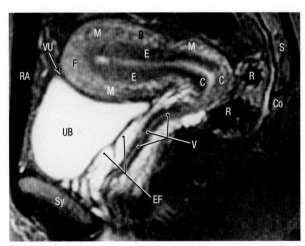

Median MRI Scan

3.69   **Median MRIs of the male and female pelvis and perineum**

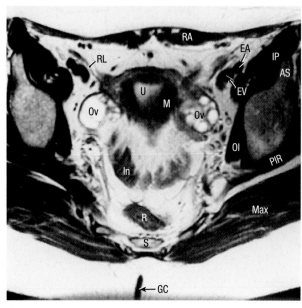

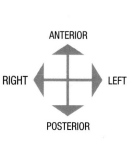

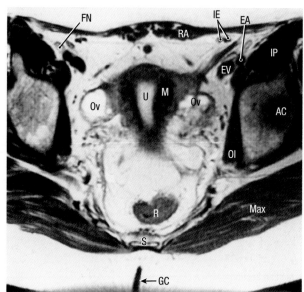

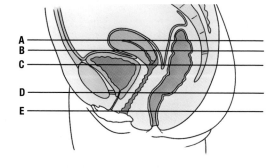

A	Anus	M	Myometrium
AC	Acetabulum	Max	Gluteus maximus
Ad	Adductor muscles	OE	Obturator externus
AS	Anterior superior iliac spine	OI	Obturator internus
BC	Body of clitoris	Ov	Ovary
CC	Crus of clitoris	OV	Obturator vessels
EA	External iliac artery	Pd	Pudendal nerve and vessels
EF	Endopelvic fascia	Pec	Pectineus
EV	External iliac vein	PIR	Piriformis
FA	Femoral artery	Pm	Perineal membrane
FN	Femoral nerve	Pu	Pubic bone
FV	Femoral vein	QF	Quadratus femoris
GC	Gluteal cleft	R	Rectum
HdF	Head of femur	RA	Rectus abdominis
I	Ilium	RF	Recto-uterine fold
IAF	Ischioanal fossa	RL	Round ligament
IE	Inferior epigastric vessels	S	Sacrum
In	Intestine	SP	Superior ramus of pubis
IP	Iliopsoas	Sy	Pubic symphysis
IPR	Ischiopubic ramus	U	Uterus
IT	Ischial tuberosity	UB	Urinary bladder
LA	Levator ani	Ur	Urethra
Lin	Linea alba	V	Vagina
LM	Labia majus	Ve	Vestibule

3.70 Transverse (axial) MRIs and sectional specimens of the female pelvis and perineum, inferior views

A–C. MRIs.

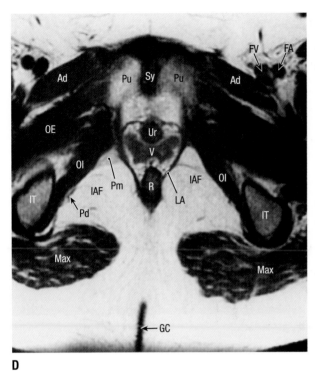

D

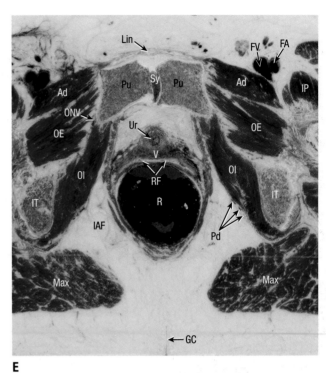

E

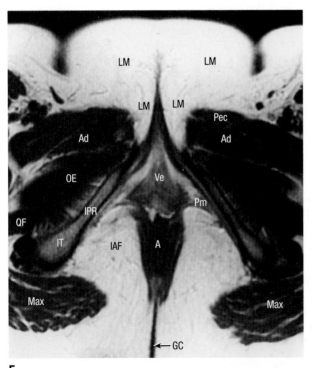

F

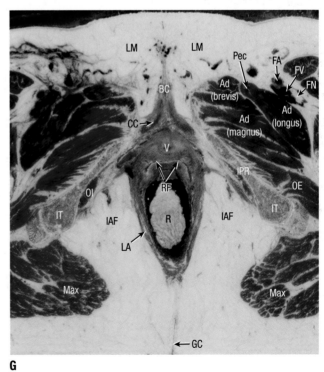

G

ANTERIOR

RIGHT ← → LEFT

POSTERIOR

3.70 Transverse (axial) MRIs and sectional specimens of the female pelvis and perineum, inferior views *(continued)*

D and F. MRIs. **E and G.** Anatomical sections.

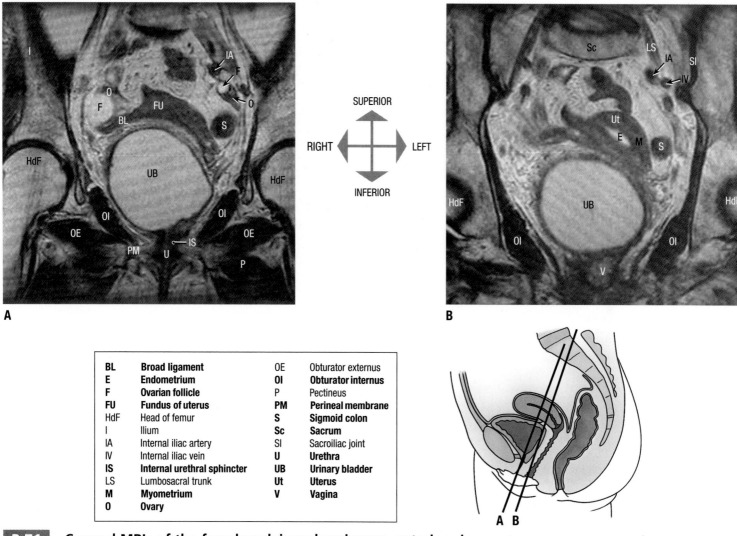

BL	**Broad ligament**	OE	Obturator externus
E	**Endometrium**	**OI**	**Obturator internus**
F	**Ovarian follicle**	P	Pectineus
FU	**Fundus of uterus**	**PM**	**Perineal membrane**
HdF	Head of femur	**S**	**Sigmoid colon**
I	Ilium	Sc	Sacrum
IA	Internal iliac artery	SI	Sacroiliac joint
IV	Internal iliac vein	**U**	**Urethra**
IS	**Internal urethral sphincter**	**UB**	**Urinary bladder**
LS	Lumbosacral trunk	**Ut**	**Uterus**
M	**Myometrium**	**V**	**Vagina**
O	**Ovary**		

3.71   Coronal MRIs of the female pelvis and perineum, anterior views

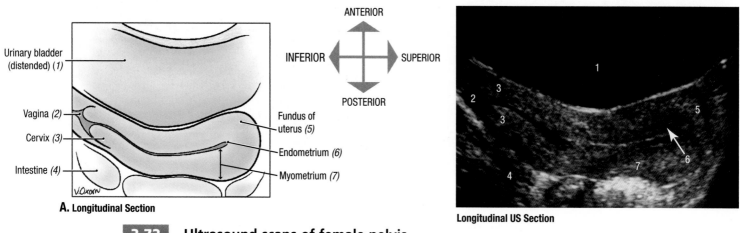

3.72   Ultrasound scans of female pelvis

A. Median (transabdominal) ultrasound scan and orientation drawing (numbers in parentheses correspond to labels on the ultrasound scan).

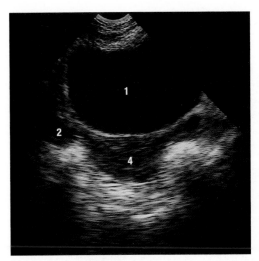

B. Transverse (Axial) Scan

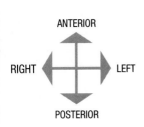

ANTERIOR

RIGHT   LEFT

POSTERIOR

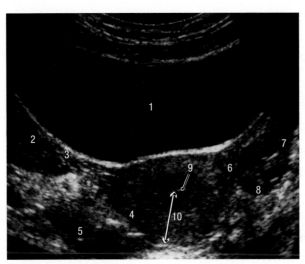

C. Transverse (Axial) Scan

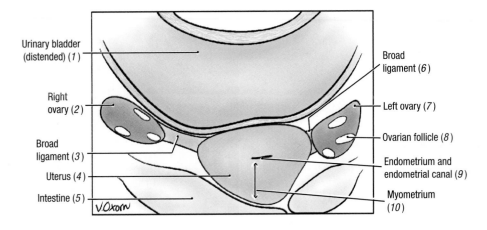

Urinary bladder (distended) (*1*)

Right ovary (*2*)

Broad ligament (*3*)

Uterus (*4*)

Intestine (*5*)

Broad ligament (*6*)

Left ovary (*7*)

Ovarian follicle (*8*)

Endometrium and endometrial canal (*9*)

Myometrium (*10*)

V.Oxorn

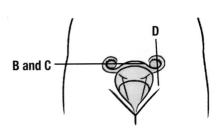

B and C

D

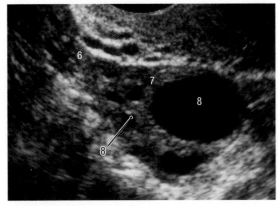

D. Sagittal Scan

3.72   **Ultrasound scans of female pelvis** *(continued)*

B and **C.** Transabdominal axial (transverse) scan through uterus and ovaries. Transabdominal US scanning requires a fully distended urinary bladder to displace the bowel loops from the pelvis and to provide an acoustical window through which to observe pelvic anatomy.

D. Transvaginal sagittal scan of left ovary (numbers in parentheses correspond to labels on the ultrasound scans). Transvaginal and transrectal ultrasonography enables the placing of the probe closer to the structures of interest, allowing increased resolution.

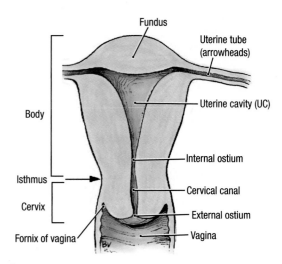

A. Coronal Section

Fundus
Uterine tube (arrowheads)
Uterine cavity (UC)
Body
Internal ostium
Isthmus
Cervical canal
Cervix
External ostium
Fornix of vagina
Vagina

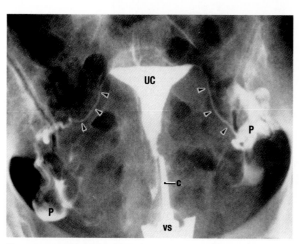

B. Hysterosalpingogram of Normal Uterus, Anteroposterior View

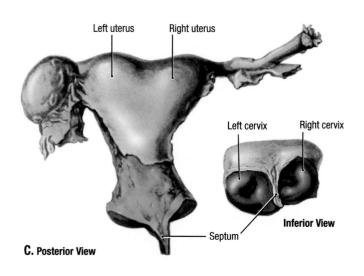

C. Posterior View

Left uterus   Right uterus
Left cervix   Right cervix
Inferior View
Septum

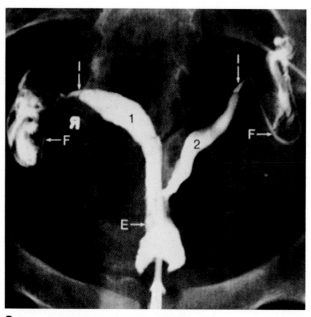

D. Hysterosalpingogram of Bicornate Uterus, Anteroposterior View

3.73   Radiograph of uterus and uterine tubes (hysterosalpingogram)

A. Coronal section of uterus. **B.** Radiopaque material was injected into the uterus through external os of the uterus. The contrast medium traveled through the triangular uterine cavity (UC) and uterine tubes (arrowheads) and passed into the pararectal fossae (P) of the peritoneal cavity. c, catheter in the cervical canal; vs, vaginal speculum. The female genital tract is in direct communication with the peritoneal cavity and is, therefore, a potential pathway for the spread of an infection from the vagina and uterus. **C.** Illustration of duplicated uterus. **D.** Hysterosalpingogram of a bicornate ("two horned") uterus. 1 and 2, uterine cavities; E, cervical canal; F, uterine tubes; I, isthmus of tubes.

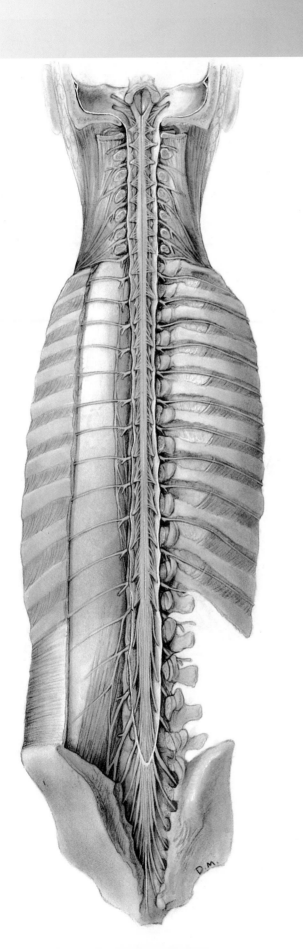

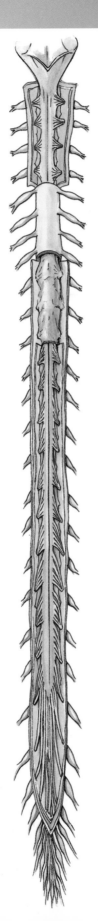

■ Overview of Vertebral Column **286**
■ Cervical Spine **294**
■ Craniovertebral Joints **298**
■ Thoracic Spine **300**
■ Lumbar Spine **302**
■ Ligaments and Intervertebral Discs **304**
■ Vertebral Venous Plexuses **309**
■ Bones, Joints, and Ligaments of Pelvic Girdle **310**
■ Anomalies of Vertebrae **318**
■ Muscles of Back **320**
■ Suboccipital Region **330**
■ Spinal Cord and Meninges **334**
■ Components of Spinal Nerves **343**
■ Dermatomes and Myotomes **348**
■ Imaging of Vertebral Column **350**

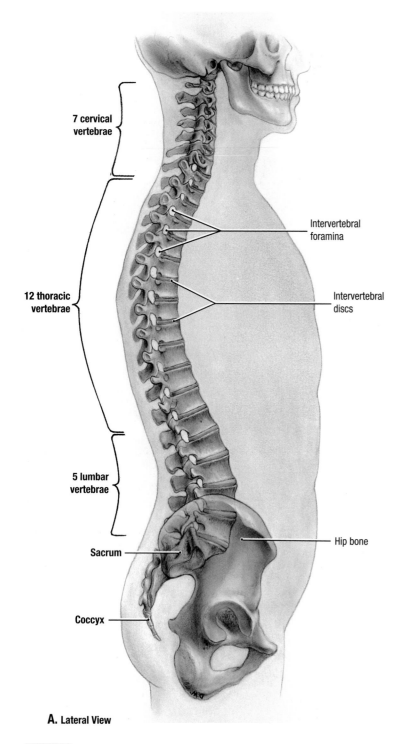

7 cervical vertebrae

Intervertebral foramina

12 thoracic vertebrae

Intervertebral discs

5 lumbar vertebrae

Hip bone

Sacrum

Coccyx

A. Lateral View

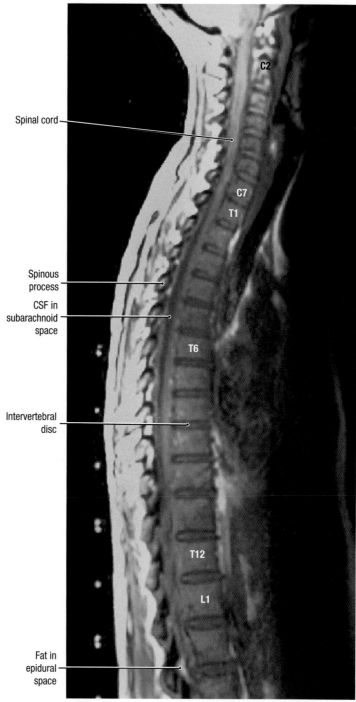

Spinal cord

C2

C7

T1

Spinous process

CSF in subarachnoid space

T6

Intervertebral disc

T12

L1

Fat in epidural space

B. Sagittal MRI

4.1 Overview of vertebral column

A. Vertebral column showing articulation with skull and hip bone.
B. Sagittal MRI, lateral view.

- The vertebral column usually consists of 24 separate (presacral) vertebrae, 5 fused vertebrae in the sacrum, and variably 4 fused or separate coccygeal vertebrae. Of the 24 separate vertebrae, 12 support ribs (thoracic), 7 are in the neck (cervical), and 5 are in the lumbar region (lumbar).

- Vertebrae contributing to the posterior walls of the thoracic and pelvic cavities are concave anteriorly; elsewhere (in the cervical and lumbar regions) they are convex anteriorly.
- The spinal nerves exit the vertebral (spinal) canal via the intervertebral foramina. There are 8 cervical, 12 thoracic, 5 lumbar, 5 sacral, and 1 to 2 coccygeal spinal nerves.
- Note the size and shape of the vertebral bodies, the direction of the spinous processes, and the spinal cord in the vertebral canal (in **B**).

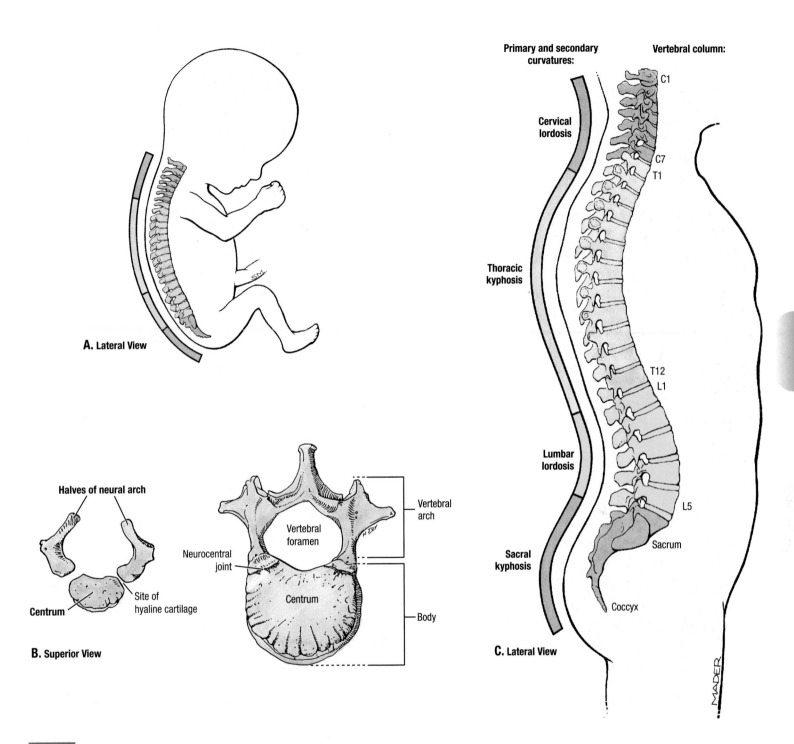

A. Lateral View

Halves of neural arch

Centrum

Site of hyaline cartilage

B. Superior View

Neurocentral joint

Vertebral foramen

Centrum

Vertebral arch

Body

Primary and secondary curvatures:

Cervical lordosis

Thoracic kyphosis

Lumbar lordosis

Sacral kyphosis

Vertebral column:

C1

C7

T1

T12

L1

L5

Sacrum

Coccyx

C. Lateral View

4.2   Curvatures of vertebral column

A. Fetus. Note the C-shaped curvature of the fetal spine, which is concave anteriorly over its entire length. **B.** Development of the vertebrae. At birth, a vertebra consists of three bony parts (two halves of the neural arch and the centrum) united by hyaline cartilage. At age 2, the halves of each neural arch begin to fuse, proceeding from the lumbar to the cervical region; at approximately age 7, the arches begin to fuse to the centrum, proceeding from the cervical to lumbar regions. **C. Adult.** The four curvatures of the adult vertebral column include the cervical lordosis, which is convex anteriorly and lies between vertebrae C1 and T2; the tho-racic kyphosis, which is concave anteriorly, between vertebrae T2 and T12; the lumbar lordosis, convex anteriorly and lying between T12 and the lumbosacral joint; and the sacral kyphosis, concave anteriorly and spanning from the lumbosacral joint to the tip of the coccyx. The anteriorly concave thoracic kyphosis and sacrococcygeal kyphosis are primary curves, and the anteriorly convex cervical lordosis and lumbar lordosis are secondary curves that develop after birth. The cervical lordosis develops when the child begins to hold the head up, and the lumbar kyphosis devel-ops when the child begins to walk.

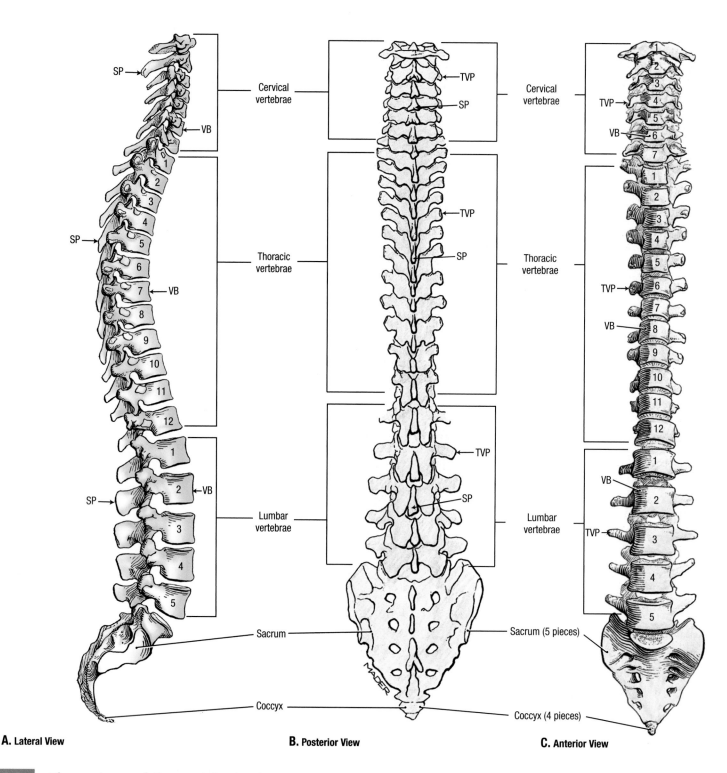

SP

VB

Cervical
vertebrae

TVP

SP

Cervical
vertebrae

TVP

VB

SP

VB

1
2
3
4
5
6
7
8
9
10
11
12

TVP

TVP

SP

Thoracic
vertebrae

Thoracic
vertebrae

TVP

VB

1
2
3
4
5
6
7
8
9
10
11
12

SP

VB

1
2
3
4
5

TVP

SP

Lumbar
vertebrae

Lumbar
vertebrae

VB

TVP

1
2
3
4
5

Sacrum

Sacrum (5 pieces)

Coccyx

Coccyx (4 pieces)

MADER

A. Lateral View   **B.** Posterior View   **C.** Anterior View

4.3   Three views of the vertebral column

- The vertebral bodies (VB) vary in size and shape.
- Transverse processes (TVP) in the cervical region are directed laterally, inferiorly and anteriorly. In the thoracic region, they are directed laterally posteriorly, and superiorly, have a facet for the tubercle of the rib, and are stout. In the lumbar region, the TVPs point laterally and are long and slender.

- Generally, spinous processes (SP) are bifid in caucasians in the cervical region, long and spinelike in the thoracic region, and stout and oblong in the lumbar region. The cervical and thoracic SPs often overlap the adjacent, inferior vertebrae.

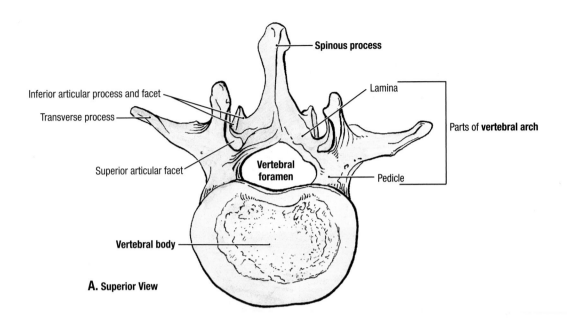

A. **Superior View**

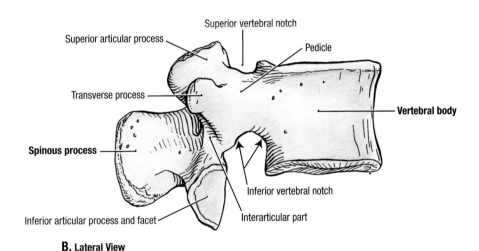

B. **Lateral View**

`4.4` **Typical vertebra**

A typical vertebra (e.g., the 2nd lumbar vertebra) consists of the following parts:

- A vertebral body, situated anteriorly, functions to support weight.
- A vertebral arch, posterior to the body, with the body, encloses the vertebral foramen. Collectively, the vertebral foramina constitute the vertebral canal, in which the spinal cord lies. The function of a vertebral arch is to protect the spinal cord. The vertebral arch consists of two rounded pedicles, one on each side, which arise from the body, and two flat plates called laminae that unite posteriorly in the midline.
- Three processes, two transverse and one spinous, provide attachment for muscles and are the levers that help move the vertebrae.
- Four articular processes, two superior and two inferior, each have an articular facet. The articular processes project superiorly and inferiorly from the vertebral arch and come into apposition with the articular facet of the corresponding processes of the vertebrae above and below. The direction of the articular facets determines the nature of the movement between adjacent vertebrae and prevents the vertebrae from slipping anteriorly.

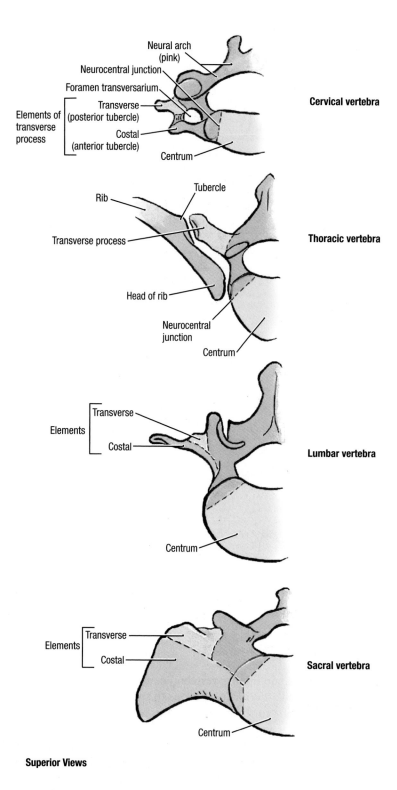

Superior Views

4.5   Homologous parts of vertebrae

A rib is a free costal element in the thoracic region; in the cervical and lumbar regions, it is represented by the anterior part of a transverse process, and in the sacrum, by the anterior part of the lateral mass. The heads of the ribs (thoracic region) articulate with the sides of the vertebral bodies posterior to the neurocentral junctions.

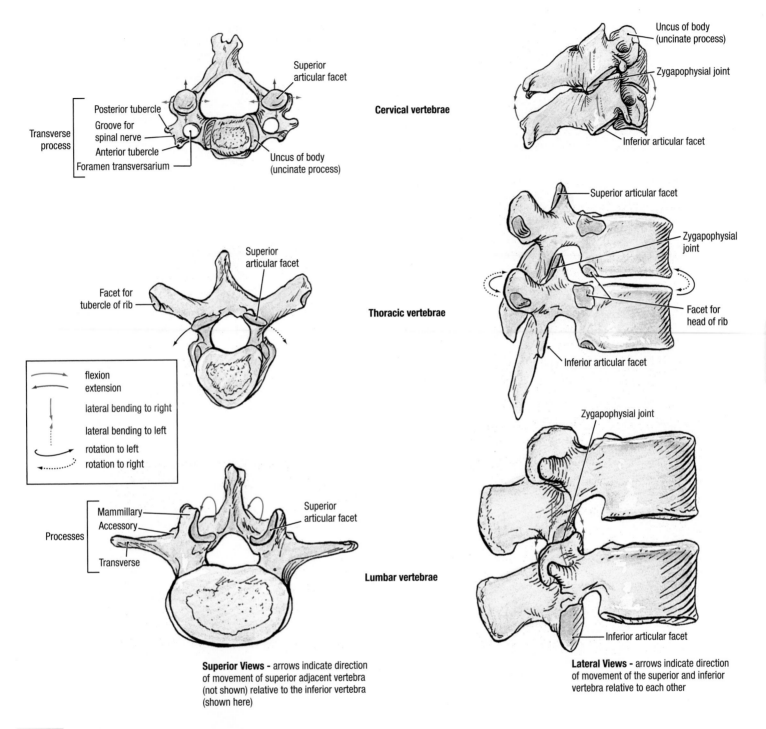

Cervical vertebrae

Transverse process
- Posterior tubercle
- Groove for spinal nerve
- Anterior tubercle
- Foramen transversarium

Superior articular facet

Uncus of body (uncinate process)

Uncus of body (uncinate process)

Zygapophysial joint

Inferior articular facet

Thoracic vertebrae

Facet for tubercle of rib

Superior articular facet

Superior articular facet

Zygapophysial joint

Inferior articular facet

Facet for head of rib

Inferior articular facet

flexion
extension
lateral bending to right
lateral bending to left
rotation to left
rotation to right

Lumbar vertebrae

Processes
- Mammillary
- Accessory
- Transverse

Superior articular facet

Zygapophysial joint

Inferior articular facet

Superior Views - arrows indicate direction of movement of superior adjacent vertebra (not shown) relative to the inferior vertebra (shown here)

Lateral Views - arrows indicate direction of movement of the superior and inferior vertebra relative to each other

| 4.6 | **Vertebral features and movements** |

Direction of movement is indicated by *arrows*.
- In the thoracic and lumbar regions, the superior articular facets lie posterior to the pedicles, and the inferior facets are anterior to the laminae. Superior articular facets in the cervical region face mainly superiorly, in the thoracic region, mainly posteriorly, and in the lumbar region, mainly medially. The change in direction is gradual from cervical to thoracic but abrupt from thoracic to lumbar.
- Although movements between adjacent vertebrae are relatively small, especially in the thoracic region, the summation of all the small movements produces a considerable range of movement of the vertebral column as a whole.

- Movements of the vertebral column are freer in the cervical and lumbar regions than in the thoracic region. Lateral bending is freest in the cervical and lumbar regions; flexion of the vertebral column is greatest in the cervical region; extension is most marked in the lumbar region, but the interlocking articular processes prevent rotation.
- The thoracic region is most stable because of the external support gained from the articulations of the ribs and costal cartilages with the sternum. The direction of the articular facets permits rotation, but flexion, extension, and lateral bending is severely restricted.

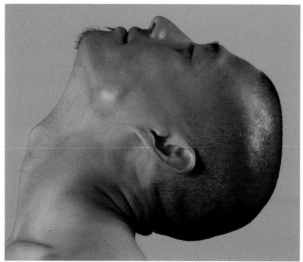

A. Lateral View

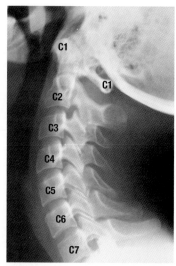

B. Lateral View

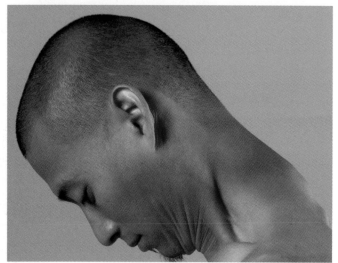

C. Lateral View

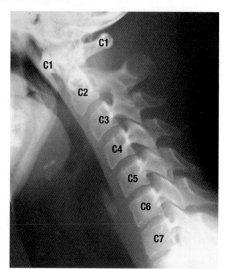

D. Lateral View

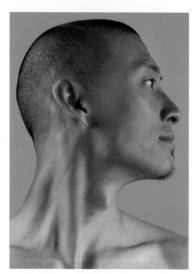

E. Anterior View

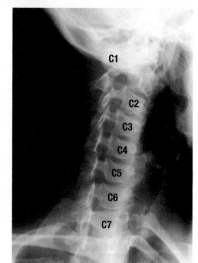

F. Oblique View

4.7   **Surface anatomy with radiographic correlation of selected movements of the cervical spine**

A. Extension of the neck. **B.** Radiograph of the extended cervical spine. **C.** Flexion of the neck. **D.** Radiograph of the flexed cervical spine. **E.** Head turned (rotated) to left. **F.** Radiograph of cervical spine rotated to left.

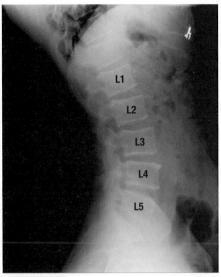

B. Lateral View

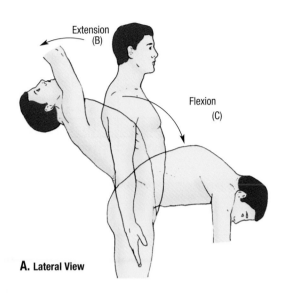

Extension
(B)

Flexion
(C)

A. Lateral View

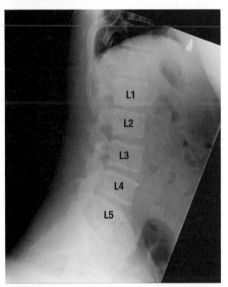

C. Lateral View

Lateral bending
(E)

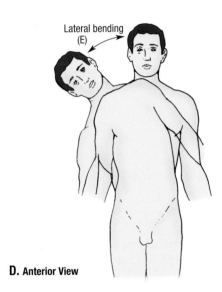

D. Anterior View

4.8 **Surface anatomy with radiographic correlation of selected movements of the lumbar spine**

A. Flexion and extension of the trunk. **B.** Radiograph of the extended lumbar spine. **C.** Radiograph of the flexed lumbar spine. **D.** Lateral bending of the trunk. **E.** Radiograph of the lumbar spine during lateral bending.

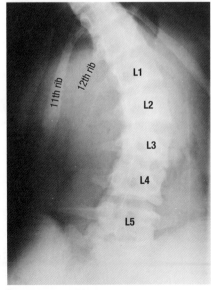

E. Anteroposterior View

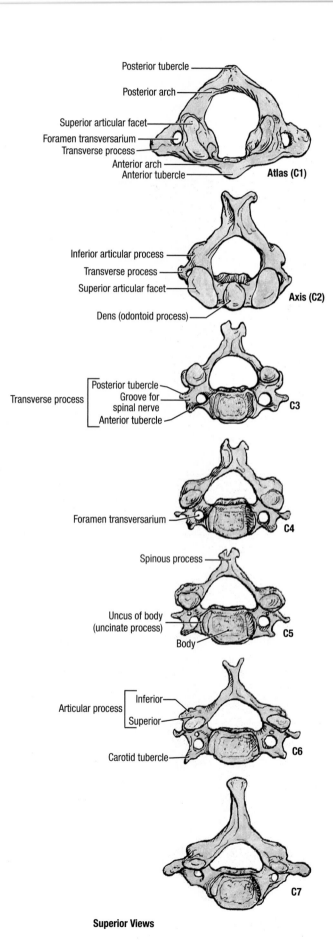

Atlas (C1)

Posterior tubercle
Posterior arch
Superior articular facet
Foramen transversarium
Transverse process
Anterior arch
Anterior tubercle

Axis (C2)

Inferior articular process
Transverse process
Superior articular facet
Dens (odontoid process)

C3

Transverse process
Posterior tubercle
Groove for spinal nerve
Anterior tubercle

C4

Foramen transversarium

C5

Spinous process
Uncus of body (uncinate process)
Body

C6

Articular process
Inferior
Superior
Carotid tubercle

C7

Superior Views

TABLE 4.1   TYPICAL CERVICAL VERTEBRAE (C3-C7)[a]

Part	Distinctive Characteristics
Body	Small and wider from side to side than anteroposteriorly; superior surface is concave with uncus of body (uncinate process); inferior surface is convex
Vertebral foramen	Large and triangular
Transverse processes	Foramina transversaria small or absent in C7; vertebral arteries and accompanying venous and sympathetic plexuses pass through foramina, except C7, which transmits only small accessory vertebral veins; anterior and posterior tubercles separated by groove for spinal nerve
Articular processes	Superior articular facets directed superoposteriorly; inferior articular facets directed inferoanteriorly; obliquely placed facets are most nearly horizontal in this region
Spinous process	Short (C3–C5) and bifid, only in Caucasians (C3–C5); process of C6 is long but that of C7 is longer; C7 is called "vertebra prominens"

[a]C1 and C2 vertebrae are atypical.

4.9   Cervical vertebrae

The bodies of the cervical vertebrae can be dislocated in neck injuries with less force than is required to fracture them. Because of the large vertebral canal in the cervical region, slight dislocation can occur without damaging the spinal cord. When a cervical vertebra is severely dislocated, it injures the spinal cord. If the dislocation does not result in "facet jumping" with locking of the displaced articular processes, the cervical vertebrae may self-reduce ("slip back into place") so that a radiograph may not indicate that the cord has been injured. MRI may reveal the resulting soft tissue damage.

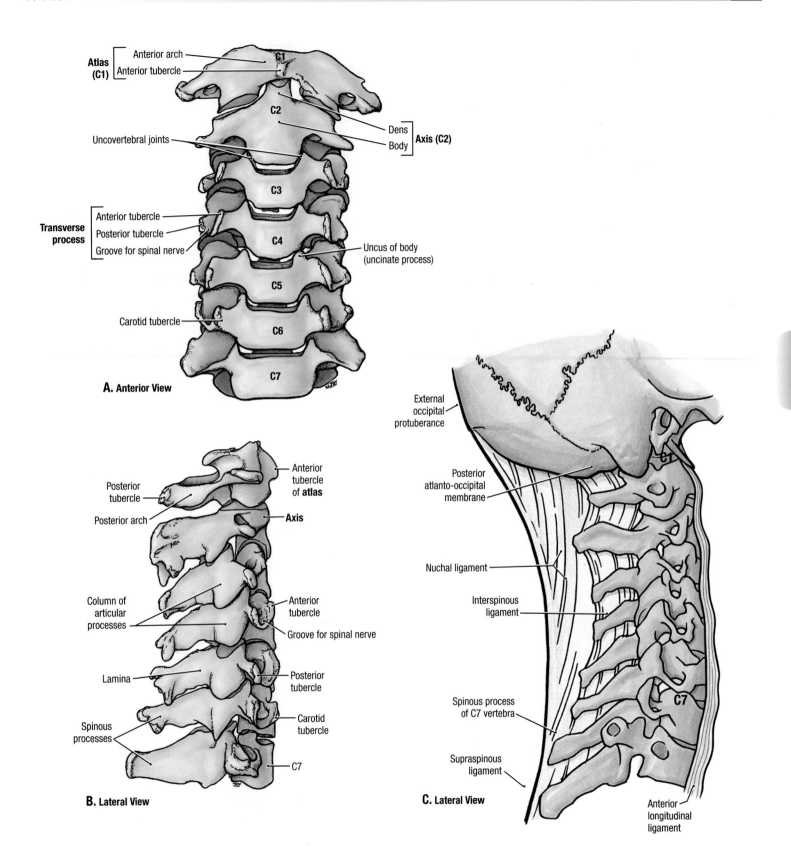

Atlas (C1)
- Anterior arch
- Anterior tubercle

C1

C2

Uncovertebral joints

Dens
Body — **Axis (C2)**

C3

Transverse process
- Anterior tubercle
- Posterior tubercle
- Groove for spinal nerve

C4

Uncus of body (uncinate process)

C5

Carotid tubercle

C6

C7

A. Anterior View

Posterior tubercle

Anterior tubercle of **atlas**

Posterior arch

Axis

Column of articular processes

Anterior tubercle

Groove for spinal nerve

Lamina

Posterior tubercle

Spinous processes

Carotid tubercle

C7

B. Lateral View

External occipital protuberance

Posterior atlanto-occipital membrane

C1

Nuchal ligament

Interspinous ligament

Spinous process of C7 vertebra

C7

Supraspinous ligament

Anterior longitudinal ligament

C. Lateral View

4.10   Cervical spine

A and **B.** Articulated cervical vertebrae. **C.** Ligaments.

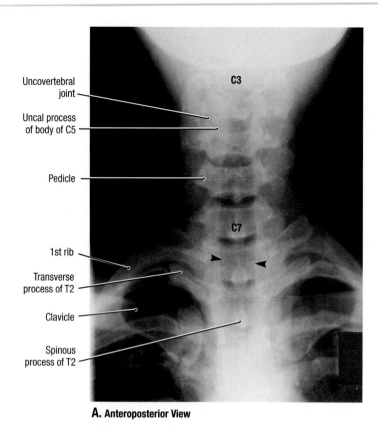

Uncovertebral joint

Uncal process of body of C5

Pedicle

1st rib

Transverse process of T2

Clavicle

Spinous process of T2

A. Anteroposterior View

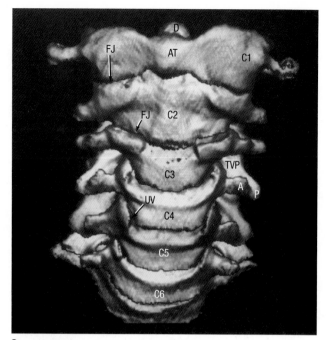

C. Anterior View

A	Anterior tubercle of transverse process	PA	Posterior arch of C1
AA	Anterior arch of C1	PT	Posterior tubercle of C1
AT	Anterior tubercle of C1	SF	Superior articular facet of C1
C1–C7	Vertebrae	SP	Spinous process
D	Dens (odontoid) process of C2	T	Foramen transversarium
FJ	Zygapophysial (facet) joint	TVP	Transverse process
La	Lamina	UV	Uncovertebral joint
P	Posterior tubercle of transverse process	VC	Vertebral canal

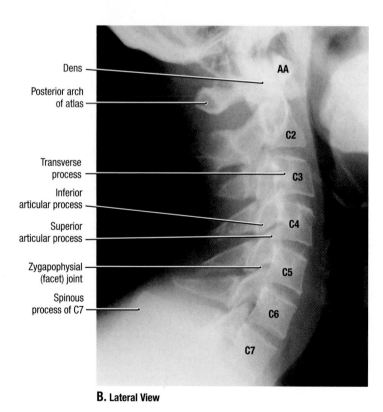

Dens

Posterior arch of atlas

Transverse process

Inferior articular process

Superior articular process

Zygapophysial (facet) joint

Spinous process of C7

B. Lateral View

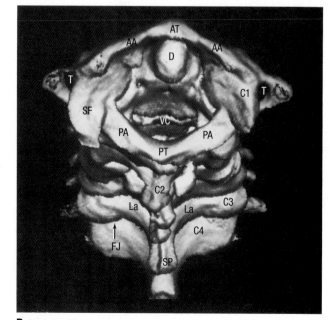

D. Posterior View

4.11   Imaging of the cervical spine

A and B. Radiographs. The arrowheads demarcate the margins of the *(black)* column of air in the trachea. **C** and **D.** Three-dimensional (3D) reconstructed computed tomographic (CT) images.

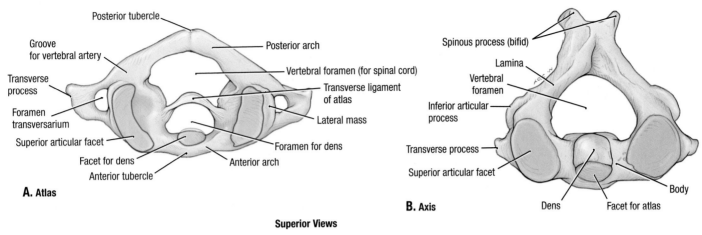

Posterior tubercle

Groove
for vertebral artery

Posterior arch

Transverse
process

Vertebral foramen (for spinal cord)

Foramen
transversarium

Transverse ligament
of atlas

Superior articular facet

Lateral mass

Facet for dens

Foramen for dens

Anterior tubercle

Anterior arch

A. Atlas

Spinous process (bifid)

Lamina

Vertebral
foramen

Inferior articular
process

Transverse process

Superior articular facet

Dens

Facet for atlas

Body

B. Axis

Superior Views

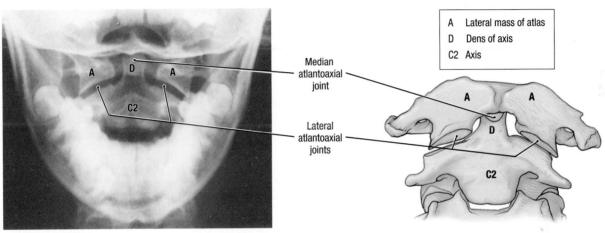

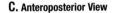

A	Lateral mass of atlas
D	Dens of axis
C2	Axis

Median
atlantoaxial
joint

Lateral
atlantoaxial
joints

C. Anteroposterior View

D. Anterior View

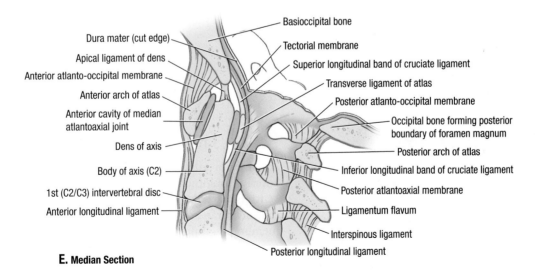

Dura mater (cut edge)

Basioccipital bone

Apical ligament of dens

Tectorial membrane

Anterior atlanto-occipital membrane

Superior longitudinal band of cruciate ligament

Anterior arch of atlas

Transverse ligament of atlas

Anterior cavity of median
atlantoaxial joint

Posterior atlanto-occipital membrane

Dens of axis

Occipital bone forming posterior
boundary of foramen magnum

Body of axis (C2)

Posterior arch of atlas

1st (C2/C3) intervertebral disc

Inferior longitudinal band of cruciate ligament

Anterior longitudinal ligament

Posterior atlantoaxial membrane

Ligamentum flavum

Interspinous ligament

Posterior longitudinal ligament

E. Median Section

4.12   **Atlas and axis and the atlantoaxial joint**

A. Atlas. **B.** Axis. **C.** Radiograph taken through the open mouth. **D.** Articulated atlas and
axis. **E.** Median section with ligaments.

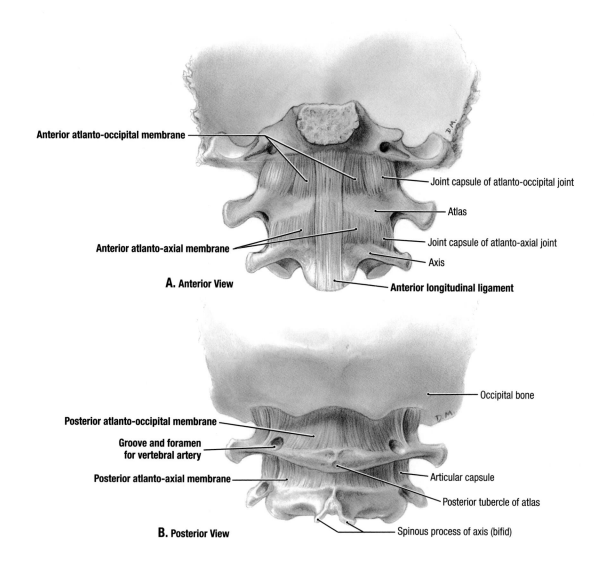

Anterior atlanto-occipital membrane

Joint capsule of atlanto-occipital joint

Atlas

Joint capsule of atlanto-axial joint

Anterior atlanto-axial membrane

Axis

Anterior longitudinal ligament

A. Anterior View

Occipital bone

Posterior atlanto-occipital membrane

Groove and foramen for vertebral artery

Posterior atlanto-axial membrane

Articular capsule

Posterior tubercle of atlas

Spinous process of axis (bifid)

B. Posterior View

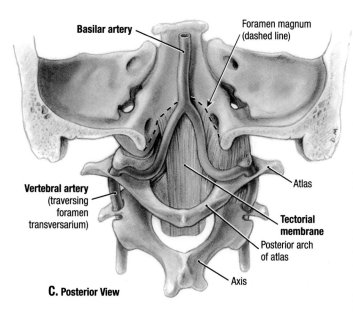

Basilar artery

Foramen magnum (dashed line)

Vertebral artery (traversing foramen transversarium)

Atlas

Tectorial membrane

Posterior arch of atlas

Axis

C. Posterior View

4.13   Craniovertebral joints and vertebral artery

A. Anterior atlanto-axial and atlanto-occipital membranes. The anterior longitudinal ligament ascends to blend with, and form a central thickening in, the anterior atlanto-axial and atlanto-occipital membranes. **B.** Posterior atlanto-axial and atlanto-occipital membranes. Inferior to the axis (C2 vertebra), ligamenta flava occur in this position. **C.** Tectorial membrane and vertebral artery. The tectorial membrane is a superior continuation of the posterior longitudinal ligament superior to the axis. After coursing through the foramina transversaria of vertebrae C6–C1, the arteries turning medially, grooving the superior aspect of the posterior arch of the atlas and piercing the posterior atlanto-occipital membrane **(B)**. The right and left vertebral arteries traverse the foramen magnum and merge to form the intracranial basilar artery.

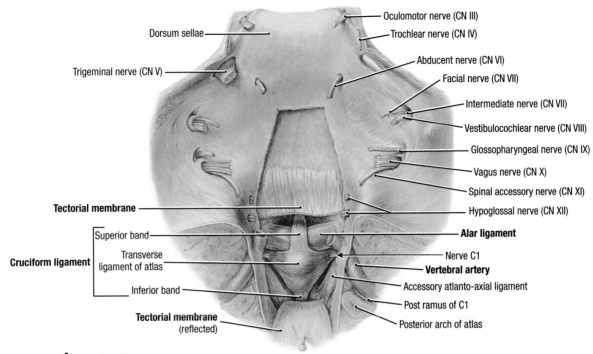

Oculomotor nerve (CN III)
Dorsum sellae
Trochlear nerve (CN IV)
Abducent nerve (CN VI)
Trigeminal nerve (CN V)
Facial nerve (CN VII)
Intermediate nerve (CN VII)
Vestibulocochlear nerve (CN VIII)
Glossopharyngeal nerve (CN IX)
Vagus nerve (CN X)
Spinal accessory nerve (CN XI)
Tectorial membrane
Hypoglossal nerve (CN XII)
Superior band
Alar ligament
Cruciform ligament Transverse ligament of atlas
Nerve C1
Vertebral artery
Inferior band
Accessory atlanto-axial ligament
Tectorial membrane (reflected)
Post ramus of C1
Posterior arch of atlas

A. Posterior View

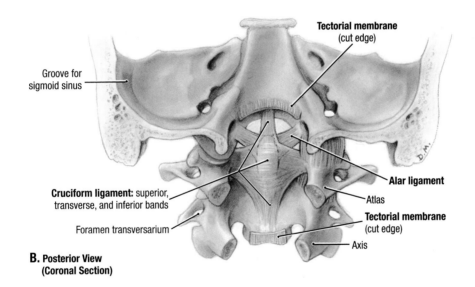

Tectorial membrane (cut edge)
Groove for sigmoid sinus
Alar ligament
Cruciform ligament: superior, transverse, and inferior bands
Atlas
Tectorial membrane (cut edge)
Foramen transversarium
Axis

B. Posterior View (Coronal Section)

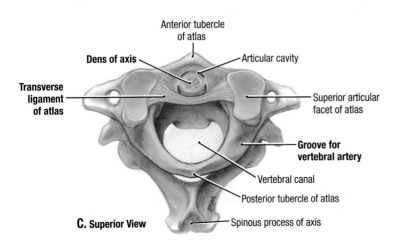

Anterior tubercle of atlas
Dens of axis
Articular cavity
Transverse ligament of atlas
Superior articular facet of atlas
Groove for vertebral artery
Vertebral canal
Posterior tubercle of atlas
C. Superior View
Spinous process of axis

4.14 Ligaments of atlanto-occipital and atlantoaxial joints

A. Cranial nerves and dura mater of posterior cranial fossa with dura mater and tentorial membrane incised and removed to reveal the medial atlanto-axial joint. **B.** The alar ligaments serve as check ligaments for the rotary movements of the atlanto-axial joints. **B** and **C.** The transverse ligament (band) of the cruciform ligament provides the posterior wall of a socket that receives the dens of the axis, forming a pivot joint.

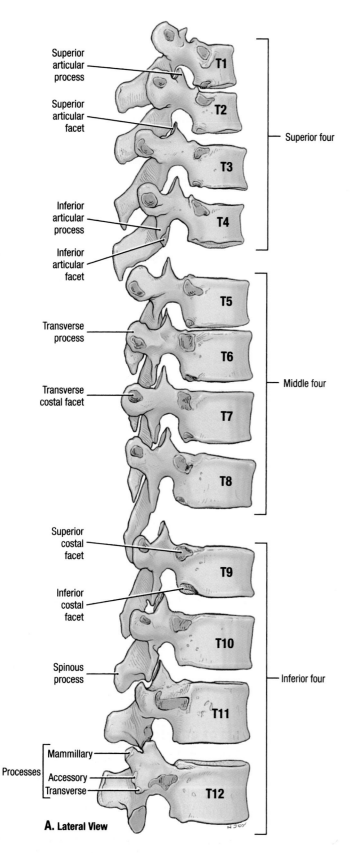

Superior articular process

Superior articular facet

Superior four

T1

T2

T3

T4

Inferior articular process

Inferior articular facet

Transverse process

T5

T6

Transverse costal facet

Middle four

T7

T8

Superior costal facet

Inferior costal facet

T9

T10

Spinous process

Inferior four

T11

Processes

Mammillary

Accessory

Transverse

T12

A. Lateral View

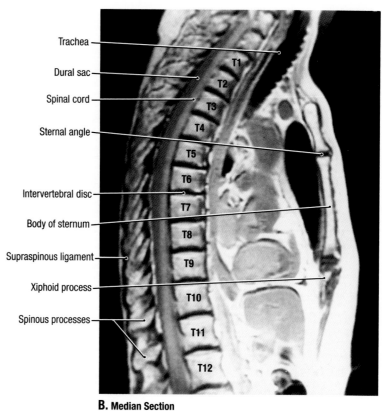

Trachea

Dural sac

Spinal cord

Sternal angle

Intervertebral disc

Body of sternum

Supraspinous ligament

Xiphoid process

Spinous processes

T1
T2
T3
T4
T5
T6
T7
T8
T9
T10
T11
T12

B. Median Section

TABLE 4.2 THORACIC VERTEBRAE

Part	Distinctive Characteristics
Body	Heart-shaped; has one or two costal facets for articulation with head of rib
Vertebral foramen	Circular and smaller than those of cervical and lumbar vertebrae
Transverse processes	Long and strong and extend posterolaterally; length diminishes from T1 to T12; T1–T10 have transverse costal facets for articulation with tubercle of a rib
Articular processes	Superior articular facets directed posteriorly and slightly laterally; inferior articular facets directed anteriorly and slightly medially
Spinous process	Long and slopes posteroinferiorly; tip extends to level of vertebral body below

4.15 **Thoracic vertebrae**

A. Features. **B.** MRI scan of thoracic spine, median section.

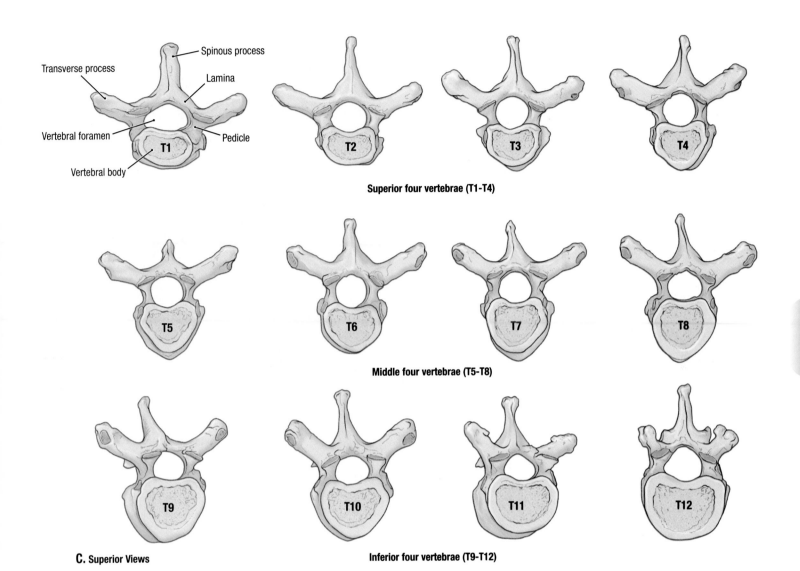

Spinous process
Transverse process
Lamina
Vertebral foramen
Pedicle
T1
Vertebral body

T2

T3

T4

Superior four vertebrae (T1-T4)

T5

T6

T7

T8

Middle four vertebrae (T5-T8)

T9

T10

T11

T12

C. Superior Views

Inferior four vertebrae (T9-T12)

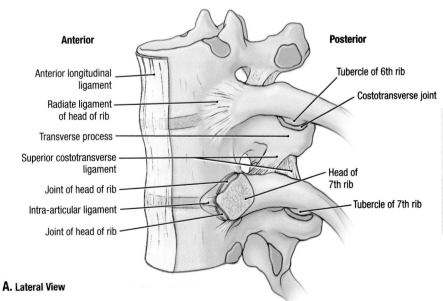

Anterior

Posterior

Anterior longitudinal ligament
Radiate ligament of head of rib
Transverse process
Superior costotransverse ligament
Joint of head of rib
Intra-articular ligament
Joint of head of rib

Tubercle of 6th rib
Costotransverse joint
Head of 7th rib
Tubercle of 7th rib

A. Lateral View

4.15 Thoracic vertebrae *(continued)*

C. Comparative anatomy. The vertebral bodies increase in size as the vertebral column descends, each bearing an increasing amount of weight transferred by the vertebra above. Although the characteristics of the superior aspect of vertebra T12 are distinctly thoracic, its inferior aspect has lumbar characteristics for articulation with vertebra L1. The abrupt transition allowing primarily rotational movements with vertebra T11 while disallowing rotational movements with vertebral L1 makes vertebra T12 especially susceptible to fracture. **D.** Intra- and extra-articular ligaments of the costovertebral articulations. Typically, the head of each rib articulates with the bodies of two adjacent vertebrae and the invertebral disc between them, and the tubercle of the rib articulates with the transverse process of the inferior vertebra.

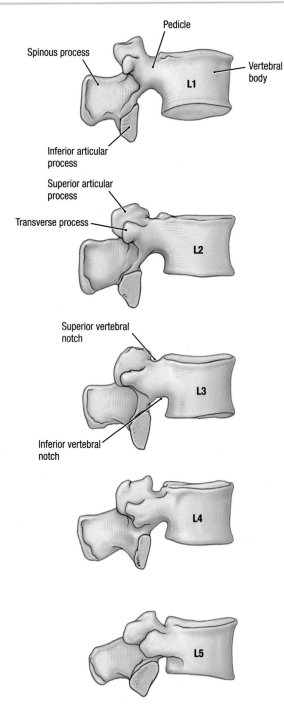

A. Lateral Views

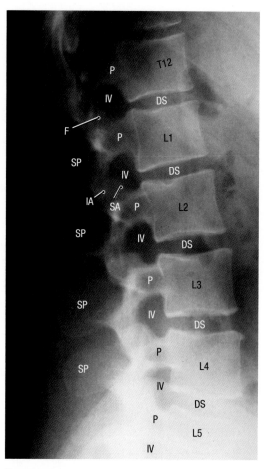

B. Lateral View

Key for B	
F	Zygapophysial (facet) joint
DS	Intervertebral disc space
IA	Inferior articular process
IV	Intervertebral foramen
P	Pedicle
SA	Superior articular process
SP	Spinous process
T12–L5	Vertebral bodies

TABLE 4.3   LUMBAR VERTEBRAE

Part	Distinctive Characteristics
Body	Massive; kidney-shaped when viewed superiorly
Vertebral foramen	Triangular; larger than in thoracic vertebrae and smaller than in cervical vertebrae
Transverse processes	Long and slender; accessory process on posterior surface of base of each transverse process
Articular processes	Superior articular facets directed posteromedially (or medially); inferior articular facets directed anterolaterally (or laterally); mamillary process on posterior surface of each superior articular process
Spinous process	Short and sturdy; thick, broad, and rectangular

4.16   **Lumbar vertebrae**

A, C, and **D.** Features. **B.** Radiograph. A laminectomy is the surgical excision of one or more spinous processes and their supporting laminae in a particular region of the vertebral column i.e., removal of most of the vertebral arch by transecting the pedicles. Laminectomies provide access to the vertebral canal to relieve pressure on the spinal cord or nerve roots, commonly caused by a tumor, herniated IV disc, or bony hypertrophy (excess growth). Laminectomies are most commonly performed in the lumbar region.

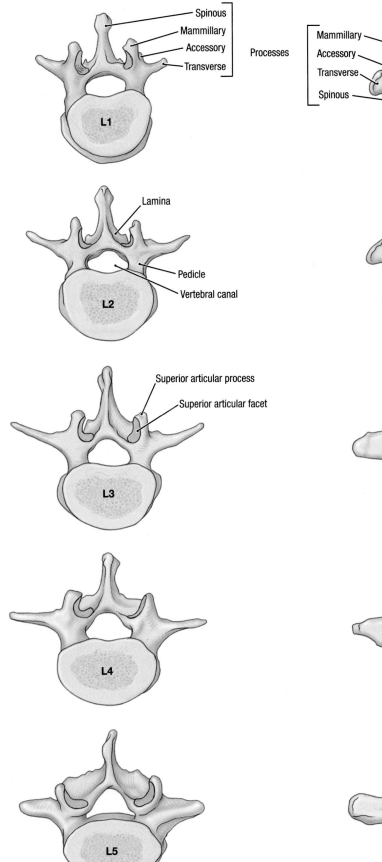

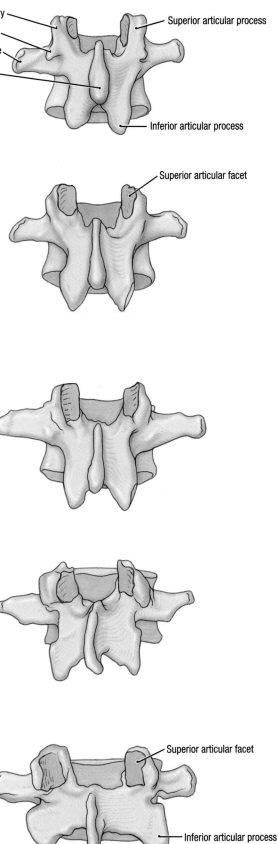

C. Superior View

D. Posterior View

4.16   Lumbar vertebrae *(continued)*

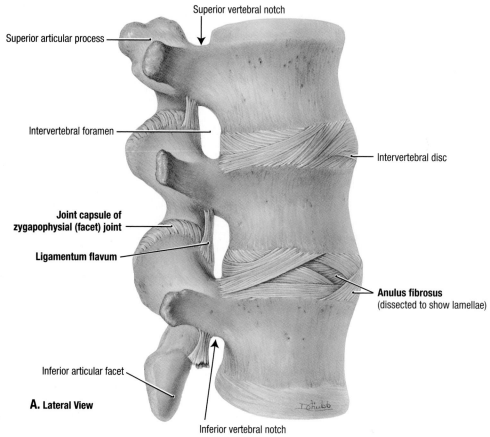

Superior vertebral notch

Superior articular process

Intervertebral foramen

Intervertebral disc

Joint capsule of zygapophysial (facet) joint

Ligamentum flavum

Anulus fibrosus (dissected to show lamellae)

Inferior articular facet

A. Lateral View

Inferior vertebral notch

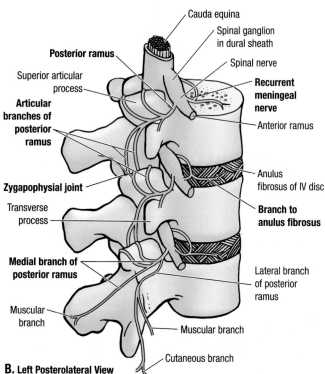

Cauda equina

Spinal ganglion in dural sheath

Posterior ramus

Spinal nerve

Superior articular process

Recurrent meningeal nerve

Articular branches of posterior ramus

Anterior ramus

Zygapophysial joint

Anulus fibrosus of IV disc

Transverse process

Branch to anulus fibrosus

Medial branch of posterior ramus

Lateral branch of posterior ramus

Muscular branch

Muscular branch

Cutaneous branch

B. Left Posterolateral View

When the zygapophyseal joints are injured or develop osteophytes during aging (osteoarthritis), the related spinal nerves are affected. This causes pain along the distribution pattern of the dermatomes and spasm in the muscles derived from the associated myotomes (a myotome consists of all the muscles or parts of muscles receiving innervation from one spinal nerve). Denervation of lumbar zygapophysial joints is a procedure that may be used for treatment of back pain caused by disease of these joints. The nerves are sectioned near the joints or are destroyed by radiofrequency percutaneous rhizolysis (root dissolution). The denervation process is directed at the articular branches of two adjacent posterior rami of the spinal nerves because each joint receives innervation from both the nerve exiting that level and the superadjacent nerve.

4.17   Structure and innervation of intervertebral discs and zygapophysial joints

A. Anulus fibrosus and intervertebral foramen. Sections have been removed from the superficial layers of the inferior intervertebral disc to show the change in direction of the fibers in the concentric layers of the anulus fibrosus. **B.** Innervation of zygapophysial joint and intervertebral disc.

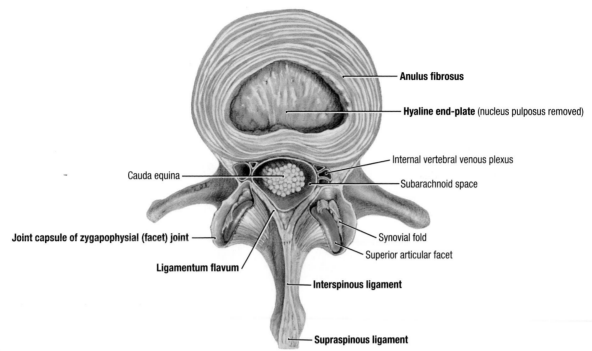

Anulus fibrosus

Hyaline end-plate (nucleus pulposus removed)

Internal vertebral venous plexus

Cauda equina

Subarachnoid space

Synovial fold

Superior articular facet

Joint capsule of zygapophysial (facet) joint

Ligamentum flavum

Interspinous ligament

Supraspinous ligament

C. Transverse Section, Superior View

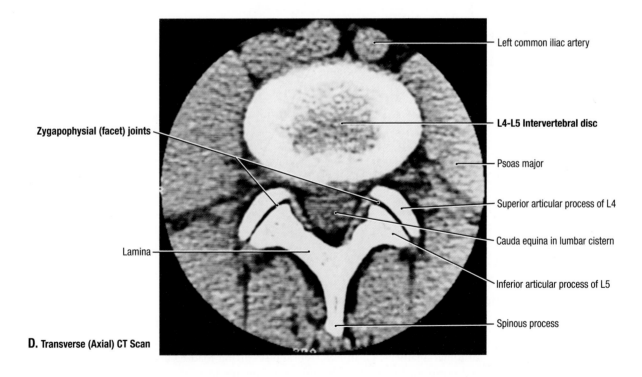

Left common iliac artery

Zygapophysial (facet) joints

L4-L5 Intervertebral disc

Psoas major

Superior articular process of L4

Cauda equina in lumbar cistern

Lamina

Inferior articular process of L5

Spinous process

D. Transverse (Axial) CT Scan

4.17   **Structure and innervation of intervertebral discs and zygapophysial joints** *(continued)*

C. Transverse section. The nucleus pulposus has been removed, and the cartilaginous epiphyseal plate exposed. There are fewer rings of the anulus fibrosus posteriorly, and consequently, this portion of the annulus fibrosus is thinner. The ligamentum flavum, interspinous, and supraspinous ligaments are continuous. **D.** CT image of L4/L5 intervertebral disc.

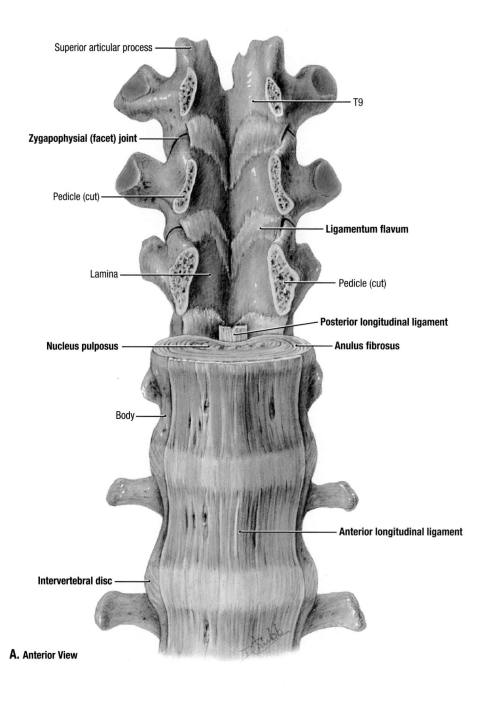

Superior articular process

T9

Zygapophysial (facet) joint

Pedicle (cut)

Ligamentum flavum

Lamina

Pedicle (cut)

Posterior longitudinal ligament

Nucleus pulposus

Anulus fibrosus

Body

Anterior longitudinal ligament

Intervertebral disc

A. Anterior View

4.18   Intervertebral discs: ligaments and movements

A. Anterior longitudinal ligament and ligamenta flava. The pedicles of T9 to T11 were sawed through, and the posterior aspect of the bodies is shown in **B.**

B. Posterior longitudinal ligament. **C.** Intervertebral disc during loading and movement.

- The anterior and posterior longitudinal ligaments are ligaments of the vertebral bodies; the ligamenta flava are ligaments of the vertebral arches.
- The anterior longitudinal ligament consists of broad, strong, fibrous bands that are attached to the intervertebral discs and vertebral bodies anteriorly and are perforated by the foramina for arteries and veins passing to and from the vertebral bodies.
- The ligamenta flava, composed of elastic fibers, extend between adjacent laminae; right and left ligaments converge in the median plane. They extend laterally to the articular processes, where they blend with the joint capsule of the zygapophysial joint.

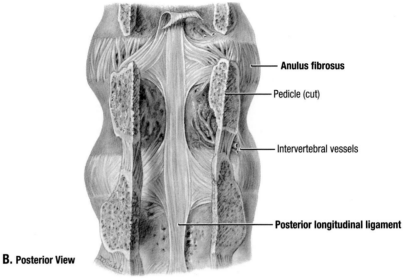

Anulus fibrosus

Pedicle (cut)

Intervertebral vessels

Posterior longitudinal ligament

B. Posterior View

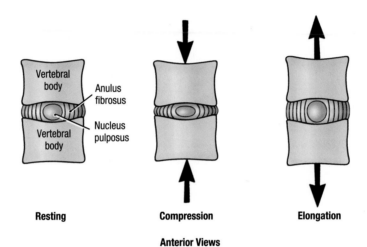

Vertebral body

Anulus fibrosus

Nucleus pulposus

Vertebral body

Resting   **Compression**   **Elongation**

Anterior Views

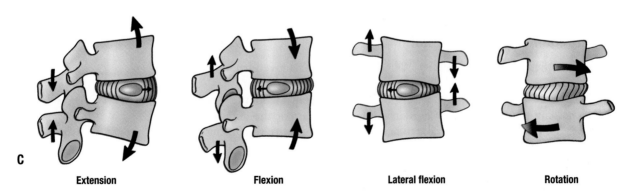

C

Extension   **Flexion**   **Lateral flexion**   **Rotation**

Lateral Views   **Anterior Views**

4.18   **Intervertebral discs: ligaments and movements *(continued)***

- The posterior longitudinal ligament is a narrow band passing from disc to disc, spanning the posterior surfaces of the vertebral bodies (in **B**). The ligament is diamond shaped posterior to each intervertebral disc, where it exchanges fibers with the anulus fibrosus; the ligament extends to the sacrum inferiorly and becomes the tectorial membrane cranially.
- The movement or loading of the intervertebral disc changes its shape and the position of the nucleus pulposus. Flexion and extension movements cause compression and elongation simultaneously.

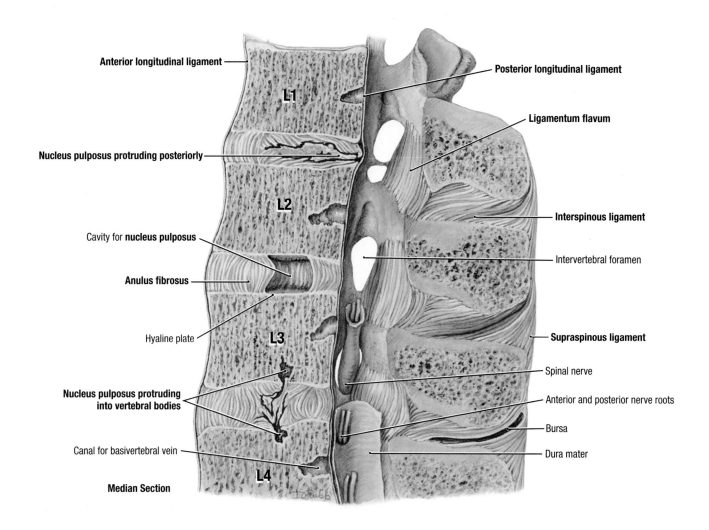

Anterior longitudinal ligament

L1

Nucleus pulposus protruding posteriorly

L2

Cavity for **nucleus pulposus**

Anulus fibrosus

Hyaline plate

L3

Nucleus pulposus protruding into vertebral bodies

Canal for basivertebral vein

L4

Median Section

Posterior longitudinal ligament

Ligamentum flavum

Interspinous ligament

Intervertebral foramen

Supraspinous ligament

Spinal nerve

Anterior and posterior nerve roots

Bursa

Dura mater

4.19 Lumbar region of vertebral column

The nucleus pulposus of the normal disc between L2 and L3 has been removed from the enclosing anulus fibrosus.

- The ligamentum flavum extends from the superior border and adjacent part of the posterior aspect of one lamina to the inferior border and adjacent part of the anterior aspect of the lamina above and extends laterally to become continuous with the fibrous capsule of the zygapophysial joint.
- The obliquely placed interspinous ligament unites the superior and inferior borders of two adjacent spines.
- The bursa between L3 and L4 spines is presumably the result of habitual hyperextension, which brings the lumbar spines into contact.

The nucleus pulposus of the disc between L1 and L2 has herniated posteriorly through the anulus. Herniation or protrusion of the gelatinous nucleus pulposus into or through the anulus fibrosus is a well-recognized cause of low back and lower limb pain. If degeneration of the posterior longitudinal ligament and wearing of the anulus fibrosus has occurred, the nucleus pulposus may herniate into the vertebral canal and compress the spinal cord or nerve roots of spinal nerves in the cauda equina. Herniations usually occur posterolaterally, where the anulus is relatively thin and does not receive support from the posterior or anterior longitudinal ligaments.

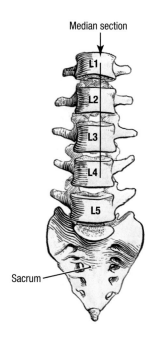

Median section

L1

L2

L3

L4

L5

Sacrum

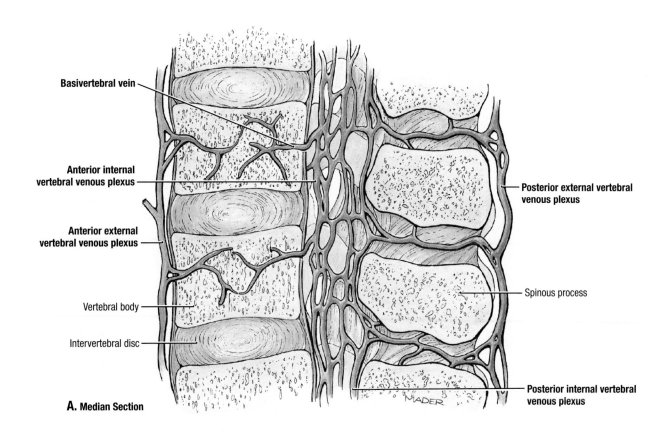

Basivertebral vein

Anterior internal
vertebral venous plexus

Anterior external
vertebral venous plexus

Vertebral body

Intervertebral disc

Posterior external vertebral
venous plexus

Spinous process

Posterior internal vertebral
venous plexus

A. Median Section

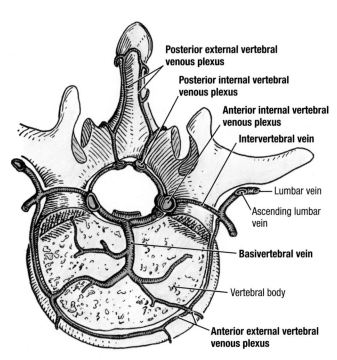

Posterior external vertebral
venous plexus

Posterior internal vertebral
venous plexus

Anterior internal vertebral
venous plexus

Intervertebral vein

Lumbar vein

Ascending lumbar
vein

Basivertebral vein

Vertebral body

Anterior external vertebral
venous plexus

B. Superior View

4.20   Vertebral venous plexuses

A. Median section of lumbar spine. **B.** Superior view of lumbar vertebra with the vertebral body sectioned transversely.

- There are internal and external vertebral venous plexuses, communicating with each other and with both systemic veins and the portal system. Infection and tumors can spread from the areas drained by the systemic and portal veins to the vertebral venous system and lodge in the vertebrae, spinal cord, brain, or skull.

- The internal vertebral venous plexus, located in the vertebral canal, consists of a plexus of thin-walled, valveless veins that surround the dura mater. Cranially, the internal venous plexus communicates through the foramen magnum with the occipital and basilar sinuses; at each spinal segment, the plexus receives veins from the spinal cord and a basivertebral vein from the vertebral body. The plexus is drained by intervertebral veins that pass through the intervertebral and sacral foramina to the vertebral, intercostal, lumbar, and lateral sacral veins.

- The anterior external vertebral venous plexus is formed by veins that course through the body of each vertebra. Veins that pass through the ligamenta flava form the posterior external vertebral venous plexus. In the cervical region, these plexuses communicate with the occipital and deep cervical veins. In the thoracic, lumbar, and pelvic regions, the azygos (or hemiazygos), ascending lumbar, and lateral sacral veins, respectively, further link segment to segment.

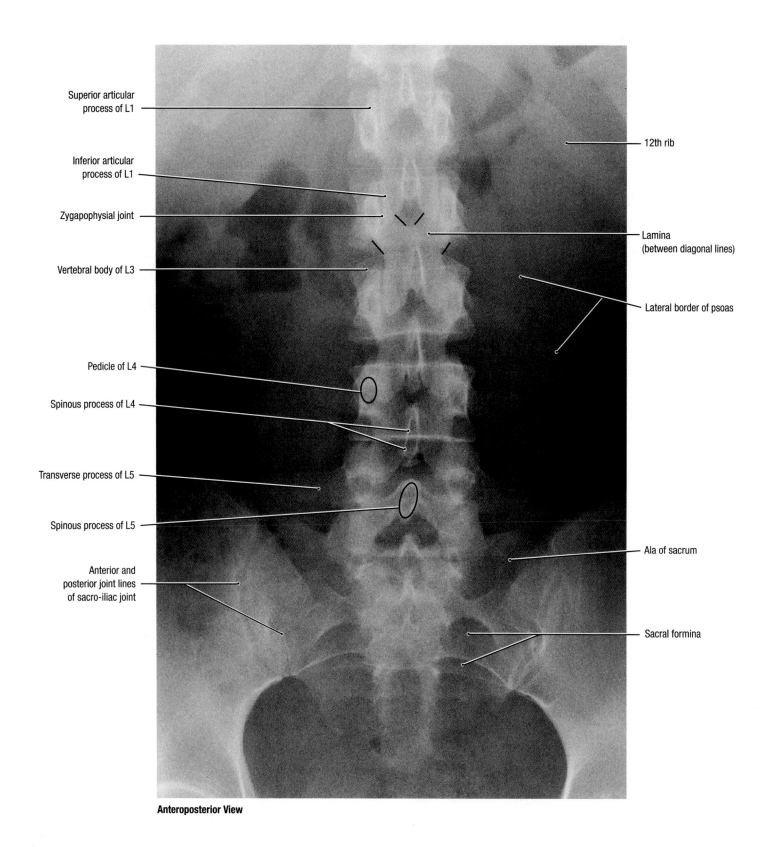

Superior articular process of L1

Inferior articular process of L1

Zygapophysial joint

Vertebral body of L3

Pedicle of L4

Spinous process of L4

Transverse process of L5

Spinous process of L5

Anterior and posterior joint lines of sacro-iliac joint

12th rib

Lamina (between diagonal lines)

Lateral border of psoas

Ala of sacrum

Sacral formina

Anteroposterior View

4.21   Radiograph of inferior thoracic and lumbosacral spine

Note the bodies and processes of the five lumbar vertebrae, the labeled spinous and transverse processes of L5, the sinuous sacro-iliac joint, the lateral margin of the right and left psoas muscles, and the 12th rib.

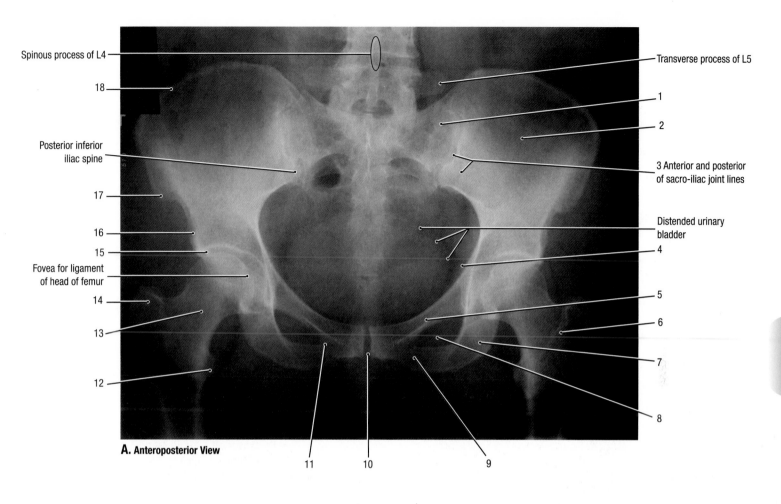

Spinous process of L4

Transverse process of L5

18

1

2

Posterior inferior iliac spine

3 Anterior and posterior of sacro-iliac joint lines

17

Distended urinary bladder

16

4

15

Fovea for ligament of head of femur

5

14

6

13

7

12

8

A. Anteroposterior View

11   10   9

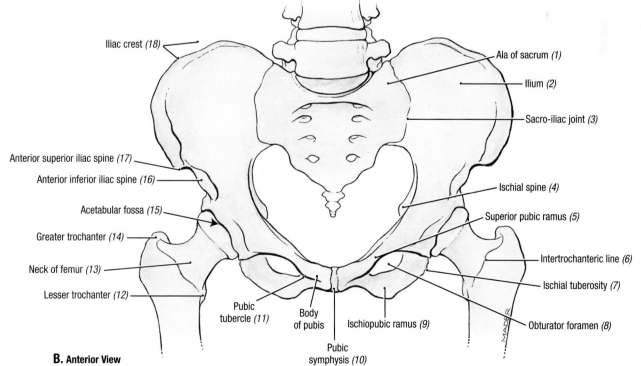

Iliac crest (18)

Ala of sacrum (1)

Ilium (2)

Sacro-iliac joint (3)

Anterior superior iliac spine (17)

Anterior inferior iliac spine (16)

Ischial spine (4)

Acetabular fossa (15)

Superior pubic ramus (5)

Greater trochanter (14)

Intertrochanteric line (6)

Neck of femur (13)

Ischial tuberosity (7)

Lesser trochanter (12)

Obturator foramen (8)

Pubic tubercle (11)

Body of pubis

Ischiopubic ramus (9)

Pubic symphysis (10)

B. Anterior View

4.22   **Pelvis**

A. Radiograph of pelvis. **B.** Bony pelvis with articulated femora.

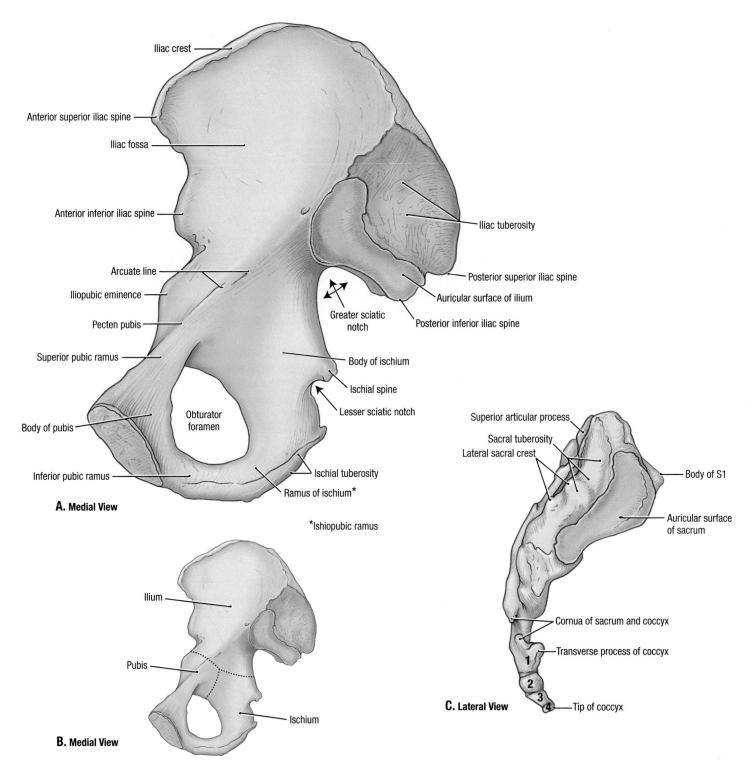

Iliac crest

Anterior superior iliac spine

Iliac fossa

Anterior inferior iliac spine

Arcuate line

Iliopubic eminence

Pecten pubis

Superior pubic ramus

Body of pubis

Obturator foramen

Inferior pubic ramus

A. Medial View

Iliac tuberosity

Posterior superior iliac spine

Auricular surface of ilium

Posterior inferior iliac spine

Greater sciatic notch

Body of ischium

Ischial spine

Lesser sciatic notch

Ischial tuberosity

Ramus of ischium*

*Ishiopubic ramus

Ilium

Pubis

Ischium

B. Medial View

Superior articular process

Sacral tuberosity

Lateral sacral crest

Body of S1

Auricular surface of sacrum

Cornua of sacrum and coccyx

Transverse process of coccyx

1

2

3

4   Tip of coccyx

C. Lateral View

4.23   Hip bone, sacrum, and coccyx

A. Features of hip bone. **B.** Ilium, ischium, and pubis. **C.** Sacrum and coccyx.

- Each hip bone consists of three bones: ilium, ischium, and pubis. The ilium is the superior, larger part of the hip bone, forming the superior part of the acetabulum, the deep socket on the lateral aspect of the hip bone that articulates with the head of the femur. The ischium forms the posteroinferior part of the acetabulum and hip bone. The pubis forms the anterior part of the acetabulum and anteromedial part of the hip bone.
- Anterosuperiorly, the auricular, ear-shaped surface of the sacrum articulates with the auricular surface of the ilium; the sacral and iliac tuberosities are for the attachment of the posterior sacro-iliac and interosseous sacro-iliac ligaments.

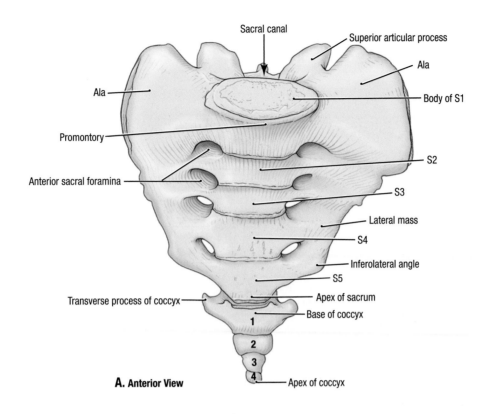

A. Anterior View

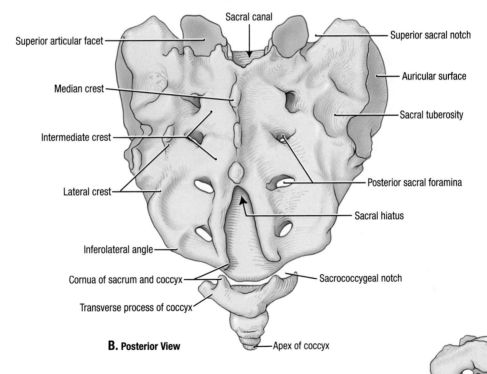

B. Posterior View

C. Anterior View

4.24   Sacrum and coccyx

A. Pelvic (anterior) surface. **B.** Dorsal (posterior surface). **C.** Sacrum in youth.

- In **A** the five sacral bodies are demarcated in the mature sacrum by four transverse lines ending laterally in four pairs of anterior sacral foramina. The coccyx has four pieces—the first having a pair of transverse processes and a pair of cornua (horns).
- The costal (lateral) elements begin to fuse around puberty. The bodies begin to fuse from inferior to superior at about the 17th to 18th year, with fusion usually completed by the 23rd year.

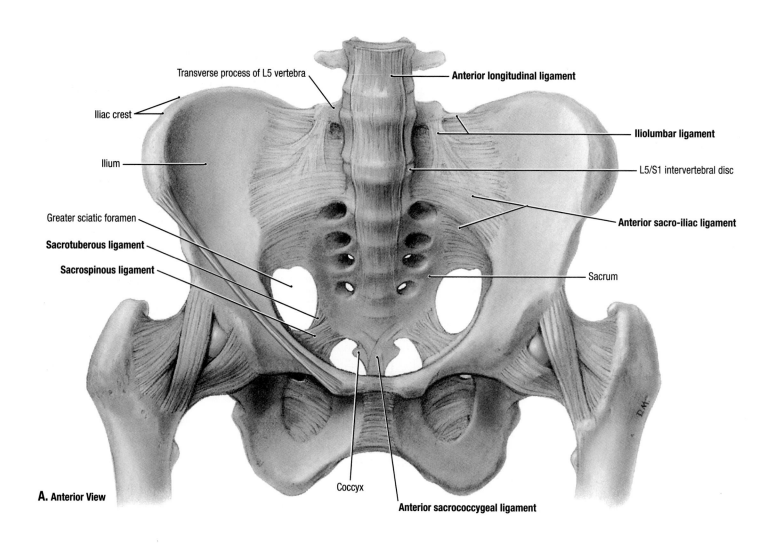

Transverse process of L5 vertebra

Iliac crest

Ilium

Greater sciatic foramen

Sacrotuberous ligament

Sacrospinous ligament

Anterior longitudinal ligament

Iliolumbar ligament

L5/S1 intervertebral disc

Anterior sacro-iliac ligament

Sacrum

Coccyx

Anterior sacrococcygeal ligament

A. Anterior View

4.25   Lumbar and pelvic ligaments

- The anterior sacro-iliac ligament is part of the fibrous capsule anteriorly and spans between the lateral aspect of the sacrum and the ilium, anterior to the auricular surfaces.

During pregnancy, the pelvic joint and ligaments relax, and pelvic movements increase. The sacro-iliac interlocking mechanism is less effective because the relaxation permits greater rotation of the pelvis and contributes to the lordotic posture often assumed during pregnancy with the change in the center of gravity. Relaxation of the sacro-iliac joints and pubic symphysis permits as much as 10–15% increase in diameters (mostly transverse), facilitating passage of the fetus through the pelvic canal. The coccyx is also allowed to move posteriorly.

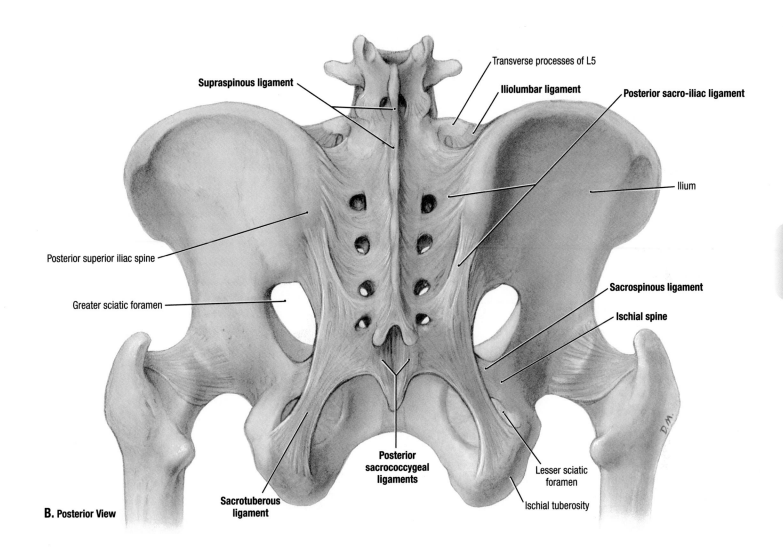

Transverse processes of L5

Supraspinous ligament

Iliolumbar ligament

Posterior sacro-iliac ligament

Ilium

Posterior superior iliac spine

Sacrospinous ligament

Greater sciatic foramen

Ischial spine

Posterior sacrococcygeal ligaments

Lesser sciatic foramen

Ischial tuberosity

Sacrotuberous ligament

B. Posterior View

`4.25`   **Lumbar and pelvic ligaments (continued)**

- The sacrotuberous ligaments attach the sacrum, ilium, and coccyx to the ischial tuberosity; the sacrospinous ligaments unite the sacrum and coccyx to the ischial spine. The sacrotuberous and sacrospinous ligaments convert the sciatic notches of the hip bones into greater and lesser sciatic foramina.
- The fibers of the posterior sacro-iliac ligament vary in obliquity; the superior fibers are shorter and lie between the ilium and superior part of the sacrum; the longer, obliquely oriented inferior fibers span between the posterior superior iliac spine and the inferior part of the sacrum, also blending with the sacrotuberous ligament.
- The interosseous sacro-iliac ligament lies deep to the posterior sacro-iliac ligament (see Fig. 4.26).
- The iliolumbar ligaments unite the ilia and transverse processes of L5; the lumbosacral portions of the ligaments descend to the alae of the sacrum and blend with the anterior sacro-iliac ligaments.

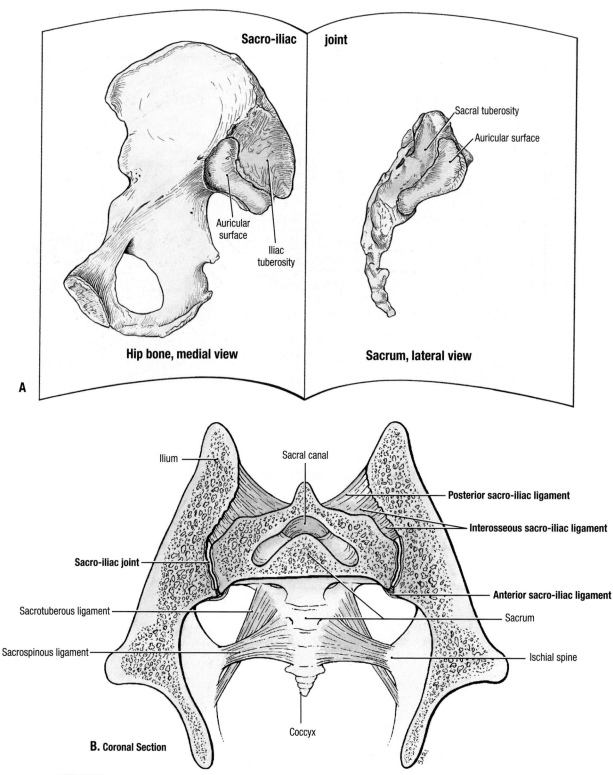

Sacro-iliac   joint

Sacral tuberosity

Auricular surface

Auricular surface

Iliac tuberosity

Hip bone, medial view

Sacrum, lateral view

A

Ilium

Sacral canal

Posterior sacro-iliac ligament

Interosseous sacro-iliac ligament

Sacro-iliac joint

Anterior sacro-iliac ligament

Sacrotuberous ligament

Sacrospinous ligament

Sacrum

Ischial spine

Coccyx

B. Coronal Section

4.26   Articular surfaces of sacro-iliac joint and ligaments

A. Articular surfaces. Note the auricular surface (articular area, *blue*) of the sacrum and hip bone and the roughened areas superior and posterior to the auricular areas *(orange)* for the attachment of the interosseous sacro-iliac ligament. **B.** Sacro-iliac ligaments. Note the sacro-iliac joints and the strong interosseous sacro-iliac ligament that lies inferior and anterior to the posterior sacro-iliac ligament. The interosseous sacro-iliac ligament consists of short fibers connecting the sacral tuberosity to the iliac tuberosity. The sacrum is suspended from the ilia by the sacro-iliac ligaments.

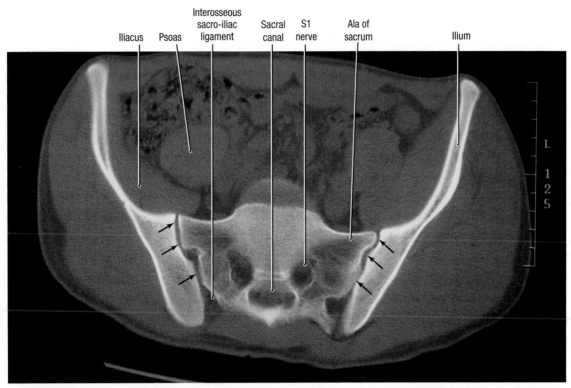

A. Transverse (axial) CT Scan

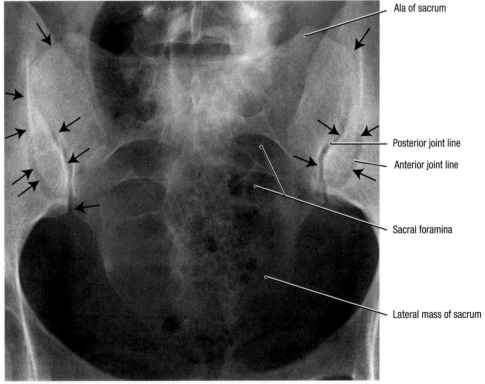

B. Anteroposterior View

4.27   **Imaging of the sacro-iliac joint**

A. CT scan. The sacro-iliac joint is indicated by *arrows*. Note that the articular surfaces of the ilium and sacrum have irregular shapes that result in partial interlocking of the bones. The sacro-iliac joint is oblique, with the anterior aspect of the joint situated lateral to the posterior aspect of the joint. **B.** Radiograph. Due to the oblique placement of the sacro-iliac joints, the anterior and posterior joint lines appear separately.

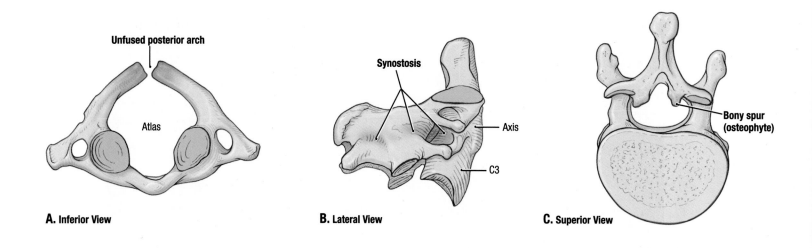

A. Inferior View

B. Lateral View

C. Superior View

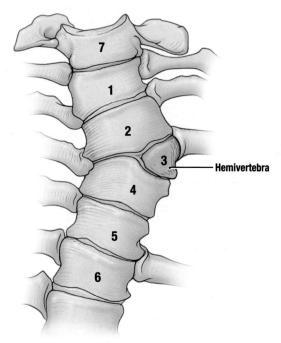

D. Anterior View

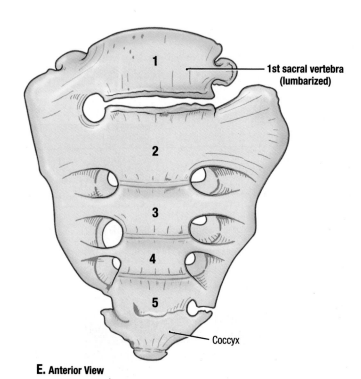

E. Anterior View

4.28 **Anomalies of the vertebrae**

A. Unfused posterior arch of the atlas. The centrum fused to the right and left halves of the neural arch, but the arch did not fuse in the midline posteriorly. **B.** Synostosis (fusion) of vertebrae C2 (axis) and C3. **C.** Bony spurs. Sharp bony spurs may grow from the laminae inferiorly into the ligamenta flava, thereby reducing the lengths of the functional portions of these ligaments. When the vertebral column is flexed, the ligaments may be torn. **D.** Hemivertebra. The entire right half of T3 and the corresponding rib are absent. The left lamina and the spine are fused with those of T4, and the left intervertebral foramen is reduced in size. Observe the associated scoliosis (lateral curvature of the spine). **E.** Transitional lumbosacral vertebra. Here, the 1st sacral vertebra is partly free (lumbarized). Not uncommonly, the 5th lumbar vertebra may be partly fused to the sacrum (sacralized).

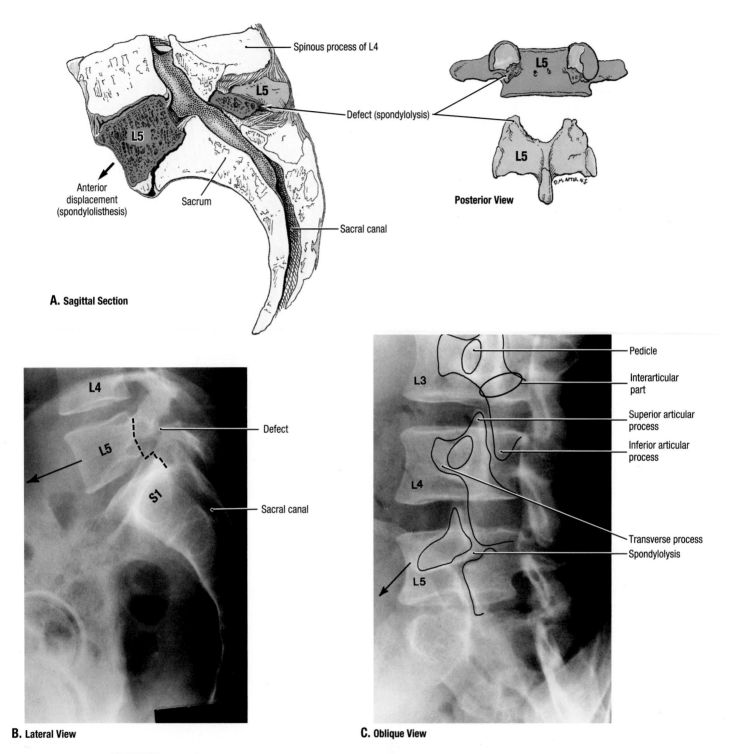

A. Sagittal Section

B. Lateral View

C. Oblique View

4.29 Spondylolysis and spondylolisthesis

A. Articulated and isolated spondylolytic L5 vertebra. The vertebra has an oblique defect (spondylolysis) through the interarticular part (pars interarticularis). The defect may be traumatic or congenital in origin. The interarticular part is the region of the lamina of a lumbar vertebra between the superior and inferior articular processes. Also, the vertebral body of L5 has slipped anteriorly (spondylolisthesis). **B** and **C.** Radiographs. In **B,** the *dotted line* following the posterior vertebral margins of L5 and the sacrum shows the anterior displacement of L5 *(arrow)*. In **C,** note the superimposed outline of a dog: the head is the transverse process, the eye is the pedicle, and the ear is the superior articular process. The lucent (dark) cleft across the "neck" of the dog is the spondylolysis; the anterior displacement *(arrow)* is the spondylolisthesis.

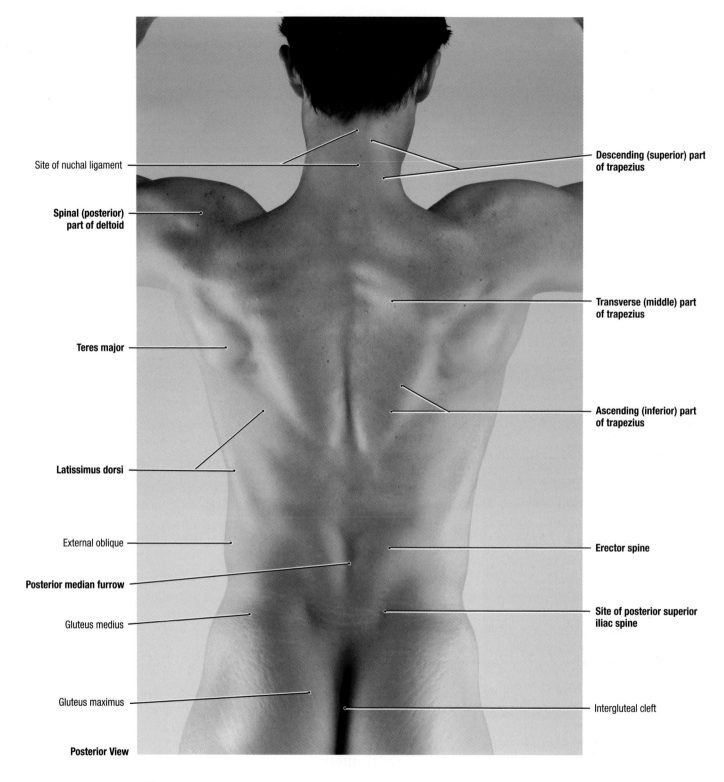

Site of nuchal ligament

Spinal (posterior) part of deltoid

Teres major

Latissimus dorsi

External oblique

Posterior median furrow

Gluteus medius

Gluteus maximus

Posterior View

Descending (superior) part of trapezius

Transverse (middle) part of trapezius

Ascending (inferior) part of trapezius

Erector spine

Site of posterior superior iliac spine

Intergluteal cleft

4.30   **Surface anatomy of back**

- The arms are abducted, so the scapulae have rotated superiorly on the thoracic wall.
- The latissimus dorsi and teres major muscles form the posterior axillary fold.
- The trapezius muscle has three parts: descending, transverse, and ascending.
- Note the deep median furrow that separates the longitudinal bulges formed by the contracted erector spinae group of muscles;
- Dimples (depressions) indicate the site of the posterior superior iliac spines, which usually lie at the level of the sacro-iliac joint.

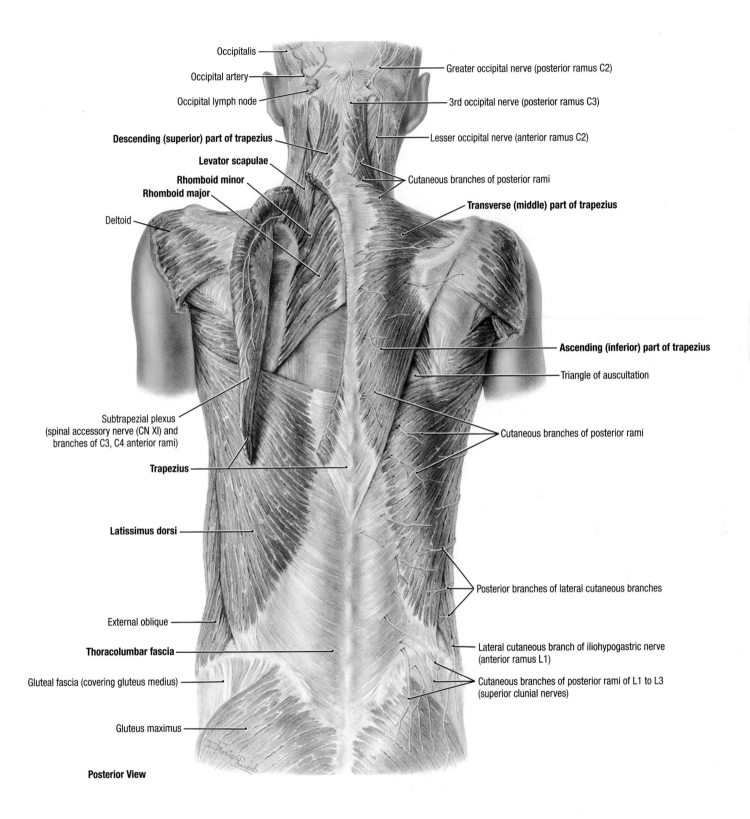

Occipitalis

Occipital artery

Occipital lymph node

Descending (superior) part of trapezius

Levator scapulae

Rhomboid minor

Rhomboid major

Deltoid

Subtrapezial plexus
(spinal accessory nerve (CN XI) and
branches of C3, C4 anterior rami)

Trapezius

Latissimus dorsi

External oblique

Thoracolumbar fascia

Gluteal fascia (covering gluteus medius)

Gluteus maximus

Posterior View

Greater occipital nerve (posterior ramus C2)

3rd occipital nerve (posterior ramus C3)

Lesser occipital nerve (anterior ramus C2)

Cutaneous branches of posterior rami

Transverse (middle) part of trapezius

Ascending (inferior) part of trapezius

Triangle of auscultation

Cutaneous branches of posterior rami

Posterior branches of lateral cutaneous branches

Lateral cutaneous branch of iliohypogastric nerve
(anterior ramus L1)

Cutaneous branches of posterior rami of L1 to L3
(superior clunial nerves)

4.31   **Superficial muscles of back**

On the *left*, the trapezius muscle is reflected. Observe two layers: the trapezius and latissimus dorsi muscles, and the levator scapulae and rhomboids minor and major. These axial
appendicular muscles help attach the upper limb to the trunk.

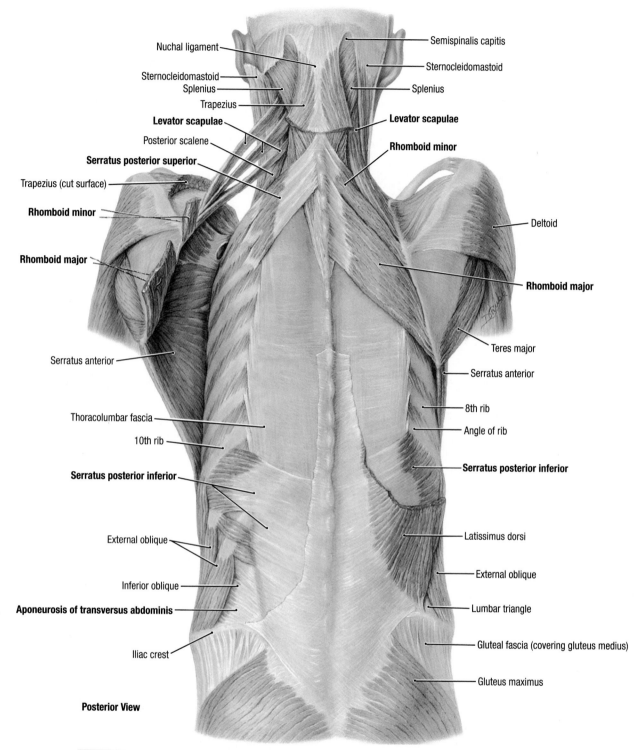

Nuchal ligament
Sternocleidomastoid
Splenius
Trapezius
Levator scapulae
Posterior scalene
Serratus posterior superior
Trapezius (cut surface)
Rhomboid minor
Rhomboid major
Serratus anterior
Thoracolumbar fascia
10th rib
Serratus posterior inferior
External oblique
Inferior oblique
Aponeurosis of transversus abdominis
Iliac crest
Posterior View

Semispinalis capitis
Sternocleidomastoid
Splenius
Levator scapulae
Rhomboid minor
Deltoid
Rhomboid major
Teres major
Serratus anterior
8th rib
Angle of rib
Serratus posterior inferior
Latissimus dorsi
External oblique
Lumbar triangle
Gluteal fascia (covering gluteus medius)
Gluteus maximus

4.32   Intermediate muscles of back

The trapezius and latissimus dorsi muscles are largely cut away on both sides. On the *left*, the rhomboid muscles have been severed, allowing the vertebral border of the scapula to be raised from the thoracic wall. The serratus posterior superior and inferior form the intermediate layer of muscles, passing from the vertebral spines to the ribs; the two muscles slope in opposite directions and are muscles of respiration. The thoracolumbar fascia extends laterally to the angles of the ribs, becoming thin superiorly and passing deep to the serratus posterior superior muscle. The fascia gives attachment to the latissimus dorsi and serratus posterior inferior muscles (see Fig. 4.34).

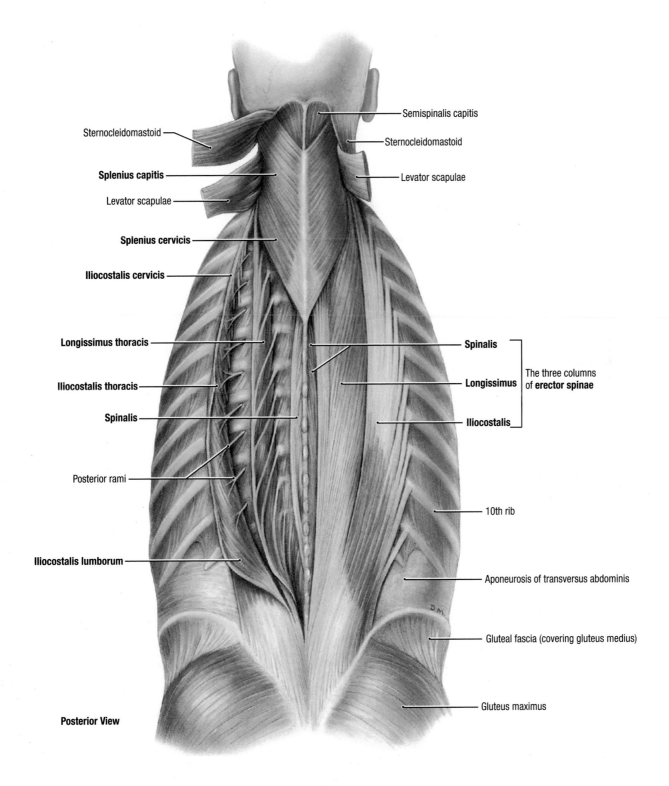

Semispinalis capitis

Sternocleidomastoid

Sternocleidomastoid

Splenius capitis

Levator scapulae

Levator scapulae

Splenius cervicis

Iliocostalis cervicis

Longissimus thoracis

Spinalis

Longissimus

The three columns of **erector spinae**

Iliocostalis thoracis

Spinalis

Iliocostalis

Posterior rami

10th rib

Iliocostalis lumborum

Aponeurosis of transversus abdominis

Gluteal fascia (covering gluteus medius)

Gluteus maximus

Posterior View

4.33   **Deep muscles of back: splenius and erector spinae**

On the *right* of the body, the erector spinae muscles are in situ, lying between the spinous processes medially and the angles of the ribs laterally. The erector spinae split into three longitudinal columns: iliocostalis laterally, longissimus in the middle, and spinalis medially. On the *left*, the longissimus muscle is pulled laterally to show the insertion into the transverse processes and ribs; not shown here are its extensions to the neck and head, longissimus cervicis and capitis.

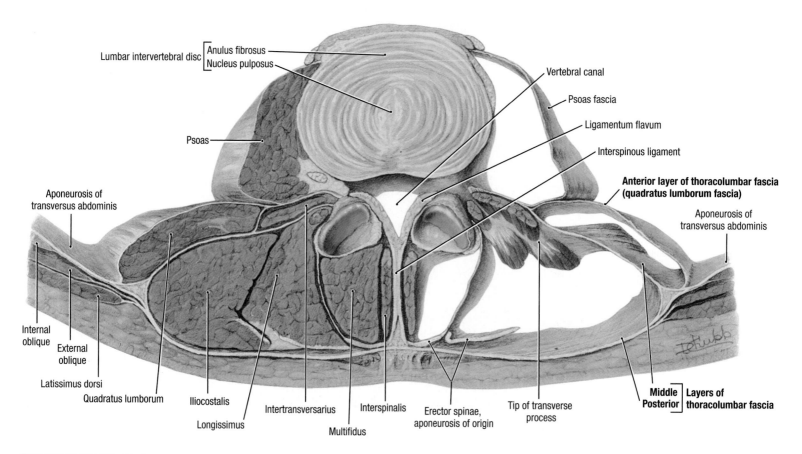

Lumbar intervertebral disc ⌈Anulus fibrosus
                          ⌊Nucleus pulposus

Psoas

Aponeurosis of
transversus abdominis

Internal
oblique

External
oblique

Latissimus dorsi

Quadratus lumborum

Iliocostalis

Longissimus

Intertransversarius

Multifidus

Interspinalis

Erector spinae,
aponeurosis of origin

Tip of transverse
process

Vertebral canal

Psoas fascia

Ligamentum flavum

Interspinous ligament

**Anterior layer of thoracolumbar fascia
(quadratus lumborum fascia)**

Aponeurosis of
transversus abdominis

Middle ⌉ Layers of
Posterior ⌋ thoracolumbar fascia

**Transverse Section (Dissected),
Superior View**

4.34   Transverse section of back muscles and thoracolumbar fascia

- On the *left*, the muscles are seen in their fascial sheaths or compartments; on the *right*, the muscles have been removed from their sheaths.
- The deep back muscles extend from the pelvis to the cranium and are enclosed in fascia. This fascia attaches medially to the nuchal ligament, the tips of the spinous processes, the supraspinous ligament, and the median crest of the sacrum. The lateral attachment of the fascia is to the cervical transverse processes, the angles of the ribs and to the aponeurosis of transversus abdominis. The thoracic and lumbar parts of the fascia are named thoracolumbar fascia.
- The aponeurosis of transversus abdominis and posterior aponeurosis of internal oblique muscles split into two strong sheets, the middle and posterior layers of the thoracolumbar

fascia. The anterior layer of thoracolumbar fascia is the deep fascia of the quadratus lumborum (quadratus lumborum fascia). The posterior layer of the thoracolumbar fascia provides proximal attachment for the latissimus dorsi muscle and, at a higher level, the serratus posterior inferior muscle.

Back strain is a common back problem that usually results from extreme movements of the vertebral column, such as extension or rotation. Back strain refers to some stretching or microscopic tearing of muscle fibers and/or ligaments of the back. The muscles usually involved are those producing movements of the lumbar IV joints.

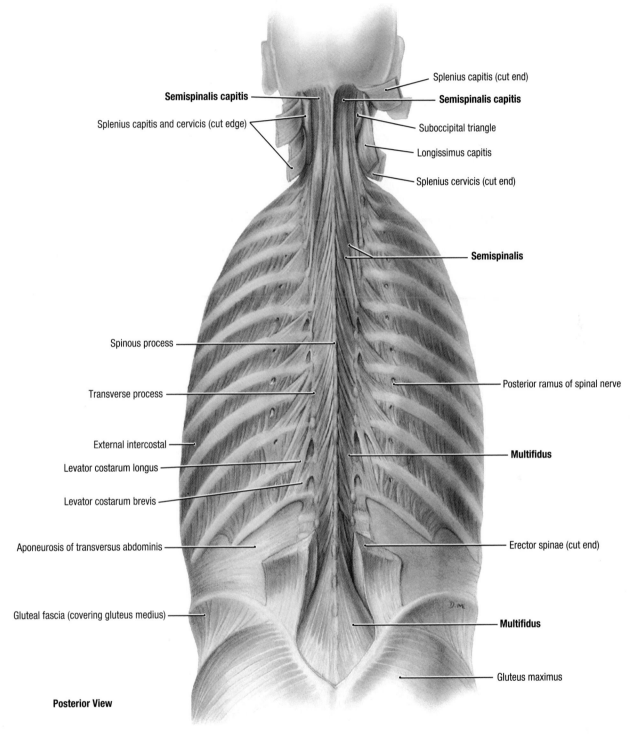

Semispinalis capitis

Splenius capitis and cervicis (cut edge)

Splenius capitis (cut end)

Semispinalis capitis

Suboccipital triangle

Longissimus capitis

Splenius cervicis (cut end)

Semispinalis

Spinous process

Transverse process

External intercostal

Levator costarum longus

Levator costarum brevis

Aponeurosis of transversus abdominis

Posterior ramus of spinal nerve

Multifidus

Erector spinae (cut end)

Gluteal fascia (covering gluteus medius)

Multifidus

Gluteus maximus

Posterior View

4.35 Deep muscles of back: semispinalis and multifidus

- The semispinalis, multifidus, and rotatores muscles constitute the transversospinalis group of deep muscles. In general, their bundles pass obliquely in a superomedial direction, from transverse processes to spinous processes in successively deeper layers. The bundles of semispinalis span approximately five interspaces, those of multifidus approximately three, and those of rotatores, one or two.
- The semispinalis (thoracis, cervicis, and capitis) muscles extend from the lower thoracic region to the skull; the semispinalis capitis, a powerful extensor muscle, originates from the lower cervical and upper thoracic vertebrae and inserts into the occipital bone between the superior and inferior nuchal lines.
- The multifidus muscle extends from the sacrum to the spine of the axis. In the lumbosacral region it emerges from the aponeurosis of the erector spinae, and extends from the sacrum, and mammillary processes of the lumbar vertebrae, to insert into spinous processes approximately three segments higher.

Posterior View

4.36   **Back: multifidus, quadratus lumborum, and thoracolumbar fascia**

Right: After removal of erector spinae at the L1 level, the middle layer of thoracolumbar fascia extends from the tip of each lumbar transverse process in a fan-shaped manner. A short lumbar rib is present at the level of L1. *Left:* After removal of the posterior and middle layers of thoracolumbar fascia, the lateral border of the quadratus lumborum muscle is oblique, and the medial border is in continuity with the intertransversarii.

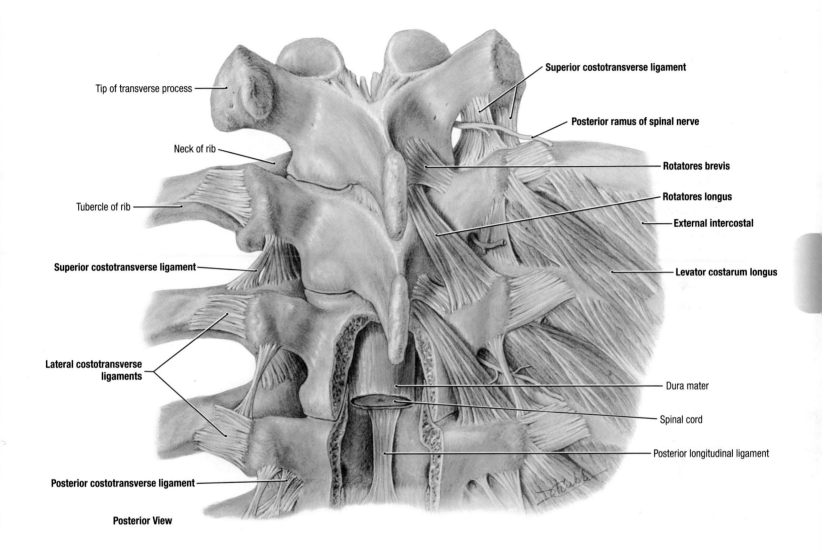

Tip of transverse process

Superior costotransverse ligament

Posterior ramus of spinal nerve

Neck of rib

Rotatores brevis

Tubercle of rib

Rotatores longus

External intercostal

Superior costotransverse ligament

Levator costarum longus

Lateral costotransverse ligaments

Dura mater

Spinal cord

Posterior longitudinal ligament

Posterior costotransverse ligament

Posterior View

4.37   Rotatores and costotransverse ligaments

- Of the three layers of transversospinalis, or oblique muscles of the back (semispinalis, multifidus, rotatores), the rotatores are the deepest and shortest. They pass from the root of one transverse process superomedially to the junction of the transverse process and lamina of the vertebra above. Rotatores longus span two vertebrae.
- The levatores costarum pass from the tip of one transverse process inferiorly to the rib below; some span two ribs.
- The superior costotransverse ligament splits laterally into two sheets, between which lie the levatores costarum and external intercostal muscles; the posterior ramus passes posterior to this ligament.
- The lateral costotransverse ligament is strong and joins the tubercle of the rib to the tip of the transverse process. It forms the posterior aspect of the joint capsule of the costotransverse joint.

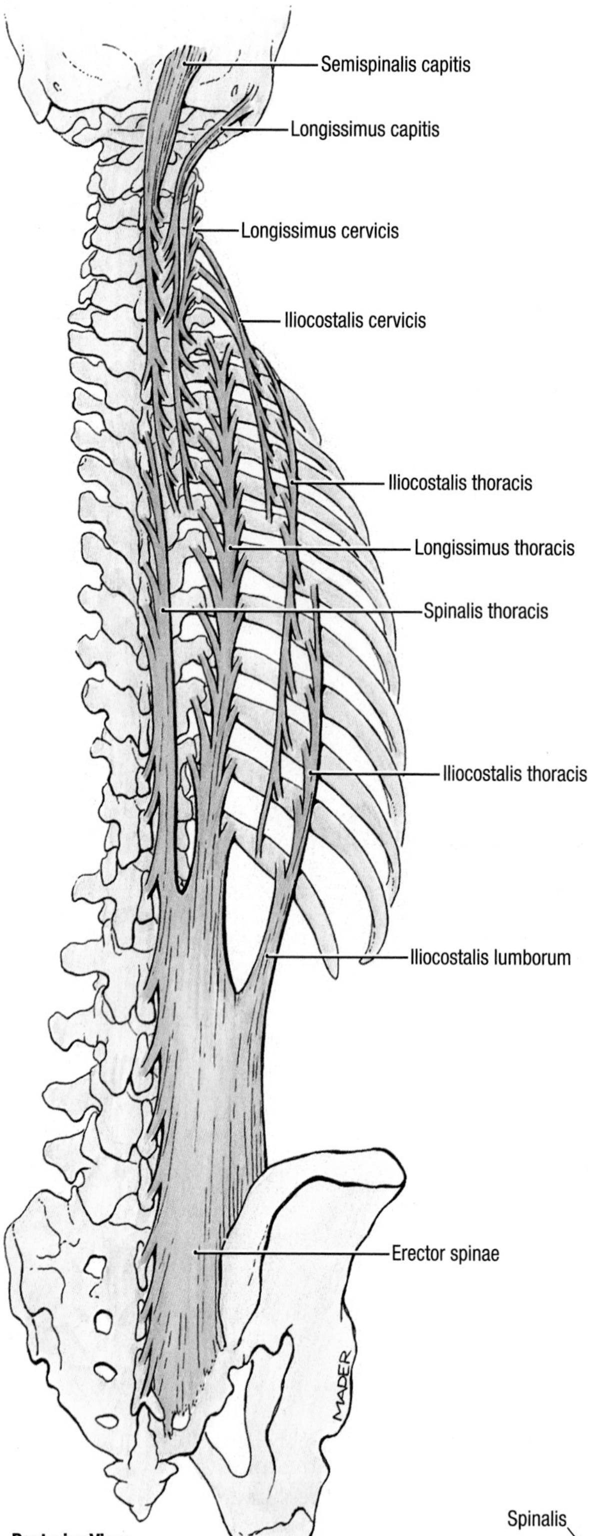

Semispinalis capitis

Longissimus capitis

Longissimus cervicis

Iliocostalis cervicis

Iliocostalis thoracis

Longissimus thoracis

Spinalis thoracis

Iliocostalis thoracis

Iliocostalis lumborum

Erector spinae

Posterior View

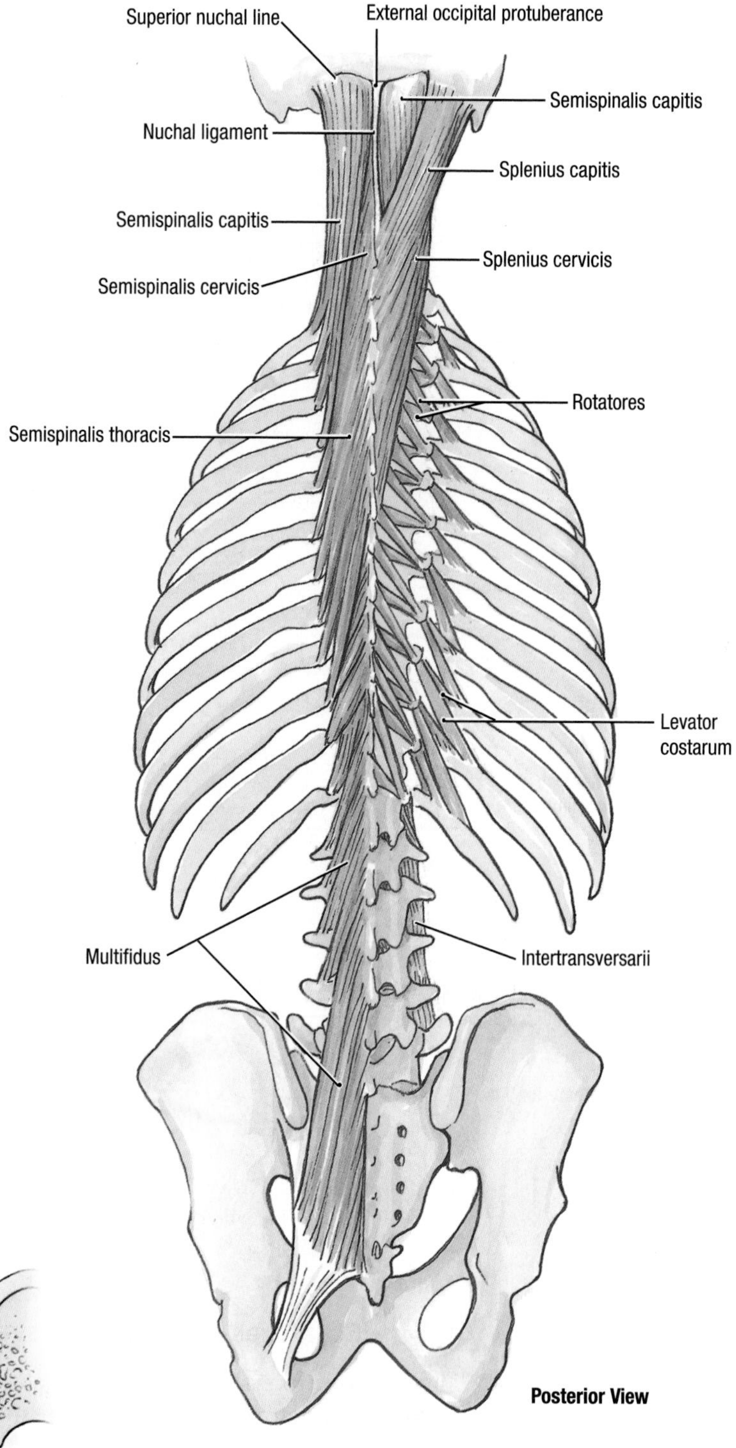

Superior nuchal line

External occipital protuberance

Nuchal ligament

Semispinalis capitis

Splenius capitis

Semispinalis capitis

Semispinalis cervicis

Splenius cervicis

Semispinalis thoracis

Rotatores

Levator costarum

Multifidus

Intertransversarii

Posterior View

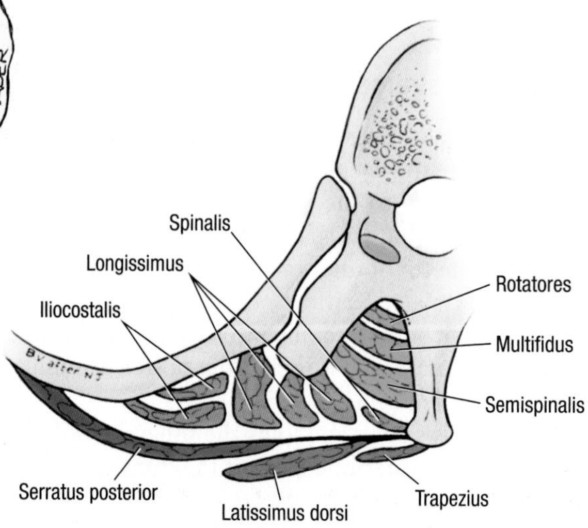

Spinalis

Longissimus

Iliocostalis

Rotatores

Multifidus

Semispinalis

Transverse Section, Superior View

Serratus posterior

Latissimus dorsi

Trapezius

■	Superficial extrinsic
■	Intermediate extrinsic
■	Erector spinae (intermediate intrinsic)
■	Transversospinal (deep intrinsic)

TABLE 4.4   INTRINSIC BACK MUSCLES[a]

MUSCLES	ORIGIN	INSERTION	NERVE SUPPLY[b]	MAIN ACTIONS
Superficial layer Splenius	Arises from nuchal ligament and spinous processes of C7–T3 or T4 vertebrae	*Splenius capitis:* fibers run superolaterally to mastoid process of temporal bone and lateral third of superior nuchal line of occipital bone *Splenius cervicis:* posterior tubercles of transverse processes of C1–C3 or C4 vertebrae	Posterior rami of spinal nerves	*Acting unilaterally:* laterally bend to side of active muscles; *Acting bilaterally:* extend head and neck
Intermediate layer Erector spinae	Arises by a broad tendon from posterior part of iliac crest, posterior surface of sacrum, sacral and inferior lumbar spinous processes, and supraspinous ligament	*Iliocostalis (lumborum, thoracis, and cervicis):* fibers run superiorly to angles of lower ribs and cervical transverse processes *Longissimus (thoracis, cervicis, and capitis):* fibers run superiorly to ribs between tubercles and angles to transverse processes in thoracic and cervical regions, and to mastoid process of temporal bone *Spinalis (thoracis, cervicis, and capitis):* fibers run superiorly to spinous processes in the upper thoracic region and to skull		*Acting unilaterally:* laterally bend vertebral column to side of active muscles; *Acting bilaterally:* extend vertebral column and head; as back is flexed, control movement by gradually lengthening their fibers
Deep layer Transversospinalis	*Semispinalis:* arises from thoracic and cervical transverse processes *Multifidus:* arises from sacrum and ilium, transverse processes of T1–L5, and articular processes of C4–C7 *Rotatores:* arise from transverse processes of vertebrae; best developed in thoracic region	*Semispinalis: thoracis, cervicis, and capitis;* fibers run superomedially and attach to occipital bone and spinous processes in thoracic and cervical regions, spanning four to six segments *Multifidus (lumborum, thoracis, and cervicis):* fibers pass superomedially to spinous processes, spanning two to four segments *Rotatores (thoracis and cervicis):* Pass superomedially and attach to junction of lamina and transverse process of vertebra of origin or into spinous process above their origin, spanning one to two segments		*Acting unilaterally:* rotate head and neck contralaterally; *Acting bilaterally:* extend head and thoracic cervical regions Stabilizes vertebrae during local movements of vertebral column Stabilize vertebrae and assist with local extension and rotary movements
Minor deep layer Interspinales	Superior surfaces of spinous processes of cervical and lumbar vertebrae	Inferior surfaces of spinous processes of vertebrae superior to vertebrae of origin	Posterior rami of spinal nerves	Aid in extension and rotation of vertebral column
Intertransversarii	Transverse processes of cervical and lumbar vertebrae	Transverse processes of adjacent vertebrae	Posterior and anterior rami of spinal nerves	Aid in lateral bending of vertebral column; *Acting bilaterally:* stabilize vertebral column
Levatores costarum	Tips of transverse processes of C7 and T1–T11 vertebrae	Pass inferolaterally and insert on rib between its tubercle and angle	Posterior rami of C8–T11 spinal nerves	Elevate ribs, assisting inspiration Assist with lateral bending of vertebral column

[a]See figures on opposite page.
[b]Most back muscles are innervated by dorsal rami of spinal nerves, but a few are innervated by anterior rami. Intertransversarii of cervical region are supplied by anterior rami.

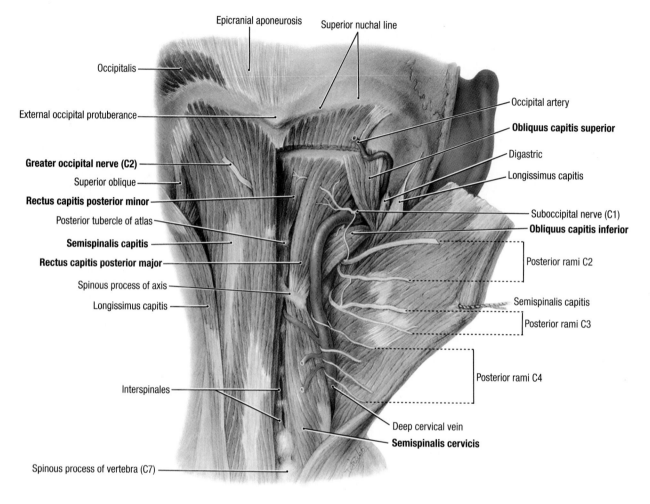

Epicranial aponeurosis

Superior nuchal line

Occipitalis

External occipital protuberance

Greater occipital nerve (C2)

Superior oblique

Rectus capitis posterior minor

Posterior tubercle of atlas

Semispinalis capitis

Rectus capitis posterior major

Spinous process of axis

Longissimus capitis

Interspinales

Spinous process of vertebra (C7)

Occipital artery

Obliquus capitis superior

Digastric

Longissimus capitis

Suboccipital nerve (C1)

Obliquus capitis inferior

Posterior rami C2

Semispinalis capitis

Posterior rami C3

Posterior rami C4

Deep cervical vein

Semispinalis cervicis

Posterior View

4.38 Suboccipital region—I

The trapezius, sternocleidomastoid, and splenius muscles are removed. The right semispinalis capitis muscle is cut and turned laterally.

- The semispinalis capitis, the great extensor muscle of the head and neck, forms the posterior wall of the suboccipital region. It is pierced by the greater occipital nerve (posterior ramus of C2) and has free medial and lateral borders at this level.
- The greater occipital nerve, when followed caudally, leads to the inferior border of the obliquus capitis inferior muscle, around which it turns. Following the inferior border of the obliquus capitis inferior muscle medially from the nerve leads to the spinous process of the axis; followed laterally, this leads to the transverse process of the atlas.
- Five muscles (all paired) are attached to the spinous process of the axis: obliquus capitis inferior, rectus capitis posterior major, semispinalis cervicis, multifidus, and interspinalis; the latter two are largely concealed by the semispinalis cervicis.

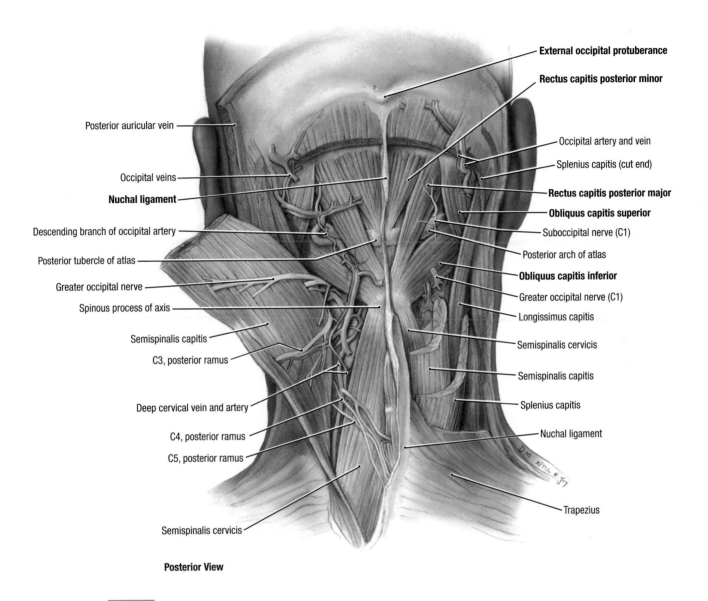

Posterior auricular vein

Occipital veins

Nuchal ligament

Descending branch of occipital artery

Posterior tubercle of atlas

Greater occipital nerve

Spinous process of axis

Semispinalis capitis

C3, posterior ramus

Deep cervical vein and artery

C4, posterior ramus

C5, posterior ramus

Semispinalis cervicis

External occipital protuberance

Rectus capitis posterior minor

Occipital artery and vein

Splenius capitis (cut end)

Rectus capitis posterior major

Obliquus capitis superior

Suboccipital nerve (C1)

Posterior arch of atlas

Obliquus capitis inferior

Greater occipital nerve (C1)

Longissimus capitis

Semispinalis cervicis

Semispinalis capitis

Splenius capitis

Nuchal ligament

Trapezius

Posterior View

4.39 **Suboccipital region—II**

The semispinalis capitis is reflected on the *left* and removed on the *right* side of the body.

- The suboccipital region contains four pairs of structures: two straight muscles, the rectus capitis posterior major and minor; two oblique muscles, the obliquus capitis superior and obliquus capitis inferior; two nerves (posterior rami), C1 suboccipital (motor) and C2 greater occipital (sensory); and two arteries, the occipital and vertebral.
- The nuchal ligament, which represents the cervical part of the supraspinous ligament, is a median, thin, fibrous partition attached to the spinous processes of cervical vertebrae and the external occipital crest; its posterior border gives origin to the trapezius muscle and extends superiorly to the external occipital protuberance.
- The suboccipital triangle is bounded by three muscles: obliquus capitis superior and inferior, and rectus capitis posterior major.
- The suboccipital nerve (posterior ramus of C1) supplies the three muscles bounding the suboccipital triangle and also the rectus capitis minor muscle and communicates with the greater occipital nerve.
- The occipital veins along with the suboccipital nerve (posterior ramus of C1) emerge through the suboccipital triangle to join the deep cervical vein.
- The posterior arch of the atlas forms the floor of the suboccipital triangle.

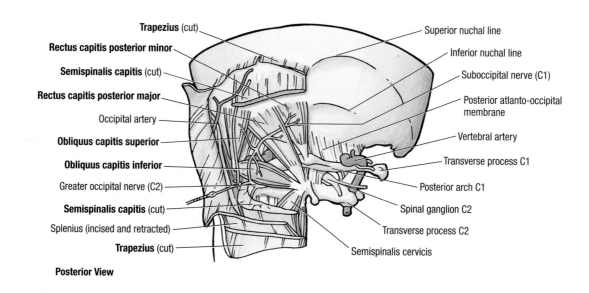

Posterior View

Lateral View

Anterior View

TABLE 4.5   MUSCLES OF THE ATLANTO-OCCIPITAL AND ATLANTOAXIAL JOINTS

MOVEMENTS OF ATLANTO-OCCIPITAL JOINTS

FLEXION	*EXTENSION*	*LATERAL BENDING*
Longus capitis Rectus capitis anterior Anterior fibers of sternocleidomastoid	Rectus capitis posterior major and minor Obliquus capitis superior Semispinalis capitis Splenius capitis Longissimus capitis Trapezius	Sternocleidomastoid Obliquus capitis superior and inferior Rectus capitis lateralis Splenius capitis

ROTATION OF ATLANTOAXIAL JOINTS[a]

IPSILATERAL[b]	*CONTRALATERAL*
Obliquus capitis inferior Rectus capitis posterior, major and minor Longissimus capitis Splenius capitis	Sternocleidomastoid Semispinalis capitis

[a]Rotation is the specialized movement at these joints. Movement of one joint involves the other.
[b]Same side to which head is rotated.

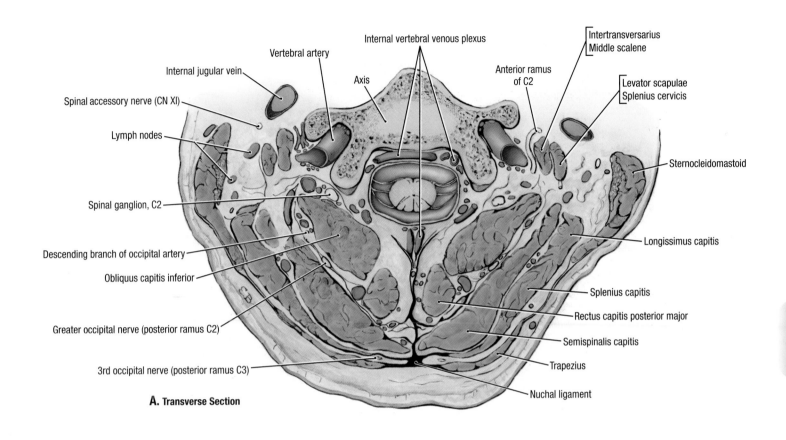

Internal vertebral venous plexus

Vertebral artery

Internal jugular vein

Spinal accessory nerve (CN XI)

Lymph nodes

Spinal ganglion, C2

Descending branch of occipital artery

Obliquus capitis inferior

Greater occipital nerve (posterior ramus C2)

3rd occipital nerve (posterior ramus C3)

Axis

Anterior ramus of C2

Intertransversarius
Middle scalene

Levator scapulae
Splenius cervicis

Sternocleidomastoid

Longissimus capitis

Splenius capitis

Rectus capitis posterior major

Semispinalis capitis

Trapezius

Nuchal ligament

A. Transverse Section

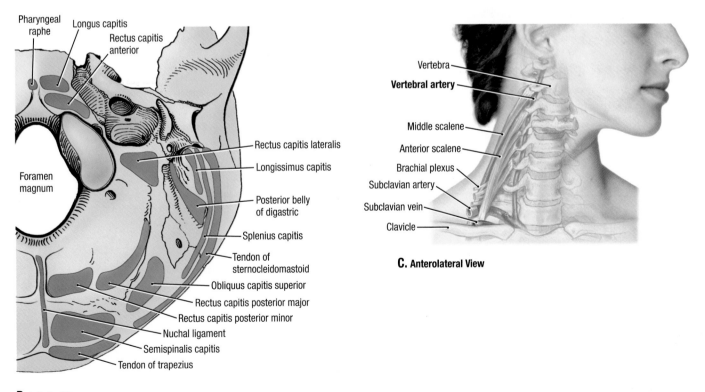

Pharyngeal raphe

Longus capitis

Rectus capitis anterior

Foramen magnum

Rectus capitis lateralis

Longissimus capitis

Posterior belly of digastric

Splenius capitis

Tendon of sternocleidomastoid

Obliquus capitis superior

Rectus capitis posterior major

Rectus capitis posterior minor

Nuchal ligament

Semispinalis capitis

Tendon of trapezius

B. Inferior View

Vertebra

Vertebral artery

Middle scalene

Anterior scalene

Brachial plexus

Subclavian artery

Subclavian vein

Clavicle

C. Anterolateral View

4.40   **Nuchal Region**

A. Transverse section at the level of the axis. **B.** Muscle attachments to inferior aspect of skull. **C.** Vertebral artery.

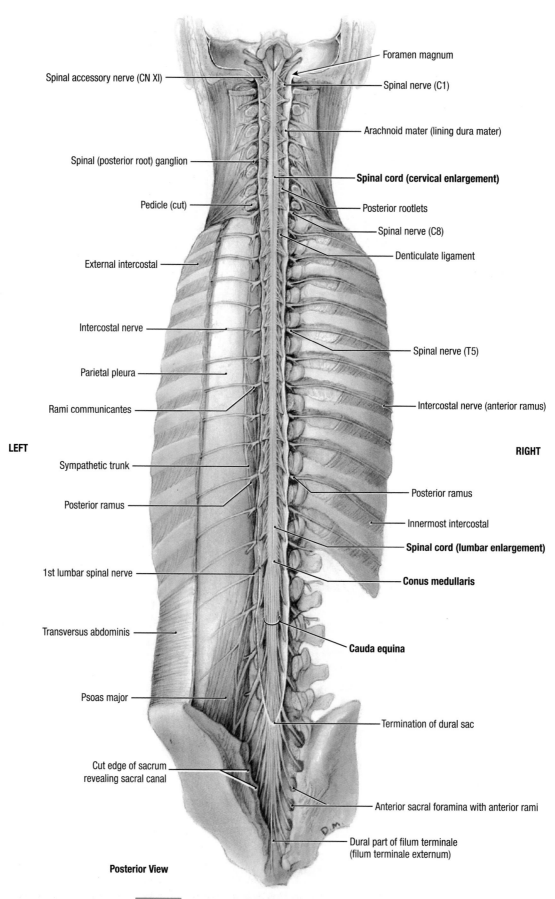

Spinal accessory nerve (CN XI)

Spinal (posterior root) ganglion

Pedicle (cut)

External intercostal

Intercostal nerve

Parietal pleura

Rami communicantes

LEFT

Sympathetic trunk

Posterior ramus

1st lumbar spinal nerve

Transversus abdominis

Psoas major

Cut edge of sacrum
revealing sacral canal

Posterior View

Foramen magnum

Spinal nerve (C1)

Arachnoid mater (lining dura mater)

Spinal cord (cervical enlargement)

Posterior rootlets

Spinal nerve (C8)

Denticulate ligament

Spinal nerve (T5)

Intercostal nerve (anterior ramus)

RIGHT

Posterior ramus

Innermost intercostal

Spinal cord (lumbar enlargement)

Conus medullaris

Cauda equina

Termination of dural sac

Anterior sacral foramina with anterior rami

Dural part of filum terminale
(filum terminale externum)

4.41   **Spinal cord in situ**

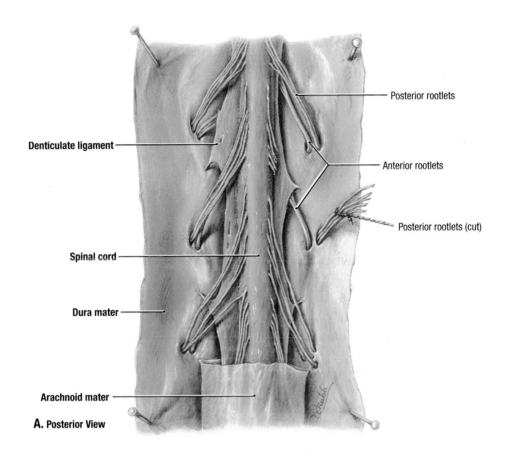

Posterior rootlets

Denticulate ligament

Anterior rootlets

Posterior rootlets (cut)

Spinal cord

Dura mater

Arachnoid mater

A. Posterior View

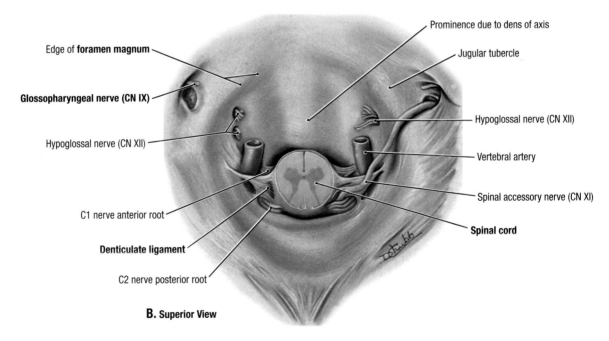

Prominence due to dens of axis

Edge of **foramen magnum**

Jugular tubercle

Glossopharyngeal nerve (CN IX)

Hypoglossal nerve (CN XII)

Hypoglossal nerve (CN XII)

Vertebral artery

Spinal accessory nerve (CN XI)

C1 nerve anterior root

Spinal cord

Denticulate ligament

C2 nerve posterior root

B. Superior View

4.42   Spinal cord and meninges

A. Dural sac cut open. The denticulate ligament anchors the cord to the dural sac between successive nerve roots by means of strong, toothlike processes. The anterior nerve roots lie anterior to the denticulate ligament, and the posterior nerve roots lie posterior to the ligament. **B.** Structures of vertebral canal seen through foramen magnum. The spinal cord, vertebral arteries, spinal accessory nerve (CN XI), and most superior part of the denticulate ligament pass through the foramen magnum within the meninges.

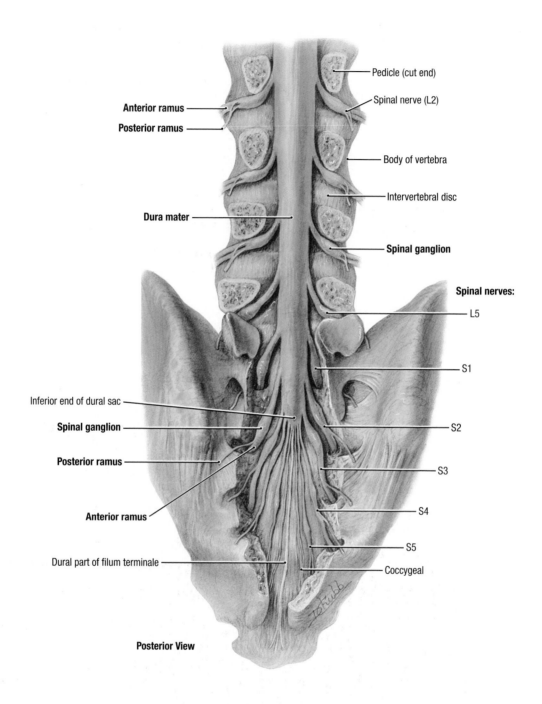

Anterior ramus

Posterior ramus

Dura mater

Inferior end of dural sac

Spinal ganglion

Posterior ramus

Anterior ramus

Dural part of filum terminale

Pedicle (cut end)

Spinal nerve (L2)

Body of vertebra

Intervertebral disc

Spinal ganglion

Spinal nerves:

L5

S1

S2

S3

S4

S5

Coccygeal

Posterior View

4.43   Inferior end of dural sac—I

The posterior parts of the lumbar vertebrae and sacrum were removed.

- The inferior limit of the dural sac is at the level of the posterior superior iliac spine (body of 2nd sacral vertebra); the dura continues as the dural part of the filum terminale (filum terminale externum).
- The lumbar spinal ganglia are in the intervertebral foramina, and the sacral spinal ganglia are somewhat asymmetrically placed within the sacral canal.
- The posterior rami are smaller than the anterior rami.

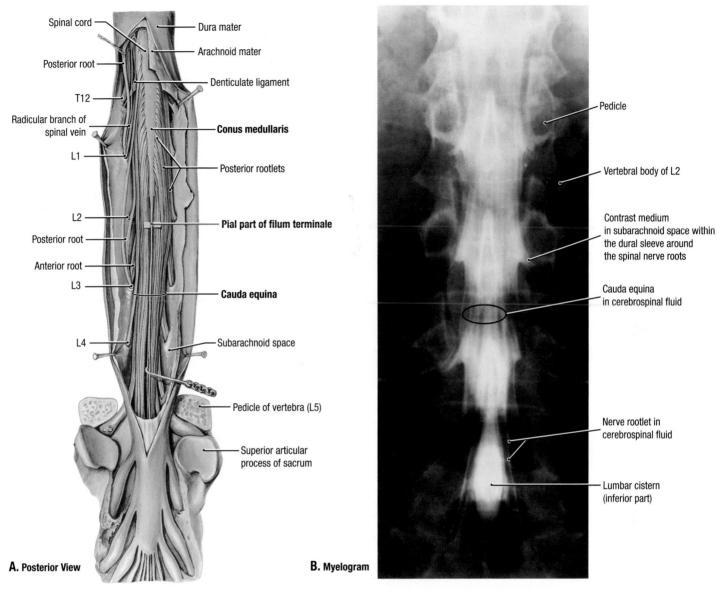

A. Posterior View   **B. Myelogram**

4.44   **Inferior end of dural sac—II**

A. Inferior dural sac and lumbar cistern of subarachnoid space, opened. **B.** Myelogram of the lumbar region of the vertebral column. Contrast medium was injected into the subarachnoid space. **C.** Termination of spinal cord, in situ, sagittal section.

- The conus medullaris, or conical lower end of the spinal cord, continues as a glistening thread, the plial part of the filum terminale (filum terminale internum), which descends with the posterior and anterior nerve roots; these constitute the cauda equina.
- In the adult, the spinal cord usually ends at the level of the disc between L1 and L2. Variations: 95% of cords end within the limits of the bodies of L1 and L2, whereas 3% end posterior to the inferior half of T12, and 2% posterior to L3.
- The subarachnoid space usually ends at the level of the disc between S1 and S2, but it can be more inferior.

To obtain a sample of CSF from the lumbar cistern, a lumbar puncture needle, fitted with a stylet, is inserted into the subarachnoid space. Flexion of the vertebral column facilitates insertion of the needle by stretching the ligamenta flava and spreading the laminae and spinous processes apart. The needle is inserted in the midline between the spinous processes of the L3 and L4 (or the L4 and L5) vertebrae. At these levels in adults, there is little danger of damaging the spinal cord.

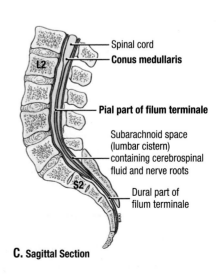

C. Sagittal Section

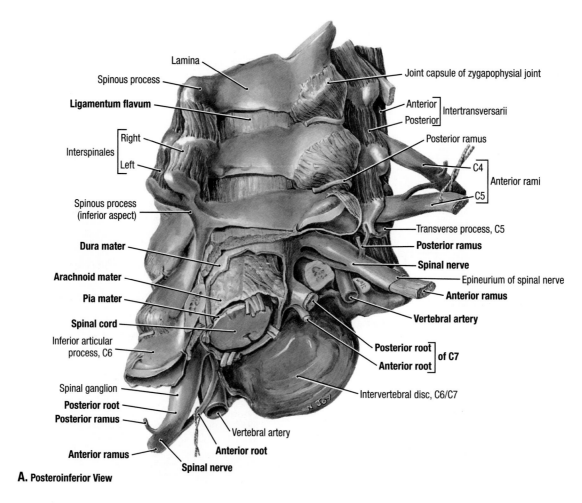

Lamina

Spinous process

Ligamentum flavum

Interspinales { Right / Left }

Spinous process
(inferior aspect)

Dura mater

Arachnoid mater

Pia mater

Spinal cord

Inferior articular
process, C6

Spinal ganglion

Posterior root
Posterior ramus

Anterior ramus

Spinal nerve

Joint capsule of zygapophysial joint

Anterior] Intertransversarii
Posterior]

Posterior ramus

C4] Anterior rami
C5]

Transverse process, C5

Posterior ramus

Spinal nerve

Epineurium of spinal nerve

Anterior ramus

Vertebral artery

Posterior root] of C7
Anterior root]

Intervertebral disc, C6/C7

Vertebral artery

Anterior root

A. Posteroinferior View

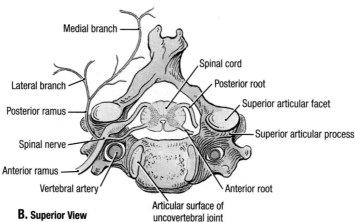

Medial branch

Spinal cord

Lateral branch

Posterior root

Posterior ramus

Superior articular facet

Spinal nerve

Superior articular process

Anterior ramus

Vertebral artery

Anterior root

Articular surface of
uncovertebral joint

B. Superior View

4.45   Lower cervical vertebrae and associated structures and nerves

A. Relationship of cervical spinal cord, spinal nerves, and coverings. The anterior and posterior roots, in a common or separate dural sleeve, unite beyond the spinal ganglion to form a spinal nerve that immediately divides into a small posterior and large anterior ramus. The roots pass anterior to the zygapophysial joints and unite as they exit the intervertebral foramina and pass posterior to the vertebral artery. The posterior ramus curves dorsally around the superior articular process, and the anterior ramus rests on the transverse process, which is grooved to support it. **B.** Transverse section of spinal cord in situ. Note the vulnerability of the vertebral artery, spinal cord, and nerve roots to arthritic expansion from articular processes and the vertebral body, particularly the lateral edge of the superior surface of the body, the uncovertebral joint (joint of Luschka).

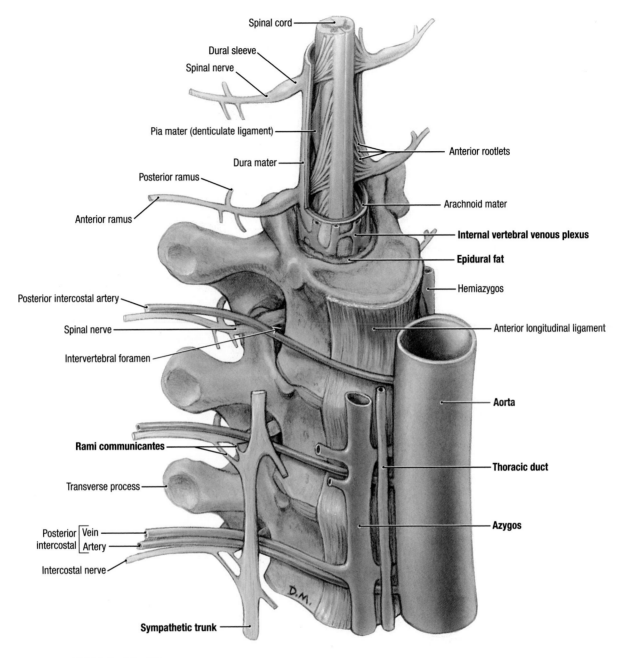

Spinal cord

Dural sleeve

Spinal nerve

Pia mater (denticulate ligament)

Dura mater

Posterior ramus

Anterior ramus

Posterior intercostal artery

Spinal nerve

Intervertebral foramen

Rami communicantes

Transverse process

Posterior intercostal { Vein / Artery }

Intercostal nerve

Sympathetic trunk

Anterior rootlets

Arachnoid mater

Internal vertebral venous plexus

Epidural fat

Hemiazygos

Anterior longitudinal ligament

Aorta

Thoracic duct

Azygos

D.M.

Right Anterolateral View

4.46   **Spinal cord and prevertebral structures**

The vertebrae have been removed superiorly to expose the spinal cord and meninges.
- The aorta descends to the left of the midline, with the thoracic duct and azygos vein to its right.
- Typically, the azygos vein is on the right side of the vertebral bodies, and the hemiazygous vein is on the left.
- The thoracic sympathetic trunk and ganglia lie lateral to the thoracic vertebrae; the rami communicantes connect the sympathetic ganglia with the spinal nerve.
- A sleeve of dura mater surrounds the spinal nerves and blends with the sheath (epineurium) of the spinal nerve.
- The dura mater is separated from the walls of the vertebral canal by epidural fat and the internal vertebral venous plexus.

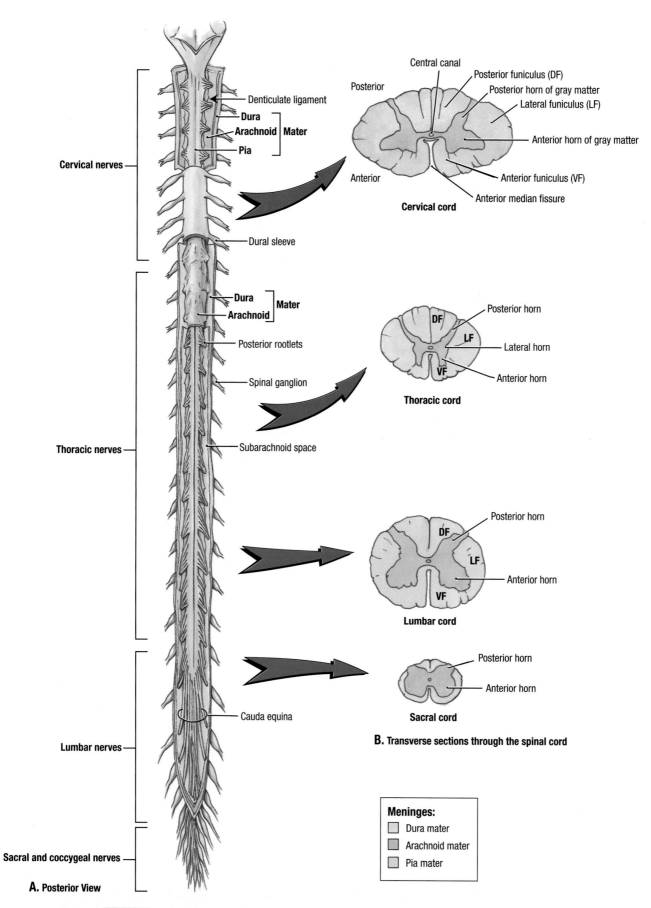

Denticulate ligament

Dura
Arachnoid } **Mater**
Pia

Cervical nerves

Dural sleeve

Dura
Arachnoid } **Mater**

Posterior rootlets

Spinal ganglion

Thoracic nerves

Subarachnoid space

Lumbar nerves

Cauda equina

Sacral and coccygeal nerves

A. Posterior View

Central canal
Posterior
Posterior funiculus (DF)
Posterior horn of gray matter
Lateral funiculus (LF)
Anterior horn of gray matter
Anterior
Anterior funiculus (VF)
Anterior median fissure
Cervical cord

Posterior horn
DF
LF
Lateral horn
VF
Anterior horn
Thoracic cord

Posterior horn
DF
LF
Anterior horn
VF
Lumbar cord

Posterior horn
Anterior horn
Sacral cord

B. Transverse sections through the spinal cord

Meninges:
☐ Dura mater
☐ Arachnoid mater
☐ Pia mater

4.47   **Isolated spinal cord and spinal nerve roots with coverings and regional sections**

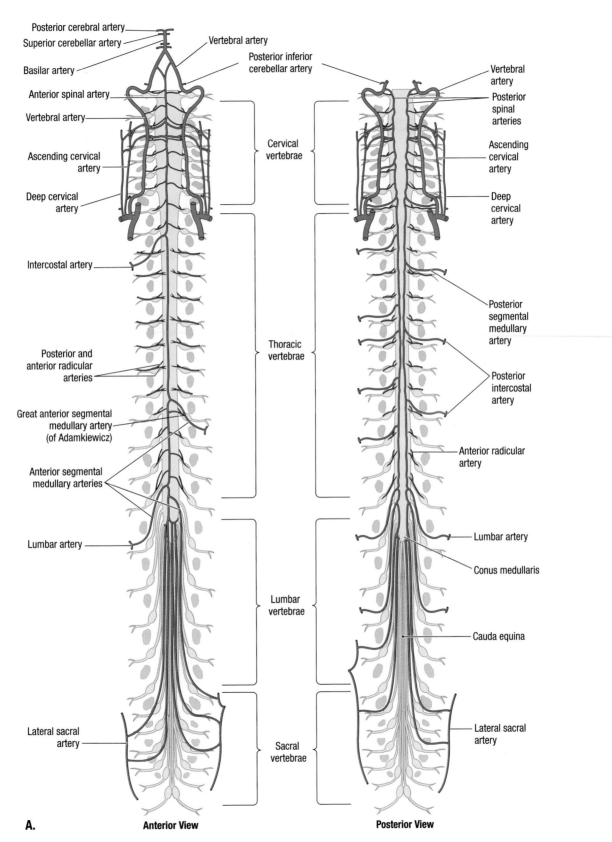

Posterior cerebral artery
Superior cerebellar artery
Basilar artery
Vertebral artery
Posterior inferior cerebellar artery
Anterior spinal artery
Vertebral artery
Ascending cervical artery
Deep cervical artery
Intercostal artery
Posterior and anterior radicular arteries
Great anterior segmental medullary artery (of Adamkiewicz)
Anterior segmental medullary arteries
Lumbar artery
Lateral sacral artery

Cervical vertebrae
Thoracic vertebrae
Lumbar vertebrae
Sacral vertebrae

Vertebral artery
Posterior spinal arteries
Ascending cervical artery
Deep cervical artery
Posterior segmental medullary artery
Posterior intercostal artery
Anterior radicular artery
Lumbar artery
Conus medullaris
Cauda equina
Lateral sacral artery

A.   **Anterior View**   **Posterior View**

4.48   **Blood supply of spinal cord**

A. Arteries of spinal cord. The segmental reinforcements of blood supply from the segmental medullary arteries are important in supplying blood to the anterior and posterior spinal arteries. Fractures, dislocations, and fracture-dislocations may interfere with the blood supply to the spinal cord from the spinal and medullary arteries. Deficiency of blood supply (ischemia) of the spinal cord affects its function and can lead to muscle weakness and paralysis. The spinal cord may also suffer circulatory impairment if the segmental medullary arteries, particularly the great anterior segmental medullary artery (of Adamkiewicz), are narrowed by obstructive arterial disease.

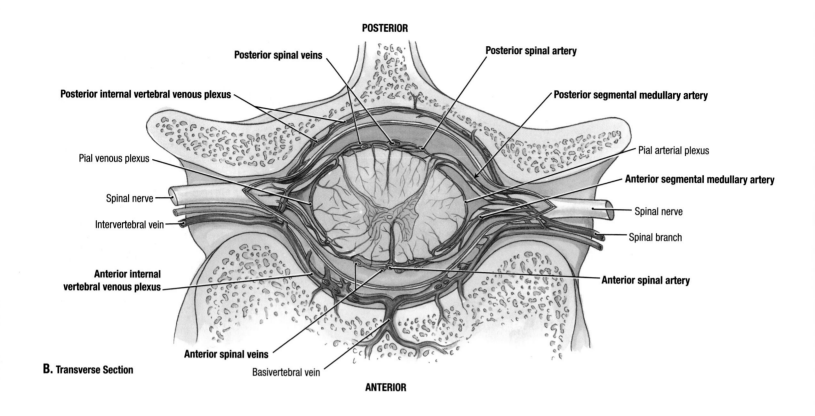

POSTERIOR

Posterior spinal veins

Posterior spinal artery

Posterior internal vertebral venous plexus

Posterior segmental medullary artery

Pial venous plexus

Pial arterial plexus

Spinal nerve

Anterior segmental medullary artery

Intervertebral vein

Spinal nerve

Spinal branch

Anterior internal vertebral venous plexus

Anterior spinal artery

Anterior spinal veins

Basivertebral vein

B. Transverse Section

ANTERIOR

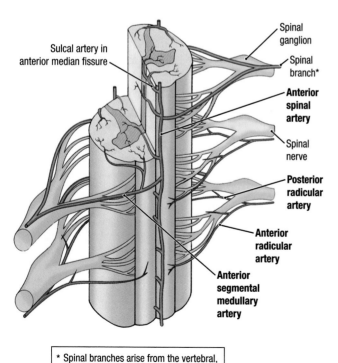

Sulcal artery in anterior median fissure

Spinal ganglion

Spinal branch*

Anterior spinal artery

Spinal nerve

Posterior radicular artery

Anterior radicular artery

Anterior segmental medullary artery

* Spinal branches arise from the vertebral, intercostal, lumbar, or sacral artery, depending on level of spinal cord.

C. Anterolateral View

| 4.48 | **Blood supply of spinal cord** *(continued)* |

B. Arterial supply and venous drainage. C. Segmental medullary and radicular arteries. Three longitudinal arteries supply the spinal cord: an anterior spinal artery, formed by the union of branches of vertebral arteries, and paired posterior spinal arteries, each of which is a branch of either the vertebral artery or the posterior inferior cerebellar artery.

- The spinal arteries run longitudinally from the medulla oblongata of the brainstem to the conus medullaris of the spinal cord. By themselves, the anterior and posterior spinal arteries supply only the short superior part of the spinal cord. The circulation to much of the spinal cord depends on segmental medullary and radicular arteries.
- The anterior and posterior segmental medullary arteries enter the intervertebral foramen to unite with the spinal arteries to supply blood to the spinal cord. The great anterior segmented medullary artery (Adamkiewicz artery) occurs on the left side in 65% of people. It reinforces the circulation to two thirds of the spinal cord.
- Posterior and anterior roots of the spinal nerves and their coverings are supplied by posterior and anterior radicular arteries, which run along the nerve roots. These vessels do not reach the posterior or anterior spinal arteries.
- The 3 anterior and 3 posterior spinal veins are arranged longitudinally; they communicate freely with each other and are drained by up to 12 anterior and posterior medullary and radicular veins. The veins draining the spinal cord join the internal vertebral plexus in the epidural space.

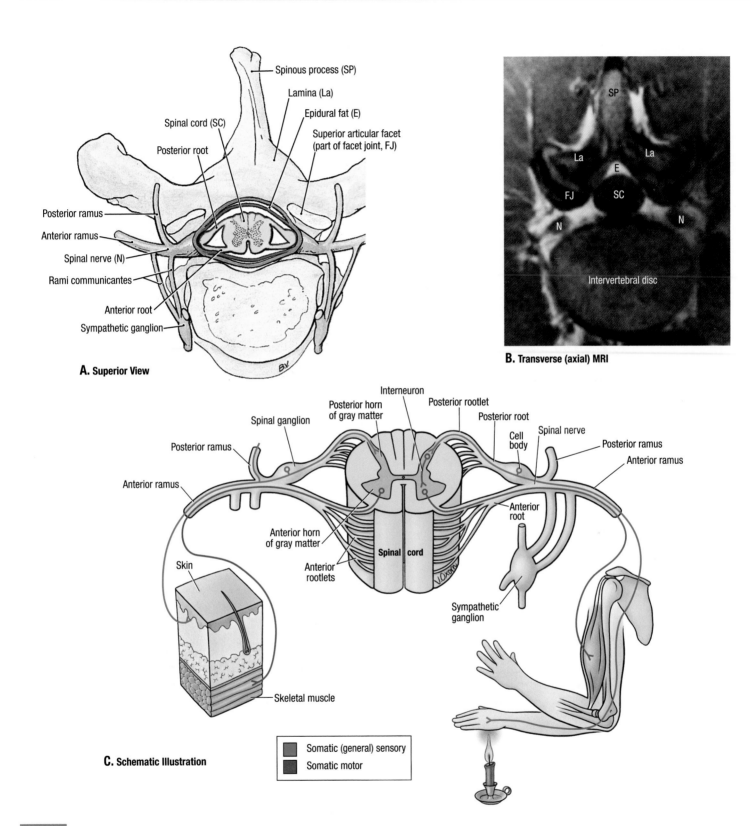

A. Superior View

B. Transverse (axial) MRI

C. Schematic Illustration

Somatic (general) sensory
Somatic motor

4.49   **Overview of somatic nervous system**

A. Spinal cord in situ in vertebral canal. **B.** T1 axial (transverse) MRI of lumbar spine. **C.** Components of typical spinal nerve. The somatic nervous system, or voluntary nervous system, composed of somatic parts of the CNS and PNS, provides general sensory and motor innervation to all parts of the body (G. *soma*), except the viscera in the body cavities, smooth muscle, and glands. The somatic (general) sensory fibers transmit sensations of touch, pain, temperature, and position from sensory receptors. The somatic motor fibers permit voluntary and reflexive movement by causing contraction of skeletal muscles, such as occurs when one touches a candle flame.

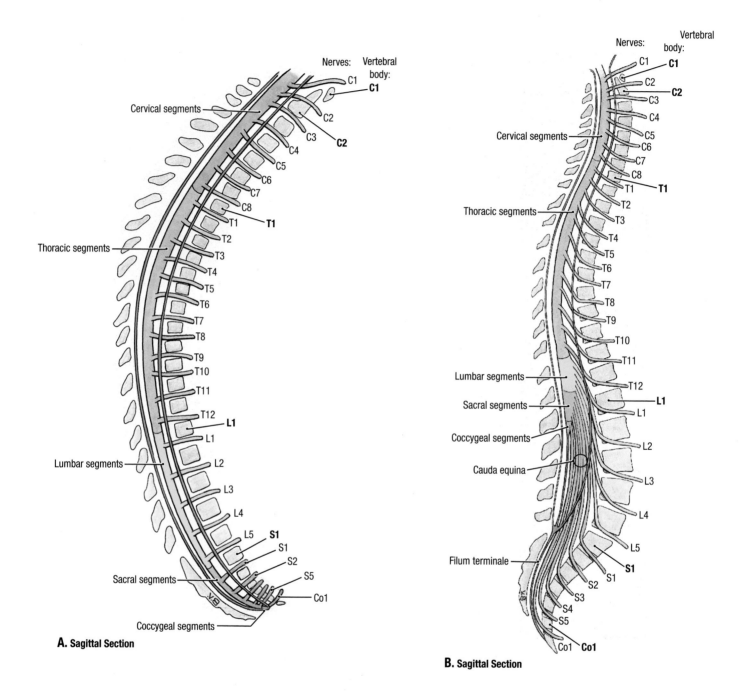

4.50 Spinal cord and spinal nerves

A. Spinal cord at 12 weeks gestation. **B.** Spinal cord of an adult.

- Early in development, the spinal cord and vertebral (spinal) canal are nearly equal in length. The canal grows longer, so spinal nerves have an increasingly longer course to reach the intervertebral foramen at the correct level for their exit. The spinal cord of adults terminates between vertebral bodies L1–L2. The remaining spinal nerves, seeking their intervertebral foramen of exit, form the cauda equina.
- All 31 pairs of spinal nerves—8 cervical (C), 12 thoracic (T), 5 lumbar (L), 5 sacral (S), and 1 coccygeal (Co)—arise from the spinal cord and exit through the intervertebral foramina in the vertebral column.

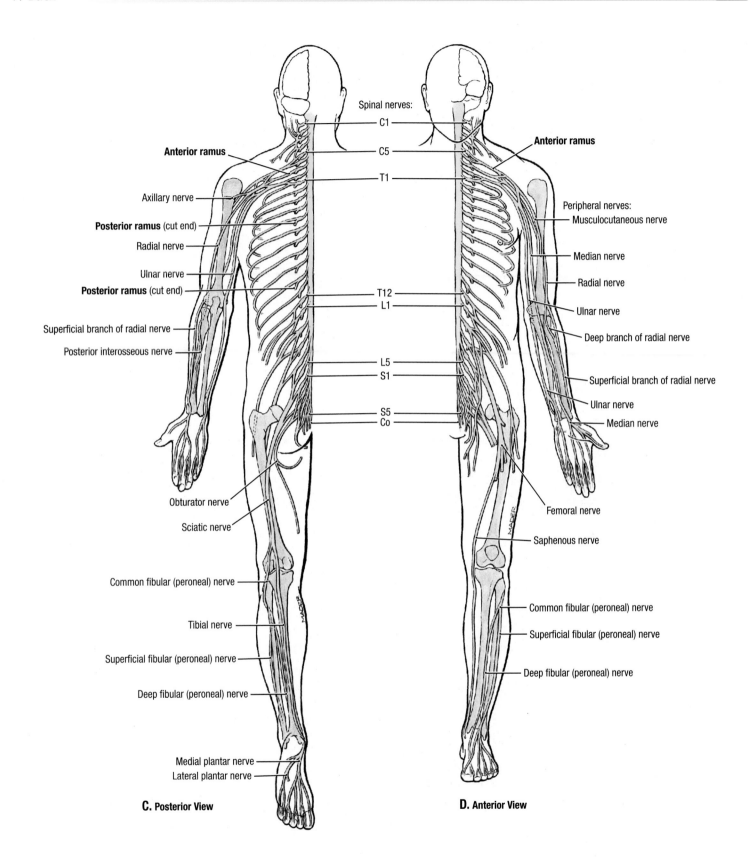

Spinal nerves:
C1
C5
T1
T12
L1
L5
S1
S5
Co

Anterior ramus

Anterior ramus

Axillary nerve

Posterior ramus (cut end)

Radial nerve

Ulnar nerve

Posterior ramus (cut end)

Superficial branch of radial nerve

Posterior interosseous nerve

Peripheral nerves:
Musculocutaneous nerve

Median nerve

Radial nerve

Ulnar nerve

Deep branch of radial nerve

Superficial branch of radial nerve

Ulnar nerve

Median nerve

Obturator nerve

Sciatic nerve

Femoral nerve

Saphenous nerve

Common fibular (peroneal) nerve

Tibial nerve

Superficial fibular (peroneal) nerve

Deep fibular (peroneal) nerve

Common fibular (peroneal) nerve

Superficial fibular (peroneal) nerve

Deep fibular (peroneal) nerve

Medial plantar nerve
Lateral plantar nerve

C. Posterior View

D. Anterior View

4.50   **Spinal cord and spinal nerves (continued)**

C and **D.** Peripheral nerves.
- The anterior rami supply nerve fibers to the anterior and lateral regions of the trunk and upper and lower limbs.

- The posterior rami supply nerve fibers to synovial joints of the vertebral column, deep muscles of the back, and overlying skin.

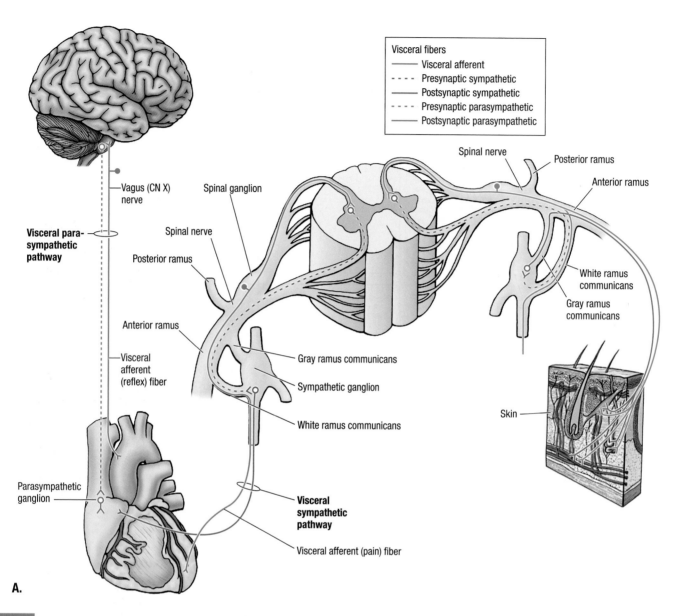

Visceral fibers
- ——— Visceral afferent
- - - - - Presynaptic sympathetic
- ——— Postsynaptic sympathetic
- - - - - Presynaptic parasympathetic
- ——— Postsynaptic parasympathetic

A.

4.51   **Visceral afferent and visceral efferent (motor) innervation**

A. Schematic illustration. Visceral afferent fibers have important relationships to the CNS, both anatomically and functionally. We are usually unaware of the sensory input of these fibers, which provides information about the condition of the body's internal environment. This information is integrated in the CNS, often triggering visceral or somatic reflexes or both. Visceral reflexes regulate blood pressure and chemistry by altering such functions as heart and respiratory rates and vascular resistance. Visceral sensation that reaches a conscious level is generally categorized as pain that is usually poorly localized and may be perceived as hunger or nausea. However, adequate stimulation may elicit true pain. Most visceral/reflex (unconscious) sensation and some pain travel in visceral afferent fibers that accompany the parasympathetic fibers retrograde. Most visceral pain impulses (from the heart and most organs of the peritoneal cavity) travel along visceral afferent fibers accompanying sympathetic fibers.

Visceral efferent (motor) innervation. The efferent nerve fibers and ganglia of the ANS are organized into two systems or divisions.
1. Sympathetic (thoracolumbar) division. In general, the effects of sympathetic stimulation are catabolic (preparing the body for "flight or fight").
2. Parasympathetic (craniosacral) division. In general, the effects of parasympathetic stimulation are anabolic (promoting normal function and conserving energy).

Conduction of impulses from the CNS to the effector organ involves a series of two neurons in both sympathetic and parasympathetic systems. The cell body of the presynaptic (preganglionic) neuron (first neuron) is located in the gray matter of the CNS. Its fiber (axon) synapses on the cell body of a postsynaptic (postganglionic) neuron, the second neuron in the series. The cell bodies of such second neurons are located in autonomic ganglia outside the CNS, and the postsynaptic fibers terminate on the effector organ (smooth muscle, modified cardiac muscle, or glands).

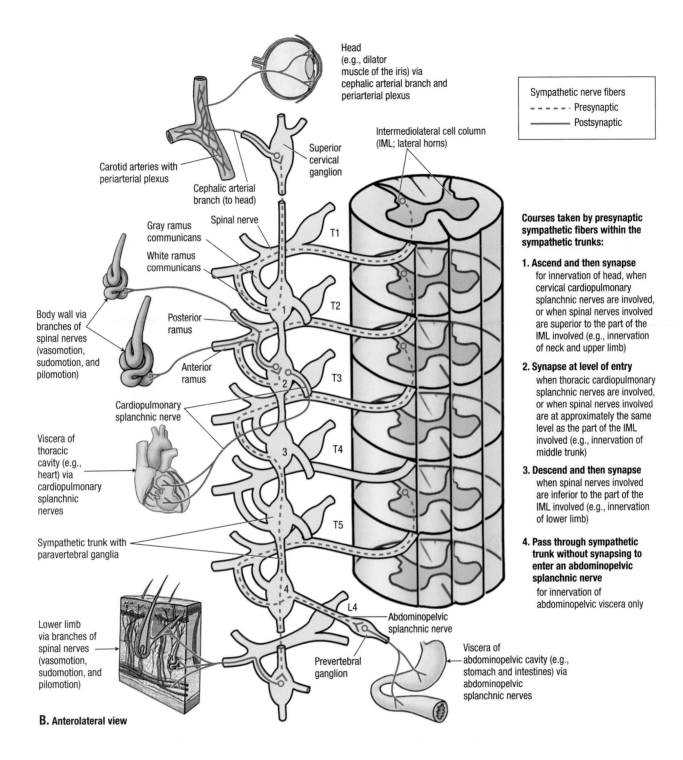

Head
(e.g., dilator
muscle of the iris) via
cephalic arterial branch and
periarterial plexus

Carotid arteries with
periarterial plexus

Cephalic arterial
branch (to head)

Superior
cervical
ganglion

Spinal nerve

Gray ramus
communicans

White ramus
communicans

Body wall via
branches of
spinal nerves
(vasomotion,
sudomotion, and
pilomotion)

Posterior
ramus

Anterior
ramus

Cardiopulmonary
splanchnic nerve

Viscera of
thoracic
cavity (e.g.,
heart) via
cardiopulmonary
splanchnic
nerves

Sympathetic trunk with
paravertebral ganglia

Lower limb
via branches of
spinal nerves
(vasomotion,
sudomotion, and
pilomotion)

Prevertebral
ganglion

Abdominopelvic
splanchnic nerve

Viscera of
abdominopelvic cavity (e.g.,
stomach and intestines) via
abdominopelvic
splanchnic nerves

Intermediolateral cell column
(IML; lateral horns)

Sympathetic nerve fibers
- - - - - Presynaptic
———— Postsynaptic

T1
T2
T3
T4
T5
L4

Courses taken by presynaptic sympathetic fibers within the sympathetic trunks:

1. Ascend and then synapse
for innervation of head, when cervical cardiopulmonary splanchnic nerves are involved, or when spinal nerves involved are superior to the part of the IML involved (e.g., innervation of neck and upper limb)

2. Synapse at level of entry
when thoracic cardiopulmonary splanchnic nerves are involved, or when spinal nerves involved are at approximately the same level as the part of the IML involved (e.g., innervation of middle trunk)

3. Descend and then synapse
when spinal nerves involved are inferior to the part of the IML involved (e.g., innervation of lower limb)

4. Pass through sympathetic trunk without synapsing to enter an abdominopelvic splanchnic nerve
for innervation of abdominopelvic viscera only

B. Anterolateral view

4.51   **Visceral afferent and visceral efferent (motor) innervation (continued)**

B. Courses taken by sympathetic motor fibers. Presynaptic fibers all follow the same course until they reach the sympathetic trunks. In the sympathetic trunks, they follow one of four possible courses. Fibers involved in providing sympathetic innervation to the body wall and limbs or viscera above the level of the diaphragm follow paths 1–3. They synapse in the paravertebral ganglia of the sympathetic trunks. Fibers involved in innervating abdominopelvic viscera follow path 4 to prevertebral ganglion via abdominopelvic splanchnic nerves.

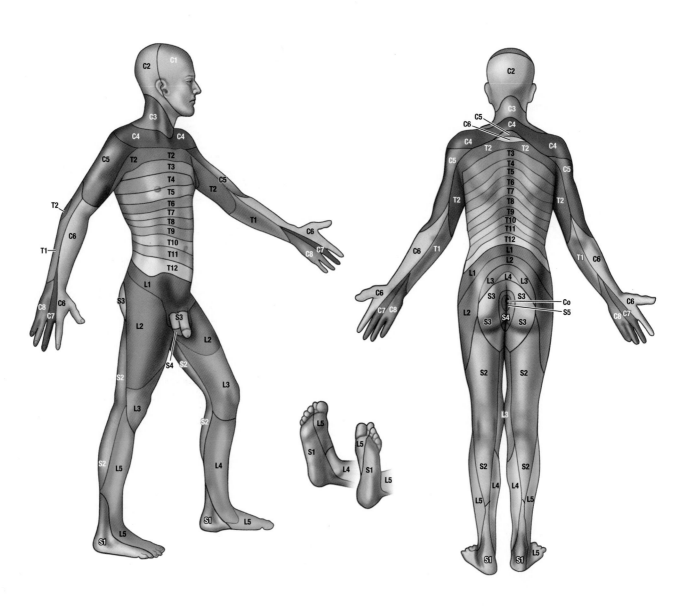

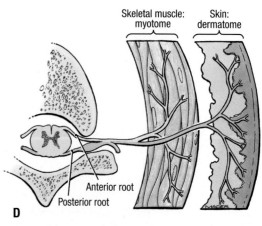

4.52   Dermatomes

A–C. Dermatome map (Foerster, 1933). The Keegan and Garrett (1948) dermatome map is not included here. The two schemes are similar in the trunk but differ in the limbs, where both are presented. **D.** Schematic illustration of a dermatome and myotome. The unilateral area of skin innervated by the general sensory fibers of a single spinal nerve is called a dermatome. From clinical studies of lesions in the posterior roots or spinal nerves, dermatome maps have been devised that indicate the typical pattens of innervation of the skin by specific spinal nerves.

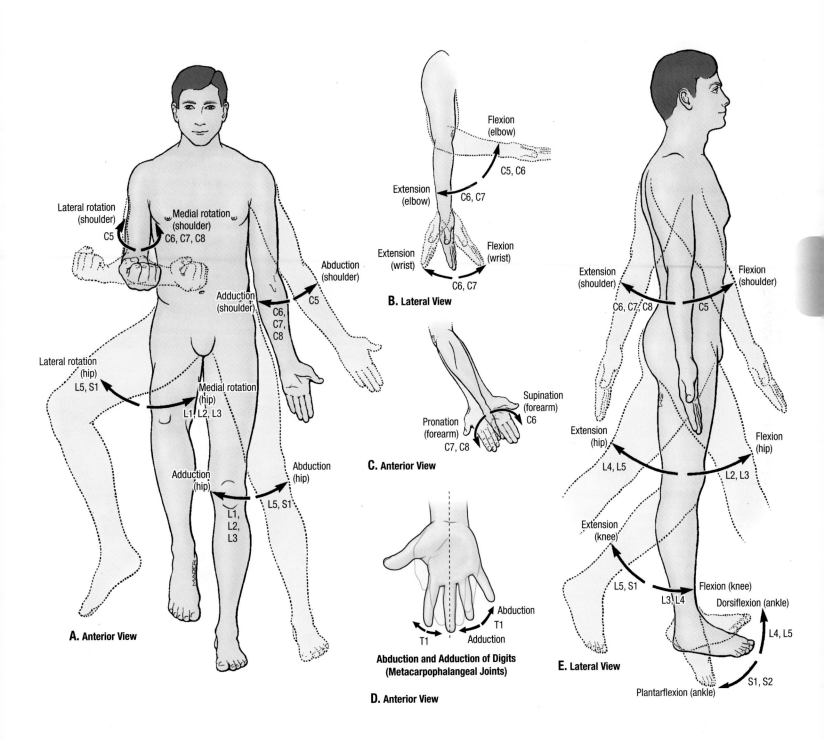

B. Lateral View

C. Anterior View

A. Anterior View

Abduction and Adduction of Digits
(Metacarpophalangeal Joints)

D. Anterior View

E. Lateral View

4.53 Myotomes

Somatic motor (general somatic efferent) fibers transmit impulses to skeletal (voluntary) muscles. The unilateral muscle mass receiving innervation from the somatic motor fibers conveyed by a single spinal nerve is a myotome. Each skeletal muscle is innervated by the somatic motor fibers of several spinal nerves; therefore, the muscle myotome will consist of several segments. The muscle myotomes have been grouped by joint movement to facilitate clinical testing. The intrinsic muscles of the hand constitute a single myotome—T1.

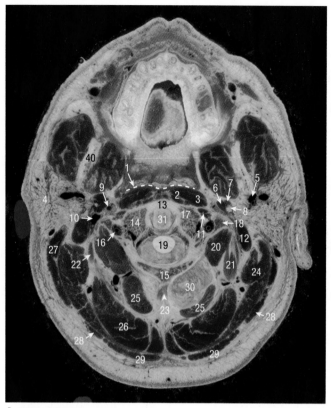

A. Inferior View

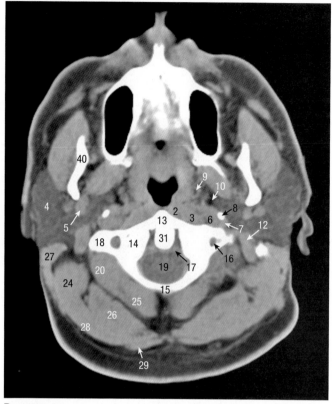

B. Inferior View

1	Site of retropharyngeal space
2	Longus colli
3	Longus capitis
4	Parotid gland
5	Retromandibular vein
6	Stylopharyngeus
7	Styloglossus
8	Stylohyoid muscle and ligament/process
9	Internal carotid artery
10	Internal jugular vein
11	Rectus capitis lateralis
12	Posterior belly of digastric
13	Anterior arch of atlas (C1)
14	Lateral mass of atlas (C1)
15	Posterior arch of atlas (C1)
16	Vertebral artery
17	Transverse ligament of atlas (C1)
18	Transverse process of atlas (C1)
19	Spinal cord
20	Rectus capitis posterior major
21	Obliquus capitis inferior
22	Obliquus capitis superior
23	Spinous process of atlas (C1)
24	Longissimus capitis
25	Rectus capitis posterior minor
26	Semispinalis capitis
27	Sternocleidomastoid
28	Splenius capitis
29	Trapezius
30	Fatty mass
31	Dens of axis (C2)
32	Anterior tubercle of atlas (C1)
33	Inferior articular facet of atlas (C1)
34	Foramen magnum
35	Foramen transversarium
36	Posterior tubercle of atlas (C1)
37	Mastoid process
38	Occipital bone of skull
39	External occipital protuberance
40	Ramus of mandible

ANTERIOR

RIGHT   LEFT

POSTERIOR

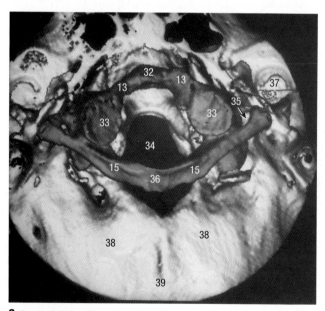

C. Posteroinferior View

4.54   **Imaging of superior nuchal region at the level of the atlas**

A. Transverse section of specimen. **B.** Transverse computed tomographic (CT) scan. **C.** Three-dimensional (3D) CT of the base of the skull and atlas.

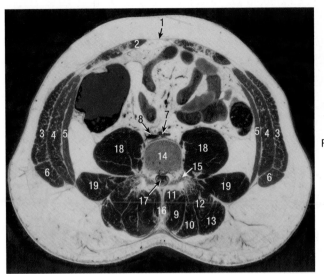

A. Inferior View

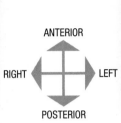

ANTERIOR

RIGHT ⊢ LEFT

POSTERIOR

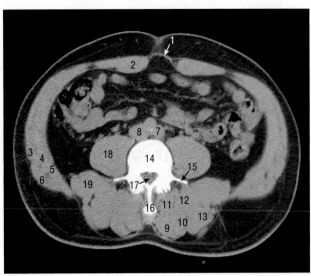

B. Inferior View

1	Linea alba	6	Latissimus dorsi	11	Multifidus	16	Spinous process
2	Rectus abdominis	7	Descending aorta	12	Rotatores	17	Cauda equina
3	External oblique	8	Inferior vena cava	13	Iliocostalis	18	Psoas major
4	Internal oblique	9	Spinalis	14	4th lumbar vertebra	19	Quadratus lumborum
5	Transversus abdominis	10	Longissimus	15	Transverse process		

4.55   **Imaging of lumbar spine at L4**

A. Transverse section of specimen. **B.** Transverse computed tomographic (CT) scan.

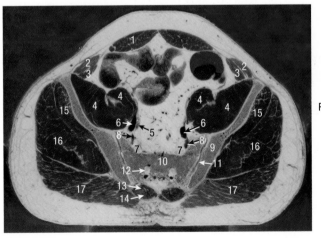

A. Inferior View

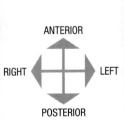

ANTERIOR

RIGHT ⊢ LEFT

POSTERIOR

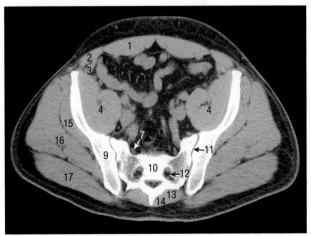

B. Inferior View

1	Rectus abdominis	6	Internal iliac vein	10	2nd sacral vertebra	14	Erector spinae
2	External oblique	7	Anterior rami	11	Sacro-iliac joint	15	Gluteus minimis
3	Internal oblique	8	Superior gluteal vessels	12	Sacral nerve root	16	Gluteus medius
4	Iliopsoas	9	Body of ilium	13	Multifidus	17	Gluteus maximus
5	Internal iliac artery						

4.56   **Imaging of sacro-iliac joint**

A. Transverse section of specimen. **B.** Transverse computed tomographic (CT) scan.

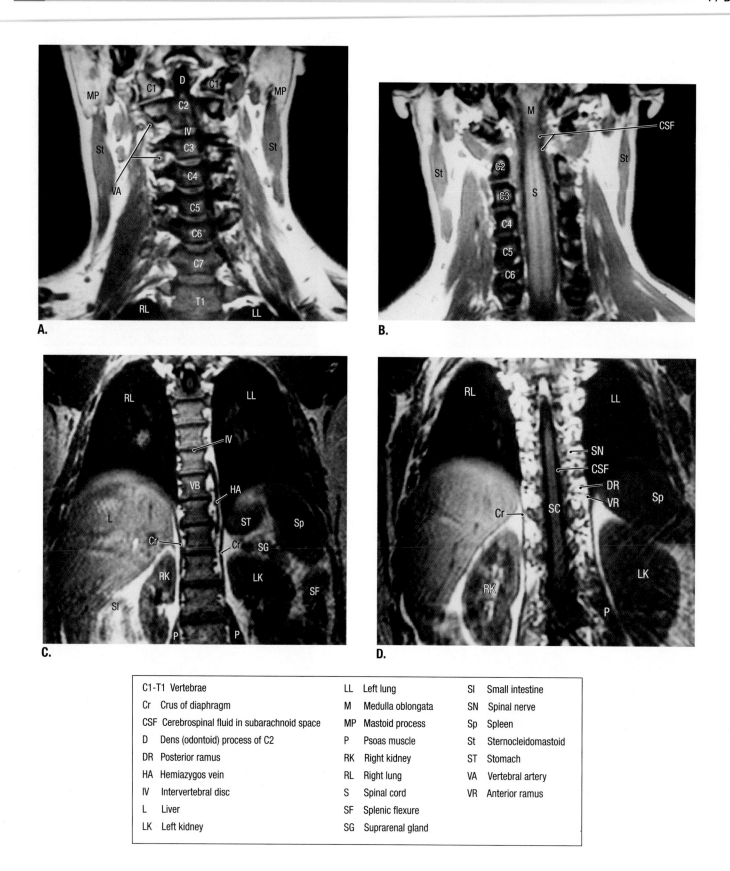

C1-T1	Vertebrae	LL	Left lung	SI	Small intestine
Cr	Crus of diaphragm	M	Medulla oblongata	SN	Spinal nerve
CSF	Cerebrospinal fluid in subarachnoid space	MP	Mastoid process	Sp	Spleen
D	Dens (odontoid) process of C2	P	Psoas muscle	St	Sternocleidomastoid
DR	Posterior ramus	RK	Right kidney	ST	Stomach
HA	Hemiazygos vein	RL	Right lung	VA	Vertebral artery
IV	Intervertebral disc	S	Spinal cord	VR	Anterior ramus
L	Liver	SF	Splenic flexure		
LK	Left kidney	SG	Suprarenal gland		

4.57   **Coronal MRI scans of cervical and thoracic spine**

A and **B.** Cervical spine. **C** and **D.** Thoracic spine.

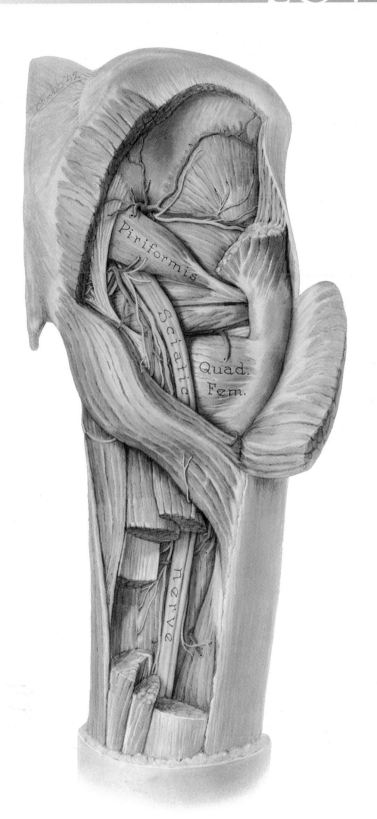

- Systemic Overview of Lower Limb **354**
  - Bones **355**
  - Nerves **356**
  - Blood Vessels **362**
  - Lymphatics **366**
  - Musculofascial Compartments **368**
- Retroinguinal Passage and Femoral Triangle **370**
- Anterior and Medial Compartments of Thigh **374**
- Lateral Thigh **383**
- Gluteal Region and Posterior Compartment of Thigh **384**
- Hip Joint **394**
- Knee Region **402**
- Knee Joint **408**
- Anterior and Lateral Compartments of Leg, Dorsum of Foot **422**
- Posterior Compartment of Leg **432**
- Tibiofibular Joints **442**
- Sole of Foot **443**
- Ankle, Subtalar, and Foot Joints **448**
- Arches of Foot **466**
- Bony Anomalies **467**
- Imaging and Sectional Anatomy **468**

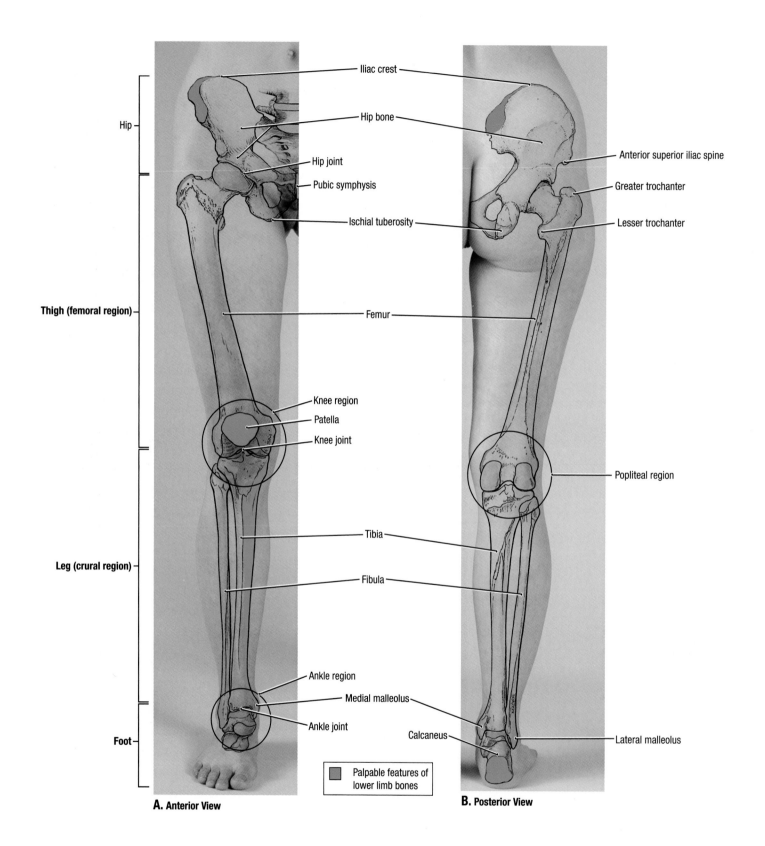

A. Anterior View

B. Posterior View

Palpable features of
lower limb bones

5.1   **Regions, bones, and major joints of lower limb**

The hip bones meet anteriorly at the symphysis pubis and articulate with the sacrum posteriorly. The femur articulates with the hip bone proximally and the tibia distally. The tibia
and fibula are the bones of the leg that join the foot at the ankle.

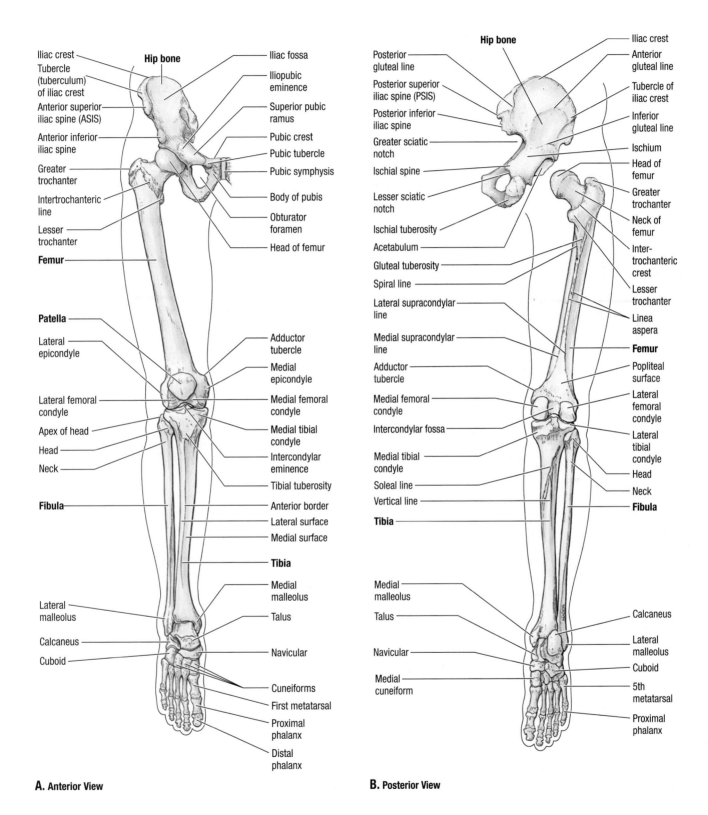

Iliac crest
Tubercle (tuberculum) of iliac crest
Anterior superior iliac spine (ASIS)
Anterior inferior iliac spine
Greater trochanter
Intertrochanteric line
Lesser trochanter
Femur

Hip bone

Iliac fossa
Iliopubic eminence
Superior pubic ramus
Pubic crest
Pubic tubercle
Pubic symphysis
Body of pubis
Obturator foramen
Head of femur

Patella
Lateral epicondyle
Lateral femoral condyle
Apex of head
Head
Neck
Fibula

Adductor tubercle
Medial epicondyle
Medial femoral condyle
Medial tibial condyle
Intercondylar eminence
Tibial tuberosity
Anterior border
Lateral surface
Medial surface
Tibia
Medial malleolus
Talus
Navicular
Cuneiforms
First metatarsal
Proximal phalanx
Distal phalanx

Lateral malleolus
Calcaneus
Cuboid

A. Anterior View

Hip bone

Posterior gluteal line
Posterior superior iliac spine (PSIS)
Posterior inferior iliac spine
Greater sciatic notch
Ischial spine
Lesser sciatic notch
Ischial tuberosity
Acetabulum
Gluteal tuberosity
Spiral line
Lateral supracondylar line
Medial supracondylar line
Adductor tubercle
Medial femoral condyle
Intercondylar fossa
Medial tibial condyle
Soleal line
Vertical line
Tibia

Iliac crest
Anterior gluteal line
Tubercle of iliac crest
Inferior gluteal line
Ischium
Head of femur
Greater trochanter
Neck of femur
Intertrochanteric crest
Lesser trochanter
Linea aspera
Femur
Popliteal surface
Lateral femoral condyle
Lateral tibial condyle
Head
Neck
Fibula

Medial malleolus
Talus
Navicular
Medial cuneiform

Calcaneus
Lateral malleolus
Cuboid
5th metatarsal
Proximal phalanx

B. Posterior View

5.2   Features of bones of lower limb

The foot is in full plantarflexion. The hip joint is disarticulated in **B** to demonstrate the acetabulum of the hip bone and the entire head of the femur.

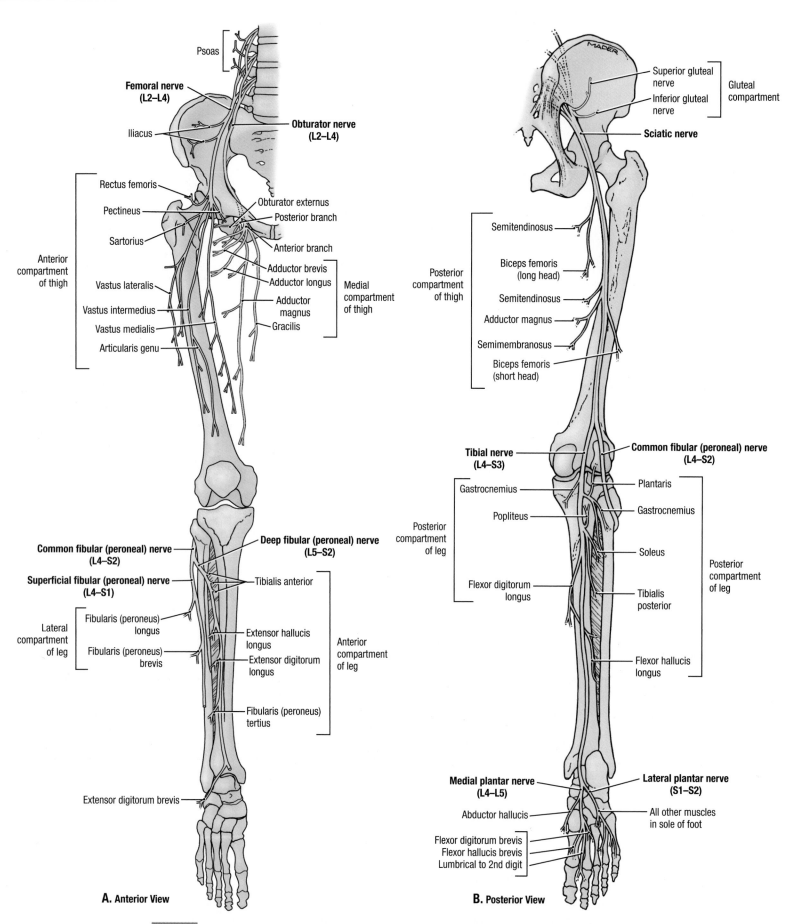

Psoas

Femoral nerve (L2–L4)

Iliacus

Obturator nerve (L2–L4)

Rectus femoris

Pectineus

Obturator externus

Posterior branch

Sartorius

Anterior branch

Adductor brevis

Adductor longus

Vastus lateralis

Adductor magnus

Vastus intermedius

Gracilis

Vastus medialis

Articularis genu

Anterior compartment of thigh

Medial compartment of thigh

Common fibular (peroneal) nerve (L4–S2)

Deep fibular (peroneal) nerve (L5–S2)

Superficial fibular (peroneal) nerve (L4–S1)

Tibialis anterior

Lateral compartment of leg

Fibularis (peroneus) longus

Extensor hallucis longus

Fibularis (peroneus) brevis

Extensor digitorum longus

Anterior compartment of leg

Fibularis (peroneus) tertius

Extensor digitorum brevis

A. Anterior View

Superior gluteal nerve

Inferior gluteal nerve

Gluteal compartment

Sciatic nerve

Semitendinosus

Biceps femoris (long head)

Semitendinosus

Adductor magnus

Semimembranosus

Biceps femoris (short head)

Posterior compartment of thigh

Tibial nerve (L4–S3)

Common fibular (peroneal) nerve (L4–S2)

Gastrocnemius

Plantaris

Popliteus

Gastrocnemius

Soleus

Posterior compartment of leg

Flexor digitorum longus

Tibialis posterior

Posterior compartment of leg

Flexor hallucis longus

Medial plantar nerve (L4–L5)

Lateral plantar nerve (S1–S2)

Abductor hallucis

All other muscles in sole of foot

Flexor digitorum brevis

Flexor hallucis brevis

Lumbrical to 2nd digit

B. Posterior View

5.3   **Overview of motor innervation of lower limb**

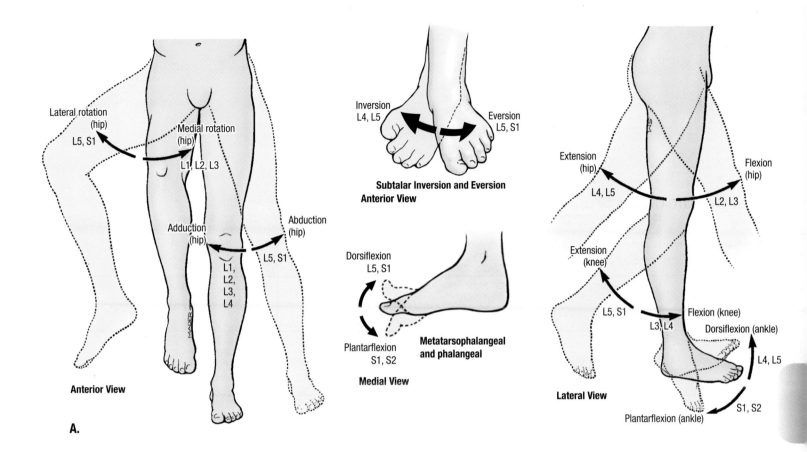

Myotatic (Deep Tendon) Reflex	Spinal Cord Segments
Quadriceps	L3/L4
Calcaneal (Achilles)	S1/S2

5.4   Myotomes and deep tendon reflexes

A. Myotomes. Somatic motor (general somatic efferent) fibers transmit impulses to skeletal (voluntary) muscles. The unilateral muscle mass receiving innervation from the somatic motor fibers conveyed by a single spinal nerve is a myotome. Each skeletal muscle is usually innervated by the somatic motor fibers of several spinal nerves; therefore, the muscle myotome will consist of several segments. The muscle myotomes have been grouped by joint movement to facilitate clinical testing.

B. Myotactic (deep tendon) reflexes. A myotatic (stretch) reflex is an involuntary contraction of a muscle in response to being stretched. Deep tendon reflexes (e.g., "knee jerk") are monosynaptic stretch reflexes that are elicited by briskly tapping the tendon with a reflex hammer. Each tendon reflex is mediated by specific spinal nerves. Stretch reflexes control muscle tone (e.g., in antigravity, muscles that keep the body upright against gravity).

TABLE 5.1 MOTOR NERVES OF LOWER LIMB

Nerve	Origin	Course	Distribution in Leg
Femoral	Lumbar plexus (L2–L4)	Passes deep to midpoint of inguinal ligament, lateral to femoral vessels, dividing into muscular and cutaneous branches in femoral triangle	Anterior thigh muscles, hip and knee joints
Obturator	Lumbar plexus (L2–L4)	Enters thigh via obturator foramen and divides; its anterior branch descends between adductor longus and adductor brevis; its posterior branch descends between adductor brevis and adductor magnus	*Anterior branch:* adductor longus, adductor brevis, gracilis, and pectineus; *posterior branch:* obturator externus, and adductor magnus
Sciatic	Sacral plexus (L4–S3)	Enters gluteal region through greater sciatic foramen, usually passing inferior to piriformis, descends in posterior compartment of thigh, bifurcating at apex of popliteal fossa into tibial and common fibular (peroneal) nerves	Muscles of posterior thigh, leg and foot; skin of posterolateral leg and foot
Tibial	Sciatic nerve	Terminal branch of sciatic nerve arising at apex of popliteal fossa; descends through popliteal fossa with popliteal vessels, continuing in deep posterior compartment of leg with posterior tibial vessels; bifurcates into medial and lateral plantar nerves	Hamstring muscles of posterior compartment of thigh, muscles of posterior compartment of leg, and sole of foot
Common fibular	Sciatic nerve	Terminal branch of sciatic nerve arising at apex of popliteal fossa; follows medial border of biceps femoris and its tendon to wind around neck of fibula deep to fibularis longus, where it bifurcates into superficial and deep fibular nerves	Short head of biceps femoris, muscles of anterior and lateral leg, and dorsum of foot
Superficial fibular	Common fibular nerve	Arises deep to fibularis longus on neck of fibula and descends in lateral compartment of the leg; pierces crural fascia in distal third of leg to become cutaneous	Fibularis longus and brevis muscles
Deep fibular	Common fibular nerve	Arises deep to fibularis longus on neck of fibula; passes through extensor digitorum longus into anterior compartment, descending on interosseous membrane; crosses ankle joint and enters dorsum of foot	Muscles of anterior compartment of leg and dorsum of foot

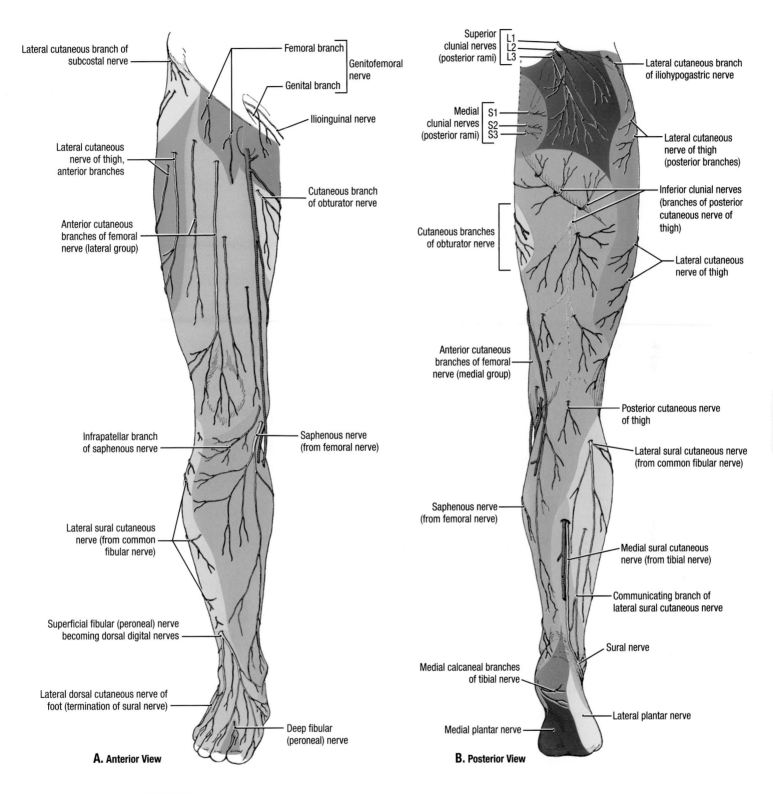

A. Anterior View

Lateral cutaneous branch of subcostal nerve

Femoral branch ⎤ Genitofemoral nerve

Genital branch ⎦

Ilioinguinal nerve

Lateral cutaneous nerve of thigh, anterior branches

Cutaneous branch of obturator nerve

Anterior cutaneous branches of femoral nerve (lateral group)

Infrapatellar branch of saphenous nerve

Saphenous nerve (from femoral nerve)

Lateral sural cutaneous nerve (from common fibular nerve)

Superficial fibular (peroneal) nerve becoming dorsal digital nerves

Lateral dorsal cutaneous nerve of foot (termination of sural nerve)

Deep fibular (peroneal) nerve

B. Posterior View

Superior clunial nerves (posterior rami) — L1, L2, L3

Medial clunial nerves (posterior rami) — S1, S2, S3

Lateral cutaneous branch of iliohypogastric nerve

Lateral cutaneous nerve of thigh (posterior branches)

Inferior clunial nerves (branches of posterior cutaneous nerve of thigh)

Lateral cutaneous nerve of thigh

Cutaneous branches of obturator nerve

Anterior cutaneous branches of femoral nerve (medial group)

Posterior cutaneous nerve of thigh

Lateral sural cutaneous nerve (from common fibular nerve)

Saphenous nerve (from femoral nerve)

Medial sural cutaneous nerve (from tibial nerve)

Communicating branch of lateral sural cutaneous nerve

Sural nerve

Medial calcaneal branches of tibial nerve

Lateral plantar nerve

Medial plantar nerve

5.5   Cutaneous nerves of lower limb

Cutaneous nerves in the subcutaneous tissue supply the skin of the lower limb. The cutaneous innervation of the lower limb reflects both the original segmental innervation of the skin via separate spinal nerves in its dermatomal pattern (Fig. 5.7) and the result of plexus formation of segmental peripheral nerves. In **B**, the medial sural cutaneous nerve (*sural* is Latin for calf) is joined between the popliteal fossa and posterior aspect of the ankle by a communicating branch of the lateral sural cutaneous nerve to form the sural nerve. The level of the junction is variable and is low in this specimen.

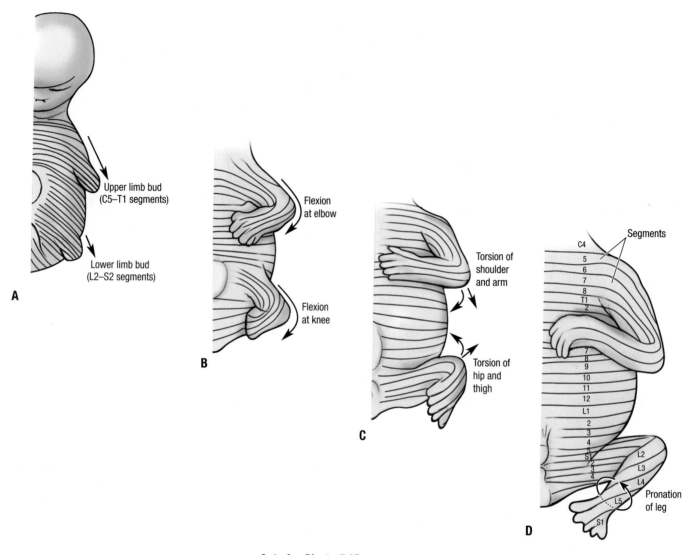

Anterior (Ventral) Views

<table>
<tr><td>**5.6**</td><td>**Rotation of limbs during development; effect on lower limb dermatome pattern**</td></tr>
</table>

A. During early development, the trunk is divided into segments (metameres) that correspond to, and receive innervation from, the corresponding spinal cord segments. During the 4th week of development, the upper limb buds appear as elevations of the C5 to T1 segments of the ventrolateral body wall. Following the cranial-to-caudal pattern of development the lower limb buds appear about a week later (5th week). The lower limb buds grow laterally from broader bases formed by the L2 to S2 segments.

B. The distal ends of the limb buds flatten into paddlelike hand plates and foot plates that are elongated in the craniocaudal axis. Initially, both the thumb and the great toe are on the cranial sides of the developing hand and foot, directed superiorly, with the palms and soles directed anteriorly. Where gaps develop between the precursors of the long bones (future elbow and knee joints), flexures occur. At first, the limbs bend anteriorly, so that the elbow and knee are directed laterally, causing the palm and sole to be directed medially (toward the trunk).

C. By the end of the 7th week, the proximal parts of the upper and lower limbs undergo a 90-degree torsion around their long axes, but in opposite directions, so that the elbow becomes directed caudally and the knee cranially.

D. In the lower limb, the torsion of the proximal limb is accompanied by a permanent pronation (twisting) of the leg, so that the foot becomes oriented with the great toe on the medial side.

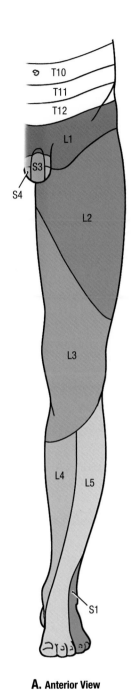

A. Anterior View

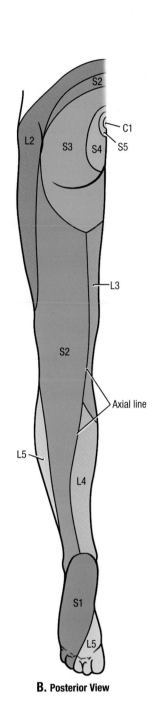

B. Posterior View

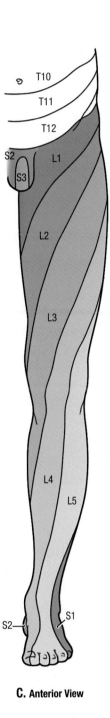

C. Anterior View

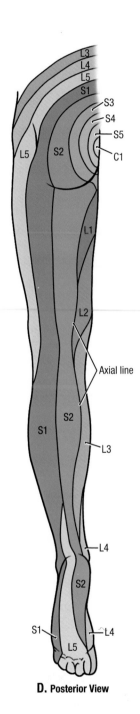

D. Posterior View

5.7   Dermatomes of lower limb

The dermatomal, or segmental, pattern of distribution of sensory nerve fibers persists despite the merging of spinal nerves in plexus formation during development. Two different dermatome maps are commonly used. **A** and **B.** The dermatome pattern of the lower limb according to Foerster (1933) is preferred by many because of its correlation with clinical findings. **C** and **D.** The dermatome pattern of the lower limb according to Keegan and Garrett (1948) is preferred by others for its aesthetic uniformity and obvious correlation with development. Although depicted as distinct zones, adjacent dermatomes overlap considerably, except along the axial line.

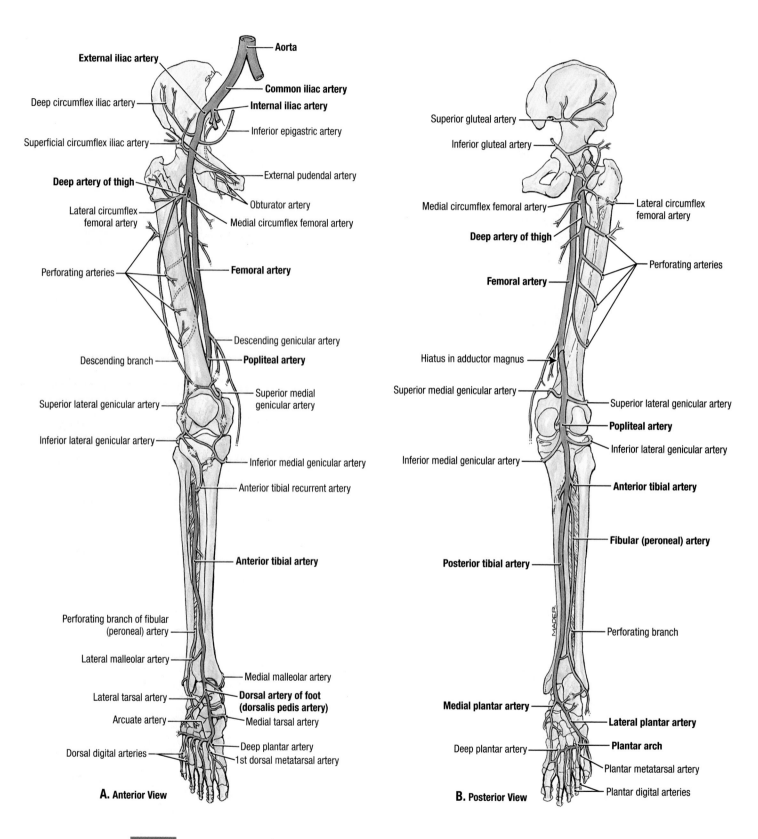

A. Anterior View

- Aorta
- External iliac artery
- Deep circumflex iliac artery
- Common iliac artery
- Internal iliac artery
- Superficial circumflex iliac artery
- Inferior epigastric artery
- External pudendal artery
- Deep artery of thigh
- Lateral circumflex femoral artery
- Obturator artery
- Medial circumflex femoral artery
- Perforating arteries
- Femoral artery
- Descending genicular artery
- Descending branch
- Popliteal artery
- Superior lateral genicular artery
- Superior medial genicular artery
- Inferior lateral genicular artery
- Inferior medial genicular artery
- Anterior tibial recurrent artery
- Anterior tibial artery
- Perforating branch of fibular (peroneal) artery
- Lateral malleolar artery
- Medial malleolar artery
- Lateral tarsal artery
- Dorsal artery of foot (dorsalis pedis artery)
- Arcuate artery
- Medial tarsal artery
- Dorsal digital arteries
- Deep plantar artery
- 1st dorsal metatarsal artery

B. Posterior View

- Superior gluteal artery
- Inferior gluteal artery
- Medial circumflex femoral artery
- Lateral circumflex femoral artery
- Deep artery of thigh
- Perforating arteries
- Femoral artery
- Hiatus in adductor magnus
- Superior medial genicular artery
- Superior lateral genicular artery
- Popliteal artery
- Inferior medial genicular artery
- Inferior lateral genicular artery
- Anterior tibial artery
- Fibular (peroneal) artery
- Posterior tibial artery
- Perforating branch
- Medial plantar artery
- Lateral plantar artery
- Plantar arch
- Deep plantar artery
- Plantar metatarsal artery
- Plantar digital arteries

5.8   Overview of arteries of lower limb

The arteries often anastomose or communicate to form networks to ensure blood supply distal to the joint throughout the range of movement. If a main channel is slowly occluded, the smaller alternate channels can usually increase in size, providing a collateral circulation that ensures the blood supply to structures distal to the blockage.

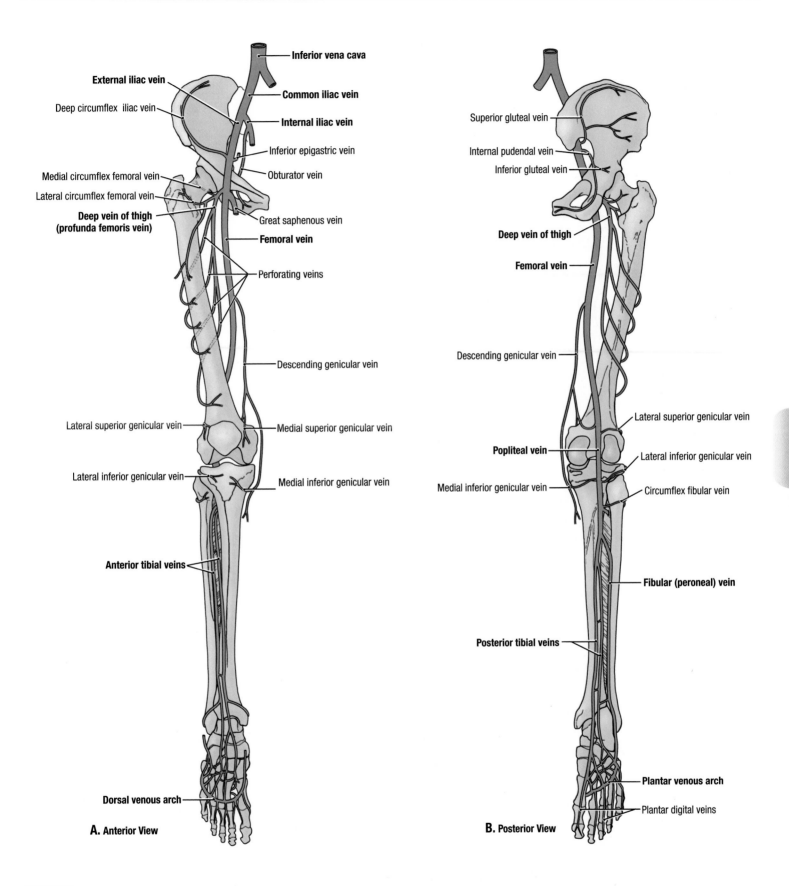

5.9   Deep veins of lower limb

Deep veins lie internal to the deep fascia. Although only the anterior and posterior tibial veins are depicted as paired structures in this schematic illustration, typically in the limbs deep veins occur as paired, continually interanastomosing accompanying veins (L., venae comitantes) surrounding and sharing the name of the artery they accompany.

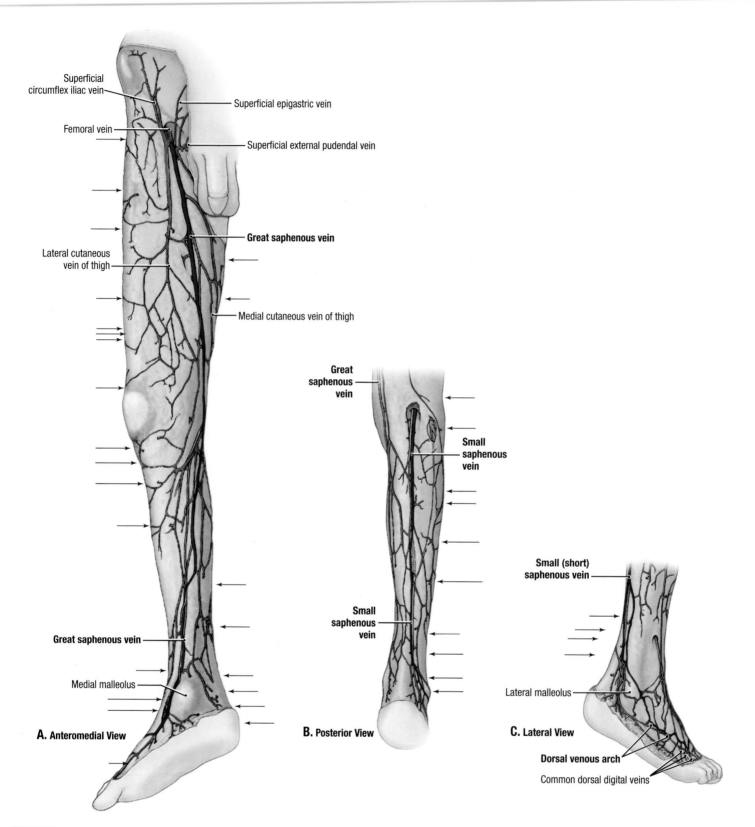

Superficial circumflex iliac vein

Superficial epigastric vein

Femoral vein

Superficial external pudendal vein

Great saphenous vein

Lateral cutaneous vein of thigh

Medial cutaneous vein of thigh

Great saphenous vein

Small saphenous vein

Great saphenous vein

Small saphenous vein

Medial malleolus

A. Anteromedial View

B. Posterior View

Small (short) saphenous vein

Lateral malleolus

C. Lateral View

Dorsal venous arch

Common dorsal digital veins

5.10   Superficial veins of lower limb

The *arrows* indicate where perforating veins penetrate the deep fascia. Blood is continuously shunted from these superficial veins in the subcutaneous tissue to deep veins via the perforating veins. Vein grafts obtained by surgically harvesting parts of the great saphenous vein are used to bypass obstructions in blood vessels (e.g., an occlusion of a coronary artery or its branches). When part of the vein is used as a bypass, it is reversed so that the valves do not obstruct blood flow. Because there are so many anastomosing leg veins, removal of the great saphenous vein rarely affects circulation seriously, provided the deep veins are intact.

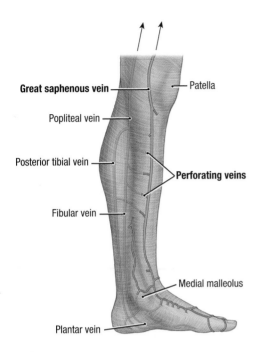

Great saphenous vein

Patella

Popliteal vein

Posterior tibial vein

Perforating veins

Fibular vein

Medial malleolus

Plantar vein

A. Medial View

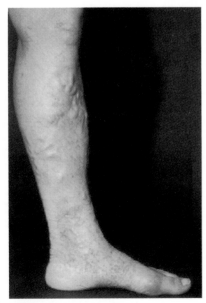

B. Medial View, Varicose Veins

Great saphenous vein

Patella

Great saphenous vein

Great saphenous vein

Medial malleolus

Dorsal venous arch

C. Anteromedial View, Normal Veins
(distended following exercise)

5.11   Drainage and surface anatomy of superficial veins of lower limb

A. Schematic diagram of drainage of superficial veins. Blood is repeatedly shunted from the superficial veins (e.g., great saphenous vein) to the deep veins (e.g., fibular and posterior tibial veins) via perforating veins that penetrate the deep fascia. Muscular compression of deep veins assists return of blood to the heart against gravity.

B. Varicose veins form when either the deep fascia or the valves of the perforating veins are incompetent. This allows the muscular compression that normally propels blood toward the heart to push blood from the deep to the superficial veins. Consequently, superficial veins become enlarged and tortuous. **C.** Normal veins, distended following exercise.

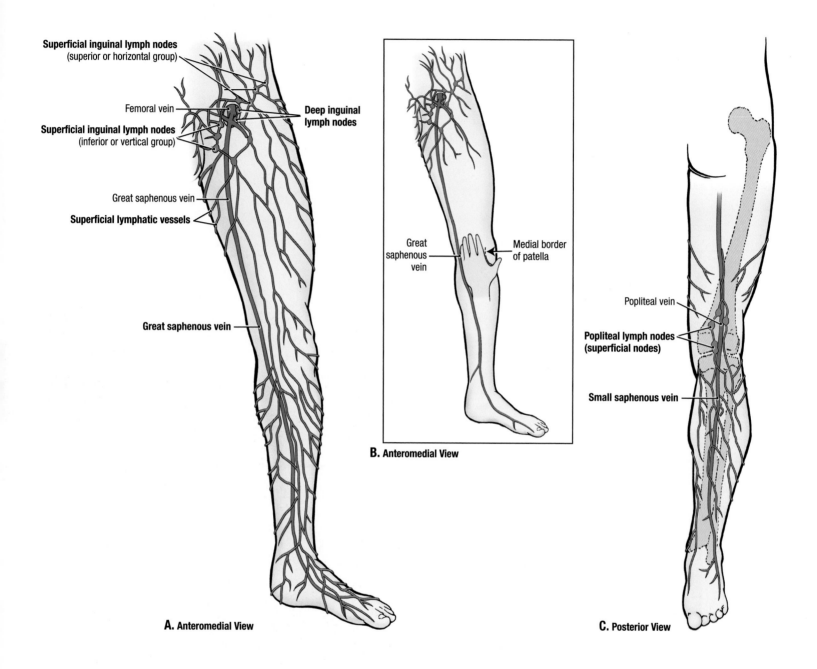

A. Anteromedial View

B. Anteromedial View

C. Posterior View

5.12   Superficial lymphatic drainage of lower limb

The superficial lymphatic vessels converge on and accompany the saphenous veins and their tributaries in the superficial fascia. The lymphatic vessels along the great saphenous vein drain into the superficial inguinal lymph nodes; those along the small saphenous vein drain into the popliteal lymph nodes. Lymph from the superficial inguinal nodes drains to the deep inguinal and external iliac nodes. Lymph from the popliteal nodes ascends through deep lymphatic vessels accompanying the deep blood vessels to the deep inguinal nodes. In **B,** note that the great saphenous vein lies anterior to the medial malleolus and a hand's breadth posterior to the medial aspect of the patella. Lymph nodes enlarge when diseased. Abrasions and minor sepsis, caused by pathogenic microorganisms or their toxins in the blood or other tissues, may produce slight enlargement of the superficial inguinal nodes (lymphadenopathy) in otherwise healthy people. Malignancies (e.g., of the external genitalia and uterus) and perineal abscesses also result in enlargement of these nodes.

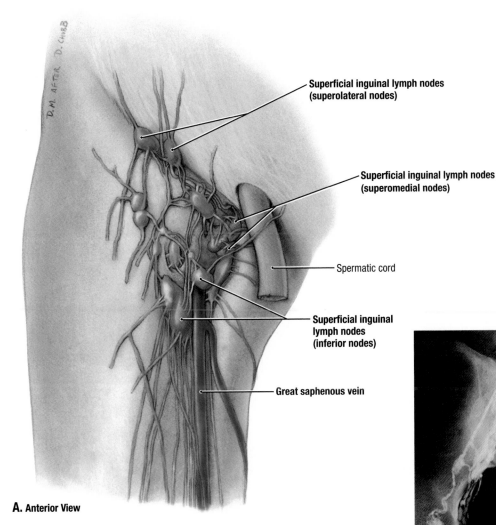

Superficial inguinal lymph nodes
(superolateral nodes)

Superficial inguinal lymph nodes
(superomedial nodes)

Spermatic cord

Superficial inguinal
lymph nodes
(inferior nodes)

Great saphenous vein

A. Anterior View

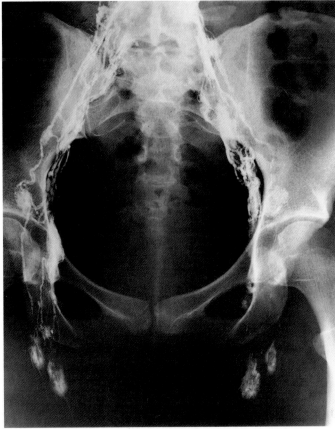

B. Anteroposterior View

5.13   **Inguinal lymph nodes**

A. Dissection. **B.** Lymphangiogram.

- Observe the arrangement of the nodes: a proximal chain parallel to the inguinal ligament (superolateral and superomedial superficial inguinal lymph nodes) and a distal chain on the sides of the great saphenous vein (inferior superficial inguinal lymph nodes). Efferent vessels leave these nodes and pass deep to the inguinal ligament to enter the external iliac nodes. Some of the lymphatic vessels traverse the femoral canal, and others ascend alongside the femoral artery and vein, some inside the femoral sheath, and some outside it.
- Note the anastomosis between the lymph vessels.

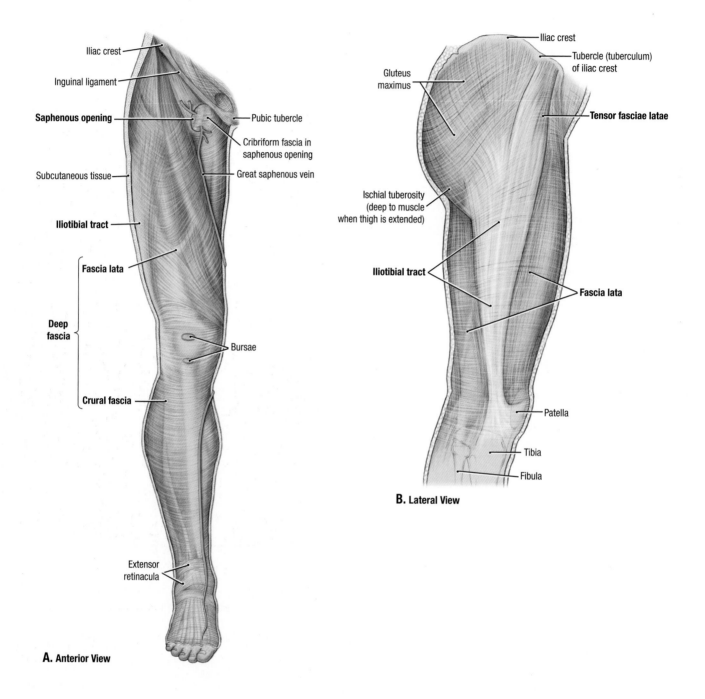

A. Anterior View

B. Lateral View

5.14   **Fascia and musculofascial compartments of lower limb**

A. Anterior skin and subcutaneous tissue have been removed to reveal the deep fascia of the thigh (fascia lata) and leg (crural fascia). **B.** Lateral skin and subcutaneous tissue have been removed to reveal the fascia lata. The fascia lata is thick laterally and forms the iliotibial tract. The iliotibial tract serves as a common aponeurosis for the gluteus maximus and tensor fasciae latae muscles.

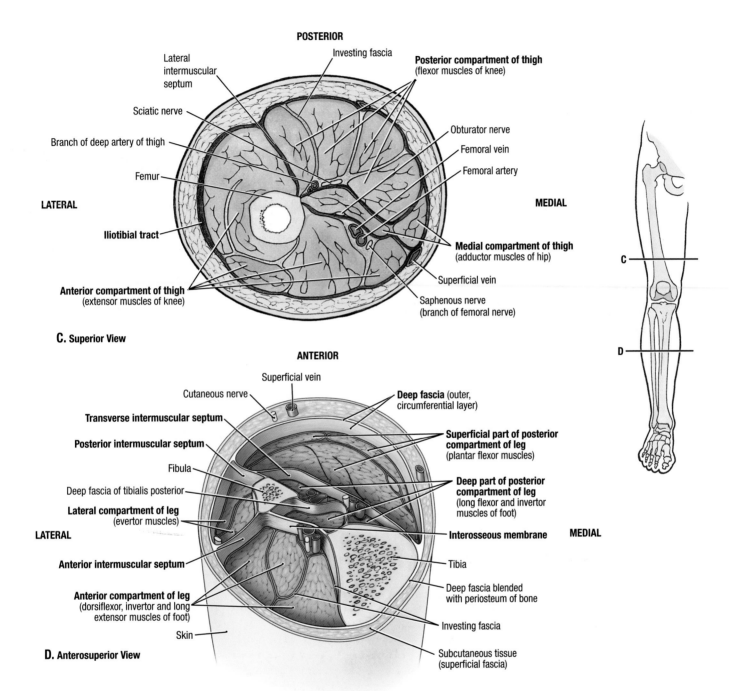

POSTERIOR

Lateral intermuscular septum

Investing fascia

Posterior compartment of thigh (flexor muscles of knee)

Sciatic nerve

Obturator nerve

Branch of deep artery of thigh

Femoral vein

Femoral artery

Femur

LATERAL

MEDIAL

Iliotibial tract

Medial compartment of thigh (adductor muscles of hip)

Superficial vein

Anterior compartment of thigh (extensor muscles of knee)

Saphenous nerve (branch of femoral nerve)

C. Superior View

ANTERIOR

Superficial vein

Cutaneous nerve

Deep fascia (outer, circumferential layer)

Transverse intermuscular septum

Superficial part of posterior compartment of leg (plantar flexor muscles)

Posterior intermuscular septum

Fibula

Deep part of posterior compartment of leg (long flexor and invertor muscles of foot)

Deep fascia of tibialis posterior

Lateral compartment of leg (evertor muscles)

LATERAL

MEDIAL

Interosseous membrane

Anterior intermuscular septum

Tibia

Anterior compartment of leg (dorsiflexor, invertor and long extensor muscles of foot)

Deep fascia blended with periosteum of bone

Skin

Investing fascia

D. Anterosuperior View

Subcutaneous tissue (superficial fascia)

C

D

5.14   **Fascia and musculofascial compartments of lower limb** (*continued*)

C and **D.** The fascial compartments of the thigh (**C**) and leg (**D**) are demonstrated in transverse section. The fascial compartments contain muscles that generally perform common functions and share common innervation, and contain the spread of infection. While both thigh and leg have anterior and posterior compartments, the thigh also includes a medial compartment and the leg a lateral compartment. Trauma to muscles and/or vessels in the compartments may product hemorrhage, edema, and inflammation of the muscles. Because the septa, deep fascia, and bony attachments firmly bound the compartments, increased volume resulting from these processes raises intracompartmental pressure. In compartment syndromes, structures within or distal to the compressed area become ischemic and may become permanently injured (e.g., compression of capillary beds results in denervation and consequent paralysis of muscles). A fasciotomy (incision of bounding fascia or septum) may be performed to relieve the pressure in the compartment and restore circulation.

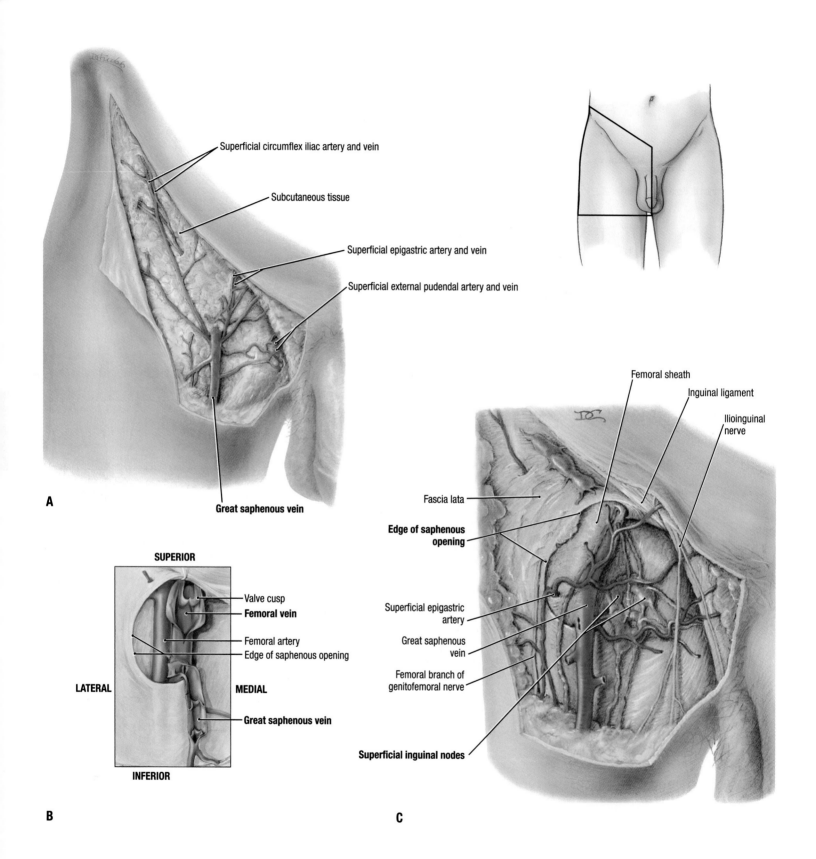

A. Superficial retroinguinal vessels. *(Labels: Superficial circumflex iliac artery and vein; Subcutaneous tissue; Superficial epigastric artery and vein; Superficial external pudendal artery and vein; Great saphenous vein)*

B. *(Labels: SUPERIOR; Valve cusp; Femoral vein; Femoral artery; Edge of saphenous opening; LATERAL; MEDIAL; Great saphenous vein; INFERIOR)*

C. *(Labels: Femoral sheath; Inguinal ligament; Ilioinguinal nerve; Fascia lata; Edge of saphenous opening; Superficial epigastric artery; Great saphenous vein; Femoral branch of genitofemoral nerve; Superficial inguinal nodes)*

5.15   Superficial inguinal vessels and saphenous opening

A. Superficial retroinguinal vessels. The arteries are branches of the femoral artery, and the veins are tributaries of the great saphenous vein. **B.** Valves of the proximal part of femoral and great saphenous veins. **C.** Saphenous opening.

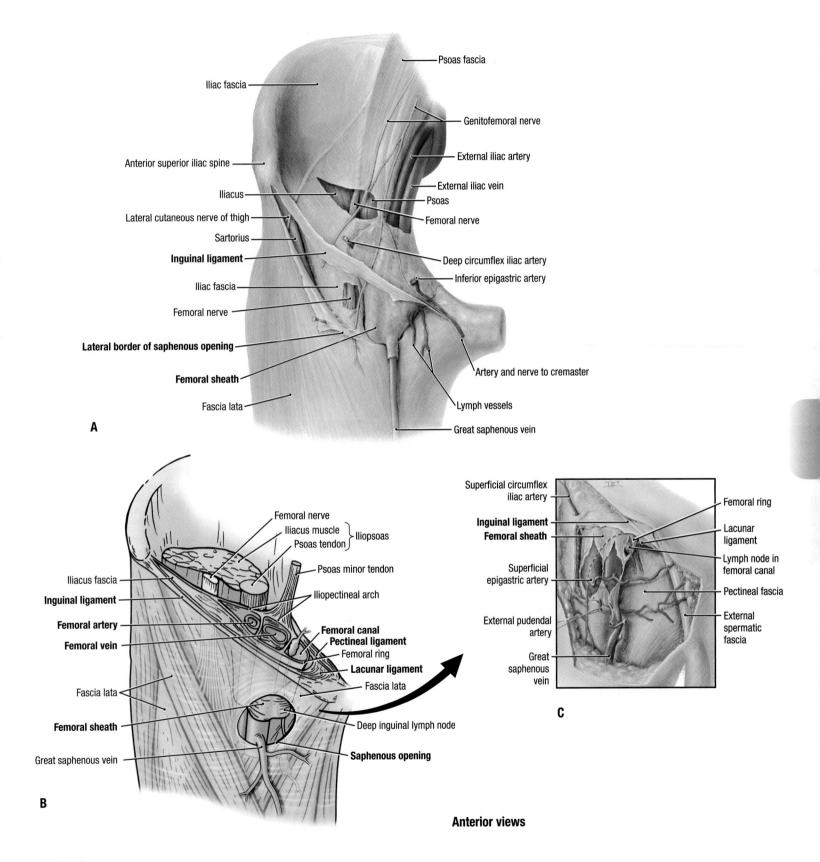

Psoas fascia

Iliac fascia

Genitofemoral nerve

External iliac artery

Anterior superior iliac spine

External iliac vein

Iliacus

Psoas

Lateral cutaneous nerve of thigh

Femoral nerve

Sartorius

Inguinal ligament

Deep circumflex iliac artery

Iliac fascia

Inferior epigastric artery

Femoral nerve

Lateral border of saphenous opening

Femoral sheath

Artery and nerve to cremaster

Fascia lata

Lymph vessels

A

Great saphenous vein

Femoral nerve
Iliacus muscle ⎫ Iliopsoas
Psoas tendon ⎭

Psoas minor tendon

Iliacus fascia

Iliopectineal arch

Inguinal ligament

Femoral artery

Femoral canal

Femoral vein

Pectineal ligament

Femoral ring

Fascia lata

Lacunar ligament

Fascia lata

Femoral sheath

Deep inguinal lymph node

Great saphenous vein

Saphenous opening

B

Superficial circumflex iliac artery

Femoral ring

Inguinal ligament

Lacunar ligament

Femoral sheath

Lymph node in femoral canal

Superficial epigastric artery

Pectineal fascia

External pudendal artery

External spermatic fascia

Great saphenous vein

C

Anterior views

5.16   Femoral sheath and inguinal ligament

A. Dissection. **B.** Schematic illustration. The femoral sheath contains the femoral artery, vein, and lymph vessels, but the femoral nerve, lying posterior to the iliacus fascia, is outside the femoral sheath. **C.** Femoral sheath and femoral ring.

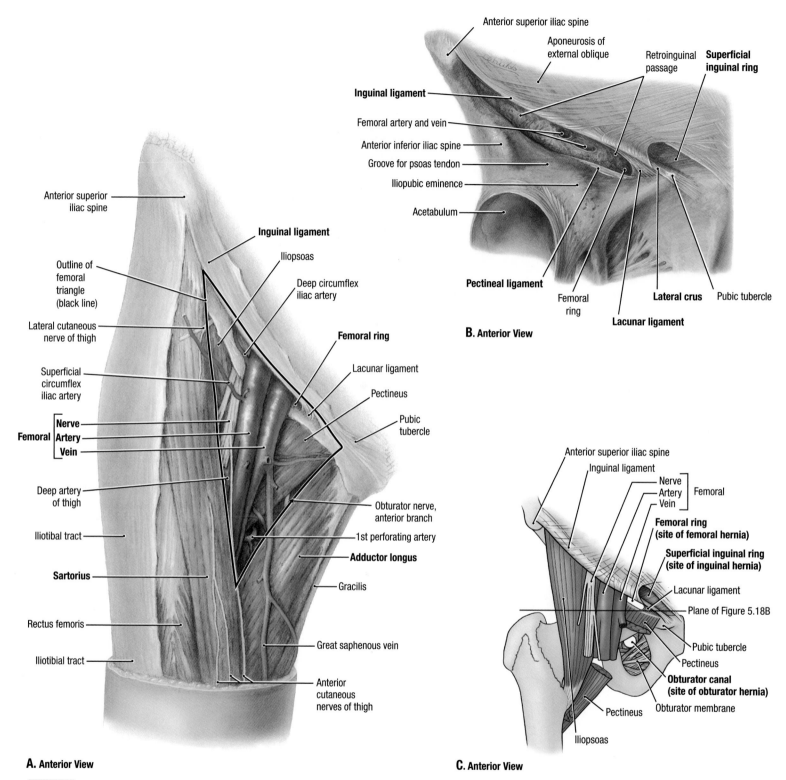

A. Anterior View

B. Anterior View

C. Anterior View

5.17 **Structures passing to/from femoral triangle via retroinguinal passage**

A. Dissection. The boundaries of the femoral triangle are the inguinal ligament superiorly (base of triangle), the medial border of the sartorius (lateral side), and the lateral border of the adductor longus (medial side). The point at which the lateral and medial sides converge inferiorly forms the apex. The femoral triangle is bisected by the femoral vessels. **B.** Retroinguinal passage between the inguinal ligament anteriorly and the bony pelvis posteriorly. **C.** The iliopsoas muscle, the femoral nerve, artery, and vein, and the lymphatic vessels draining the inguinal nodes pass deep to the inguinal ligament to enter the anterior thigh or return to the trunk. Three potential sites for hernia formation are indicated. Pulsations of the femoral artery can be felt distal to the inguinal ligament, midway between the anterior superior iliac spine and the pubic tubercle.

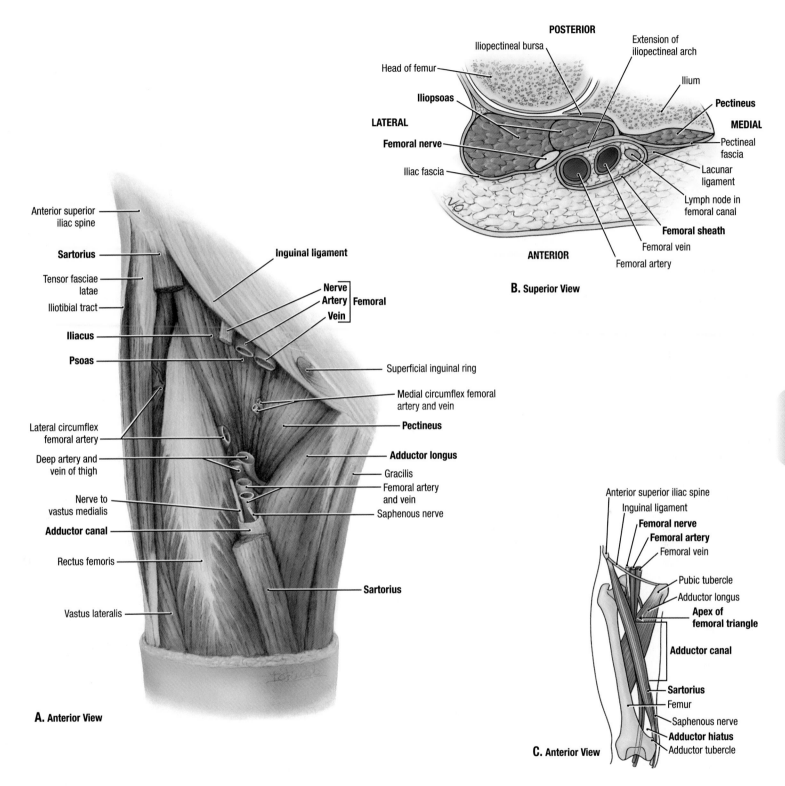

5.18   **Floor of femoral canal and retroinguinal passage**

A. Dissection. Portions of the sartorius muscle, femoral vessels, and femoral nerve have been removed revealing the floor of the femoral triangle, formed by the iliopsoas laterally and the pectineus medially. At the apex of the triangle the femoral vessels, saphenous nerve, and the nerve to the vastus medialis pass deep to the sartorius into the adductor (subsartorial) canal. **B.** Transverse section of the femoral triangle at the level of head of femur. (Level of section is indicated in Fig. 5.17**C**.) The iliopsoas and femoral nerve traverse the retroinguinal passage and femoral triangle in a fascial sheath separate from the femoral vessels, which are contained within the femoral sheath. **C.** Schematic illustration of course of femoral vessels. The adductor canal extends from the triangle's apex to the adductor hiatus, by which the vessels enter and leave the popliteal fossa.

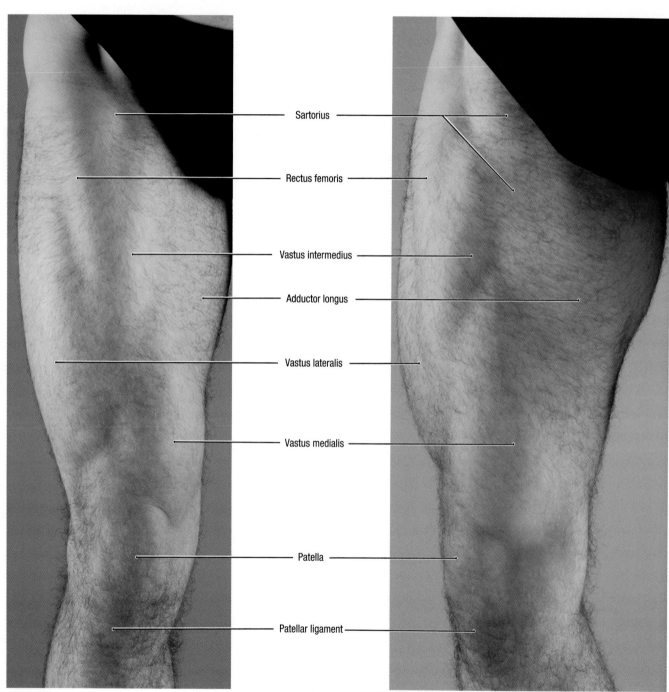

Sartorius

Rectus femoris

Vastus intermedius

Adductor longus

Vastus lateralis

Vastus medialis

Patella

Patellar ligament

A. Anterior View

B. Anteromedial View

5.19   **Surface anatomy of anterior and medial aspects of thigh**

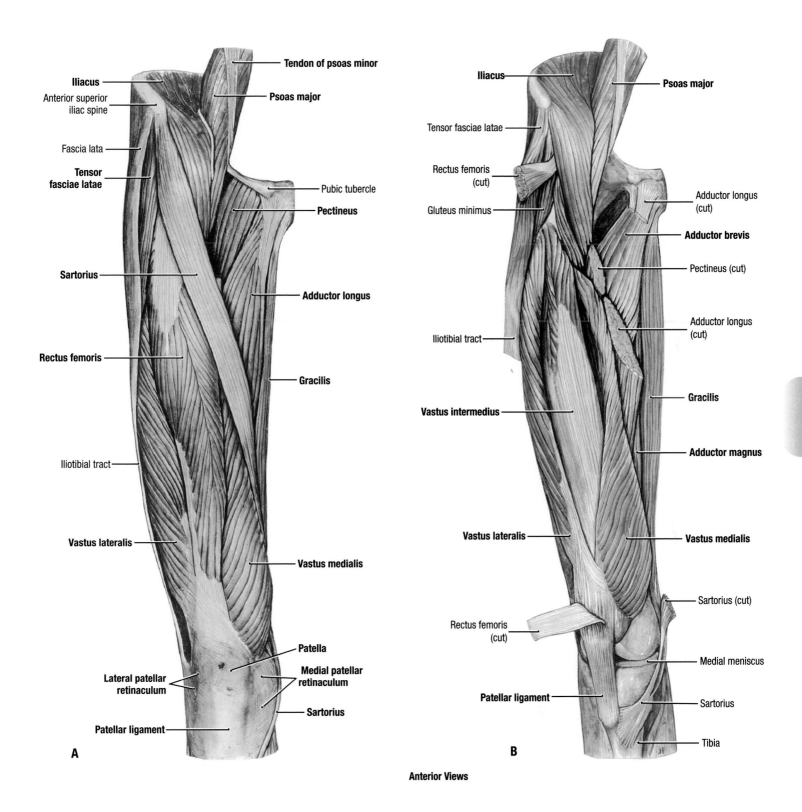

Iliacus
Anterior superior iliac spine
Fascia lata
Tensor fasciae latae
Sartorius
Rectus femoris
Iliotibial tract
Vastus lateralis
Lateral patellar retinaculum
Patellar ligament

Tendon of psoas minor
Psoas major
Pubic tubercle
Pectineus
Adductor longus
Gracilis
Vastus medialis
Patella
Medial patellar retinaculum
Sartorius

A

Iliacus
Tensor fasciae latae
Rectus femoris (cut)
Gluteus minimus
Iliotibial tract
Vastus intermedius
Vastus lateralis
Rectus femoris (cut)
Patellar ligament

Psoas major
Adductor longus (cut)
Adductor brevis
Pectineus (cut)
Adductor longus (cut)
Gracilis
Adductor magnus
Vastus medialis
Sartorius (cut)
Medial meniscus
Sartorius
Tibia

B

Anterior Views

5.20   Anterior and medial thigh muscles

A. Superficial dissection. **B.** Deep dissection. The central portions of the muscle bellies of the sartorius, rectus femoris, pectineus, and adductor longus muscles have been removed. Weakness of the vastus medialis or vastus lateralis, resulting from arthritis or trauma to the knee joint, for example, can result in abnormal patellar movement and loss of joint stability.

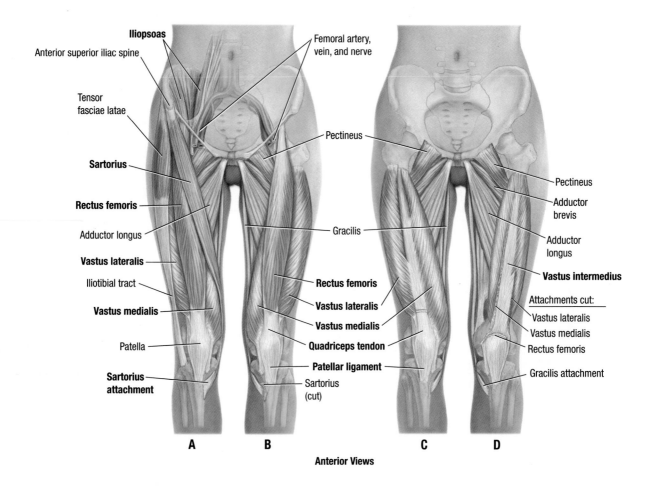

Iliopsoas

Anterior superior iliac spine

Tensor fasciae latae

Sartorius

Rectus femoris

Adductor longus

Vastus lateralis

Iliotibial tract

Vastus medialis

Patella

Sartorius attachment

Femoral artery, vein, and nerve

Pectineus

Gracilis

Rectus femoris

Vastus lateralis

Vastus medialis

Quadriceps tendon

Patellar ligament

Sartorius (cut)

Pectineus

Adductor brevis

Adductor longus

Vastus intermedius

Attachments cut:

Vastus lateralis

Vastus medialis

Rectus femoris

Gracilis attachment

A   B   C   D

Anterior Views

Table 5.2   **Anterior and medial thigh muscles, in situ.**

A to **D.** Sequential dissection from superficial to deep.

A "hip pointer," which is a contusion of the iliac crest, usually occurs at its anterior part (e.g., where the sartorius attaches to the anterior superior iliac spine). This is one of the most common injuries to the hip region, usually occurring in association with collision sports. Contusions cause bleeding from ruptured capillaries and infiltration of blood into the muscles, tendons, and other soft tissues. The term hip pointer may also refer to avulsion of bony muscle attachments, for example, of the sartorius or rectus femoris from the anterior iliac spines or of the iliopsoas from the lesser trochanter of the femur. However, these injuries should be called avulsion fractures.

A person with a paralyzed quadriceps cannot extend the leg against resistance and usually presses on the distal end of the thigh during walking to prevent inadvertent flexion of the knee joint.

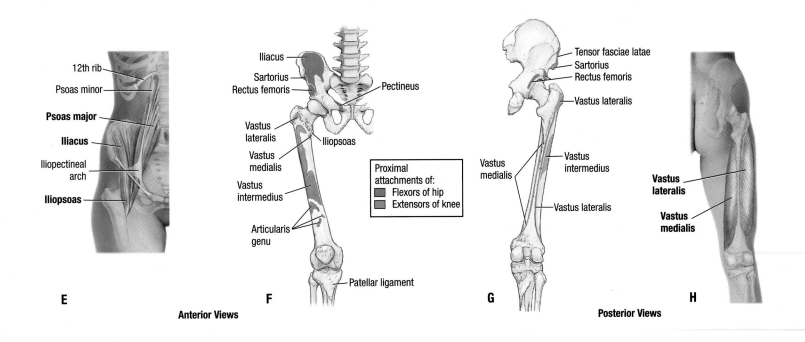

TABLE 5.2 MUSCLES OF ANTERIOR THIGH

Muscle	Proximal Attachment[d]	Distal Attachment[d]	Innervation[a]	Main Actions
Iliopsoas				
Psoas major	Lateral aspects of T12–L5 vertebrae and IV discs; transverse processes of all lumbar vertebrae	Lesser trochanter of femur	Anterior rami of lumbar nerves (**L1, L2,** and L3)	Flexes thigh at hip joint and stabilizes this joint[b]
Iliacus	Iliac crest, iliac fossa, ala of sacrum and anterior sacro-iliac ligaments	Tendon of psoas major, lesser trochanter, and femur distal to it	Femoral nerve (L2 and L3)	
Tensor fasciae latae	Anterior superior iliac spine and anterior part of iliac crest	Iliotibial tract that attaches to lateral condyle of tibia	Superior gluteal (L4 and L5)	Abducts, medially rotates, and flexes thigh; helps to keep knee extended; steadies trunk on thigh
Sartorius	Anterior superior iliac spine and superior part of notch inferior to it	Superior part of medial surface of tibia	Femoral nerve (L2 and L3)	Flexes, abducts, and laterally rotates thigh at hip joint; flexes leg at knee joint[c]
Quadriceps femoris				
Rectus femoris	Anterior inferior iliac spine and ilium superior to acetabulum	Base of patella and by patellar ligament to tibial tuberosity; medial and lateral vasti also attach to tibia and patella via aponeuroses (medial and lateral patellar	Femoral nerve (L2, **L3,** and **L4**)	Extends leg at knee joint; rectus femoris also steadies hip joint and helps iliopsoas to flex thigh
Vastus lateralis	Greater trochanter and lateral lip of linea aspera of femur			
Vastus medialis	Intertrochanteric line and medial lip of linea aspera of femur			
Vastus intermedius	Anterior and lateral surfaces of body of femur			

[a]Numbers indicate spinal cord segmental innervation of nerves (e.g., L1, L2, and L3 indicate that nerves supplying psoas major are derived from first three lumbar segments of the spinal cord; boldface type [**L1, L2**] indicates main segmental innervation). Damage to one or more of these spinal cord segments or to motor nerve roots arising from these segments results in paralysis of the muscles concerned.
[b]Psoas major is also a postural muscle that helps control deviation of trunk and is active during standing.
[c]Four actions of sartorius (L. *sartor,* tailor) produce the once common cross-legged sitting position used by tailors—hence the name.
[d]See also Figure 5.22 for muscle attachments.

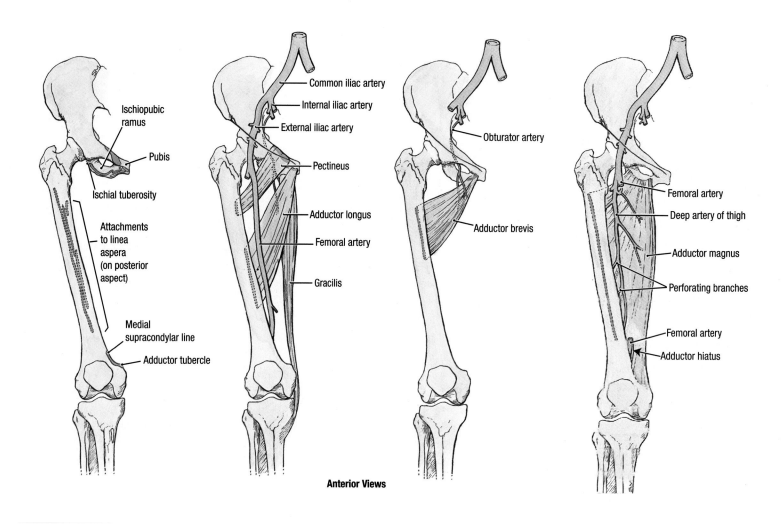

Anterior Views

TABLE 5.3 MUSCLES OF MEDIAL THIGH

Muscle	Proximal Attachment	Distal Attachment[a]	Innervation[b]	Main Actions
Pectineus	Superior pubic ramus	Pectineal line of femur, just inferior to lesser trochanter	Femoral nerve (**L2** and L3) may receive a branch from obturator nerve	Adducts and flexes thigh; assists with medial rotation of thigh
Adductor longus	Body of pubis inferior to pubic crest	Middle third of linea aspera of femur	Obturator nerve, anterior branch (L2, **L3**, and L4)	Adducts thigh
Adductor brevis	Body of pubis and inferior pubic ramus	Pectineal line and proximal part of linea aspera of femur	Obturator nerve (L2, **L3**, and L4)	Adducts thigh and, to some extent, flexes it
Adductor magnus	Inferior pubic ramus, ramus of ischium (adductor part), and ischial tuberosity	Gluteal tuberosity, linea aspera, medial supracondylar line (adductor part), and adductor tubercle of femur (hamstring part)	*Adductor part:* obturator nerve (L2, **L3**, and L4) *Hamstring part:* tibial part of sciatic nerve (**L4**)	Adducts thigh; its adductor part also flexes thigh, and its hamstring part extends it
Gracilis	Body of pubis and inferior pubic ramus	Superior part of medial surface of tibia	Obturator nerve (**L2** and L3)	Adducts thigh, flexes leg, and helps rotate it medially
Obturator externus	Margins of obturator foramen and obturator membrane	Trochanteric fossa of femur	Obturator nerve (L3 and **L4**)	Laterally rotates thigh; steadies head of femur in acetabulum

Collectively, the first five muscles listed are the adductors of the thigh, but their actions are more complex (e.g., they act as flexors of the hip joint during flexion of the knee joint and are active during walking).

[a]See Figure 5.22 for muscle attachments.

[b]See Table 5.1 for explanation of segmental innervation.

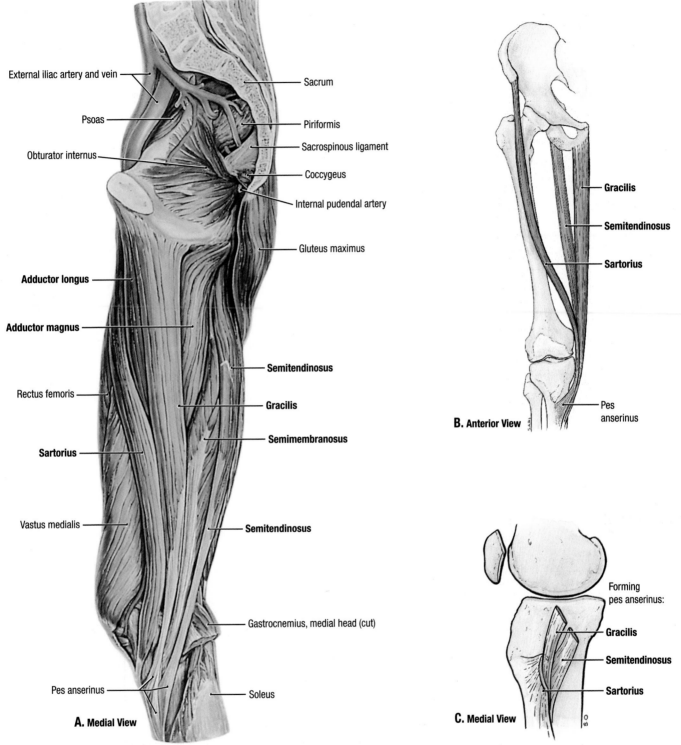

External iliac artery and vein

Psoas

Obturator internus

Adductor longus

Adductor magnus

Rectus femoris

Sartorius

Vastus medialis

Pes anserinus

A. Medial View

Sacrum

Piriformis

Sacrospinous ligament

Coccygeus

Internal pudendal artery

Gluteus maximus

Semitendinosus

Gracilis

Semimembranosus

Semitendinosus

Gastrocnemius, medial head (cut)

Soleus

Gracilis

Semitendinosus

Sartorius

Pes anserinus

B. Anterior View

Forming pes anserinus:

Gracilis

Semitendinosus

Sartorius

C. Medial View

5.21   **Muscles of medial aspect of thigh**

A. Dissection. **B.** Muscular tripod. The sartorius, gracilis, and semitendinosus muscles form an inverted tripod arising from three different components of the hip bone. These muscles course within three different compartments, perform three different functions, and are innervated by three different nerves yet share a common distal attachment. **C.** Distal attachment of sartorius, gracilis, and semitendinosus muscles. All three tendons become thin and aponeurotic and are collectively referred to as the pes anserinus. The gracilis is a relatively weak member of the adductor group and hence can be removed without noticeable loss of its actions on the leg. Surgeons often transplant the gracilis, or part of it, with its nerve and blood vessels to replace a damaged muscle in the hand, for example.

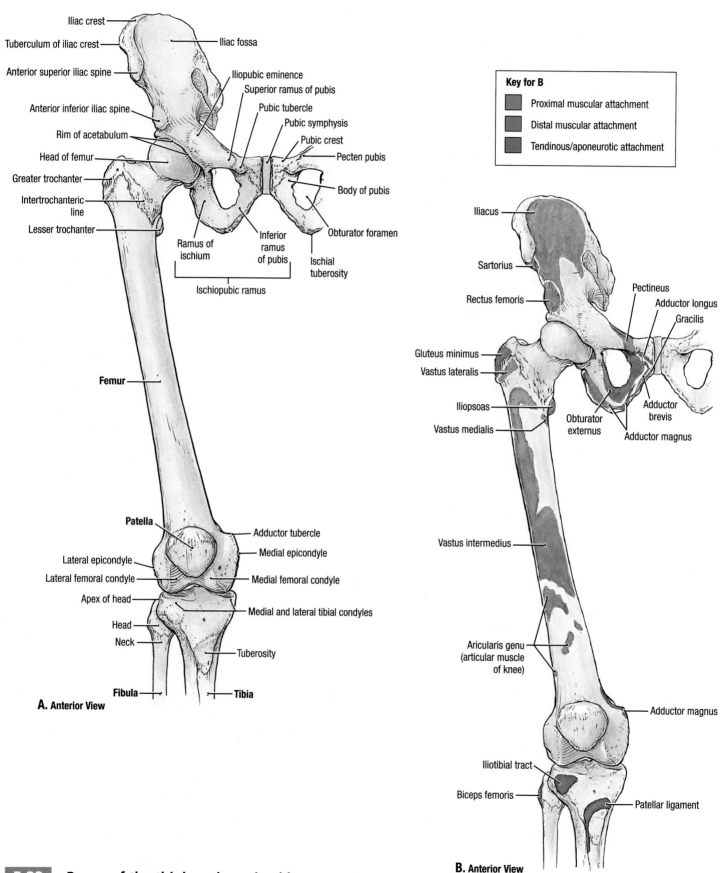

Key for B

Proximal muscular attachment

Distal muscular attachment

Tendinous/aponeurotic attachment

A. Anterior View

B. Anterior View

5.22 **Bones of the thigh and proximal leg**

A. Bony features. B. Muscle attachment sites.

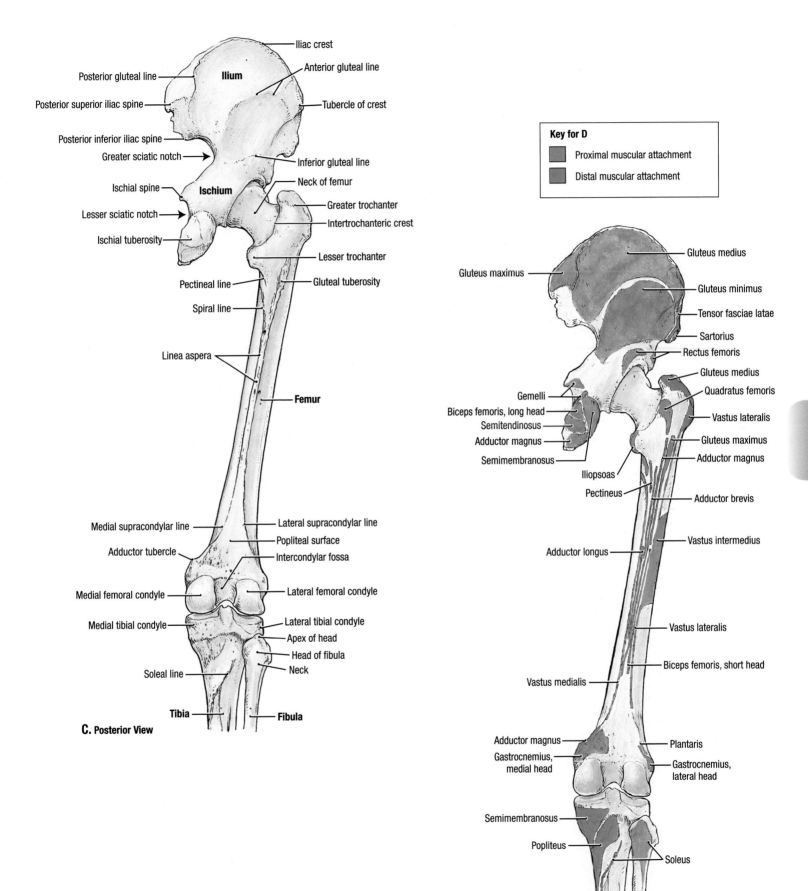

Iliac crest

Posterior gluteal line

Ilium

Anterior gluteal line

Posterior superior iliac spine

Tubercle of crest

Posterior inferior iliac spine

Greater sciatic notch

Inferior gluteal line

Neck of femur

Ischial spine

Ischium

Lesser sciatic notch

Greater trochanter

Ischial tuberosity

Intertrochanteric crest

Lesser trochanter

Pectineal line

Gluteal tuberosity

Spiral line

Linea aspera

Femur

Medial supracondylar line

Lateral supracondylar line

Adductor tubercle

Popliteal surface

Intercondylar fossa

Medial femoral condyle

Lateral femoral condyle

Medial tibial condyle

Lateral tibial condyle

Apex of head

Head of fibula

Neck

Soleal line

Tibia

Fibula

C. Posterior View

Key for D

Proximal muscular attachment

Distal muscular attachment

Gluteus medius

Gluteus maximus

Gluteus minimus

Tensor fasciae latae

Sartorius

Rectus femoris

Gluteus medius

Gemelli

Quadratus femoris

Biceps femoris, long head

Semitendinosus

Vastus lateralis

Adductor magnus

Gluteus maximus

Semimembranosus

Adductor magnus

Iliopsoas

Pectineus

Adductor brevis

Vastus intermedius

Adductor longus

Vastus lateralis

Biceps femoris, short head

Vastus medialis

Adductor magnus

Plantaris

Gastrocnemius, medial head

Gastrocnemius, lateral head

Semimembranosus

Popliteus

Soleus

D. Posterior View

5.22   **Bones of the thigh and proximal leg (continued)**

C. Bony features. **D.** Muscle attachment sites.

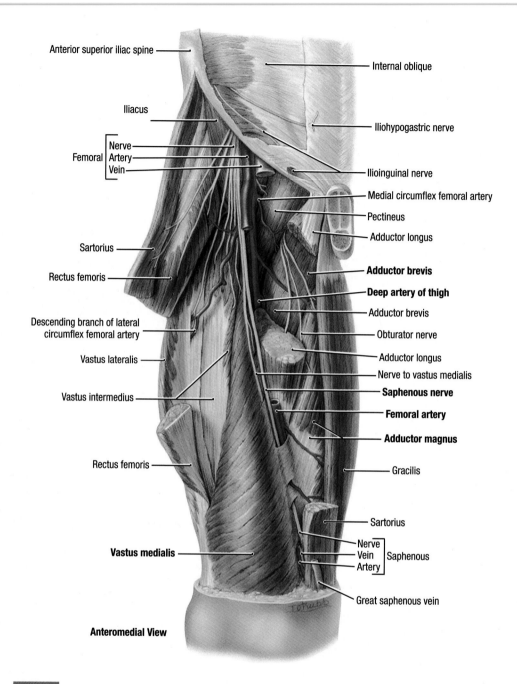

Anterior superior iliac spine

Iliacus

Femoral { Nerve
Artery
Vein

Sartorius

Rectus femoris

Descending branch of lateral
circumflex femoral artery

Vastus lateralis

Vastus intermedius

Rectus femoris

Vastus medialis

Internal oblique

Iliohypogastric nerve

Ilioinguinal nerve

Medial circumflex femoral artery

Pectineus

Adductor longus

Adductor brevis

Deep artery of thigh

Adductor brevis

Obturator nerve

Adductor longus

Nerve to vastus medialis

Saphenous nerve

Femoral artery

Adductor magnus

Gracilis

Sartorius

Saphenous { Nerve
Vein
Artery

Great saphenous vein

Anteromedial View

5.23 Anteromedial aspect of thigh

- The limb is rotated laterally.
- The femoral nerve breaks up into several nerves on entering the thigh.
- The femoral artery lies between two motor territories: that of the obturator nerve, which is medial, and that of the femoral nerve, which is lateral. No motor nerve crosses anterior to the femoral artery, but the twig to the pectineus muscle crosses posterior to the femoral artery.
- The nerve to the vastus medialis muscle and the saphenous nerve accompany the femoral artery into the adductor canal. The saphenous nerve and artery and their anastomotic accompanying vein emerge from the canal distally between the sartorius and gracilis muscles.
- The deep artery of the thigh arises approximately 4 cm distal to the inguinal ligament, lies posterior to the femoral artery, and disappears posterior to the adductor longus muscle. It supplies the thigh through the medial and lateral circumflex femoral branches and the perforating arteries that pass through the adductor magnus muscle on their way to the posterior aspect of the thigh.

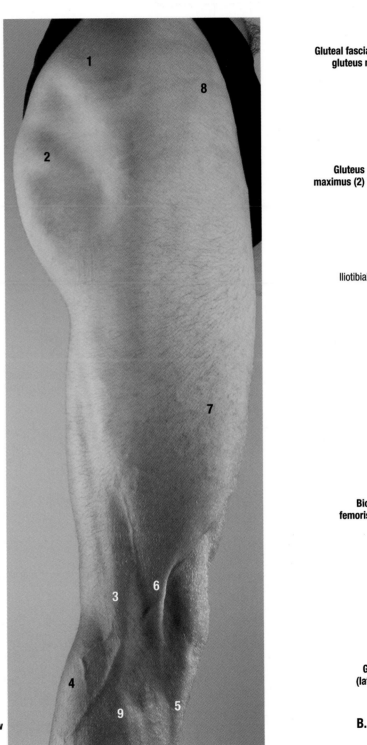

A. Lateral View

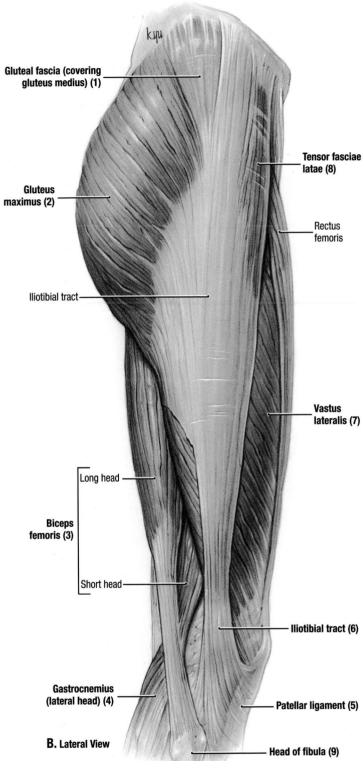

Gluteal fascia (covering gluteus medius) (1)

Tensor fasciae latae (8)

Gluteus maximus (2)

Rectus femoris

Iliotibial tract

Vastus lateralis (7)

Long head

Biceps femoris (3)

Short head

Iliotibial tract (6)

Gastrocnemius (lateral head) (4)

Patellar ligament (5)

B. Lateral View

Head of fibula (9)

5.24   **Lateral aspect of thigh**

A. Surface anatomy (*numbers* refer to structures in **B**). **B.** Dissection showing the iliotibial tract, a thickening of the fascia lata, which serves as a tendon for the gluteus maximus and tensor fasciae latae. The iliotibial tract attaches to the anterolateral (Gerdy) tubercle of the lateral condyle of the tibia. The biceps femoris tendon attaches on the head of the fibula.

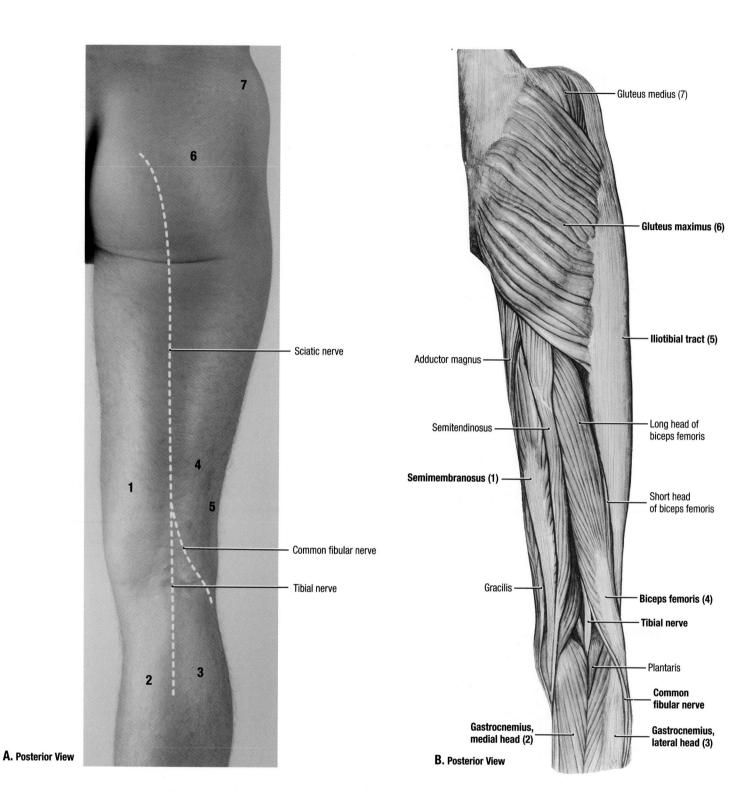

A. Posterior View

Sciatic nerve

Common fibular nerve

Tibial nerve

Gluteus medius (7)

Gluteus maximus (6)

Iliotibial tract (5)

Adductor magnus

Semitendinosus

Long head of biceps femoris

Semimembranosus (1)

Short head of biceps femoris

Gracilis

Biceps femoris (4)

Tibial nerve

Plantaris

Common fibular nerve

Gastrocnemius, medial head (2)

Gastrocnemius, lateral head (3)

B. Posterior View

5.25   Muscles of the gluteal region and posterior aspect of thigh—I

A. Surface anatomy (*numbers* refer to structures in **B**). **B.** Superficial dissection of muscles of gluteal region and posterior thigh (hamstring muscles consisting of semimembranosus, semitendinosus, and biceps femoris). Hamstring strains (pulled and/or torn hamstrings) are common in running, jumping, and quick-start sports. The muscular exertion required to excel in these sports may tear part of the proximal attachments of the hamstrings from the ischial tuberosity.

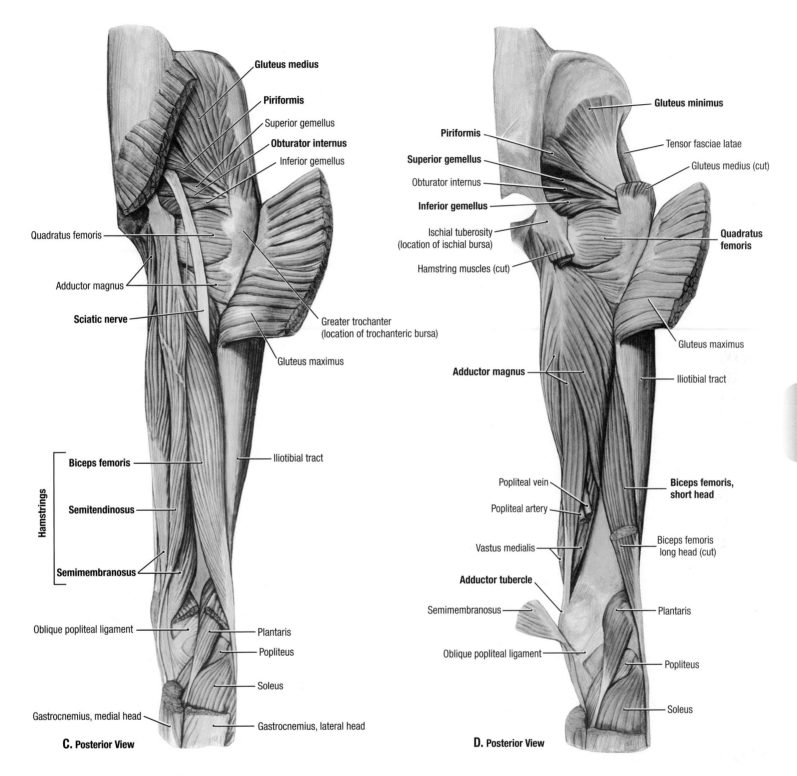

5.25 **Muscles of gluteal region and posterior aspect of thigh—**
(continued)—II and III

C. Muscles of gluteal region and posterior thigh with gluteus maximus reflected.
D. Adductor magnus muscle. The adductor magnus is a large muscle with two parts: one belongs to the adductor group and the other to the hamstring group. The adductor part is innervated by the obturator nerve and the hamstring part by the tibial portion of the sciatic nerve. The trochanteric bursa separates the superior fibers of the gluteus maximus from the greater trochanter of the femur.

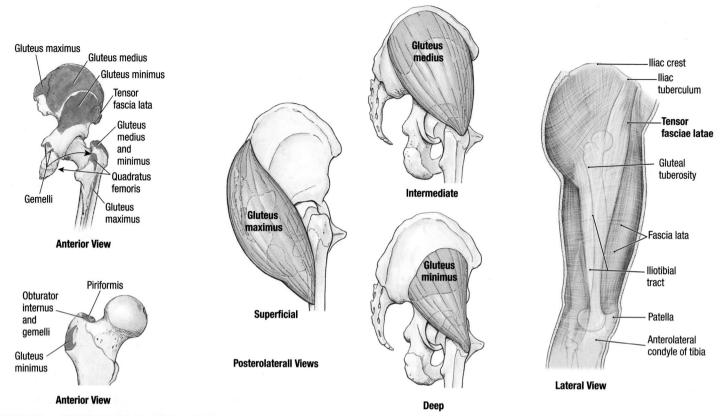

Anterior View

Anterior View

Superficial

Posterolaterall Views

Intermediate

Deep

Lateral View

TABLE 5.4 MUSCLES OF GLUTEAL REGION

Muscle	Proximal Attachment[a] (red)	Distal Attachment[a] (blue)	Innervation[b]	Main Actions
Gluteus maximus	Ilium posterior to posterior gluteal line, dorsal surface of sacrum and coccyx, sacro-tuberous ligament	Iliotibial tract that inserts into lateral condyle of tibia; some fibers to gluteal tuberosity	Inferior gluteal nerve (L5, **S1**, **S2**)	Extends thigh and assists in lateral rotation; steadies thigh and assists in raising trunk from flexed position
Gluteus medius	External surface of ilium between anterior and posterior gluteal lines; gluteal fascia	Lateral surface of greater trochanter of femur	Superior gluteal nerve (**L5**, S1)	Abducts and medially rotates thigh; keeps pelvis level when opposite leg is off ground and advances pelvis during swing phase of gait; TFL also contributes to stability of extended knee
Gluteus minimus	External surface of ilium between anterior and inferior gluteal lines	Anterior surface of greater trochanter of femur		
Tensor fasciae latae (TFL)	Anterior superior iliac spine and iliac crest	Iliotibial tract that attaches to lateral condyle (Gerdy tubercle) of tibia		
Piriformis	Anterior surface of sacrum and sacrotuberous ligament	Superior border of greater trochanter of femur	Anterior rami of S1 and S2	Laterally rotate extended thigh and abduct flexed thigh; steady femoral head in acetabulum
Obturator internus	Pelvic surface of obturator membrane and surrounding bones	Medial surface of greater trochanter of femur by common tendons	Nerve to obturator internus (L5, S1) Nerve to quadratus femoris (L5, S1)	
Superior gemellus	Ischial spine			
Inferior gemellus	Ischial tuberosity			
Quadratus femoris	Lateral border of ischial tuberosity	Quadrate tubercle on intertrochanteric crest of femur		Laterally rotates thigh,[c] steadies femoral head in acetabulum

[a]See Figure 5.22 for muscle attachments.
[b]See Table 5.1 for explanation of segmental innervation.
[c]There are six lateral rotators of the thigh: piriformis, obturator internus, gemelli (superior and inferior), quadratus femoris, and obturator externus. These muscles also stabilize the hip joint.

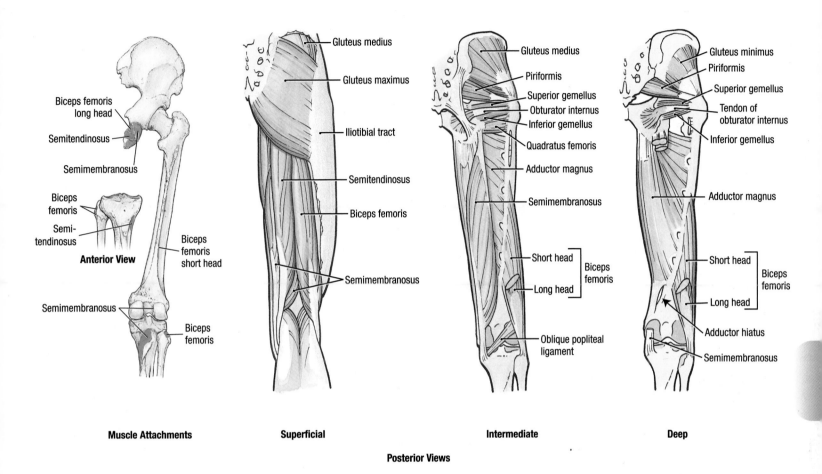

Muscle Attachments   **Superficial**   **Intermediate**   **Deep**

Posterior Views

TABLE 5.5 MUSCLES OF POSTERIOR THIGH (HAMSTRING)

Muscle[a]	Proximal Attachment[a] *(red)*	Distal Attachment[a] *(blue)*	Innervation[b]	Main Actions
Semitendinosus	Ischial tuberosity	Medial surface of superior part of tibia	Tibial division of sciatic nerve (**L5**, **S1**, and S2)	Extend thigh; flex leg and rotate it medially; when thigh and leg are flexed, can extend trunk
Semimembranosus		Posterior part of medial condyle of tibia; reflected attachment forms oblique popliteal ligament to lateral femoral condyle		
Biceps femoris	*Long head:* ischial tuberosity; *Short head:* linea aspera and lateral supracondylar line of femur	Lateral side of head of fibula; tendon is split at this site by fibular collateral ligament of knee	*Long head:* tibial division of sciatic nerve (L5, **S1**, and S2); *Short head:* common fibular (peroneal) division of sciatic nerve (L5, **S1**, and S2)	Flexes leg and rotates it laterally; extends thigh (e.g., when initiating a walking gait)

[a]See Figure 5.22 for muscle attachments.
[b]See Table 5.1 for explanation of segmental innervation.

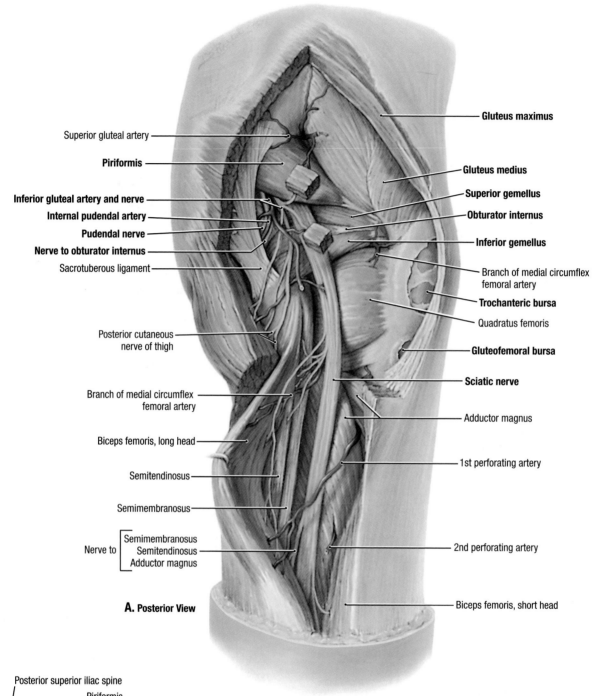

Gluteus maximus

Superior gluteal artery

Piriformis

Gluteus medius

Superior gemellus

Inferior gluteal artery and nerve

Obturator internus

Internal pudendal artery

Pudendal nerve

Inferior gemellus

Nerve to obturator internus

Sacrotuberous ligament

Branch of medial circumflex femoral artery

Trochanteric bursa

Quadratus femoris

Posterior cutaneous nerve of thigh

Gluteofemoral bursa

Sciatic nerve

Branch of medial circumflex femoral artery

Adductor magnus

Biceps femoris, long head

1st perforating artery

Semitendinosus

Semimembranosus

Nerve to Semimembranosus / Semitendinosus / Adductor magnus

2nd perforating artery

A. Posterior View

Biceps femoris, short head

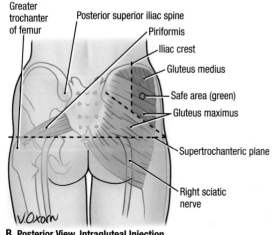

Greater trochanter of femur

Posterior superior iliac spine

Piriformis

Iliac crest

Gluteus medius

Safe area (green)

Gluteus maximus

Supertrochanteric plane

Right sciatic nerve

V.Oxorn

B. Posterior View, Intragluteal Injection

5.26   Muscles of gluteal region and posterior aspect of thigh—IV

A. Dissection. The gluteus maximus muscle is split superiorly and inferiorly, and the middle part is excised; two cubes remain to identify its nerve. The gluteus maximus is the only muscle to cover the greater trochanter; it is aponeurotic and has underlying bursae where it glides on the trochanter (trochanteric bursa) and the aponeurosis of the vastus lateralis muscle (gluteofemoral bursa). Diffuse deep pain in the lateral thigh region, especially during stair climbing or rising from a seated position, may be caused by trochanteric bursitis. This type of friction bursitis is characterized by point tenderness over the greater trochanter; however, the pain radiates along the iliotibial tract. **B. Intragluteal injection.** Injections can be made safely only into the superolateral part of the buttock, avoiding injury to the sciatic and gluteal nerves.

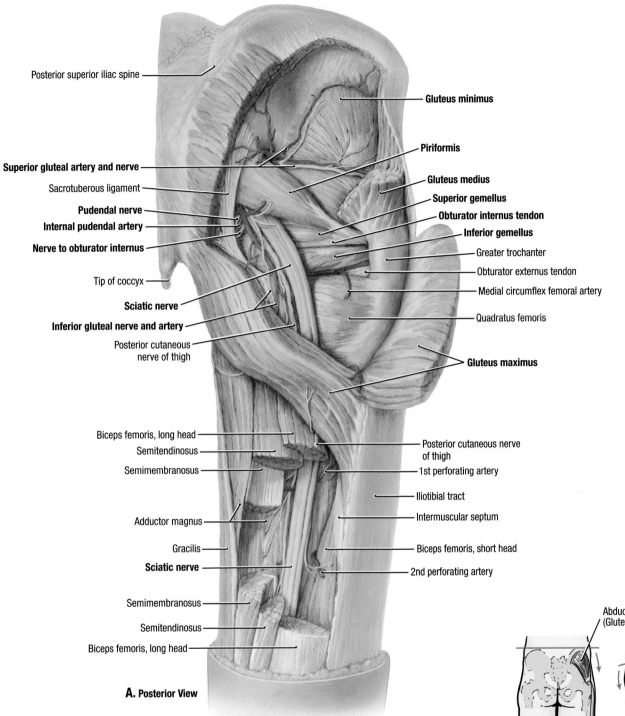

Posterior superior iliac spine

Gluteus minimus

Piriformis

Superior gluteal artery and nerve

Gluteus medius

Sacrotuberous ligament

Superior gemellus

Pudendal nerve

Obturator internus tendon

Internal pudendal artery

Inferior gemellus

Nerve to obturator internus

Greater trochanter

Obturator externus tendon

Tip of coccyx

Medial circumflex femoral artery

Sciatic nerve

Quadratus femoris

Inferior gluteal nerve and artery

Posterior cutaneous
nerve of thigh

Gluteus maximus

Biceps femoris, long head

Posterior cutaneous nerve
of thigh

Semitendinosus

1st perforating artery

Semimembranosus

Iliotibial tract

Intermuscular septum

Adductor magnus

Biceps femoris, short head

Gracilis

2nd perforating artery

Sciatic nerve

Semimembranosus

Semitendinosus

Biceps femoris, long head

A. Posterior View

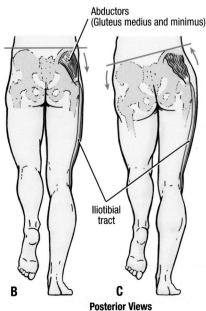

Abductors
(Gluteus medius and minimus)

Iliotibial
tract

B   C

Posterior Views

5.27   **Muscles of gluteal region and posterior aspect of thigh—V**

A. The proximal three quarters of the gluteus maximus muscle is reflected, and parts of the gluteus medius and the three hamstring muscles are excised. The superior gluteal vessels and nerves emerge superior to the piriformis muscle; all other vessels and nerves emerge inferior to it. **B.** When the weight is borne by one limb, the muscles on the supported side fix the pelvis so that it does not sag to the unsupported side, keeping the pelvis level. **C.** When the right abductors are paralyzed, owing to a lesion of the right superior gluteal nerve, fixation by these muscles is lost and the pelvis tilts to the unsupported left side (positive Trendelenburg sign).

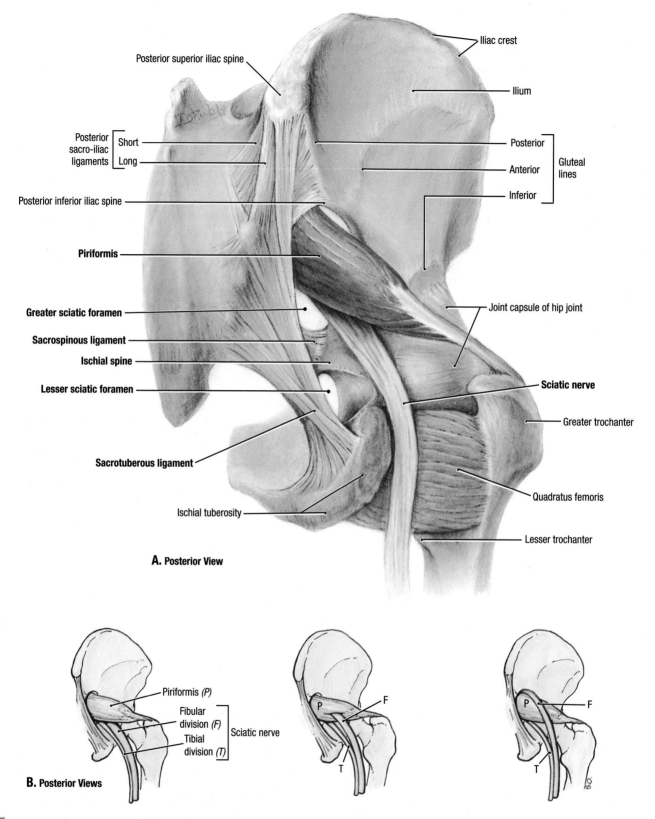

Posterior superior iliac spine

Iliac crest

Ilium

Posterior sacro-iliac ligaments { Short / Long }

Posterior

Anterior   } Gluteal lines

Inferior

Posterior inferior iliac spine

Piriformis

Joint capsule of hip joint

Greater sciatic foramen

Sacrospinous ligament

Ischial spine

Sciatic nerve

Lesser sciatic foramen

Greater trochanter

Sacrotuberous ligament

Quadratus femoris

Ischial tuberosity

Lesser trochanter

A. Posterior View

Piriformis *(P)*

Fibular division *(F)*

Tibial division *(T)*   } Sciatic nerve

P   F

T

P   F

T

B. Posterior Views

5.28   Lateral rotators of hip, sciatic nerve, and ligaments of gluteal region

A. Piriformis and quadratus femoris. In the anatomical position the tip of the coccyx lies superior to the level of the ischial tuberosity and inferior to that of the ischial spine. The lateral border of the sciatic nerve lies midway between the lateral surface of the greater trochanter and the medial surface of the ischial tuberosity.

B. Relationship of sciatic nerve to piriformis muscle. Of 640 limbs studied in Dr. Grant's laboratory, in 87%, the tibial and fibular (peroneal) divisions passed inferior to the piriformis *(left)*; in 12.2%, the fibular (peroneal) division passed through the piriformis *(center)*; and in 0.5% the fibular (peroneal) division passed superior to the piriformis *(right)*.

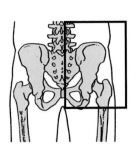

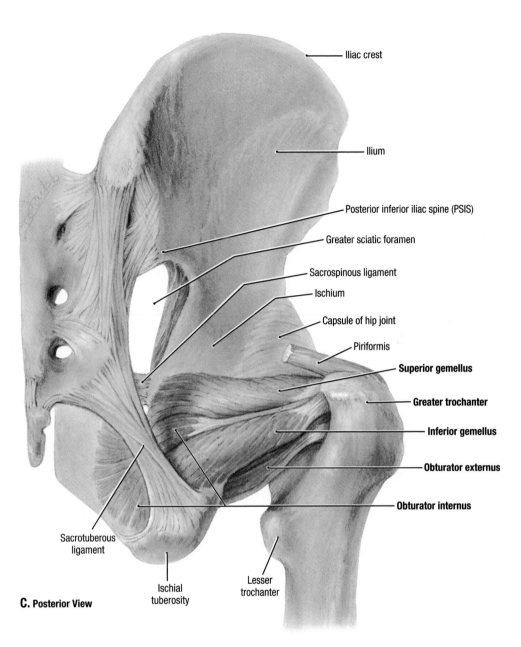

Iliac crest

Ilium

Posterior inferior iliac spine (PSIS)

Greater sciatic foramen

Sacrospinous ligament

Ischium

Capsule of hip joint

Piriformis

Superior gemellus

Greater trochanter

Inferior gemellus

Obturator externus

Obturator internus

Sacrotuberous
ligament

Ischial
tuberosity

Lesser
trochanter

C. Posterior View

5.28 **Lateral rotators of hip, sciatic nerve, and ligaments of gluteal region (continued)**

C. Obturator internus, obturator externus, and superior and inferior gemelli.

- The obturator internus is located partly in the pelvis, where it covers most of the lateral wall of the lesser pelvis. It leaves the pelvis through the lesser sciatic foramen, makes a right-angle turn, becomes tendinous, and receives the distal attachments of the gemelli before attaching to the medial surface of the greater trochanter (trochanteric fossa).

- The obturator externus extends from the external surface of the obturator membrane and surrounding bone of the pelvis to the posterior aspect of the greater trochanter, passing directly under the acetabulum and neck of the femur.

- Sensation conveyed by the sciatic nerve can be blocked by injecting an anesthetic agent a few centimeters inferior to the midpoint of the line joining the PSIS and the superior border of the greater trochanter. Paresthesia radiates to the foot because of anesthesia of the plantar nerves, which are terminal branches of the tibial nerve derived from the sciatic nerve.

- In the approximately 12% of people in whom the common fibular division of the sciatic nerve passes through the piriformis, this muscle may compress the nerve.

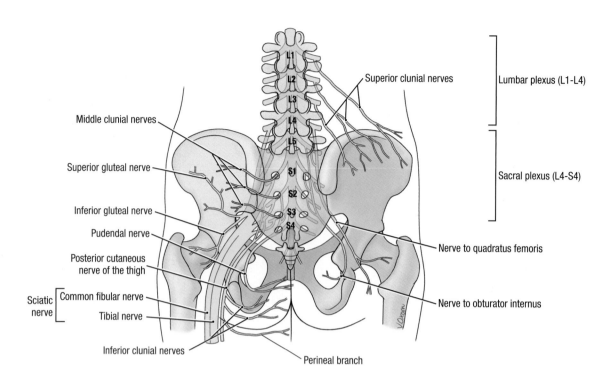

TABLE 5.6 NERVES OF GLUTEAL REGION

Nerve	Origin	Course	Distribution in Gluteal Region
Clunial (superior, middle, and inferior)	*Superior:* posterior rami of L1–L3 nerves *Middle:* posterior rami of S1–S3 nerves *Inferior:* posterior cutaneous nerve of thigh	*Superior nerves* cross iliac crest; *middle nerves* exit through posterior sacral foramina and enter gluteal region; *inferior nerves* curve around inferior border of gluteal maximus	Gluteal region as far laterally as greater trochanter
Sciatic	Sacral plexus (L4–S3)	Exits pelvis via greater sciatic foramen inferior to piriformis to enter gluteal region	No muscles in gluteal region
Posterior cutaneous nerve of thigh	Sacral plexus (S1–S3)	Exits pelvis via greater sciatic foramen inferior to piriformis, emerges from inferior border of gluteus maximus coursing deep to fascia lata	Skin of buttock via inferior cluneal branches, skin over posterior thigh and popliteal fossa; skin of lateral perineum and upper medial thigh via perineal branch
Superior gluteal	Anterior rami of L4–S1 nerves	Exits pelvis via greater sciatic foramen superior to piriformis; courses between gluteus medius and minimus	Gluteus medius, gluteus minimus, and tensor fasciae latae
Inferior gluteal	Anterior rami of L5–S2 nerves	Exits pelvis via greater sciatic foramen inferior to piriformis, dividing into multiple branches	Gluteus maximus
Nerve to quadratus femoris	Anterior rami of L4–S1 nerves	Exits pelvis via greater sciatic foramen deep to sciatic nerve	Posterior hip joint, inferior gemellus, and quadratus femoris
Pudendal	Anterior rami of S2–S4 nerves	Exits pelvis via greater sciatic foramen inferior to piriformis; descends posterior to sacrospinous ligament; enters perineum (pudendal canal) through lesser sciatic foramen	No structures in gluteal region (supplies most of perineum)
Nerve to obturator internus	Anterior rami of L5–S2 nerves	Exits pelvis via greater sciatic foramen inferior to piriformis; descends posterior to ischial spine; enters lesser sciatic foramen and passes to obturator internus	Superior gemellus and obturator internus

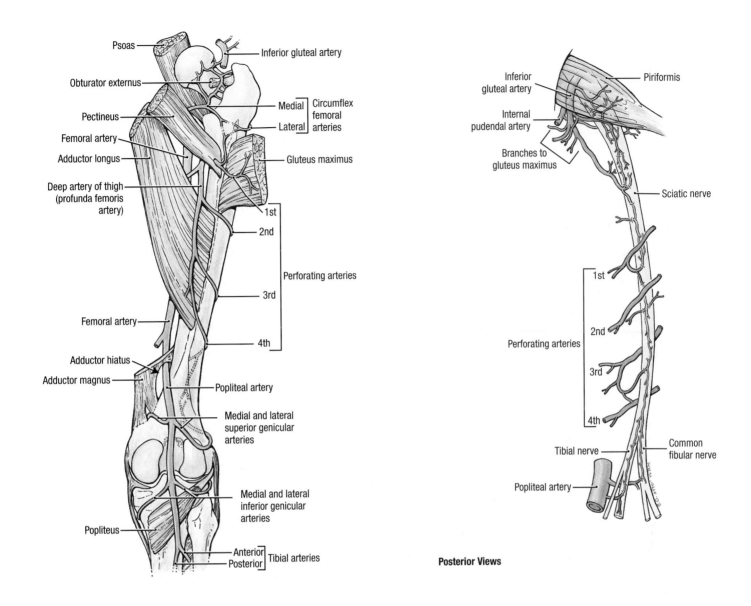

Posterior Views

TABLE 5.7 ARTERIES OF GLUTEAL REGION AND POSTERIOR THIGH

Artery	Course	Distribution/Structures Supplied
Superior gluteal	Enters gluteal region through greater sciatic foramen superior to piriformis; divides into superficial and deep branches; anastomoses with inferior gluteal and medial circumflex femoral arteries	*Superficial branch:* superior gluteus maximus *Deep branch:* runs between gluteus medius and minimus, supplying both and tensor fasciae latae
Inferior gluteal	Enters gluteal region through greater sciatic foramen inferior to piriformis; descends on medial side of sciatic nerve; anastomoses with superior gluteal artery and participates in cruciate anastomosis of thigh	Inferior gluteus maximus, obturator internus, quadratus femoris, and superior parts of hamstring muscles
Internal pudendal	Enters gluteal region through greater sciatic foramen; descends posterior to ischial spine; exits gluteal region via lesser sciatic foramen to perineum	No structures in gluteal region (supplies external genitalia and muscles in perineal region)
Perforating arteries (from deep femoral artery)	Perforate aponeurotic portion of adductor magnus attachment and medial intermuscular septum to enter and supply muscular branches to posterior compartment; then pierce lateral intermuscular septum to enter posterolateral aspect of anterior compartment	Majority (central portions) of hamstring muscles in posterior compartment; posterior portion of vastus lateralis in anterior compartment; femur (via femoral nutrient arteries); reinforce arterial supply of sciatic nerve

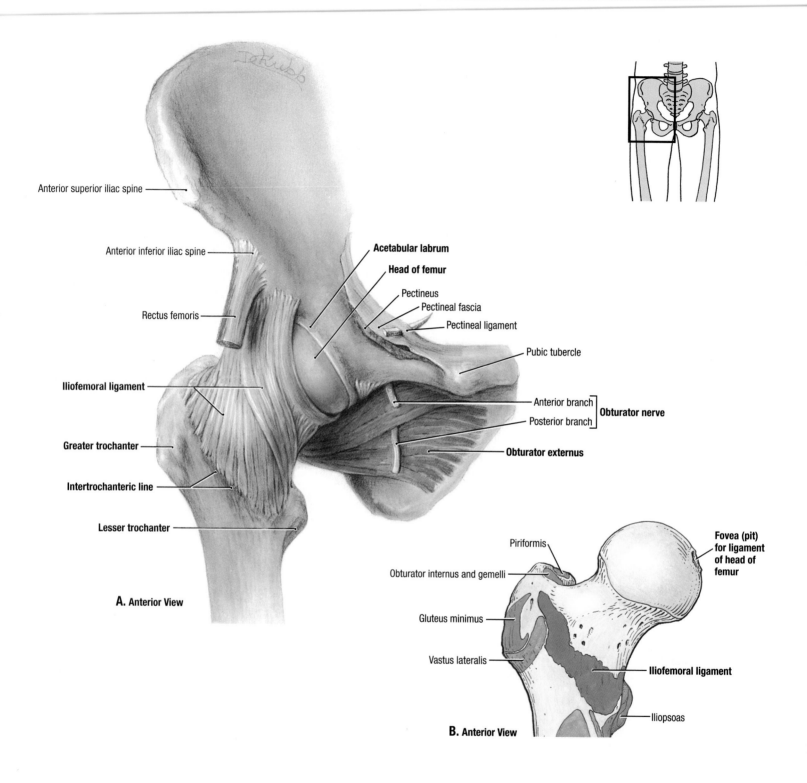

Anterior superior iliac spine

Anterior inferior iliac spine

Rectus femoris

Iliofemoral ligament

Greater trochanter

Intertrochanteric line

Lesser trochanter

A. Anterior View

Acetabular labrum

Head of femur

Pectineus

Pectineal fascia

Pectineal ligament

Pubic tubercle

Anterior branch ⎤
                  ⎬ **Obturator nerve**
Posterior branch ⎦

Obturator externus

Piriformis

Obturator internus and gemelli

Gluteus minimus

Vastus lateralis

**Fovea (pit)
for ligament
of head of
femur**

Iliofemoral ligament

Iliopsoas

B. Anterior View

5.29   Hip joint

A. Iliofemoral ligament. **B.** Muscle attachments of anterior aspect of the proximal femur.
In **A**:

- The head of the femur is exposed just medial to the iliofemoral ligament and faces superiorly, medially, and anteriorly. At the site of the subtendinous bursa of psoas, the capsule is weak or (as in this specimen) partially deficient, but it is guarded by the psoas tendon.
- The iliofemoral ligament, shaped like an inverted "Y." Superiorly it is attached deep to the rectus femoris muscle; the ligament becomes tight on medial rotation of the femur.
- The pectineus muscle is thin, and its fascia blends with the pectineal ligament.

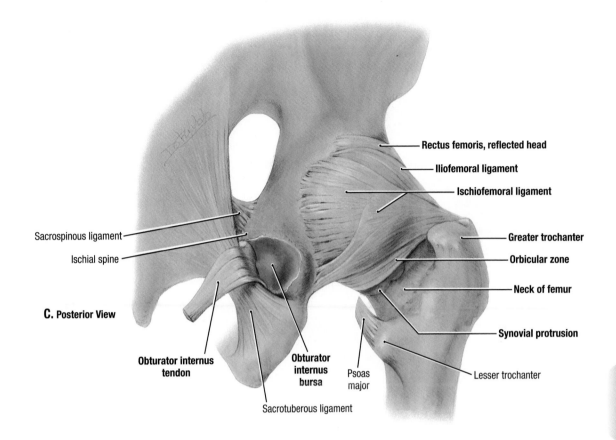

C. Posterior View

Rectus femoris, reflected head

Iliofemoral ligament

Ischiofemoral ligament

Sacrospinous ligament

Ischial spine

Greater trochanter

Orbicular zone

Neck of femur

Synovial protrusion

Obturator internus
tendon

Obturator
internus
bursa

Psoas
major

Lesser trochanter

Sacrotuberous ligament

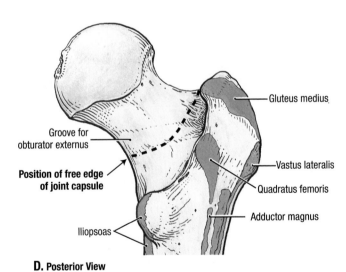

Gluteus medius

Groove for
obturator externus

Position of free edge
of joint capsule

Vastus lateralis

Quadratus femoris

Adductor magnus

Iliopsoas

D. Posterior View

5.29   Hip joint *(continued)*

C. Ischiofemoral ligament. **D.** Muscle attachments onto the posterior aspect of proximal femur. In **C:**

- The fibers of the capsule spiral to become taut during extension and medial rotation of the femur.
- The synovial membrane protrudes inferior to the fibrous capsule and forms a bursa for the tendon of the obturator externus muscle. Note the large subtendinous bursa of the obturator internus at the lesser sciatic notch, where the tendon turns 90° to attach to the greater trochanter.

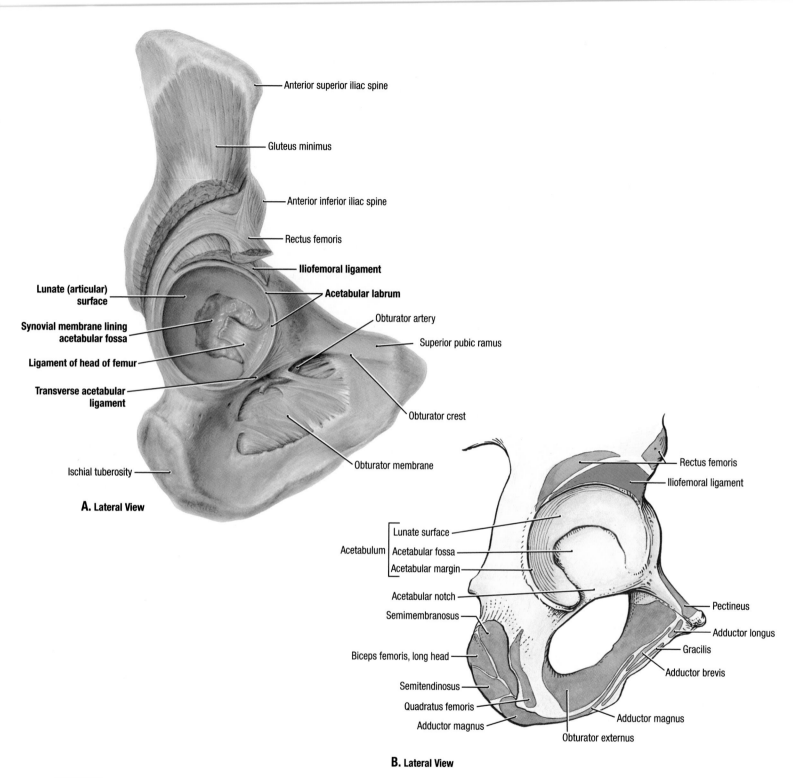

Anterior superior iliac spine

Gluteus minimus

Anterior inferior iliac spine

Rectus femoris

Iliofemoral ligament

Lunate (articular) surface

Acetabular labrum

Obturator artery

Synovial membrane lining acetabular fossa

Superior pubic ramus

Ligament of head of femur

Transverse acetabular ligament

Obturator crest

Ischial tuberosity

Obturator membrane

A. Lateral View

Rectus femoris

Iliofemoral ligament

Acetabulum
— Lunate surface
— Acetabular fossa
— Acetabular margin

Acetabular notch

Semimembranosus

Biceps femoris, long head

Semitendinosus

Quadratus femoris

Adductor magnus

Obturator externus

Adductor magnus

Pectineus

Adductor longus

Gracilis

Adductor brevis

B. Lateral View

5.30   Acetabular region

A. Dissection of acetabulum. **B.** Muscle attachments of acetabular region.

In **A**:

• The transverse acetabular ligament bridges the acetabular notch.
• The acetabular labrum is attached to the acetabular rim and transverse acetabular ligament and forms a complete ring around the head of the femur.
• The ligament of the head of the femur lies between the head of the femur and the acetabulum. These fibers are attached superiorly to the pit (fovea) on the head of the femur and inferiorly to the transverse acetabular ligament and the margins of the acetabular notch. The artery of the ligament of the head of the femur passes through the acetabular notch and into the ligament of the head of the femur.

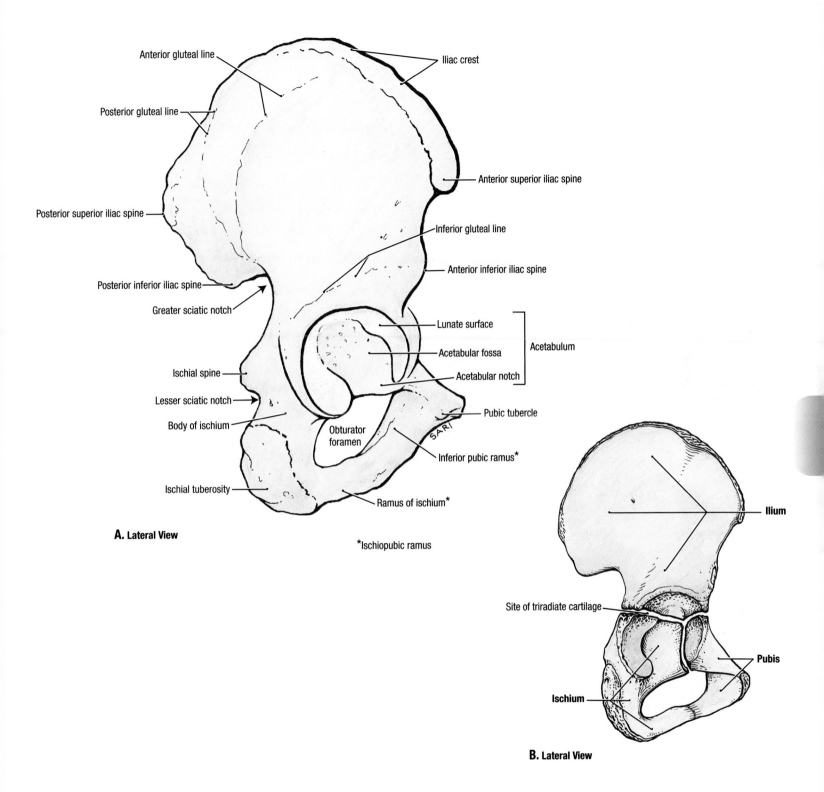

Anterior gluteal line

Posterior gluteal line

Posterior superior iliac spine

Iliac crest

Anterior superior iliac spine

Posterior inferior iliac spine

Greater sciatic notch

Inferior gluteal line

Anterior inferior iliac spine

Lunate surface

Acetabular fossa

Acetabulum

Acetabular notch

Ischial spine

Lesser sciatic notch

Body of ischium

Obturator foramen

SARI

Pubic tubercle

Inferior pubic ramus*

Ischial tuberosity

Ramus of ischium*

A. Lateral View

*Ischiopubic ramus

Site of triradiate cartilage

Ilium

Pubis

Ischium

B. Lateral View

5.31 **Hip bone**

A. Features of the lateral aspect. In the anatomical position, the anterior superior iliac spine and pubic tubercle are in the same coronal plane, and the ischial spine and superior end of the pubic symphysis are in the same horizontal plane; the internal aspect of the body of the pubis faces superiorly, and the acetabulum faces inferolaterally. **B.** Hip bone in youth. The three parts of the hip bone (ilium, ischium, and pubis) meet in the acetabulum at the triradiate synchondrosis. One or more primary centers of ossification appear in the triradiate cartilage at approximately the 12th year. Secondary centers of ossification appear along the length of the iliac crest, at the anterior inferior iliac spine, the ischial tuberosity, and the symphysis pubis at about puberty; fusion is usually complete by age 23.

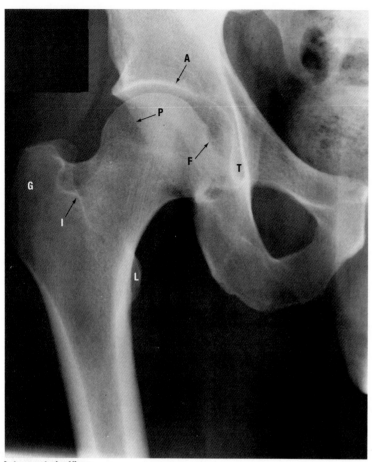

A. Anteroposterior View

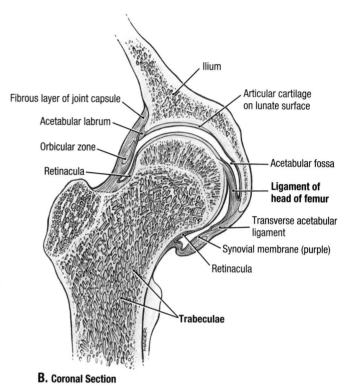

B. Coronal Section

5.32   **Radiograph and coronal section of hip joint**

A. Radiograph. On the femur, note the greater *(G)* and lesser *(L)* trochanters, the intertrochanteric crest *(I)*, and the pit or fovea *(F)* for the ligament of the head. On the pelvis, note the roof *(A)* and posterior rim *(P)* of the acetabulum and the "teardrop" appearance *(T)* caused by the superimposition of structures at the inferior margin of the acetabulum. **B.** Coronal section. Observe the bony trabeculae projecting into the head of the femur. The ligament of the head of the femur becomes taut during adduction of the hip joint, such as when crossing the legs. **C.** Hip replacement. The hip joint is subject to severe traumatic injury and degenerative disease. Osteoarthritis of the hip joint, characterized by pain, edema, limitation of motion, and erosion of articular cartilage, is a common cause of disability. During hip replacement, a metal prosthesis anchored to the person's femur by bone cement replaces the femoral head and neck. A plastic socket is cemented to the hip bone to replace the acetabulum. See Figure 5.34 blue box.

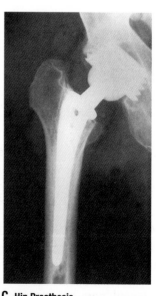

C. Hip Prosthesis

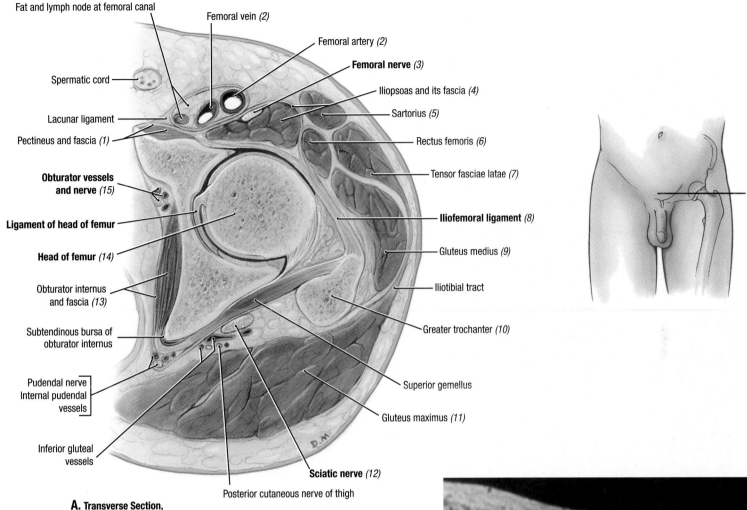

Fat and lymph node at femoral canal

Femoral vein (2)

Femoral artery (2)

Femoral nerve (3)

Spermatic cord

Iliopsoas and its fascia (4)

Sartorius (5)

Lacunar ligament

Pectineus and fascia (1)

Rectus femoris (6)

Tensor fasciae latae (7)

Obturator vessels and nerve (15)

Iliofemoral ligament (8)

Ligament of head of femur

Gluteus medius (9)

Head of femur (14)

Iliotibial tract

Obturator internus and fascia (13)

Subtendinous bursa of obturator internus

Greater trochanter (10)

Pudendal nerve
Internal pudendal vessels

Superior gemellus

Gluteus maximus (11)

Inferior gluteal vessels

Sciatic nerve (12)

Posterior cutaneous nerve of thigh

A. Transverse Section, Inferior View

5.33   Transverse section through thigh at level of hip joint

A. Transverse section. **B.** MRI (*numbers* refer to structures in A).
In **A**:

- The fibrous capsule of the joint is thick where it forms the iliofemoral ligament and thin posterior to the subtendinous bursa of psoas and tendon.
- The femoral sheath, enclosing the femoral artery, vein, lymph node, lymph vessels, and fat, is free, except posteriorly where, between the psoas and pectineus muscles, it is attached to the capsule of the hip joint.
- The femoral vein is located at the interval between the psoas and pectineus muscles. The femoral nerve lies between the iliacus muscle and fascia.

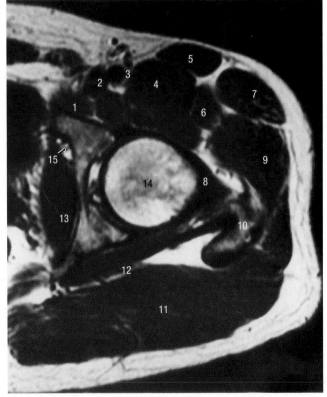

B. Transverse MRI

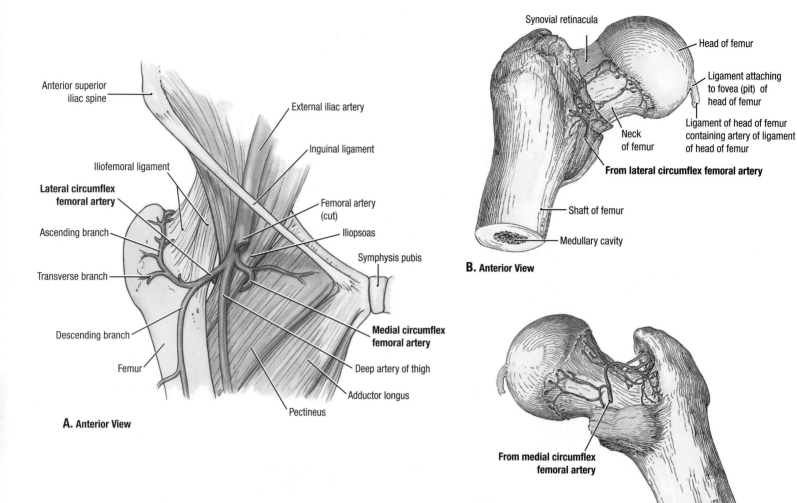

Anterior superior iliac spine

Iliofemoral ligament

Lateral circumflex femoral artery

Ascending branch

Transverse branch

Descending branch

Femur

A. Anterior View

External iliac artery

Inguinal ligament

Femoral artery (cut)

Iliopsoas

Symphysis pubis

Medial circumflex femoral artery

Deep artery of thigh

Adductor longus

Pectineus

Synovial retinacula

Head of femur

Ligament attaching to fovea (pit) of head of femur

Ligament of head of femur containing artery of ligament of head of femur

Neck of femur

From lateral circumflex femoral artery

Shaft of femur

Medullary cavity

B. Anterior View

From medial circumflex femoral artery

C. Posteroinferior View

5.34   Blood supply to head of femur

A. Medial and lateral circumflex femoral arteries in femoral triangle. **B.** Branches of lateral circumflex femoral artery. **C.** Branches of medial circumflex femoral artery.

- Branches of the medial and lateral circumflex femoral arteries ascend on the posterosuperior and posteroinferior parts of the neck of the femur. The vessels ascend in synovial retinacula—reflections of synovial membrane along the neck of the femur. The retinacula (in **B** and **C**) have been mostly removed; thus, the vessels can be clearly visualized.
- The branches of the medial and lateral circumflex femoral arteries perforate the bone just distal to the head of the femur, where they anastomose with branches from the artery of the ligament of the head of the femur and with medullary branches located within the shaft of the femur.
- The ligament of the head of the femur usually contains the artery of the ligament of the head of the femur, a branch of the obturator artery. The artery enters the head of the femur only when the center of the ossification has extended to the pit (fovea) for the ligament of the head (12th to 14th year). When present, this anastomosis persists even in advanced age; however, in 20% of persons, it is never established.

Fractures of the femoral neck often disrupt the blood supply to the head of the femur. The medial circumflex femoral artery supplies most of the blood to the head and neck of the femur and is often torn when the femoral neck is fractured. In some cases, the blood supplied by the artery of the ligament of the head may be the only blood received by the proximal fragment of the femoral head, which may be inadequate. If the blood vessels are ruptured, the fragment of bone may receive no blood and undergo aseptic necrosis.

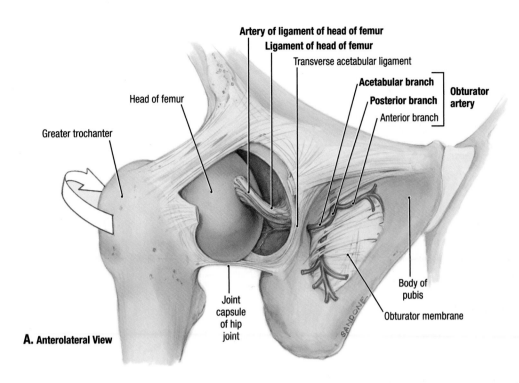

A. Anterolateral View

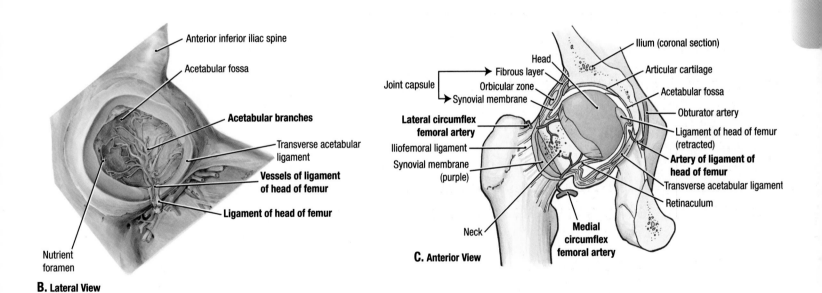

B. Lateral View

C. Anterior View

5.35 Blood vessels of acetabular fossa and ligament of head of femur

A. Obturator artery. The hip joint has been dislocated to reveal the ligament of the head of the femur. The obturator artery divides into anterior and posterior branches, and the acetabular branch arises from the posterior branch. The artery of the ligament of the head of the femur is a branch of the acetabular artery and can be seen traveling in the ligament to the head of the femur. **B.** Acetabular artery and vein. The acetabular branches (artery and vein) pass through the acetabular foramen and enter the acetabular fossa, where they diverge in the fatty areolar tissue. The branches radiate to the margin of the fossa, where they enter nutrient foramina. **C.** Blood supply of the head and neck of the femur. A section of bone has been removed from the femoral neck.

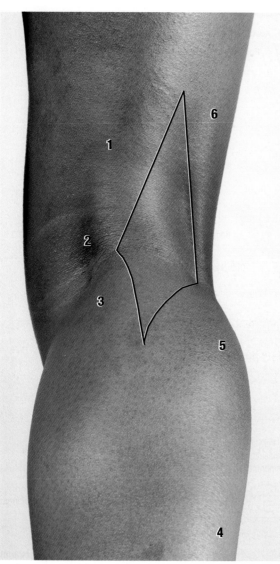

A. Posterior View

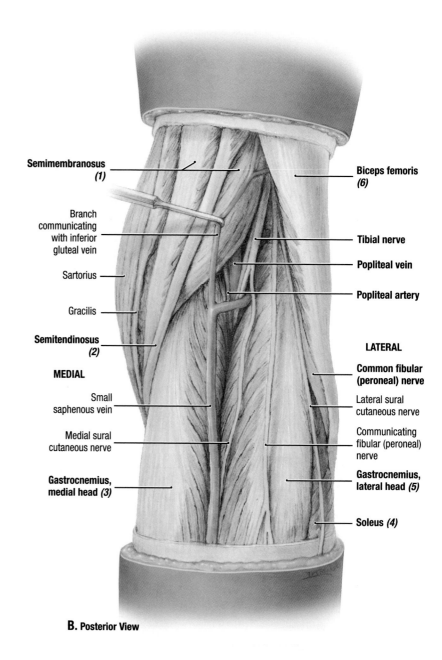

Semimembranosus *(1)*

Branch communicating with inferior gluteal vein

Sartorius

Gracilis

Semitendinosus *(2)*

MEDIAL

Small saphenous vein

Medial sural cutaneous nerve

Gastrocnemius, medial head *(3)*

Biceps femoris *(6)*

Tibial nerve

Popliteal vein

Popliteal artery

LATERAL

Common fibular (peroneal) nerve

Lateral sural cutaneous nerve

Communicating fibular (peroneal) nerve

Gastrocnemius, lateral head *(5)*

Soleus *(4)*

B. Posterior View

5.36   **Popliteal fossa**

A. Surface anatomy (*numbers* refer to structures in B). **B.** Superficial dissection.

- The two heads of the gastrocnemius muscle are embraced on the medial side by the semimembranosus muscle, which is overlaid by the semitendinosus muscle, and on the lateral side by the biceps femoris muscle.
- The small saphenous vein runs between the two heads of the gastrocnemius muscle. Deep to this vein is the medial sural cutaneous nerve, which, followed proximally, leads to the tibial nerve. The tibial nerve is superficial to the popliteal vein, which, in turn, is superficial to the popliteal artery.

Because the popliteal artery is deep in the popliteal fossa, it may be difficult to feel the popliteal pulse. Palpation of this pulse is commonly performed by placing the person in the prone position with the knee flexed to relax the popliteal fascia and hamstrings. The pulsations are best felt in the inferior part of the fossa. Weakening or loss of the popliteal pulse is a sign of femoral artery obstruction.

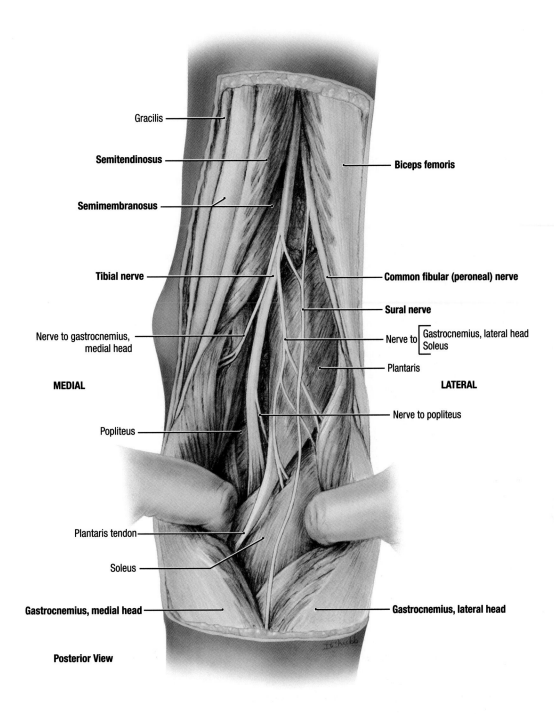

Gracilis

Semitendinosus

Semimembranosus

Biceps femoris

Tibial nerve

Common fibular (peroneal) nerve

Sural nerve

Nerve to gastrocnemius, medial head

Nerve to [Gastrocnemius, lateral head / Soleus]

Plantaris

MEDIAL

LATERAL

Nerve to popliteus

Popliteus

Plantaris tendon

Soleus

Gastrocnemius, medial head

Gastrocnemius, lateral head

Posterior View

5.37   **Nerves of popliteal fossa**

The two heads of the gastrocnemius muscle are separated.

- A cutaneous branch of the tibial nerve joins a cutaneous branch of the common fibular (peroneal) nerve to form the sural nerve. In this specimen, the junction is high; usually it is 5 to 8 cm proximal to the ankle.

All motor branches in this region emerge from the tibial nerve, one branch from its medial side and the others from its lateral side; hence, it is safer to dissect on the medial side.

Gracilis

Semitendinosus

Semimembranosus

Biceps femoris, long head

Biceps femoris, short head

Popliteal vein

Tibial nerve

MEDIAL

Popliteal artery

Superior medial genicular artery

Lateral intermuscular septum

Common fibular (peroneal) nerve

Femur

Biceps femoris

Superior lateral genicular artery

Semitendinosus

Semimembranosus

Semimembranosus bursa

Gastrocnemius,
medial head

LATERAL

Gastrocnemius, lateral head

Plantaris

Inferior lateral genicular artery

Popliteus

Inferior medial genicular artery

Nerve to popliteus

Popliteus fascia

Soleus

Plantaris

Gastrocnemius

Posterior View

5.38 Deep dissection of popliteal fossa

The common fibular (peroneal) nerve follows the posterior border of the biceps femoris muscle and, in this specimen, gives off two cutaneous branches. The popliteal artery lies on the floor of the popliteal fossa. The floor is formed by the femur, capsule of the knee joint, and popliteus muscle and fascia. The popliteal artery gives off genicular branches that also lie on the floor of the fossa. A popliteal aneurysm (abnormal dilation of all or part of the popliteal artery) usually causes edema (swelling) and pain in the popliteal fossa. If the femoral artery has to be ligated, blood can bypass the occlusion through the genicular anastomosis and reach the popliteal artery distal to the ligation.

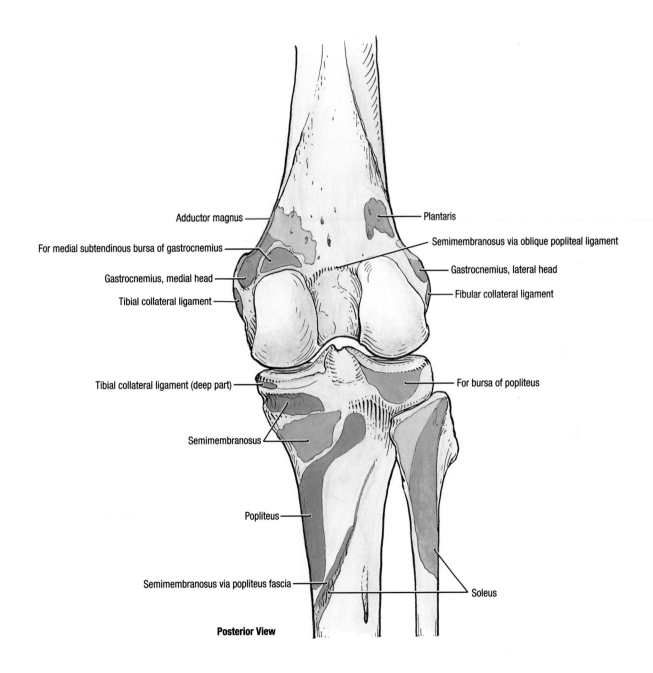

Adductor magnus

Plantaris

For medial subtendinous bursa of gastrocnemius

Semimembranosus via oblique popliteal ligament

Gastrocnemius, medial head

Gastrocnemius, lateral head

Tibial collateral ligament

Fibular collateral ligament

Tibial collateral ligament (deep part)

For bursa of popliteus

Semimembranosus

Popliteus

Semimembranosus via popliteus fascia

Soleus

Posterior View

5.39   **Attachment of muscles of popliteal region**

Lighter tones are secondary attachments.

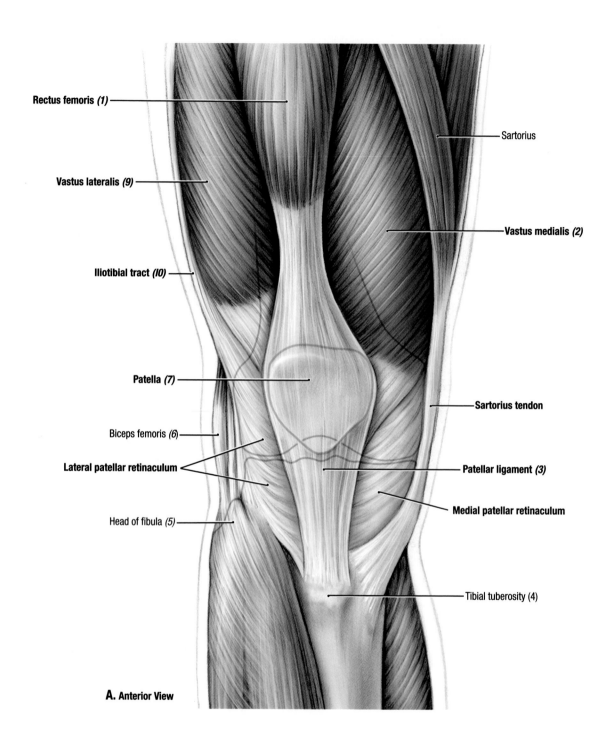

Rectus femoris *(1)*

Sartorius

Vastus lateralis *(9)*

Vastus medialis *(2)*

Iliotibial tract *(10)*

Patella *(7)*

Sartorius tendon

Biceps femoris *(6)*

Patellar ligament *(3)*

Lateral patellar retinaculum

Medial patellar retinaculum

Head of fibula *(5)*

Tibial tuberosity (4)

A. Anterior View

5.40   Anterior aspect of knee

A. Distal thigh and knee regions.

Note that the tendons of the four parts of the quadriceps unite to form the quadriceps tendon, a broad band that attaches to the patella. The patellar ligament, a continuation of the quadriceps tendon, attaches the patella to the tibial tuberosity. The lateral and medial patellar retinacula, formed largely by continuation of the iliotibial tract, and investing fascia of the vasti muscles, maintains alignment of the patella and patellar ligament. The retinacula also form the anterolateral and anteromedial portions of the fibrous layer of the joint capsule of the knee.

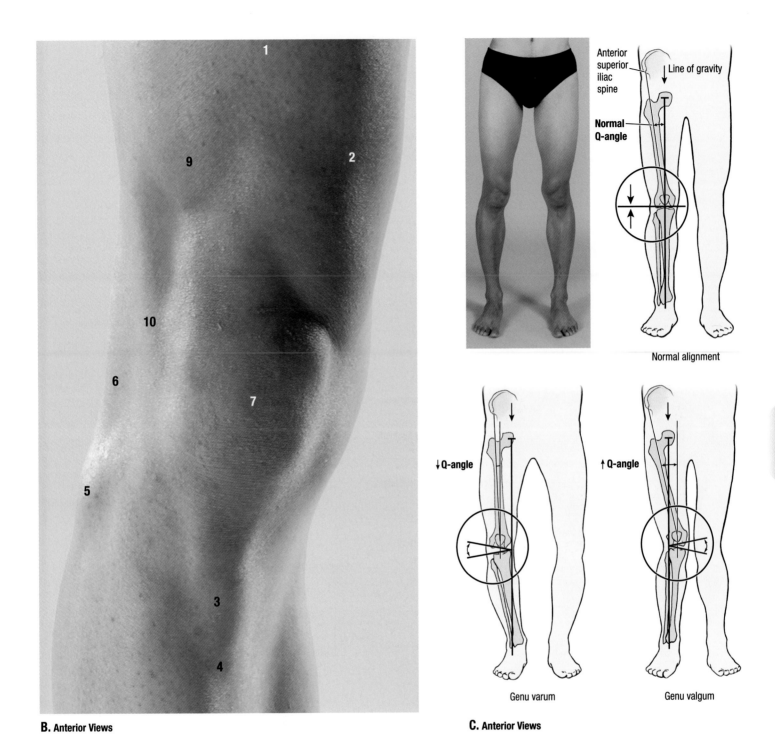

B. Anterior Views

C. Anterior Views

5.40   Anterior aspect of knee (continued)

B. Surface anatomy (numbers refer to structures in **A**). The femur is placed diagonally within the thigh, whereas the tibia is almost vertical within the leg, creating an angle at the knee between the long axes of the bones. The angle between the two bones, referred to clinically as the Q-angle, is assessed by drawing a line from the anterior superior iliac spine to the middle of the patella and extrapolating a second (vertical) line passing through the middle of the patella and tibial tuberosity. The Q-angle is typically greater in adult females, owing to their wider pelves. **C.** Genu val-

gum and genu varum. A medial angulation of the leg in relation to the thigh, in which the femur is abnormally vertical and the Q-angle is small, is a deformity called genu varum (bowleg) that causes unequal weight bearing resulting in arthrosis (destruction of knee cartilages), and an overstressed fibular collateral ligament. A lateral angulation of the leg (large Q-angle, >17°) in relation to the thigh is called genu valgum (knock-knee). This results in excess stress and degeneration of the lateral structures of the knee joint.

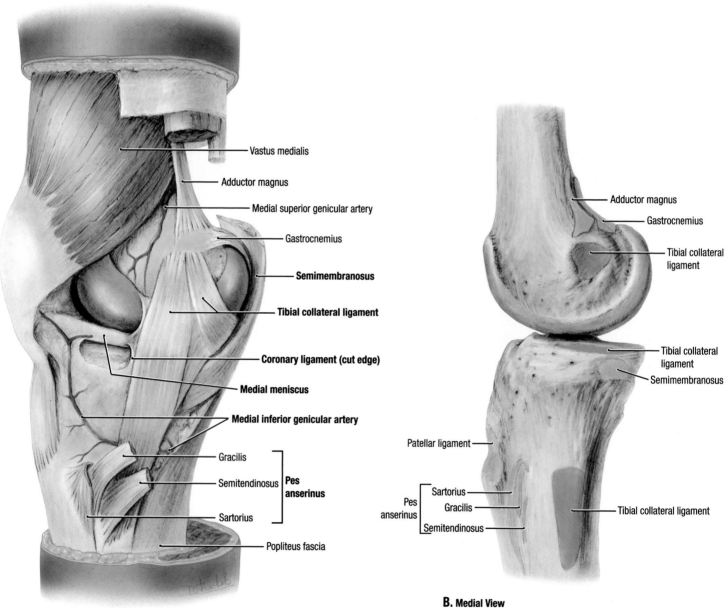

Vastus medialis

Adductor magnus

Medial superior genicular artery

Gastrocnemius

Semimembranosus

Tibial collateral ligament

Coronary ligament (cut edge)

Medial meniscus

Medial inferior genicular artery

Gracilis
Semitendinosus **Pes anserinus**
Sartorius

Popliteus fascia

A. Medial View

Adductor magnus
Gastrocnemius
Tibial collateral ligament

Tibial collateral ligament
Semimembranosus

Patellar ligament

Pes anserinus Sartorius
Gracilis
Semitendinosus

Tibial collateral ligament

B. Medial View

5.41   **Medial aspect of knee**

A. Dissection. The bandlike part of the tibial collateral ligament attaches to the medial epicondyle of the femur, bridges superficial to the insertion of the semimembranosus muscle,
and crosses the medial inferior genicular artery. Distally, the ligament is crossed by the three
tendons forming the pes anserinus (sartorius, gracilis, and semitendinosus). **B.** Bones, showing muscle and ligament attachment sites.

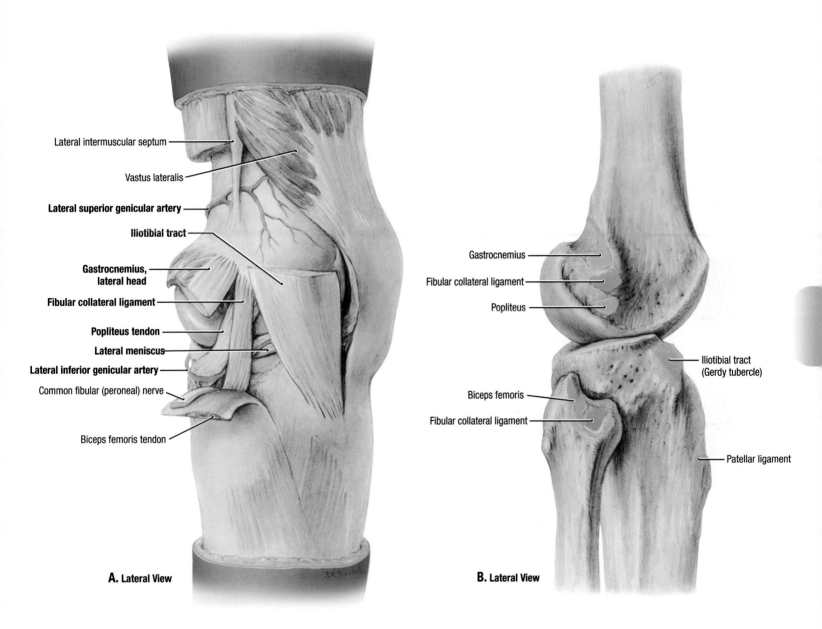

Lateral intermuscular septum

Vastus lateralis

Lateral superior genicular artery

Iliotibial tract

Gastrocnemius, lateral head

Fibular collateral ligament

Popliteus tendon

Lateral meniscus

Lateral inferior genicular artery

Common fibular (peroneal) nerve

Biceps femoris tendon

A. Lateral View

Gastrocnemius

Fibular collateral ligament

Popliteus

Iliotibial tract (Gerdy tubercle)

Biceps femoris

Fibular collateral ligament

Patellar ligament

B. Lateral View

5.42 Lateral aspect of knee

A. Dissection. **B.** Bones, showing muscle and ligament attachments.

Three structures arise from the lateral epicondyle and are uncovered by reflecting the biceps muscle: the gastrocnemius muscle is posterosuperior; the popliteus muscle is anteroinferior; and the fibular collateral ligament is in between, crossing superficial to the popliteus muscle. The lateral inferior genicular artery courses along the lateral meniscus.

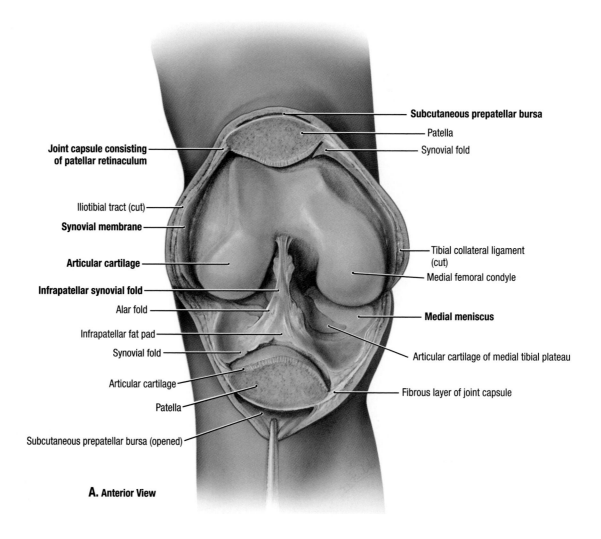

Subcutaneous prepatellar bursa
Patella
Synovial fold

**Joint capsule consisting
of patellar retinaculum**

Iliotibial tract (cut)
Synovial membrane

Articular cartilage

Infrapatellar synovial fold
Alar fold
Infrapatellar fat pad
Synovial fold
Articular cartilage
Patella
Subcutaneous prepatellar bursa (opened)

Tibial collateral ligament
(cut)
Medial femoral condyle

Medial meniscus

Articular cartilage of medial tibial plateau

Fibrous layer of joint capsule

A. Anterior View

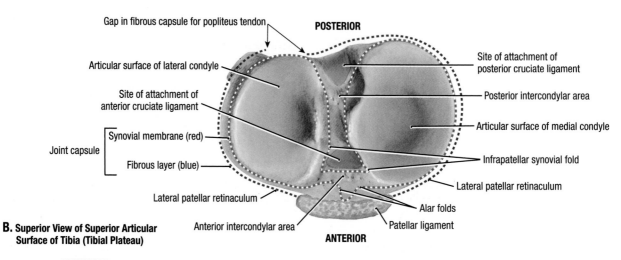

Gap in fibrous capsule for popliteus tendon
POSTERIOR

Articular surface of lateral condyle

Site of attachment of
anterior cruciate ligament

Joint capsule
   Synovial membrane (red)
   Fibrous layer (blue)

Lateral patellar retinaculum
Anterior intercondylar area
ANTERIOR

Site of attachment of
posterior cruciate ligament

Posterior intercondylar area

Articular surface of medial condyle

Infrapatellar synovial fold

Lateral patellar retinaculum

Alar folds
Patellar ligament

**B. Superior View of Superior Articular
Surface of Tibia (Tibial Plateau)**

5.43   **Fibrous layer and synovial membrane of joint capsule**

A. Dissection. **B.** Attachment of the layers of the joint capsule to the tibia. The fibrous layer (blue dotted line) and synovial membrane (red dotted line) are adjacent on each side, but they part company centrally to accommodate intercondylar and infrapatellar structures that are intracapsular (inside the fibrous layer) but extra-articular (excluded from the articular cavity by synovial membrane).

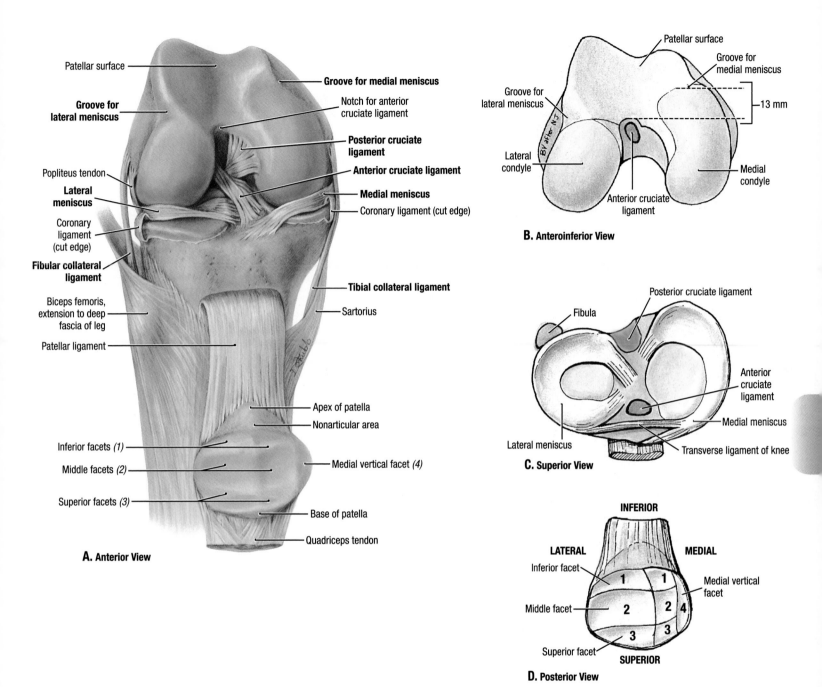

5.44   **Articular surfaces and ligaments of knee joint**

A. Flexed knee joint with patella reflected. There are indentations on the sides of the femoral condyles at the junction of the patellar and tibial articular areas. The lateral tibial articular area is shorter than the medial one. The notch at the anterolateral part of the intercondylar notch is for the anterior cruciate ligament on full extension. **B.** Distal femur. **C.** Tibial plateaus. **D.** Articular surfaces of patella. The three paired facets (superior, middle, and inferior) on the posterior surface of the patella articulate with the patellar surface of the femur successively during *(1)* extension, *(2)* slight flexion, *(3)* flexion, and the most medial vertical facet on the patella *(4)* articulates during full flexion with the cresenteric facet on the medial margin of the intercondylar notch of the femur.

When the patella is dislocated, it nearly always dislocates laterally. The tendency toward lateral dislocation is normally counterbalanced by the medial, more horizontal pull of the powerful vastus medialis. In addition, the more anterior projection of the lateral femoral condyle and deeper slope for the large lateral patellar facet provides a mechanical deterrent to lateral dislocation. An imbalance of the lateral pull and the mechanisms resisting it result in abnormal tracking of the patella within the patellar groove and chronic patellar pain, even if actual dislocation does not occur. See Figure 5.49 blue box.

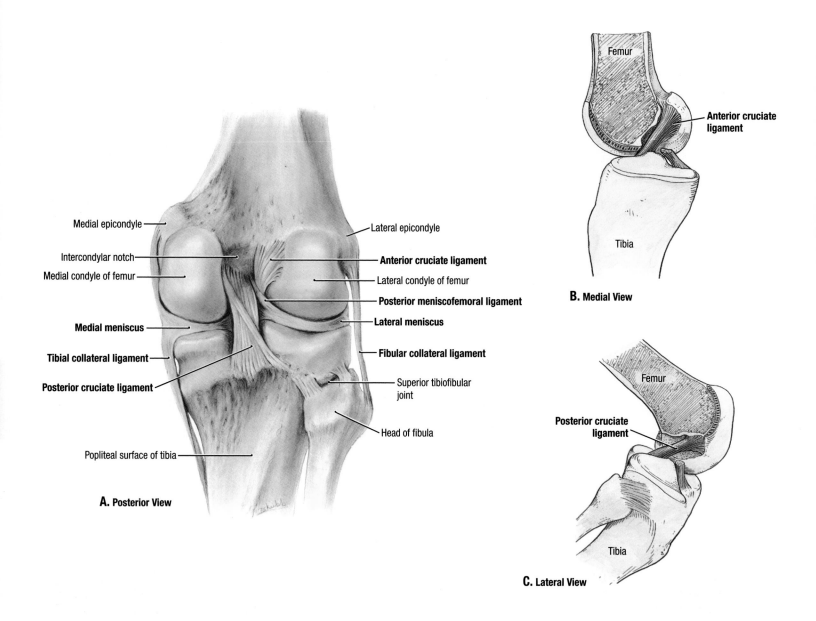

Medial epicondyle

Intercondylar notch

Medial condyle of femur

Medial meniscus

Tibial collateral ligament

Posterior cruciate ligament

Popliteal surface of tibia

A. Posterior View

Lateral epicondyle

Anterior cruciate ligament

Lateral condyle of femur

Posterior meniscofemoral ligament

Lateral meniscus

Fibular collateral ligament

Superior tibiofibular joint

Head of fibula

Femur

Anterior cruciate ligament

Tibia

B. Medial View

Femur

Posterior cruciate ligament

Tibia

C. Lateral View

5.45   Ligaments of knee joint

A. Posterior aspect of joint. The bandlike tibial (medial) collateral ligament is attached to the medial meniscus, and the cordlike fibular (lateral) collateral ligament is separated from the lateral meniscus by the width of the popliteus tendon (removed). The posterior cruciate ligament is joined by a cord from the lateral meniscus called the posterior meniscofemoral ligament. The posterior meniscofemoral ligament attaches to the medial condyle of the femur just posterior to the attachment of the posterior cruciate ligament. **B.** Anterior cruciate ligament. **C.** Posterior cruciate ligament. In each illustration, half the femur is sagittally sectioned and removed with the proximal part of the corresponding cruciate ligament. Note that the posterior cruciate ligament prevents the femur from sliding anteriorly on the tibia, particularly when the

knee is flexed. The anterior cruciate ligament prevents the femur from sliding posteriorly on the tibia, preventing hyperextension of the knee, and limits medial rotation of the femur when the foot is on the ground (i.e., when the leg is fixed). Injury to the knee joint is frequently caused by a blow to the lateral side of the extended knee or excessive lateral twisting of the flexed knee, which disrupts the tibial collateral ligament and concomitantly tears and/or detaches the medial meniscus from the joint capsule. This injury is common in athletes who twist their flexed knees while running (e.g., in football and soccer). The anterior cruciate ligament, which serves as a pivot for rotary movements of the knee, is taut during flexion and may also tear subsequent to the rupture of the tibial collateral ligament, creating an "unhappy triad" of knee injuries.

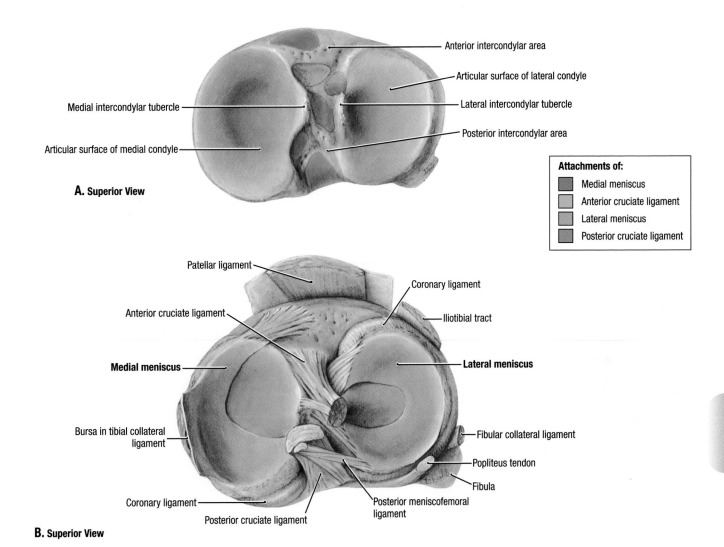

Anterior intercondylar area

Articular surface of lateral condyle

Medial intercondylar tubercle

Lateral intercondylar tubercle

Posterior intercondylar area

Articular surface of medial condyle

A. Superior View

Attachments of:
- Medial meniscus
- Anterior cruciate ligament
- Lateral meniscus
- Posterior cruciate ligament

Patellar ligament

Coronary ligament

Anterior cruciate ligament

Iliotibial tract

Medial meniscus

Lateral meniscus

Bursa in tibial collateral ligament

Fibular collateral ligament

Popliteus tendon

Fibula

Coronary ligament

Posterior meniscofemoral ligament

Posterior cruciate ligament

B. Superior View

5.46   Cruciate ligaments and menisci

A. Attachments sites on tibia. **B.** Menisci in situ.

- The lateral tibial condyle is flatter, shorter from anterior to posterior, and more circular. The medial condyle is concave, longer from anterior to posterior, and more oval.

Arthroscopy is an endoscopic examination that allows visualization of the interior of the knee joint cavity with minimal disruption of tissue. The arthroscope and one (or more) additional canula(e) are inserted through tiny incisions, known as portals. The second canula is for passage of specialized tools (e.g., manipulative probes or forceps) or equipment for trimming, shaping, or removing damaged tissue. This technique allows removal of torn menisci, loose bodies in the joint such as bone chips, and debridement (the excision of devitalized articular cartilaginous material in advanced cases of arthritis). Ligament repair or replacement may also be performed using an arthroscope.

- The menisci conform to the shapes of the surfaces on which they rest. Because the horns of the lateral meniscus are attached close together and its coronary ligament is slack, this meniscus can slide anteriorly and posteriorly on the (flat) condyle; because the horns of the medial meniscus are attached further apart, its movements on the (concave) condyle are restricted.

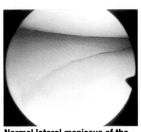

Normal lateral meniscus of the knee

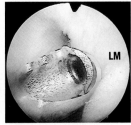

LM

Trimming of a torn lateral meniscus (LM)

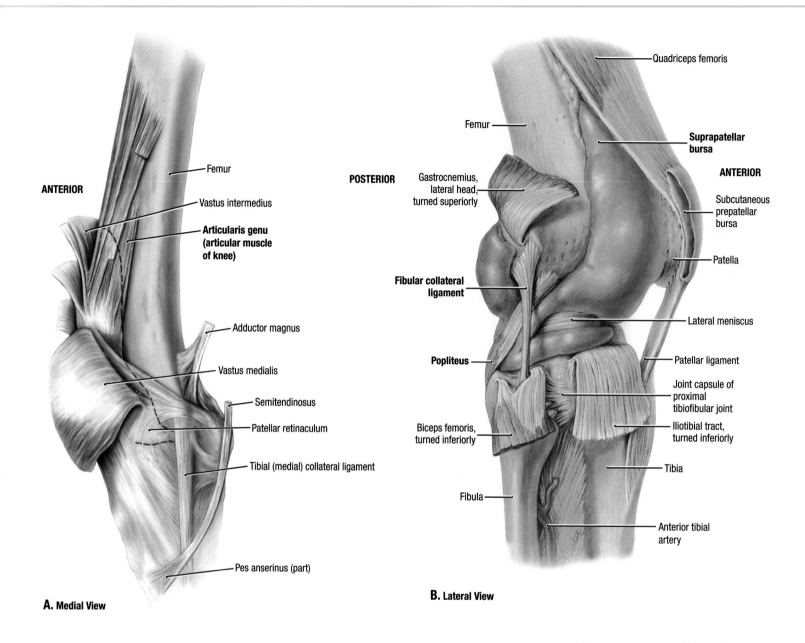

ANTERIOR

Femur

Vastus intermedius

Articularis genu (articular muscle of knee)

Adductor magnus

Vastus medialis

Semitendinosus

Patellar retinaculum

Tibial (medial) collateral ligament

Pes anserinus (part)

A. Medial View

POSTERIOR

Quadriceps femoris

Femur

Gastrocnemius, lateral head, turned superiorly

Fibular collateral ligament

Popliteus

Biceps femoris, turned inferiorly

Fibula

Suprapatellar bursa

ANTERIOR

Subcutaneous prepatellar bursa

Patella

Lateral meniscus

Patellar ligament

Joint capsule of proximal tibiofibular joint

Iliotibial tract, turned inferiorly

Tibia

Anterior tibial artery

B. Lateral View

5.47 **Articularis genu and suprapatellar bursa**

A. Articularis genu (articular muscle of the knee). This muscle lies deep to the vastus intermedius muscle and consists of fibers arising from the anterior surface of the femur proximally and attaching into the synovial membrane distally. The articularis genu pulls the synovial membrane of the suprapatellar bursa (*dotted line*) superiorly during extension of the knee so that it will not be caught between the patella and femur within the knee joint. **B.** Lateral aspect of knee. Latex was injected into the articular cavity and fixed with acetic acid. The distended synovial membrane was exposed and cleaned. The gastrocnemius muscle was reflected proximally, and the biceps femoris muscle and the iliotibial tract were reflected distally. The extent of the synovial capsule: superiorly, it rises superior to the patella, where it rests on a

layer of fat that allows it to glide freely with movements of the joint; this superior part is called the suprapatellar bursa; posteriorly, it rises as high as the origin of the gastrocnemius muscle; laterally, it curves inferior to the lateral femoral epicondyle, where the popliteus tendon and fibular collateral ligament are attached; and inferiorly, it bulges inferior to the lateral meniscus, overlapping the tibia (the coronary ligament is removed to show this). Prepatellar bursitis (housemaid's knee) is usually a friction bursitis caused by friction between the skin and the patella. The suprapatellar bursa communicates with the articular cavity of the knee joint; consequently, abrasions or penetrating wounds superior to the patella may result in suprapatellar bursitis caused by bacteria entering the bursa from the torn skin. The infection may spread to the knee joint.

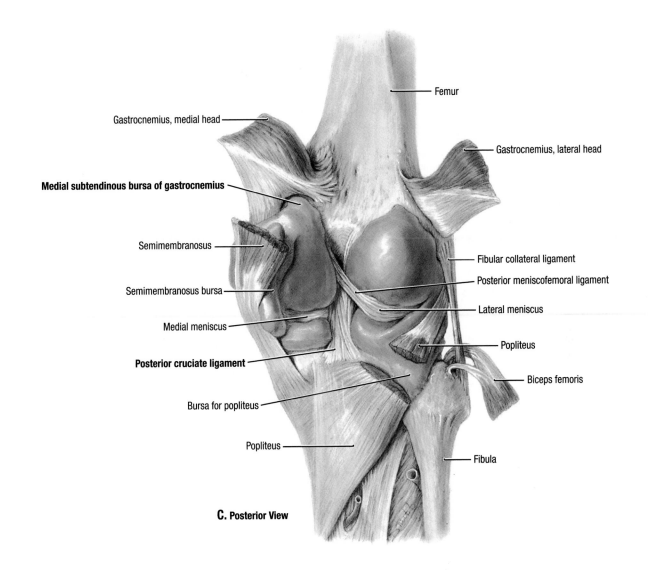

Femur

Gastrocnemius, medial head

Gastrocnemius, lateral head

Medial subtendinous bursa of gastrocnemius

Semimembranosus

Fibular collateral ligament

Posterior meniscofemoral ligament

Semimembranosus bursa

Lateral meniscus

Medial meniscus

Popliteus

Posterior cruciate ligament

Biceps femoris

Bursa for popliteus

Popliteus

Fibula

C. Posterior View

5.47 **Distended knee joint (continued)**

TABLE 5.8 BURSAE AROUND KNEE

Bursa	Location	Structural Features or Functions
Suprapatellar	Between femur and tendon of quadriceps femoris	Held in position by articular muscle of knee; communicates freely with synovial cavity of knee joint
Popliteus	Between tendon of popliteus and lateral condyle of tibia	Opens into synovial cavity of knee joint, inferior to lateral meniscus
Anserine	Separates tendons of sartorius, gracilis, and semi-tendinosus from tibia and tibial collateral ligament	Area where tendons of these muscles attach to tibia resembles the foot of a goose (L. *pes*, foot; L. *anser*, goose)
Medial subtendinous bursa of gastrocnemius	Lies deep to proximal attachment of tendon of medial head of gastrocnemius	This bursa is an extension of synovial cavity of knee joint
Semimembranosus	Located between medial head of gastrocnemius and semimembranosus tendon	Related to the distal attachment of semimembranosus
Subcutaneous prepatellar	Lies between skin and anterior surface of patella	Allows free movement of skin over patella during movements of leg
Subcutaneous infrapatellar	Located between skin and tibial tuberosity	Helps knee to withstand pressure when kneeling
Deep infrapatellar	Lies between patellar ligament and anterior surface of tibia	Separated from knee joint by infrapatellar fat-pad

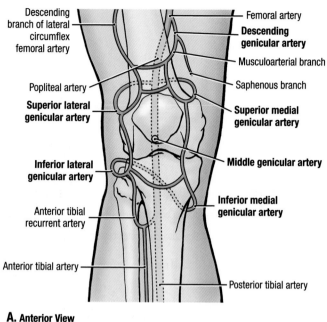

A. Anterior View

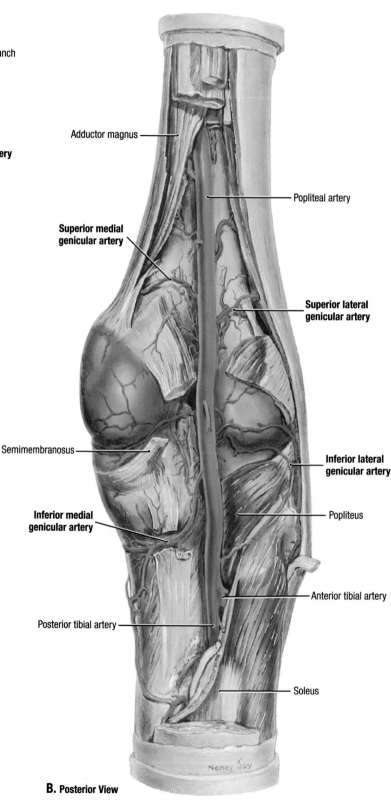

B. Posterior View

5.48   Anastomoses around knee

A. Genicular anastomosis on the anterior aspect of the knee.
B. Popliteal artery in popliteal fossa.

- The popliteal artery runs from the adductor hiatus (in the adductor magnus muscle) proximally to the inferior border of the popliteus muscle distally, where it bifurcates into the anterior and posterior tibial arteries.
- The three anterior relations of the popliteal artery include the femur (fat intervening), the joint capsule of the knee; and the popliteus muscle.
- Five genicular branches of the popliteal artery supply the capsule and ligaments of the knee joint. The genicular arteries are the superior lateral, superior medial, middle, inferior lateral, and inferior medial genicular arteries.

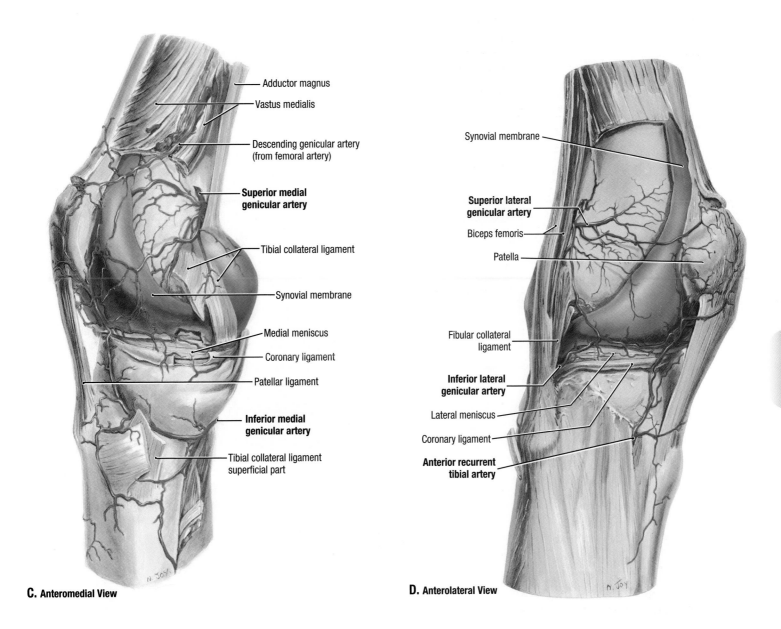

C. Anteromedial View

- Adductor magnus
- Vastus medialis
- Descending genicular artery (from femoral artery)
- **Superior medial genicular artery**
- Tibial collateral ligament
- Synovial membrane
- Medial meniscus
- Coronary ligament
- Patellar ligament
- **Inferior medial genicular artery**
- Tibial collateral ligament superficial part

D. Anterolateral View

- Synovial membrane
- **Superior lateral genicular artery**
- Biceps femoris
- Patella
- Fibular collateral ligament
- **Inferior lateral genicular artery**
- Lateral meniscus
- Coronary ligament
- **Anterior recurrent tibial artery**

5.48   **Anastomoses around knee *(continued)***

C. Medial aspect of the knee showing superior and inferior medial genicular arteries. **D.** Lateral aspect of the knee showing superior and inferior lateral genicular arteries.

The genicular arteries participate in the formation of the periarticular genicular anastomosis, a network of vessels surrounding the knee that provides collateral circulation capable of maintaining blood supply to the leg during full knee flexion, which may kink the popliteal artery. Other contributors to this important anastomosis are the descending genicular artery, a branch of the femoral artery, superomedially; descending branch of the lateral circumflex femoral artery, superolaterally; and anterior tibial recurrent artery, a branch of the anterior tibial artery, inferolaterally.

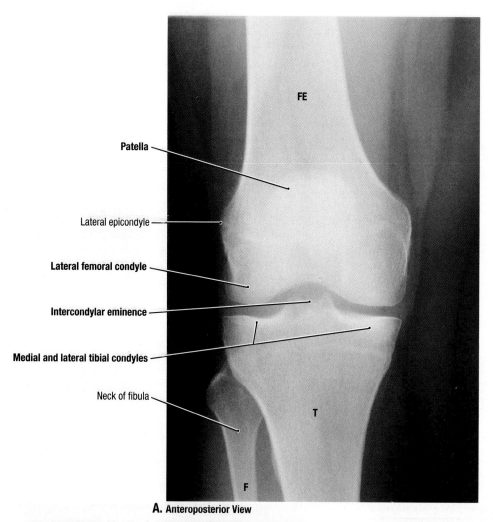

Patella

Lateral epicondyle

Lateral femoral condyle

Intercondylar eminence

Medial and lateral tibial condyles

Neck of fibula

A. Anteroposterior View

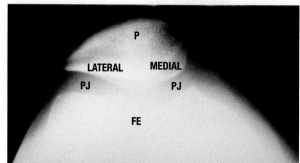

B. Skyline View (Knee in Flexion)

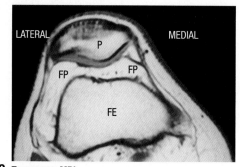

C. Transverse MRI

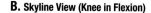

5.49   Imaging of the knee and patellofemoral articulation

A. Anteroposterior radiograph of knee. **B.** Radiograph of patella (knee joint flexed). *FE*, femur; *FP*, fat pad; *P*, patella; *PJ*, patellofemoral joint. **C.** Transverse MRI showing the patellofemoral joint.

Pain deep to the patella often results from excessive running, especially downhill; hence, this type of pain is often called "runner's knee." The pain results from repetitive microtrauma caused by abnormal tracking of the patella relative to the patellar surface of the femur, a condition known as the patellofemoral syndrome. This syndrome may also result from a direct blow to the patella and from osteoarthritis of the patellofemoral compartment (degenerative wear and tear of articular cartilages). In some cases, strengthening of the vastus medialis corrects patellofemoral dysfunction. This muscle tends to prevent lateral dislocation of the patella resulting from the Q-angle because the vastus medialis attaches to and pulls on the medial border of the patella. Hence, weakness of the vastus medialis predisposes the individual to patellofemoral dysfunction and patellar dislocation.

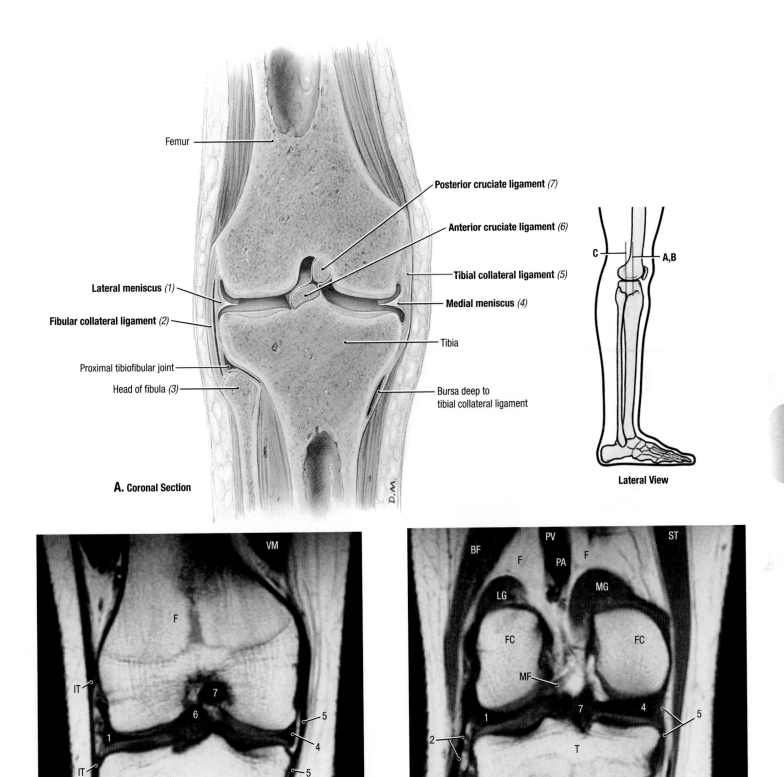

A. Coronal Section

- Femur
- Posterior cruciate ligament *(7)*
- Anterior cruciate ligament *(6)*
- Lateral meniscus *(1)*
- Fibular collateral ligament *(2)*
- Tibial collateral ligament *(5)*
- Medial meniscus *(4)*
- Tibia
- Proximal tibiofibular joint
- Head of fibula *(3)*
- Bursa deep to tibial collateral ligament

Lateral View

B. Coronal MRI

C. Coronal MRI

5.50   Coronal section and MRIs of knee

A. Section through intercondylar notch of femur, tibia, and fibula. **B.** MRI through intercondylar notch of femur and tibia. **C.** MRI through femoral condyles tibia and fibula. *Numbers* in MRIs refer to structures in **A.** *VM,* vastus medialis; *EL,* epiphyseal line; *IT,* iliotibial tract; *FC,* femoral condyle; *BF,* biceps femoris; *ST,* semitendinosus; *LG,* lateral head of gastrocnemius; *MG,* medial head of gastrocnemius; *PV,* popliteal vein; *PA,* popliteal artery; *F,* fat in popliteal fossa; *MF,* meniscofemoral ligament.

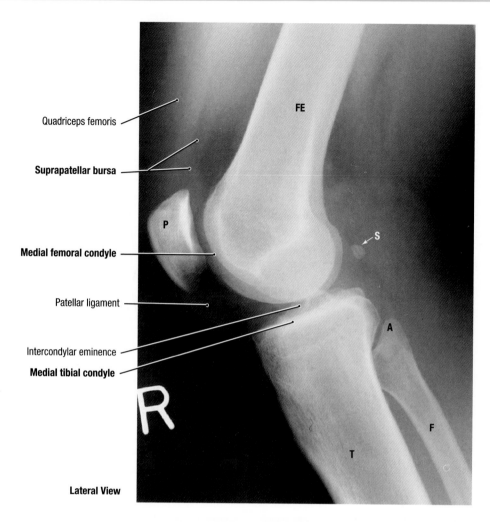

Quadriceps femoris

Suprapatellar bursa

Medial femoral condyle

Patellar ligament

Intercondylar eminence

Medial tibial condyle

Lateral View

5.51 **Radiograph of knee**

Lateral radiograph of flexed knee. *FE*, femur; *T*, tibia; *F*, fibula; *A*, apex of fibula; *S*, fabella; *P*, patella. The fabella is a sesamoid bone in the lateral head of gastrocnemius muscle.

5.52 **Sagittal section and MRIs of knee**

A. *(Opposite page)*. Section through lateral aspect of intercondylar notch of femur. **B.** MRI through medial aspect of intercondylar notch of femur showing cruciate ligaments. **C.** MRI through medial femoral and tibial condyles. *Numbers* in MRIs refer to structures in **A.** *SM*, semimembranosus; *ST*, semitendinosus; *MG*, medial head of gastrocnemius; *VM*, vastus medialis; *PF*, prefemoral fat; *SF*, suprapatellar fat; *AM*, anterior horn of medial meniscus; *PM*, posterior horn of medial meniscus; *PV*, popliteal vessels.

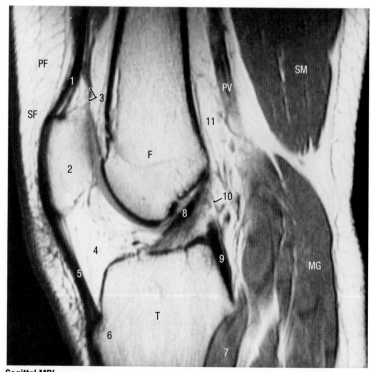

B. Sagittal MRI

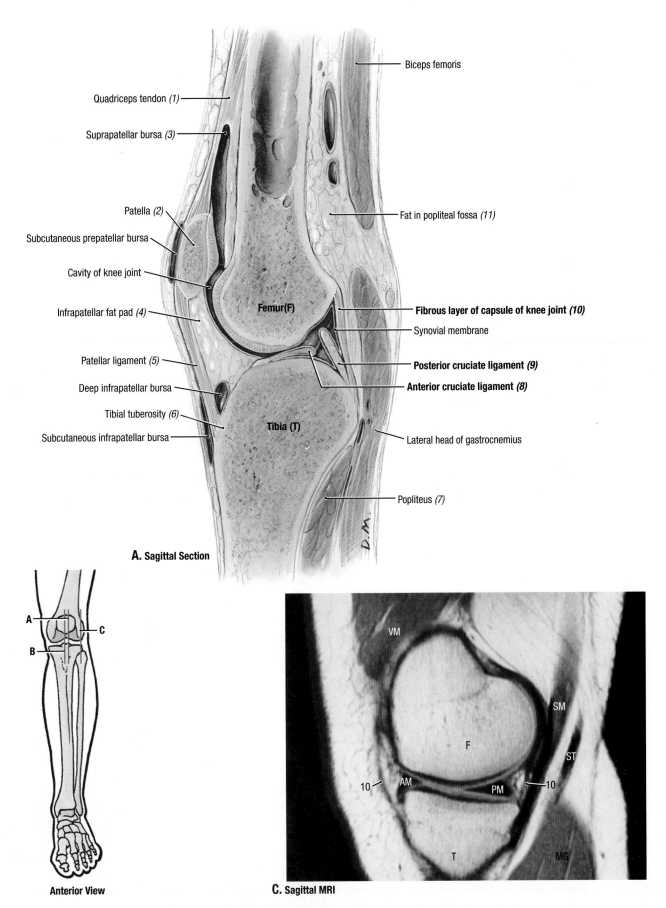

Biceps femoris

Quadriceps tendon (1)

Suprapatellar bursa (3)

Fat in popliteal fossa (11)

Patella (2)

Subcutaneous prepatellar bursa

Cavity of knee joint

Femur(F)

Fibrous layer of capsule of knee joint (10)

Infrapatellar fat pad (4)

Synovial membrane

Patellar ligament (5)

Posterior cruciate ligament (9)

Deep infrapatellar bursa

Anterior cruciate ligament (8)

Tibial tuberosity (6)

Tibia (T)

Subcutaneous infrapatellar bursa

Lateral head of gastrocnemius

Popliteus (7)

A. Sagittal Section

Anterior View

VM

SM

F

ST

10

AM

PM

10

T

MG

C. Sagittal MRI

5.52 **Sagittal section and MRIs of knee (continued)**

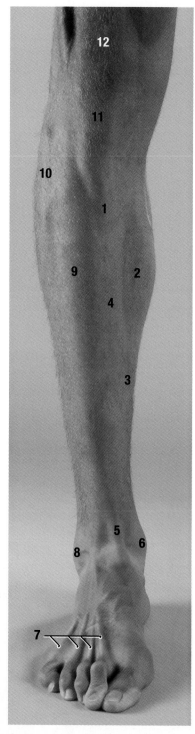

A. Anterior View

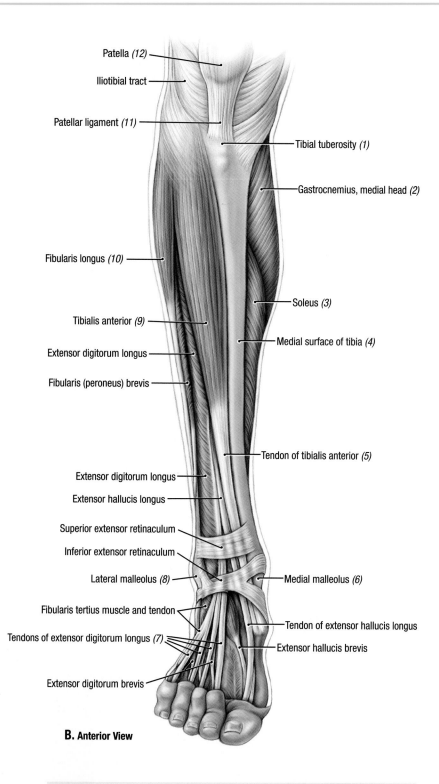

Patella (12)
Iliotibial tract
Patellar ligament (11)
Tibial tuberosity (1)
Gastrocnemius, medial head (2)
Fibularis longus (10)
Soleus (3)
Tibialis anterior (9)
Medial surface of tibia (4)
Extensor digitorum longus
Fibularis (peroneus) brevis
Tendon of tibialis anterior (5)
Extensor digitorum longus
Extensor hallucis longus
Superior extensor retinaculum
Inferior extensor retinaculum
Lateral malleolus (8)
Medial malleolus (6)
Fibularis tertius muscle and tendon
Tendon of extensor hallucis longus
Tendons of extensor digitorum longus (7)
Extensor hallucis brevis
Extensor digitorum brevis

B. Anterior View

5.53   Anterior leg—superficial muscles

A. Surface anatomy (*numbers* refer to structures labeled in **B**). **B.** Dissection.

The muscles of the anterior compartment are ankle dorsiflexors/toe extensors. They are active in walking as they concentrically contract to raise the forefoot to clear the ground during the swing phase of the gait cycle and eccentrically contract to lower the forefoot to the ground after the heel strike of the stance phase.

Shin splints, edema, and pain in the area of the distal third of the tibia, result from repetitive microtrauma of the anterior compartment muscles, especially the tibialis anterior. This produces a mild form of anterior compartment syndrome. The pain commonly occurs during traumatic injury or athletic overexertion of the muscles. Edema and muscle-tendon inflammation causes swelling that reduces blood flow to the muscles. The swollen ischemic muscles are painful and tender to pressure.

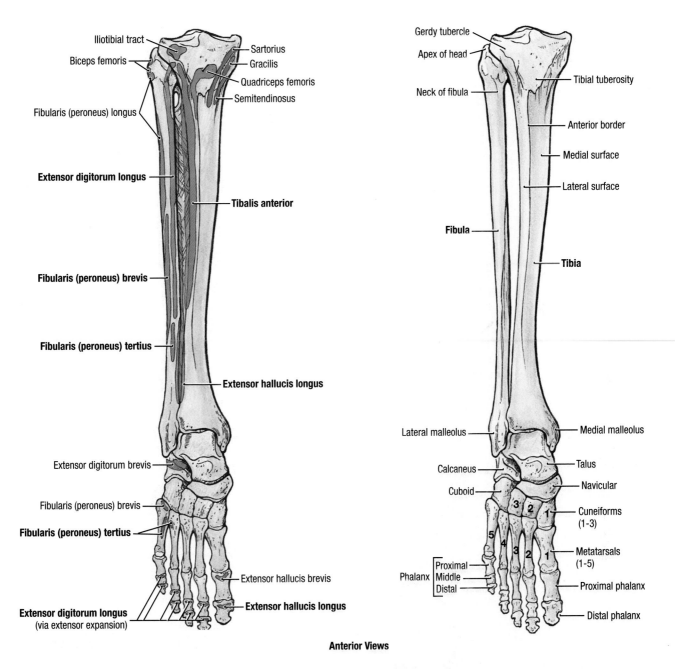

Iliotibial tract
Biceps femoris
Sartorius
Gracilis
Quadriceps femoris
Semitendinosus
Fibularis (peroneus) longus
Extensor digitorum longus
Tibialis anterior
Fibularis (peroneus) brevis
Fibularis (peroneus) tertius
Extensor hallucis longus
Extensor digitorum brevis
Fibularis (peroneus) brevis
Fibularis (peroneus) tertius
Extensor hallucis brevis
Extensor hallucis longus
Extensor digitorum longus
(via extensor expansion)

Gerdy tubercle
Apex of head
Neck of fibula
Tibial tuberosity
Anterior border
Medial surface
Lateral surface
Fibula
Tibia
Lateral malleolus
Medial malleolus
Calcaneus
Talus
Cuboid
Navicular
Cuneiforms (1-3)
Metatarsals (1-5)
Phalanx { Proximal / Middle / Distal }
Proximal phalanx
Distal phalanx

Anterior Views

TABLE 5.9 MUSCLES OF THE ANTERIOR COMPARTMENT OF LEG

Muscle	Proximal Attachment	Distal Attachment	Innervation[a]	Main Actions
Tibialis anterior	Lateral condyle and superior half of lateral surface of tibia	Medial and inferior surfaces of medial cuneiform and base of first metatarsal	Deep fibular (peroneal) nerve (**L4**–L5)	Dorsiflexes ankle and inverts foot
Extensor hallucis longus	Middle part of anterior surface of fibula and interosseous membrane	Dorsal aspect of base of distal phalanx of great toe (hallux)		Extends great toe and dorsiflexes ankle
Extensor digitorum longus	Lateral condyle of tibia and superior three fourths of anterior surface of interosseous membrane	Middle and distal phalanges of lateral four digits	Deep fibular (peroneal) nerve (L5–S1)	Extends lateral four digits and dorsiflexes ankle
Fibularis (peroneus) tertius	Inferior third of anterior surface of fibula and interosseus membrane	Dorsum of base of fifth metatarsal		Dorsiflexes ankle and aids in eversion of foot

[a]See Table 5.1 for explanation of segmental innervation.

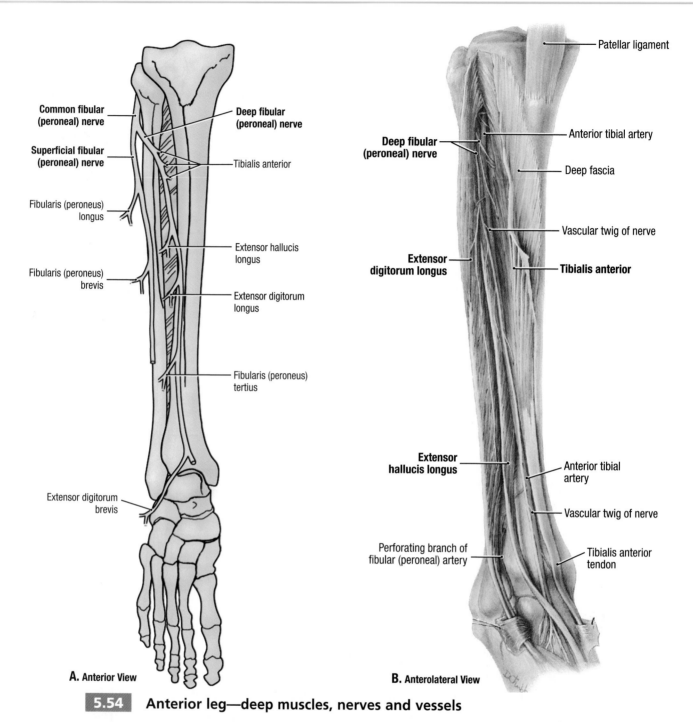

A. Anterior View

B. Anterolateral View

5.54   Anterior leg—deep muscles, nerves and vessels

TABLE 5.10 COMMON, SUPERFICIAL, AND DEEP FIBULAR NERVES

Nerve	Origin	Course	Distribution/Structure(s) Supplied
Common fibular	Sciatic nerve	Forms as sciatic nerve bifurcates at apex of popliteal fossa and follows medial border of biceps femoris; winds around neck of fibula, dividing into superficial and deep fibular nerves	Skin on lateral part of posterior aspect of leg via the lateral sural nerve; lateral aspect of knee joint via its articular branch
Superficial fibular	Common fibular nerve	Arises deep to fibularis longus and descends in lateral compartment of leg; pierces crural fascia at distal third of leg to become cutaneous	Fibularis longus and brevis and skin on distal third of anterolateral surface of leg and dorsum of foot
Deep fibular	Common fibular nerve	Arises deep to fibularis longus; passes through extensor digitorum longus, descends on interosseous membrane, and enters dorsum of foot	Anterior muscles of leg, dorsum of foot, and skin of first interdigital cleft; dorsal aspect of joints crossed via articular branches

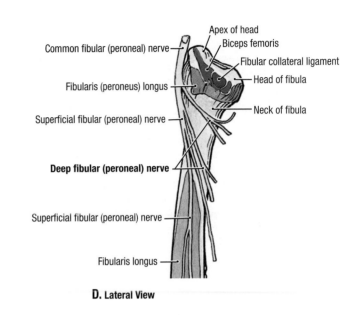

Apex of head
Common fibular (peroneal) nerve
Biceps femoris
Fibular collateral ligament
Fibularis (peroneus) longus
Head of fibula
Superficial fibular (peroneal) nerve
Neck of fibula
Deep fibular (peroneal) nerve
Superficial fibular (peroneal) nerve
Fibularis longus

D. Lateral View

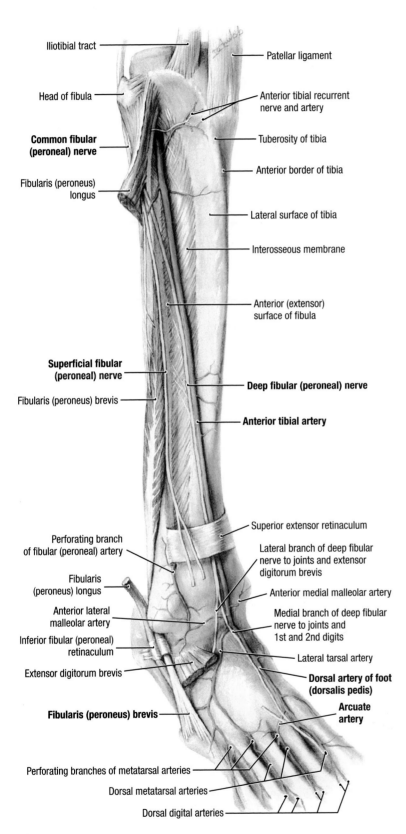

Iliotibial tract
Patellar ligament
Head of fibula
Anterior tibial recurrent nerve and artery
Common fibular (peroneal) nerve
Tuberosity of tibia
Fibularis (peroneus) longus
Anterior border of tibia
Lateral surface of tibia
Interosseous membrane
Anterior (extensor) surface of fibula
Superficial fibular (peroneal) nerve
Deep fibular (peroneal) nerve
Fibularis (peroneus) brevis
Anterior tibial artery
Superior extensor retinaculum
Perforating branch of fibular (peroneal) artery
Lateral branch of deep fibular nerve to joints and extensor digitorum brevis
Anterior medial malleolar artery
Fibularis (peroneus) longus
Anterior lateral malleolar artery
Medial branch of deep fibular nerve to joints and 1st and 2nd digits
Inferior fibular (peroneal) retinaculum
Extensor digitorum brevis
Lateral tarsal artery
Dorsal artery of foot (dorsalis pedis)
Fibularis (peroneus) brevis
Arcuate artery
Perforating branches of metatarsal arteries
Dorsal metatarsal arteries
Dorsal digital arteries

C. Anterolateral View

5.54   **Anterior leg—deep muscles, nerves and vessels (continued)**

A. Overview of motor innervation. **B.** Deep dissection of the anterior compartment of the leg. The muscles are separated to display the anterior tibial artery and deep fibular nerve. **C.** Neurovascular structures. **D.** Relations of common fibular nerve and branches to the proximal fibula.

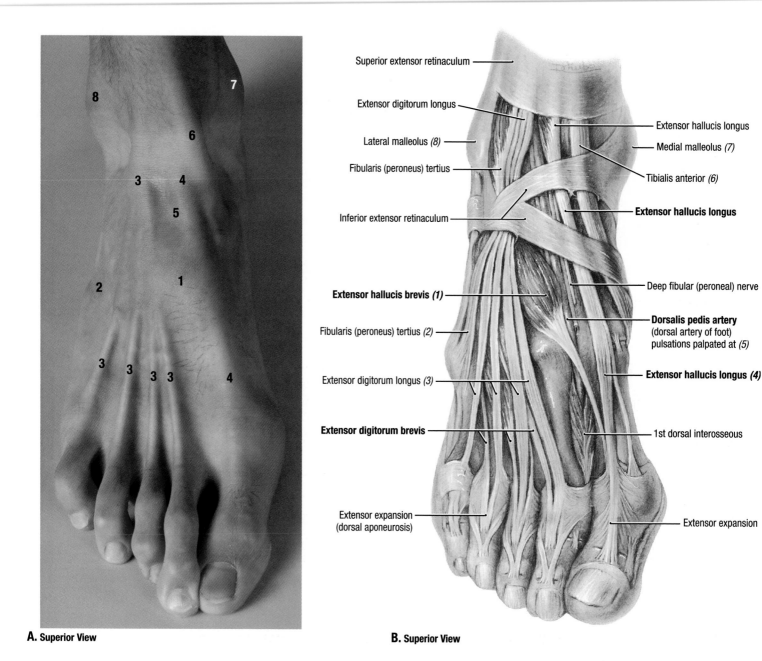

A. Superior View

B. Superior View

Labels in B (clockwise from top):
- Superior extensor retinaculum
- Extensor digitorum longus
- Lateral malleolus (8)
- Fibularis (peroneus) tertius
- Inferior extensor retinaculum
- **Extensor hallucis brevis (1)**
- Fibularis (peroneus) tertius (2)
- Extensor digitorum longus (3)
- **Extensor digitorum brevis**
- Extensor expansion (dorsal aponeurosis)
- Extensor hallucis longus
- Medial malleolus (7)
- Tibialis anterior (6)
- **Extensor hallucis longus**
- Deep fibular (peroneal) nerve
- **Dorsalis pedis artery** (dorsal artery of foot) pulsations palpated at (5)
- **Extensor hallucis longus (4)**
- 1st dorsal interosseous
- Extensor expansion

5.55   Dorsum of foot

A. Surface anatomy (*numbers* refer to structures labeled in **B**). **B.** Dissection. The dorsal vein of foot and deep fibular nerve are cut. At the ankle, the dorsalis pedis artery (dorsal artery of foot) and deep fibular nerve lie midway between the malleoli. On the dorsum of the foot, the dorsal artery of foot is crossed by the extensor hallucis brevis muscle and disappears between the two heads of the first dorsal interosseous muscle.

Clinically, knowing the location of the belly of the extensor digitorum brevis is important for distinguishing this muscle from abnormal edema. Contusion and tearing of the muscle fibers and associated blood vessels result in a hematoma, producing edema anteromedial to the lateral malleolus. Most people who have not seen this inflamed muscle assume they have a severely sprained ankle.

Dorsalis pedis pulses may be palpated with the feet slightly dorsiflexed. The pulses are usually easy to palpate because the dorsal arteries of the foot are subcutaneous and pass along a line from the extensor retinaculum to a point just lateral to the extensor hallucis longus tendon. A diminished or absent dorsalis pedis pulse usually suggests vascular insufficiency resulting from arterial disease.

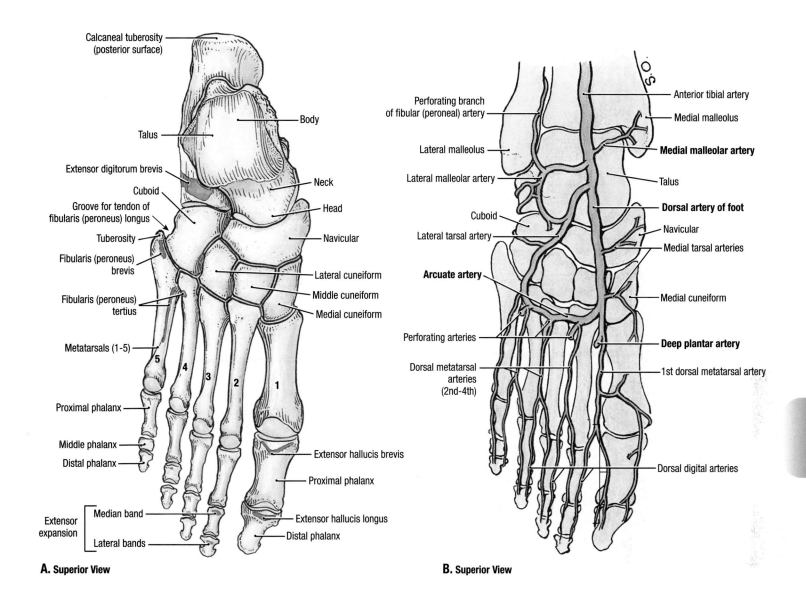

A. Superior View

B. Superior View

5.56 **Attachments of muscles and arteries of the dorsum of foot**

A. Attachments. **B.** Arterial supply.

TABLE 5.11 ARTERIAL SUPPLY TO DORSUM OF FOOT

Artery	Origin	Course and Distribution
(L. *dorsalis pedis*) **Dorsal artery of foot**	Continuation of anterior tibial artery distal to talocrural joint	Descends anteromedially to 1st interosseous space and divides into plantar and arcuate arteries
Lateral tarsal artery	Dorsal artery of foot	Runs an arched course laterally beneath extensor digitorum brevis to anastomose with branches of arcuate artery
Arcuate artery		Runs laterally from 1st interosseous space across bases of lateral four metatarsals, deep to extensor tendons
Deep plantar artery		Passes to sole of foot and joins plantar arch
Metatarsal arteries **1st**	Deep plantar artery	Run between metatarsals to clefts of toes where each vessel divides into two dorsal digital arteries.
2nd to 4th	Arcuate artery	Perforating arteries connect to plantar arch and plantar metatarsal arteries.
Dorsal digital arteries	Metatarsal arteries	Pass to sides of adjoining toes

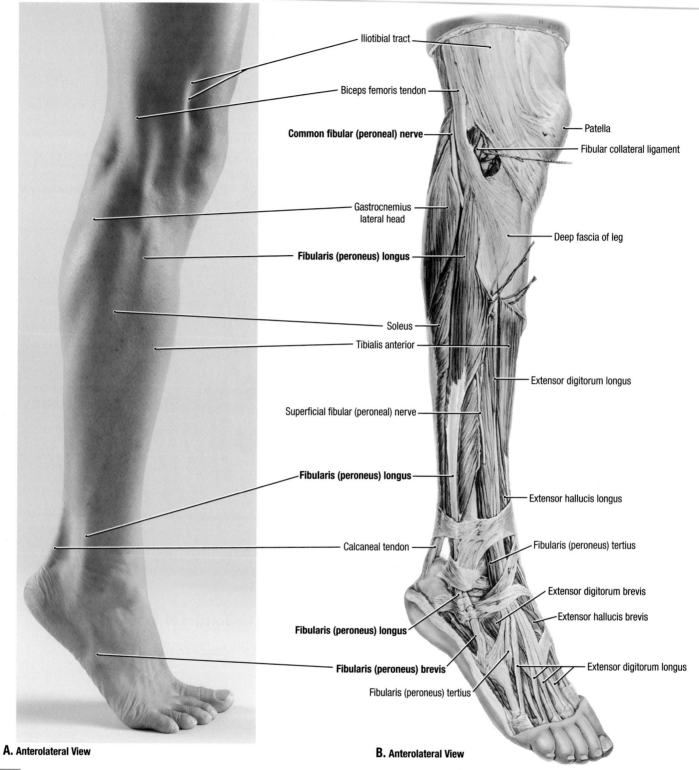

Iliotibial tract

Biceps femoris tendon

Common fibular (peroneal) nerve

Patella

Fibular collateral ligament

Gastrocnemius
lateral head

Deep fascia of leg

Fibularis (peroneus) longus

Soleus

Tibialis anterior

Extensor digitorum longus

Superficial fibular (peroneal) nerve

Fibularis (peroneus) longus

Extensor hallucis longus

Fibularis (peroneus) tertius

Calcaneal tendon

Extensor digitorum brevis

Extensor hallucis brevis

Fibularis (peroneus) longus

Extensor digitorum longus

Fibularis (peroneus) brevis

Fibularis (peroneus) tertius

A. Anterolateral View

B. Anterolateral View

5.57 Muscles of lateral aspect of leg and foot

A. Surface anatomy. **B.** Dissection
- The two fibular (peroneal) muscles both attach to two thirds of the fibula, the fibularis (peroneus) longus muscle to the proximal two thirds, and the fibularis (peroneus) brevis muscle to the distal two thirds. Where they overlap, the fibularis brevis muscle lies anteriorly.
- The fibularis (peroneus) longus muscle enters the foot by

hooking around the cuboid and traveling medially to the base of the first metatarsal and medial cuneiform.

The common fibular (peroneal) nerve is in contact with the neck of the fibula deep to the fibularis longus muscle. Here it is vulnerable to injury with serious implications; because it supplies the extensor and everter muscle groups, loss of function results in foot-drop (inability to dorsiflex the ankle) and difficulty in everting the foot.

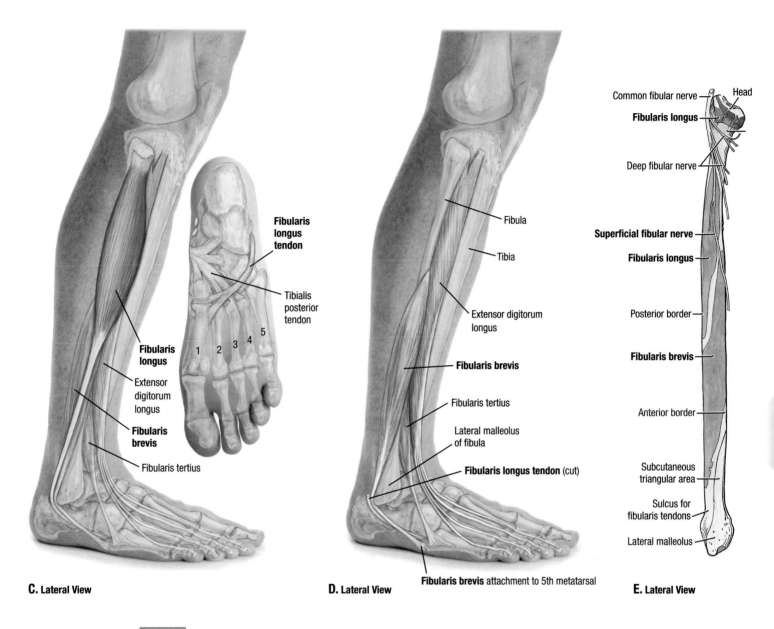

C. Lateral View   **D.** Lateral View   **Fibularis brevis** attachment to 5th metatarsal   **E.** Lateral View

5.57   **Muscles of lateral aspect of leg and foot** *(continued)*

C. Fibularis (peroneus) longus. **D.** Fibularis (peroneus) brevis. **E.** Attachments sites on fibula.

TABLE 5.12 MUSCLES OF THE LATERAL COMPARTMENT OF LEG

Muscle	Proximal Attachment	Distal Attachment	Innervation[a]	Main Actions
Fibularis (peroneus) longus	Head and superior two thirds of lateral surface of fibula	Base of first metatarsal and medial cuneiform	Superficial fibular (peroneal) nerve (**L5, S1,** and **S2**)	Evert foot and weakly plantarflex ankle
Fibularis (peroneus) brevis	Inferior two thirds of lateral surface of fibula	Dorsal surface of tuberosity on lateral side of base of fifth metatarsal		

[a]See Table 5.1 for explanation of segmental innervation

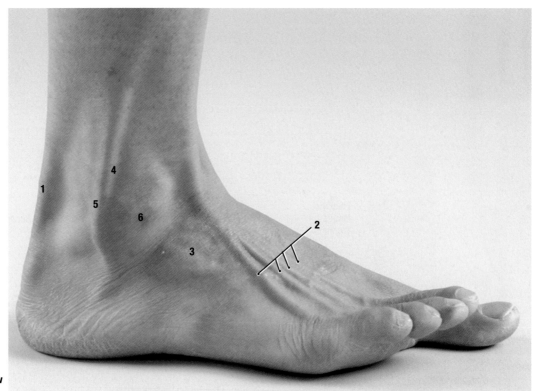

A. Lateral View

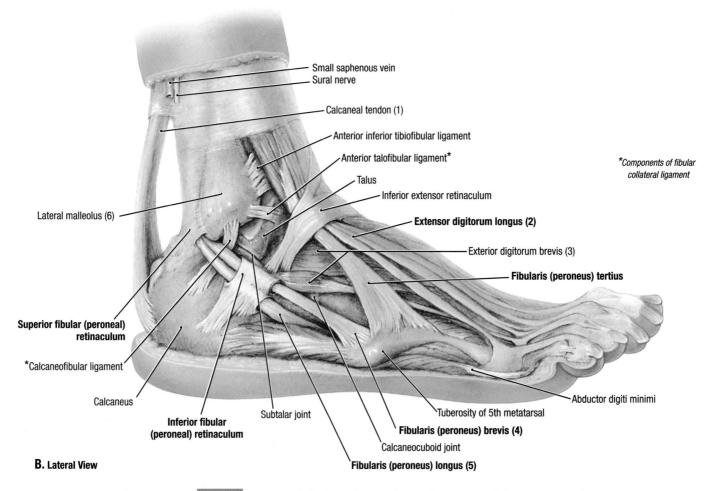

Small saphenous vein
Sural nerve
Calcaneal tendon (1)
Anterior inferior tibiofibular ligament
Anterior talofibular ligament*
Talus
Inferior extensor retinaculum
Extensor digitorum longus (2)
Exterior digitorum brevis (3)
Fibularis (peroneus) tertius

*Components of fibular
collateral ligament

Lateral malleolus (6)

**Superior fibular (peroneal)
retinaculum**

*Calcaneofibular ligament

Calcaneus

**Inferior fibular
(peroneal) retinaculum**

Subtalar joint

Abductor digiti minimi

Tuberosity of 5th metatarsal

Fibularis (peroneus) brevis (4)

Calcaneocuboid joint

Fibularis (peroneus) longus (5)

B. Lateral View

5.58 **Synovial sheaths and tendons at ankle**

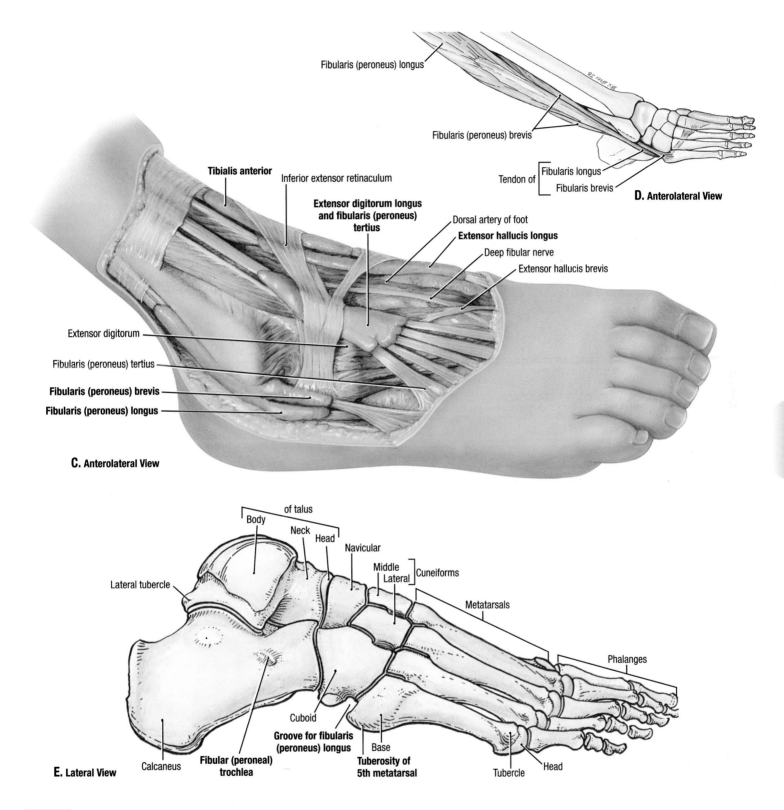

Fibularis (peroneus) longus

Fibularis (peroneus) brevis

Tendon of
Fibularis longus
Fibularis brevis

D. Anterolateral View

Tibialis anterior

Inferior extensor retinaculum

**Extensor digitorum longus
and fibularis (peroneus)
tertius**

Dorsal artery of foot

Extensor hallucis longus

Deep fibular nerve

Extensor hallucis brevis

Extensor digitorum

Fibularis (peroneus) tertius

Fibularis (peroneus) brevis

Fibularis (peroneus) longus

C. Anterolateral View

of talus

Body

Neck   Head

Navicular

Middle
Lateral   Cuneiforms

Lateral tubercle

Metatarsals

Phalanges

Cuboid

**Groove for fibularis
(peroneus) longus**

Base

**Tuberosity of
5th metatarsal**

Head

Tubercle

Calcaneus   **Fibular (peroneal)
trochlea**

E. Lateral View

5.58   **Synovial sheaths and tendons at ankle *(continued)***

A. Surface anatomy (*numbers* refer to structures labeled in **B**). **B.** Tendons at the lateral aspect of the ankle. **C.** Synovial sheaths of tendons on the anterolateral aspect of the ankle. The tendons of the fibularis (peroneus) longus and fibularis (peroneus) brevis muscles are enclosed in a common synovial sheath posterior to the lateral malleolus. This sheath splits into two, one for each tendon, posterior to the fibular (peroneal) trochlea. **D.** Schematic illustration of fibularis longus and brevis. **E.** Lateral aspect of bones of foot.

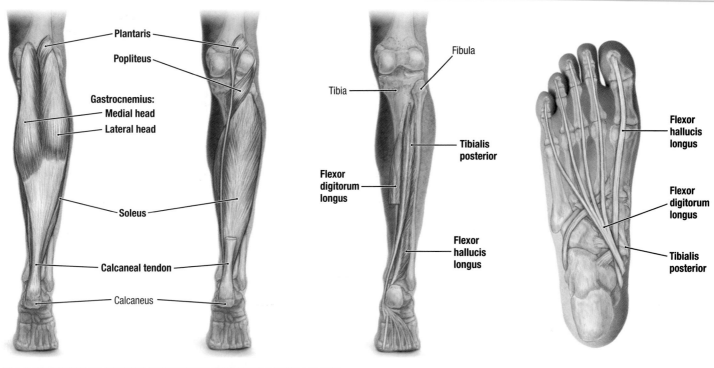

TABLE 5.13 MUSCLES OF THE POSTERIOR COMPARTMENT OF LEG

Muscle	Proximal Attachment	Distal Attachment	Innervation[a]	Main Actions
Superficial muscles				
Gastrocnemius	*Lateral head:* lateral aspect of lateral condyle of femur	Posterior surface of calcaneus with calcaneal tendon (tendocalcaneus)	Tibial nerve (S1 and S2)	Plantarflexes ankle when knee is extended; raises heel during walking, and flexes leg at knee joint
	Medial head: popliteal surface of femur, superior to medial condyle to medial condyle			
Soleus	Posterior aspect of head of fibula, superior fourth of posterior surface of fibula, soleal lne and medial border of tibia			Plantarflexes ankle (independent of knee position) and steadies leg on foot
Plantaris	Inferior end of lateral supracondylar supracondylar line of femur and oblique popliteal ligament			Weakly assists gastrocnemius in plantarflexing ankle and flexing knee
Deep muscles				
Popliteus	Lateral surface of lateral condyle of femur and lateral meniscus	Posterior surface of tibia, superior to soleal line	Tibial nerve (**L4,** L5, and S1)	Unlocks fully extended knee (laterally rotates femur 5° on planted tibia); weakly flexes knee
Flexor hallucis longus	Inferior two thirds of posterior surface of fibula and inferior part of interosseous membrane	Base of distal phalanx of great toe (hallux)		Flexes great toe at all joints and plantarflexes ankle; supports medial longitudinal arch of foot
Flexor digitorum longus	Medial part of posterior surface of tibia inferior to soleal line, and by a broad tendon to fibula	Bases of distal phalanges of lateral four digits	Tibial nerve (**S2** and S3)	Flexes lateral four digits and plantarflexes ankle; supports longitudinal arches of foot
Tibialis posterior	Interosseous membrane, posterior surface of tibia inferior to soleal line and posterior surface of fibula	Tuberosity of navicular, cuneiform, and cuboid and bases of metatarsals 2–4	Tibial nerve (L4 and L5)	Plantarflexes ankle and inverts foot

[a]See Table 5.1 for explanation of segmental innervation.

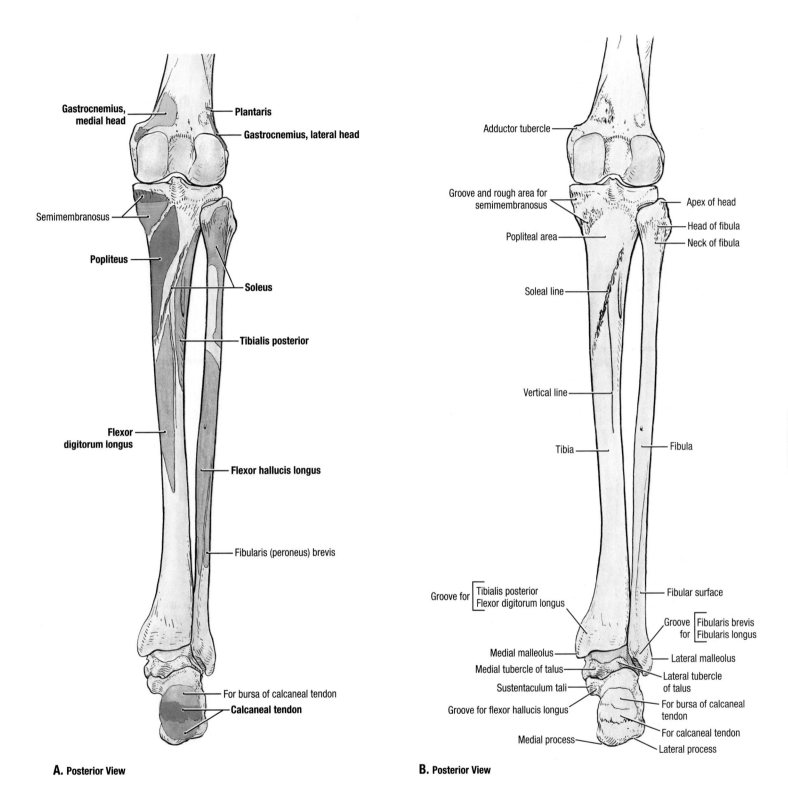

A. Posterior View

- Gastrocnemius, medial head
- Plantaris
- Gastrocnemius, lateral head
- Semimembranosus
- Popliteus
- Soleus
- Tibialis posterior
- Flexor digitorum longus
- Flexor hallucis longus
- Fibularis (peroneus) brevis
- For bursa of calcaneal tendon
- Calcaneal tendon

B. Posterior View

- Adductor tubercle
- Groove and rough area for semimembranosus
- Apex of head
- Head of fibula
- Popliteal area
- Neck of fibula
- Soleal line
- Vertical line
- Tibia
- Fibula
- Groove for | Tibialis posterior / Flexor digitorum longus
- Fibular surface
- Groove for | Fibularis brevis / Fibularis longus
- Medial malleolus
- Lateral malleolus
- Medial tubercle of talus
- Lateral tubercle of talus
- Sustentaculum tali
- For bursa of calcaneal tendon
- Groove for flexor hallucis longus
- For calcaneal tendon
- Medial process
- Lateral process

5.59 **Bones of the posterior aspect of leg**

A. Muscle attachments. **B.** Features of bones.

The tibial shaft is narrowest at the junction of its middle and inferior thirds, which is the most frequent site of fracture. Unfortunately, this area of the bone also has the poorest blood supply.

Fibular fractures commonly occur 2–6 cm proximal to the distal end of the lateral malleolus and are often associated with fracture/dislocations of the ankle joint, which are combined with tibial fractures. When a person slips and the foot is forced into an excessively inverted position, the ankle ligaments tear, forcibly tilting the talus against the lateral malleolus and shearing it off.

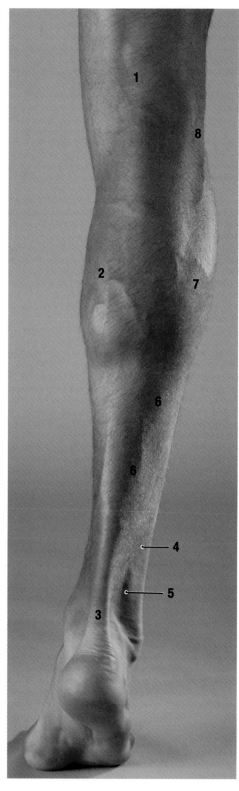

A. Posterior View

Semitendinosus

Semimembranosus *(1)*

Gracilis

Sartorius

Gastrocnemius, medial head *(2)*

Flexor digitorum longus

Tibialis posterior

Flexor retinaculum

Biceps femoris *(8)*

Tibial nerve

Common fibular (peroneal) nerve

Medial sural cutaneous nerve

Gastrocnemius, lateral head *(7)*

Soleus *(6)*

Fibularis (peroneus) longus *(4)*

Fibularis (peroneus) brevis *(5)*

Calcaneal tendon *(3)*

Superior fibular (peroneal) retinaculum

B. Posterior View

| 5.60 | **Posterior leg, superficial muscles of posterior compartment** |

A. Surface anatomy (*numbers* refer to structures labeled in **B**). **B.** Dissection. Gastrocnemius strain(tennis leg) is a painful calf injury resulting from partial tearing of the medial belly of the muscle at or near its musculotendinous junction. It is caused by overstretching the muscle during simultaneous full extension of the knee and dorsiflexion of the ankle.

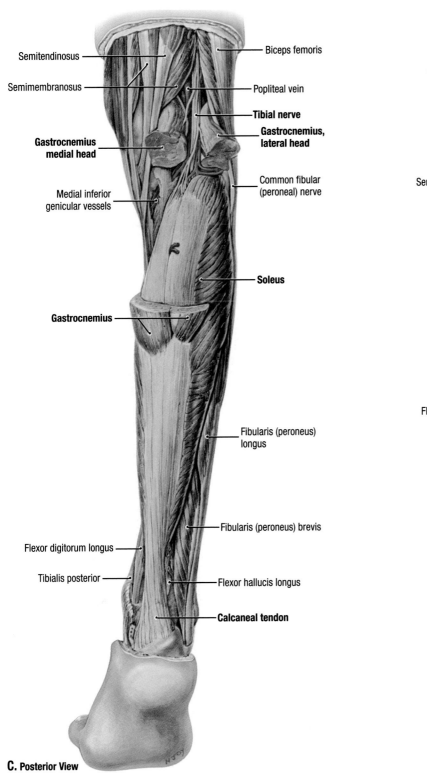

C. Posterior View

Semitendinosus

Semimembranosus

Gastrocnemius medial head

Medial inferior genicular vessels

Gastrocnemius

Flexor digitorum longus

Tibialis posterior

Biceps femoris

Popliteal vein

Tibial nerve

Gastrocnemius, lateral head

Common fibular (peroneal) nerve

Soleus

Fibularis (peroneus) longus

Fibularis (peroneus) brevis

Flexor hallucis longus

Calcaneal tendon

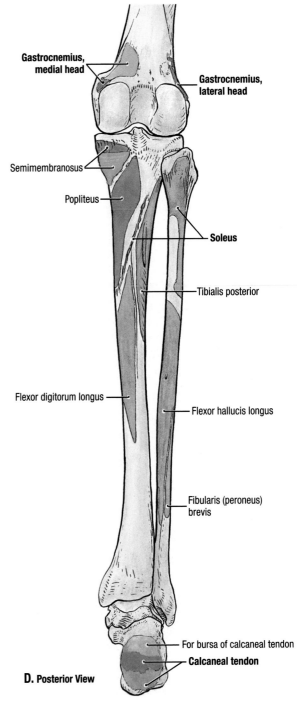

D. Posterior View

Gastrocnemius, medial head

Gastrocnemius, lateral head

Semimembranosus

Popliteus

Soleus

Tibialis posterior

Flexor digitorum longus

Flexor hallucis longus

Fibularis (peroneus) brevis

For bursa of calcaneal tendon

Calcaneal tendon

5.60   **Posterior leg, superficial muscles of posterior compartment (continued)**

C. Dissection revealing soleus. **D.** Bones of leg showing muscle attachments. Inflammation of the calcaneal tendon due to microscopic tears of collagen fibers in the tendon, particularly just superior to its attachment to the calcaneus, results in tendinitis, which causes pain during walking. Calcaneal tendon rupture is probably the most severe acute muscular problem of the leg. Following complete rupture of the tendon, passive dorsiflexion is excessive, and the person cannot plantarflex against resistance.

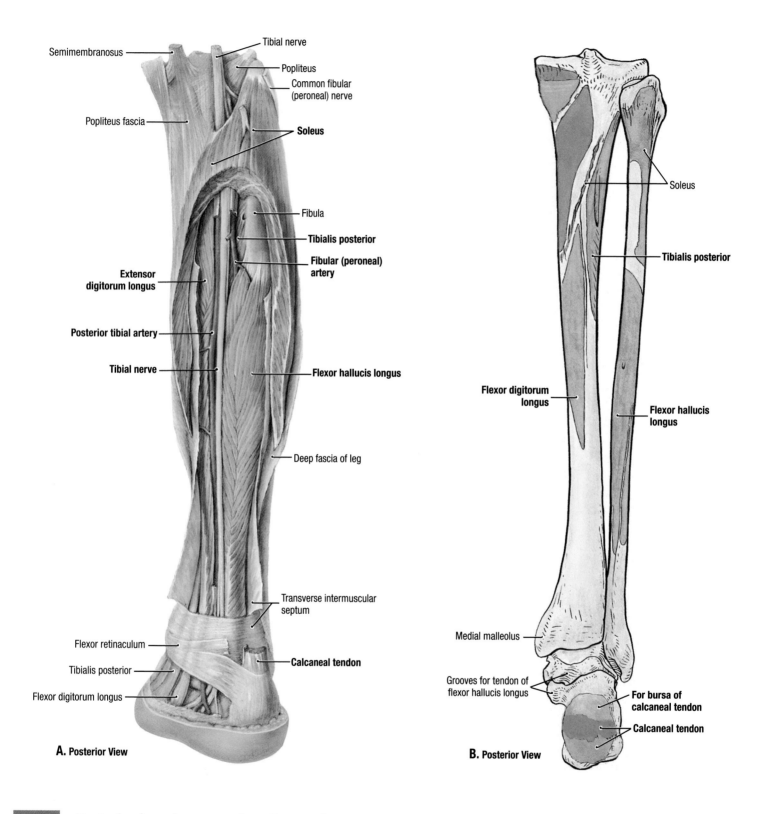

Semimembranosus

Tibial nerve

Popliteus

Common fibular (peroneal) nerve

Popliteus fascia

Soleus

Fibula

Tibialis posterior

Fibular (peroneal) artery

Extensor digitorum longus

Posterior tibial artery

Tibial nerve

Flexor hallucis longus

Deep fascia of leg

Transverse intermuscular septum

Flexor retinaculum

Tibialis posterior

Calcaneal tendon

Flexor digitorum longus

A. Posterior View

Soleus

Tibialis posterior

Flexor digitorum longus

Flexor hallucis longus

Medial malleolus

Grooves for tendon of flexor hallucis longus

For bursa of calcaneal tendon

Calcaneal tendon

B. Posterior View

5.61   **Posterior leg, deep muscles of posterior compartment**

A. Superficial dissection. The calcaneal tendon (Achilles tendon) is cut, the gastrocnemius muscle is removed, and only a horseshoe-shaped proximal part of the soleus muscle remains in place. **B.** Bones of leg showing muscle attachments. Calcaneal bursitis results from inflammation of the bursa of the calcaneal tendon located between the calcaneal tendon and the superior part of the posterior surface of the calcaneus. Calcaneal bursitis causes pain posterior to the heel and occurs commonly during long-distance running, basketball, and tennis. It is caused by excessive friction on the bursa as the calcaneal tendon continuously slides over it.

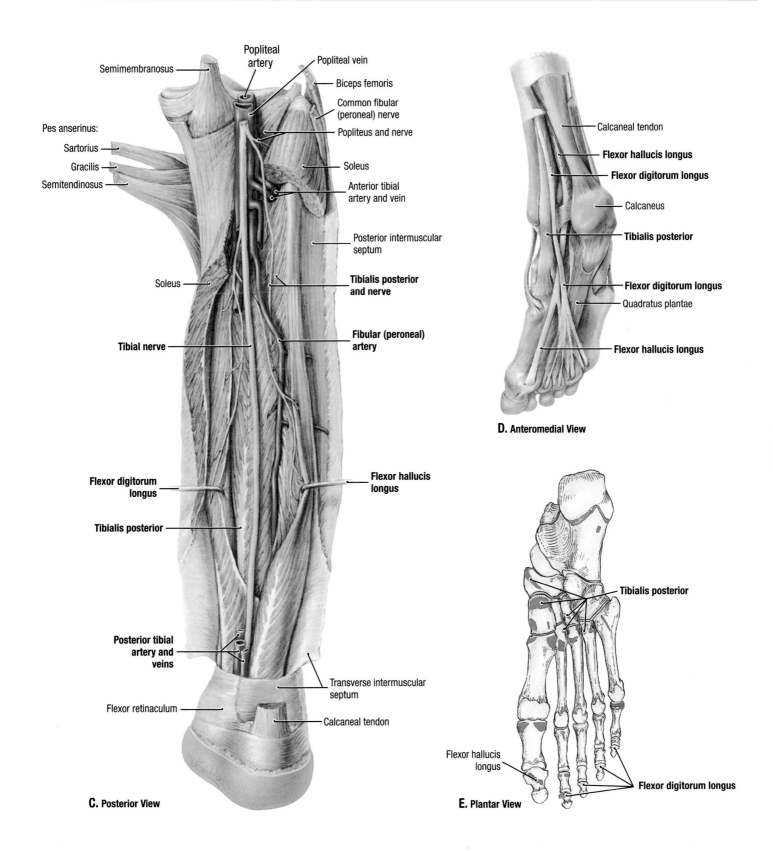

Popliteal
artery

Semimembranosus

Popliteal vein

Biceps femoris

Common fibular
(peroneal) nerve

Popliteus and nerve

Pes anserinus:

Sartorius

Gracilis

Semitendinosus

Soleus

Anterior tibial
artery and vein

Posterior intermuscular
septum

Soleus

**Tibialis posterior
and nerve**

Tibial nerve

**Fibular (peroneal)
artery**

**Flexor digitorum
longus**

**Flexor hallucis
longus**

Tibialis posterior

**Posterior tibial
artery and
veins**

Transverse intermuscular
septum

Flexor retinaculum

Calcaneal tendon

C. Posterior View

Calcaneal tendon

Flexor hallucis longus

Flexor digitorum longus

Calcaneus

Tibialis posterior

Flexor digitorum longus

Quadratus plantae

Flexor hallucis longus

D. Anteromedial View

Tibialis posterior

Flexor hallucis
longus

Flexor digitorum longus

E. Plantar View

5.61   **Posterior leg, deep muscles of posterior compartment *(continued)***

C. Deeper dissection. The flexor hallucis longus and flexor digitorum longus are pulled apart, and the posterior tibial artery is partly excised. The tibialis posterior lies deep to the two long digital flexors. **D.** Crossing of muscles (tendons) of the deep compartment superoposterior to the medial malleolus and into the sole of the foot. **E.** Bones of foot showing muscle attachments.

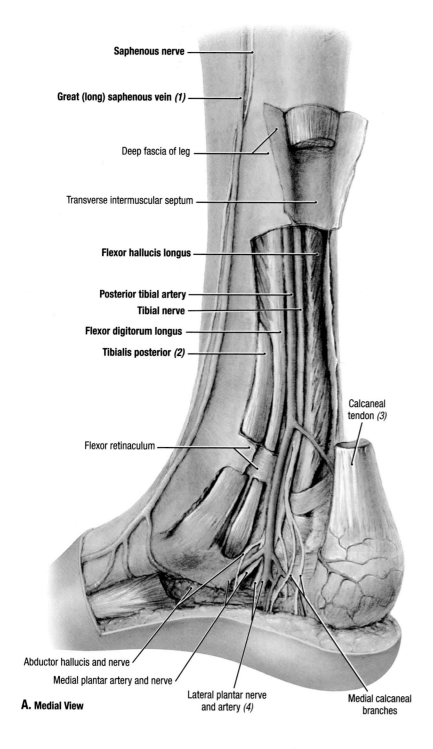

Saphenous nerve

Great (long) saphenous vein *(1)*

Deep fascia of leg

Transverse intermuscular septum

Flexor hallucis longus

Posterior tibial artery

Tibial nerve

Flexor digitorum longus

Tibialis posterior *(2)*

Calcaneal
tendon *(3)*

Flexor retinaculum

Abductor hallucis and nerve

Medial plantar artery and nerve

Lateral plantar nerve
and artery *(4)*

Medial calcaneal
branches

A. Medial View

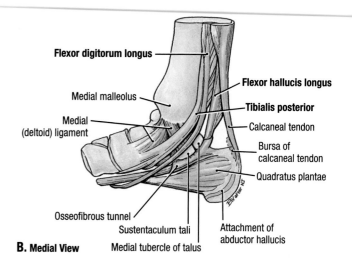

Flexor digitorum longus

Medial malleolus

Medial
(deltoid) ligament

Flexor hallucis longus

Tibialis posterior

Calcaneal tendon

Bursa of
calcaneal tendon

Quadratus plantae

Osseofibrous tunnel

Sustentaculum tali

Medial tubercle of talus

Attachment of
abductor hallucis

B. Medial View

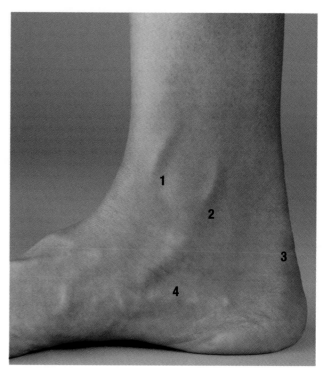

C. Medial View

5.62   **Medial ankle region**

A. Dissection. The calcaneal tendon and posterior part of the abductor hallucis were excised. **B.** Schematic illustration of the tendons passing posterior to medial malleolus. **C.** Surface anatomy (*numbers* refer to structures labeled in **A**).

- The posterior tibial artery and the tibial nerve lie between the flexor digitorum longus and flexor hallucis longus muscles and divide into medial and lateral plantar branches.

- The tibialis posterior and flexor digitorum longus tendons occupy separate osseofibrous tunnels posterior to the medial malleolus.

- The posterior tibial pulse can usually be palpated between the posterior surface of the medial malleolus and the medial border of the calcaneal tendon.

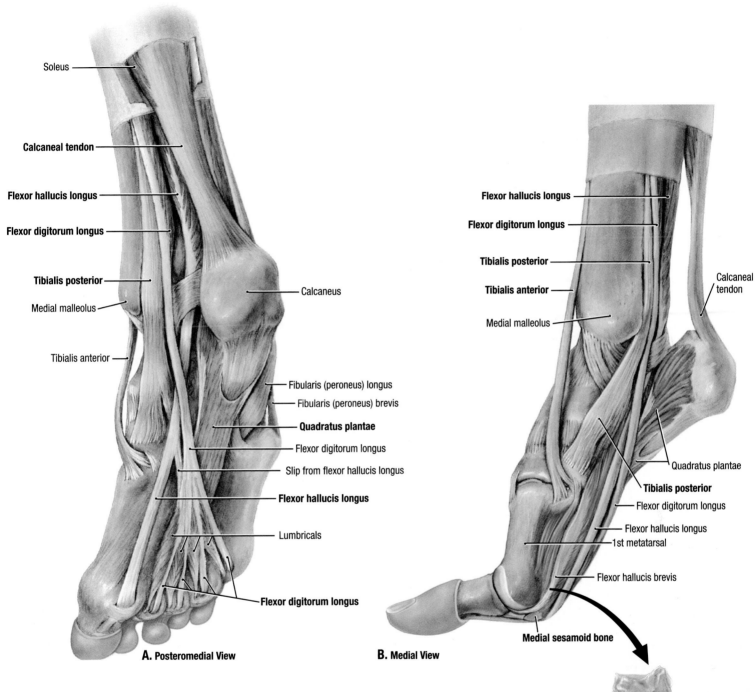

A. Posteromedial View

B. Medial View

C. Plantar Surface

5.63   **Medial ankle and foot**

A. Tendons of deep compartment of the leg traced to their distal attachments in the sole of the foot. **B.** Foot raised as in walking and sesamoid bones of the great toe. The sesamoid bones of the great toe are located on each side of a bony ridge on the 1st metatarsal.

- The sesamoid bones are a "footstool" for the first metatarsal, giving it increased height.
- By inserting into the flexor digitorum longus muscle, the quadratus plantae muscle modifies the oblique pull of the flexor tendons.
- The flexor hallucis longus muscle uses three pulleys: a groove on the posterior aspect of the distal end of the tibia, a groove on the posterior aspect of the talus, and a groove inferior to the sustentaculum tali.
- The flexor digitorum longus muscle crosses superficial to the tibialis posterior, superoposterior to the medial malleolus.

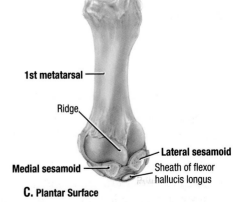

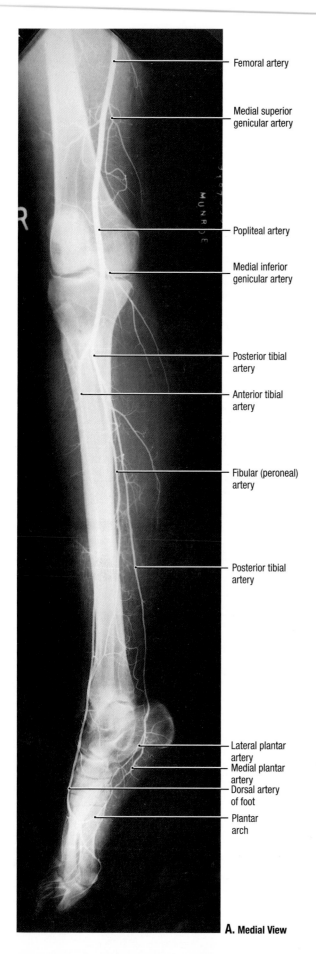

Femoral artery

Medial superior
genicular artery

Popliteal artery

Medial inferior
genicular artery

Posterior tibial
artery

Anterior tibial
artery

Fibular (peroneal)
artery

Posterior tibial
artery

Lateral plantar
artery
Medial plantar
artery
Dorsal artery
of foot
Plantar
arch

A. Medial View

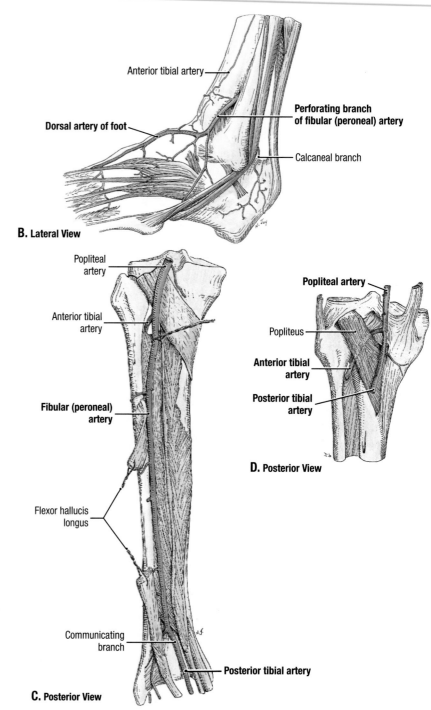

Anterior tibial artery

Dorsal artery of foot

**Perforating branch
of fibular (peroneal) artery**

Calcaneal branch

B. Lateral View

Popliteal
artery

Anterior tibial
artery

**Fibular (peroneal)
artery**

Flexor hallucis
longus

Communicating
branch

Posterior tibial artery

C. Posterior View

Popliteal artery

Popliteus

**Anterior tibial
artery**

**Posterior tibial
artery**

D. Posterior View

5.64 Popliteal arteriogram and arterial anomalies

A. Popliteal arteriogram. The femoral artery becomes the popliteal artery at the adductor hiatus. The anterior tibial artery continues as the dorsalis pedis (dorsal artery of the foot). The posterior tibial artery terminates as the medial and lateral plantar arteries; its major branch is the fibular artery. **B.** Anomalous dorsal artery of the foot. The perforating branch of the fibular artery rarely continues as the dorsal artery of the foot, but when it does, the anterior tibial artery ends proximal to the ankle or is a slender vessel. **C.** Absence of posterior tibial artery. Compensatory enlargement of the fibular artery was found to occur in approximately 5% of limbs. **D.** High division of popliteal artery. Along with the anterior tibial artery descending anterior to the popliteus muscle; this anomaly was found to occur in approximately 2% of limbs.

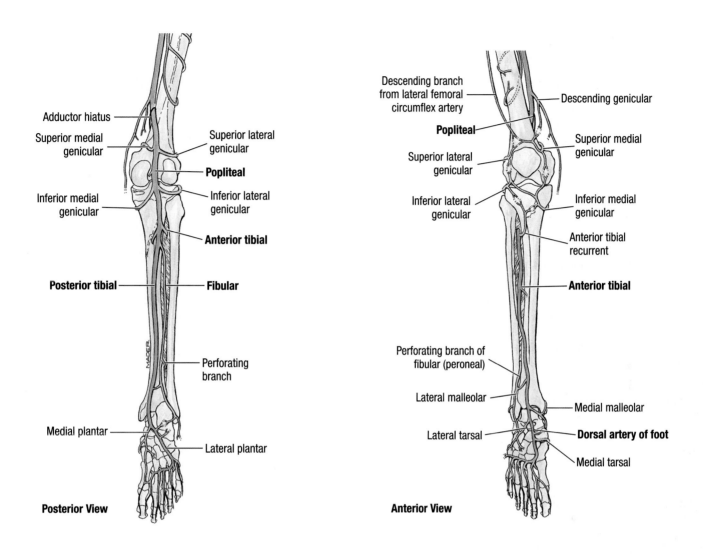

Posterior View

Anterior View

TABLE 5.14 ARTERIAL SUPPLY OF LEG AND FOOT

Artery	Origin	Course	Distribution in Leg
Popliteal	Continuation of femoral artery at adductor hiatus	Passes through popliteal fossa to leg; divides into anterior and posterior tibial arteries at lower border of popliteus	Lateral and medial aspects of knee via genicular arteries
Anterior tibial	Popliteal	Passes between tibia and fibula into anterior compartment through gap superior to inter- osseous membrane; descends between tibialis anterior and extensor digitorum longus muscles	Anterior compartment
Dorsal artery of foot (dorsalis pedis)	Continuation of anterior tibial artery distal to talocrural joint	Descends to first interosseous space; divides into plantar and arcuate arteries	Muscles on dorsum of foot; pierces first dorsal interosseous muscle as deep plantar artery; joins deep plantar arch
Posterior tibial	Popliteal	Passes through posterior compartment; divides into medial and lateral plantar arteries posterior to medial malleolus	Posterior and lateral compartments, nutrient artery passes to tibia
Fibular (peroneal)	Posterior tibial	Descends in posterior compartment adjacent to posterior intermuscular septum	Posterior compartment: perforating branches supply lateral compartment
Medial plantar		In foot between abductor hallucis and flexor digitorum brevis muscles	Supplies mainly muscles of great toe and skin on medial side of sole of foot
Lateral plantar	Posterior tibial	Runs anterolaterally deep to abductor hallucis and flexor digitorum brevis, then arches medially to form deep plantar arch	Supplies remainder (lateral aspect) of sole of foot

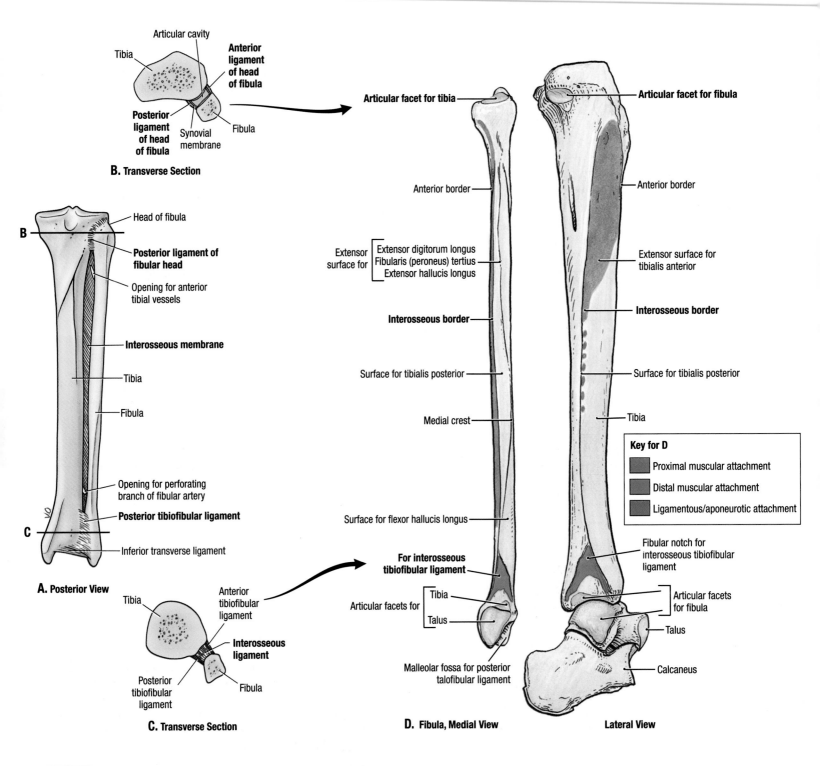

B. Transverse Section

- Articular cavity
- Tibia
- **Anterior ligament of head of fibula**
- **Posterior ligament of head of fibula**
- Synovial membrane
- Fibula

A. Posterior View

- Head of fibula
- **Posterior ligament of fibular head**
- Opening for anterior tibial vessels
- **Interosseous membrane**
- Tibia
- Fibula
- Opening for perforating branch of fibular artery
- **Posterior tibiofibular ligament**
- Inferior transverse ligament

C. Transverse Section

- Tibia
- Anterior tibiofibular ligament
- **Interosseous ligament**
- Posterior tibiofibular ligament
- Fibula

D. Fibula, Medial View

- Articular facet for tibia
- Anterior border
- Extensor surface for: Extensor digitorum longus, Fibularis (peroneus) tertius, Extensor hallucis longus
- **Interosseous border**
- Surface for tibialis posterior
- Medial crest
- Surface for flexor hallucis longus
- **For interosseous tibiofibular ligament**
- Articular facets for: Tibia, Talus
- Malleolar fossa for posterior talofibular ligament

Lateral View

- Articular facet for fibula
- Anterior border
- Extensor surface for tibialis anterior
- **Interosseous border**
- Surface for tibialis posterior
- Tibia
- Fibular notch for interosseous tibiofibular ligament
- Articular facets for fibula
- Talus
- Calcaneus

Key for D
- Proximal muscular attachment
- Distal muscular attachment
- Ligamentous/aponeurotic attachment

5.65   Superior tibiofibular joint and tibiofibular syndesmosis

A. Tibiofibular joints. **B.** Superior tibiofibular joint. **C.** Tibiofibular syndesmosis. **D.** Tibia and fibula, disarticulated.

- The superior tibiofibular joint (proximal tibiofibular joint) is a plane type of synovial joint between the flat facet on the fibular head and a similar facet located posterolaterally on the lateral tibial condyle. The tense joint capsule surrounds the joint and attaches to the margins of the articular surfaces of the fibula and tibia.

- The tibiofibular syndesmosis is a compound fibrous joint. This articulation is essential for stability of the ankle joint because it keeps the lateral malleolus firmly against the lateral surface of the talus. The strong interosseous tibiofibular ligament is continuous superiorly with the interosseous membrane and forms the principal connection between the distal ends of the tibia and fibula.

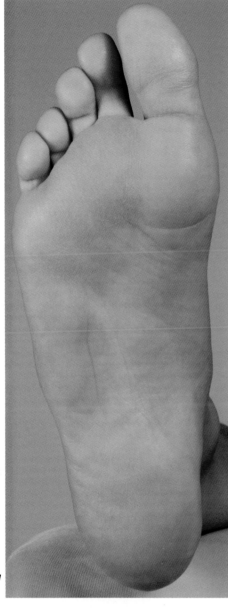

A. Plantar View

Flexor digitorum longus

Fibrous digital sheaths

Superficial transverse
metatarsal ligament

Flexor hallucis longus

Plantar digital
nerves and arteries

Plantar aponeurosis

Plantar fascia

Plantar fascia

Cutaneous branches
of lateral plantar
vessels and nerves

Cutaneous branches
of medial plantar
nerve and artery

Medial calcaneal branches
of tibial nerve and
calcaneal branches
of posterior tibial artery

Fat pad

B. Plantar View

Sesamoid bones of 1st metatarsal

Heads of 2nd to 5th metatarsals

Tuberosity of calcaneus

C. Plantar View

5.66 Sole of foot, superficial

A. Surface anatomy. **B.** Dissection. Plantar aponeurosis and fascia, with neurovascular structures. **C.** Weight-bearing areas.

- The weight of the body is transmitted to the talus from the tibia and fibula. It is then transmitted to the tuberosity of the calcaneus, the heads of the second to fifth metatarsals, and the sesamoid bones of the first digit.

- Straining and inflammation of the plantar aponeurosis, a condition called plantar fasciitis, may result from running and high-impact aerobics, especially when inappropriate footwear is worn. It causes pain on the plantar surface of the heel and on the medial aspect of the foot. Point tenderness is located at the proximal attachment of the plantar aponeurosis to the medial tubercle of the calcaneus and on the medial surface of this bone. The pain increases with passive extension of the great toe and may be further exacerbated by dorsiflexion of the ankle and/or weight bearing.

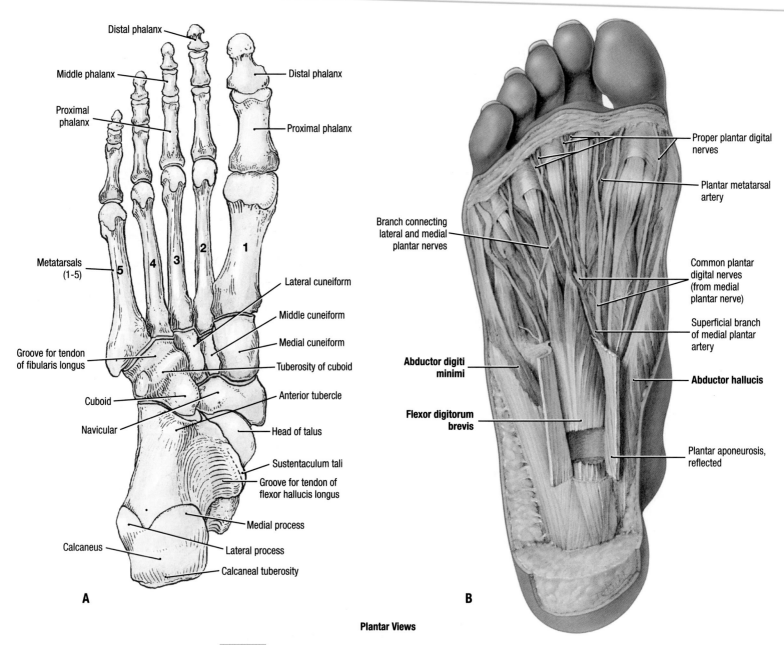

Plantar Views

5.67 **First layer of muscles of sole of foot**

A. Bones. **B.** Dissection. Muscles and neurovascular structures.

TABLE 5.15 MUSCLES IN SOLE OF FOOT—FIRST LAYER

Muscle	Proximal Attachment	Distal Attachment	Innervation	Actions[a]
Abductor hallucis	Medial process of tuberosity of calcaneus, flexor retinaculum, and plantar aponeurosis	Medial side of base of proximal phalanx of first digit	Medial plantar nerve (S2–S3)	Abducts and flexes
Flexor digitorum brevis	Medial process of tuberosity of calcaneus, plantar aponeurosis, and intermuscular septa	Both sides of middle phalanges of lateral four digits		Flexes lateral four digits
Abductor digiti minim	Medial and lateral processes of tuberosity of calcaneus, plantar aponeurosis, and intermuscular septa	Lateral side of base of proximal phalanx of fifth digit	Lateral plantar nerve (S2–S3)	Abducts and flexes fifth digit

[a]Although individual actions are described, the primary function of the intrinsic muscles of the foot is to act collectively to resist forces that stress (attempt to flatten) the arches of the foot.

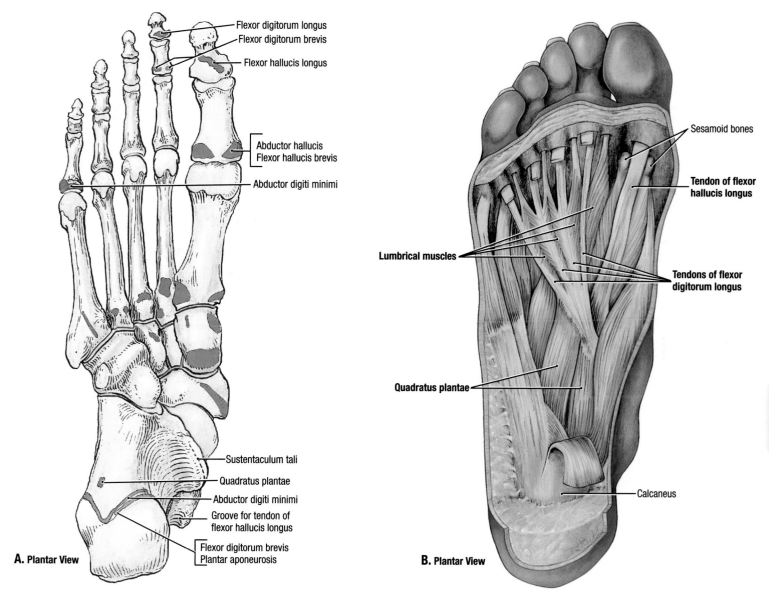

A. Plantar View

Flexor digitorum longus
Flexor digitorum brevis
Flexor hallucis longus

Abductor hallucis
Flexor hallucis brevis

Abductor digiti minimi

Sustentaculum tali
Quadratus plantae
Abductor digiti minimi
Groove for tendon of
flexor hallucis longus
Flexor digitorum brevis
Plantar aponeurosis

B. Plantar View

Sesamoid bones

Tendon of flexor
hallucis longus

Lumbrical muscles

Tendons of flexor
digitorum longus

Quadratus plantae

Calcaneus

5.68   **Second layer of muscles of sole of foot**

A. Bony attachments. **B.** Dissection. Muscles.

TABLE 5.16 MUSCLES IN SOLE OF FOOT—SECOND LAYER

Muscle	Proximal Attachment	Distal Attachment	Innervation	Actions[a]
Quadratus plantae	Medial surface and lateral margin of plantar surface of calcaneus	Posterolateral margin of tendon of flexor digitorum longus	Lateral plantar nerve (S2–**S3**)	Assists flexor digitorum longus in flexing lateral four digits
Lumbricals	Tendons of flexor digitorum longus	Medial aspect of extensor expansion over lateral four digits	*Medial one:* medial plantar nerve (S2–**S3**); *Lateral three:* lateral plantar nerve (S2–**S3**)	Flex proximal phalanges and extend middle and distal phalanges of lateral four digits

[a]Although individual actions are described, the primary function of the intrinsic muscles of the foot is to act collectively to resist forces that stress (attempt to flatten) the arches of the foot.

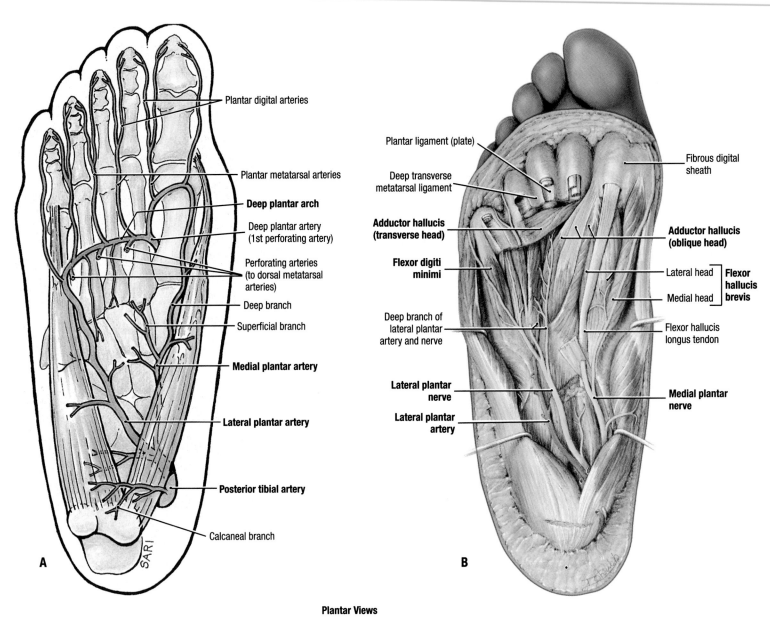

Plantar Views

5.69 **Third layer of muscles and arterial supply of sole of foot**

A. Arterial supply. **B.** Dissection. Muscles and neurovascular structures.

TABLE 5.17 MUSCLES IN SOLE OF FOOT—THIRD LAYER

Muscle	Proximal Attachment	Distal Attachment	Innervation	Actions[a]
Flexor hallucis brevis	Plantar surfaces of cuboid and lateral cuneiforms	Both sides of base of proximal phalanx of first digit	Medial plantar nerve (S2 –**S3**)	Flexes proximal phalanx of first digit
Adductor hallucis	*Oblique head:* bases of metatarsals 2–4; *Transverse head:* plantar ligaments of metatarsophalangeal joints	Tendons of both heads attach to lateral side of base of proximal phalanx of first digit	Deep branch of lateral plantar nerve (S2–**S3**)	Adducts first digit; assists in maintaining transverse arch of foot
Flexor digiti minimi	Base of fifth metatarsal	Base of proximal phalanx of fifth digit	Superficial branch of lateral plantar nerve (S2–**S3**)	Flexes proximal phalanx of fifth digit, thereby assisting with its flexion

[a]Although individual actions are described, the primary function of the intrinsic muscles of the foot is to act collectively to resist forces that stress (attempt to flatten) the arches of the foot.

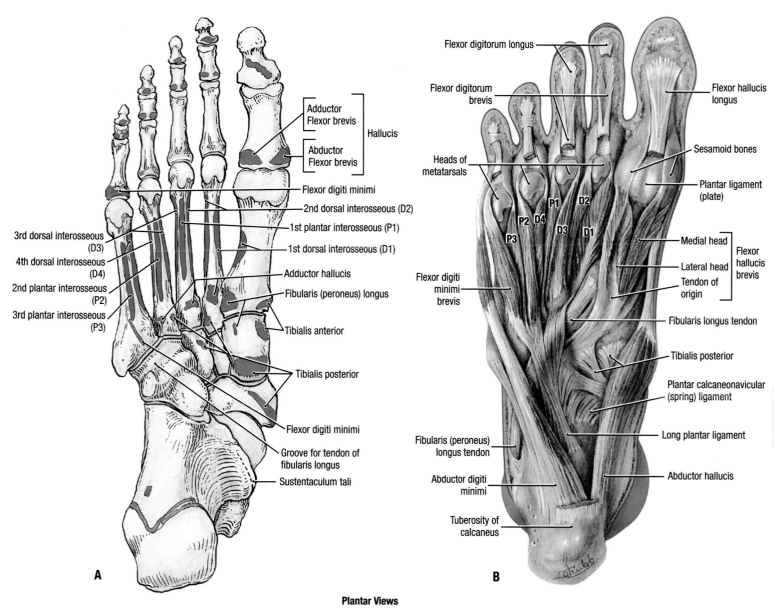

Plantar Views

5.70   **Fourth layer of muscles of sole of foot**

A. Bony attachments. **B.** Dissection. Muscles and ligaments.

TABLE 5.18 MUSCLES IN SOLE OF FOOT—FOURTH LAYER

Muscle	Proximal Attachment	Distal Attachment	Innervation	Actions[a]
Plantar interossei (three muscles; P1–P3)	Bases and medial sides of metatarsals 3–5	Medial sides of bases of proximal phalanges of third to fifth digits	Lateral plantar nerve (S2–S3)	Adduct digits (3–5) and flex metatarsophalangeal joints
Dorsal interossei (four muscles; D1–D4)	Adjacent sides of metatarsals 1–5	First: medial side of proximal phalanx of second digit Second to fourth: lateral sides of second to fourth digits		Abduct digits (2–4) and flex metatarsophalangeal joints

[a]Although individual actions are described, the primary function of the intrinsic muscles of the foot is to act collectively to resist forces that stress (attempt to flatten) the arches of the foot.

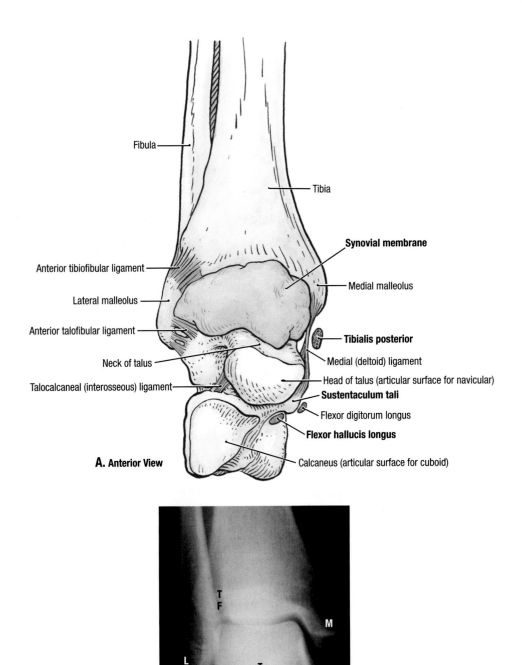

Fibula

Tibia

Synovial membrane

Anterior tibiofibular ligament

Medial malleolus

Lateral malleolus

Anterior talofibular ligament

Tibialis posterior

Neck of talus

Medial (deltoid) ligament

Head of talus (articular surface for navicular)

Talocalcaneal (interosseous) ligament

Sustentaculum tali

Flexor digitorum longus

Flexor hallucis longus

A. Anterior View

Calcaneus (articular surface for cuboid)

B. Anteroposterior View

5.71 **Joint cavity of ankle joint**

A. Ankle joint with joint cavity distended with injected latex.
B. Radiograph of joints of ankle region. *L*, lateral malleolus; *M*, medial malleolus; *T*, talus; *TF*, tibiofibular syndesmosis.

- The anterior articular surfaces of the calcaneus and head of the talus are each convex from side to side; thus the foot can be inverted and everted at the transverse tarsal joint.

- Note the relations of the tendons to the sustentaculum tali: the flexor hallucis longus inferior to it, flexor digitorum longus along its medial aspect, and tibialis posterior superior to it and in contact with the medial (deltoid) ligament.

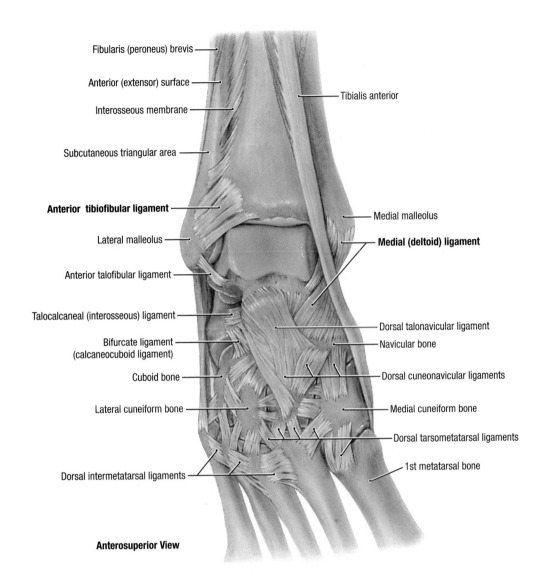

Fibularis (peroneus) brevis

Anterior (extensor) surface

Interosseous membrane

Subcutaneous triangular area

Anterior tibiofibular ligament

Lateral malleolus

Anterior talofibular ligament

Talocalcaneal (interosseous) ligament

Bifurcate ligament
(calcaneocuboid ligament)

Cuboid bone

Lateral cuneiform bone

Dorsal intermetatarsal ligaments

Tibialis anterior

Medial malleolus

Medial (deltoid) ligament

Dorsal talonavicular ligament

Navicular bone

Dorsal cuneonavicular ligaments

Medial cuneiform bone

Dorsal tarsometatarsal ligaments

1st metatarsal bone

Anterosuperior View

5.72 Ankle joint and ligaments of dorsum of foot

Dissection. The ankle joint is plantarflexed, and its anterior capsular fibers are removed.

- All muscles attached to the fibula except the biceps femoris pull inferiorly on the bone during contraction. The oblique fibers of the interosseous membrane and ligaments uniting the fibula to the tibia resist this inferior pull but allow the fibula to be forced superiorly during full dorsiflexion of the ankle.

- The anterior talofibular ligament (part of the lateral ligament of the ankle) is a weak band that is easily torn (see the legend for Fig. 5.77).

- The bifurcate ligament, a Y-shaped ligament consisting of calcaneocuboid and calcaneonavicular ligaments, and the talonavicular ligament are the primary dorsal ligaments of the transverse tarsal joint (Fig. 5.83).

- A Pott fracture-dislocation of the ankle occurs when the foot is forcibly everted. This action pulls on the extremely strong medial (deltoid) ligament, often avulsing the medial malleolus and compressing the lateral malleolus against the talus, shearing off the malleolus or, more often, fracturing the fibula superior to the tibiofibular syndesmosis.

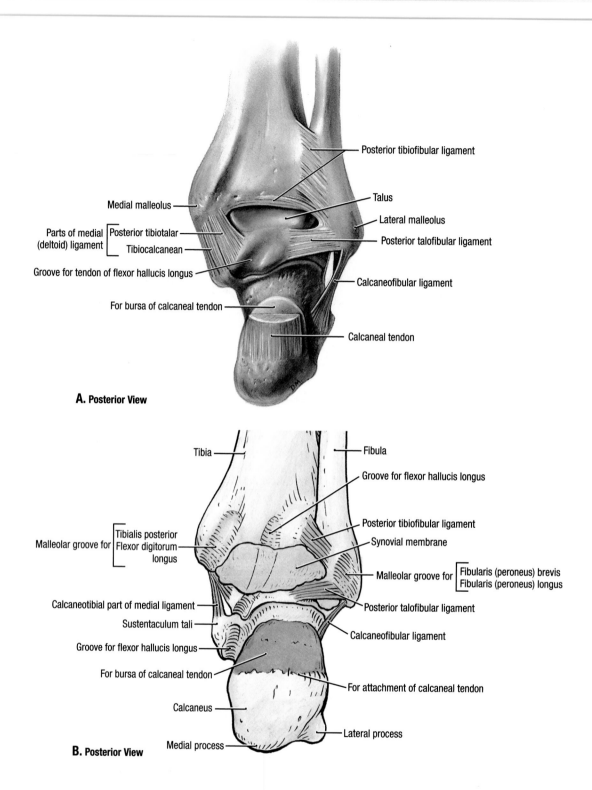

Posterior tibiofibular ligament

Talus

Lateral malleolus

Medial malleolus

Parts of medial (deltoid) ligament — Posterior tibiotalar / Tibiocalcanean

Posterior talofibular ligament

Groove for tendon of flexor hallucis longus

Calcaneofibular ligament

For bursa of calcaneal tendon

Calcaneal tendon

A. Posterior View

Tibia

Fibula

Groove for flexor hallucis longus

Posterior tibiofibular ligament

Malleolar groove for — Tibialis posterior / Flexor digitorum longus

Synovial membrane

Malleolar groove for — Fibularis (peroneus) brevis / Fibularis (peroneus) longus

Calcaneotibial part of medial ligament

Posterior talofibular ligament

Sustentaculum tali

Calcaneofibular ligament

Groove for flexor hallucis longus

For bursa of calcaneal tendon

For attachment of calcaneal tendon

Calcaneus

Lateral process

Medial process

B. Posterior View

5.73   **Posterior aspect of ankle joint**

A. Dissection. **B.** Ankle joint with joint cavity distended with latex. Observe the grooves for the flexor hallucis longus muscle, which crosses the middle of the ankle joint posteriorly, the two tendons posterior to the medial malleolus, and the two tendons posterior to the lateral malleolus.

- The posterior aspect of the ankle joint is strengthened by the transversely oriented posterior tibiofibular and posterior talofibular ligaments.

- The calcaneofibular ligament stabilizes the joint laterally, and the posterior tibiotalar and tibiocalcanean parts of the medial (deltoid) ligament stabilize it medially.
- The groove for the flexor hallucis tendon is between the medial and lateral tubercles of the talus and continues inferior to the sustentaculum tali.

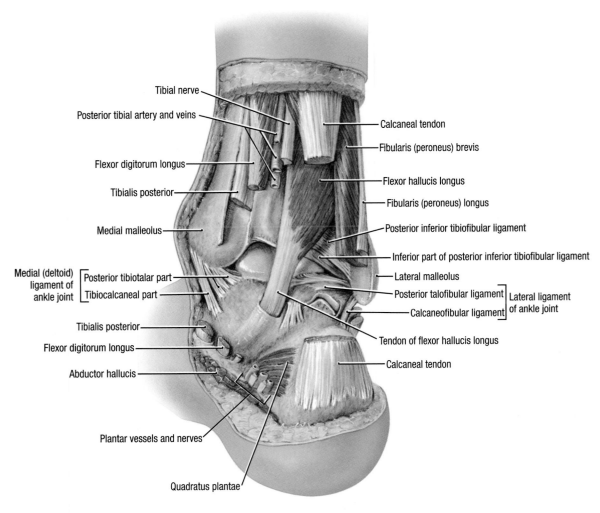

Tibial nerve

Posterior tibial artery and veins

Flexor digitorum longus

Tibialis posterior

Medial malleolus

Medial (deltoid) ligament of ankle joint
- Posterior tibiotalar part
- Tibiocalcaneal part

Tibialis posterior

Flexor digitorum longus

Abductor hallucis

Plantar vessels and nerves

Quadratus plantae

Calcaneal tendon

Fibularis (peroneus) brevis

Flexor hallucis longus

Fibularis (peroneus) longus

Posterior inferior tibiofibular ligament

Inferior part of posterior inferior tibiofibular ligament

Lateral malleolus

Posterior talofibular ligament ⎤ Lateral ligament
Calcaneofibular ligament ⎦ of ankle joint

Tendon of flexor hallucis longus

Calcaneal tendon

Posteromedial View

   Posteromedial ankle

- The flexor hallucis longus muscle is midway between the medial and lateral malleoli; the tendons of the flexor digitorum and tibialis posterior are medial to it, and the tendons of the fibularis longus and brevis are lateral to it.
- The posterior tibial artery and the tibial nerve lie medial to the flexor hallucis longus muscle proximally and distally, after bifurcating posterolateral to it.
- The strongest parts of the ligaments of the ankle are those that prevent anterior displacement of the leg bones, namely, the posterior part of the medial ligament (posterior tibiotalar), the posterior talofibular, the tibiocalcanean, and the calcaneofibular.

- Entrapment and compression of the tibial nerve (tarsal tunnel syndrome) occurs when there is edema and tightness in the ankle involving the synovial sheaths of the tendons of muscles in the posterior compartment of the leg. The area involved is from the medial malleolus to the calcaneus. The heel pain results from compression of the tibial nerve by the flexor retinaculum.

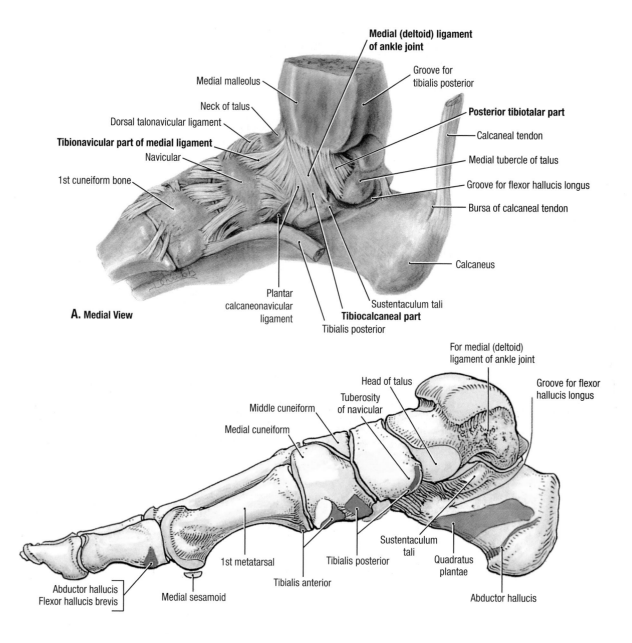

Medial (deltoid) ligament
of ankle joint

Medial malleolus

Neck of talus

Dorsal talonavicular ligament

Tibionavicular part of medial ligament

Navicular

1st cuneiform bone

Groove for
tibialis posterior

Posterior tibiotalar part

Calcaneal tendon

Medial tubercle of talus

Groove for flexor hallucis longus

Bursa of calcaneal tendon

Calcaneus

Plantar
calcaneonavicular
ligament

Tibialis posterior

Sustentaculum tali

Tibiocalcaneal part

A. Medial View

For medial (deltoid)
ligament of ankle joint

Head of talus

Tuberosity
of navicular

Middle cuneiform

Medial cuneiform

Groove for flexor
hallucis longus

1st metatarsal

Tibialis anterior

Tibialis posterior

Sustentaculum
tali

Quadratus
plantae

Abductor hallucis

Abductor hallucis
Flexor hallucis brevis

Medial sesamoid

B

5.75   Medial ligaments of ankle region

A. Dissection. **B.** Bones. The joint capsule of the ankle joint is reinforced medially by the large, strong medial ligament of the ankle (deltoid ligament) that attaches proximally to the medial malleolus and fans out from it to attach distally to the talus, calcaneus, and navicular via four adjacent and continuous parts: the tibionavicular part, the tibiocalcaneal part, and the anterior and posterior tibiotalar parts. The medial ligament stabilizes the ankle joint during eversion of the foot and prevents subluxation (partial dislocation) of the ankle joint.

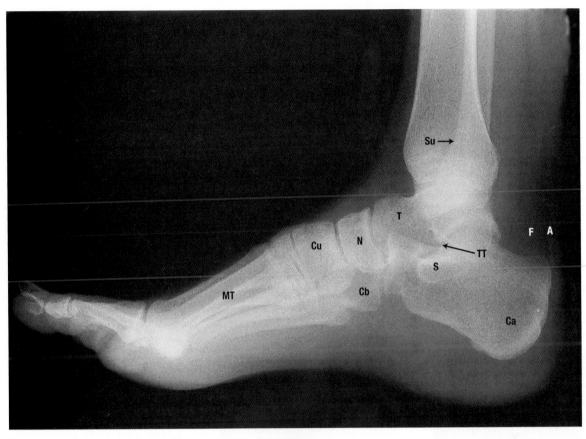

A.

Medial Views

A	Calcaneal (Achilles) tendon
Ca	Calcaneus
Cb	Cuboid
Cu	Cuneiforms
F	Fat
L	Lateral malleolus
MT	Metatarsal
N	Navicular
S	Sustentaculum tali
Su	Superimposed tibia and fibula
T	Talus
TT	Tarsal sinus

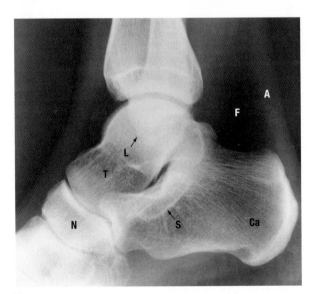

B.

5.76   Radiographs of ankle and foot

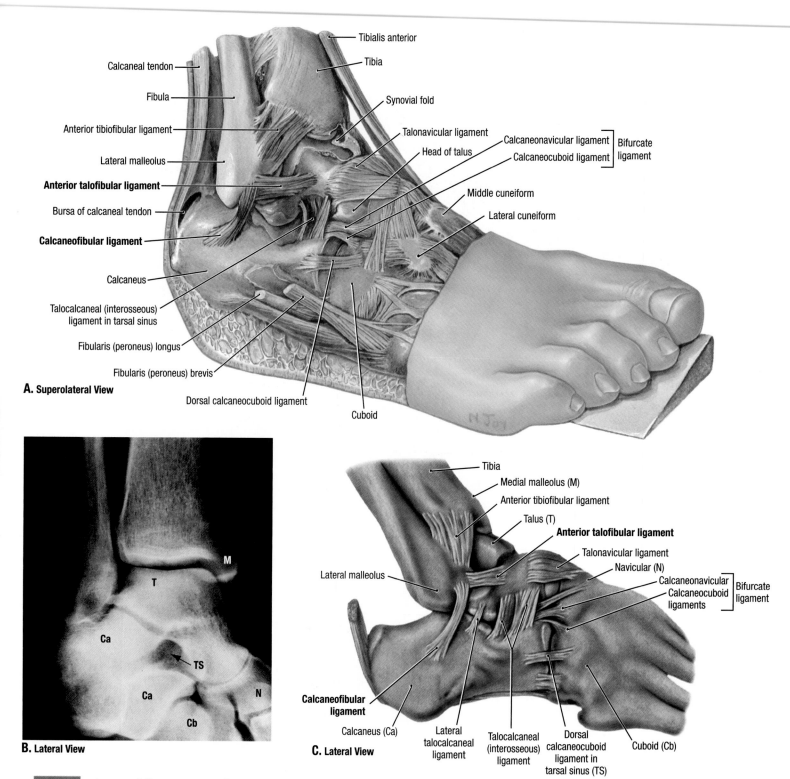

A. Superolateral View

Tibialis anterior
Calcaneal tendon
Tibia
Fibula
Synovial fold
Anterior tibiofibular ligament
Talonavicular ligament
Lateral malleolus
Head of talus
Calcaneonavicular ligament ⎤ Bifurcate
Calcaneocuboid ligament ⎦ ligament
Anterior talofibular ligament
Middle cuneiform
Bursa of calcaneal tendon
Lateral cuneiform
Calcaneofibular ligament
Calcaneus
Talocalcaneal (interosseous) ligament in tarsal sinus
Fibularis (peroneus) longus
Fibularis (peroneus) brevis
Dorsal calcaneocuboid ligament
Cuboid

B. Lateral View

M
T
Ca
TS
Ca
N
Cb

C. Lateral View

Tibia
Medial malleolus (M)
Anterior tibiofibular ligament
Talus (T)
Anterior talofibular ligament
Talonavicular ligament
Navicular (N)
Lateral malleolus
Calcaneonavicular ⎤ Bifurcate
Calcaneocuboid ⎦ ligament
ligaments
Calcaneofibular ligament
Calcaneus (Ca)
Lateral talocalcaneal ligament
Talocalcaneal (interosseous) ligament
Dorsal calcaneocuboid ligament in tarsal sinus (TS)
Cuboid (Cb)

5.77   Lateral ligaments of ankle region

A. Dissection with foot inverted by underlying wedge. **B.** Lateral radiograph. **C.** Dissection. (Abbreviations following some labels refer to structures identified in **B.**)

The ankle joint is reinforced laterally by the lateral ligament of the ankle, which consists of three separate ligaments: (1) anterior talofibular ligament, a flat, weak band; (2) calcaneofibular ligament, a round cord directed posteroinferiorly; and (3) posterior talofibular ligament, a strong, medially-directed horizontal ligament (see Fig. 5.74).

Ankle sprains (partial or fully torn ligaments) are common injuries. Ankle sprains nearly always result from forceful inversion of the weight-bearing plantarflexed foot. The anterior talofibular ligament is most commonly injured, resulting in instability of the ankle. The calcaneofibular is also often torn.

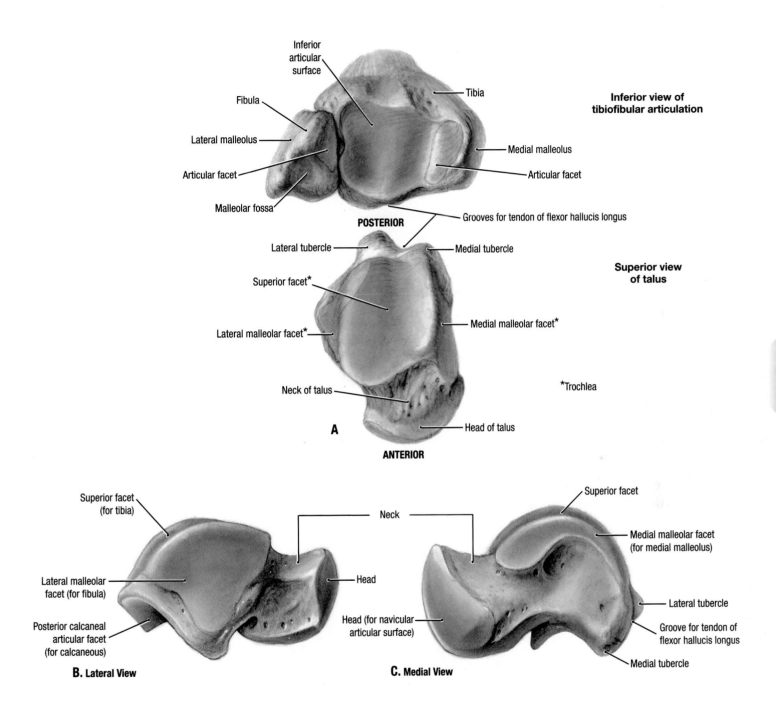

Inferior
articular
surface

Tibia

Fibula

Lateral malleolus

Medial malleolus

Articular facet

Articular facet

Malleolar fossa

POSTERIOR

Grooves for tendon of flexor hallucis longus

**Inferior view of
tibiofibular articulation**

Lateral tubercle

Medial tubercle

**Superior view
of talus**

Superior facet*

Medial malleolar facet*

Lateral malleolar facet*

Neck of talus

*Trochlea

A

Head of talus

ANTERIOR

Superior facet
(for tibia)

Neck

Superior facet

Medial malleolar facet
(for medial malleolus)

Lateral malleolar
facet (for fibula)

Head

Lateral tubercle

Posterior calcaneal
articular facet
(for calcaneous)

Head (for navicular
articular surface)

Groove for tendon of
flexor hallucis longus

B. Lateral View

C. Medial View

Medial tubercle

5.78   Articular surfaces of ankle joint

A. Superior aspect of talus separated from distal ends of tibia and fibula. The superior articular surface of the talus is broader anteriorly than posteriorly; hence the medial and lateral malleoli, which grasp the sides of the talus, tend to be forced apart in dorsiflexion. The fully dorsiflexed position is stable compared with the fully plantar flexed position. In plantar flexion, when the tibia and fibula articulate with the narrower posterior part of the supe- rior articular surface of the talus, some side-to-side movement of the joint is allowed, accounting for the instability of the joint in this position. **B.** Lateral aspect of talus. The lateral, triangular articular area is for articulation with the lateral malleolus. **C.** Medial aspect of talus. The comma-shaped articular area is for articulation with the medial malleolus.

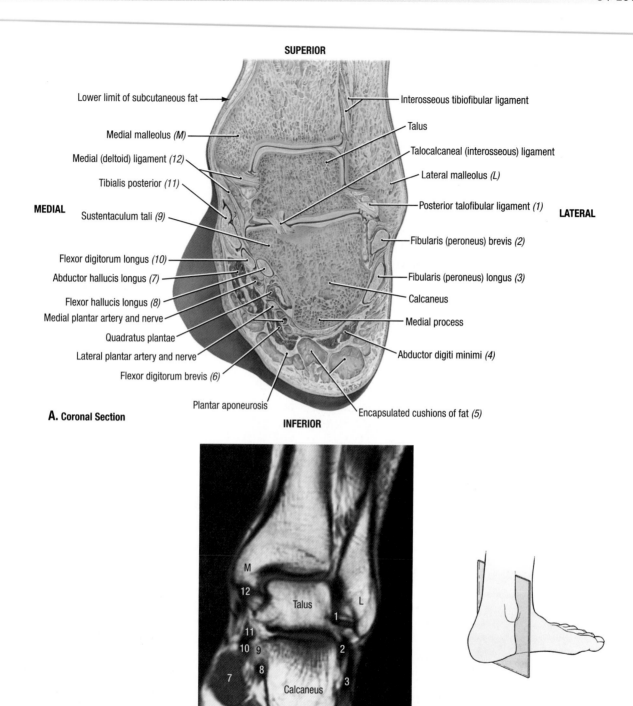

SUPERIOR

Lower limit of subcutaneous fat

Medial malleolus *(M)*

Medial (deltoid) ligament *(12)*

Tibialis posterior *(11)*

MEDIAL

Sustentaculum tali *(9)*

Flexor digitorum longus *(10)*

Abductor hallucis longus *(7)*

Flexor hallucis longus *(8)*

Medial plantar artery and nerve

Quadratus plantae

Lateral plantar artery and nerve

Flexor digitorum brevis *(6)*

Plantar aponeurosis

A. Coronal Section

INFERIOR

Interosseous tibiofibular ligament

Talus

Talocalcaneal (interosseous) ligament

Lateral malleolus *(L)*

Posterior talofibular ligament *(1)*

LATERAL

Fibularis (peroneus) brevis *(2)*

Fibularis (peroneus) longus *(3)*

Calcaneus

Medial process

Abductor digiti minimi *(4)*

Encapsulated cushions of fat *(5)*

B. Coronal MRI

5.79 Coronal section and MRI through ankle

A. Coronal section. **B.** Coronal MRI (*numbers* in **B** refer to structures labeled in **A**).

- The tibia rests on the talus, and the talus rests on the calcaneus; between the calcaneus and the skin are several encapsulated cushions of fat.
- The lateral malleolus descends farther inferiorly than the medial malleolus.

- The talocalcaneal (interosseous) ligament between the talus and calcaneus separates the subtalar, or posterior, talocalcanean joint from the talocalcaneonavicular joint.
- The sustentaculum tali acts as a pulley for the flexor hallucis longus muscle and gives attachment to the calcaneotibial part of the medial (deltoid) ligament.

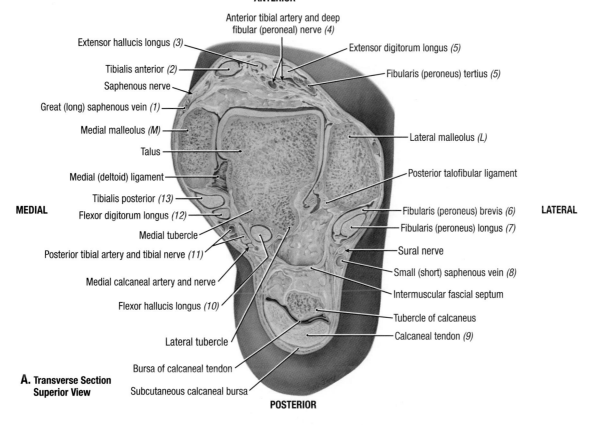

ANTERIOR

Anterior tibial artery and deep fibular (peroneal) nerve (4)

Extensor hallucis longus (3)

Tibialis anterior (2)

Saphenous nerve

Great (long) saphenous vein (1)

Medial malleolus (M)

Talus

Medial (deltoid) ligament

Tibialis posterior (13)

Flexor digitorum longus (12)

Medial tubercle

Posterior tibial artery and tibial nerve (11)

Medial calcaneal artery and nerve

Flexor hallucis longus (10)

Lateral tubercle

Bursa of calcaneal tendon

Subcutaneous calcaneal bursa

MEDIAL

A. Transverse Section
Superior View

Extensor digitorum longus (5)

Fibularis (peroneus) tertius (5)

Lateral malleolus (L)

Posterior talofibular ligament

Fibularis (peroneus) brevis (6)

Fibularis (peroneus) longus (7)

Sural nerve

Small (short) saphenous vein (8)

Intermuscular fascial septum

Tubercle of calcaneus

Calcaneal tendon (9)

LATERAL

POSTERIOR

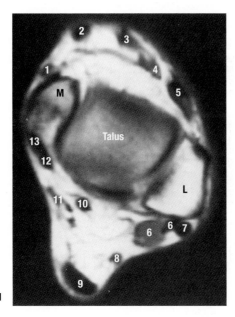

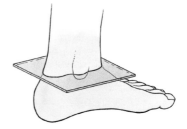

B. Transverse MRI

5.80   **Transverse section and MRI through ankle**

A. Transverse section. **B.** Transverse MRI (*numbers* in **B** refer to structures labeled in **A**).

- The body of the talus is wedge shaped and positioned between the malleoli, which are bound to it by the medial (deltoid) and posterior talofibular ligaments.

- The flexor hallucis longus muscle lies within its osseofibrous sheath between the medial and lateral tubercles of the talus.
- There is a small, inconstant subcutaneous bursa superficial to the calcaneal tendon and a large, constant bursa of calcaneal tendon deep to it.

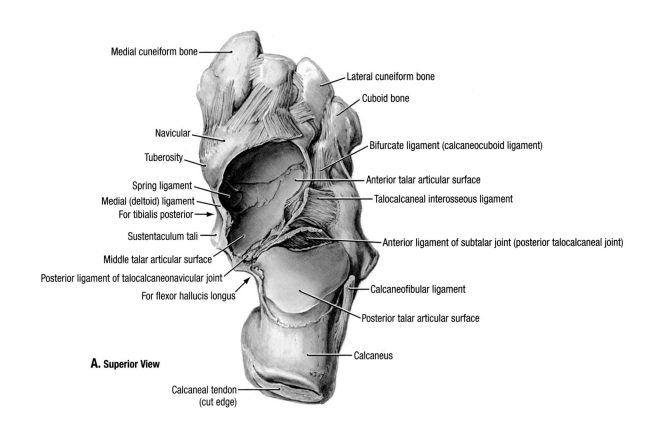

Medial cuneiform bone

Lateral cuneiform bone

Cuboid bone

Navicular

Bifurcate ligament (calcaneocuboid ligament)

Tuberosity

Anterior talar articular surface

Spring ligament

Talocalcaneal interosseous ligament

Medial (deltoid) ligament

For tibialis posterior

Sustentaculum tali

Anterior ligament of subtalar joint (posterior talocalcaneal joint)

Middle talar articular surface

Posterior ligament of talocalcaneonavicular joint

Calcaneofibular ligament

For flexor hallucis longus

Posterior talar articular surface

Calcaneus

A. Superior View

Calcaneal tendon
(cut edge)

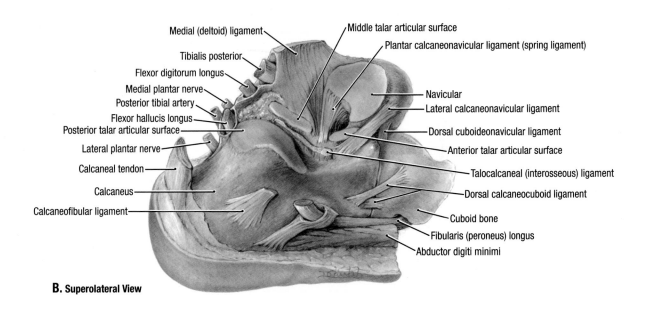

Medial (deltoid) ligament

Middle talar articular surface

Tibialis posterior

Plantar calcaneonavicular ligament (spring ligament)

Flexor digitorum longus

Medial plantar nerve

Posterior tibial artery

Navicular

Flexor hallucis longus

Lateral calcaneonavicular ligament

Posterior talar articular surface

Dorsal cuboideonavicular ligament

Lateral plantar nerve

Anterior talar articular surface

Calcaneal tendon

Talocalcaneal (interosseous) ligament

Calcaneus

Dorsal calcaneocuboid ligament

Calcaneofibular ligament

Cuboid bone

Fibularis (peroneus) longus

Abductor digiti minimi

B. Superolateral View

5.81   Joints of inversion and eversion

The joints of inversion and eversion are the subtalar (posterior talocalcanean) joint, talo-calcaneonavicular joint, and transverse tarsal (combined calcaneocuboid and talonavicular) joint. **A.** Posterior and middle parts of foot with talus removed. **B.** Posterior part of foot with talus removed. The convex posterior talar facet is separated from the concave middle, and anterior facets by the talocalcaneal (interosseous) ligament within the tarsal sinus.

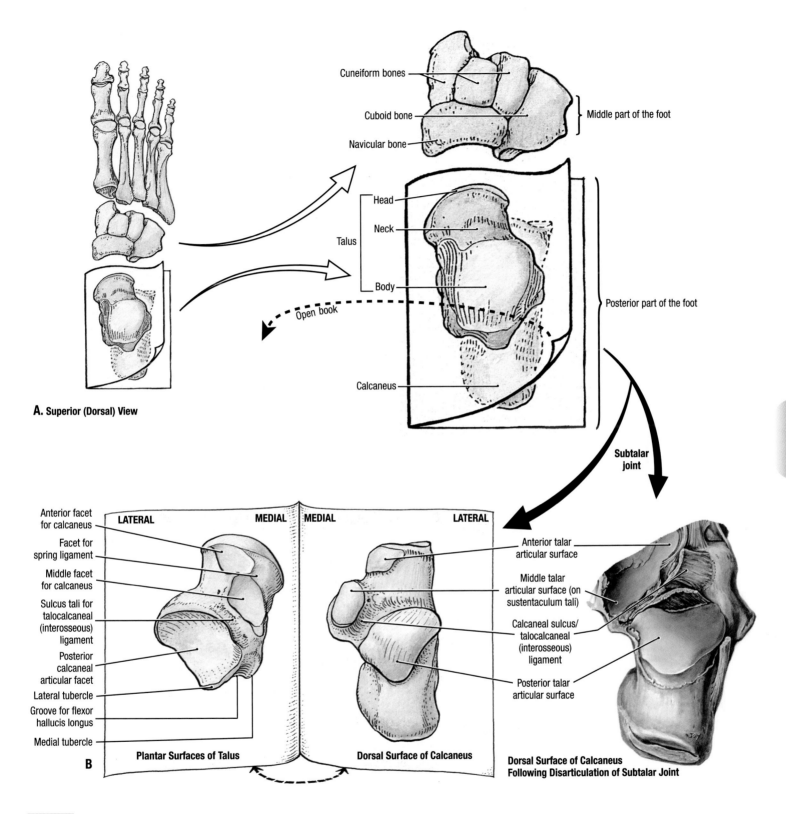

A. **Superior (Dorsal) View**

Cuneiform bones

Cuboid bone

Navicular bone

Middle part of the foot

Talus

Head

Neck

Body

Calcaneus

Open book

Posterior part of the foot

Subtalar joint

Anterior facet for calcaneus

Facet for spring ligament

Middle facet for calcaneus

Sulcus tali for talocalcaneal (interosseous) ligament

Posterior calcaneal articular facet

Lateral tubercle

Groove for flexor hallucis longus

Medial tubercle

LATERAL   MEDIAL   MEDIAL   LATERAL

Plantar Surfaces of Talus

Dorsal Surface of Calcaneus

Anterior talar articular surface

Middle talar articular surface (on sustentaculum tali)

Calcaneal sulcus/ talocalcaneal (interosseous) ligament

Posterior talar articular surface

Dorsal Surface of Calcaneus Following Disarticulation of Subtalar Joint

B

5.82   Talocalcanean joint

A. Bones of foot, dorsal view. **B.** Bony surfaces of talocalcanean joints. The plantar surface of the talus and dorsal surface of the calcaneus are displayed as pages in a book.

- The joints of inversion and eversion are the subtalar (posterior talocalcanean) joint, talocalcaneonavicular joint, and transverse tarsal (combined calcaneocuboid and talonavicular) joint.

- The talus is part of the ankle joint, of the posterior and anterior talocalcanean joints, and of the talonavicular joint.
- The posterior and anterior talocalcanean joints are separated from each other by the sulcus tarsi and calcaneal sulcus, which, when the talus and calcaneus are in articulation, become the tarsal sinus.

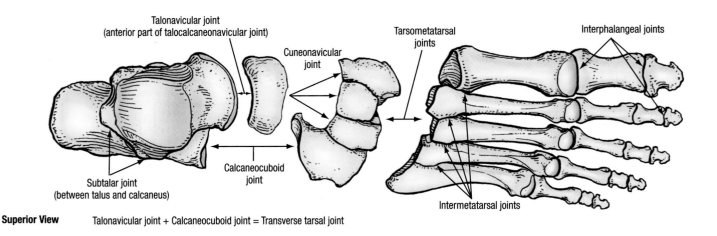

Superior View   Talonavicular joint + Calcaneocuboid joint = Transverse tarsal joint

TABLE 5.19 JOINTS OF FOOT

Joint	Type	Articular Surface	Joint Capsule	Ligaments	Movements
Subtalar	Synovial (plane) joint	Inferior surface of body of talus articulates with superior surface of calcaneus	Attached to margins of articular surfaces	Medial, lateral, and posterior talocalcaneal ligaments support capsule; talocalcaneal (interosseous) ligament binds bones together	Inversion and eversion of foot
Talocalcaneo-navicular	Synovial joint; talonavicular part is ball-and-socket type	Head of talus articulates with calcaneus and navicular bones	Incompletely encloses joint	Plantar calcaneonavicular ("spring") ligament supports head of talus	Gliding and rotary movements
Calcaneocuboid	Synovial (plane) joint	Anterior end of calcaneus articulates with posterior surface of cuboid	Encloses joint	Dorsal calcaneocuboid ligament, plantar calcaneocuboid ligament, and long plantar ligament support fibrous capsule	Inversion and eversion of foot
Cuneonavicular	Synovial (plane) joint	Anterior navicular articulates with posterior surface of cuneiforms	Common joint capsule	Dorsal and plantar ligaments	Little movement
Tarsometatarsal	Synovial (plane) joint	Anterior tarsal bones articulate with bases of metatarsal bones	Encloses joint	Dorsal, plantar, and interosseous ligaments	Gliding or sliding
Intermetatarsal	Synovial (plane) joint	Bases of metatarsal bones articulate with each other	Encloses each joint	Dorsal, plantar, and interosseous ligaments bind bones together	Little individual movement
Metatarsophalangeal	Synovial (condyloid) joint	Heads of metatarsal bones articulate with bases of proximal phalanges	Encloses each joint ligament supports	Collateral ligaments support capsule on each side; plantar and circumduction plantar part of capsule	Flexion, extension, and some abduction, adduction,
Interphalangeal	Synovial (hinge) joint	Head of proximal or middle phalanx articulates with base of phalanx distal to it	Encloses each joint	Collateral and plantar ligaments support joints	Flexion and extension

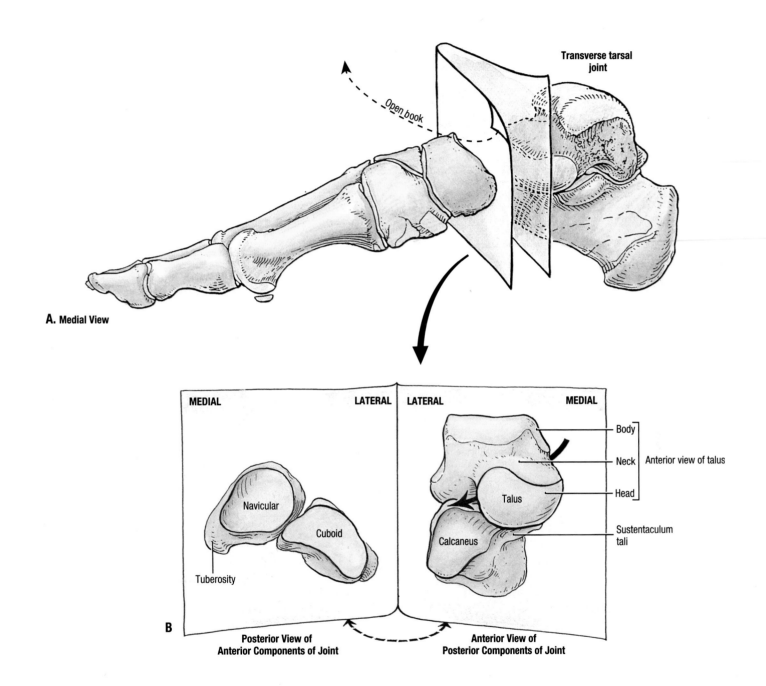

Transverse tarsal joint

Open book

A. Medial View

MEDIAL   LATERAL   LATERAL   MEDIAL

Body
Neck   Anterior view of talus
Head

Navicular

Cuboid

Talus

Calcaneus

Sustentaculum tali

Tuberosity

B

Posterior View of
Anterior Components of Joint

Anterior View of
Posterior Components of Joint

5.83   **Transverse tarsal joint**

A. Bones of foot, medial view. **B.** Articular surfaces of transverse tarsal joint. This compound joint includes the talonavicular and calcaneocuboid articulations. The posterior surfaces of the navicular and cuboid bones and the anterior surfaces of the talus and calcaneus are displayed as pages in a book. The *black arrow* traverses the tarsal sinus, in which the talocalcaneal (interosseous) ligament is located.

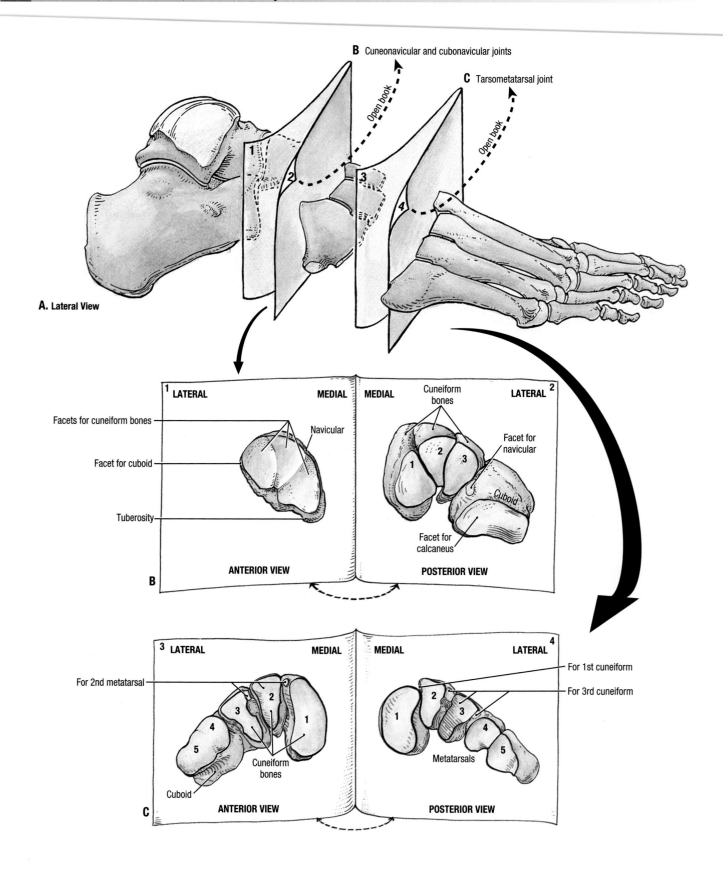

B Cuneonavicular and cubonavicular joints

C Tarsometatarsal joint

Open book

Open book

A. Lateral View

1 LATERAL   MEDIAL

Facets for cuneiform bones

Facet for cuboid

Navicular

Tuberosity

ANTERIOR VIEW

B

MEDIAL   **2** LATERAL

Cuneiform bones

Facet for navicular

Cuboid

Facet for calcaneus

POSTERIOR VIEW

3 LATERAL   MEDIAL

For 2nd metatarsal

Cuneiform bones

Cuboid

ANTERIOR VIEW

C

MEDIAL   **4** LATERAL

For 1st cuneiform

For 3rd cuneiform

Metatarsals

POSTERIOR VIEW

5.84   **Cuneonavicular, cubonavicular, and tarsometatarsal joints**

A. Bones of foot, lateral view. **B.** Bony surfaces of the cuneonavicular and cubonavicular joints. **C.** Bony surfaces of the tarsometatarsal joints.

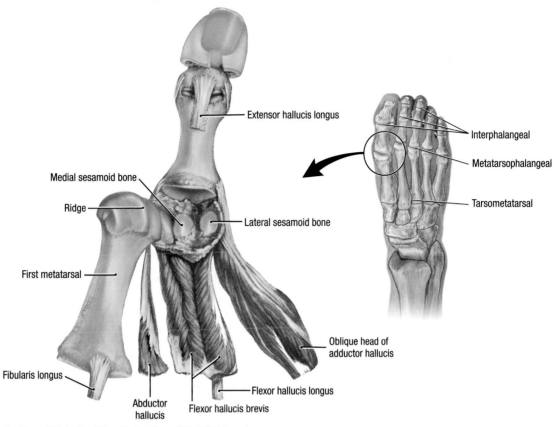

Extensor hallucis longus

Interphalangeal

Metatarsophalangeal

Medial sesamoid bone

Tarsometatarsal

Ridge

Lateral sesamoid bone

First metatarsal

Oblique head of
adductor hallucis

Fibularis longus

Flexor hallucis longus

Abductor
hallucis

Flexor hallucis brevis

A. Superior View of Right Great Toe, Medial View of First Metetarsal

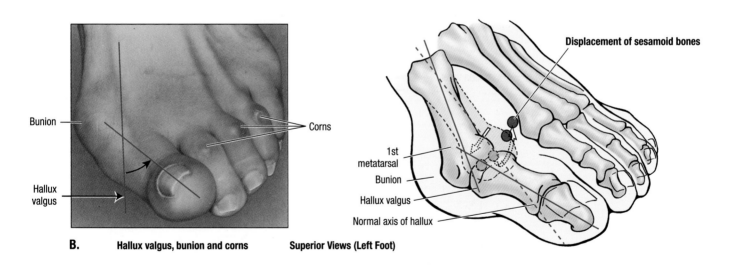

Bunion

Corns

Displacement of sesamoid bones

1st
metatarsal

Bunion

Hallux
valgus

Hallux valgus

Normal axis of hallux

B.   **Hallux valgus, bunion and corns**   **Superior Views (Left Foot)**

5.85   Metatarsophalangeal joint of great toe

A. First metatarsal and sesamoid bones of the right great toe. The sesamoid bones of the great toe (hallux) are bound together and located on each side of a bony ridge on the first metatarsal. **B.** Hallux valgus. Hallux valgus is a foot deformity caused by pressure from footwear and degenerative joint disease; it is characterized by lateral deviation of the great toe (L. *hallux*). In some people, the deviation is so great that the 1st toe overlaps the 2nd toe. These individuals are unable to move their 1st digit away from their 2nd digit because the sesamoid bones under the head of the 1st metatarsal are displaced and lie in the space between the heads of the 1st and 2nd metatarsals. In addition, a subcutaneous bursa may form owing to pressure and friction against the shoe. When tender and inflamed, the bursa is called a bunion.

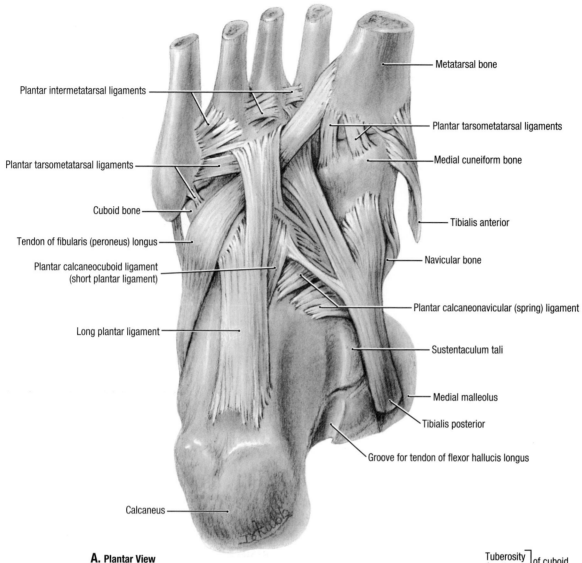

A. Plantar View

Plantar intermetatarsal ligaments

Plantar tarsometatarsal ligaments

Cuboid bone

Tendon of fibularis (peroneus) longus

Plantar calcaneocuboid ligament
(short plantar ligament)

Long plantar ligament

Calcaneus

Metatarsal bone

Plantar tarsometatarsal ligaments

Medial cuneiform bone

Tibialis anterior

Navicular bone

Plantar calcaneonavicular (spring) ligament

Sustentaculum tali

Medial malleolus

Tibialis posterior

Groove for tendon of flexor hallucis longus

5.86   Ligaments of sole of foot

A. Dissection of superficial ligaments. **B.** Bones lying deep to ligaments of **A**. In **A**:

- The head of the talus is exposed between the sustentaculum tali of the calcaneus and the navicular.
- Note the insertions of three long tendons: fibularis (peroneus) longus, tibialis anterior, and tibialis posterior.
- The tendon of the fibularis (peroneus) longus muscle crosses the sole of the foot in the groove anterior to the ridge of the cuboid, is bridged by some fibers of the long plantar ligament, and inserts into the base of the first metatarsal.
- Observe the slips of the tibialis posterior tendon extending to the bones anterior to the transverse tarsal joint.

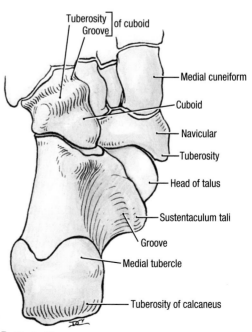

Tuberosity ⎤
Groove ⎦ of cuboid

Medial cuneiform

Cuboid

Navicular

Tuberosity

Head of talus

Sustentaculum tali

Groove

Medial tubercle

Tuberosity of calcaneus

B. Plantar View

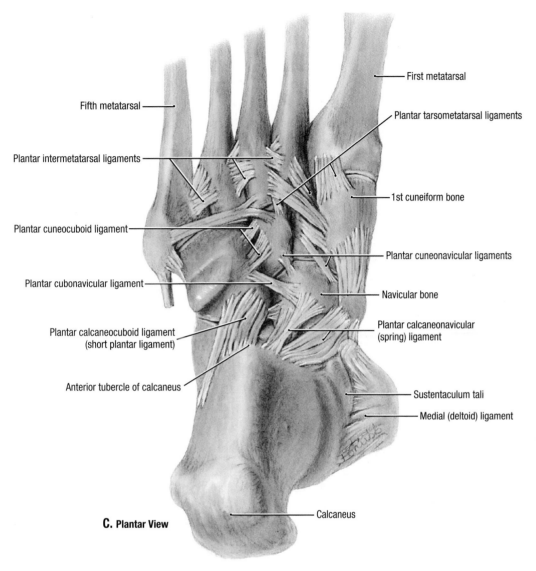

First metatarsal

Fifth metatarsal

Plantar tarsometatarsal ligaments

Plantar intermetatarsal ligaments

1st cuneiform bone

Plantar cuneocuboid ligament

Plantar cuneonavicular ligaments

Plantar cubonavicular ligament

Navicular bone

Plantar calcaneocuboid ligament
(short plantar ligament)

Plantar calcaneonavicular
(spring) ligament

Anterior tubercle of calcaneus

Sustentaculum tali

Medial (deltoid) ligament

Calcaneus

C. Plantar View

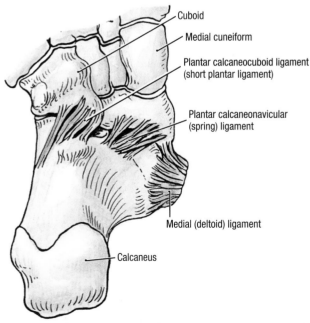

Cuboid

Medial cuneiform

Plantar calcaneocuboid ligament
(short plantar ligament)

Plantar calcaneonavicular
(spring) ligament

Medial (deltoid) ligament

Calcaneus

D. Plantar View

 5.86   **Ligaments of sole of foot** *(continued)*

C. Dissection of the deep ligaments. **D.** Support for head of talus. The head of the talus is supported by the plantar calcaneonavicular ligament (spring ligament) and the tendon of the tibialis posterior.

- The plantar calcaneocuboid (short plantar) and plantar calcaneonavicular (spring) ligaments are the primary plantar ligaments of the transverse tarsal joint .

- The ligaments of the anterior foot diverge laterally and posteriorly from each side of the long axis of the third metatarsal and third cuneiform; hence a posterior thrust received by the first metatarsal, as when rising on the big toe while in walking, is transmitted directly to the navicular and talus by the first cuneiform and indirectly by the second metatarsal, second cuneiform, third metatarsal, and third cuneiform.

- A posterior thrust received by the fourth and fifth metatarsals is transmitted directly to the cuboid and calcaneus.

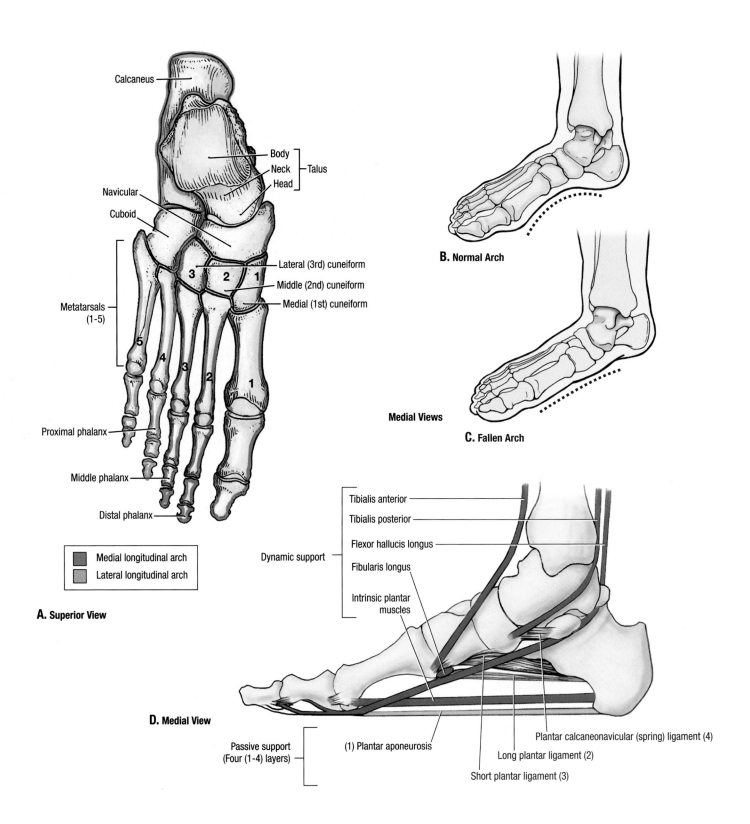

Calcaneus

Body ⎤
Neck ⎬ Talus
Head ⎦

Navicular

Cuboid

Lateral (3rd) cuneiform
Middle (2nd) cuneiform
Medial (1st) cuneiform

Metatarsals
(1-5)

Proximal phalanx

Middle phalanx

Distal phalanx

■ Medial longitudinal arch
■ Lateral longitudinal arch

A. Superior View

B. Normal Arch

Medial Views

C. Fallen Arch

Tibialis anterior
Tibialis posterior
Flexor hallucis longus
Fibularis longus
Intrinsic plantar
muscles

Dynamic support

Passive support
(Four (1-4) layers)

(1) Plantar aponeurosis

Plantar calcaneonavicular (spring) ligament (4)
Long plantar ligament (2)
Short plantar ligament (3)

D. Medial View

5.87   Arches of foot

A. Medial and lateral longitudinal arches. **B.** Normal arch. **C.** Fallen arch. **D.** Supports of the longitudinal arches.

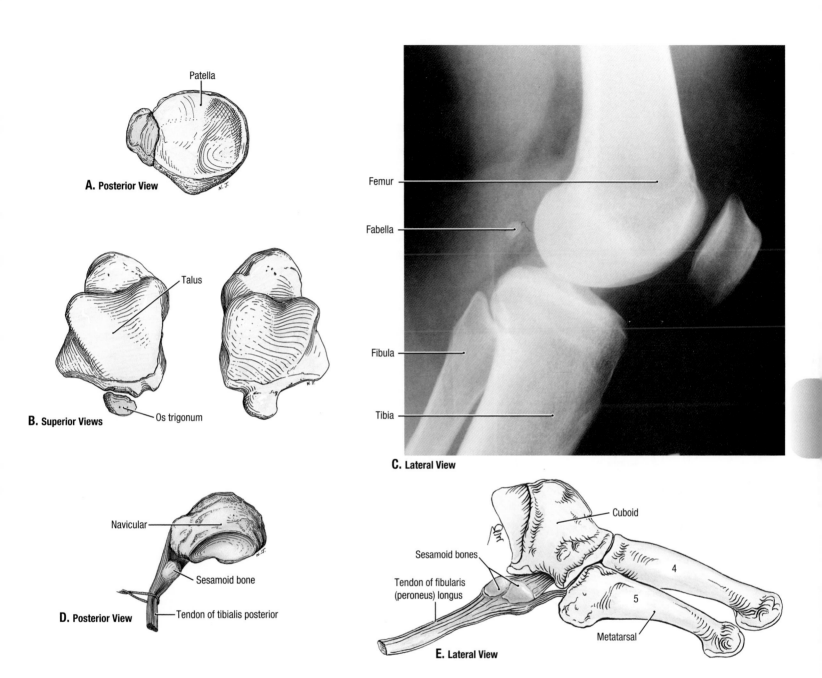

A. Posterior View

Patella

B. Superior Views

Talus

Os trigonum

D. Posterior View

Navicular

Sesamoid bone

Tendon of tibialis posterior

C. Lateral View

Femur

Fabella

Fibula

Tibia

E. Lateral View

Cuboid

Sesamoid bones

Tendon of fibularis (peroneus) longus

4

5

Metatarsal

5.88   Bony anomalies

A. Bipartite patella. Occasionally, the superolateral angle of the patella ossifies independently and remains discrete. **B.** Os trigonum. The lateral (posterior) tubercle of the talus has a separate center of ossification that appears from the ages of 7 to 13 years; when this fails to fuse with the body of the talus, as in the left bone of this pair, it is called an *os trigonum*. It was found in 7.7% of 558 adult feet; 22 were paired, and 21 were unpaired. **C.** Fabella. A sesamoid bone in the lateral head of the gastrocnemius muscle was present in 21.6% of 116 limbs. **D.** Sesamoid bone in the tendon of tibialis posterior. A sesamoid bone was found in 23% of 348 adults. **E.** Sesamoid bone in the tendon of fibularis (peroneus) longus. A sesamoid bone was found in 26% of 92 feet. In this specimen, it is bipartite, and the fibularis (peroneus) longus muscle has an additional attachment to the 5th metatarsal bone.

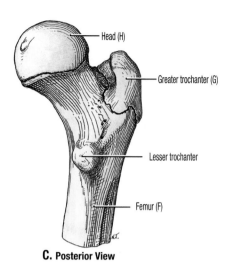

Head (H)

Greater trochanter (G)

Lesser trochanter

Femur (F)

C. Posterior View

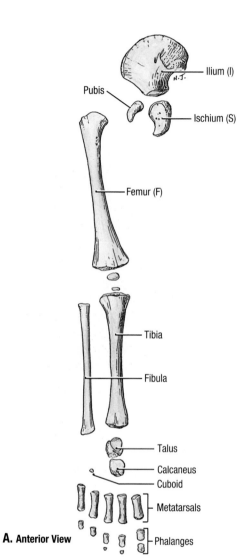

Ilium (I)

Pubis

Ischium (S)

Femur (F)

Tibia

Fibula

Talus

Calcaneus

Cuboid

Metatarsals

Phalanges

A. Anterior View

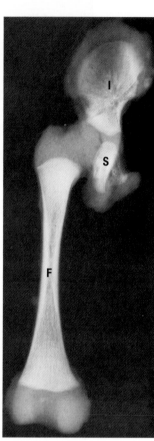

B. Anteroposterior View

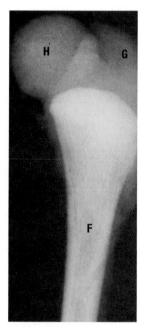

H

G

F

D. Anteroposterior View

5.89   Postnatal lower limb development

A. Bones of lower limb at birth. The hip bone can be divided into three primary parts: ilium, ischium, and pubis. The diaphyses (bodies) of the long bones are well ossified. Some epiphyses (growth plates) and tarsal bones have begun to ossify, including the distal epiphysis of the femur, proximal epiphysis of the tibia, calcaneus, talus, and cuboid. **B** and **D.** Anteroposterior radiographs of postmortem specimens of newborns show the bony *(white)* and cartilaginous *(gray)* components of the femur and hip bone. **C.** Epiphyses at proximal end of femur. The epiphysis of the head of the femur begins to ossify during the 1st year, that of the greater trochanter before the 5th year, and that of the lesser trochanter before the 14th year. These usually fuse completely with the body (shaft) before the end of the 18th year.

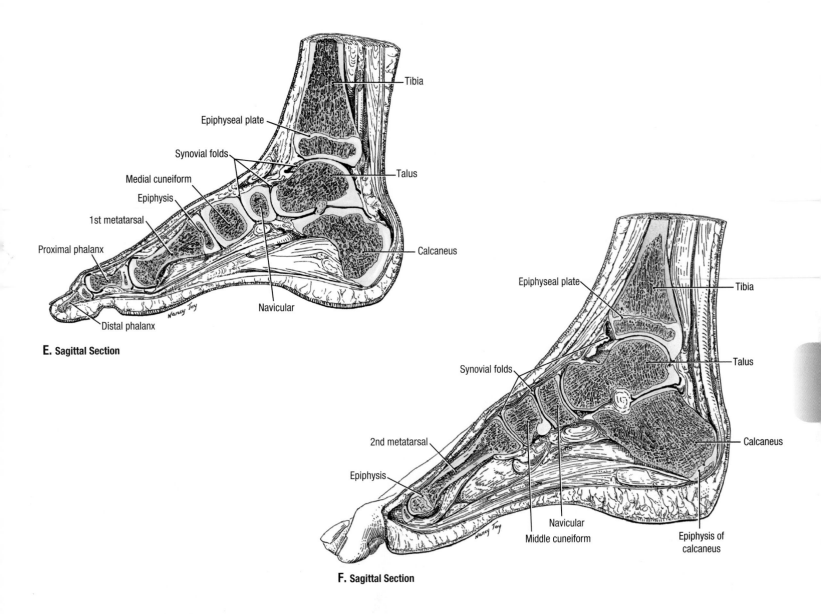

E. Sagittal Section

F. Sagittal Section

5.89   **Postnatal lower limb development** *(continued)*

E. Foot of child age 4. **F.** Foot of child age 10.
- In the foot of the younger child **(E)**, epiphyses of long bones (tibia, metatarsals, and phalanges) ossify like short bones, with the ossification centers being enveloped in cartilage. Ossification has already extended to the surface of the larger tarsal bones.
- In the foot of the older child **(F)**, ossification has spread to the dorsal and plantar surfaces of all tarsal bones in view, and cartilage persists on the articular surfaces only.
- The traction epiphysis of the calcaneus for the calcaneal tendon and plantar aponeurosis begins to ossify from the ages of 6 to 10 years.
- The first metatarsal bone is similar to a phalanx in that its epiphysis is at the base instead of the head, as in the second and other metatarsal bones.
- The tuberosity of the calcaneus and the sesamoid bones of the first and the heads of the second to fifth metatarsals (here the second) support the longitudinal arch of the foot; the medial part of the longitudinal arch is higher and more mobile than the lateral.

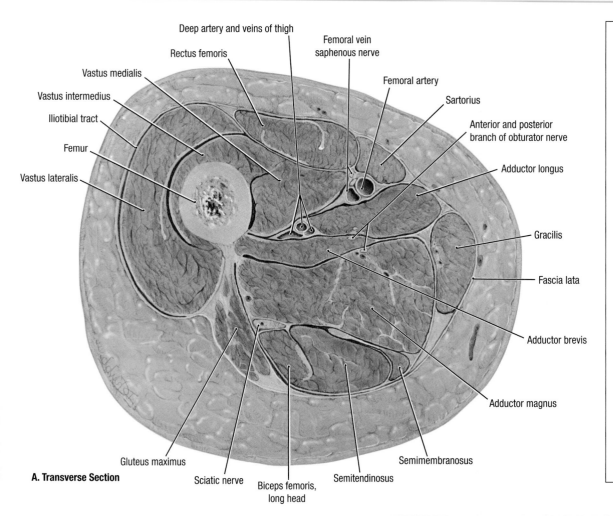

Deep artery and veins of thigh
Rectus femoris
Vastus medialis
Vastus intermedius
Iliotibial tract
Femur
Vastus lateralis
Femoral vein
saphenous nerve
Femoral artery
Sartorius
Anterior and posterior
branch of obturator nerve
Adductor longus
Gracilis
Fascia lata
Adductor brevis
Adductor magnus
Gluteus maximus
Sciatic nerve
Biceps femoris,
long head
Semitendinosus
Semimembranosus

A. Transverse Section

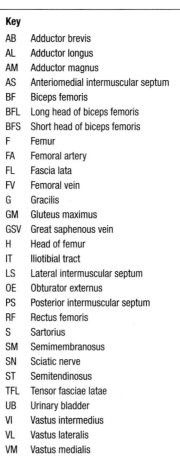

Key

AB	Adductor brevis
AL	Adductor longus
AM	Adductor magnus
AS	Anteriomedial intermuscular septum
BF	Biceps femoris
BFL	Long head of biceps femoris
BFS	Short head of biceps femoris
F	Femur
FA	Femoral artery
FL	Fascia lata
FV	Femoral vein
G	Gracilis
GM	Gluteus maximus
GSV	Great saphenous vein
H	Head of femur
IT	Iliotibial tract
LS	Lateral intermuscular septum
OE	Obturator externus
PS	Posterior intermuscular septum
RF	Rectus femoris
S	Sartorius
SM	Semimembranosus
SN	Sciatic nerve
ST	Semitendinosus
TFL	Tensor fasciae latae
UB	Urinary bladder
VI	Vastus intermedius
VL	Vastus lateralis
VM	Vastus medialis

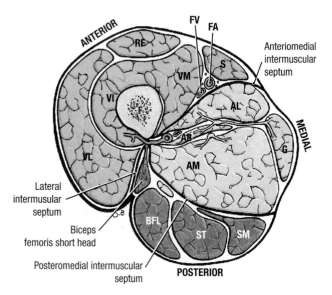

B. Transverse Section

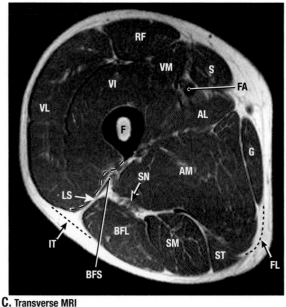

C. Transverse MRI

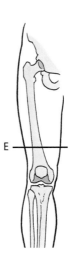

5.90   Transverse sections and MRIs of thigh

A. Anatomical section. **B.** Compartments of thigh. **C.** T1 transverse (axial) MRIs. The thigh has three compartments, each with its own nerve supply and primary function: anterior group extends the knee and is supplied by the femoral nerve; medial group adducts the hip and is supplied by the obturator nerve; posterior group flexes the knee and is supplied by the sciatic nerve.

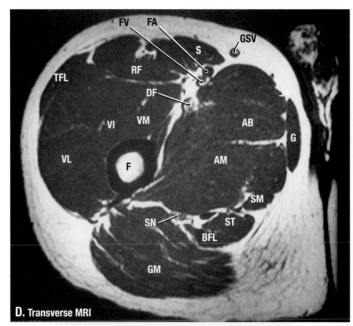

D. Transverse MRI

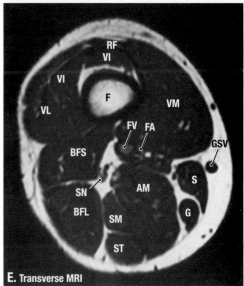

E. Transverse MRI

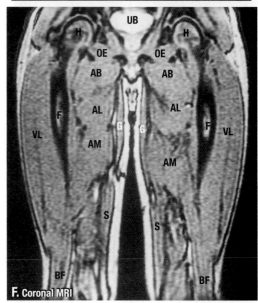

F. Coronal MRI

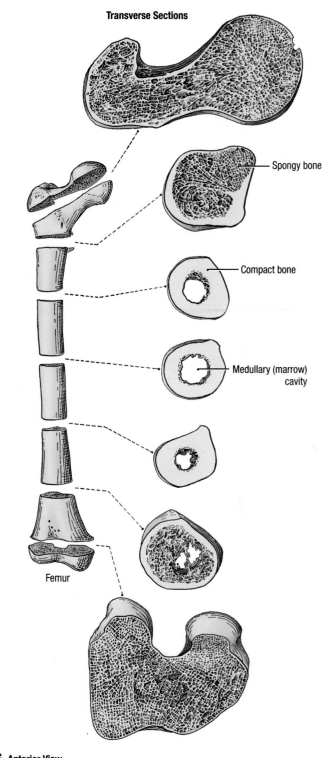

Transverse Sections

Spongy bone

Compact bone

Medullary (marrow) cavity

Femur

G. Anterior View

5.90 **Transverse sections and MRIs of thigh** *(continued)*

D and **E.** T1 transverse MRIs. **F.** T1 coronal MRI. **G.** Transverse sections of femur. Note the differences in thickness of the compact and spongy bone and in the width of the medullary (marrow) cavity.

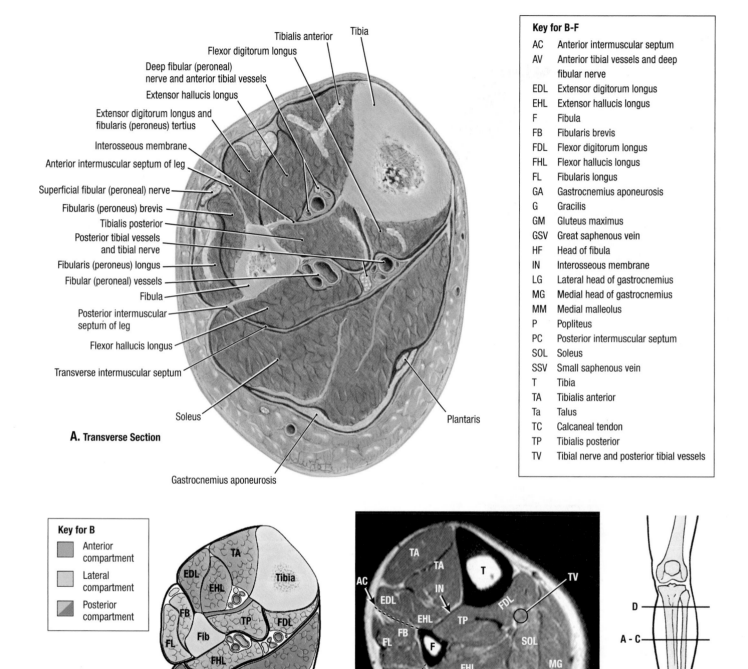

Key for B-F

AC	Anterior intermuscular septum
AV	Anterior tibial vessels and deep fibular nerve
EDL	Extensor digitorum longus
EHL	Extensor hallucis longus
F	Fibula
FB	Fibularis brevis
FDL	Flexor digitorum longus
FHL	Flexor hallucis longus
FL	Fibularis longus
GA	Gastrocnemius aponeurosis
G	Gracilis
GM	Gluteus maximus
GSV	Great saphenous vein
HF	Head of fibula
IN	Interosseous membrane
LG	Lateral head of gastrocnemius
MG	Medial head of gastrocnemius
MM	Medial malleolus
P	Popliteus
PC	Posterior intermuscular septum
SOL	Soleus
SSV	Small saphenous vein
T	Tibia
TA	Tibialis anterior
Ta	Talus
TC	Calcaneal tendon
TP	Tibialis posterior
TV	Tibial nerve and posterior tibial vessels

A. Transverse Section

Key for B

- ■ Anterior compartment
- ■ Lateral compartment
- ■ Posterior compartment

B. Transverse Section

C. Transverse Section

5.91   Transverse sections and MRI of leg

A. Anatomical section. **B.** Compartments of leg. **C.** T1 transverse (axial) MRI. The anterior compartment is bounded by the tibia, interosseous membrane, fibula, anterior intermuscular septum, and crural fascia. The lateral compartment is bounded by the fibula, anterior and posterior intermuscular septa, and the crural fascia.

The posterior compartment is bounded by the tibia, interosseous membrane, fibula, posterior intermuscular septum, and crural fascia. This compartment is subdivided by the transverse intermuscular septum into superficial and deep subcompartments.

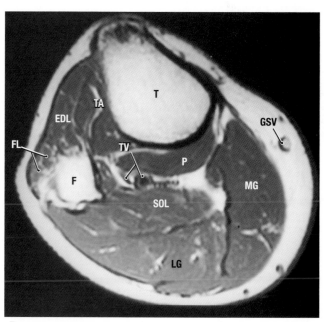

D. Transverse MRI

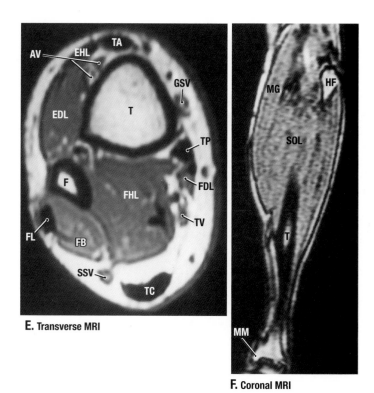

E. Transverse MRI

F. Coronal MRI

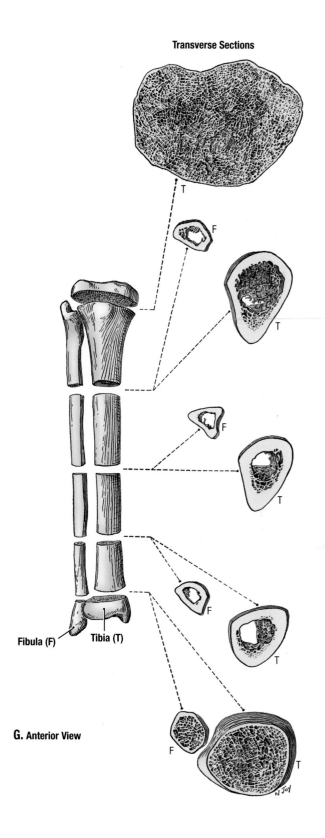

Transverse Sections

Fibula (F)   Tibia (T)

G. Anterior View

5.91   **Transverse sections and MRI of leg *(continued)***

D and **E.** T1 transverse (axial) MRIs. **F.** T1 coronal MRI. **G.** Transverse sections of tibia and fibula.

CHAPTER 6

UPPER LIMB

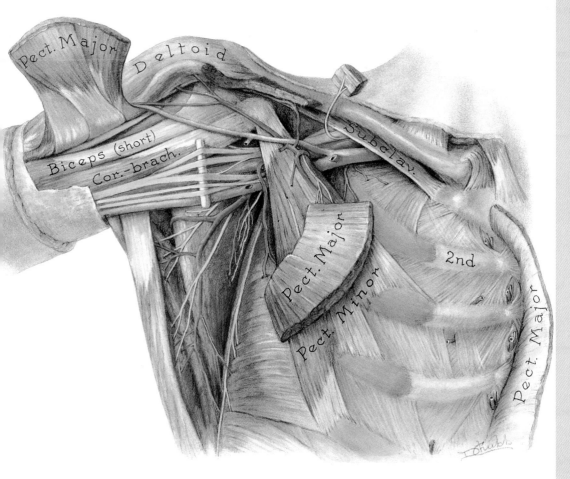

- Systemic Overview of Upper Limb **476**
  - Bones **476**
  - Nerves **480**
  - Blood Vessels **486**
  - Musculofascial Compartments **492**
- Pectoral Region **494**
- Axilla, Axillary Vessels, and Brachial Plexus **501**
- Scapular Region and Superficial Back **512**
- Arm and Rotator Cuff **516**
- Joints of Shoulder Region **530**
- Elbow Region **538**
- Elbow Joint **544**
- Anterior Aspect of Forearm **550**
- Anterior Aspect of Wrist and Palm of Hand **558**
- Posterior Aspect of Forearm **574**
- Posterior Aspect of Wrist and Dorsum of Hand **578**
- Lateral Aspect of Wrist and Hand **584**
- Medial Aspect of Wrist and Hand **587**
- Bones and Joints of Wrist and Hand **588**
- Function of Hand: Grips, Pinches, and Thumb Movements **596**
- Imaging and Sectional Anatomy **598**

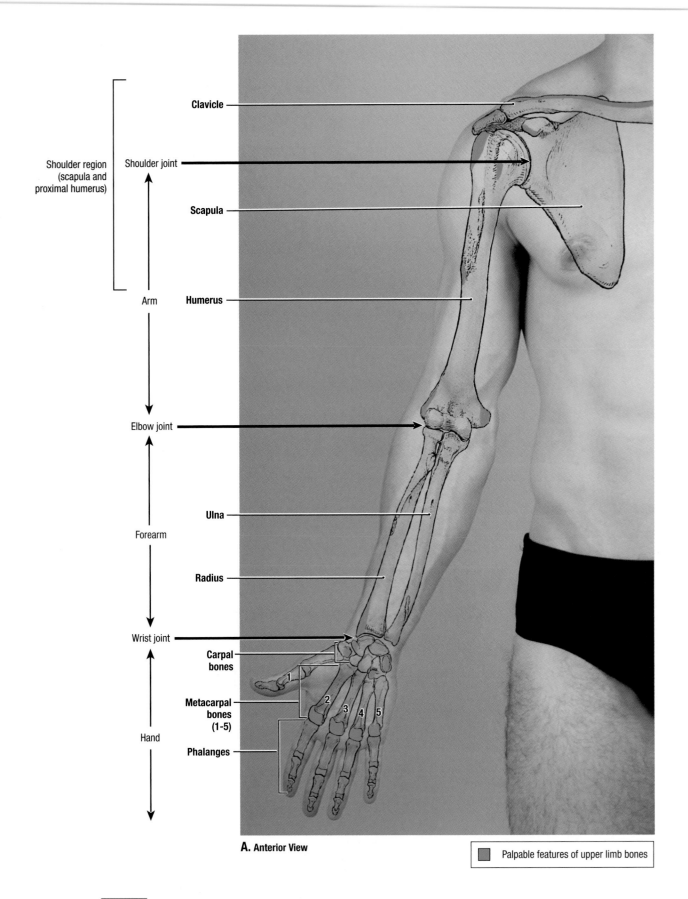

Shoulder region
(scapula and
proximal humerus)

Arm

Forearm

Hand

Clavicle

Shoulder joint

Scapula

Humerus

Elbow joint

Ulna

Radius

Wrist joint

Carpal
bones

Metacarpal
bones
(1-5)

Phalanges

A. Anterior View

Palpable features of upper limb bones

6.1   **Regions, bones, and major joints of upper limb**

The joints divide the upper limb into four main regions: the shoulder, arm, forearm, and hand.

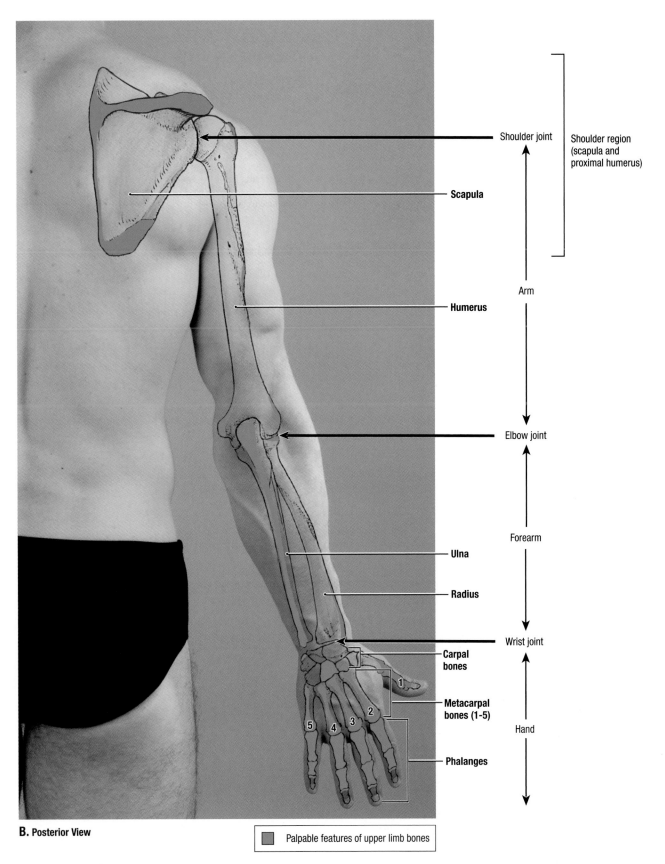

B. Posterior View

☐ Palpable features of upper limb bones

6.1   **Regions, bones, and major joints of upper limb** *(continued)*

The pectoral (shoulder) girdle is an incomplete ring of bones formed by the right and left scapulae and clavicles and is joined medially to the manubrium of the sternum.

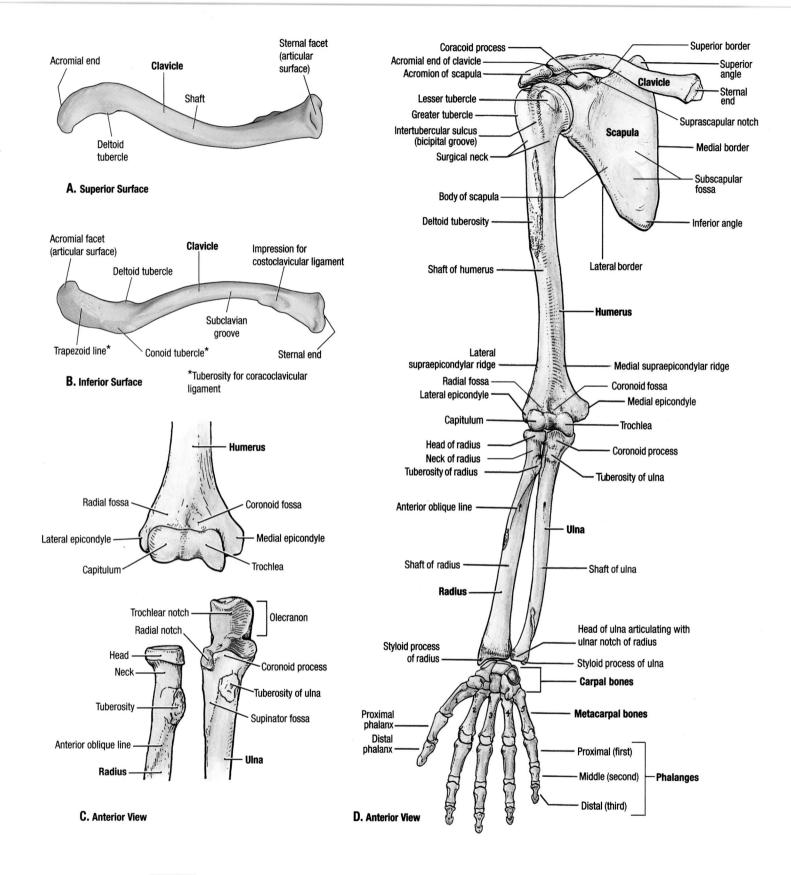

Acromial end

Clavicle

Shaft

Sternal facet (articular surface)

Deltoid tubercle

A. Superior Surface

Acromial facet (articular surface)

Deltoid tubercle

Clavicle

Impression for costoclavicular ligament

Subclavian groove

Trapezoid line*

Conoid tubercle*

Sternal end

B. Inferior Surface

*Tuberosity for coracoclavicular ligament

Humerus

Radial fossa

Coronoid fossa

Lateral epicondyle

Medial epicondyle

Capitulum

Trochlea

C. Anterior View

Trochlear notch

Olecranon

Radial notch

Head

Neck

Coronoid process

Tuberosity

Tuberosity of ulna

Supinator fossa

Anterior oblique line

Radius

Ulna

Coracoid process

Superior border

Acromial end of clavicle

Superior angle

Acromion of scapula

Clavicle

Sternal end

Lesser tubercle

Greater tubercle

Suprascapular notch

Intertubercular sulcus (bicipital groove)

Scapula

Surgical neck

Medial border

Body of scapula

Subscapular fossa

Deltoid tuberosity

Inferior angle

Shaft of humerus

Lateral border

Humerus

Lateral supraepicondylar ridge

Medial supraepicondylar ridge

Radial fossa

Coronoid fossa

Lateral epicondyle

Medial epicondyle

Capitulum

Trochlea

Head of radius

Coronoid process

Neck of radius

Tuberosity of radius

Tuberosity of ulna

Anterior oblique line

Ulna

Shaft of radius

Shaft of ulna

Radius

Head of ulna articulating with ulnar notch of radius

Styloid process of radius

Styloid process of ulna

Carpal bones

Proximal phalanx

Metacarpal bones

Distal phalanx

Proximal (first)

Middle (second)

Phalanges

Distal (third)

D. Anterior View

6.2   **Features of bones of upper limb**

A and **B.** Clavicle. **C.** Anterior aspect of disarticulated distal end of humerus and proximal end of radius and ulna. **D.** Anterior aspect of articulated upper limb.

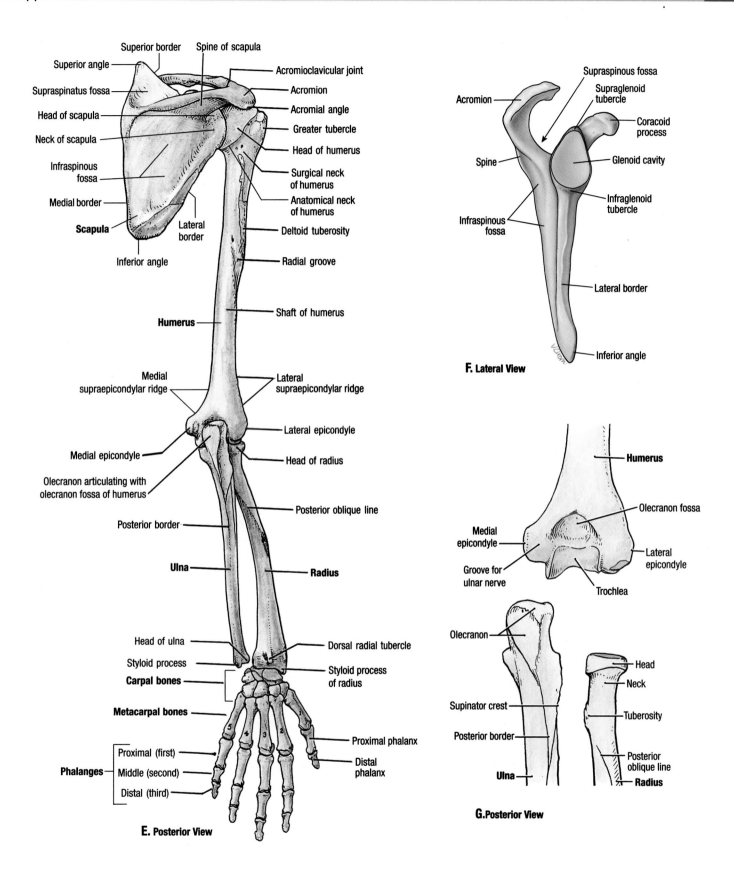

6.2   **Features of bones of upper limb (continued)**

E. Posterior aspect of articulated upper limb bones. **F.** Lateral aspect of scapula. **G.** Posterior aspect of disarticulated distal end of humerus and proximal ends of radius and ulna.

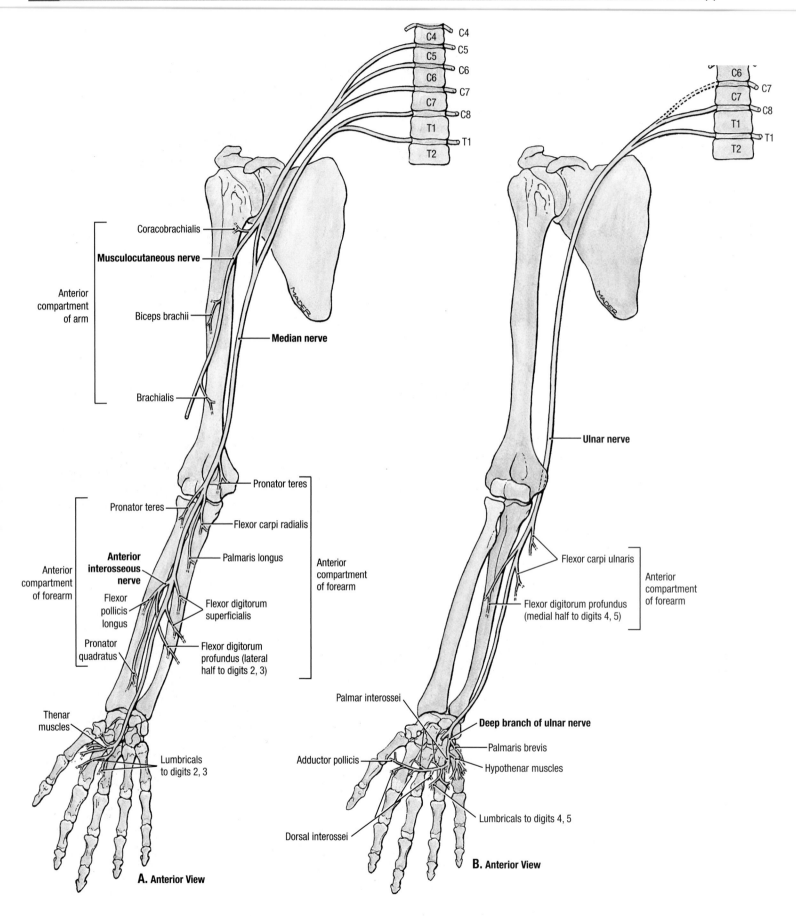

A. Anterior View

B. Anterior View

6.3   **Overview of motor innervation of upper limb**

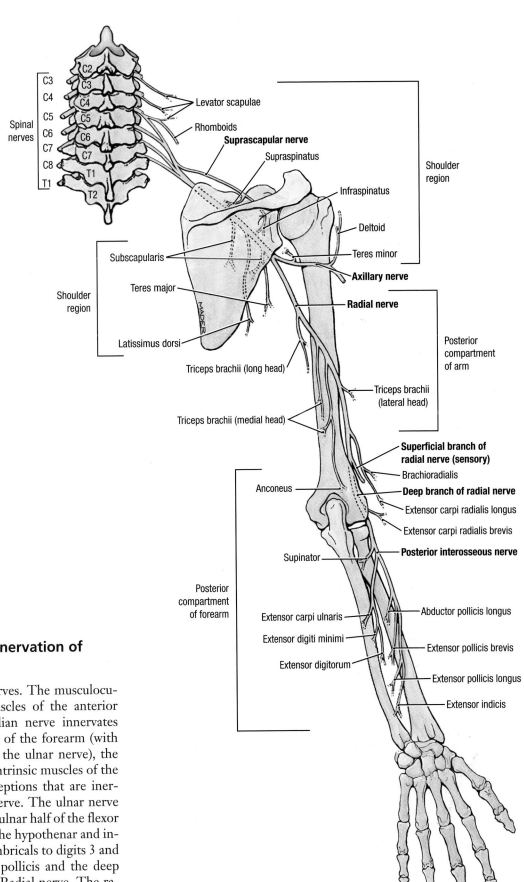

Spinal nerves

C3
C4
C5
C6
C7
C8
T1

C2
C3
C4
C5
C6
C7
C8
T1
T2

Levator scapulae

Rhomboids

Suprascapular nerve

Supraspinatus

Infraspinatus

Deltoid

Teres minor

Axillary nerve

Radial nerve

Shoulder region

Subscapularis

Teres major

Shoulder region

Latissimus dorsi

Triceps brachii (long head)

Triceps brachii (medial head)

Triceps brachii (lateral head)

Posterior compartment of arm

Superficial branch of radial nerve (sensory)

Brachioradialis

Deep branch of radial nerve

Extensor carpi radialis longus

Extensor carpi radialis brevis

Anconeus

Supinator

Posterior interosseous nerve

Posterior compartment of forearm

Extensor carpi ulnaris

Extensor digiti minimi

Extensor digitorum

Abductor pollicis longus

Extensor pollicis brevis

Extensor pollicis longus

Extensor indicis

C. Posterior View

6.3   Overview of motor innervation of upper limb

A. Musculocutaneous and median nerves. The musculocutaneous nerve innervates all the muscles of the anterior compartment of the arm. The median nerve innervates muscles of the anterior compartment of the forearm (with 1½ exceptions that are innervated by the ulnar nerve), the lumbricals to digits 2 and 3, and the intrinsic muscles of the thumb (thenar muscles) with 1½ exceptions that are inervated by the ulnar nerve. **B.** Ulnar nerve. The ulnar nerve innervates the flexor carpi ulnaris and ulnar half of the flexor digitorum profundus in the forearm, the hypothenar and interosseus muscles of the hand, the lumbricals to digits 3 and 4, and 1½ thenar muscles (adductor pollicis and the deep head of the flexor pollicis brevis). **C.** Radial nerve. The radial nerve innervates all muscles of the posterior compartments of the arm and forearm.

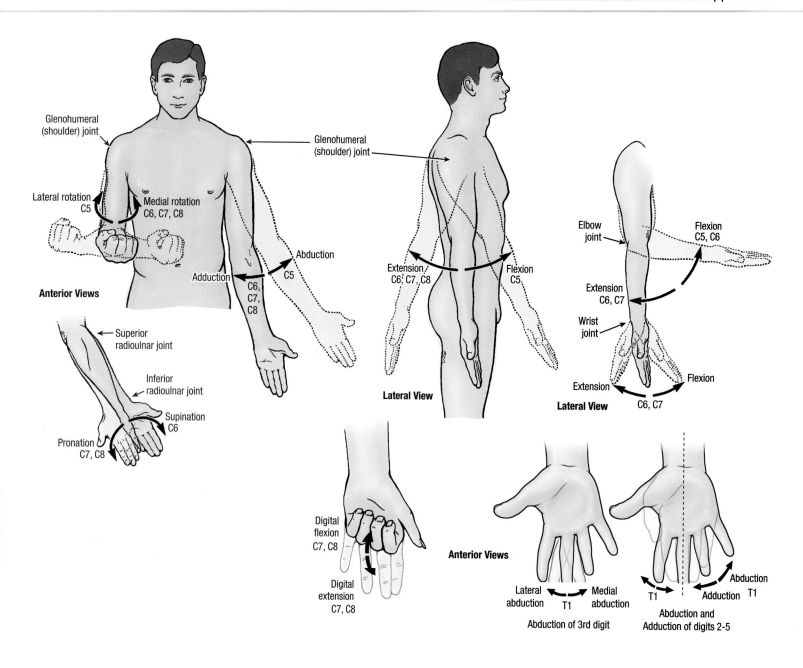

Myotatic (deep tendon) reflex	Spinal cord segments
Biceps	C5/C6
Brachioradialis	C5/C6
Triceps	C6/C7

6.4   Myotomes and myotatic (deep tendon stretch) reflexes

A. Myotomes. Somatic motor (general somatic efferent) fibers transmit impulses to skeletal (voluntary) muscles. The unilateral muscle mass receiving information from the somatic motor fibers conveyed by a single spinal nerve is a myotome. The intrinsic muscles of the hand constitute a single myotome—myotome T1. **B.** Myotatic reflexes. A myotatic reflex (deep tendon or stretch re-

flex) is an involuntary contraction of a muscle in response to sudden stretching. Myotatic reflexes are monosynaptic stretch reflexes that are elicited by briskly tapping the tendon with a reflex hammer. Each tendon reflex is mediated by specific spinal nerves. Stretch reflexes control muscle tone.

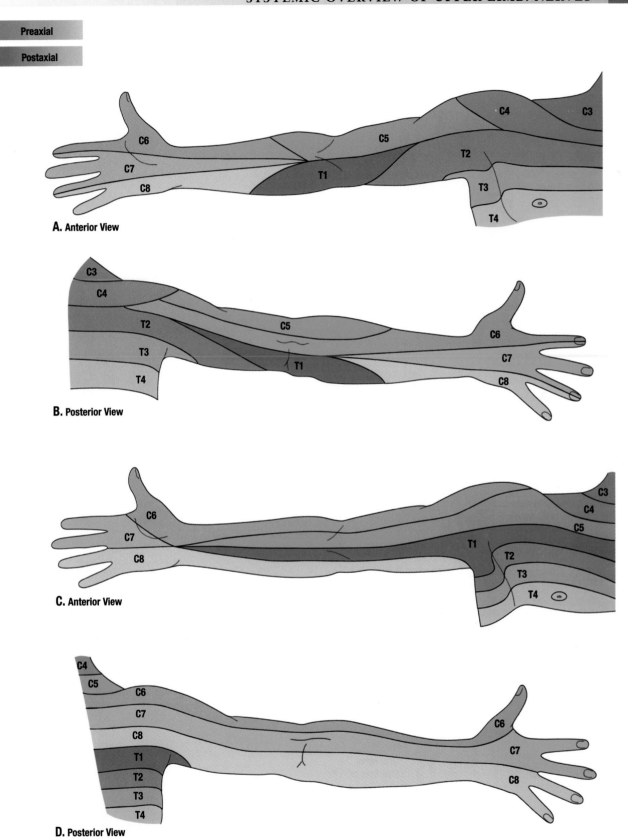

Preaxial

Postaxial

A. Anterior View

B. Posterior View

C. Anterior View

D. Posterior View

6.5 Dermatomes of upper limb

The dermatomal or segmental pattern of distribution of sensory nerve fibers persists despite the merging of spinal nerves in plexus formation during development. Two different dermatome maps are commonly used. **A** and **B**. The dermatome pattern of the upper limb according to Foerster (1933) is preferred by many because of its correlation with clinical findings. In the Foerster schema, dermatomes C6–T1 are displaced from the trunk to limbs. **C** and **D**. The dermatome pattern of the upper limb according to Keegan and Garrett (1948) is preferred by others for its correlation with development. Although depicted as distinct zones, adjacent dermatomes overlap considerably except along the axial line.

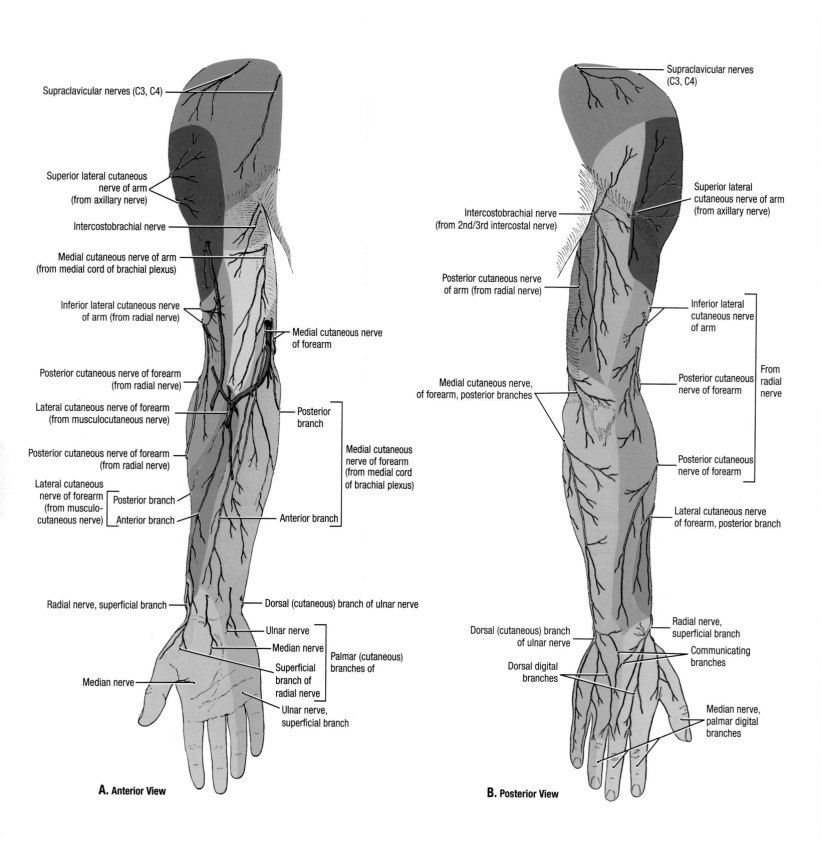

Supraclavicular nerves (C3, C4)

Superior lateral cutaneous
nerve of arm
(from axillary nerve)

Intercostobrachial nerve

Medial cutaneous nerve of arm
(from medial cord of brachial plexus)

Inferior lateral cutaneous nerve
of arm (from radial nerve)

Posterior cutaneous nerve of forearm
(from radial nerve)

Lateral cutaneous nerve of forearm
(from musculocutaneous nerve)

Posterior cutaneous nerve of forearm
(from radial nerve)

Lateral cutaneous
nerve of forearm
(from musculo-
cutaneous nerve)   Posterior branch

                        Anterior branch

Radial nerve, superficial branch

Median nerve

Medial cutaneous nerve
of forearm

Posterior
branch

Medial cutaneous
nerve of forearm
(from medial cord
of brachial plexus)

Anterior branch

Dorsal (cutaneous) branch of ulnar nerve

Ulnar nerve

Median nerve

Superficial
branch of
radial nerve

Palmar (cutaneous)
branches of

Ulnar nerve,
superficial branch

A. Anterior View

Supraclavicular nerves
(C3, C4)

Intercostobrachial nerve
(from 2nd/3rd intercostal nerve)

Posterior cutaneous nerve
of arm (from radial nerve)

Medial cutaneous nerve,
of forearm, posterior branches

Dorsal (cutaneous) branch
of ulnar nerve

Dorsal digital
branches

Superior lateral
cutaneous nerve of arm
(from axillary nerve)

Inferior lateral
cutaneous nerve
of arm

Posterior cutaneous
nerve of forearm

Posterior cutaneous
nerve of forearm

From
radial
nerve

Lateral cutaneous nerve
of forearm, posterior branch

Radial nerve,
superficial branch

Communicating
branches

Median nerve,
palmar digital
branches

B. Posterior View

6.6   Cutaneous nerves of upper limb

TABLE 6.1 CUTANEOUS NERVES OF UPPER LIMB

Nerve	Spinal Nerve components	Source	Course/Distribution
Supraclavicular nerves	C3–C4	Cervical plexus	Pass anterior to clavicle, immediately deep to platysma, and supply the skin over the clavicle and superolateral aspect of the pectoralis major muscle
Superior lateral cutaneous nerve of arm	C5–C6	Axillary nerve (posterior cord of brachial plexus)	Emerges from posterior margin of deltoid to supply skin over lower part of this muscle and the lateral side of the midarm
Inferior lateral cutaneous nerve of arm		Radial nerve (posterior cord of brachial plexus)	Arises with the posterior cutaneous nerve of forearm; pierces lateral head of triceps brachii to supply skin over the inferolateral aspect of the arm
Posterior cutaneous nerve of arm			Arises in axilla and supplies skin on posterior surface of the arm to olecranon
Posterior cutaneous nerve of forearm	C5–C8		Arises with the inferior lateral cutaneous nerve of the arm; pieces lateral head of triceps brachii to supply skin over the posterior aspect of the arm
Superficial branch of radial nerve			Arises in cubital fossa; supplies lateral (radial) half of the dorsal aspect of hand and thumb, and proximal portion of the dorsal aspects of digits 2 and 3, and the lateral (radial) half of dorsal aspect of digit 4
Lateral cutaneous nerve of forearm	C6–C7	Musculocutaneous nerve (lateral cord of brachial plexus)	Arises between biceps brachii and brachialis muscle as continuation of musculocutaneous nerve distal to branch to brachialis; emerges in cubital fossa lateral to biceps tendon and median cubital vein; supplies skin along radial (lateral) border of forearm to base of thenar eminence
Median nerve	C6–C7 (via lateral root); C8–T1 (via medial root)	Lateral and medial cords of brachial plexus	Courses with brachial artery in arm and deep to flexor digitorum superficialis in forearm; distal to origin of palmar cutaneous branch, traverses carpal tunnel to supply skin of palmar aspect of radial 3½ digits and adjacent palm, plus distal dorsal aspects of same, including nail beds
Ulnar nerve	(C7), C8–T1	Medial cord of brachial plexus	Courses with brachial, superior ulnar collateral, and ulnar arteries; supplies skin of palmar and dorsal aspects of medial (ulnar) 1½ digits and palm and dorsum of hand proximal to those digits
Medial cutaneous nerve of forearm	C8–T1		Pierces deep fascia with basilic vein in midarm; divides into anterior and posterior branches supplying skin over anterior and medial surfaces of forearm to wrist
Medial cutaneous nerve of arm	C8–T2		Smallest and most medial branch of brachial plexus; communicates with intercostobrachial nerve, then descends medial to brachial artery and basilic vein to innervate skin of distal medial arm
Intercostobrachial nerve	T2	Lateral cutaneous branch of 2nd intercostal nerve	Arises distal to angle of 2nd rib; supplies skin of axilla and proximal medial arm

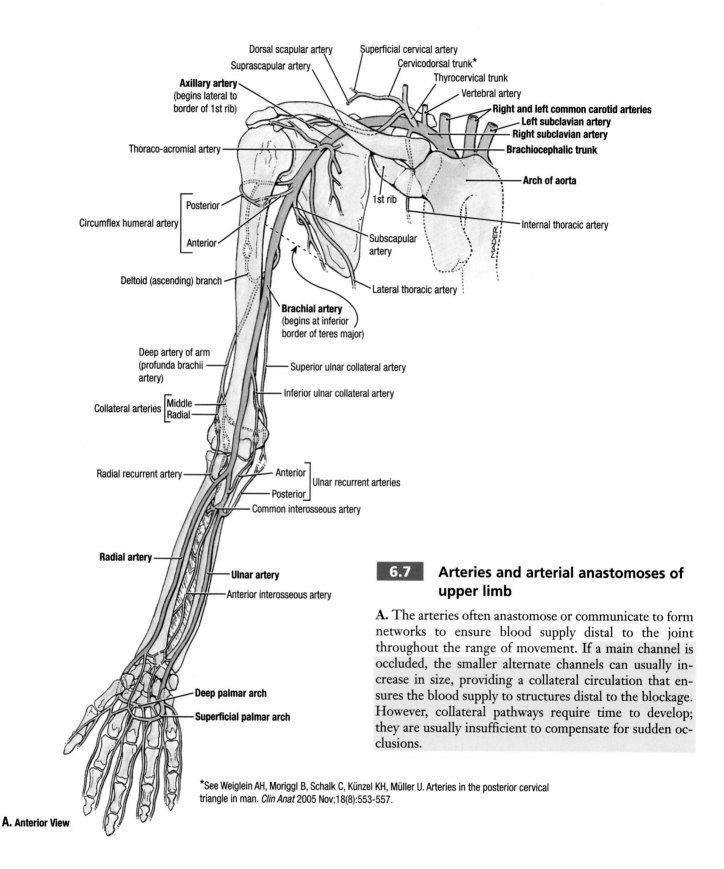

Dorsal scapular artery

Suprascapular artery

Axillary artery
(begins lateral to
border of 1st rib)

Thoraco-acromial artery

Circumflex humeral artery — Posterior / Anterior

Deltoid (ascending) branch

Brachial artery
(begins at inferior
border of teres major)

Deep artery of arm
(profunda brachii
artery)

Collateral arteries { Middle / Radial }

Radial recurrent artery

Common interosseous artery

Radial artery

Ulnar artery

Anterior interosseous artery

Deep palmar arch

Superficial palmar arch

A. Anterior View

Superficial cervical artery

Cervicodorsal trunk*

Thyrocervical trunk

Vertebral artery

Right and left common carotid arteries

Left subclavian artery

Right subclavian artery

Brachiocephalic trunk

Arch of aorta

1st rib

Internal thoracic artery

Subscapular artery

Lateral thoracic artery

Superior ulnar collateral artery

Inferior ulnar collateral artery

Anterior / Posterior } Ulnar recurrent arteries

MADER

6.7   Arteries and arterial anastomoses of upper limb

A. The arteries often anastomose or communicate to form networks to ensure blood supply distal to the joint throughout the range of movement. If a main channel is occluded, the smaller alternate channels can usually increase in size, providing a collateral circulation that ensures the blood supply to structures distal to the blockage. However, collateral pathways require time to develop; they are usually insufficient to compensate for sudden occlusions.

*See Weiglein AH, Moriggl B, Schalk C, Künzel KH, Müller U. Arteries in the posterior cervical triangle in man. *Clin Anat* 2005 Nov;18(8):553-557.

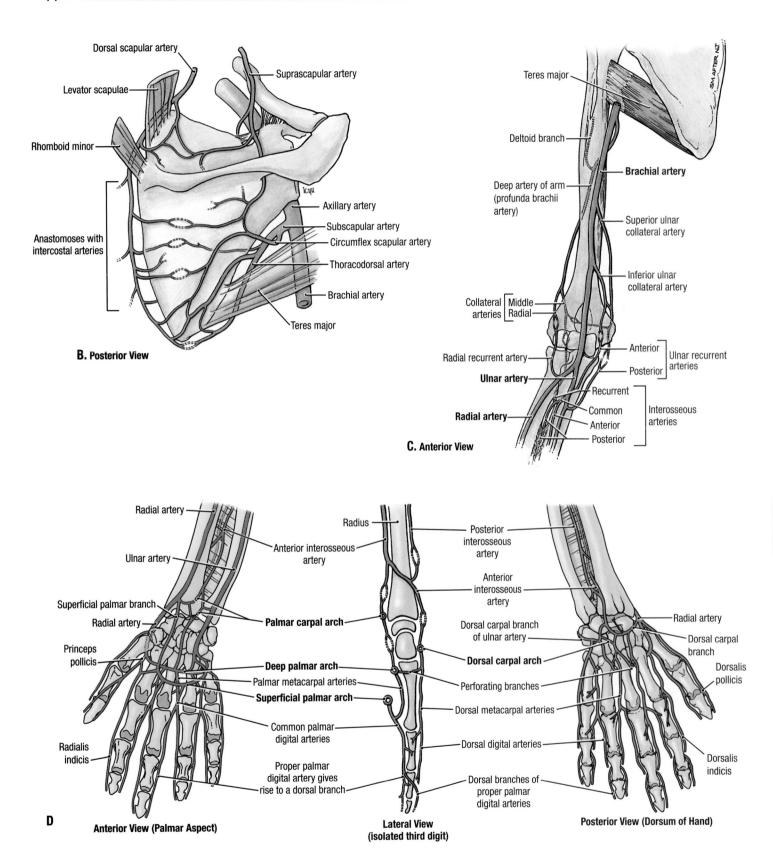

B. Posterior View

C. Anterior View

D

Anterior View (Palmar Aspect)   **Lateral View (isolated third digit)**   **Posterior View (Dorsum of Hand)**

6.7   **Arteries and periarterial anastomoses of upper limb** *(continued)*

B. Scapular anastomoses. **C.** Anastomoses of the elbow. **D.** Anastomoses of the hand. Joints receive blood from articular arteries that arise from vessels around joints.

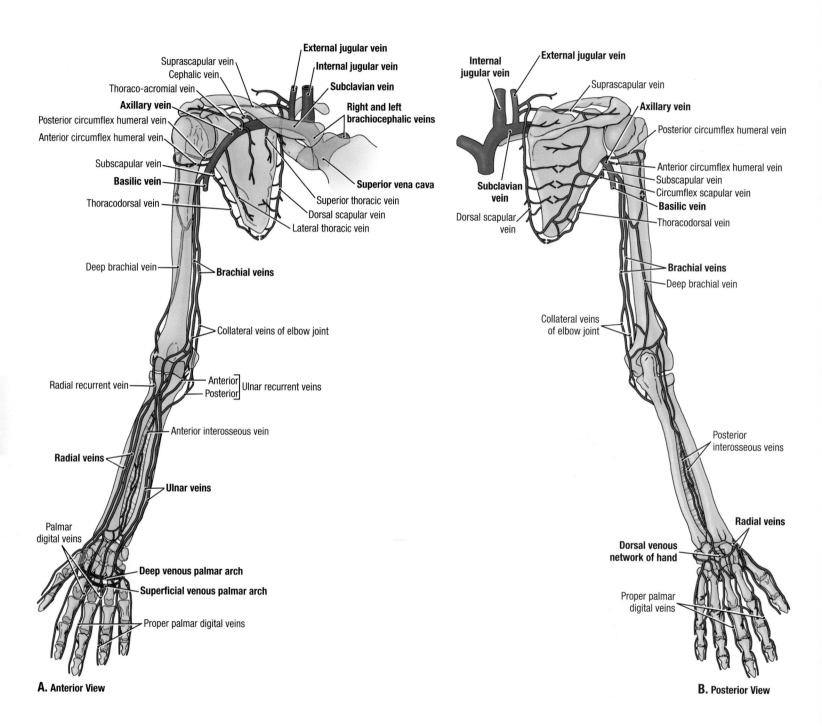

A. Anterior View

B. Posterior View

6.8   **Overview of the deep veins of the upper limb**

Deep veins lie internal to the deep fascia and occur as paired, continually interanastomosing "accompanying veins" (L., *venae comitantes*) surrounding and sharing the name of the artery they accompany.

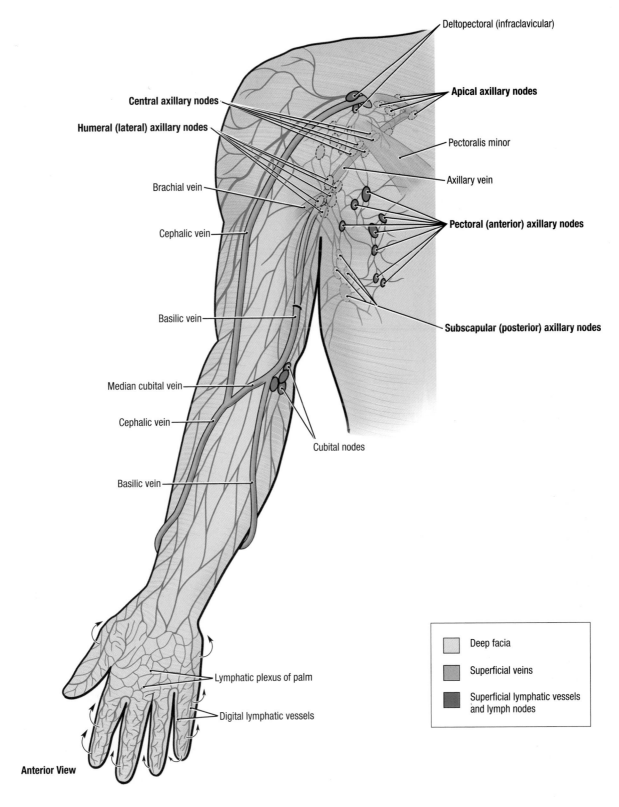

Deltopectoral (infraclavicular)

Apical axillary nodes

Central axillary nodes

Humeral (lateral) axillary nodes

Pectoralis minor

Brachial vein

Axillary vein

Cephalic vein

Pectoral (anterior) axillary nodes

Basilic vein

Subscapular (posterior) axillary nodes

Median cubital vein

Cephalic vein

Cubital nodes

Basilic vein

Lymphatic plexus of palm

Digital lymphatic vessels

Anterior View

	Deep facia
	Superficial veins
	Superficial lymphatic vessels and lymph nodes

6.9   **Superficial venous and lymphatic drainage of upper limb**

Superficial lymphatic vessels arise from lymphatic plexuses in the digits, palm, and dorsum of the hand and ascend with the superficial veins of the upper limb. The superficial lymphatic vessels ascend through the forearm and arm, converging toward the cephalic and especially to the basilic vein to reach the axillary lymph nodes. Some lymph passes through the cubital nodes at the elbow and the deltopectoral (infraclavicular) nodes at the shoulder. Deep lymphatic vessels accompany the neurovascular bundles of the upper limb and end primarily in the humeral (lateral) and central axillary lymph nodes.

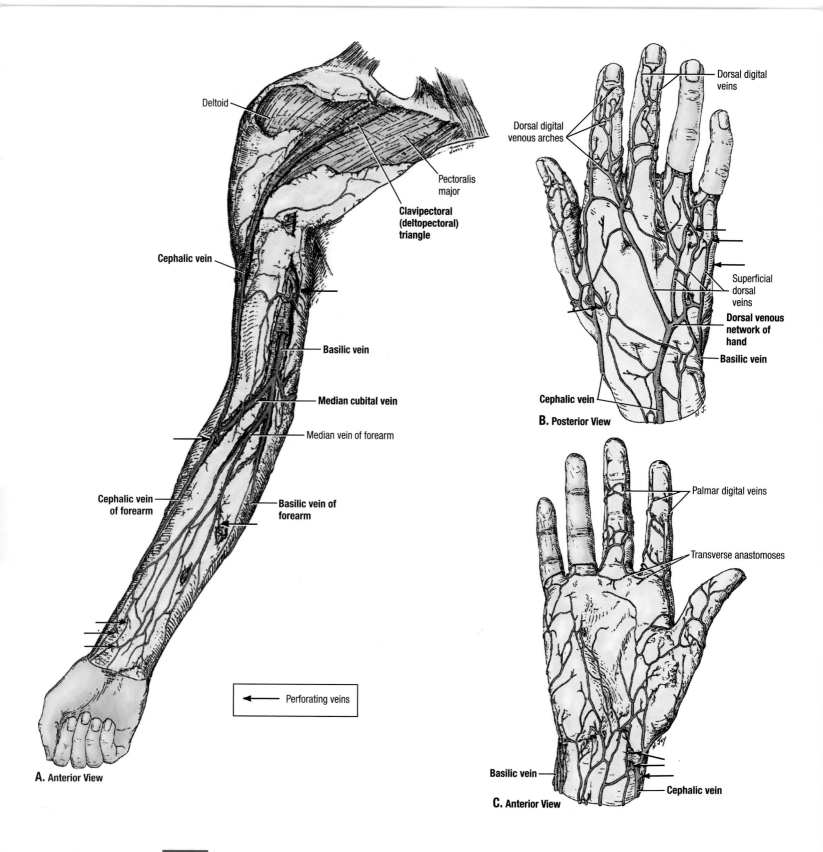

Deltoid

Pectoralis major

Clavipectoral (deltopectoral) triangle

Cephalic vein

Basilic vein

Median cubital vein

Median vein of forearm

Cephalic vein of forearm

Basilic vein of forearm

Perforating veins

A. Anterior View

Dorsal digital veins

Dorsal digital venous arches

Superficial dorsal veins

Dorsal venous network of hand

Basilic vein

Cephalic vein

B. Posterior View

Palmar digital veins

Transverse anastomoses

Basilic vein

Cephalic vein

C. Anterior View

6.10   Superficial venous drainage of upper limb

A. Forearm, arm, and pectoral region. **B.** Dorsal surface of hand. **C.** Palmar surface of hand. The *arrows* indicate where perforating veins penetrate the deep fascia. Blood is continuously shunted from these superficial veins in the subcutaneous tissue to deep veins via the perforating veins.

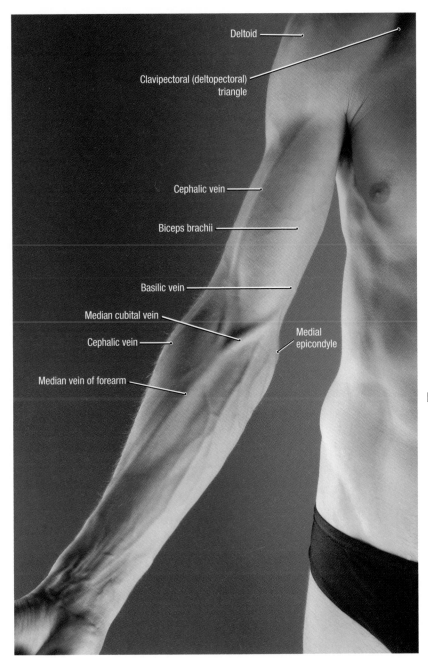

Deltoid

Clavipectoral (deltopectoral) triangle

Cephalic vein

Biceps brachii

Basilic vein

Median cubital vein

Cephalic vein

Median vein of forearm

Medial epicondyle

D. Anterior View

Superficial dorsal veins

Cephalic vein

Dorsal venous network of hand

E. Posterior View

6.10   **Superficial venous drainage of upper limb (continued)**

D. Surface anatomy of veins of forearm and arm. **E.** Surface anatomy of veins of the dorsal surface of hand.

Because of the prominence and accessibility of the superficial veins, they are commonly used for venipuncture (puncture of a vein to draw blood or inject a solution). By applying a tourniquet to the arm, the venous return is occluded, and the veins distend and usually are visible and/or palpable. Once a vein is punctured, the tourniquet is removed so that when the needle is removed the vein will not bleed extensively. The median cubital vein is commonly used for venipuncture. The veins forming the dorsal venous network of the hand and the cephalic and basilic veins arising from it are commonly used for long-term introduction of fluids (intravenous feeding). The cubital veins are also a site for the introduction of cardiac catheters to secure blood samples from the great vessels and chambers of the heart.

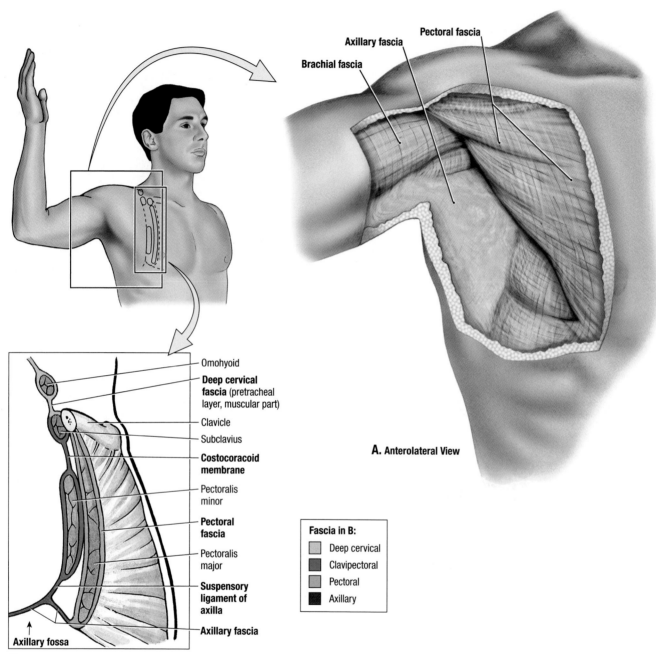

Pectoral fascia

Axillary fascia

Brachial fascia

A. Anterolateral View

Omohyoid

Deep cervical fascia (pretracheal layer, muscular part)

Clavicle

Subclavius

Costocoracoid membrane

Pectoralis minor

Pectoral fascia

Pectoralis major

Suspensory ligament of axilla

Axillary fascia

Axillary fossa

B. Sagittal Section

Fascia in B:

▢	Deep cervical
▨	Clavipectoral
▨	Pectoral
▨	Axillary

6.11   Deep fascia of upper limb—axillary and clavipectoral fascia

A. Axillary fascia. The axillary fascia forms the floor of the axillary fossa and is continuous with the pectoral fascia covering the pectoralis major muscle and the brachial fascia of the arm. **B.** Clavipectoral fascia. The clavipectoral fascia extends from the axillary fascia to enclose the pectoralis minor and subclavius muscles and then attaches to the clavicle. The part of the clavipectoral fascia superior to the pectoralis minor is the costocoracoid membrane and the part of the clavipectoral fascia inferior to the pectoralis minor is the suspensory ligament of the axilla. The suspensory ligament of the axilla, an extension of the axillary fascia, supports the axillary fascia and pulls the axillary fascia and the skin inferior to it superiorly when the arm is abducted, forming the axillary fossa or "armpit."

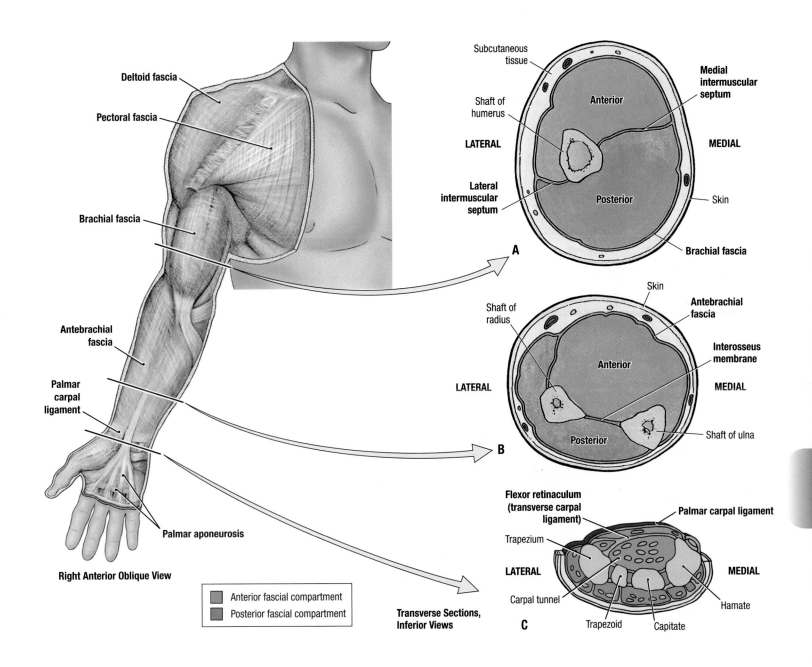

6.12   Deep fascia of upper limb—brachial and antebrachial fascia

A. Brachial fascia. The brachial fascia is the deep fascia of the arm and is continuous superiorly with the pectoral and axillary layers of fascia. Medial and lateral intermuscular septa extend from the deep aspect of the brachial fascia to the humerus, dividing the arm into anterior and posterior musculofascial compartments. **B.** Antebrachial fascia. The antebrachial fascia surrounds the forearm and is continuous with the brachial fascia and deep fascia of the hand. The interosseous membrane separates the forearm into anterior and posterior musculofascial compartments. Distally the fascia thickens to form the palmar carpal ligament, which is continuous with the flexor retinaculum and dorsally with the extensor expansion. The deep fascia of the hand is continuous with the antebrachial fascia, and on the palmar surface of the hand it thickens to form the palmar aponeurosis. **C.** Flexor retinaculum (transverse carpal ligament). The flexor retinaculum extends between the medial and lateral carpal bones to form the carpal tunnel.

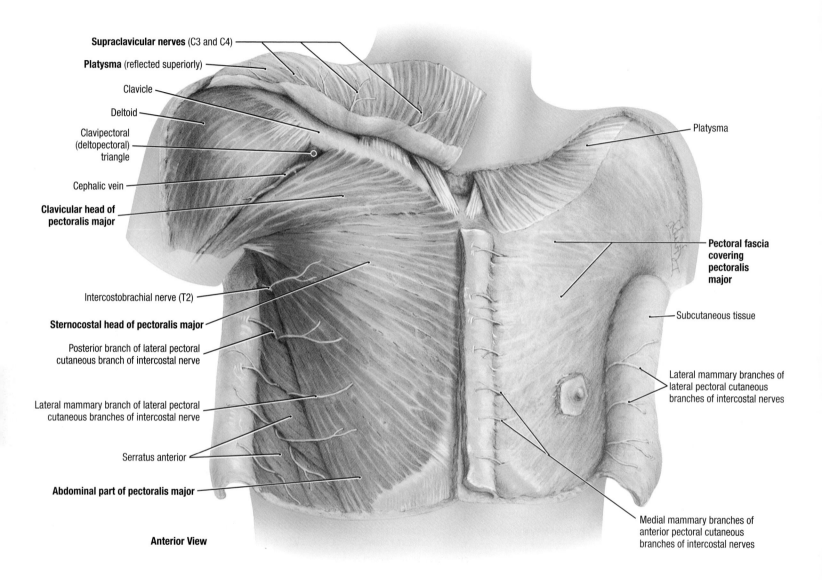

Supraclavicular nerves (C3 and C4)

Platysma (reflected superiorly)

Clavicle

Deltoid

Clavipectoral (deltopectoral) triangle

Cephalic vein

Clavicular head of pectoralis major

Intercostobrachial nerve (T2)

Sternocostal head of pectoralis major

Posterior branch of lateral pectoral cutaneous branch of intercostal nerve

Lateral mammary branch of lateral pectoral cutaneous branches of intercostal nerve

Serratus anterior

Abdominal part of pectoralis major

Platysma

Pectoral fascia covering pectoralis major

Subcutaneous tissue

Lateral mammary branches of lateral pectoral cutaneous branches of intercostal nerves

Medial mammary branches of anterior pectoral cutaneous branches of intercostal nerves

Anterior View

6.13   **Superficial dissection, male pectoral region**

- The platysma muscle, which usually descends to the 2nd or 3rd rib, is cut short on the right side and, together with the supraclavicular nerves, is reflected on the left side.
- The exposed intermuscular bony strip of the clavicle is subcutaneous and subplatysmal.
- The cephalic vein passes deeply to join the axillary vein in the clavipectoral (deltopectoral) triangle.
- The cutaneous innervation of the pectoral region by the supraclavicular nerves (C3 and C4) and upper thoracic nerves (T2 to T6); the brachial plexus (C5–T1) does not supply cutaneous branches to the pectoral region.

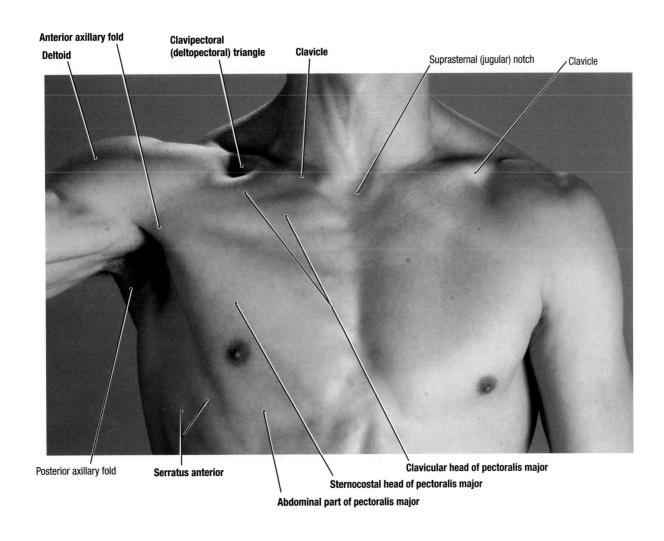

Anterior axillary fold
Deltoid
Clavipectoral (deltopectoral) triangle
Clavicle
Suprasternal (jugular) notch
Clavicle
Posterior axillary fold
Serratus anterior
Clavicular head of pectoralis major
Sternocostal head of pectoralis major
Abdominal part of pectoralis major

6.14   Surface anatomy, male pectoral region

The **clavipectoral** (deltopectoral) **triangle** is the depressed area just inferior to the lateral part of the clavicle. The clavipectoral triangle is bounded by the clavicle superiorly, the deltoid laterally, and the clavicular head of pectoralis major medially. When the arm is abducted and then adducted against resistance, the two heads of the pectoralis major are visible and palpable. As this mus-cle extends from the thoracic wall to the arm, it forms the anterior axillary fold. Digitations of the serratus anterior appear inferolat-eral to the pectoralis major. The coracoid process of the scapula is covered by the anterior part of deltoid; however, the tip of the process can be felt on deep palpation in the clavipectoral triangle. The deltoid forms the contour of the shoulder.

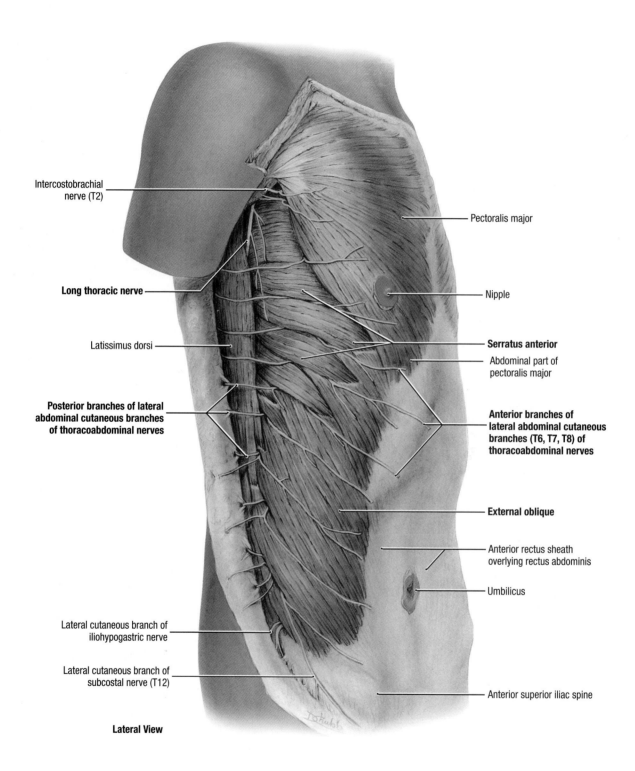

Intercostobrachial
nerve (T2)

Long thoracic nerve

Latissimus dorsi

**Posterior branches of lateral
abdominal cutaneous branches
of thoracoabdominal nerves**

Lateral cutaneous branch of
iliohypogastric nerve

Lateral cutaneous branch of
subcostal nerve (T12)

Pectoralis major

Nipple

Serratus anterior

Abdominal part of
pectoralis major

**Anterior branches of
lateral abdominal cutaneous
branches (T6, T7, T8) of
thoracoabdominal nerves**

External oblique

Anterior rectus sheath
overlying rectus abdominis

Umbilicus

Anterior superior iliac spine

Lateral View

6.15   Superficial dissection of trunk

- The slips of the serratus anterior interdigitate with the external oblique.
- The long thoracic nerve (nerve to serratus anterior) lies on the lateral (superficial) aspect of the serratus anterior; this nerve is vulnerable to damage from stab wounds and during surgery (e.g., radical mastectomy).
- The anterior and posterior branches of the lateral thoracic and abdominal cutaneous branches of intercostal and thoracoabdominal nerves are dissected.

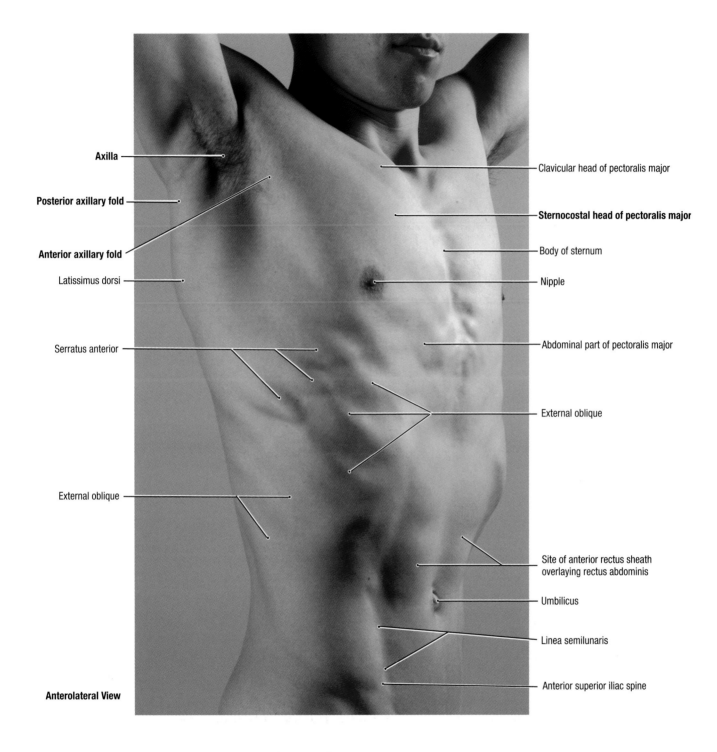

Axilla

Posterior axillary fold

Anterior axillary fold

Latissimus dorsi

Serratus anterior

External oblique

Clavicular head of pectoralis major

Sternocostal head of pectoralis major

Body of sternum

Nipple

Abdominal part of pectoralis major

External oblique

Site of anterior rectus sheath overlaying rectus abdominis

Umbilicus

Linea semilunaris

Anterior superior iliac spine

Anterolateral View

6.16   **Surface anatomy of anterolateral aspect of the trunk**

When the arm is abducted and then adducted against resistance, the sternocostal part of the pectoralis major can be seen and palpated. If the anterior axillary fold bounding the axilla is grasped between the fingers and thumb, the inferior border of the sternocostal head of the pectoralis major can be felt. Several digitations of the serratus anterior are visible inferior to the anterior axillary fold. The posterior axillary fold is composed of skin and muscular tissue (latissimus dorsi and teres major) bounding the axilla posteriorly.

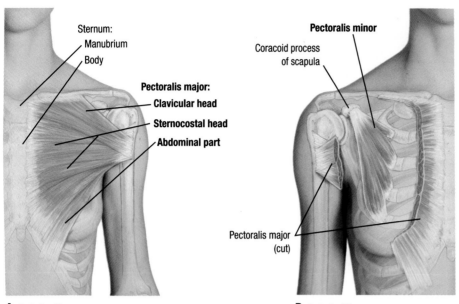

Sternum:
Manubrium
Body

Pectoralis major:
Clavicular head
Sternocostal head
Abdominal part

A. Anterior View

Pectoralis minor
Coracoid process
of scapula

Pectoralis major
(cut)

B. Anterior View

Clavicle
Subclavius

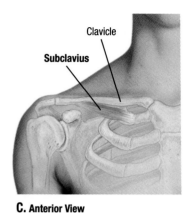

C. Anterior View

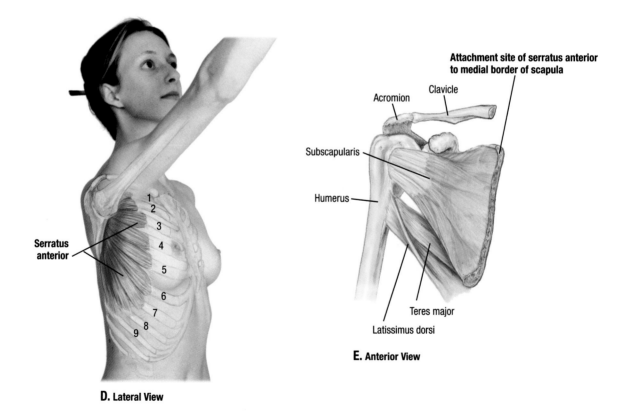

D. Lateral View

Serratus
anterior

1
2
3
4
5
6
7
8
9

Attachment site of serratus anterior
to medial border of scapula

Acromion   Clavicle

Subscapularis

Humerus

Teres major
Latissimus dorsi

E. Anterior View

6.17   **Pectoralis major and minor and serratus anterior**

A. Pectoralis major. **B.** Pectoralis minor. **C.** Subclavius. **D** and **E.** Serratus anterior and its scapular attachment.

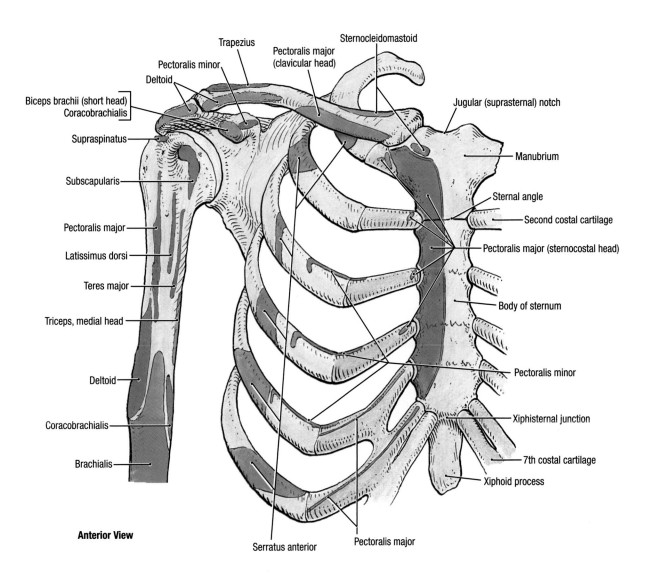

Anterior View

TABLE 6.2 ANTERIOR AXIOAPPENDICULAR MUSCLES

Muscle	Proximal Attachment (red)	Distal Attachment (blue)	Innervation[a]	Main Actions
Pectoralis major	*Clavicular head:* anterior surface of medial half of clavicle *Sternocostal head:* anterior surface of sternum, superior six costal cartilages *Abdominal part:* aponeurosis of external oblique muscle	Crest of greater tubercle of intertubercular sulcus (lateral lip of bicipital groove)	Lateral and medial pectoral nerves; clavicular head (C5 and **C6**), sternocostal head (**C7**, **C8**, and T1)	Adducts and medially rotates humerus; draws scapula anteriorly and inferiorly Acting alone: clavicular head flexes humerus and sternocostal head extends it from the flexed position
Pectoralis minor	3rd to 5th ribs near their costal cartilages	Medial border and superior surface of coracoid process of scapula	Medial pectoral nerve (C8 and T1)	Stabilizes scapula by drawing it inferiorly and anteriorly against thoracic wall
Subclavius	Junction of 1st rib and its costal cartilage	Inferior surface of middle third of clavicle	Nerve to subclavius (**C5** and C6)	Anchors and depresses clavicle
Serratus anterior	External surfaces of lateral parts of 1st to 8th–9th ribs	Anterior surface of medial border of scapula	Long thoracic nerve (C5, **C6**, and **C7**)	Protracts scapula and holds it against thoracic wall; rotates scapula

[a]Numbers indicate spinal cord segmental innervation (e.g., C5 and C6 indicate that nerves supplying the clavicular head of pectoralis major are derived from 5th and 6th cervical segments of spinal cord). Boldface numbers indicate the main segmental innervation. Damage to these segments or to motor nerve roots arising from them results in paralysis of the muscles concerned.

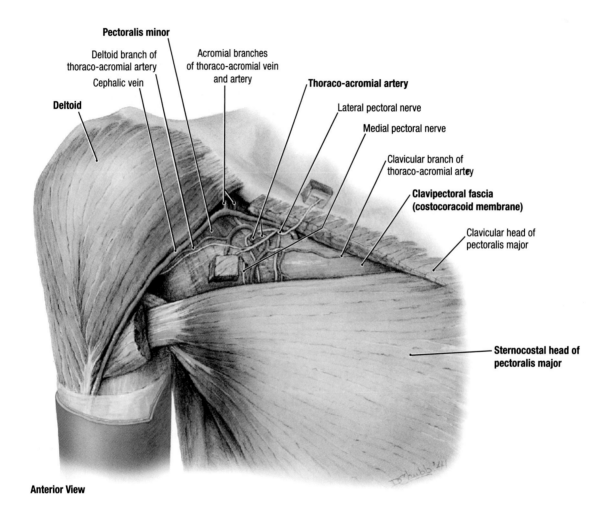

Anterior View

6.18   Anterior wall of axilla and clavipectoral fascia

A. Anterior wall of axilla. The clavicular head of the pectoralis major is excised, except for two cubes of muscle that remain to identify the branches of the lateral pectoral nerve.

- The clavipectoral fascia superior to the pectoralis minor (costocoracoid membrane) is pierced by the cephalic vein, the lateral pectoral nerve, and the thoraco-acromial vessels.
- The pectoralis minor and clavipectoral fascia are pierced by the medial pectoral nerve.
- Observe the trilaminar insertion of the pectoralis major from deep to superficial: inferior part of the sternocostal head, superior part of the sternocostal head, and clavicular head.

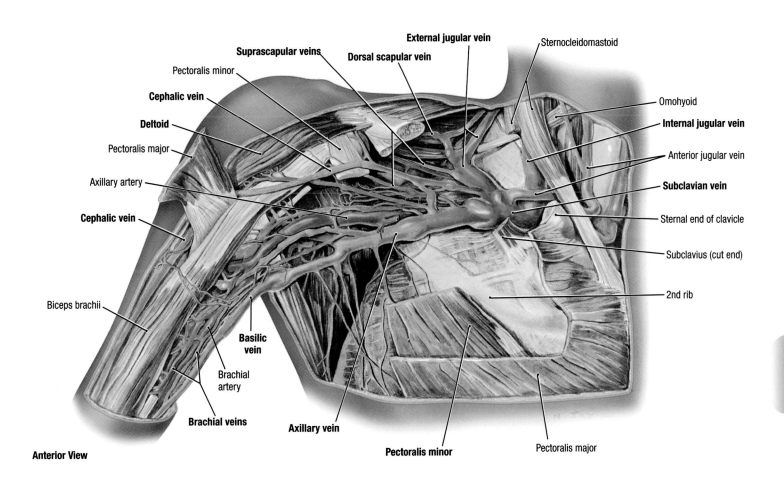

External jugular vein

Suprascapular veins

Dorsal scapular vein

Sternocleidomastoid

Pectoralis minor

Cephalic vein

Omohyoid

Deltoid

Internal jugular vein

Pectoralis major

Anterior jugular vein

Axillary artery

Subclavian vein

Cephalic vein

Sternal end of clavicle

Subclavius (cut end)

2nd rib

Biceps brachii

Basilic vein

Brachial artery

Brachial veins

Axillary vein

Pectoralis minor

Pectoralis major

Anterior View

6.19 Veins of axilla

- The basilic vein joins the brachial veins to become the axillary vein near the inferior border of teres major, the axillary vein becomes the subclavian vein at the lateral border of the 1st rib, and the subclavian joins the internal jugular to become the brachiocephalic vein posterior to the sternal end of the clavicle.
- Numerous valves, enlargements in the vein, are shown.
- The cephalic vein in this specimen bifurcates to end in the axillary and external jugular veins.

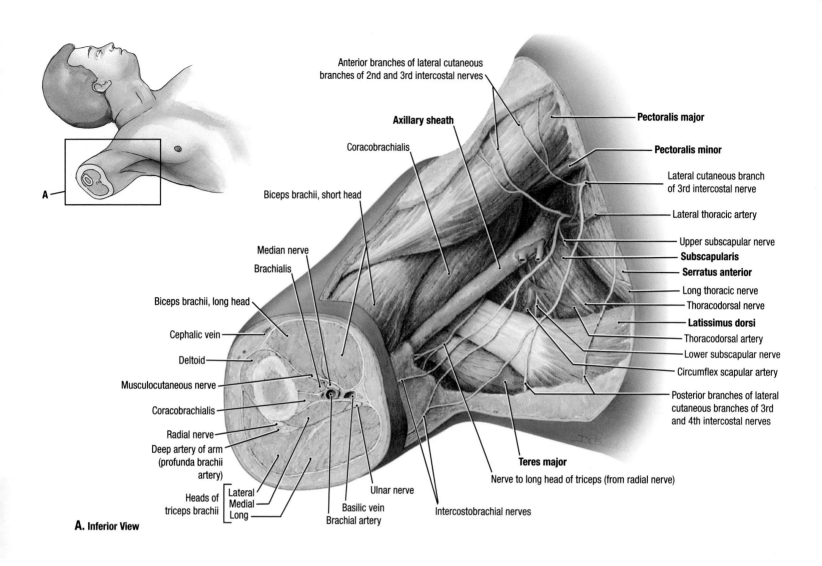

Anterior branches of lateral cutaneous
branches of 2nd and 3rd intercostal nerves

Axillary sheath

Coracobrachialis

Biceps brachii, short head

Median nerve

Brachialis

Biceps brachii, long head

Cephalic vein

Deltoid

Musculocutaneous nerve

Coracobrachialis

Radial nerve

Deep artery of arm
(profunda brachii
artery)

Heads of ⎱ Lateral
triceps brachii ⎰ Medial
             Long

A. Inferior View

Ulnar nerve

Basilic vein
Brachial artery

Intercostobrachial nerves

Teres major

Nerve to long head of triceps (from radial nerve)

Pectoralis major

Pectoralis minor

Lateral cutaneous branch
of 3rd intercostal nerve

Lateral thoracic artery

Upper subscapular nerve

Subscapularis

Serratus anterior

Long thoracic nerve

Thoracodorsal nerve

Latissimus dorsi

Thoracodorsal artery

Lower subscapular nerve

Circumflex scapular artery

Posterior branches of lateral
cutaneous branches of 3rd
and 4th intercostal nerves

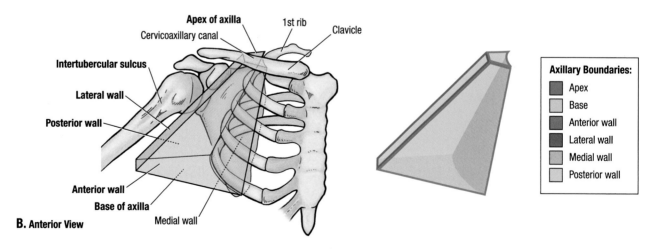

Apex of axilla   1st rib   Clavicle

Cervicoaxillary canal

Intertubercular sulcus

Lateral wall

Posterior wall

Anterior wall

Base of axilla

Medial wall

B. Anterior View

Axillary Boundaries:

Apex

Base

Anterior wall

Lateral wall

Medial wall

Posterior wall

6.20   **Walls and contents of the axilla**

A. Dissection. **B.** Location and walls of axilla, schematic diagram.
- The walls of the axilla are: anterior (formed by the pectoralis major, pectoralis minor, and subclavius muscles), posterior (formed by subscapularis, latissimus dorsi, and teres major muscles), medial (formed by the serratus anterior muscle), and lateral (formed by the intertubercular sulcus [bicipital groove] of the humerus [concealed by the biceps and coracobrachialis muscles]).
- The axillary sheath surrounds the nerves and vessels (neurovascular bundle) of the upper limb.

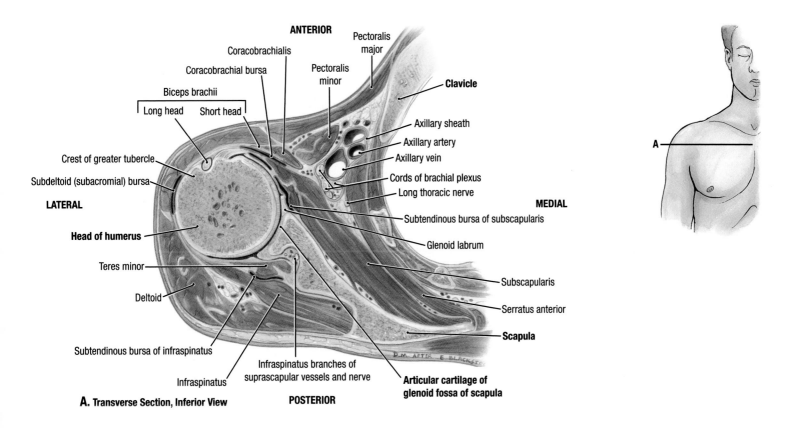

ANTERIOR

Coracobrachialis

Coracobrachial bursa

Biceps brachii
Long head   Short head

Pectoralis major

Pectoralis minor

Clavicle

Axillary sheath

Axillary artery

Axillary vein

Cords of brachial plexus

Long thoracic nerve

Crest of greater tubercle

Subdeltoid (subacromial) bursa

LATERAL

MEDIAL

Subtendinous bursa of subscapularis

Head of humerus

Glenoid labrum

Teres minor

Subscapularis

Deltoid

Serratus anterior

Scapula

Subtendinous bursa of infraspinatus

Infraspinatus

Infraspinatus branches of suprascapular vessels and nerve

Articular cartilage of glenoid fossa of scapula

D.M. AFTER E. BLACKSTONE

A. Transverse Section, Inferior View

POSTERIOR

A

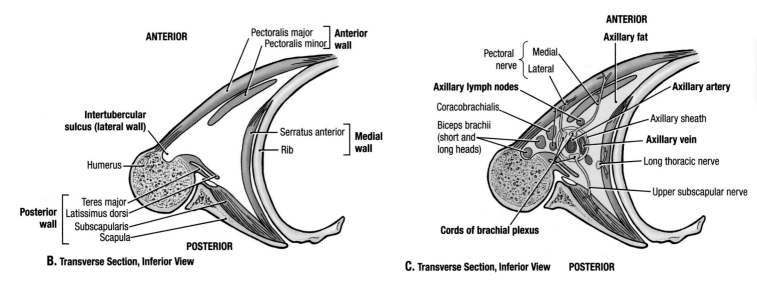

ANTERIOR

Pectoralis major
Pectoralis minor

Anterior wall

Intertubercular sulcus (lateral wall)

Serratus anterior

Rib

Medial wall

Humerus

Teres major
Latissimus dorsi
Subscapularis
Scapula

Posterior wall

POSTERIOR

B. Transverse Section, Inferior View

ANTERIOR

Axillary fat

Pectoral nerve
Medial
Lateral

Axillary lymph nodes

Coracobrachialis

Biceps brachii (short and long heads)

Axillary artery

Axillary sheath

Axillary vein

Long thoracic nerve

Upper subscapular nerve

Cords of brachial plexus

C. Transverse Section, Inferior View   POSTERIOR

6.21   Transverse sections through the shoulder joint and axilla

A. Anatomical section. **B.** Walls of axilla, schematic illustration. **C.** Walls and contents of axilla, schematic illustration.

- The intertubercular sulcus (bicipital groove) containing the tendon of the long head of the biceps brachii muscle is directed anteriorly; the short head of the biceps muscle and the coracobrachialis and pectoralis minor muscles are sectioned just inferior to their attachments to the coracoid process.
- The small glenoid cavity is deepened by the glenoid labrum.

- Bursae include the subdeltoid (subacromial) bursa, between the deltoid and greater tubercle; the subtendinous bursa of subscapularis, between the subscapularis tendon and scapula; and coracobrachial bursa, between the coracobrachialis and subscapularis.
- The axillary sheath encloses the axillary artery and vein and the three cords of the brachial plexus to form a neurovascular bundle, surrounded by axillary fat.

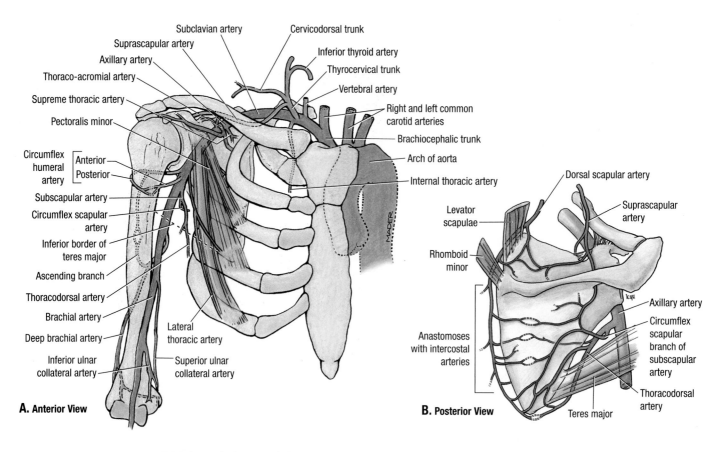

Subclavian artery
Suprascapular artery
Axillary artery
Thoraco-acromial artery
Supreme thoracic artery
Pectoralis minor
Circumflex humeral artery — Anterior / Posterior
Subscapular artery
Circumflex scapular artery
Inferior border of teres major
Ascending branch
Thoracodorsal artery
Brachial artery
Deep brachial artery
Inferior ulnar collateral artery

Cervicodorsal trunk
Inferior thyroid artery
Thyrocervical trunk
Vertebral artery
Right and left common carotid arteries
Brachiocephalic trunk
Arch of aorta
Internal thoracic artery

Lateral thoracic artery
Superior ulnar collateral artery

A. Anterior View

Dorsal scapular artery
Suprascapular artery
Levator scapulae
Rhomboid minor
Anastomoses with intercostal arteries
Axillary artery
Circumflex scapular branch of subscapular artery
Thoracodorsal artery
Teres major

B. Posterior View

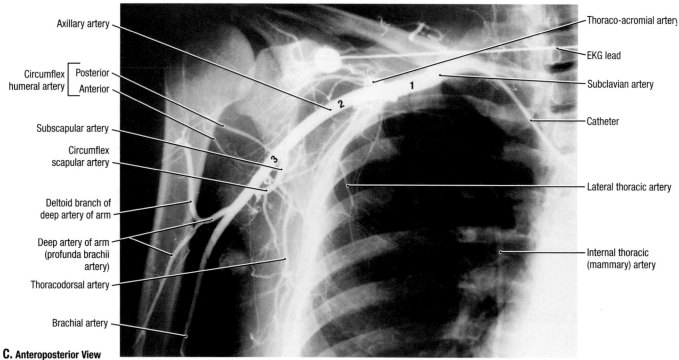

Axillary artery
Circumflex humeral artery — Posterior / Anterior
Subscapular artery
Circumflex scapular artery
Deltoid branch of deep artery of arm
Deep artery of arm (profunda brachii artery)
Thoracodorsal artery
Brachial artery

Thoraco-acromial artery
EKG lead
Subclavian artery
Catheter
Lateral thoracic artery
Internal thoracic (mammary) artery

C. Anteroposterior View

1: First part of the axillary artery is located between the lateral border of the 1st rib and the medial border of pectoralis minor.
2: Second part of the axillary artery lies posterior to pectoralis minor.
3: Third part of the axillary artery extends from the lateral border of pectoralis minor to the inferior border of teres major, where it becomes the brachial artery.

6.22   Arteries of the proximal upper limb

A and **B.** Schematic illustrations. **C.** Axillary arteriogram.

TABLE 6.3 ARTERIES OF PROXIMAL UPPER LIMB (SHOULDER REGION AND ARM)

Artery	Origin	Course
Internal thoracic	Subclavian artery	Descends, inclining anteromedially, posterior to sternal end of clavicle and first costal cartilage; enters thorax to descend in parasternal plane; gives rise to perforating branches, anterior intercostal, musculophrenic, and superior epigastric arteries
Thyrocervical trunk		Ascends as a short, wide trunk, often giving rise to the suprascapular artery and/or cervicodorsal trunk and terminating by bifurcating into the ascending cervical and inferior thyroid arteries
Suprascapular	Cervicodorsal trunk from thyrocervical trunk (or as direct branch of subclavian artery[a])	Passes inferolaterally over anterior scalene muscle and phrenic nerve, subclavian artery and brachial plexus running laterally posterior and parallel to clavicle; next passes over transverse scapular ligament to supraspinous fossa, then lateral to scapular spine (deep to acromion) to infraspinous fossa
Supreme thoracic	1st part (as only branch)	Runs anteromedially along superior border of pectoralis minor; then passes between it and pectoralis major to thoracic wall; helps supply 1st and 2nd intercostal spaces and superior part of serratus anterior
Thoraco-acromial	2nd part (medial branch)	Curls around superomedial border of pectoralis minor, pierces costocaracoid membrane (clavipectoral fascia), and divides into four branches: pectoral, deltoid, acromial, and clavicular
Lateral thoracic	2nd part (lateral branch) — Axillary artery	Descends along axillary border of pectoralis minor; follows it onto thoracic wall, supplying lateral aspect of breast
Circumflex humeral (anterior and posterior)	3rd part (sometimes via a common trunk)	Encircle surgical neck of humerus, anastomosing with each other laterally; larger posterior branch traverses quadrangular space
Subscapular	3rd part (largest branch)	Descends from level of inferior border of subscapularis along lateral border of scapula, dividing within 2-3 cm into terminal branches, the circumflex scapular and thoracodorsal arteries
Circumflex scapular	Subscapular artery	Curves around lateral border of scapula to enter infraspinous fossa, anastomosing with subscapular artery
Thoracodorsal	Near its origin	Continuation course of subscapular artery; accompanies thoracodorsal nerve to enter latissimus dorsi
Deep brachial	Near middle of arm — Brachial artery	Accompanies radial nerve through radial groove of humerus, supplying posterior compartment of arm and participating in periarticular arterial anastomosis around elbow joint
Superior ulnar collateral	Superior to medial epicondyle of humerus	Accompanies ulnar nerve to posterior aspect of elbow; anastomoses with posterior ulnar recurrent artery
Inferior ulnar collateral		Passes anterior to medial epicondyle of humerus to anastomose with anterior ulnar collateral artery around elbow joint

[a] See Weiglein AH, Moriggl B, Schalk C, et al. Arteries in the posterior cervical triangle. Clinical Anatomy 2005;18:533–537.

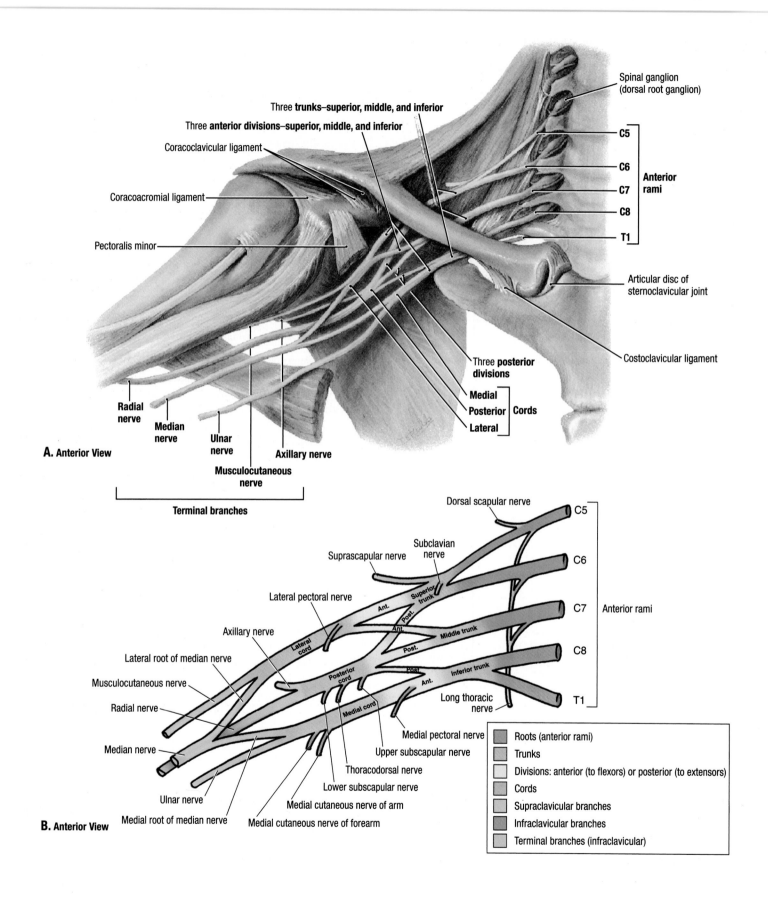

6.23 **Brachial plexus**

A. Dissection. **B.** Schematic illustration.

TABLE 6.4 AXILLA, AXILLARY VESSELS, AND BRACHIAL PLEXUS

Nerve	Origin	Course	Distribution/Structure(s) Supplied
Supraclavicular branches			
Dorsal scapular	Anterior ramus of C5 with a frequent contribution from C4	Pierces scalenus medius, descends deep to levator scapulae, and enters deep surface of rhomboids	Rhomboids and occasionally supplies levator scapulae
Long thoracic	Anterior rami of C5–C7	Descends posterior to C8 and T1 rami and passes distally on external surface of serratus anterior	Serratus anterior
Subclavian	Superior trunk receiving fibers from C5 and C6 and often C4	Descends posterior to clavicle and anterior to brachial plexus and subclavian artery	Subclavius and sternoclavicular joint
Suprascapular	Superior trunk receiving fibers from C5 and C6 and often C4	Passes laterally across posterior triangle of neck, through suprascapular notch deep to superior transverse scapular ligament	Supraspinatus, infraspinatus, and glenohumeral (shoulder) joint
Infraclavicular branches			
Lateral pectoral	Lateral cord receiving fibers from C5–C7	Pierces clavipectoral fascia to reach deep surface of pectoral muscles	Primarily pectoralis major but sends a loop to medial pectoral nerve that innervates pectoralis minor
Musculocutaneous	Lateral cord receiving fibers from C5–C7	Enters deep surface of coracobrachialis and descends between biceps brachii and brachialis	Coracobrachialis, biceps brachii, and brachialis; continues as lateral cutaneous nerve of forearm
Median	Lateral root of median nerve is a terminal branch of lateral cord (C6, C7); medial root of median nerve is a terminal branch of medial cord (C8, T1)	Lateral and medial roots merge to form median nerve lateral to axillary artery; crosses anterior to brachial artery to lie medial to artery in cubital fossa	Flexor muscles in forearm (except flexor carpi ulnaris, ulnar half of flexor digitorum profundus, and five hand muscles) and skin of palm and 3½ digits lateral to a line bisecting 4th digit and the dorsum of the distal halves of these digits
Medial pectoral	Medial cord receiving fibers from C8, T1	Passes between axillary artery and vein and enters deep surface of pectoralis minor	Pectoralis minor and part of pectoralis major
Medial cutaneous nerve of arm	Medial cord receiving fibers from C8, T1	Runs along the medial side of axillary vein and communicates with intercosto-brachial nerve	Skin on medial side of arm
Medial cutaneous nerve of forearm	Medial cord receiving fibers from C8, T1	Runs between axillary artery and vein	Skin over medial side of forearm
Ulnar	A terminal branch of medial cord receiving fibers from C8, T1 and often C7	Passes down medial aspect of arm and runs posterior to medial epicondyle to enter forearm	Innervates 1½ flexor muscles in forearm, most small muscles in hand, and skin of hand medial to a line bisecting 4th digit (ring finger) anteriorly and posteriorly
Upper subscapular	Branch of posterior cord receiving fibers from C5	Passes posteriorly and enters subscapularis	Superior portion of subscapularis
Thoracodorsal	Branch of posterior cord receiving fibers from C6–C8	Arises between upper and lower subscapular nerves and runs inferolaterally to latissimus dorsi	Latissimus dorsi
Lower subscapular	Branch of posterior cord receiving fibers from C6	Passes inferolaterally, deep to subscapular artery and vein, to subscapularis and teres major	Inferior portion of subscapularis and teres major
Axillary	Terminal branch of posterior cord receiving fibers from C5 and C6	Passes to posterior aspect of arm through quadrangular space in company with posterior circumflex humeral artery and then winds around surgical neck of humerus; gives rise to lateral cutaneous nerve of arm	Teres minor and deltoid, glenohumeral (shoulder) joint, and skin of superolateral part of arm
Radial	Terminal branch of posterior cord receiving fibers from C5–T1	Descends posterior to axillary artery; enters radial groove to pass between long and medial heads of triceps	Triceps brachii, anconeus, brachioradialis, and extensor muscles of forearm; supplies skin on posterior aspect of arm and forearm and dorsum of hand lateral to axial line of digit 4

[a] Quadrangular space is bounded superiorly by subscapularis and teres minor, inferiorly by teres major, medially by long head of triceps, and laterally by humerus.

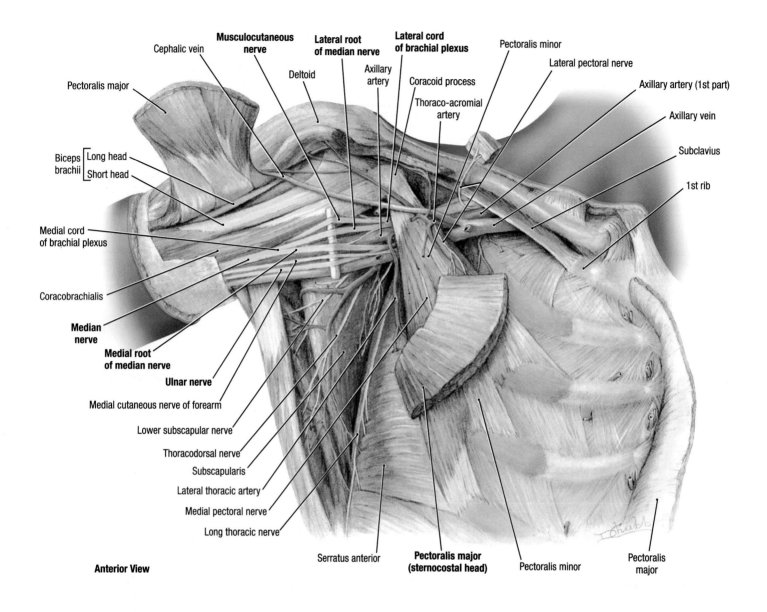

Cephalic vein

Musculocutaneous nerve

Lateral root of median nerve

Lateral cord of brachial plexus

Pectoralis minor

Pectoralis major

Deltoid

Axillary artery

Coracoid process

Lateral pectoral nerve

Axillary artery (1st part)

Thoraco-acromial artery

Axillary vein

Biceps brachii [Long head / Short head]

Subclavius

1st rib

Medial cord of brachial plexus

Coracobrachialis

Median nerve

Medial root of median nerve

Ulnar nerve

Medial cutaneous nerve of forearm

Lower subscapular nerve

Thoracodorsal nerve

Subscapularis

Lateral thoracic artery

Medial pectoral nerve

Long thoracic nerve

Serratus anterior

Pectoralis major (sternocostal head)

Pectoralis minor

Pectoralis major

Anterior View

6.24   Structures of axilla: Deep dissection I

- The pectoralis major muscle is reflected, and the clavipectoral fascia is removed; the cube of muscle superior to the clavicle is cut from the clavicular head of the pectoralis major muscle.
- The subclavius and pectoralis minor are the two deep muscles of the anterior wall.
- The 2nd part axillary artery passes posterior to the pectoralis minor muscle, a finger-breadth from the tip of the coracoid process; the axillary vein lies anterior and then medial to the axillary artery.
- The median nerve, followed proximally, leads by its lateral root to the lateral cord and musculocutaneous nerve and by its medial root to the medial cord and ulnar nerve. These four nerves and the medial cutaneous nerve of the forearm are derived from the anterior division of the brachial plexus and are raised on a stick. The lateral root of the median nerve may occur as several strands.
- The musculocutaneous nerve enters the flexor compartment of the arm by piercing the coracobrachialis muscle.

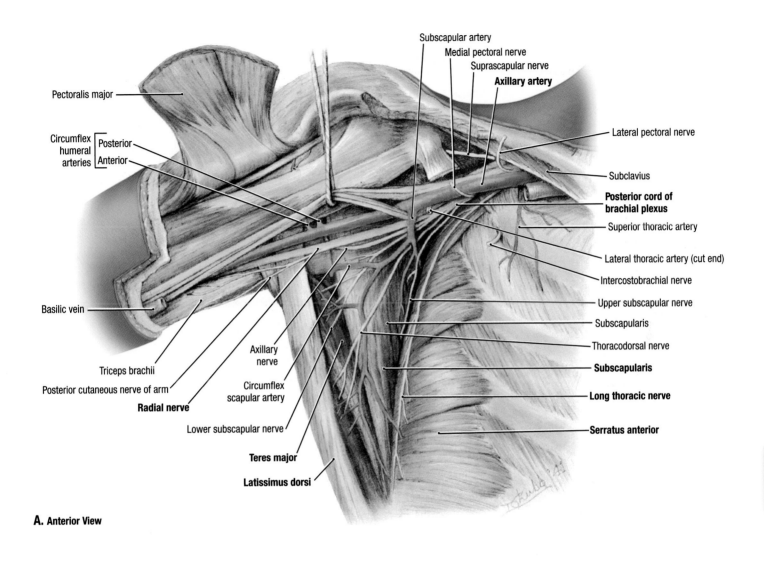

A. Anterior View

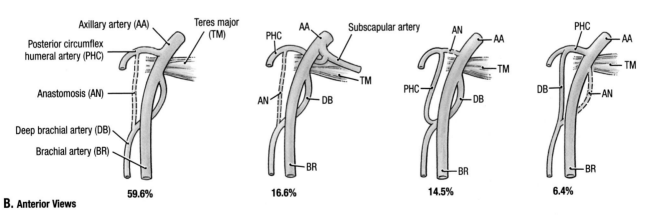

B. Anterior Views

6.25 Posterior and medial walls of axilla: Deep dissection II

A. Dissection. The pectoralis minor muscle is excised, the lateral and medial cords of the brachial plexus are retracted, and the axillary vein is removed. **B.** Variations of the posterior circumflex humeral artery and deep artery of arm. Percentages are based on 235 specimens.

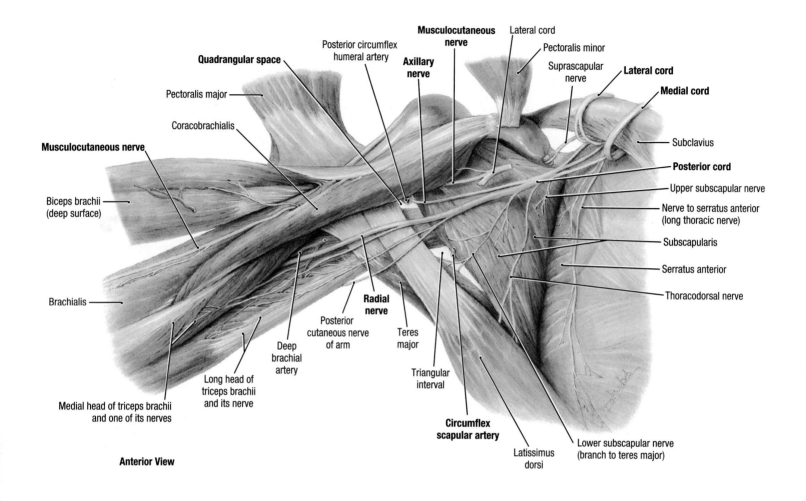

Anterior View

6.26   Posterior wall of axilla, musculocutaneous nerve, and posterior cord: Deep dissection III

- The pectoralis major and minor muscles are reflected laterally, the lateral and medial cords of the brachial plexus are reflected superiorly, and the arteries, veins, and median and ulnar nerves are removed.
- Coracobrachialis arises with the short head of the biceps brachii muscle from the tip of the coracoid process and attaches halfway down the medial aspect of the humerus.
- The musculocutaneous nerve pierces the coracobrachialis muscle and supplies it, the biceps, and the brachialis before becoming the lateral cutaneous nerve of the forearm.
- The posterior cord of the plexus is formed by the union of the three posterior divisions; it supplies the three muscles of the posterior wall of the axilla and then bifurcates into the radial and axillary nerves.
- In the axilla, the radial nerve gives off the nerve to the long head of the triceps brachii muscle and a cutaneous branch; in this specimen, it also gives off a branch to the medial head of the triceps. It then enters the radial groove of the humerus with the deep brachial (profunda brachii) artery.
- The axillary nerve passes through the quadrangular space along with the posterior circumflex humeral artery. The borders of the quadrangular space are superiorly, the lateral border of the scapula; inferiorly, the teres major; laterally, the humerus (surgical neck); and medially, the long head of triceps brachii. The circumflex scapular artery traverses the triangular interval.

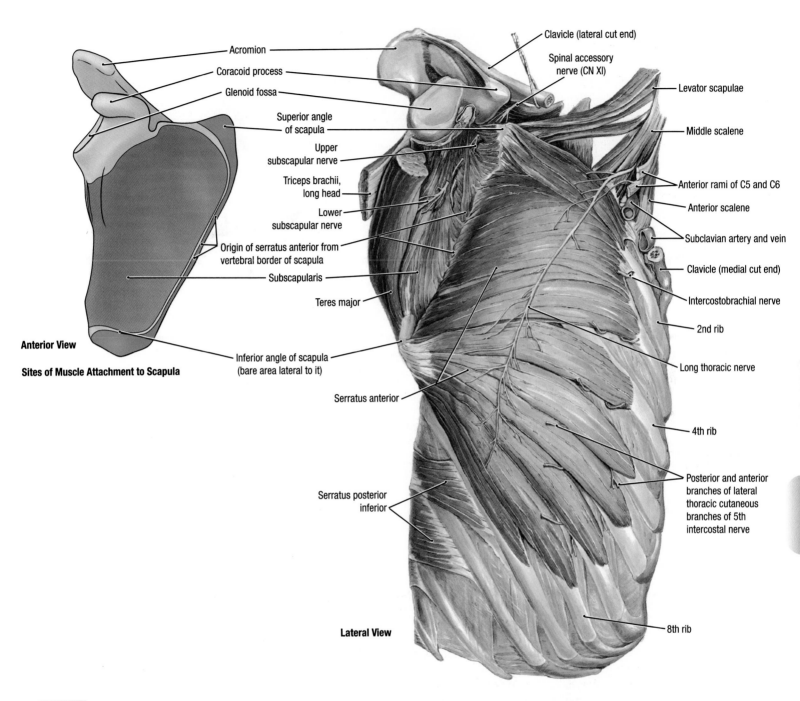

Anterior View

Sites of Muscle Attachment to Scapula

- Acromion
- Coracoid process
- Glenoid fossa
- Superior angle of scapula
- Upper subscapular nerve
- Triceps brachii, long head
- Lower subscapular nerve
- Origin of serratus anterior from vertebral border of scapula
- Subscapularis
- Teres major
- Inferior angle of scapula (bare area lateral to it)
- Serratus anterior
- Serratus posterior inferior

- Clavicle (lateral cut end)
- Spinal accessory nerve (CN XI)
- Levator scapulae
- Middle scalene
- Anterior rami of C5 and C6
- Anterior scalene
- Subclavian artery and vein
- Clavicle (medial cut end)
- Intercostobrachial nerve
- 2nd rib
- Long thoracic nerve
- 4th rib
- Posterior and anterior branches of lateral thoracic cutaneous branches of 5th intercostal nerve
- 8th rib

Lateral View

6.27   **Serratus anterior and subscapularis**

The serratus anterior muscle, which forms the medial wall of the axilla, has a fleshy belly extending from the superior 8 or 9 ribs in the midclavicular line *(right)* to the medial border of the scapula *(left)*.

- The fibers of the serratus anterior muscle from the 1st rib and the tendinous arch between the 1st and 2nd ribs (see Table 6.2) converge on the superior angle of the scapula; those from the 2nd and 3rd ribs diverge to spread thinly along the medial border; and the remainder (from the 4th to 9th ribs), which form the bulk of the muscle, converge on the inferior angle via a tendinous insertion.
- The long thoracic nerve to serratus anterior arises from spinal nerves C5, C6, and C7 and courses externally along most of the muscle's length.

- When the serratus anterior is paralyzed because of injury to the long thoracic nerve, the medial border of the scapula moves laterally and posteriorly, away from the thoracic wall. When the arm is abducted, the medial border and the inferior angle of the scapula pull away from the posterior thoracic wall, a deformation known as a winged scapula. In addition, the arm cannot be abducted above the horizontal position because the serratus anterior is unable to rotate the glenoid cavity superiorly.

- The trunks of the brachial plexus and the subclavian artery emerge between the anterior and middle scalene muscles (scalene triangle); the subclavian vein is separated from the artery by the anterior scalene muscle.

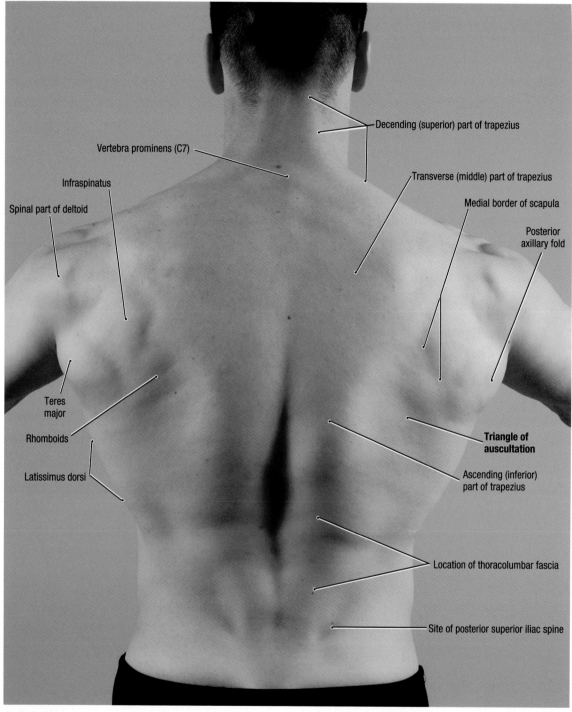

Posterior View

6.28   **Surface anatomy of superficial back**

The superior border of the latissimus dorsi and a part of the rhomboid major are overlapped by the trapezius. The area formed by the superior border of latissimus dorsi, the medial border of the scapula, and the inferolateral border of the trapezius is called the triangle of auscultation. This gap in the thick back muscula- ture is a good place to examine posterior segments of the lungs with a stethoscope. When the scapulae are drawn anteriorly by folding the arms across the thorax and the trunk is flexed, the auscultatory triangle enlarges. The teres major forms a raised oval area on the inferolateral third of the posterior aspect of the scapula when the arm is adducted against resistance. The poste- rior axillary fold is formed by the teres major and the tendon of the latissimus dorsi.

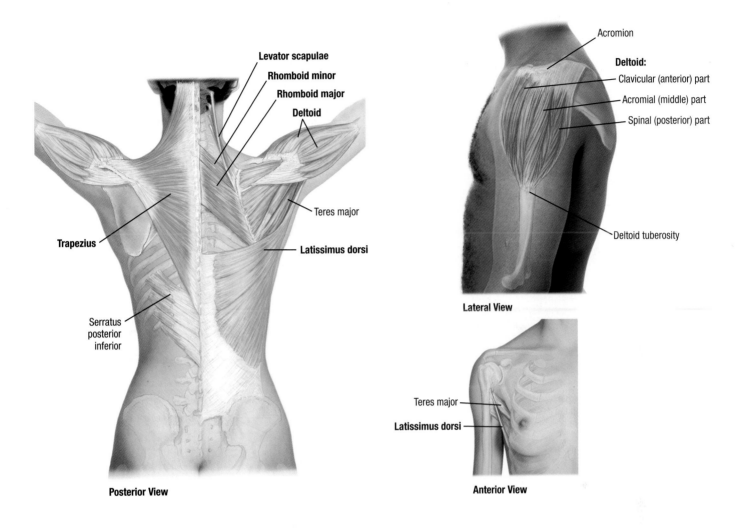

Posterior View

Lateral View

Anterior View

TABLE 6.5 SUPERFICIAL BACK (POSTERIOR AXIOAPPENDICULAR) AND DELTOID MUSCLES

Muscle	Proximal Attachment	Distal Attachment	Innervation	Main Actions
Trapezius	Medial third of superior nuchal line; external occipital protuberance, nuchal ligament, and spinous processes of T7–T12	Lateral third of clavicle, acromion, and spine of scapula	Spinal accessory nerve (CN XI) and cervical nerves (C3–C4)	Elevates, retracts, and rotates scapula; *descending part* elevates, *transverse part* retracts, and *ascending part* depresses scapula; descending and ascending part act together in superior rotation of scapula
Latissimus dorsi	Spinous processes of inferior six thoracic vertebrae, thoracolumbar fascia, iliac crest, and inferior three or four ribs	Intertubercular sulcus (bicipital groove) of humerus	Thoracodorsal nerve (C6–C8)	Extends, adducts, and medially rotates humerus; raises body toward arms during climbing
Levator scapulae	Posterior tubercles of transverse processes of C1–C4 vertebrae	Superior part of medial border of scapula	Dorsal scapular (C5) and cervical (C3–C4) nerves	Elevates scapula and tilts its glenoid cavity inferiorly by rotating scapula
Rhomboid minor and major	*Minor:* nuchal ligament and spinous processes of C7 and T1 vertebrae *Major:* spinous processes of T2–T5 vertebrae	Medial border of scapula from level of spine to inferior angle	Dorsal scapular nerve (C4–C5)	Retracts scapula and rotates it to depress glenoid cavity; fixes scapula to thoracic wall
Deltoid	Lateral third of clavicle (*clavicular part*), acromion (*acromial part*), and spine (*spinal part*) of scapula	Deltoid tuberosity of humerus	Axillary nerve (C5–C6)	*Clavicular (anterior) part:* flexes and medially rotates arm; *acromial (middle) part:* abducts arm; *spinal (posterior) part:* extends and laterally rotates arm

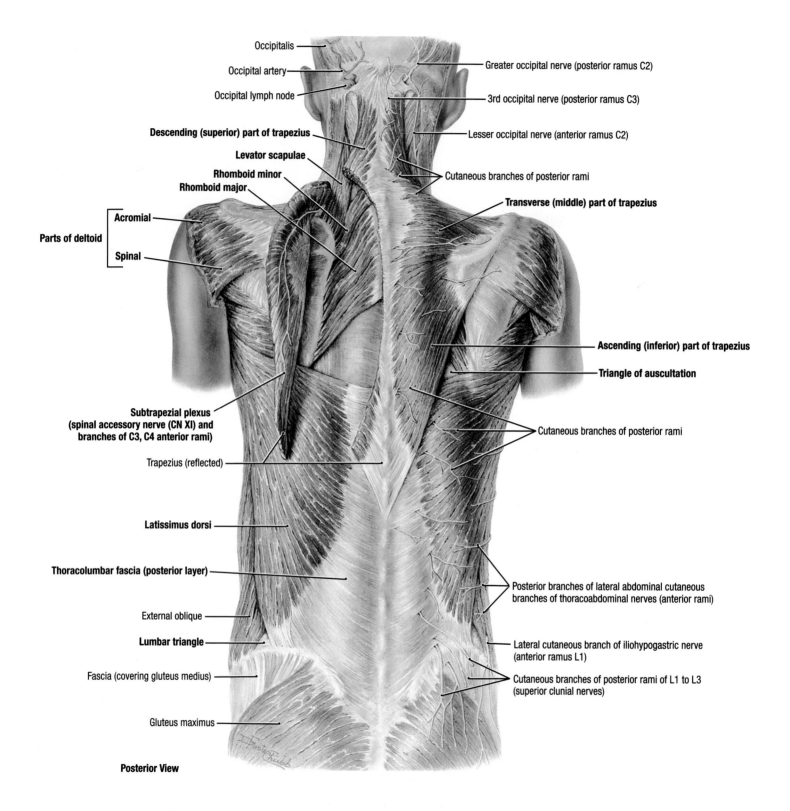

Occipitalis

Occipital artery

Occipital lymph node

Descending (superior) part of trapezius

Levator scapulae

Rhomboid minor

Rhomboid major

Acromial

Parts of deltoid

Spinal

Subtrapezial plexus (spinal accessory nerve (CN XI) and branches of C3, C4 anterior rami)

Trapezius (reflected)

Latissimus dorsi

Thoracolumbar fascia (posterior layer)

External oblique

Lumbar triangle

Fascia (covering gluteus medius)

Gluteus maximus

Posterior View

Greater occipital nerve (posterior ramus C2)

3rd occipital nerve (posterior ramus C3)

Lesser occipital nerve (anterior ramus C2)

Cutaneous branches of posterior rami

Transverse (middle) part of trapezius

Ascending (inferior) part of trapezius

Triangle of auscultation

Cutaneous branches of posterior rami

Posterior branches of lateral abdominal cutaneous branches of thoracoabdominal nerves (anterior rami)

Lateral cutaneous branch of iliohypogastric nerve (anterior ramus L1)

Cutaneous branches of posterior rami of L1 to L3 (superior clunial nerves)

6.29   **Cutaneous nerves of superficial back and posterior axioapendicular muscles**

The trapezius muscle is cut and reflected on the left side. A superficial or first muscle layer consists of the trapezius and latissimus dorsi muscles, and a second layer of the levator scapulae and rhomboids. Cutaneous branches of posterior rami penetrate but do not supply the superficial muscles.

TABLE 6.6 MOVEMENTS OF SCAPULA

Boldface indicates prime movers. In the *middle* and *right columns* the *dotted outlines* represent the starting position for each movement.

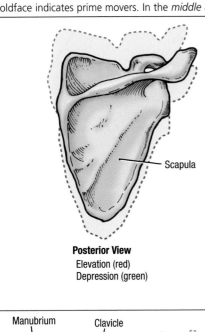

Posterior View
Elevation (red)
Depression (green)

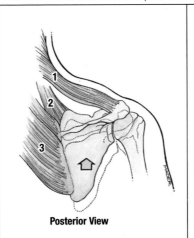

Posterior View

Elevation:
Trapezius, superior part (1)
Levator scapulae (2)
Rhomboids (3)

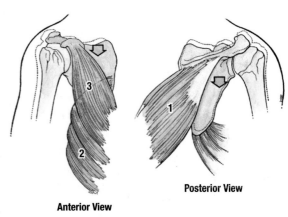

Anterior View   **Posterior View**

Depression:
Trapezius, inferior part (1)
Serratus anterior, inferior part
Pectoralis minor

Also: Gravity, Latissimus dorsi,
Inferior sternocostal head of
pectoralis major

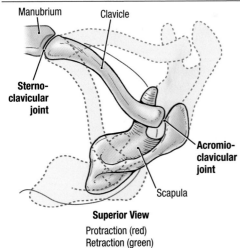

Superior View
Protraction (red)
Retraction (green)

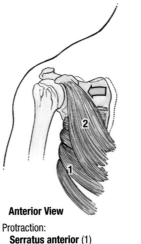

Anterior View

Protraction:
Serratus anterior (1)
Pectoralis minor (2)
Also: Pectoralis major

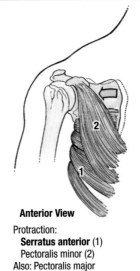

Posterior View

Retraction:
Trapezius, middle part (1)
Rhomboids(2)
Latissimus dorsi (3)

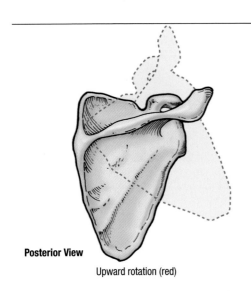

Posterior View

Upward rotation (red)

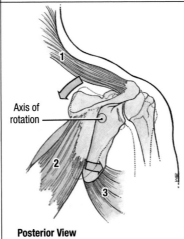

Posterior View

Upward rotation
Trapezius, superior part (1)
Trapezius, inferior part (2)
Serratus anterior, inferior part(3)

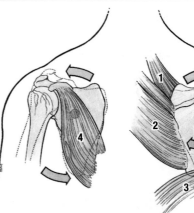

Anterior View   **Posterior View**

Downward rotation
Levator scapulae (1)
Rhomboids (2)
Latissimus dorsi (3)
Pectoralis minor (4)

Also: Gravity, Inferior sternocostal
head of pectoralis major

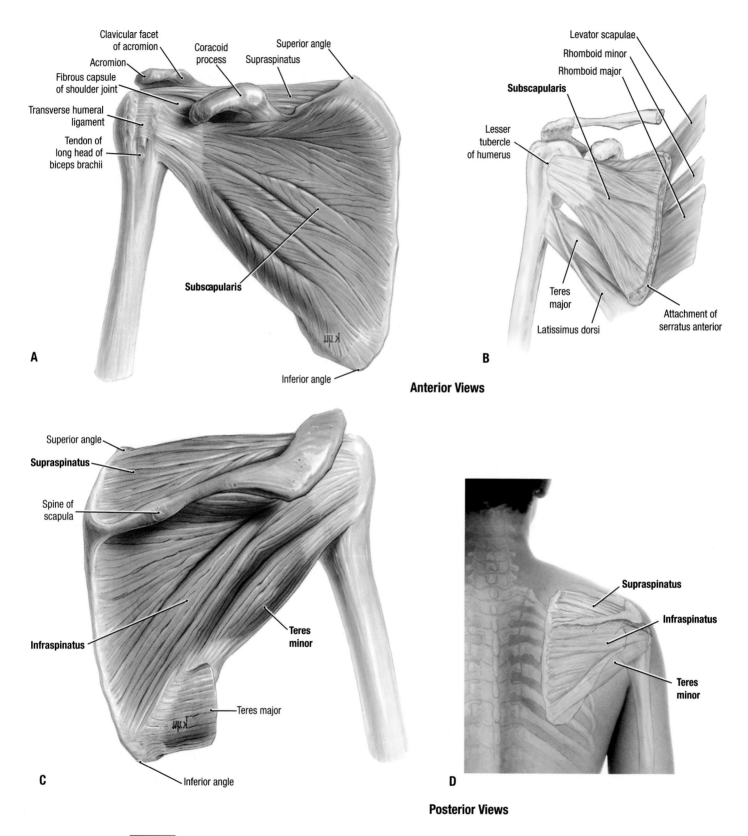

Anterior Views

Posterior Views

6.30 Rotator cuff

A and **B.** Subscapularis. **C** and **D.** Supraspinatus, infraspinatus, and teres minor.

Four of the scapulohumeral muscles—supraspinatus, infraspinatus, teres minor, and subscapularis—are called rotator cuff muscles because they form a musculotendinous rotator cuff around the glenohumeral joint. All except the supraspinatus are rotators of the humerus.

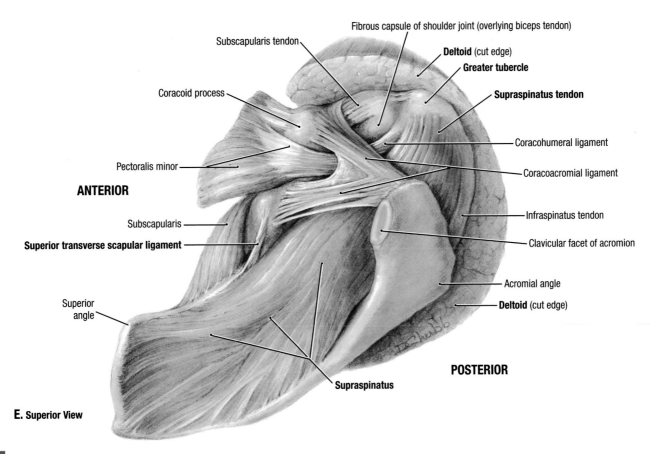

E. Superior View

6.30   Rotator cuff (continued)

E. Supraspinatus and supraspinatus tendon.

The supraspinatus, besides being part of the rotator cuff, initiates and assists the deltoid in the first 15° of abduction of the arm. The tendons of the rotator cuff muscles blend with the joint capsule of the glenohumeral joint, reinforcing it as the musculotendinous rotator cuff, which protects the joint and gives it stability.

Injury or disease may damage the rotator cuff, producing instability of the glenohumeral joint. Rupture or tear of the supraspinatus tendon is the most common injury of the rotator cuff. Degenerative tendinitis of the rotator cuff is common, especially in older people.

TABLE 6.7 DEEP SCAPULOHUMERAL/SHOULDER MUSCLES

Muscle	Proximal Attachment	Distal Attachment	Innervation	Main Actions
Supraspinatus (S)	Supraspinous fossa of scapula	Superior facet on greater tubercle of humerus	Suprascapular nerve (C4, C5, and C6)	Helps deltoid to abduct arm and acts with rotator cuff muscles[a]
Infraspinatus (I)	Infraspinous fossa of scapula	Middle facet on greater tubercle of humerus	Suprascapular nerve (C5 and C6)	Laterally rotates arm; helps to hold humeral head in glenoid cavity of scapula
Teres minor (T)	Superior part of lateral border of scapula	Inferior facet on greater tubercle of humerus	Axillary nerve (C5 and C6)	
Subscapularis(S)	Subscapular fossa	Lesser tubercle of humerus	Upper and lower subscapular nerves (C5, C6, and C7)	Medially rotates arm and adducts it; helps to hold humeral head in glenoid cavity
Teres major[b]	Posterior surface of inferior angle of scapula	Crest of lesser tubercle (medial lip) of humerus	Lower subscapular nerve (C6 and C7)	Adducts and medially rotates arm

[a]Collectively, the supraspinatus, infraspinatus, teres minor, and subscapularis muscles are referred to as the rotator cuff muscles or "SITS" muscles. They function together during all movements of the shoulder joint to hold the head of the humerus in the glenoid cavity of scapula.
[b]Not a rotator cuff muscle.

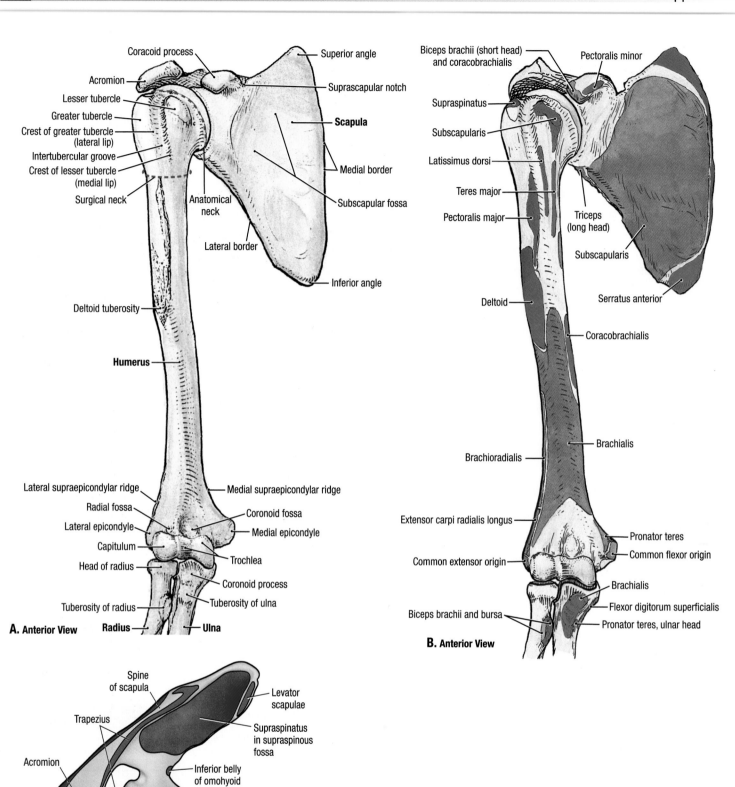

A. Anterior View

Coracoid process
Acromion
Lesser tubercle
Greater tubercle
Crest of greater tubercle (lateral lip)
Intertubercular groove
Crest of lesser tubercle (medial lip)
Surgical neck
Deltoid tuberosity
Humerus
Lateral supraepicondylar ridge
Radial fossa
Lateral epicondyle
Capitulum
Head of radius
Tuberosity of radius
Radius
Ulna
Superior angle
Suprascapular notch
Scapula
Medial border
Subscapular fossa
Anatomical neck
Lateral border
Inferior angle
Medial supraepicondylar ridge
Coronoid fossa
Medial epicondyle
Trochlea
Coronoid process
Tuberosity of ulna

B. Anterior View

Biceps brachii (short head) and coracobrachialis
Supraspinatus
Subscapularis
Latissimus dorsi
Teres major
Pectoralis major
Deltoid
Brachioradialis
Extensor carpi radialis longus
Common extensor origin
Biceps brachii and bursa
Pectoralis minor
Subscapularis
Serratus anterior
Coracobrachialis
Brachialis
Pronator teres
Common flexor origin
Brachialis
Flexor digitorum superficialis
Pronator teres, ulnar head
Triceps (long head)

C. Superior View

Spine of scapula
Trapezius
Acromion
Deltoid
Coracobrachialis and short head of biceps brachii
Coracoid process
Levator scapulae
Supraspinatus in supraspinous fossa
Inferior belly of omohyoid
Scapula
Clavicle
Sternocleidomastoid (SCM)
Pectoralis major

6.31 Bones of proximal upper limb

A. Bony features, anterior aspect. **B.** Muscle attachment sites, anterior aspect. **C.** Muscle attachment sites, clavicle and scapula.

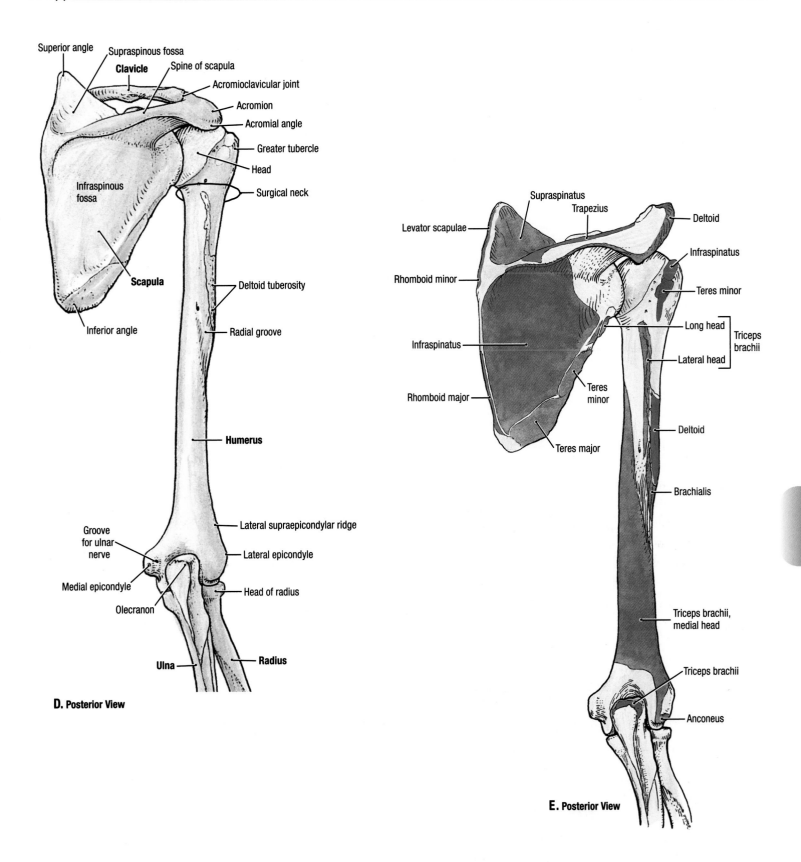

Superior angle
Suprraspinous fossa
Clavicle
Spine of scapula
Acromioclavicular joint
Acromion
Acromial angle
Greater tubercle
Head
Surgical neck
Infraspinous fossa
Scapula
Deltoid tuberosity
Inferior angle
Radial groove
Humerus
Lateral supraepicondylar ridge
Groove for ulnar nerve
Lateral epicondyle
Medial epicondyle
Head of radius
Olecranon
Ulna
Radius

D. Posterior View

Levator scapulae
Supraspinatus
Trapezius
Deltoid
Rhomboid minor
Infraspinatus
Teres minor
Infraspinatus
Long head
Lateral head
} Triceps brachii
Rhomboid major
Teres minor
Teres major
Deltoid
Brachialis
Triceps brachii, medial head
Triceps brachii
Anconeus

E. Posterior View

6.31   **Bones of proximal upper limb (continued)**

D. Bony features, posterior aspect. **E.** Muscle attachment sites, posterior aspect.

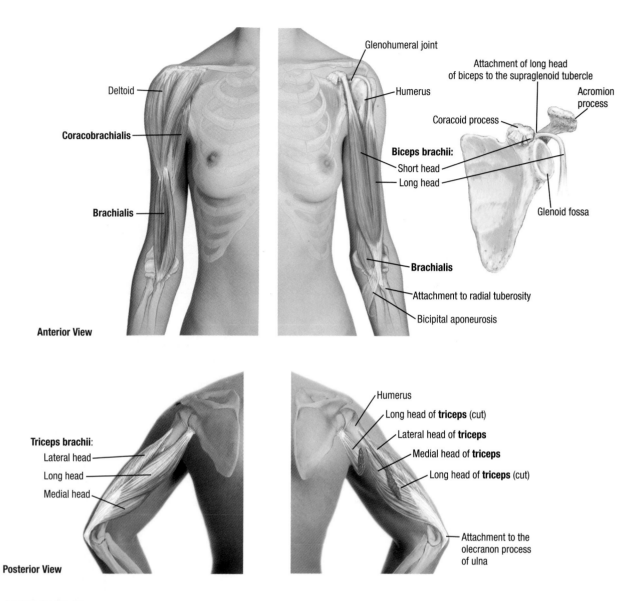

Anterior View

Posterior View

TABLE 6.8 ARM MUSCLES

Muscle	Proximal Attachment	Distal Attachment	Innervation	Main Actions
Biceps brachii	*Short head:* tip of coracoid process of scapula *Long head:* supraglenoid tubercle of scapula	Tuberosity of radius and fascia of forearm through bicipital aponeurosis	Musculocutaneous nerve (C5–C6)	Supinates forearm and, when forearm is supine, flexes forearm
Brachialis	Distal half of anterior surface of humerus	Coronoid process and tuberosity of ulna		Flexes forearm in all positions
Coracobrachialis	Tip of coracoid process of scapula	Middle third of medial surface of humerus	Musculocutaneous nerve (C5–C7)	Assists with flexion and adduction of arm
Triceps brachii	*Long head:* infraglenoid tubercle of scapula *Lateral head:* posterior surface of humerus, superior to radial groove *Medial head:* posterior surface of humerus, inferior to radial groove	Proximal end of olecranon of ulna and fascia of forearm	Radial nerve (C6–C8)	Extends the forearm; long head steadies head of abducted humerus
Anconeus	Lateral epicondyle of humerus	Lateral surface of olecranon and superior part of posterior surface of ulna	Radial nerve (C7–T1)	Assists triceps in extending forearm; stabilizes elbow joint; abducts ulna during pronation

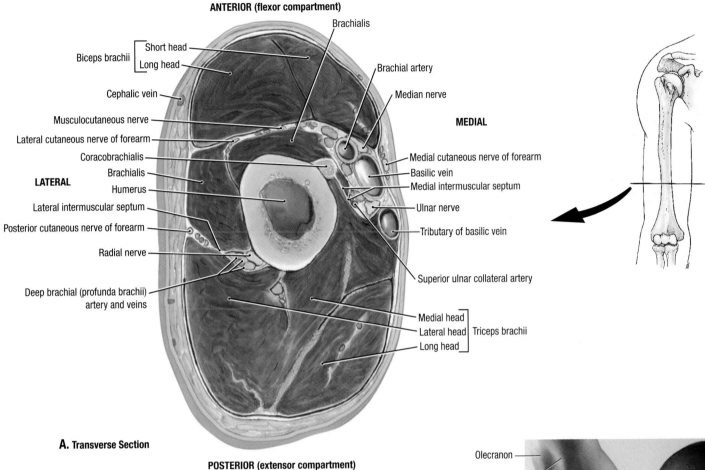

ANTERIOR (flexor compartment)

Biceps brachii
- Short head
- Long head

Brachialis

Brachial artery

Median nerve

Cephalic vein

Musculocutaneous nerve

Lateral cutaneous nerve of forearm

MEDIAL

Coracobrachialis

LATERAL

Brachialis

Humerus

Lateral intermuscular septum

Posterior cutaneous nerve of forearm

Radial nerve

Deep brachial (profunda brachii) artery and veins

Medial cutaneous nerve of forearm

Basilic vein

Medial intermuscular septum

Ulnar nerve

Tributary of basilic vein

Superior ulnar collateral artery

Medial head
Lateral head — Triceps brachii
Long head

A. Transverse Section

POSTERIOR (extensor compartment)

6.32 Anterior and posterior compartments of arm

A. Anatomical section. **B.** Surface anatomy.

- Three muscles, the biceps, brachialis, and coracobrachialis, lie in the anterior compartment of the arm; the triceps brachii lies in the posterior compartment.
- The medial and lateral intermuscular septum separates these two muscle groups.
- The radial nerve and deep brachial artery and veins serving the posterior compartment lie in contact with the radial groove of the humerus.
- The musculocutaneous nerve serving the anterior compartment lies in the plane between the biceps and the brachialis muscles.
- The median nerve crosses to the medial side of the brachial artery.
- The ulnar nerve passes posteriorly onto the medial side of the triceps muscle.
- The basilic vein (appearing here as two vessels) has pierced the deep fascia.

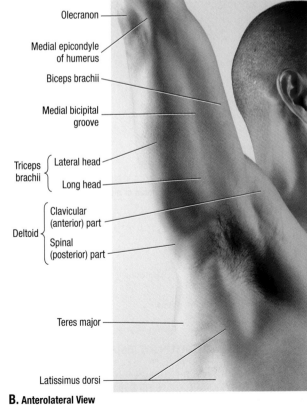

Olecranon

Medial epicondyle of humerus

Biceps brachii

Medial bicipital groove

Triceps brachii
- Lateral head
- Long head

Deltoid
- Clavicular (anterior) part
- Spinal (posterior) part

Teres major

Latissimus dorsi

B. Anterolateral View

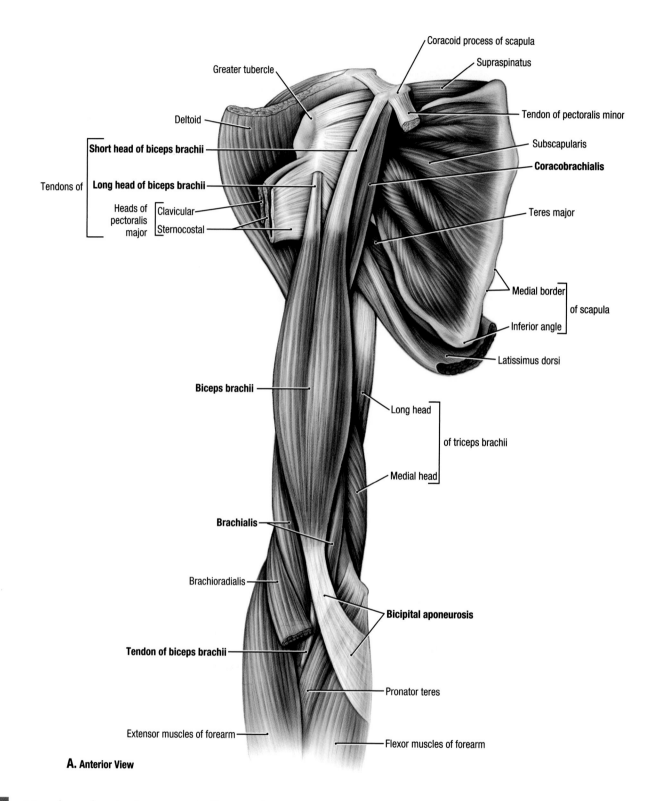

Coracoid process of scapula

Greater tubercle

Supraspinatus

Deltoid

Tendon of pectoralis minor

Short head of biceps brachii

Subscapularis

Coracobrachialis

Tendons of | **Long head of biceps brachii**

Heads of pectoralis major { Clavicular / Sternocostal }

Teres major

Medial border | of scapula

Inferior angle

Latissimus dorsi

Biceps brachii

Long head | of triceps brachii

Medial head

Brachialis

Brachioradialis

Bicipital aponeurosis

Tendon of biceps brachii

Pronator teres

Extensor muscles of forearm

Flexor muscles of forearm

A. Anterior View

6.33   **Muscles of anterior aspect of arm—I**

- The biceps brachii has two heads: a long head and a short head.
- However, when the elbow is flexed approximately 90° the biceps is a flexor from the supinated position of the forearm but a very powerful supinator from the pronated position.

- A triangular membranous band, the bicipital aponeurosis runs from the biceps tendon across the cubital fossa and merges with the antebrachial (deep) fascia covering the flexor muscles on the medial side of the forearm.

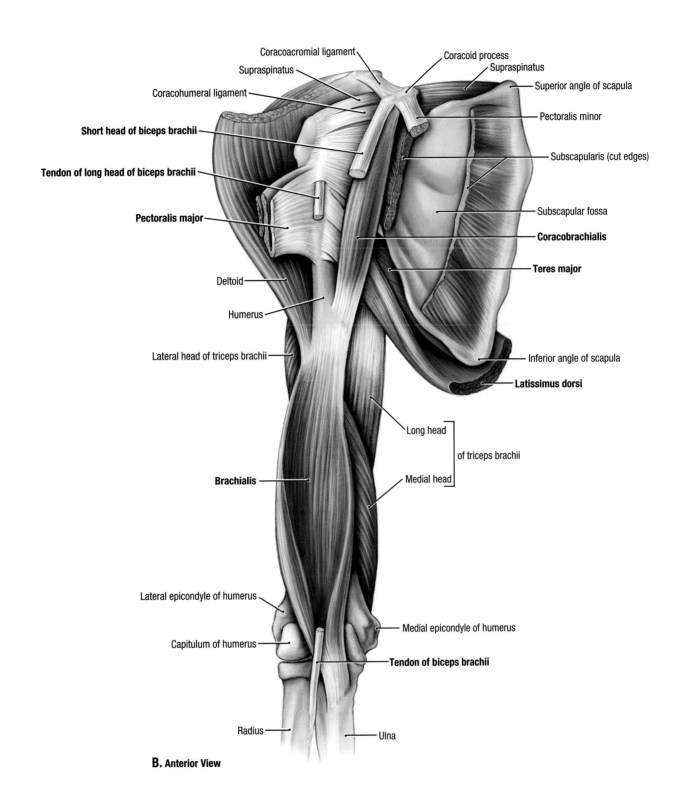

Coracoacromial ligament

Coracoid process

Supraspinatus

Supraspinatus

Superior angle of scapula

Coracohumeral ligament

Pectoralis minor

Short head of biceps brachii

Tendon of long head of biceps brachii

Subscapularis (cut edges)

Pectoralis major

Subscapular fossa

Coracobrachialis

Deltoid

Teres major

Humerus

Lateral head of triceps brachii

Inferior angle of scapula

Latissimus dorsi

Long head

of triceps brachii

Medial head

Brachialis

Lateral epicondyle of humerus

Medial epicondyle of humerus

Capitulum of humerus

Tendon of biceps brachii

Radius

Ulna

B. Anterior View

6.33 Muscles of anterior aspect of arm—II

- The **brachialis**, a flattened fusiform muscle, lies posterior (deep) to the biceps that produce the greatest amount of flexion force.
- The **coracobrachialis**, an elongated muscle in the superomedial part of the arm, is pierced by the musculocutaneous nerve. It helps flex and adduct the arm.

Rupture of the tendon of the long head of the biceps usually results from wear and tear of an inflamed tendon (*biceps tendinitis*). Normally, the tendon is torn from its attachment to the supraglenoid tubercle of the scapula. The detached muscle belly forms a ball near the center of the distal part of the anterior aspect of the arm.

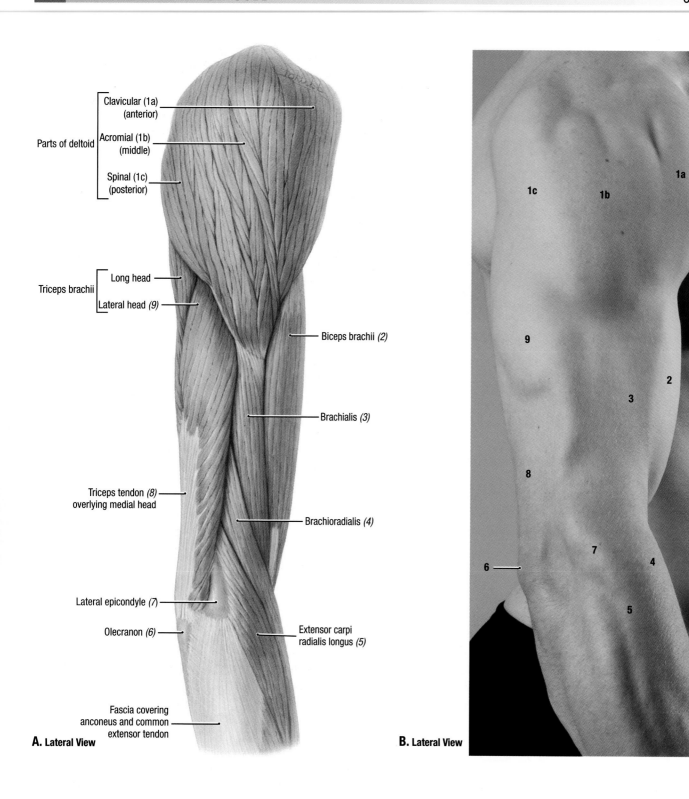

Parts of deltoid
Clavicular (1a) (anterior)
Acromial (1b) (middle)
Spinal (1c) (posterior)

Triceps brachii
Long head
Lateral head (9)

Biceps brachii (2)

Brachialis (3)

Triceps tendon (8) overlying medial head

Brachioradialis (4)

Lateral epicondyle (7)

Olecranon (6)

Extensor carpi radialis longus (5)

Fascia covering anconeus and common extensor tendon

A. Lateral View

B. Lateral View

6.34   Lateral aspect of arm

A. Dissection (*numbers* in parentheses refer to structures in **B**). **B.** Surface anatomy.

Atrophy of the deltoid occurs when the axillary nerve (C5 and C6) is severely damaged (e.g., as might occur when the surgical neck of the humerus is fractured). As the deltoid atrophies, the rounded contour of the shoulder disappears. This gives the shoulder a flattened appearance and produces a slight hollow inferior to the acromion. A loss of sensation may occur over the lateral side of the proximal part of the arm, the area supplied by the superior lateral cutaneous nerve of the arm. To test the deltoid (or the function of the axillary nerve) the arm is abducted, against resistance, starting from approximately 15°. Supraspinatus initiates abduction.

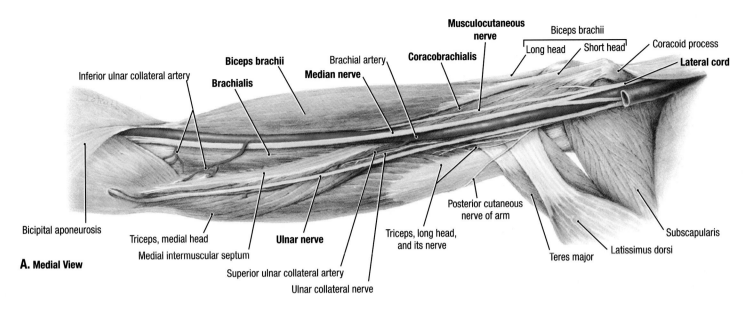

A. Medial View

Labels (clockwise from upper left): Inferior ulnar collateral artery, **Biceps brachii**, **Brachialis**, Brachial artery, **Median nerve**, **Coracobrachialis**, **Musculocutaneous nerve**, Biceps brachii, Long head, Short head, Coracoid process, **Lateral cord**, Subscapularis, Latissimus dorsi, Teres major, Posterior cutaneous nerve of arm, Triceps, long head, and its nerve, Ulnar collateral nerve, Superior ulnar collateral artery, **Ulnar nerve**, Medial intermuscular septum, Triceps, medial head, Bicipital aponeurosis

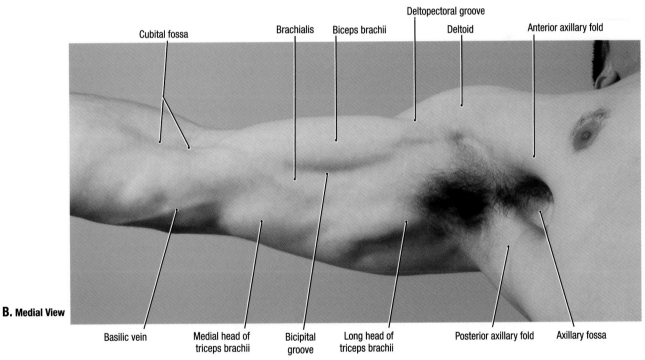

B. Medial View

Labels: Cubital fossa, Brachialis, Biceps brachii, Deltopectoral groove, Deltoid, Anterior axillary fold, Basilic vein, Medial head of triceps brachii, Bicipital groove, Long head of triceps brachii, Posterior axillary fold, Axillary fossa

6.35   Medial aspect of arm

A. Dissection. **B.** Surface anatomy.

- The axillary artery passes just inferior to the tip of the coracoid process and courses posterior to the coracobrachialis. At the inferior border of the teres major, the axillary artery changes names to become the brachial artery and continues distally on the anterior aspect of the brachialis.

- Although collateral pathways confer some protection against gradual temporary and partial occlusion, sudden complete occlusion or laceration of the brachial artery creates a surgical emergency because paralysis of muscles results from ischemia within a few hours.

- The median nerve lies adjacent to the axillary and brachial arteries and then crosses the artery from lateral to medial.
- Proximally, the ulnar nerve is adjacent to the medial side of the artery, passes posterior to the medial intermuscular septum, and descends on the medial head of triceps to pass posterior to the medial epicondyle; here, the ulnar nerve is palpable.
- The superior ulnar collateral artery and ulnar collateral branch of the radial nerve (to medial head of the triceps) accompany the ulnar nerve in the arm.

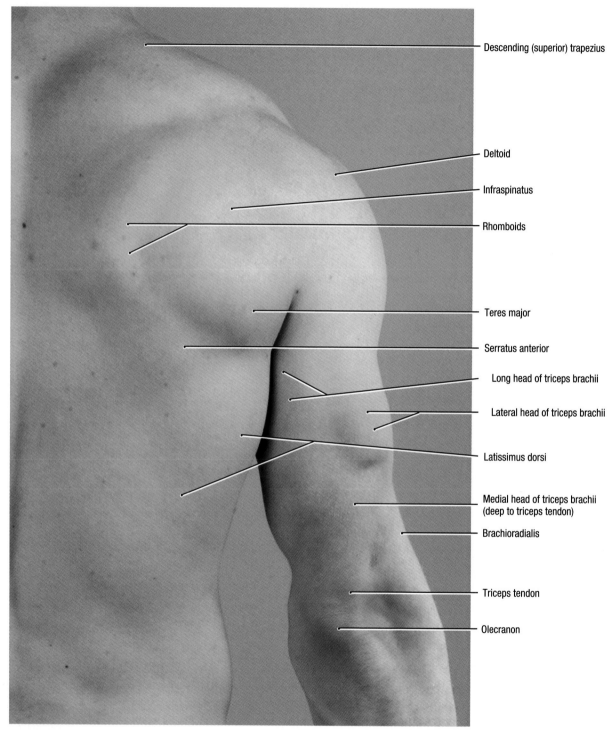

Descending (superior) trapezius

Deltoid

Infraspinatus

Rhomboids

Teres major

Serratus anterior

Long head of triceps brachii

Lateral head of triceps brachii

Latissimus dorsi

Medial head of triceps brachii
(deep to triceps tendon)

Brachioradialis

Triceps tendon

Olecranon

Posterior View

6.36 **Surface anatomy of the scapular region and posterior aspect of arm**

The three heads of the triceps form a bulge on the posterior aspect of the arm and are identifiable when the forearm is extended from the flexed position against resistance.

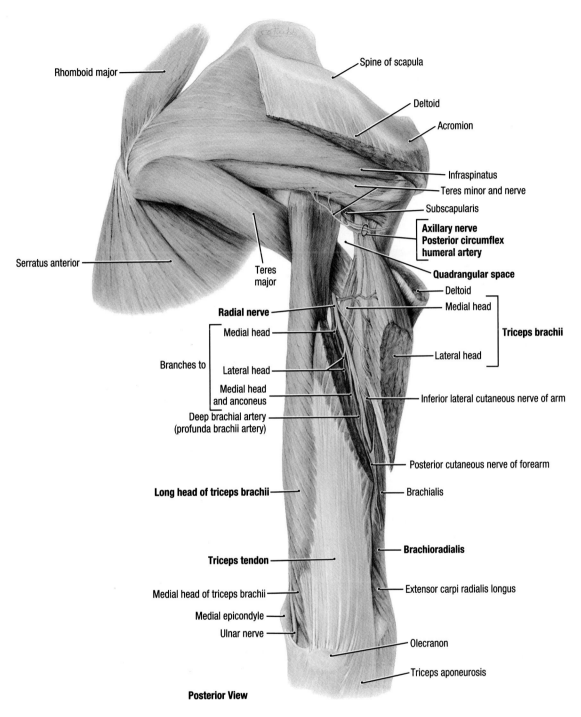

Posterior View

Labels:
Rhomboid major
Spine of scapula
Deltoid
Acromion
Infraspinatus
Teres minor and nerve
Subscapularis
Axillary nerve
Posterior circumflex humeral artery
Quadrangular space
Deltoid
Medial head
Triceps brachii
Lateral head
Serratus anterior
Teres major
Radial nerve
Medial head
Branches to
Lateral head
Medial head and anconeus
Inferior lateral cutaneous nerve of arm
Deep brachial artery (profunda brachii artery)
Posterior cutaneous nerve of forearm
Long head of triceps brachii
Brachialis
Brachioradialis
Triceps tendon
Extensor carpi radialis longus
Medial head of triceps brachii
Medial epicondyle
Ulnar nerve
Olecranon
Triceps aponeurosis

6.37   Triceps brachii and related nerves

- The lateral head is reflected laterally, and the medial head is attached to the deep surface of the triceps tendon, which attaches to the olecranon.
- The radial nerve and deep brachial artery pass between the proximal attachments of the long and medial heads of the triceps brachii in the middle third of the arm, directly contacting the radial groove of the humerus.
- The middle third of the arm is a common site for fractures of the humerus, often with associated radial nerve trauma. When the radial nerve is injured in the radial groove, the triceps brachii muscle typically is only weakened because only the medial head is affected. However, the muscles in the posterior compartment of the forearm, supplied by more distal branches of the radial nerve, are paralyzed. The characteristic clinical sign of radial nerve injury is wrist drop (inability to extend the wrist and fingers at the metacarpophalangeal joints).
- The axillary nerve passes through the quadrangular space along with the posterior humeral circumflex artery.
- The ulnar nerve follows the medial border of the triceps then passes posterior to the medial epicondyle.

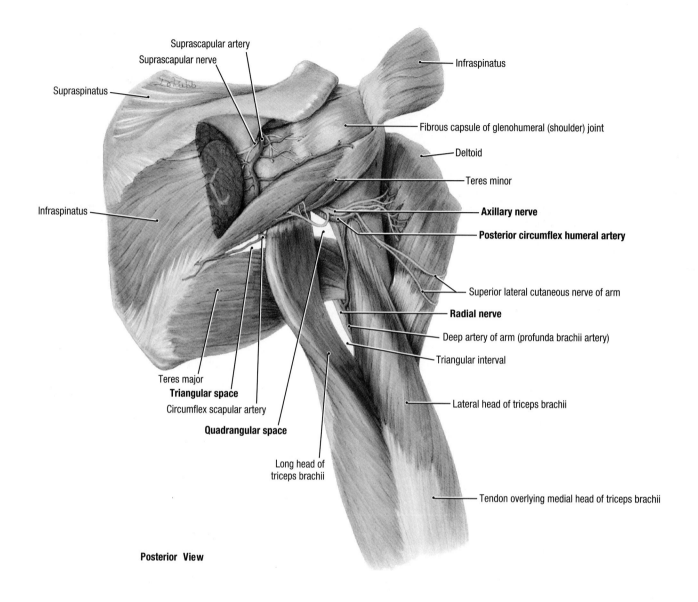

Suprascapular artery
Suprascapular nerve
Supraspinatus
Infraspinatus
Infraspinatus
Teres major
Triangular space
Circumflex scapular artery
Quadrangular space
Long head of triceps brachii

Infraspinatus
Fibrous capsule of glenohumeral (shoulder) joint
Deltoid
Teres minor
Axillary nerve
Posterior circumflex humeral artery
Superior lateral cutaneous nerve of arm
Radial nerve
Deep artery of arm (profunda brachii artery)
Triangular interval
Lateral head of triceps brachii
Tendon overlying medial head of triceps brachii

Posterior View

6.38   Dorsal scapular and subdeltoid regions

- The infraspinatus muscle, aided by the teres minor and spinal (posterior) fibers of the deltoid muscle, rotates the humerus laterally.
- The long head of the triceps muscle passes between the teres minor (a lateral rotator) and teres major (a medial rotator) muscles.
- The long head of the triceps muscle separates the quadrangular space from the triangular space.
- Regarding the distribution of the suprascapular and axillary nerves, each comes from C5 and C6; each supplies two muscles—the suprascapular nerve innervates the supraspinatus and infraspinatus, and the axillary nerve innervates the teres minor and deltoid muscles. Both nerves supply the shoulder joint, but only the axillary nerve has a cutaneous branch.

- The axillary nerve may be injured when the glenohumeral joint dislocates because of its close relation to the inferior part of the joint capsule of this joint. The subglenoid displacement of the head of the humerus into the quadrangular space damages the axillary nerve. Axillary nerve injury is indicated by paralysis of the deltoid.

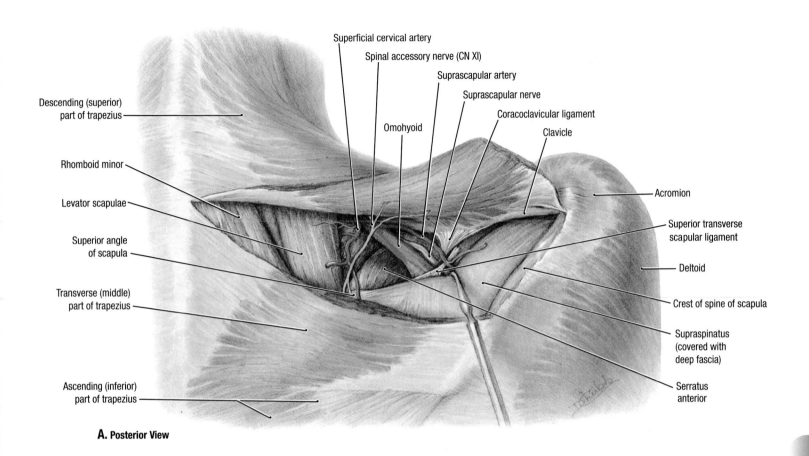

A. Posterior View

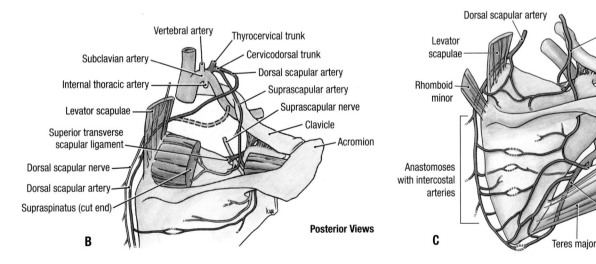

Posterior Views

B

C

6.39 **Suprascapular region**

A. Dissection. At the level of the superior angle of the scapula, the transverse part of the trapezius muscle is reflected. **B.** Suprascapular and dorsal scapular arteries. **C.** Scapular anastomosis.

Several arteries join to form anastomoses on the anterior and posterior surfaces of the scapula. The importance of the collateral circulation made possible by these anastomoses becomes apparent when ligation of a lacerated subclavian or axillary artery is necessary or there is occlusion of these vessels. The direction of blood flow in the subscapular artery is then reversed, enabling blood to reach the third part of the axillary artery. In contrast to a sudden occlusion, slow occlusion of an artery often enables sufficient lateral circulation to develop, preventing ischemia (deficiency of blood).

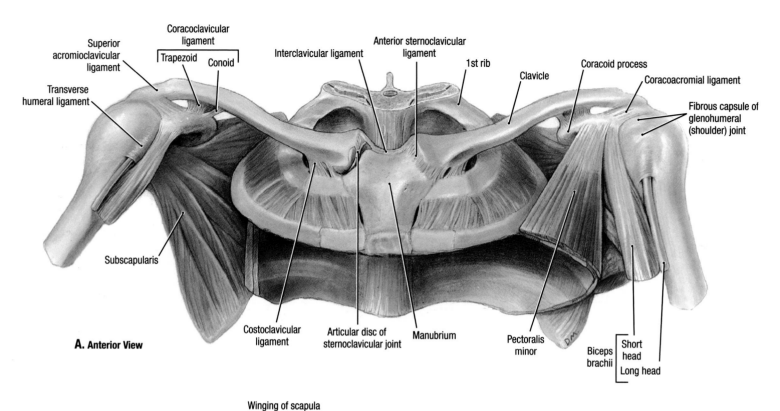

A. Anterior View

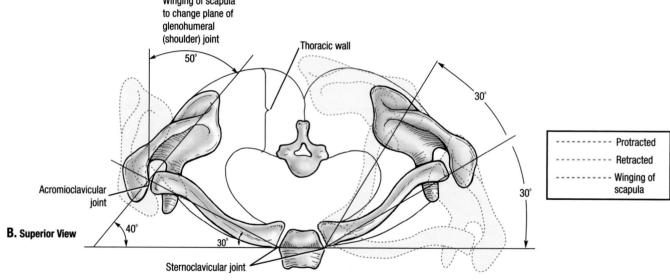

B. Superior View

6.40 Pectoral girdle

A. Dissection. **B.** Clavicular movements at the sternoclavicular and acromioclavicular joints during rotation, protraction, and retraction of the scapula on the thoracic wall *(left side)* and winging of the scapula *(right side)*.
- The shoulder region includes the sternoclavicular, acromioclavicular, and shoulder (glenohumeral) joints; the mobility of the clavicle is essential to the movement of the upper limb.
- The sternoclavicular joint is the only joint connecting the upper limb (appendicular skeleton) to the trunk (axial skeleton). The articular disc of the sternoclavicular joint divides the

joint cavity into two parts and attaches superiorly to the clavicle and inferiorly to the first costal cartilage; the disc resists superior and medial displacement of the clavicle.

In **B**, note that when the serratus anterior is paralyzed because of injury to the long thoracic nerve, the medial border of the scapula moves laterally and posteriorly away from the thoracic wall, giving the scapula the appearance of a wing. The arm cannot be abducted beyond the horizontal position because the serratus anterior cannot rotate the glenoid cavity superiorly to allow complete abduction of the arm.

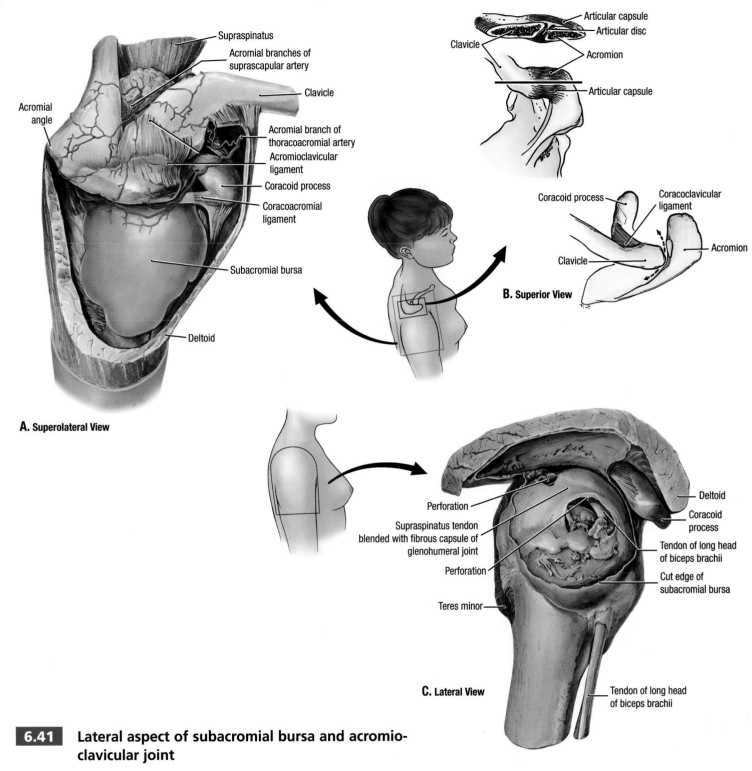

A. Superolateral View

- Supraspinatus
- Acromial branches of suprascapular artery
- Acromial angle
- Clavicle
- Acromial branch of thoracoacromial artery
- Acromioclavicular ligament
- Coracoid process
- Coracoacromial ligament
- Subacromial bursa
- Deltoid

B. Superior View

- Articular capsule
- Articular disc
- Clavicle
- Acromion
- Articular capsule
- Coracoid process
- Coracoclavicular ligament
- Clavicle
- Acromion

C. Lateral View

- Perforation
- Supraspinatus tendon blended with fibrous capsule of glenohumeral joint
- Perforation
- Teres minor
- Deltoid
- Coracoid process
- Tendon of long head of biceps brachii
- Cut edge of subacromial bursa
- Tendon of long head of biceps brachii

6.41   Lateral aspect of subacromial bursa and acromio-clavicular joint

A. Subacromial bursa. The bursa has been injected with purple latex. **B.** Acromioclavicular joint. **C.** Attrition of supraspinatus tendon. As a result of wearing away of the supraspinatus tendon and underlying capsule, the subacromial bursa and shoulder joint come into communication. The intracapsular part of the tendon of the long head of biceps muscle becomes frayed, leaving it adherent to the intertubercular groove. Of 95 dissecting room subjects, none of the 18 younger than 50 years of age had a perforation, but 4 of the 19 who were 50 to 60 years and 23 of the 57 older than 60 years had perforations. The perforation was bilateral in 11 subjects and unilateral in 14.

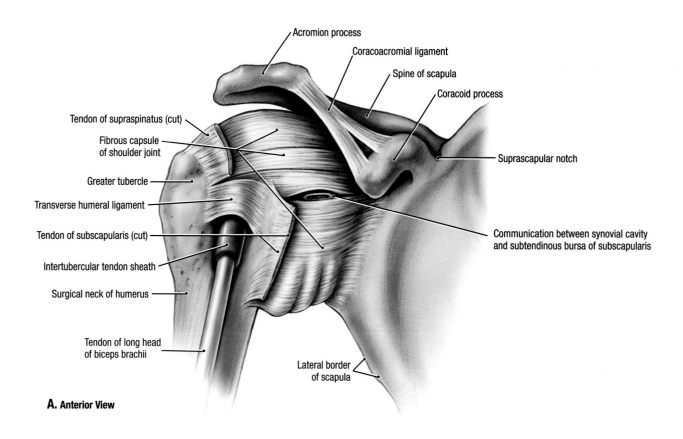

Acromion process
Coracoacromial ligament
Spine of scapula
Coracoid process

Tendon of supraspinatus (cut)

Fibrous capsule
of shoulder joint

Greater tubercle

Transverse humeral ligament

Tendon of subscapularis (cut)

Intertubercular tendon sheath

Surgical neck of humerus

Suprascapular notch

Communication between synovial cavity
and subtendinous bursa of subscapularis

Tendon of long head
of biceps brachii

Lateral border
of scapula

A. Anterior View

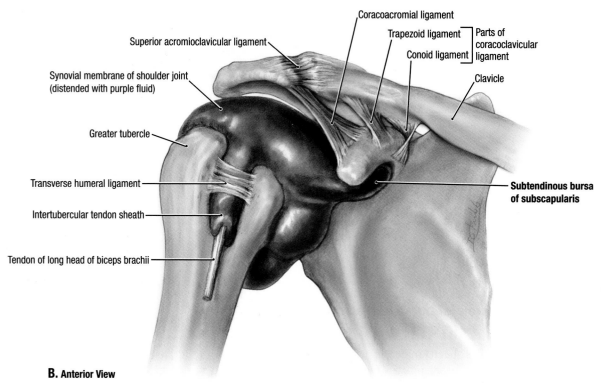

Coracoacromial ligament
Trapezoid ligament   Parts of
Conoid ligament   coracoclavicular
                         ligament

Superior acromioclavicular ligament

Clavicle

Synovial membrane of shoulder joint
(distended with purple fluid)

Greater tubercle

Transverse humeral ligament

Intertubercular tendon sheath

Tendon of long head of biceps brachii

**Subtendinous bursa
of subscapularis**

B. Anterior View

6.42   Ligaments and articular capsule of glenohumeral (shoulder) joint

A. Fibrous capsule.
- The loose fibrous capsule is attached to the margin of the glenoid cavity and to the anatomical neck of the humerus.
- The strong coracoclavicular ligament provides stability to the acromioclavicular joint and prevents the scapula from being driven medially and the acromion from being driven inferior to the clavicle.
- The coracoacromial ligament prevents superior displacement of the head of the humerus.

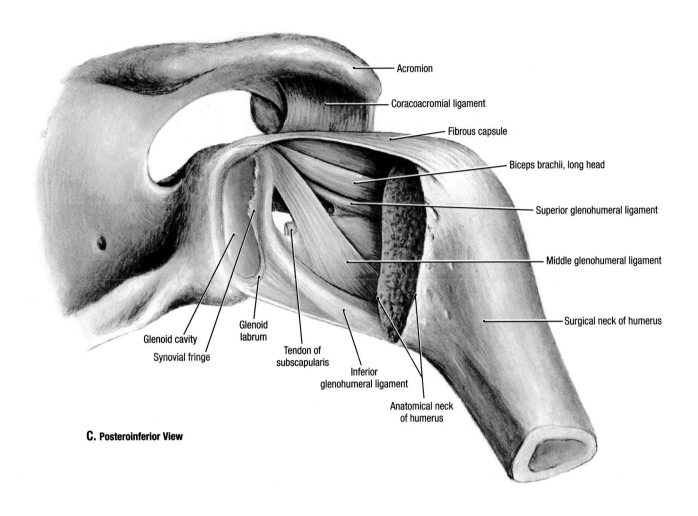

Acromion

Coracoacromial ligament

Fibrous capsule

Biceps brachii, long head

Superior glenohumeral ligament

Middle glenohumeral ligament

Surgical neck of humerus

Glenoid cavity

Synovial fringe

Glenoid labrum

Tendon of subscapularis

Inferior glenohumeral ligament

Anatomical neck of humerus

C. Posteroinferior View

6.42   **Ligaments and articular capsule of glenohumeral (shoulder) joint** *(continued)*

B. Synovial membrane of joint capsule. The synovial membrane lines the fibrous capsule and has two prolongations: (1) where it forms a synovial sheath for the tendon of the long head of the biceps muscle in its osseofibrous tunnel and (2) inferior to the coracoid process, where it forms a bursa between the subscapularis tendon and margin of the glenoid cavity—the subtendinous bursa of the subscapularis. **C.** Glenohumeral ligaments viewed from the interior of the shoulder joint.

- The joint is exposed from the posterior aspect by cutting away the thinner posteroinferior part of the capsule and sawing off the head of the humerus.
- The glenohumeral ligaments are visible from within the joint but are not easily seen externally.
- The glenohumeral ligaments and tendon of the long head of biceps brachii muscle converge on the supraglenoid tubercle.

- The slender superior glenohumeral ligament lies parallel to the tendon of the long head of biceps brachii. The middle ligament is free medially because the subtendinous bursa of subscapularis communicates with the joint cavity, usually there is only a single site of communication. In this individual there are openings on both sides of the ligament.

Because of its freedom of movement and instability, the glenohumeral joint is commonly dislocated by direct or indirect injury. Most dislocations of the humeral head occur in the downward (inferior) direction but are described clinically as anterior or (more rarely) posterior dislocations, indicating whether the humeral head has descended anterior or posterior to the infraglenoid tubercle and the long head of triceps. Anterior dislocation of the glenohumeral joint occurs most often in young adults, particularly athletes. It is usually caused by excessive extension and lateral rotation of the humerus.

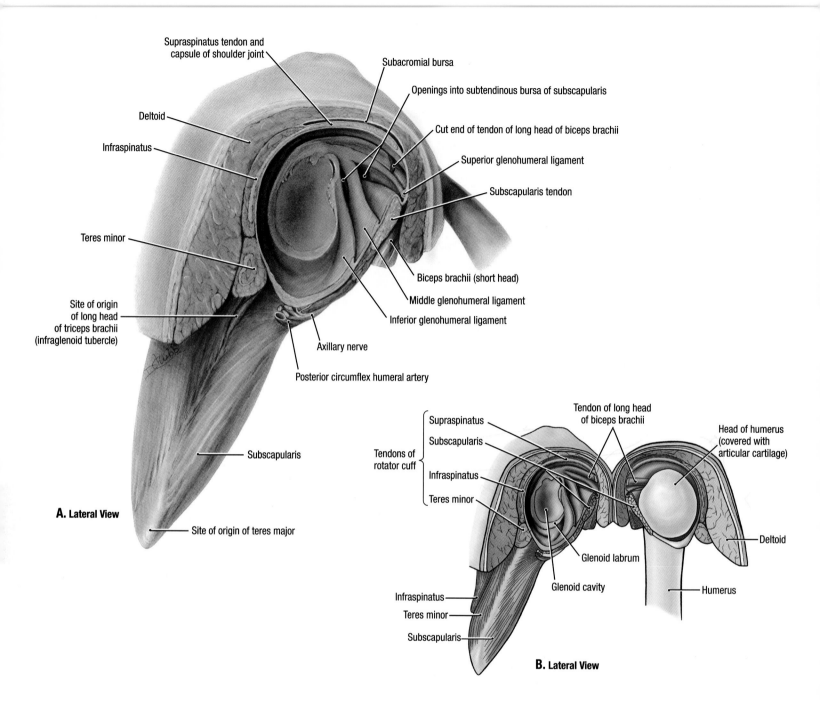

Supraspinatus tendon and
capsule of shoulder joint

Subacromial bursa

Openings into subtendinous bursa of subscapularis

Deltoid

Cut end of tendon of long head of biceps brachii

Infraspinatus

Superior glenohumeral ligament

Subscapularis tendon

Teres minor

Biceps brachii (short head)

Middle glenohumeral ligament

Inferior glenohumeral ligament

Site of origin
of long head
of triceps brachii
(infraglenoid tubercle)

Axillary nerve

Posterior circumflex humeral artery

Subscapularis

A. Lateral View

Site of origin of teres major

Supraspinatus

Tendon of long head
of biceps brachii

Subscapularis

Head of humerus
(covered with
articular cartilage)

Tendons of
rotator cuff

Infraspinatus

Teres minor

Deltoid

Glenoid labrum

Glenoid cavity

Humerus

Infraspinatus

Teres minor

Subscapularis

B. Lateral View

6.43   **Interior of the glenohumeral (shoulder) joint and relationship of rotator cuff**

A. Dissection. **B.** Schematic illustration.
- The fibrous capsule of the joint is thickened anteriorly by the three glenohumeral ligaments.
- The subacromial bursa is between the acromion and deltoid superiorly and the tendon of supraspinatus inferiorly.
- The four short rotator cuff muscles (supraspinatus, infraspinatus, teres minor, and subscapularis) cross the joint and blend with the capsule.
- The axillary nerve and posterior circumflex humeral artery are in contact with the capsule inferiorly and may be injured when the glenohumeral joint dislocates.

- Inflammation and calcification of the subacromial bursa result in pain, tenderness, and limitation of movement of the glenohumeral joint. This condition is also known as calcific scapulohumeral bursitis. Deposition of calcium in the supraspinatus tendon may irritate the overlying subacromial bursa, producing an inflammatory reaction, subacromial bursitis.

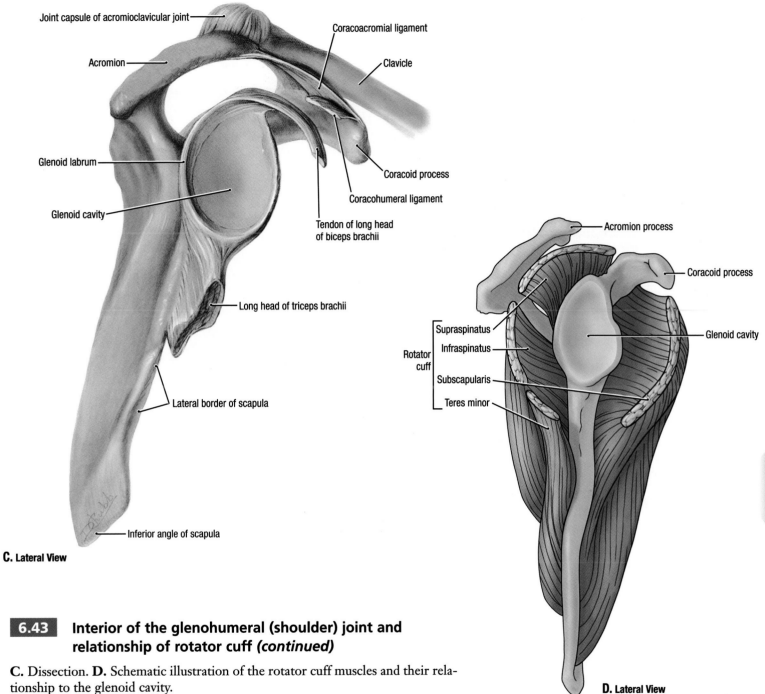

Joint capsule of acromioclavicular joint

Coracoacromial ligament

Acromion

Clavicle

Glenoid labrum

Coracoid process

Coracohumeral ligament

Glenoid cavity

Tendon of long head
of biceps brachii

Long head of triceps brachii

Lateral border of scapula

Inferior angle of scapula

C. Lateral View

Acromion process

Coracoid process

Supraspinatus

Rotator
cuff

Infraspinatus

Glenoid cavity

Subscapularis

Teres minor

D. Lateral View

**6.43   Interior of the glenohumeral (shoulder) joint and
relationship of rotator cuff (continued)**

C. Dissection. **D.** Schematic illustration of the rotator cuff muscles and their relationship to the glenoid cavity.

- The coracoacromial arch (coracoid process, coracoacromial ligament, and
acromion) prevents superior displacement of the head of the humerus.
- The long head of the triceps brachii muscle arises just inferior to the glenoid
cavity; the long head of biceps just superior to it.
- The main function of the musculotendinous rotator cuff is to hold the large
head of the humerus in the smaller and shallow glenoid cavity of the scapula,
both during the relaxed state (by tonic contraction) and during active abduction.

Tearing of the fibrocartilaginous glenoid labrum commonly occurs in the athletes
who throw (e.g., a baseball) and in those who have shoulder instability and subluxation (partial dislocation) of the glenohumeral joint. The tear often results from
sudden contraction of the biceps or forceful subluxation of the humeral head over
the glenoid labrum. Usually a tear occurs in the anterosuperior part of the labrum.

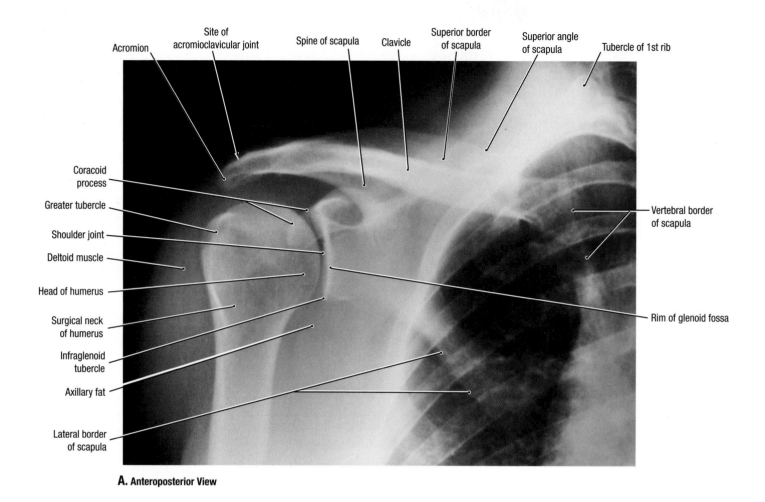

Acromion

Site of acromioclavicular joint

Spine of scapula

Clavicle

Superior border of scapula

Superior angle of scapula

Tubercle of 1st rib

Coracoid process

Greater tubercle

Shoulder joint

Deltoid muscle

Head of humerus

Surgical neck of humerus

Infraglenoid tubercle

Axillary fat

Lateral border of scapula

Vertebral border of scapula

Rim of glenoid fossa

A. Anteroposterior View

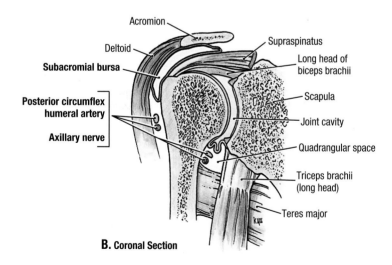

Acromion

Deltoid

Subacromial bursa

Posterior circumflex humeral artery

Axillary nerve

Supraspinatus

Long head of biceps brachii

Scapula

Joint cavity

Quadrangular space

Triceps brachii (long head)

Teres major

B. Coronal Section

6.44   **Imaging of glenohumeral (shoulder) joint**

A. Radiograph. **B.** Sectioned joint to show location of subacromial bursa and joint cavity.

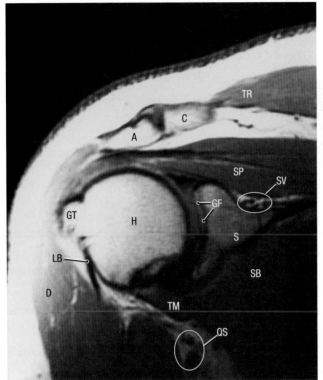

C. Coronal MRI

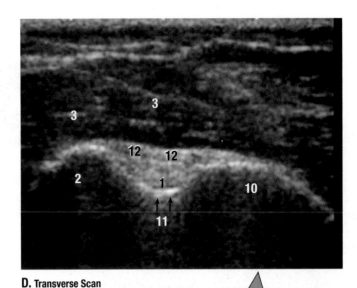

D. Transverse Scan

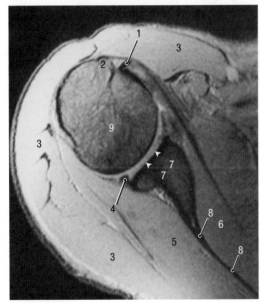

E. Transverse MRI

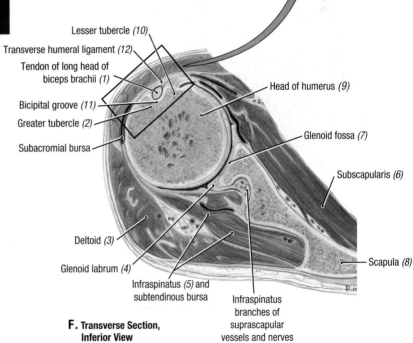

Lesser tubercle *(10)*

Transverse humeral ligament *(12)*

Tendon of long head of biceps brachii *(1)*

Bicipital groove *(11)*

Greater tubercle *(2)*

Subacromial bursa

Head of humerus *(9)*

Glenoid fossa *(7)*

Subscapularis *(6)*

Scapula *(8)*

Deltoid *(3)*

Glenoid labrum *(4)*

Infraspinatus *(5)* and subtendinous bursa

Infraspinatus branches of suprascapular vessels and nerves

F. Transverse Section, Inferior View

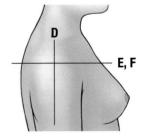

6.44   **Imaging of glenohumeral (shoulder) joint** *(continued)*

C. Coronal MRI. *A,* acromion; *C,* clavicle; *D,* deltoid; *GF,* glenoid cavity; *GT,* crest of greater tubercle; *H,* head of humerus; *LB,* long head of biceps brachii; *QS,* quadrangular space; *S,* scapula; *SB,* subscapularis; *SP,* supraspinatus; *SV,* suprascapular vessels and nerve; *TM,* teres minor; *TR,* trapezius. **D.** Transverse ultrasound scan of area indicated in **F. E.** Transverse MRI. **F.** Transverse section (*numbers* in **F** refer to structures labeled in **D** and **E**).

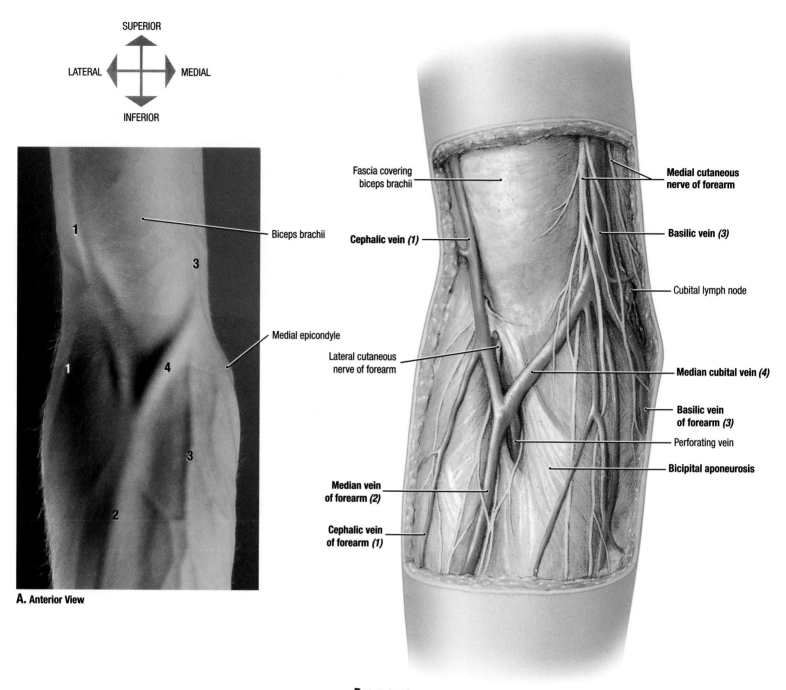

SUPERIOR

LATERAL ← → MEDIAL

INFERIOR

A. Anterior View

Fascia covering biceps brachii

Cephalic vein *(1)*

Lateral cutaneous nerve of forearm

Median vein of forearm *(2)*

Cephalic vein of forearm *(1)*

Biceps brachii

Medial epicondyle

Medial cutaneous nerve of forearm

Basilic vein *(3)*

Cubital lymph node

Median cubital vein *(4)*

Basilic vein of forearm *(3)*

Perforating vein

Bicipital aponeurosis

B. Anterior View

6.45 Cubital fossa: Surface anatomy and superficial dissection

A. Surface anatomy. **B.** Cutaneous nerves and superficial veins (*numbers* in parentheses refer to structures in **A**).
- The cubital fossa is a triangular space (compartment) inferior to the elbow crease, roofed by deep fascia.
- In the forearm, the superficial veins (cephalic, median, basilic, and their connecting veins) make a variable, M-shaped pattern.
- The cephalic and basilic veins occupy the bicipital grooves, one on each side of the biceps brachii. In the lateral bicipital groove,

the lateral cutaneous nerve of the forearm appears just superior to the elbow crease; in the medial bicipital groove, the medial cutaneous nerve of the forearm becomes cutaneous at approximately the midpoint of the arm.

- The cubital fossa is the common site for sampling and transfusion of blood and intravenous injections because of the prominence and accessibility of veins. Usually, the median cubital vein or basilic vein is selected.

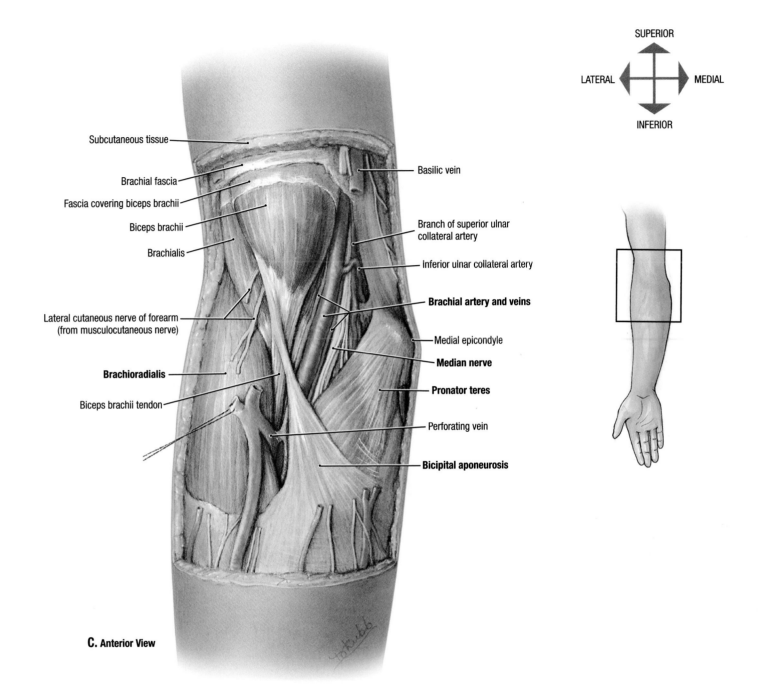

SUPERIOR

LATERAL ← → MEDIAL

INFERIOR

Subcutaneous tissue

Brachial fascia

Fascia covering biceps brachii

Biceps brachii

Brachialis

Lateral cutaneous nerve of forearm
(from musculocutaneous nerve)

Brachioradialis

Biceps brachii tendon

Basilic vein

Branch of superior ulnar
collateral artery

Inferior ulnar collateral artery

Brachial artery and veins

Medial epicondyle

Median nerve

Pronator teres

Perforating vein

Bicipital aponeurosis

C. Anterior View

6.45 Cubital fossa: Deep dissection I

C. Boundaries and contents of the cubital fossa.
- The cubital fossa is bound laterally by the brachioradialis and medially by the pronator teres and superiorly by a line joining the medial and lateral epicondyles.
- The three chief contents of the cubital fossa are the biceps brachii tendon, brachial artery, and median nerve.
- The biceps brachii tendon, on approaching its insertion, rotates through 90°, and the bicipital aponeurosis extends medially from the proximal part of the tendon.

- A fracture of the distal part of the humerus, near the supraepicondylar ridges, is called a *supraepicondylar fracture*. The distal bone fragment may be displaced anteriorly or posteriorly. Any of the nerves or branches of the brachial vessels related to the humerus may be injured by a displaced bone fragment.

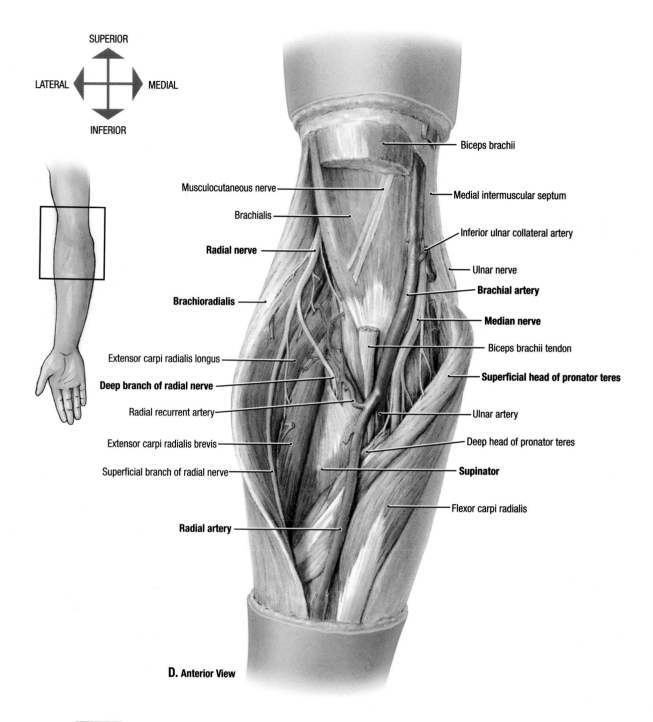

D. Anterior View

6.45   **Cubital fossa: Deep dissection II**

D. Floor of the cubital fossa.
- Part of the biceps brachii muscle is excised, and the cubital fossa is opened widely, exposing the brachialis and supinator muscles in the floor of the fossa.
- The deep branch of the radial nerve pierces the supinator.
- The brachial artery lies between the biceps tendon and median nerve and divides into two branches, the ulnar and radial arteries.
- The median nerve supplies the flexor muscles. With the exception of the twig to the deep head of pronator teres, its motor branches arise from its medial side.
- The radial nerve supplies the extensor muscles. With the exception of the twig to brachioradialis, its motor branches arise from its lateral side. In this specimen, the radial nerve has been displaced laterally, so here its lateral branches appear to run medially.

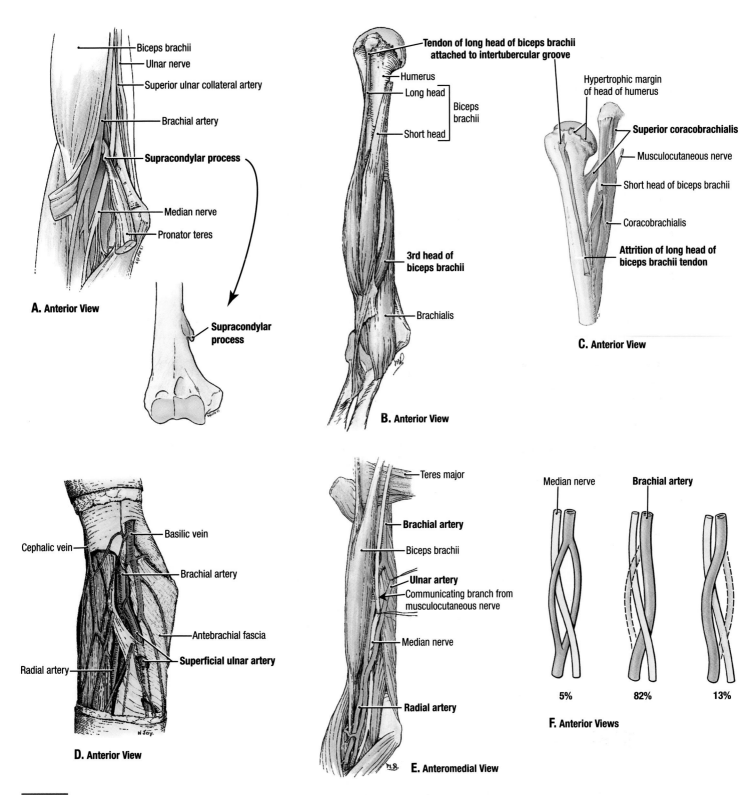

A. Anterior View

Biceps brachii
Ulnar nerve
Superior ulnar collateral artery
Brachial artery
Supracondylar process
Median nerve
Pronator teres

Supracondylar process

B. Anterior View

Tendon of long head of biceps brachii attached to intertubercular groove
Humerus
Long head
Short head
Biceps brachii
3rd head of biceps brachii
Brachialis

C. Anterior View

Hypertrophic margin of head of humerus
Superior coracobrachialis
Musculocutaneous nerve
Short head of biceps brachii
Coracobrachialis
Attrition of long head of biceps brachii tendon

D. Anterior View

Cephalic vein
Basilic vein
Brachial artery
Antebrachial fascia
Superficial ulnar artery
Radial artery

E. Anteromedial View

Teres major
Brachial artery
Biceps brachii
Ulnar artery
Communicating branch from musculocutaneous nerve
Median nerve
Radial artery

F. Anterior Views

Median nerve   **Brachial artery**

5%   82%   13%

6.46   Anomalies

A. Supracondylar process of humerus. A fibrous band, from which the pronator teres muscle arises, joins this supraepicondylar process to the medial epicondyle. The median nerve, often accompanied by the brachial artery, passes through the foramen formed by this band. This may be a cause of nerve entrapment. **B.** Third head of biceps brachii. In this case, there is also attrition of the biceps tendon. **C.** Attrition of the tendon of the long head of biceps brachii and presence of a coracobrachialis.

D. Superficial ulnar artery. **E.** Anomalous division of brachial artery. In this case, the median nerve passes between the radial and ulnar arteries, which arise high in the arm. **F.** Relationship of median nerve and brachial artery. The variable relationship of these two structures can be explained developmentally. In a study of 307 limbs, portions of both primitive brachial arteries persisted in 5%, the posterior in 82%, and the anterior in 13%.

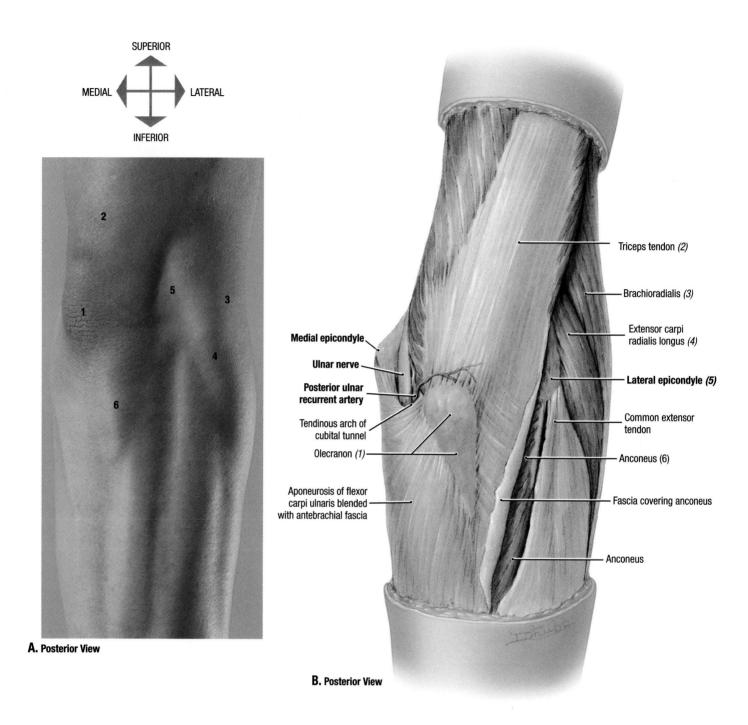

SUPERIOR

MEDIAL ← → LATERAL

INFERIOR

A. Posterior View

Triceps tendon *(2)*

Brachioradialis *(3)*

Extensor carpi
radialis longus *(4)*

Lateral epicondyle *(5)*

Common extensor
tendon

Anconeus (6)

Fascia covering anconeus

Anconeus

Medial epicondyle

Ulnar nerve

**Posterior ulnar
recurrent artery**

Tendinous arch of
cubital tunnel

Olecranon *(1)*

Aponeurosis of flexor
carpi ulnaris blended
with antebrachial fascia

B. Posterior View

6.47   Posterior aspect of elbow–I

A. Surface anatomy. **B.** Superficial dissection (*numbers* in parentheses refer to structures in **A**).

- The triceps brachii is attached distally to the superior surface of the olecranon and, through the deep fascia covering the anconeus, into the lateral border of olecranon.
- The posterior surfaces of the medial epicondyle, lateral epicondyle, and olecranon are subcutaneous and palpable.
- The ulnar nerve, also palpable, runs subfascially posterior to the medial epicondyle; distal to this point, it disappears deep to the two heads of the flexor carpi ulnaris.

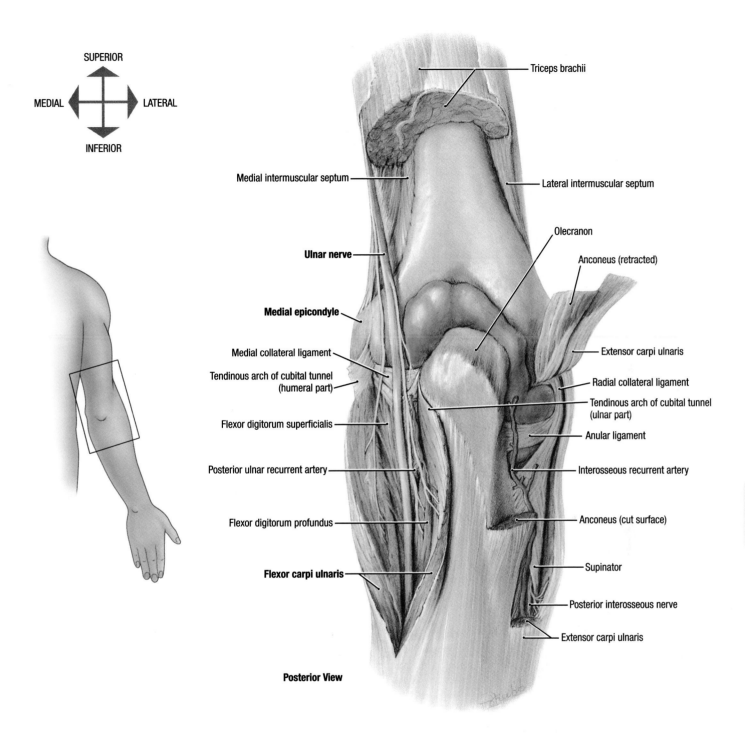

SUPERIOR

MEDIAL   LATERAL

INFERIOR

Triceps brachii

Medial intermuscular septum

Lateral intermuscular septum

Olecranon

Ulnar nerve

Anconeus (retracted)

Medial epicondyle

Extensor carpi ulnaris

Medial collateral ligament

Radial collateral ligament

Tendinous arch of cubital tunnel (humeral part)

Tendinous arch of cubital tunnel (ulnar part)

Flexor digitorum superficialis

Anular ligament

Posterior ulnar recurrent artery

Interosseous recurrent artery

Flexor digitorum profundus

Anconeus (cut surface)

Supinator

Flexor carpi ulnaris

Posterior interosseous nerve

Extensor carpi ulnaris

Posterior View

6.48   **Posterior aspect of elbow–II**

C. Deep dissection. The distal portion of the triceps brachii muscle was removed.

• The ulnar nerve descends subfascially within the posterior compartment of the arm, passing posterior to the medial epicondyle in the groove for the ulnar nerve. Next it passes posterior to the ulnar collateral ligament of the elbow joint and then between the flexor carpi ulnaris and flexor digitorum profundus muscles.

Ulnar nerve injury occurs most commonly where the nerve passes posterior to the medial epicondyle of the humerus. The injury results when the medial part of the elbow hits a hard surface, fracturing the medial epicondyle. The ulnar nerve may be compressed in the cubital tunnel (cubital tunnel syndrome) formed by the tendinous arch joining the humeral and ulnar heads of attachment of the flexor carpi ulnaris muscle. Ulnar nerve injury can result in extensive motor and sensory loss to the hand.

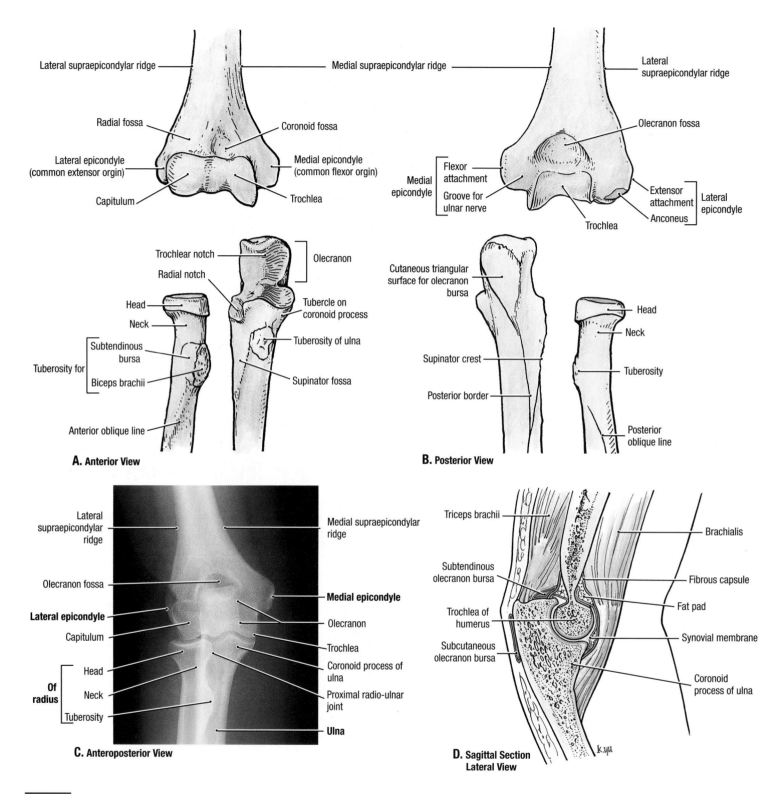

6.49   Bones and imaging of elbow region

A. Anterior bony features. **B.** Posterior bony features. **C.** Radiograph of elbow joint. **D.** Section of humero-ulnar joint.

The subcutaneous olecranon bursa is exposed to injury during falls on the elbow and to infection from abrasions of the skin covering the olecranon. Repeated excessive pressure and friction produces a friction subcutaneous olecranon bursitis (e.g., "student's elbow"). Subtendinous olecranon bursitis results from excessive friction between the triceps tendon and the olecranon, for example, resulting from repeated flexion-extension of the forearm as occurs during certain assembly-line jobs. The pain is severe during flexion of the forearm because of pressure exerted on the inflamed subtendinous olecranon bursa by the triceps tendon.

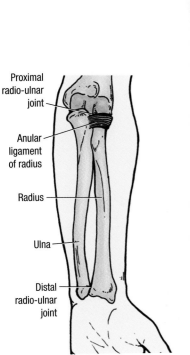

Proximal radio-ulnar joint

Anular ligament of radius

Radius

Ulna

Distal radio-ulnar joint

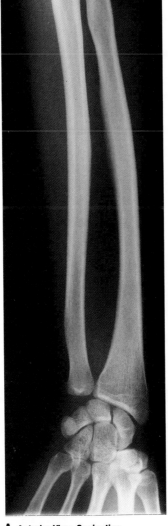

A. Anterior View, Supination

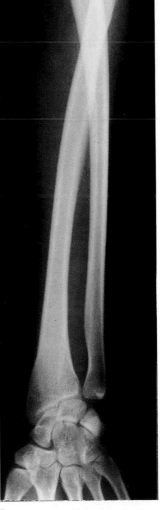

B. Anterior View, Pronation

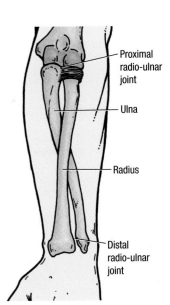

Proximal radio-ulnar joint

Ulna

Radius

Distal radio-ulnar joint

6.50   **Supination and pronation at superior, middle, and inferior radio-ulnar joints**

A. Radiograph of forearm in supination. **B.** Radiograph of forearm in pronation. The radius crosses the ulna when the forearm is pronated. The superior and inferior radio-ulnar joints are synovial joints; the middle radio-ulnar joint is a syndesmosis (fibrous joint) in which the interosseous ligament connects the forearm bones.

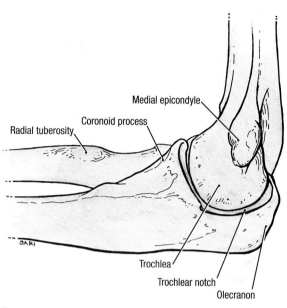

A. Medial View

Radial tuberosity

Coronoid process

Medial epicondyle

Trochlea

Trochlear notch

Olecranon

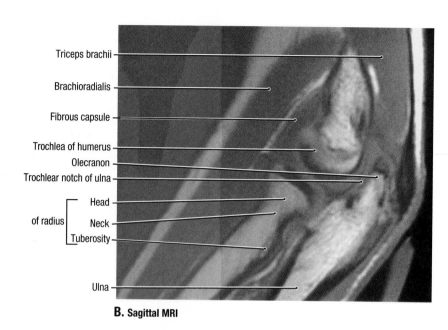

B. Sagittal MRI

Triceps brachii

Brachioradialis

Fibrous capsule

Trochlea of humerus

Olecranon

Trochlear notch of ulna

of radius — Head

Neck

Tuberosity

Ulna

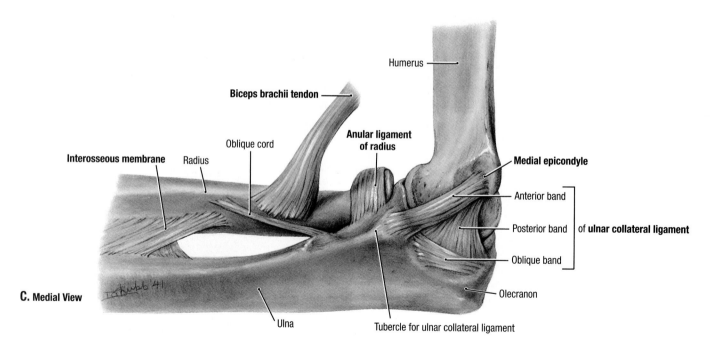

C. Medial View

Humerus

Biceps brachii tendon

Oblique cord

Anular ligament of radius

Interosseous membrane

Radius

Medial epicondyle

Anterior band

Posterior band — of **ulnar collateral ligament**

Oblique band

Olecranon

Ulna

Tubercle for ulnar collateral ligament

6.51 **Medial aspect of bones and ligaments of elbow region**

A. Bony features. **B.** MRI of elbow joint. **C.** Ligaments. The anterior band of the ulnar (medial) collateral ligament is a strong, round cord that is taut when the elbow joint is extended. The posterior band is a weak fan that is taut in flexion of the joint. The oblique fibers deepen the socket for the trochlea of the humerus.

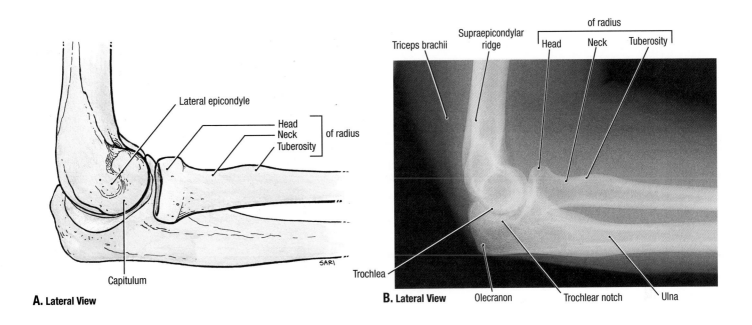

Lateral epicondyle

Head
Neck
Tuberosity
of radius

Capitulum

A. Lateral View

Triceps brachii

Supraepicondylar ridge

of radius
Head   Neck   Tuberosity

Trochlea

B. Lateral View   Olecranon   Trochlear notch   Ulna

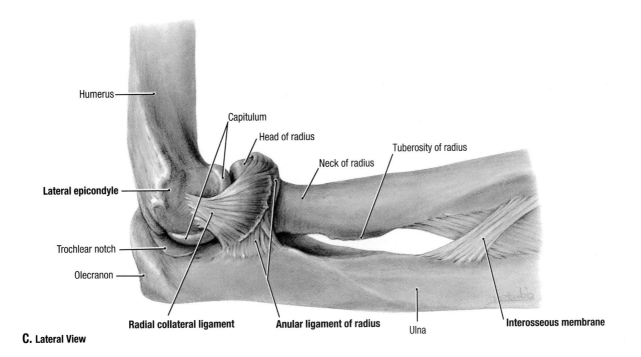

Humerus

Capitulum

Head of radius

Neck of radius

Tuberosity of radius

Lateral epicondyle

Trochlear notch

Olecranon

Radial collateral ligament   **Anular ligament of radius**   Ulna   **Interosseous membrane**

C. Lateral View

6.52   **Lateral aspect of bones and ligaments of elbow region**

A. Bony features. **B.** Lateral radiograph. **C.** Ligaments. The fan-shaped radial (lateral) collateral ligament is primarily attached to the anular ligament of the radius; superficial fibers of the lateral ligament blend with the fibrous capsule and continue onto the radius.

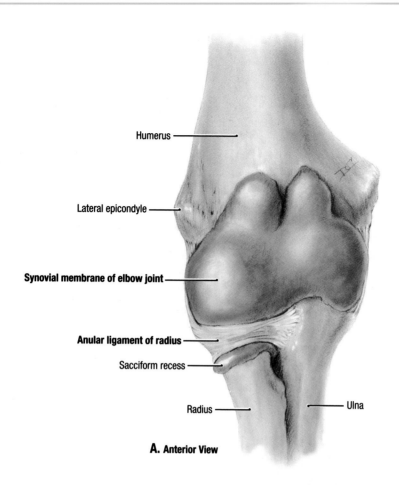

Humerus

Lateral epicondyle

Synovial membrane of elbow joint

Anular ligament of radius

Sacciform recess

Radius

Ulna

A. Anterior View

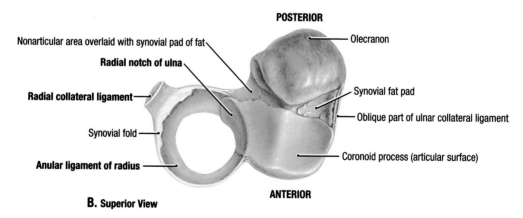

POSTERIOR

Olecranon

Nonarticular area overlaid with synovial pad of fat

Radial notch of ulna

Synovial fat pad

Radial collateral ligament

Oblique part of ulnar collateral ligament

Synovial fold

Anular ligament of radius

Coronoid process (articular surface)

ANTERIOR

B. Superior View

6.53   Synovial capsule of elbow joint and anular ligament

A. Synovial capsule of elbow and proximal radio-ulnar joints. The cavity of the elbow was injected with purple fluid (wax). The fibrous capsule was removed, and the synovial membrane remains. **B.** Anular ligament.

• The anular ligament secures the head of the radius to the radial notch of the ulna and with it forms a tapering columnar socket (i.e., wide superiorly, narrow inferiorly).

• The anular ligament is bound to the humerus by the radial collateral ligament of the elbow.

A common childhood injury is subluxation and dislocation of the head of the radius after traction on a pronated forearm (e.g., when lifting a child onto a bus). The sudden pulling of the upper limb tears or stretches the distal attachment of the less tapering anular ligament of a child. The radial head then moves distally, partially out of the anular ligament. The proximal part of the torn ligament may become trapped between the head of the radius and the capitulum of the humerus. The source of pain is the pinched anular ligament.

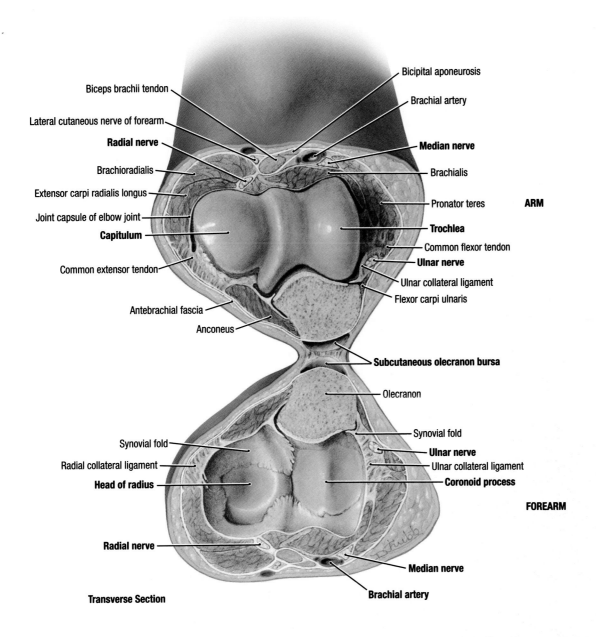

Transverse Section

- Biceps brachii tendon
- Lateral cutaneous nerve of forearm
- **Radial nerve**
- Brachioradialis
- Extensor carpi radialis longus
- Joint capsule of elbow joint
- **Capitulum**
- Common extensor tendon
- Antebrachial fascia
- Anconeus
- Synovial fold
- Radial collateral ligament
- **Head of radius**
- **Radial nerve**

- Bicipital aponeurosis
- Brachial artery
- **Median nerve**
- Brachialis
- Pronator teres
- **Trochlea**
- Common flexor tendon
- **Ulnar nerve**
- Ulnar collateral ligament
- Flexor carpi ulnaris
- **Subcutaneous olecranon bursa**
- Olecranon
- Synovial fold
- **Ulnar nerve**
- Ulnar collateral ligament
- **Coronoid process**
- **Median nerve**
- **Brachial artery**

ARM

FOREARM

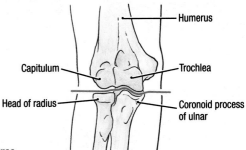

- Humerus
- Capitulum
- Trochlea
- Head of radius
- Coronoid process of ulnar

6.54   Articular surfaces of elbow joint

The tissue surrounding the condyles of the humerus has been sectioned in a transverse plane, followed by disarticulation of the elbow joint, revealing the articular surfaces. Compare the forearm (inferior) component with Fig. 6.53B.

- Synovial folds containing fat overlie the periphery of the head of the radius and the nonarticular indentations on the trochlear notch of the ulna.
- The radial nerve is in contact with the joint capsule, the ulnar nerve is in contact with the ulnar collateral ligament, and the median nerve is separated from the joint capsule by the brachialis muscle.

TABLE 6.9 ARTERIES OF FOREARM

Radial artery

Origin:
In cubital fossa, as smaller terminal division of brachial artery

Course/Distribution:
Runs distally under brachioradialis, lateral to flexor carpi radialis, defining boundary between the flexor and extensor compartments and supplying the radial aspect of both. Gives rise to a superficial palmar branch near the radio-carpal joint; it then transverses the anatomical snuff box to pass between the heads of the 1st dorsal interosseous muscle joining the deep branch of the ulnar artery to form the deep palmar arch

Ulanr artery

Origin:
In cubital fossa, as larger terminal division of brachial artery

Course/Distribution:
Passes distally between 2nd and 3rd layers of forearm flexor muscles, supplying ulnar aspect of flexor compartment; passes superficial to flexor retinaculum at wrist, continuing as the superficial palmar arch (with superficial branch of ra-dial) after its deep palmar branch joins the deep palmar arch

Radial recurrent artery

Origin:
In cubital fossa, as 1st (lateral) branch of radial artery

Course/Distribution:
Courses proximally, superficial to supinator, passing between brachioradialis and brachialis to anastomose with radial collateral artery

Anterior and posterior ulnar recurrent arteries

Origin:
In and immediately distal to cubital fossa, as 1st and 2nd medial branches of ulnar artery

Course/Distribution:
Course proximally to anastomose with the inferior and superior ulnar collateral arteries, respectively, forming collateral pathways anterior and posterior to the medial epicondyle of the humerus

Common interosseous artery

Origin:
Immediately distal to the cubital fossa, as 1st lateral branch of ulnar artery

Course/Distribution:
Terminates almost immediately, dividing into anterior and posterior in-terosseous arteries

Anterior and posterior interosseous arteries

Origin:
Distal to radial tubercle, as terminal branches of common interosseous

Course/Distribution:
Pass to opposite sides of interosseous membrane; anterior artery runs on in-terosseous membrane; posterior artery runs between superficial and deep lay-ers of extensor muscles as primary artery of compartment

Interosseous recurrent artery

Origin:
Initial part of posterior interosseous artery

Course/Distribution:
Courses proximally between lateral epicondyle and olecranon, deep to an-coneus, to anastomose with middle collateral artery

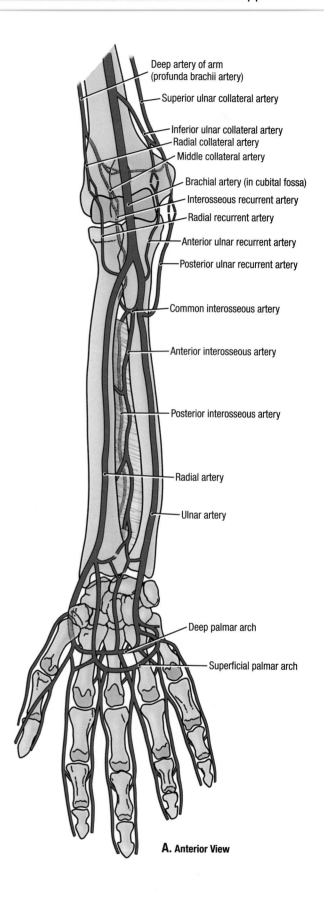

Deep artery of arm (profunda brachii artery)
Superior ulnar collateral artery
Inferior ulnar collateral artery
Radial collateral artery
Middle collateral artery
Brachial artery (in cubital fossa)
Interosseous recurrent artery
Radial recurrent artery
Anterior ulnar recurrent artery
Posterior ulnar recurrent artery
Common interosseous artery
Anterior interosseous artery
Posterior interosseous artery
Radial artery
Ulnar artery
Deep palmar arch
Superficial palmar arch

A. Anterior View

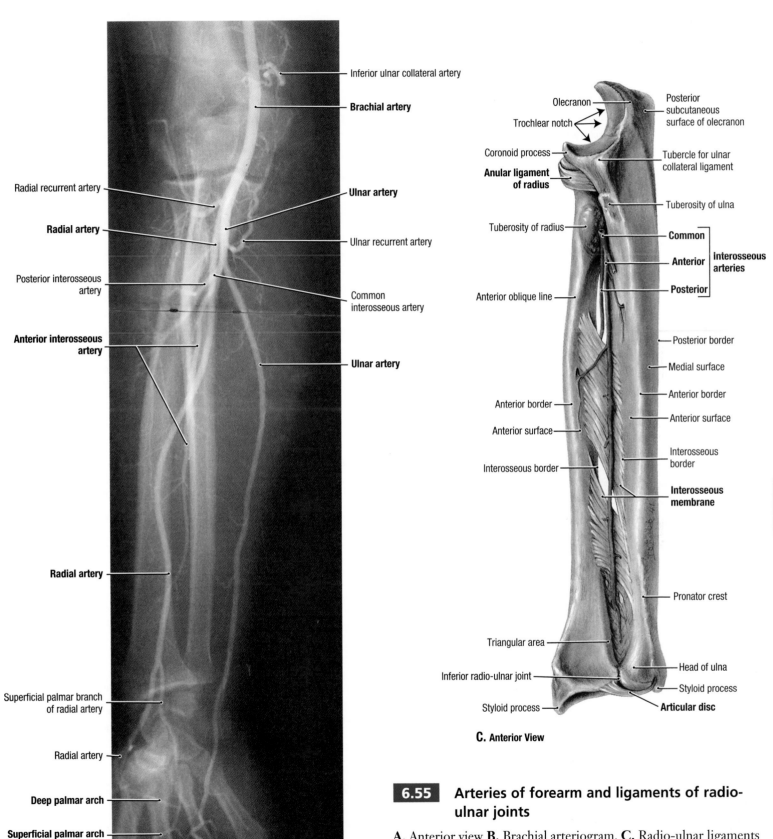

Inferior ulnar collateral artery

Brachial artery

Radial recurrent artery

Radial artery

Ulnar artery

Ulnar recurrent artery

Posterior interosseous artery

Common interosseous artery

Anterior interosseous artery

Ulnar artery

Radial artery

Superficial palmar branch of radial artery

Radial artery

Deep palmar arch

Superficial palmar arch

B. Anteroposterior View

Olecranon

Posterior subcutaneous surface of olecranon

Trochlear notch

Coronoid process

Tubercle for ulnar collateral ligament

Anular ligament of radius

Tuberosity of ulna

Tuberosity of radius

Common

Anterior — Interosseous arteries

Posterior

Anterior oblique line

Posterior border

Medial surface

Anterior border

Anterior border

Anterior surface

Anterior surface

Interosseous border

Interosseous border

Interosseous membrane

Pronator crest

Triangular area

Head of ulna

Inferior radio-ulnar joint

Styloid process

Styloid process

Articular disc

C. Anterior View

6.55 **Arteries of forearm and ligaments of radio-ulnar joints**

A. Anterior view **B.** Brachial arteriogram. **C.** Radio-ulnar ligaments and interosseous arteries. The ligament maintaining the proximal radio-ulnar joint is the anular ligament, that for the distal joint is the articular disc, and that for the middle joint is the interosseous membrane. The interosseous membrane is attached to the interosseous borders of the radius and ulna, but it also spreads onto their surfaces.

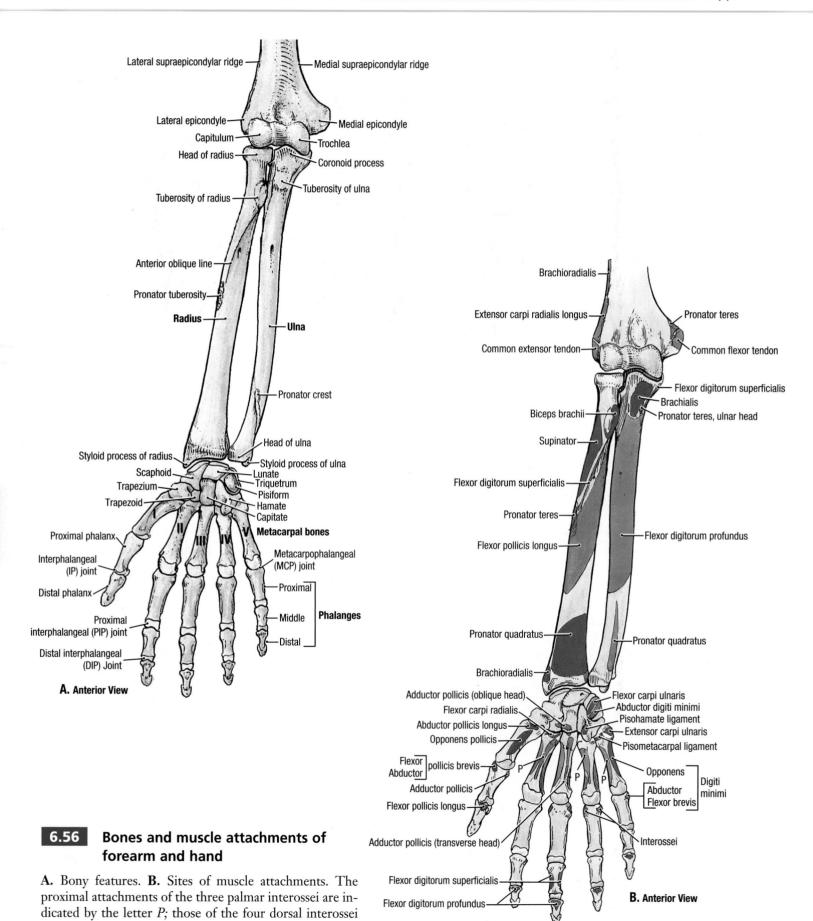

Lateral supraepicondylar ridge
Medial supraepicondylar ridge
Lateral epicondyle
Medial epicondyle
Capitulum
Trochlea
Head of radius
Coronoid process
Tuberosity of radius
Tuberosity of ulna
Anterior oblique line
Pronator tuberosity
Radius
Ulna
Pronator crest
Head of ulna
Styloid process of radius
Styloid process of ulna
Scaphoid
Lunate
Trapezium
Triquetrum
Trapezoid
Pisiform
Hamate
Capitate
Metacarpal bones
Proximal phalanx
Interphalangeal (IP) joint
Metacarpophalangeal (MCP) joint
Distal phalanx
Proximal
Proximal interphalangeal (PIP) joint
Middle **Phalanges**
Distal interphalangeal (DIP) Joint
Distal

A. Anterior View

Brachioradialis
Extensor carpi radialis longus
Pronator teres
Common extensor tendon
Common flexor tendon
Flexor digitorum superficialis
Brachialis
Biceps brachii
Pronator teres, ulnar head
Supinator
Flexor digitorum superficialis
Pronator teres
Flexor digitorum profundus
Flexor pollicis longus
Pronator quadratus
Pronator quadratus
Brachioradialis
Adductor pollicis (oblique head)
Flexor carpi ulnaris
Flexor carpi radialis
Abductor digiti minimi
Abductor pollicis longus
Pisohamate ligament
Opponens pollicis
Extensor carpi ulnaris
Pisometacarpal ligament
Flexor Abductor pollicis brevis
Opponens
Adductor pollicis
Abductor Flexor brevis
Digiti minimi
Flexor pollicis longus
Interossei
Adductor pollicis (transverse head)
Flexor digitorum superficialis
Flexor digitorum profundus

B. Anterior View

6.56 **Bones and muscle attachments of forearm and hand**

A. Bony features. **B.** Sites of muscle attachments. The proximal attachments of the three palmar interossei are indicated by the letter *P*; those of the four dorsal interossei are indicated by color only.

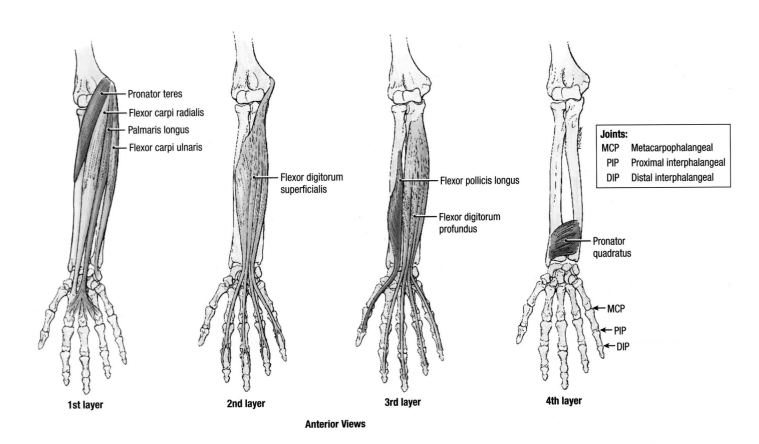

1st layer

Pronator teres
Flexor carpi radialis
Palmaris longus
Flexor carpi ulnaris

2nd layer

Flexor digitorum superficialis

3rd layer

Flexor pollicis longus
Flexor digitorum profundus

4th layer

Pronator quadratus

MCP
PIP
DIP

Joints:
MCP   Metacarpophalangeal
PIP   Proximal interphalangeal
DIP   Distal interphalangeal

Anterior Views

TABLE 6.10 MUSCLES OF ANTERIOR SURFACE OF FOREARM

Muscle	Proximal Attachment	Distal Attachment	Innervation	Main Actions
Pronator teres	Medial epicondyle of humerus and coronoid process of ulna	Middle of lateral surface of radius (pronator tuberosity)	Median nerve (C6–**C7**)	Pronates forearm and flexes elbow
Flexor carpi radialis	Medial epicondyle of humerus	Base of 2nd metacarpal	Median nerve (C7–**C8**)	Flexes wrist and abducts hand
Palmaris longus		Distal half of flexor retinaculum and palmar aponeurosis		Flexes wrist and tightens palmar aponeurosis
Flexor carpi ulnaris	*Humeral head:* medial epicondyle of humerus; *Ulnar head:* olecranon and posterior border of ulna	Pisiform, hook of hamate, and 5th metacarpal	Ulnar nerve (C7–**C8**)	Flexes wrist and adducts hand
Flexor digitorum superficialis	*Humeroulnar head:* medial epicondyle of humerus, ulnar collateral ligament, and coronoid process of ulna *Radial head:* superior half of anterior border of radius	Bodies of middle phalanges of medial four digits	Median nerve (C7, **C8**, and T1)	Flexes PIPs of medial four digits; acting more strongly, it flexes MCPs and hand
Flexor digitorum profundus	Proximal three quarters of medial and anterior surfaces of ulna and interosseous membrane	Bases of distal phalanges of medial four digits	*Medial part:* ulnar nerve (**C8**–T1) *Lateral part:* median nerve (**C8**–T1)	Flexes DIPs of medial four digits; assists with flexion of wrist
Flexor pollicis longus	Anterior surface of radius and adjacent interosseous membrane	Base of distal phalanx of thumb	Anterior interosseous nerve from median (**C8**–T1)	Flexes phalanges of 1st digit (thumb)
Pronator quadratus	Distal fourth of anterior surface of ulna	Distal fourth of anterior surface of radius		Pronates forearm; deep fibers bind radius and ulna together

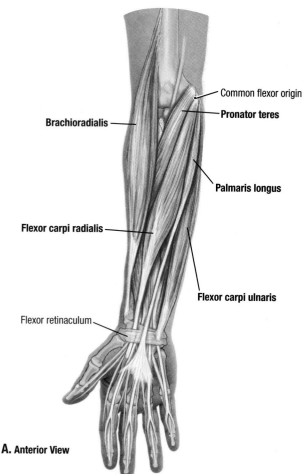

Brachioradialis

Common flexor origin

Pronator teres

Palmaris longus

Flexor carpi radialis

Flexor carpi ulnaris

Flexor retinaculum

A. Anterior View

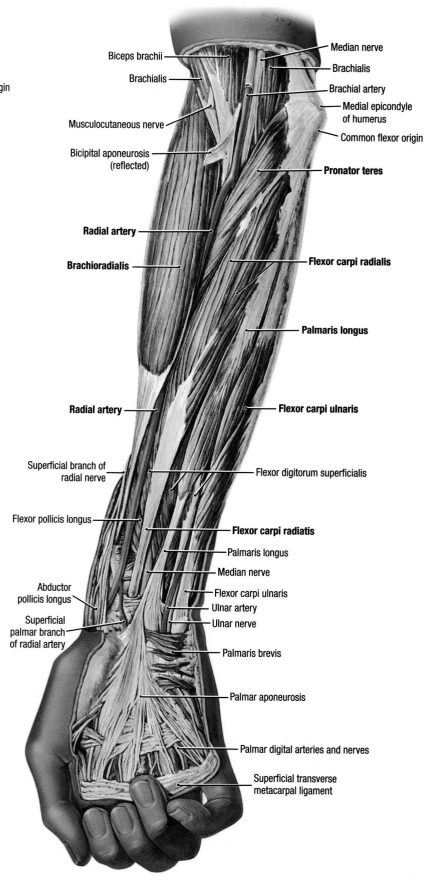

Biceps brachii

Brachialis

Musculocutaneous nerve

Bicipital aponeurosis
(reflected)

Radial artery

Brachioradialis

Radial artery

Superficial branch of
radial nerve

Flexor pollicis longus

Abductor
pollicis longus

Superficial
palmar branch
of radial artery

Median nerve

Brachialis

Brachial artery

Medial epicondyle
of humerus

Common flexor origin

Pronator teres

Flexor carpi radialis

Palmaris longus

Flexor carpi ulnaris

Flexor digitorum superficialis

Flexor carpi radiatis

Palmaris longus

Median nerve

Flexor carpi ulnaris

Ulnar artery

Ulnar nerve

Palmaris brevis

Palmar aponeurosis

Palmar digital arteries and nerves

Superficial transverse
metacarpal ligament

B. Anterior View

6.57   **Superficial muscles of the forearm
and palmar aponeurosis**

- At the elbow, the brachial artery lies between the biceps tendon and median nerve. It then bifurcates into the radial and ulnar arteries.
- At the wrist, the radial artery is lateral to the flexor carpi radialis tendon, and the ulnar artery is lateral to flexor carpi ulnaris tendon.
- In the forearm, the radial artery lies between the flexor and extensor compartments. The muscles lateral to the artery are supplied by the radial nerve, and those medial to it by the median and ulnar nerves; thus, no motor nerve crosses the radial artery.
- The brachioradialis muscle slightly overlaps the radial artery, which is otherwise superficial.
- The four superficial muscles (pronator teres, flexor carpi radialis, palmaris longus, and flexor carpi ulnaris) all attach proximally to the medial epicondyle of the humerus (common flexor origin).
- The palmaris longus muscle, in this specimen, has an anomalous distal belly; this muscle usually has a small belly at the common flexor origin and a long tendon that is continued into the palm as the palmar aponeurosis. The palmaris longus is absent in approximately 14% of limbs.

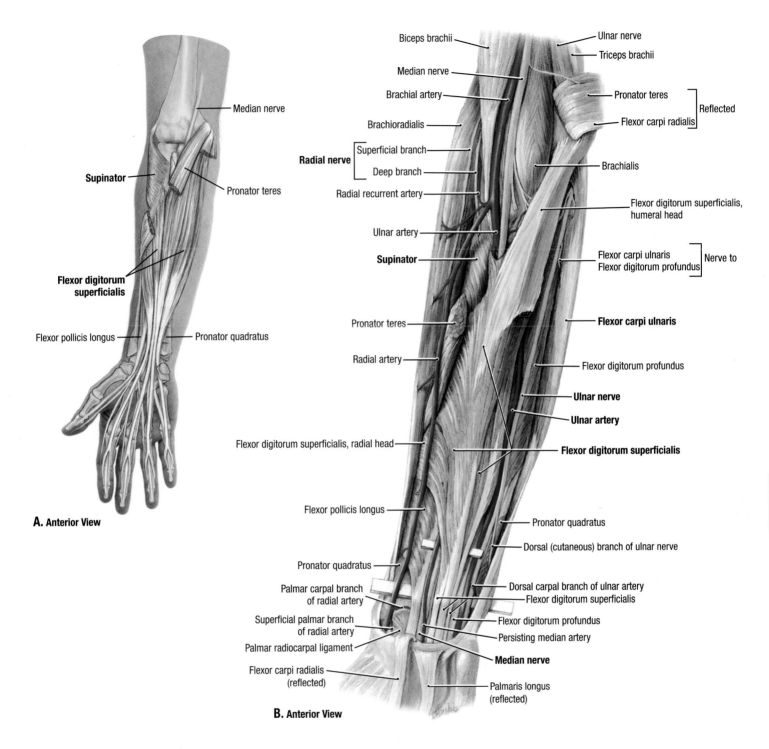

A. Anterior View

Median nerve

Supinator

Pronator teres

Flexor digitorum superficialis

Flexor pollicis longus

Pronator quadratus

B. Anterior View

Biceps brachii

Median nerve

Brachial artery

Brachioradialis

Radial nerve
Superficial branch
Deep branch

Radial recurrent artery

Ulnar artery

Supinator

Pronator teres

Radial artery

Flexor digitorum superficialis, radial head

Flexor pollicis longus

Pronator quadratus

Palmar carpal branch of radial artery

Superficial palmar branch of radial artery

Palmar radiocarpal ligament

Flexor carpi radialis (reflected)

Ulnar nerve

Triceps brachii

Pronator teres
Flexor carpi radialis
Reflected

Brachialis

Flexor digitorum superficialis, humeral head

Flexor carpi ulnaris
Flexor digitorum profundus
Nerve to

Flexor carpi ulnaris

Flexor digitorum profundus

Ulnar nerve

Ulnar artery

Flexor digitorum superficialis

Pronator quadratus

Dorsal (cutaneous) branch of ulnar nerve

Dorsal carpal branch of ulnar artery
Flexor digitorum superficialis

Flexor digitorum profundus
Persisting median artery

Median nerve

Palmaris longus (reflected)

6.58 Flexor digitorum superficialis and related structures

- The flexor digitorum superficialis muscle is attached proximally to the humerus, ulna, and radius.
- The ulnar artery passes obliquely posterior to the flexor digitorum superficialis; at the medial border of the muscle, the ulnar artery joins the ulnar nerve.
- The ulnar nerve lies between the flexor digitorum profundus and flexor carpi ulnaris.
- The median nerve descends vertically posterior to the flexor digitorum superficialis and appears distally at its lateral border.
- The median artery of this specimen is a variation resulting from persistence of an embryologic vessel that usually disappears.

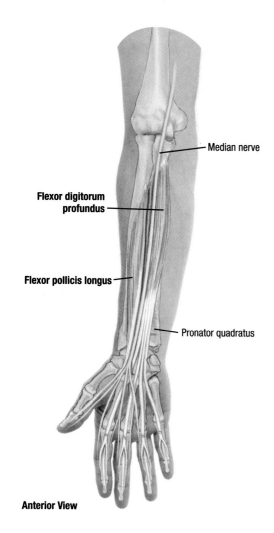

Anterior View

Median nerve

Flexor digitorum profundus

Flexor pollicis longus

Pronator quadratus

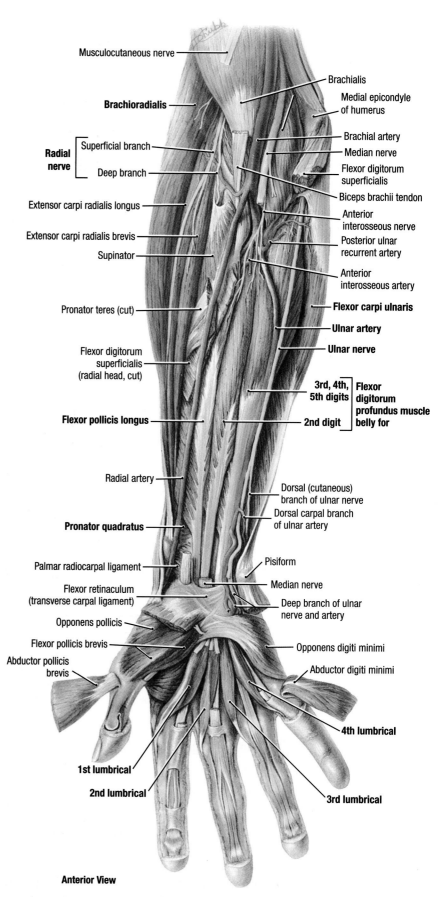

Musculocutaneous nerve

Brachioradialis

Radial nerve
Superficial branch
Deep branch

Extensor carpi radialis longus

Extensor carpi radialis brevis

Supinator

Pronator teres (cut)

Flexor digitorum superficialis (radial head, cut)

Flexor pollicis longus

Radial artery

Pronator quadratus

Palmar radiocarpal ligament

Flexor retinaculum (transverse carpal ligament)

Opponens pollicis

Flexor pollicis brevis

Abductor pollicis brevis

1st lumbrical

2nd lumbrical

Brachialis

Medial epicondyle of humerus

Brachial artery

Median nerve

Flexor digitorum superficialis

Biceps brachii tendon

Anterior interosseous nerve

Posterior ulnar recurrent artery

Anterior interosseous artery

Flexor carpi ulnaris

Ulnar artery

Ulnar nerve

3rd, 4th, 5th digits | Flexor digitorum profundus muscle belly for
2nd digit |

Dorsal (cutaneous) branch of ulnar nerve

Dorsal carpal branch of ulnar artery

Pisiform

Median nerve

Deep branch of ulnar nerve and artery

Opponens digiti minimi

Abductor digiti minimi

4th lumbrical

3rd lumbrical

Anterior View

6.59 Deep flexors of the digits and related structures

- The two deep digital flexor muscles, flexor pollicis longus and flexor digitorum profundus, arise from the flexor aspects of the radius, interosseous membrane, and ulna between the origin of flexor digitorum superficialis proximally and pronator quadratus distally.
- The ulnar nerve enters the forearm posterior to the medial epicondyle, then descends between the flexor digitorum profundus and flexor carpi ulnaris and is joined by the ulnar artery. At the wrist the ulnar nerve and artery pass anterior to the flexor retinaculum and lateral to the pisiform to enter the palm.
- At the elbow, the ulnar nerve supplies the flexor carpi ulnaris and the medial half of the flexor digitorum profundus muscles; superior to the wrist, it gives off the dorsal (cutaneous) branch.
- The four lumbricals arise from the flexor digitorum profundus tendons.

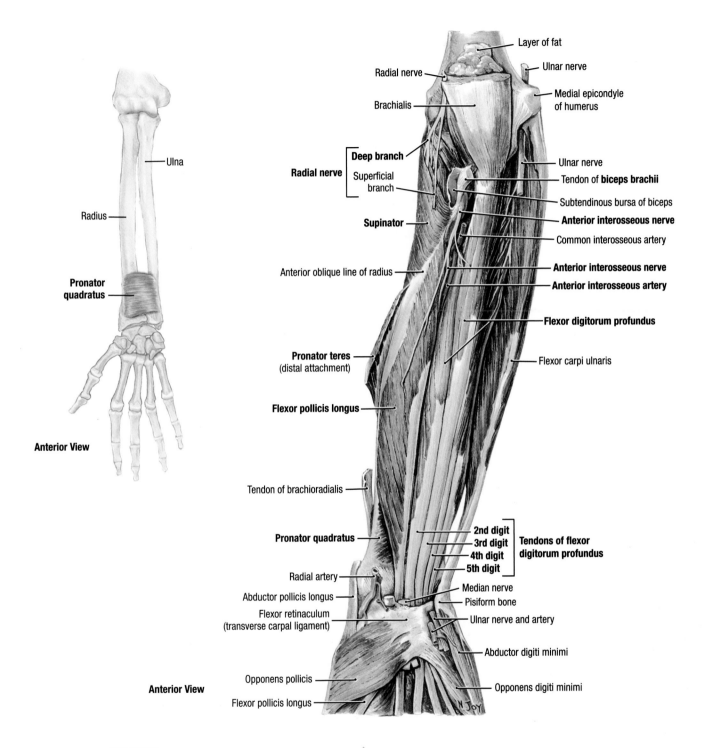

Anterior View

Anterior View

6.60 Deep flexors of the digits and supinator

- The five tendons of the deep digital flexors (flexor pollicis longus and flexor digitorum profundus) lie side by side as they enter the carpal tunnel.
- The biceps brachii muscle attaches to the medial aspect of the radius; hence, it can supinate the forearm, whereas the pronator teres muscle, by attaching to the lateral surface, can pronate the forearm.
- The deep branch of the radial nerve pierces and innervates the supinator muscle.
- The anterior interosseous nerve and artery disappear between the flexor pollicis longus and flexor digitorum profundus muscles to lie on the interosseous membrane.

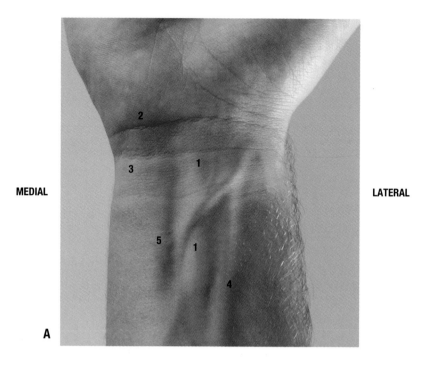

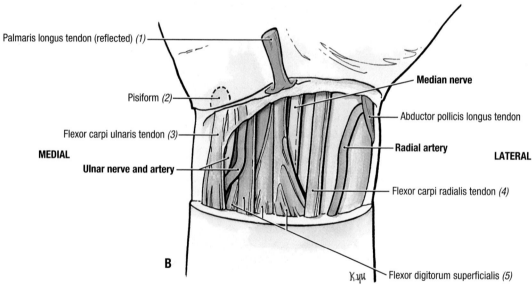

Anterior Views of Right Hand and Wrist

Palmaris longus tendon (reflected) *(1)*

Pisiform *(2)*

Flexor carpi ulnaris tendon *(3)*

MEDIAL

Ulnar nerve and artery

Median nerve

Abductor pollicis longus tendon

Radial artery

LATERAL

Flexor carpi radialis tendon *(4)*

Flexor digitorum superficialis *(5)*

6.61   Structures of anterior aspect of wrist

A. Surface anatomy. **B.** Schematic illustration. **C.** Dissection.

- The distal skin incision follows the transverse skin crease at the wrist. The incision crosses the pisiform, to which the flexor carpi ulnaris muscle attaches, and the tubercle of the scaphoid, to which the tendon of flexor carpi radialis muscle is a guide.
- The palmaris longus tendon bisects the transverse skin crease; deep to its lateral margin is the median nerve.

- The radial artery passes deep to the tendon of the abductor pollicis longus muscle.
- The flexor digitorum superficialis tendons to the 3rd and 4th digits become anterior to those of the 2nd and 5th digits.
- The recurrent branch of the median nerve to the thenar muscles lies within a circle whose center is 2.5 to 4 cm distal to the tubercle of the scaphoid.

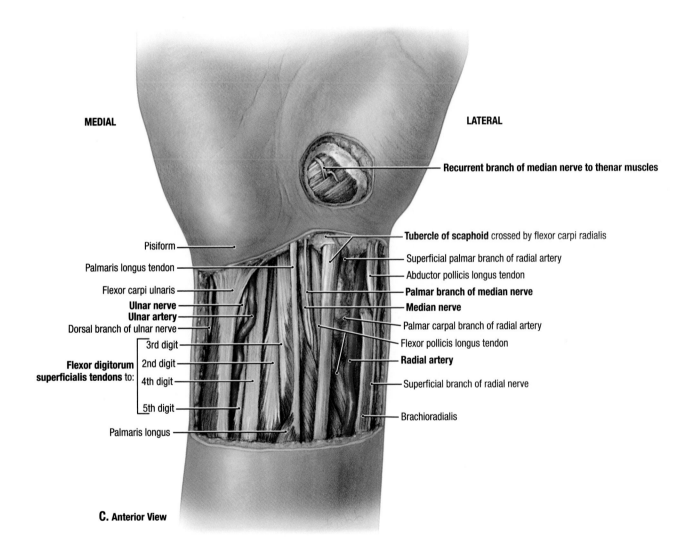

MEDIAL

LATERAL

Recurrent branch of median nerve to thenar muscles

Pisiform

Palmaris longus tendon

Flexor carpi ulnaris

Ulnar nerve
Ulnar artery

Dorsal branch of ulnar nerve

3rd digit
Flexor digitorum 2nd digit
superficialis tendons to:
4th digit

5th digit

Palmaris longus

Tubercle of scaphoid crossed by flexor carpi radialis

Superficial palmar branch of radial artery

Abductor pollicis longus tendon

Palmar branch of median nerve

Median nerve

Palmar carpal branch of radial artery

Flexor pollicis longus tendon

Radial artery

Superficial branch of radial nerve

Brachioradialis

C. Anterior View

6.61   **Structures of anterior aspect of wrist (continued)**

Lesions of the median nerve usually occur in two places: the fore-arm and wrist. The most common site is where the nerve passes though the carpal tunnel. Lacerations of the wrist often cause median nerve injury because this nerve is relatively close to the surface. This results in paralysis of the thenar muscles and the first two lumbricals. Hence opposition of the thumb is not possible and fine control movements of the 2nd and 3rd digits are impaired. Sensation is also lost over the thumb and adjacent two and a half fingers.

Median nerve injury resulting from a perforating wound in the elbow region results in loss of flexion of the proximal and distal interphalangeal joints of the 2nd and 3rd digits. The ability to flex the metacarpophalangeal joints of these digits is also affected because digital branches of the median nerve supply the 1st and 2nd lumbricals. The palmar cutaneous branch of the median nerve does not traverse the carpal tunnel. It supplies the skin of the central palm, which remains sensitive in carpal tunnel syndrome.

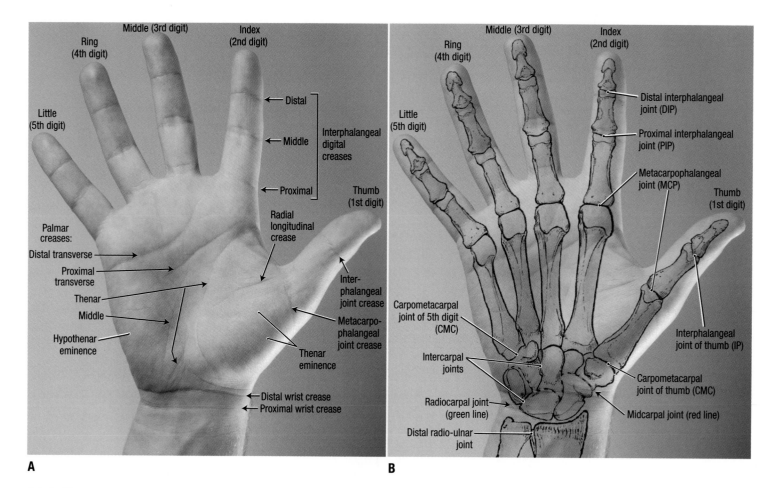

A. Skin creases of wrist and hand. **B.** Surface projection of joints of wrist and hand. Note relationship of bones and joints to features of the hand.

Anterior Views

6.62   **Surface anatomy of skeleton of hand and wrist**

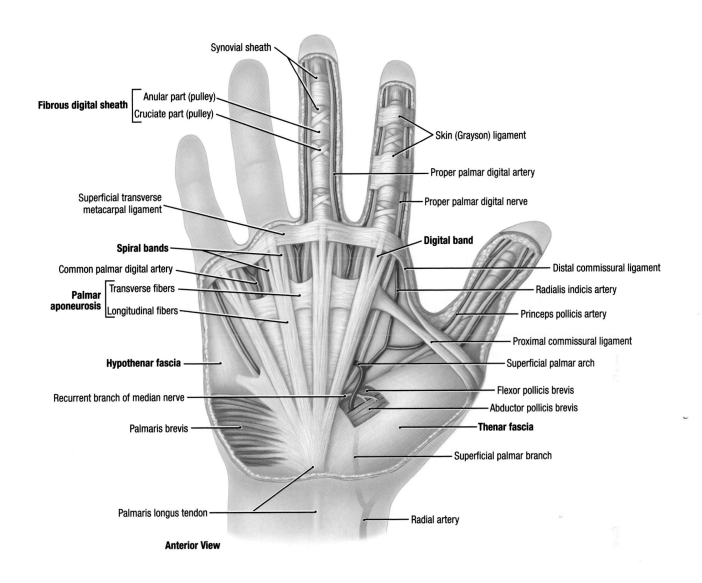

Synovial sheath

Fibrous digital sheath [Anular part (pulley)

Cruciate part (pulley)

Skin (Grayson) ligament

Proper palmar digital artery

Proper palmar digital nerve

Superficial transverse metacarpal ligament

Digital band

Spiral bands

Common palmar digital artery

Distal commissural ligament

Radialis indicis artery

Palmar aponeurosis [Transverse fibers

Longitudinal fibers

Princeps pollicis artery

Proximal commissural ligament

Hypothenar fascia

Superficial palmar arch

Flexor pollicis brevis

Recurrent branch of median nerve

Abductor pollicis brevis

Thenar fascia

Palmaris brevis

Superficial palmar branch

Palmaris longus tendon

Radial artery

Anterior View

6.63   Palmar (deep) fascia: palmar aponeurosis, thenar and hypothenar fascia

- The palmar fascia is thin over the thenar and hypothenar eminences, but thick centrally, where it forms the palmar aponeurosis, and in the digits, where it forms the fibrous digital sheaths.

- At the distal end (base) of the palmar aponeurosis, four bundles of digital and spiral bands continue to the bases and fibrous digital sheaths of digits 2–5.

- Dupuytren contracture is a disease of the palmar fascia resulting in progressive shortening, thickening, and fibrosis of the palmar fascia and palmar aponeurosis. The fibrous degeneration of the longitudinal digital bands of the aponeurosis on the medial side

of the hand pulls the 4th and 5th fingers into partial flexion at the metacarpophalangeal and proximal interphalangeal joints. The contracture is frequently bilateral. Treatment of Dupuytren contracture usually involves surgical excision of all fibrotic parts of the palmar fascia to free the fingers.

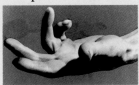

Dupuytren contracture

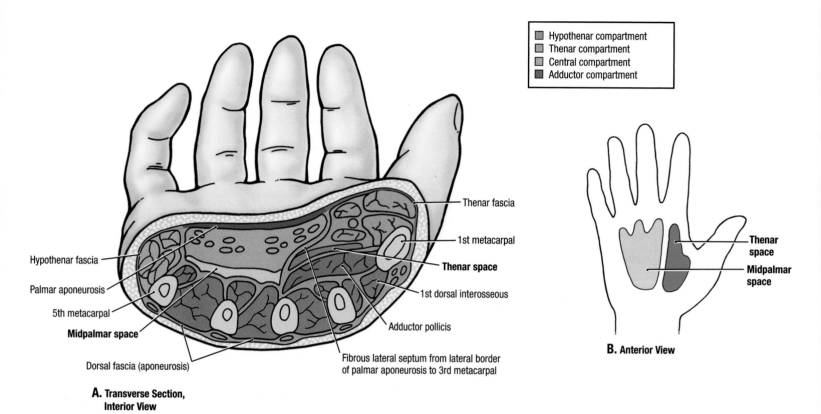

Hypothenar compartment
Thenar compartment
Central compartment
Adductor compartment

Thenar fascia

1st metacarpal

Thenar space

Hypothenar fascia

Palmar aponeurosis

5th metacarpal

Midpalmar space

Dorsal fascia (aponeurosis)

1st dorsal interosseous

Adductor pollicis

Fibrous lateral septum from lateral border
of palmar aponeurosis to 3rd metacarpal

**A. Transverse Section,
Interior View**

Thenar
space

Midpalmar
space

B. Anterior View

6.64   Compartments, spaces, and fascia of the palm

A. Transverse section through the middle of the palm showing the fascial compartments for the musculotendinous structures of the hand. **B.** Potential fascial spaces of palm.

- The potential midpalmar space lies posterior to the central compartment, is bounded medially by the hypothenar compartment, and is related distally to the synovial sheath of the 3rd, 4th, and 5th digits.
- The potential thenar space lies posterior to the thenar compartment and is related distally to the synovial sheath of the index finger.
- The potential midpalmar and thenar spaces are separated by a septum that passes from the palmar aponeurosis to the third metacarpal.

Because the palmar fascia is thick and strong, swellings resulting from hand infections usually appear on the dorsum of the hand where the fascia is thinner. The potential fascial spaces of the palm are important because they may become infected. The fascial spaces determine the extent and direction of the spread of pus formed in the infected areas. Depending on the site of infection, pus will accumulate in the thenar, hypothenar, or adductor compartments. Antibiotic therapy has made infections that spread beyond one of these fascial compartments rare, but an untreated infection can spread proximally through the carpal tunnel into the forearm anterior to the pronator quadratus and its fascia.

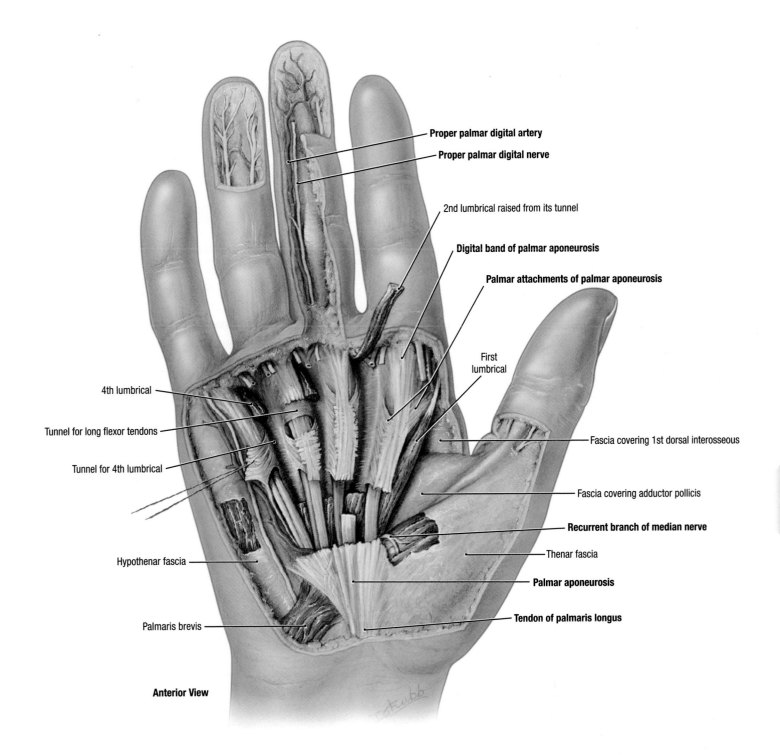

Proper palmar digital artery

Proper palmar digital nerve

2nd lumbrical raised from its tunnel

Digital band of palmar aponeurosis

Palmar attachments of palmar aponeurosis

First
lumbrical

Fascia covering 1st dorsal interosseous

Fascia covering adductor pollicis

Recurrent branch of median nerve

Thenar fascia

Palmar aponeurosis

Tendon of palmaris longus

4th lumbrical

Tunnel for long flexor tendons

Tunnel for 4th lumbrical

Hypothenar fascia

Palmaris brevis

Anterior View

6.65   **Attachments of palmar aponeurosis, digital vessels, and nerves**

- From the palmar aponeurosis, four longitudinal digital bands enter the fingers; the other fibers form extensive fibroareolar septa that pass posteriorly to the palmar ligaments (see Fig. 6.71) and, more proximally, to the fascia covering the interossei. Thus, two sets of tunnels exist in the distal half of the palm: (1) tunnels for long flexor tendons and (2) tunnels for lumbricals, digital vessels, and digital nerves.
- In the dissected middle finger, note the absence of fat deep to the skin creases of the fingers.

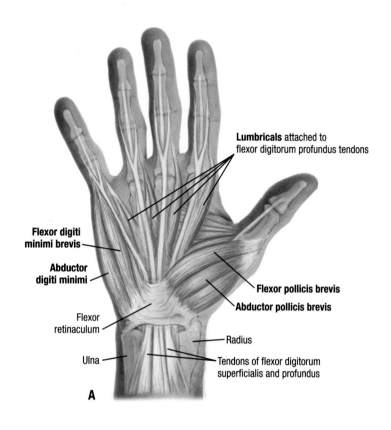

Lumbricals attached to
flexor digitorum profundus tendons

Flexor digiti
minimi brevis

Abductor
digiti minimi

Flexor
retinaculum

Ulna

Flexor pollicis brevis

Abductor pollicis brevis

Radius

Tendons of flexor digitorum
superficialis and profundus

A

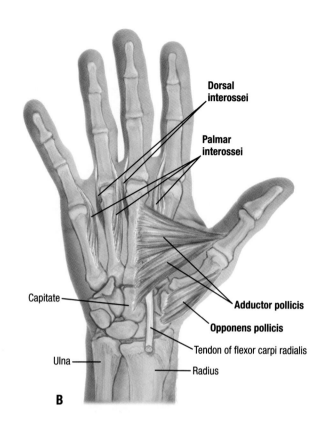

Dorsal
interossei

Palmar
interossei

Capitate

Ulna

Adductor pollicis

Opponens pollicis

Tendon of flexor carpi radialis

Radius

B

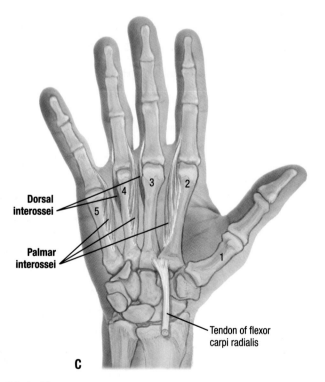

Dorsal
interossei

Palmar
interossei

4   3   2

5

1

Tendon of flexor
carpi radialis

C

Anterior Views

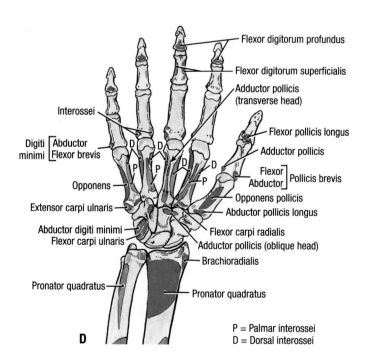

Interossei

Digiti ⎡ Abductor
minimi ⎣ Flexor brevis

Opponens

Extensor carpi ulnaris

Abductor digiti minimi
Flexor carpi ulnaris

Pronator quadratus

Flexor digitorum profundus

Flexor digitorum superficialis

Adductor pollicis
(transverse head)

Flexor pollicis longus

Adductor pollicis

Flexor ⎤ Pollicis brevis
Abductor ⎦

Opponens pollicis

Abductor pollicis longus

Flexor carpi radialis

Adductor pollicis (oblique head)

Brachioradialis

Pronator quadratus

P = Palmar interossei
D = Dorsal interossei

D

6.66   Muscular layers of palm

A. Lumbricals. **B.** Adductor pollicis. **C.** Dorsal and palmar interossei. **D.** Bony attachments.

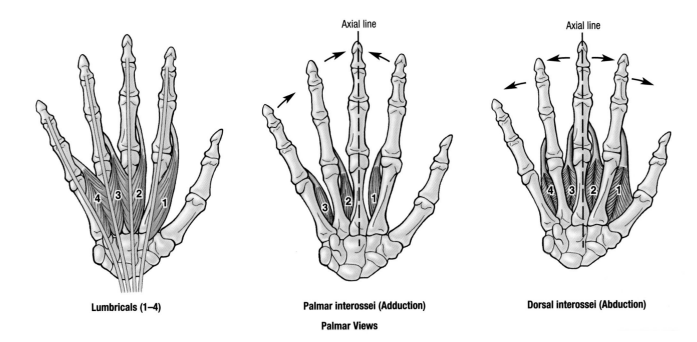

Lumbricals (1–4)   Palmar interossei (Adduction)   Dorsal interossei (Abduction)

Palmar Views

TABLE 6.11 MUSCLES OF HAND

Muscle	Proximal Attachment	Distal Attachment	Innervation	Main Actions
Abductor pollicis brevis	Flexor retinaculum and tubercles of scaphoid and trapezium	Lateral side of base of proximal phalanx of thumb	Recurrent branch of median nerve (**C8** and T1)	Abducts thumb and helps oppose it
Flexor pollicis brevis	Flexor retinaculum (transverse carpal ligament) and tubercle of trapezium			Flexes thumb
Opponens pollicis		Lateral side of first metacarpal		Opposes thumb toward center of palm and rotates it medially
Adductor pollicis	*Oblique head:* bases of second and third metacarpals, capitate, and adjacent carpal bones *Transverse head:* anterior surface of body of third metacarpal	Medial side of base of proximal phalanx of thumb	Deep branch of ulnar nerve (C8 and **T1**)	Adducts thumb toward middle digit
Abductor digiti minimi	Pisiform	Medial side of base of proximal phalanx of digit 5	Deep branch of ulnar nerve (C8 and T1)	Abducts digit 5
Flexor digiti minimi brevis	Hook of hamate and flexor retinaculum (transverse carpal ligament)	Medial border of fifth metacarpal		Flexes proximal phalanx of digit 5
Opponens digiti minimi				Draws fifth metacarpal anteriorly and rotates it, bringing digit 5 into opposition with thumb
Lumbricals 1 and 2	Lateral two tendons of flexor digitorum profundus	Lateral sides of extensor expansions of digits 2–5	Median nerve (C8 and **T1**)	Flex digits at metacarpophalangeal joints and extend interphalangeal joints
Lumbricals 3 and 4	Medial three tendons of flexor digitorum profundus		Deep branch of ulnar nerve (C8 and **T1**)	
Dorsal interossei 1–4	Adjacent sides of two metacarpals	Extensor expansions and bases of proximal phalanges of digits 2–4		Abduct digits 2–5 and assist lumbricals
Palmar interossei 1–3	Palmar surfaces of second, fourth, and fifth metacarpals	Extensor expansions of digits and bases of proximal phalanges of digits 2, 4, and 5		Adduct digits 2, 4, and 5 and assist lumbricals

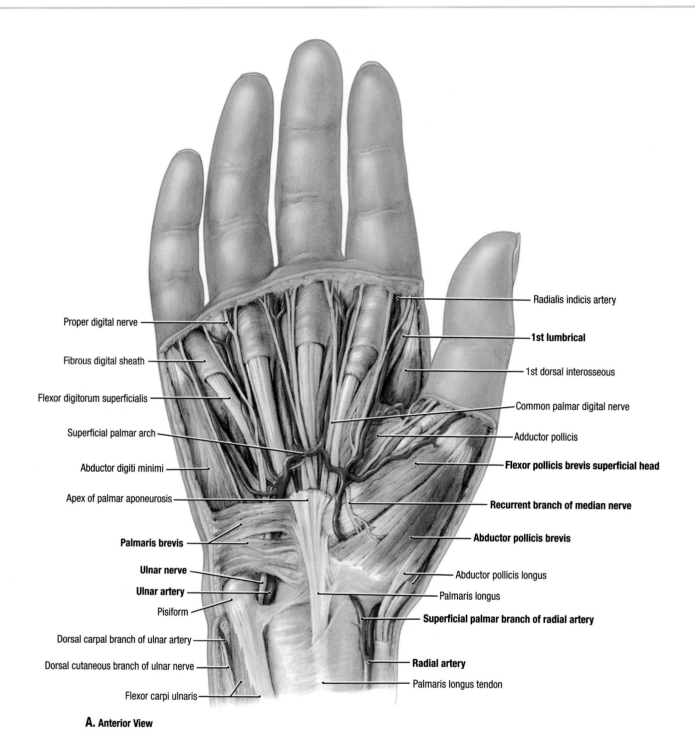

Proper digital nerve

Fibrous digital sheath

Flexor digitorum superficialis

Superficial palmar arch

Abductor digiti minimi

Apex of palmar aponeurosis

Palmaris brevis

Ulnar nerve

Ulnar artery

Pisiform

Dorsal carpal branch of ulnar artery

Dorsal cutaneous branch of ulnar nerve

Flexor carpi ulnaris

Radialis indicis artery

1st lumbrical

1st dorsal interosseous

Common palmar digital nerve

Adductor pollicis

Flexor pollicis brevis superficial head

Recurrent branch of median nerve

Abductor pollicis brevis

Abductor pollicis longus

Palmaris longus

Superficial palmar branch of radial artery

Radial artery

Palmaris longus tendon

A. Anterior View

6.67 **Superficial dissection of palm, ulnar, and median nerves**

A. Superficial palmar arch and digital nerves and vessels.
- The skin, superficial fascia, palmar aponeurosis, and thenar and hypothenar fasciae have been removed.
- The superficial palmar arch is formed by the ulnar artery and completed by the superficial palmar branch of the radial artery.

Bleeding is usually profuse when the palmar (arterial) arches are lacerated. It may not be sufficient to ligate (tie off) only one forearm artery when the arches are lacerated, because these vessels usually have numerous communications in the forearm and hand and thus bleed from both ends.

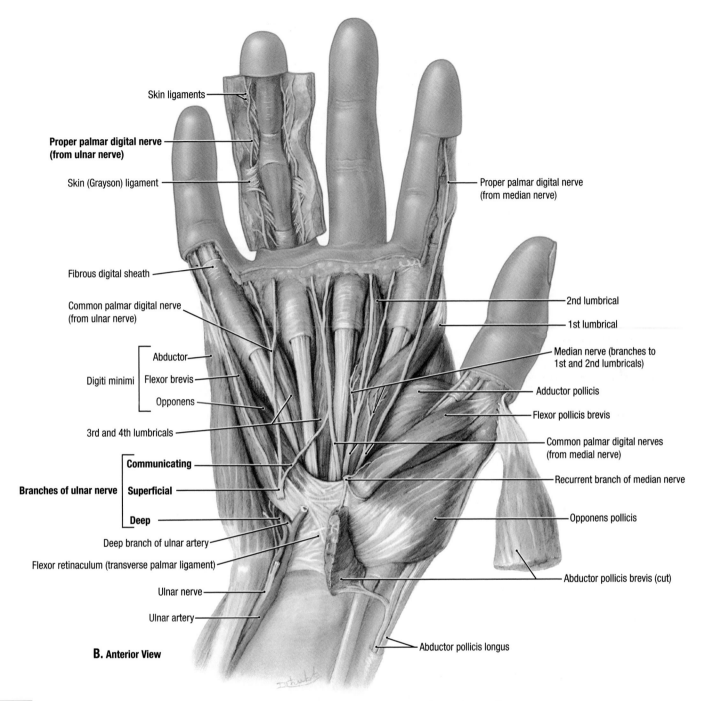

Skin ligaments

Proper palmar digital nerve (from ulnar nerve)

Skin (Grayson) ligament

Fibrous digital sheath

Common palmar digital nerve (from ulnar nerve)

Digiti minimi { Abductor — Flexor brevis — Opponens

3rd and 4th lumbricals

Branches of ulnar nerve { **Communicating** — **Superficial** — **Deep**

Deep branch of ulnar artery

Flexor retinaculum (transverse palmar ligament)

Ulnar nerve

Ulnar artery

B. Anterior View

Proper palmar digital nerve (from median nerve)

2nd lumbrical

1st lumbrical

Median nerve (branches to 1st and 2nd lumbricals)

Adductor pollicis

Flexor pollicis brevis

Common palmar digital nerves (from medial nerve)

Recurrent branch of median nerve

Opponens pollicis

Abductor pollicis brevis (cut)

Abductor pollicis longus

6.67   **Superficial dissection of palm, ulnar, and median nerves** *(continued)*

B. Ulnar and median nerves.

Carpal tunnel syndrome results from any lesion that significantly reduces the size of the carpal tunnel or, more commonly, increases the size of some of the structures (or their coverings) that pass though it (e.g., inflammation of the synovial sheaths). The median nerve is the most sensitive structure in the carpal tunnel. The median nerve has two terminal sensory branches that supply the skin of the hand; hence paresthesia (tingling), hypothesia (diminished sensation), or anesthesia (absence of tactile sensation) may occur in the lateral three and a half digits. Recall, however, that the palmar cutaneous branch of the median nerve

arises proximal to and does not pass through the carpal tunnel; thus sensation in the central palm remains unaffected. This nerve also has one terminal motor branch, the recurrent branch, which innervates the three thenar muscles. Wasting of the thenar eminence and progressive loss of coordination and strength in the thumb may occur. To relieve the compression and resulting symptoms, partial or complete surgical division of the flexor retinaculum, a procedure called **carpal tunnel release**, may be necessary. The incision for carpal tunnel release is made toward the medial side of the wrist and flexor retinaculum to avoid possible injury to the recurrent branch of the median nerve.

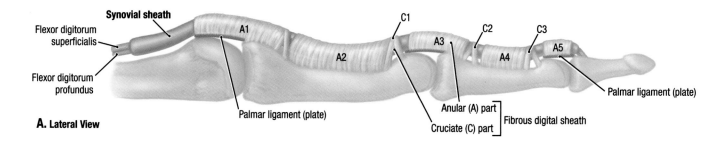

Synovial sheath

Flexor digitorum superficialis

Flexor digitorum profundus

C1   C2   C3

A1   A2   A3   A4   A5

Palmar ligament (plate)

Anular (A) part

Cruciate (C) part

Fibrous digital sheath

Palmar ligament (plate)

A. Lateral View

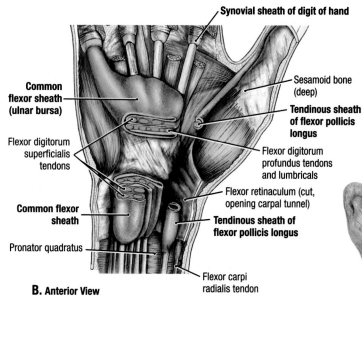

Synovial sheath of digit of hand

Common flexor sheath (ulnar bursa)

Flexor digitorum superficialis tendons

Common flexor sheath

Pronator quadratus

Sesamoid bone (deep)

Tendinous sheath of flexor pollicis longus

Flexor digitorum profundus tendons and lumbricals

Flexor retinaculum (cut, opening carpal tunnel)

Tendinous sheath of flexor pollicis longus

Flexor carpi radialis tendon

B. Anterior View

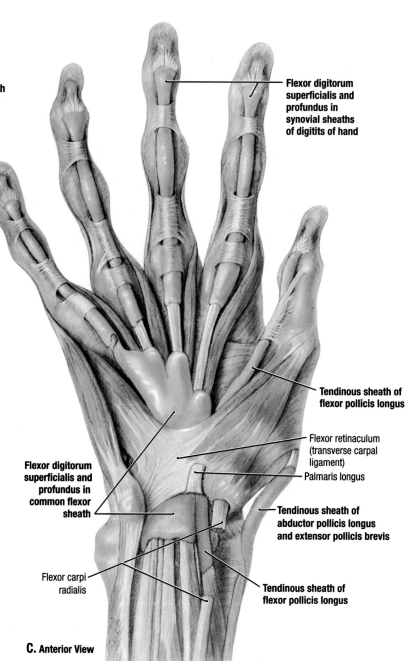

Flexor digitorum superficialis and profundus in synovial sheaths of digitits of hand

Tendinous sheath of flexor pollicis longus

Flexor retinaculum (transverse carpal ligament)

Palmaris longus

Tendinous sheath of abductor pollicis longus and extensor pollicis brevis

Flexor digitorum superficialis and profundus in common flexor sheath

Flexor carpi radialis

Tendinous sheath of flexor pollicis longus

C. Anterior View

6.68   Synovial sheaths of palm of hand

A. Anular and cruciate parts (pulleys) of the fibrous digital sheath. **B.** Common flexor sheath. **C.** Tendinous (synovial) sheaths of long flexor tendons of the digits.

Injuries such as puncture of a finger by a rusty nail can cause infection of the digital synovial sheaths. When inflammation of the tendon and synovial sheath (tenosynovitis) occurs, the digit swells and movement becomes painful. Because the tendons of the 2nd–4th digits nearly always have separate synovial sheaths, the infection usually is confined to the infected digits. If the infection is untreated, however, the proximal ends of these sheaths may rupture, allowing the infection to spread to the midpalmar space. Because the synovial sheath of the little finger is usually continuous with the common flexor sheath, tenosynovitis in this finger may spread to the common flexor sheath and thus through the palm and carpal tunnel to the anterior forearm. Likewise, tenosynovitis in the thumb may spread through the continuous tendinous sheath of flexor pollicis longus.

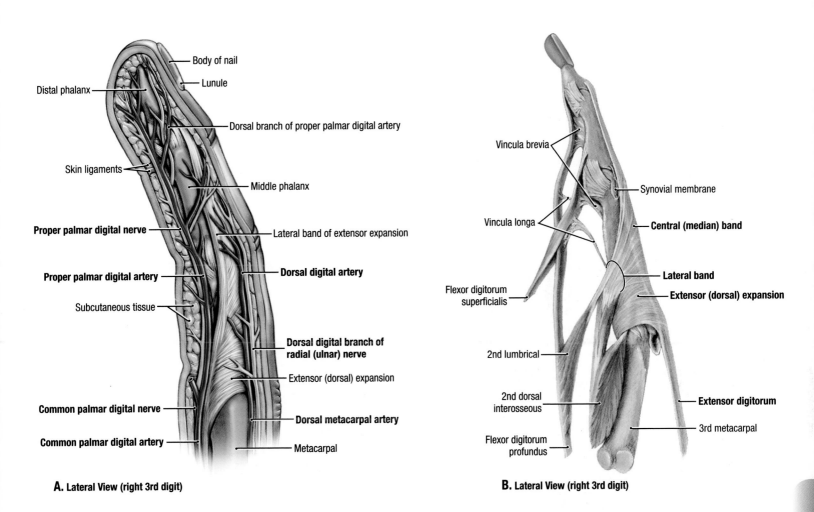

Body of nail

Lunule

Distal phalanx

Dorsal branch of proper palmar digital artery

Skin ligaments

Middle phalanx

Proper palmar digital nerve

Lateral band of extensor expansion

Proper palmar digital artery

Dorsal digital artery

Subcutaneous tissue

Dorsal digital branch of radial (ulnar) nerve

Extensor (dorsal) expansion

Common palmar digital nerve

Dorsal metacarpal artery

Common palmar digital artery

Metacarpal

A. Lateral View (right 3rd digit)

Vincula brevia

Synovial membrane

Vincula longa

Central (median) band

Flexor digitorum superficialis

Lateral band

Extensor (dorsal) expansion

2nd lumbrical

2nd dorsal interosseous

Extensor digitorum

3rd metacarpal

Flexor digitorum profundus

B. Lateral View (right 3rd digit)

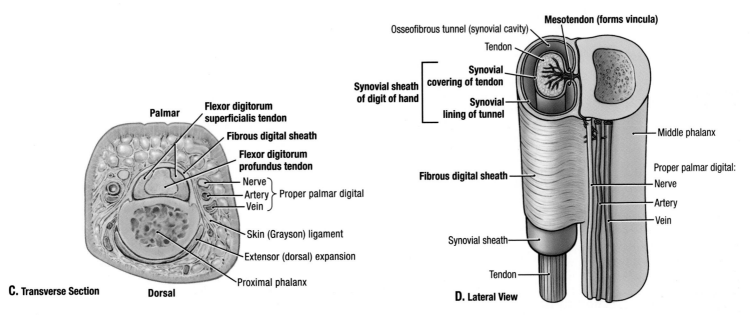

Osseofibrous tunnel (synovial cavity)

Mesotendon (forms vincula)

Tendon

Synovial covering of tendon

Synovial sheath of digit of hand

Synovial lining of tunnel

Middle phalanx

Palmar

Flexor digitorum superficialis tendon

Fibrous digital sheath

Flexor digitorum profundus tendon

Nerve

Artery   } Proper palmar digital

Vein

Proper palmar digital:

Nerve

Artery

Vein

Fibrous digital sheath

Skin (Grayson) ligament

Extensor (dorsal) expansion

Synovial sheath

Proximal phalanx

Tendon

C. Transverse Section   **Dorsal**

D. Lateral View

6.69   Digital tendons, vessels, and nerves

A. Digital vessels and nerves. **B.** Extensor expansion of the 3rd (middle) digit. **C.** Transverse section through the proximal phalanx. **D.** Osseofibrous tunnel and tendinous (synovial) sheath.

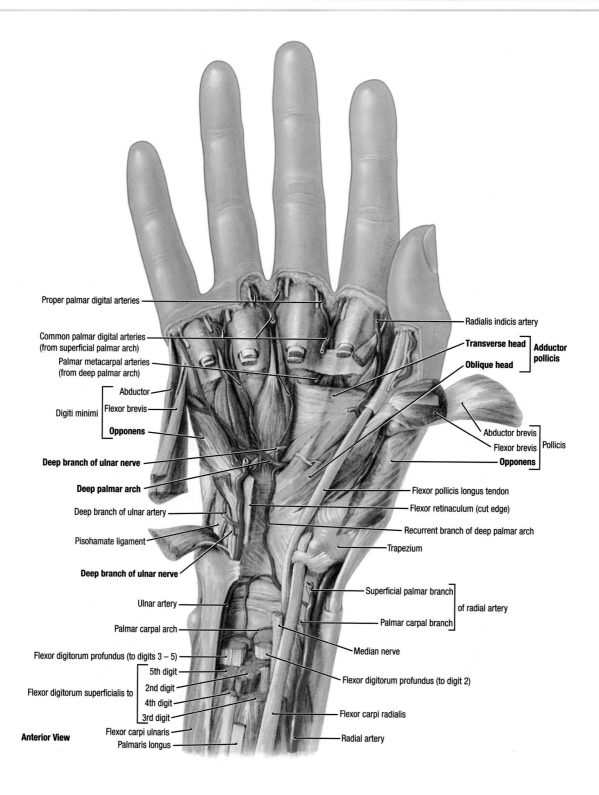

Proper palmar digital arteries

Common palmar digital arteries
(from superficial palmar arch)

Palmar metacarpal arteries
(from deep palmar arch)

Abductor

Digiti minimi — Flexor brevis

Opponens

Deep branch of ulnar nerve

Deep palmar arch

Deep branch of ulnar artery

Pisohamate ligament

Deep branch of ulnar nerve

Ulnar artery

Palmar carpal arch

Flexor digitorum profundus (to digits 3 – 5)

5th digit
2nd digit
Flexor digitorum superficialis to
4th digit
3rd digit

Anterior View — Flexor carpi ulnaris

Palmaris longus

Radialis indicis artery

Transverse head } **Adductor**
Oblique head } **pollicis**

Abductor brevis } Pollicis
Flexor brevis }
Opponens

Flexor pollicis longus tendon

Flexor retinaculum (cut edge)

Recurrent branch of deep palmar arch

Trapezium

Superficial palmar branch]
] of radial artery
Palmar carpal branch]

Median nerve

Flexor digitorum profundus (to digit 2)

Flexor carpi radialis

Radial artery

6.70   Deep dissection of palm

- The deep branch of the ulnar artery joins the radial artery to form the deep palmar arch.

Compression of the ulnar nerve may occur at the wrist where it passes between the pisiform and the hook of hamate. The depression between these bones is converted by the pisohamate ligament into an osseofibrous ulnar canal (Guyon canal). Ulnar canal syndrome is manifest by hypoesthesia in the medial one and one half fingers and weakness of the intrinsic hand muscles. Clawing of the 4th and 5th fingers may occur, but in contrast to proximal nerve injury, their ability to flex is unaffected and there is no radical deviation of the hand.

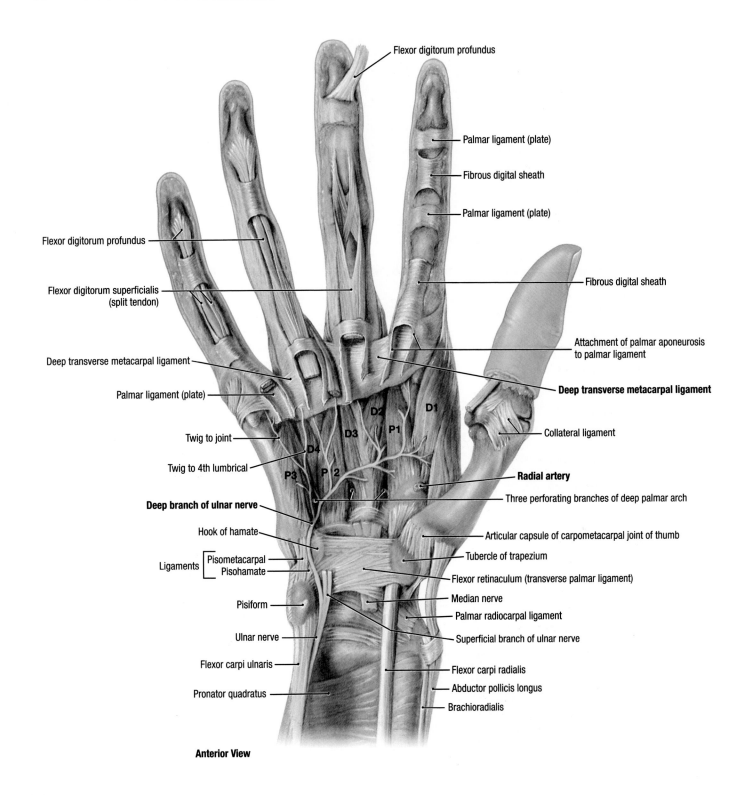

Flexor digitorum profundus

Palmar ligament (plate)

Fibrous digital sheath

Palmar ligament (plate)

Fibrous digital sheath

Flexor digitorum profundus

Flexor digitorum superficialis
(split tendon)

Attachment of palmar aponeurosis
to palmar ligament

Deep transverse metacarpal ligament

Deep transverse metacarpal ligament

Palmar ligament (plate)

Collateral ligament

D2   D1

D3   P1

Twig to joint

D4

Radial artery

Twig to 4th lumbrical

P3   P 2

Three perforating branches of deep palmar arch

Deep branch of ulnar nerve

Articular capsule of carpometacarpal joint of thumb

Hook of hamate

Tubercle of trapezium

Ligaments [Pisometacarpal
Pisohamate]

Flexor retinaculum (transverse palmar ligament)

Median nerve

Pisiform

Palmar radiocarpal ligament

Ulnar nerve

Superficial branch of ulnar nerve

Flexor carpi ulnaris

Flexor carpi radialis

Pronator quadratus

Abductor pollicis longus

Brachioradialis

Anterior View

6.71   Deep dissection of palm and digits with deep branch of ulnar nerve

- Three unipennate palmar *(P1–3)* and four bipennate dorsal *(D1–4)* interosseous muscles are illustrated; the palmar interossei adduct the fingers, and the dorsal interossei abduct the fingers in relation to the axial line, an imaginary line drawn through the long axis of the 3rd digit (see Table 6.11).
- The deep transverse metacarpal ligaments unite the palmar ligaments; the lumbricals pass anterior to the deep transverse metacarpal ligament, and the interossei pass posterior to the ligament.
- Note the ulnar (Guyon) canal through which the ulnar vessels and nerve pass medial to the pisiform.

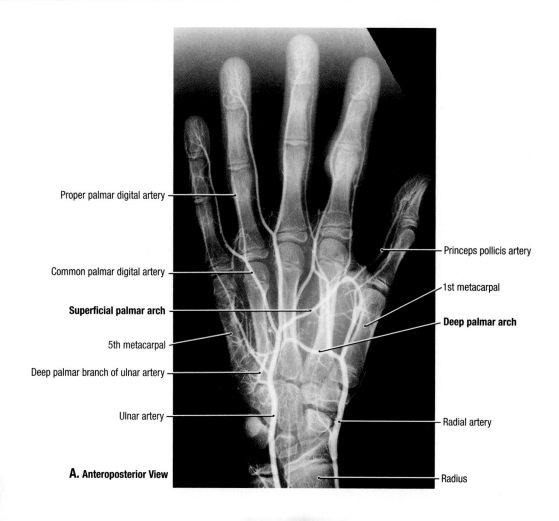

Proper palmar digital artery

Common palmar digital artery

Superficial palmar arch

5th metacarpal

Deep palmar branch of ulnar artery

Ulnar artery

Princeps pollicis artery

1st metacarpal

Deep palmar arch

Radial artery

Radius

A. Anteroposterior View

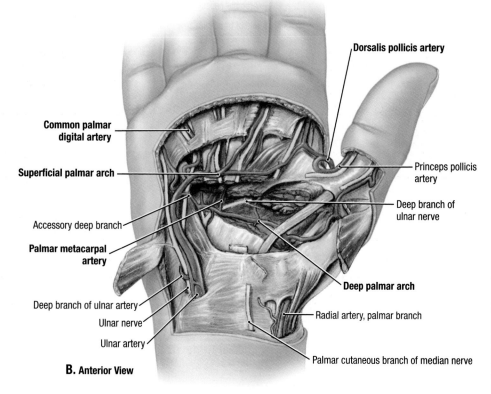

Common palmar digital artery

Superficial palmar arch

Accessory deep branch

Palmar metacarpal artery

Deep branch of ulnar artery

Ulnar nerve

Ulnar artery

Dorsalis pollicis artery

Princeps pollicis artery

Deep branch of ulnar nerve

Deep palmar arch

Radial artery, palmar branch

Palmar cutaneous branch of median nerve

B. Anterior View

6.72   Arterial supply of hand

A. Arteriogram of the hand. **B.** Dissection of palmar arterial arches.

• The superficial palmar arch is usually completed by the superficial palmar branch of the radial artery, but in this specimen the dorsalis pollicis artery completes the arch.

The superficial and deep palmar (arterial) arches are not palpable, but their surface markings are visible. The superficial palmar arch occurs at the level of the distal border of the fully extended thumb. The deep palmar arch lies approximately 1 cm proximal to the superficial palmar arch. The location of these arches should be borne in mind in wounds of the palm and when palmar incisions are made.

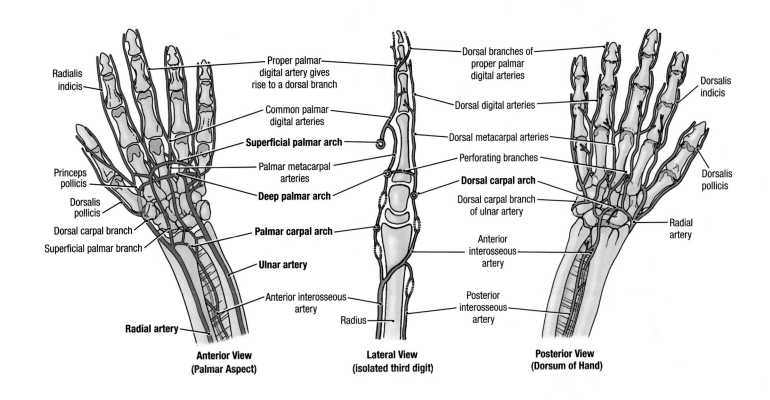

**Anterior View
(Palmar Aspect)**

**Lateral View
(isolated third digit)**

**Posterior View
(Dorsum of Hand)**

TABLE 6.12 ARTERIES OF HAND

Artery	Origin	Course
Superficial palmar arch	Direct continuation of ulnar artery; arch is completed on lateral side by superficial branch of radial artery or another of its branches	Curves laterally deep to palmar aponeurosis and superficial to long flexor tendons; curve of arch lies across palm at level of distal border of extended thumb
Deep palmar arch	Direct continuation of radial artery; arch is completed on medial side by deep branch of ulnar artery	Curves medially, deep to long flexor tendons and is in contact with bases of metacarpals
Common palmar digitals	Superficial palmar arch	Pass directly on lumbricals to webbings of digits
Proper palmar digitals	Common palmar digital arteries	Run along sides of digits 2–5
Princeps pollicis	Radial artery as it turns into palm	Descends on palmar aspect of first metacarpal and divides at the base of proximal phalanx into two branches that run along sides of thumb
Radialis indicis	Radial artery, but may arise from princeps pollicis artery	Passes along lateral side of index finger to its distal end
Dorsal carpal arch	Radial and ulnar arteries	Arches within fascia on dorsum of hand

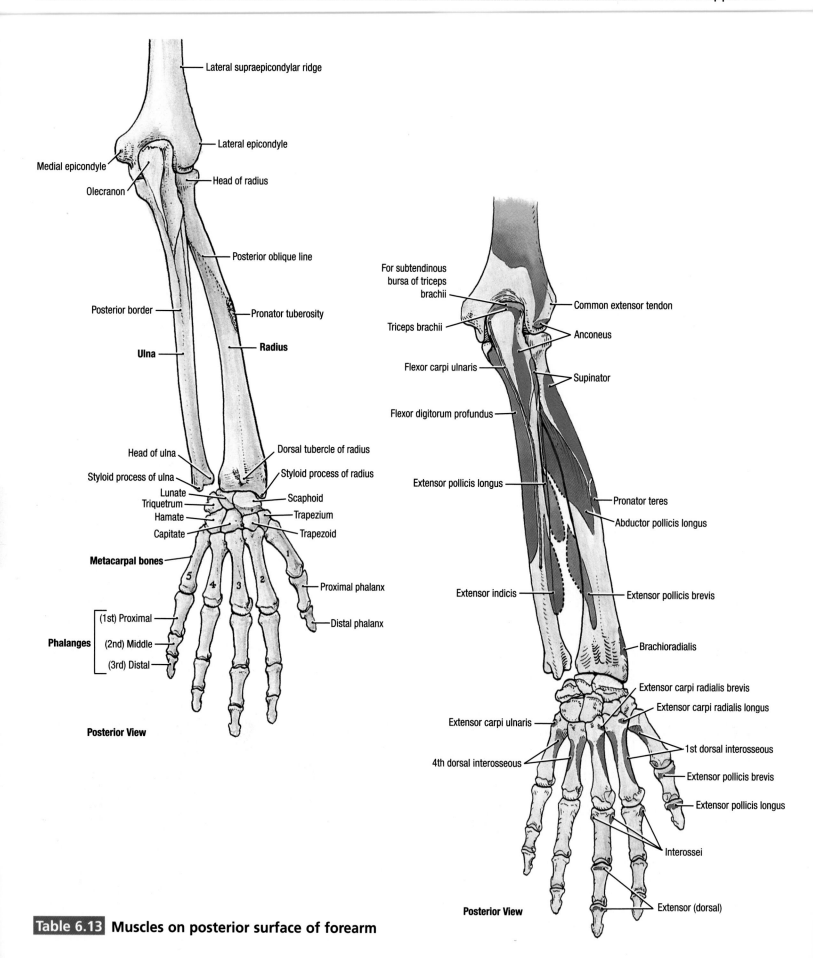

Lateral supraepicondylar ridge

Lateral epicondyle

Medial epicondyle

Head of radius

Olecranon

Posterior oblique line

Posterior border

Pronator tuberosity

Ulna

Radius

Head of ulna

Dorsal tubercle of radius

Styloid process of ulna

Styloid process of radius

Lunate

Scaphoid

Triquetrum

Hamate

Trapezium

Capitate

Trapezoid

Metacarpal bones

1

5 4 3 2

Proximal phalanx

(1st) Proximal

Distal phalanx

Phalanges

(2nd) Middle

(3rd) Distal

Posterior View

For subtendinous bursa of triceps brachii

Common extensor tendon

Triceps brachii

Anconeus

Flexor carpi ulnaris

Supinator

Flexor digitorum profundus

Extensor pollicis longus

Pronator teres

Abductor pollicis longus

Extensor indicis

Extensor pollicis brevis

Brachioradialis

Extensor carpi radialis brevis

Extensor carpi radialis longus

Extensor carpi ulnaris

1st dorsal interosseous

4th dorsal interosseous

Extensor pollicis brevis

Extensor pollicis longus

Interossei

Extensor (dorsal)

Posterior View

Table 6.13 **Muscles on posterior surface of forearm**

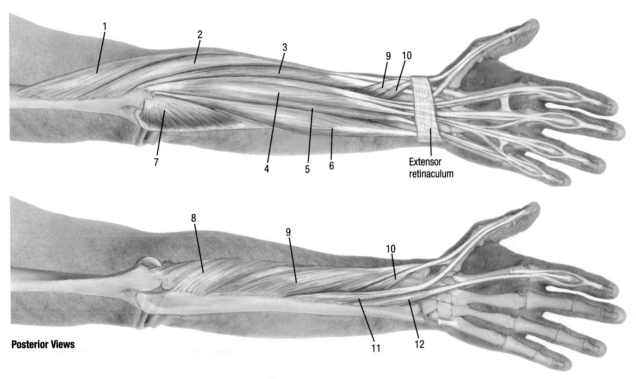

Extensor retinaculum

Posterior Views

TABLE 6.13 MUSCLES OF POSTERIOR SURFACE OF FOREARM

Muscle	Proximal Attachment	Distal Attachment	Innervation	Main Actions
Brachioradialis (1)	Proximal two thirds of lateral supraepicondylar ridge of humerus	Lateral surface of distal end of radius	Radial nerve (C5, **C6**, and C7)	Flexes forearm
Extensor carpi radialis longus (2)	Lateral supraepicondylar ridge of humerus	Base of second metacarpal bone	Radial nerve (C6 and C7)	Extend and abduct hand at wrist joint
Extensor carpi radialis brevis (3)		Base of third metacarpal bone	Deep branch of radial nerve (**C7** and C8)	
Extensor digitorum (4)	Lateral epicondyle of humerus	Extensor expansions of medial four digits	Posterior interosseous nerve (C7 and C8), a branch of the radial nerve	Extends medial four digits at metacarpophalangeal joints; extends hand at wrist joint
Extensor digiti minimi (5)		Extensor expansion of fifth digit		Extends fifth digit at metacarpophalangeal and interphalangeal joints
Extensor carpi ulnaris (6)	Lateral epicondyle of humerus and posterior border of ulna	Base of fifth metacarpal bone		Extends and adducts hand at wrist joint
Anconeus (7)	Lateral epicondyle of humerus	Lateral surface of olecranon and superior part of posterior surface of ulna	Radial nerve (C7, C8, and T1)	Assists triceps in extending elbow joint; stabilizes elbow joint; abducts ulna during pronation
Supinator (8)	Lateral epicondyle of humerus, radial collateral and anular ligaments, supinator fossa, and crest of ulna	Lateral, posterior, and anterior surfaces of proximal third of radius	Deep branch of radial nerve (C5 and **C6**)	Supinates forearm
Abductor pollicis longus (9)	Posterior surface of ulna, radius, and interosseous membrane	Base of first metacarpal bone	Posterior interosseous nerve (C7 and **C8**)	Abducts thumb and extends it at carpometacarpal joint
Extensor pollicis brevis (10)	Posterior surface of radius and interosseous membrane	Base of proximal phalanx of thumb		Extends proximal phalanx of thumb at metacarpophalangeal **joint**
Extensor pollicis longus (11)	Posterior surface of middle third of ulna and interosseous membrane	Base of distal phalanx of thumb		Extends distal phalanx of thumb at metacarpophalangeal and interphalangeal joints
Extensor indicis (12)	Posterior surface of ulna and interosseous membrane	Extensor expansion of second digit		Extends second digit and helps to extend hand

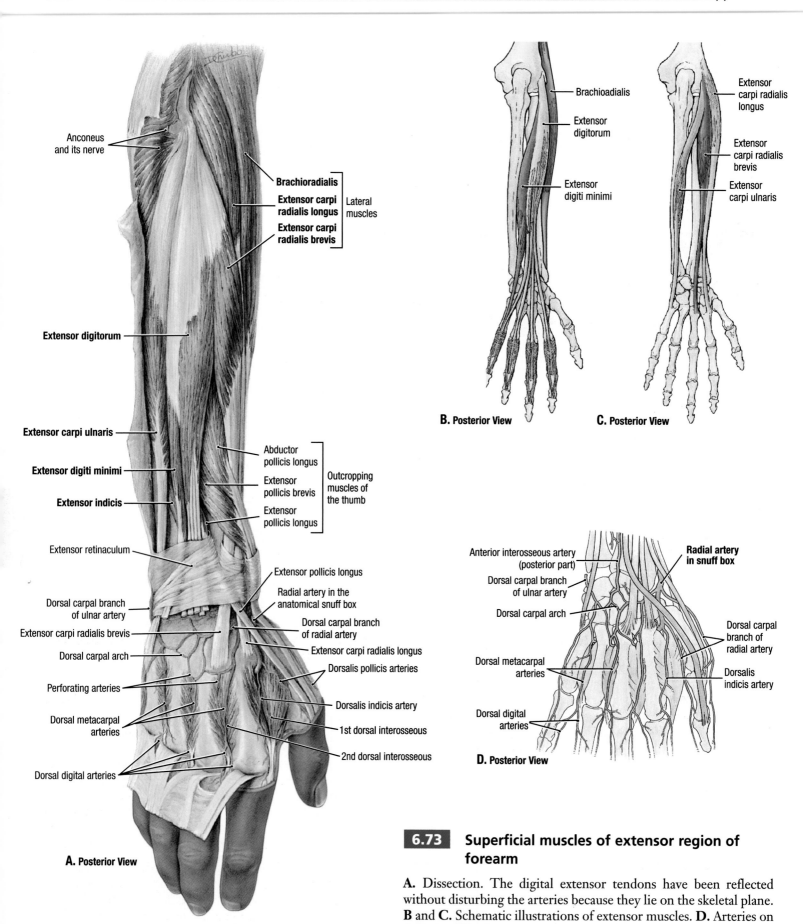

Anconeus and its nerve

Brachioradialis
Extensor carpi radialis longus
Extensor carpi radialis brevis
} Lateral muscles

Extensor digitorum

Extensor carpi ulnaris

Extensor digiti minimi

Extensor indicis

Abductor pollicis longus
Extensor pollicis brevis
Extensor pollicis longus
} Outcropping muscles of the thumb

Extensor retinaculum

Dorsal carpal branch of ulnar artery

Extensor carpi radialis brevis

Dorsal carpal arch

Perforating arteries

Dorsal metacarpal arteries

Dorsal digital arteries

Extensor pollicis longus
Radial artery in the anatomical snuff box
Dorsal carpal branch of radial artery
Extensor carpi radialis longus
Dorsalis pollicis arteries
Dorsalis indicis artery
1st dorsal interosseous
2nd dorsal interosseous

A. Posterior View

Brachioadialis
Extensor digitorum
Extensor digiti minimi

B. Posterior View

Extensor carpi radialis longus
Extensor carpi radialis brevis
Extensor carpi ulnaris

C. Posterior View

Anterior interosseous artery (posterior part)
Dorsal carpal branch of ulnar artery
Dorsal carpal arch
Dorsal metacarpal arteries
Dorsal digital arteries

Radial artery in snuff box
Dorsal carpal branch of radial artery
Dorsalis indicis artery

D. Posterior View

6.73 **Superficial muscles of extensor region of forearm**

A. Dissection. The digital extensor tendons have been reflected without disturbing the arteries because they lie on the skeletal plane. **B** and **C.** Schematic illustrations of extensor muscles. **D.** Arteries on dorsum of hand.

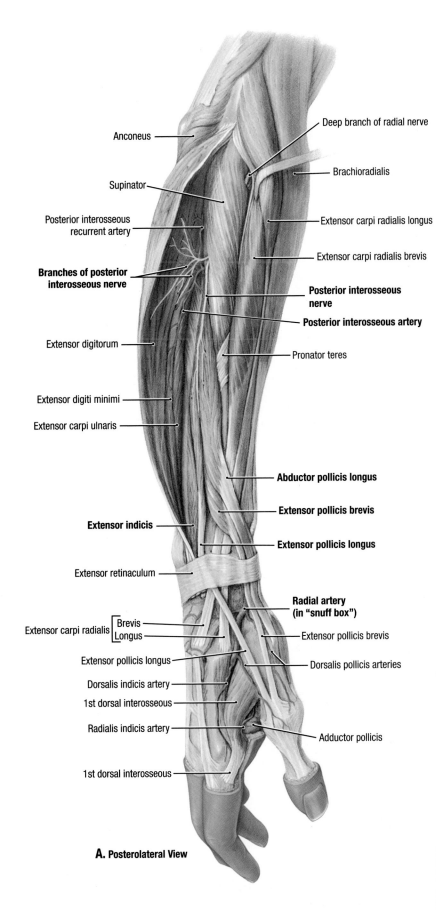

Anconeus

Deep branch of radial nerve

Supinator

Brachioradialis

Posterior interosseous
recurrent artery

Extensor carpi radialis longus

Extensor carpi radialis brevis

**Branches of posterior
interosseous nerve**

**Posterior interosseous
nerve**

Posterior interosseous artery

Extensor digitorum

Pronator teres

Extensor digiti minimi

Extensor carpi ulnaris

Abductor pollicis longus

Extensor pollicis brevis

Extensor indicis

Extensor pollicis longus

Extensor retinaculum

**Radial artery
(in "snuff box")**

Extensor carpi radialis ⎡ Brevis
                   ⎣ Longus

Extensor pollicis brevis

Extensor pollicis longus

Dorsalis pollicis arteries

Dorsalis indicis artery

1st dorsal interosseous

Radialis indicis artery

Adductor pollicis

1st dorsal interosseous

A. Posterolateral View

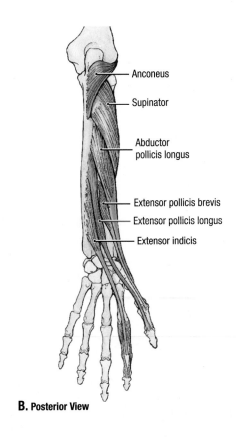

Anconeus

Supinator

Abductor
pollicis longus

Extensor pollicis brevis

Extensor pollicis longus

Extensor indicis

B. Posterior View

6.74   **Deep structures on extensor aspect of
forearm**

A. Dissection. **B.** Schematic illustration.

- Three "outcropping" muscles of the thumb (abductor pollicis longus, extensor pollicis brevis, and extensor pollicis longus) emerge between the extensor carpi radialis brevis and the extensor digitorum.
- The laterally retracted brachioradialis and extensor carpi radialis longus and brevis muscles and supinator muscles are innervated by the deep branch of the radial nerve; the other extensor muscles are supplied by the posterior interosseous nerve, which is a continuation of the deep branch of the radial nerve that pierced the supinator.

Severance of the deep branch of the radial nerve results in an inability to extend the thumb and the metacarpophalangeal joints of the other digits. Loss of sensation does not occur because the deep branch is entirely muscular and articular in distribution.

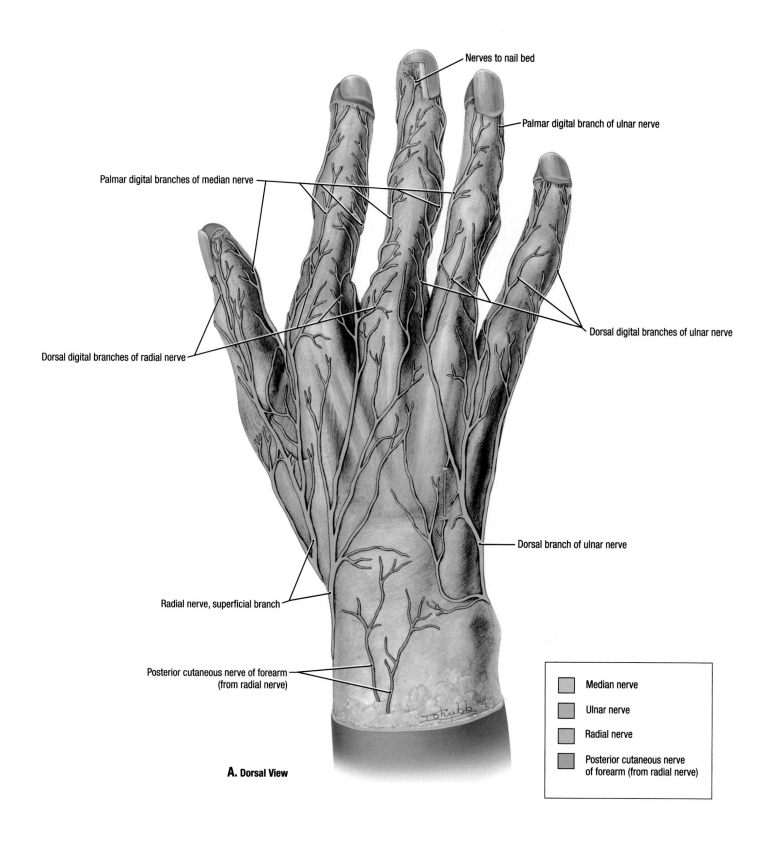

Nerves to nail bed

Palmar digital branch of ulnar nerve

Palmar digital branches of median nerve

Dorsal digital branches of ulnar nerve

Dorsal digital branches of radial nerve

Dorsal branch of ulnar nerve

Radial nerve, superficial branch

Posterior cutaneous nerve of forearm
(from radial nerve)

Median nerve

Ulnar nerve

Radial nerve

Posterior cutaneous nerve
of forearm (from radial nerve)

A. Dorsal View

6.75 Cutaneous innervation of hand

A. Dissection of nerves of dorsum of hand.

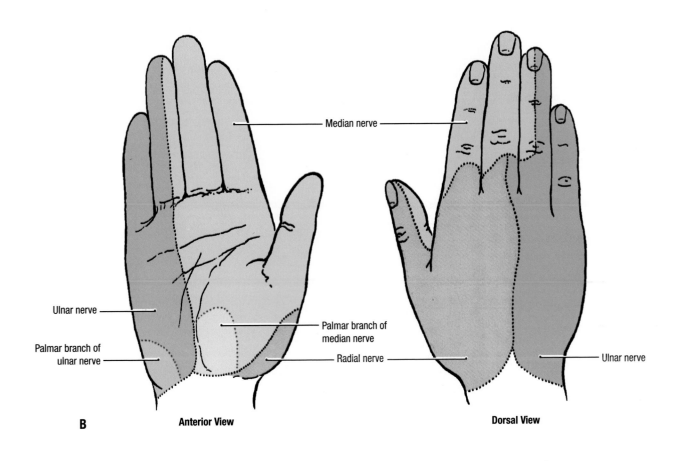

Median nerve

Ulnar nerve

Palmar branch of median nerve

Palmar branch of ulnar nerve

Radial nerve

Ulnar nerve

B   **Anterior View**

Dorsal View

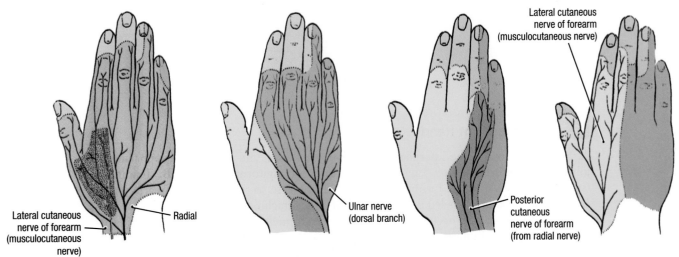

Lateral cutaneous nerve of forearm (musculocutaneous nerve)

Radial

Ulnar nerve (dorsal branch)

Lateral cutaneous nerve of forearm (musculocutaneous nerve)

Posterior cutaneous nerve of forearm (from radial nerve)

C. Dorsal Views

6.75   **Cutaneous innervation of hand** *(continued)*

B. Distribution of the cutaneous nerves to the palm and dorsum of the hand, schematic illustration. **C.** Variations in pattern of cutaneous nerves in dorsum of hand.

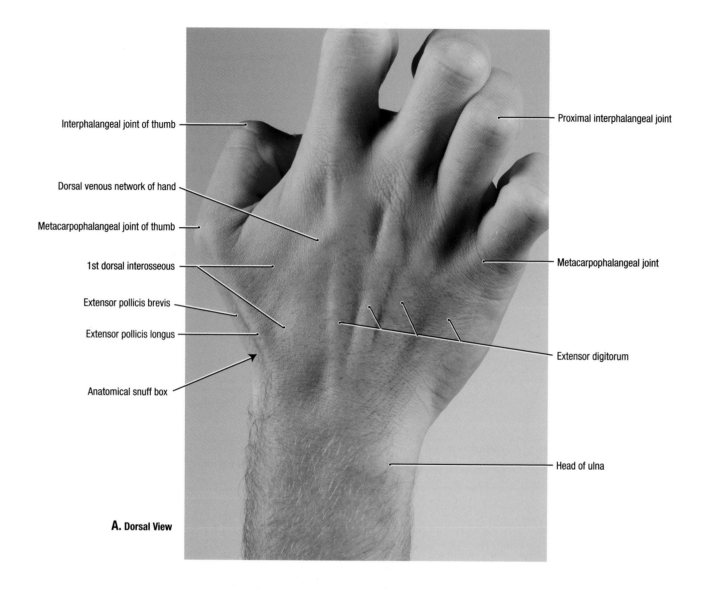

Interphalangeal joint of thumb

Dorsal venous network of hand

Metacarpophalangeal joint of thumb

1st dorsal interosseous

Extensor pollicis brevis

Extensor pollicis longus

Anatomical snuff box

Proximal interphalangeal joint

Metacarpophalangeal joint

Extensor digitorum

Head of ulna

A. Dorsal View

6.76 **Dorsum of hand**

A. Surface anatomy. The interphalangeal joints are flexed, and the metacarpophalangeal joints are hyperextended to demonstrate the extensor digitorum tendons. **B.** Tendinous (synovial) sheaths distended with blue fluid. **C.** Transverse section of distal forearm (*numbers* refer to structures labeled in B). **D.** Sites of bony attachments.

- Six tendinous sheaths occupy the six osseofibrous tunnels deep to the extensor retinaculum. They contain nine tendons: tendons for the thumb in sheaths 1 and 3, tendons for the extensors of the wrist in sheaths 2 and 6, and tendons for the extensors of the wrist and fingers in sheaths 4 and 5.
- The tendon of the extensor pollicis longus hooks around the dorsal tubercle of radius to pass obliquely across the tendons of the extensor carpi radialis longus and brevis to the thumb.

The tendons of the abductor pollicis longus and extensor pollicis brevis are in the same tendinous sheath on the dorsum of the wrist. Excessive friction of these tendons results in fibrous thickening of the sheath and stenosis of the osseofibrous tunnel, Quervain tenovaginitis stenosans. This condition causes pain in the wrist that radiates proximally to the forearm and distally to the thumb.

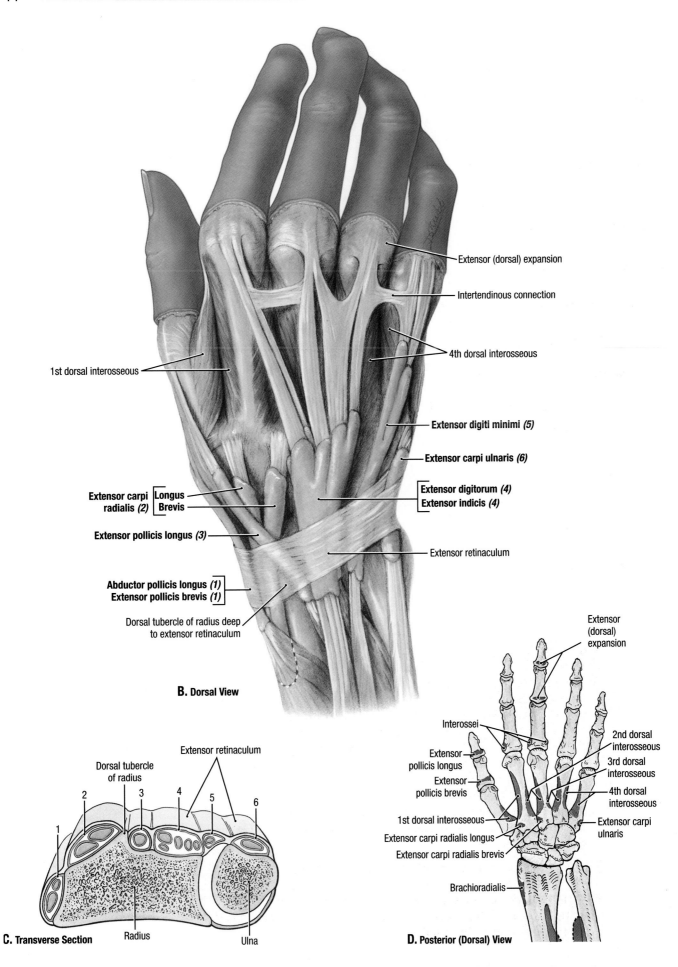

Extensor (dorsal) expansion

Intertendinous connection

4th dorsal interosseous

1st dorsal interosseous

Extensor digiti minimi *(5)*

Extensor carpi ulnaris *(6)*

Extensor carpi radialis *(2)* | **Longus** / **Brevis**

Extensor digitorum *(4)*
Extensor indicis *(4)*

Extensor pollicis longus *(3)*

Extensor retinaculum

Abductor pollicis longus *(1)*
Extensor pollicis brevis *(1)*

Dorsal tubercle of radius deep to extensor retinaculum

B. Dorsal View

Extensor retinaculum

Dorsal tubercle of radius

2   3   4   5   6

1

C. Transverse Section   Radius   Ulna

Extensor (dorsal) expansion

Interossei

Extensor pollicis longus

Extensor pollicis brevis

1st dorsal interosseous

Extensor carpi radialis longus

Extensor carpi radialis brevis

Brachioradialis

2nd dorsal interosseous

3rd dorsal interosseous

4th dorsal interosseous

Extensor carpi ulnaris

D. Posterior (Dorsal) View

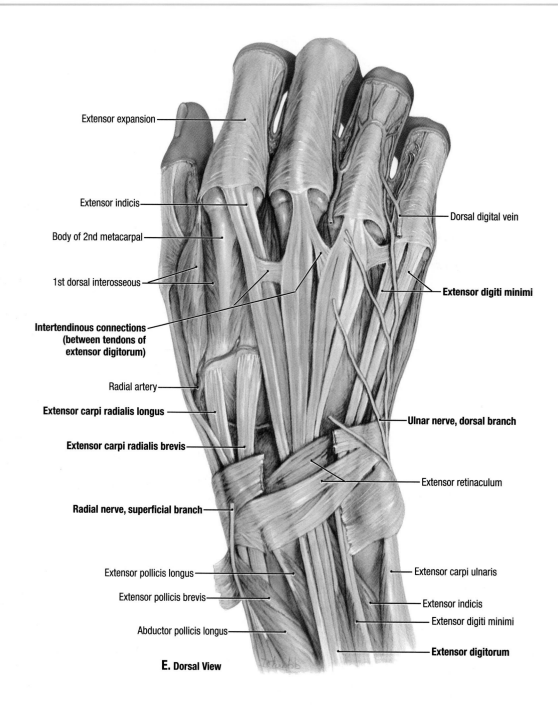

Extensor expansion

Extensor indicis

Body of 2nd metacarpal

1st dorsal interosseous

Intertendinous connections
(between tendons of
extensor digitorum)

Radial artery

Extensor carpi radialis longus

Extensor carpi radialis brevis

Radial nerve, superficial branch

Extensor pollicis longus

Extensor pollicis brevis

Abductor pollicis longus

Dorsal digital vein

Extensor digiti minimi

Ulnar nerve, dorsal branch

Extensor retinaculum

Extensor carpi ulnaris

Extensor indicis

Extensor digiti minimi

Extensor digitorum

E. Dorsal View

6.76   Dorsum of hand (continued)

E. Tendons on dorsum of hand and extensor retinaculum.
- The deep fascia is thickened to form the extensor retinaculum.
- Proximal to the knuckles, intertendinous connections extend between the tendons of the digital extensors and, thereby, restrict the independent action of the fingers.

Sometimes a nontender cystic swelling appears on the hand, most commonly on the dorsum of the wrist. The thin-walled cyst contains clear mucinous fluid. Clinically, this type of swelling is called a "ganglion" (G. swelling or knot). These synovial cysts are close to and often communicate with the synovial sheaths. The distal attachment of the extensor carpi radialis brevis tendon is a common site for such a cyst.

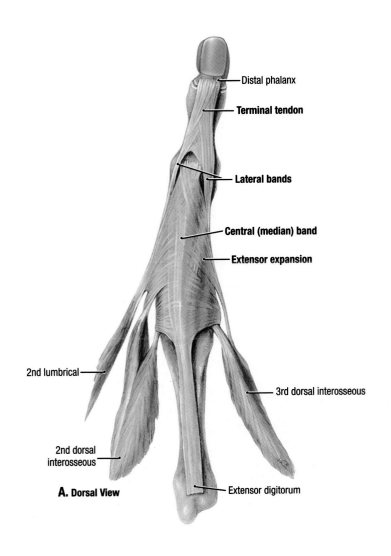

Distal phalanx

Terminal tendon

Lateral bands

Central (median) band

Extensor expansion

2nd lumbrical

3rd dorsal interosseous

2nd dorsal interosseous

A. Dorsal View   Extensor digitorum

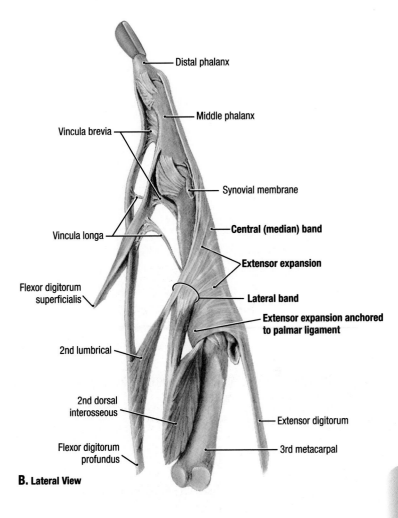

Distal phalanx

Middle phalanx

Vincula brevia

Synovial membrane

Central (median) band

Vincula longa

Extensor expansion

Flexor digitorum superficialis

Lateral band

Extensor expansion anchored to palmar ligament

2nd lumbrical

2nd dorsal interosseous

Extensor digitorum

Flexor digitorum profundus

3rd metacarpal

B. Lateral View

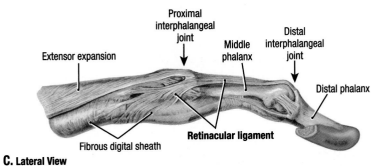

Proximal interphalangeal joint

Middle phalanx

Distal interphalangeal joint

Extensor expansion

Distal phalanx

Fibrous digital sheath

Retinacular ligament

C. Lateral View

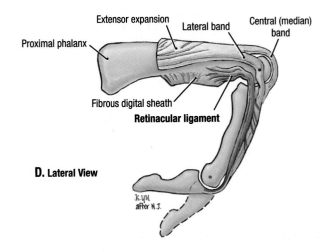

Extensor expansion

Lateral band

Central (median) band

Proximal phalanx

Fibrous digital sheath

Retinacular ligament

K.YU after N.T.

D. Lateral View

6.77   Extensor (dorsal) expansion of 3rd digit

A. Dorsal aspect. **B.** Lateral aspect. **C.** Retinacular ligaments of extended digit. **D.** Retinacular ligaments of flexed digit.

- The hood covering the head of the metacarpal is attached to the palmar ligament.
- Contraction of the muscles attaching to the lateral band will produce flexion of the metacarpophalangeal joint and extension of the interphalangeal joints.

- The retinacular ligament is a fibrous band that runs from the proximal phalanx and fibrous digital sheath obliquely across the middle phalanx and two interphalangeal joints to join the extensor (dorsal) expansion, and then to the distal phalanx.
- On flexion of the distal interphalangeal joint, the retinacular ligament becomes taut and pulls the proximal joint into flexion; on extension of the proximal joint, the distal joint is pulled by the ligament into nearly complete extension.

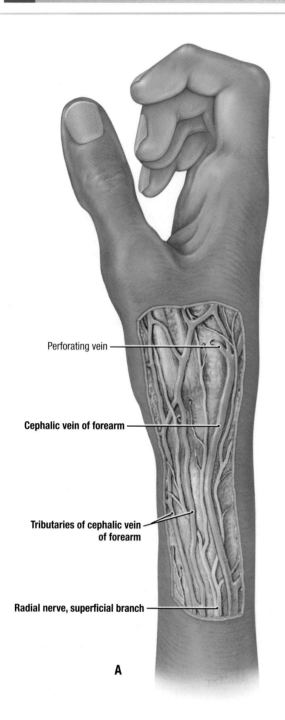

Perforating vein

Cephalic vein of forearm

Tributaries of cephalic vein of forearm

Radial nerve, superficial branch

A

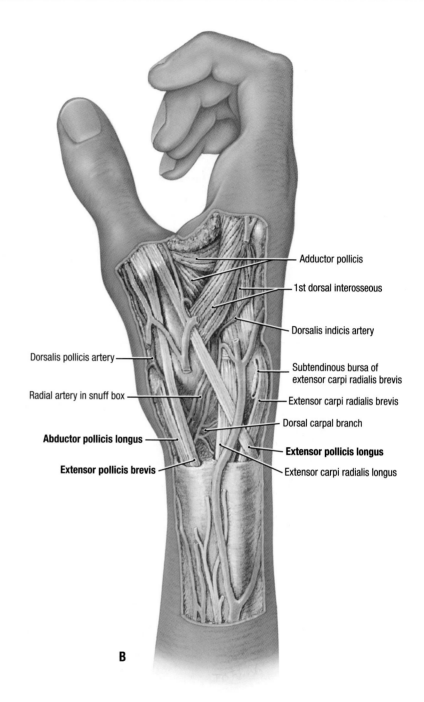

Adductor pollicis

1st dorsal interosseous

Dorsalis indicis artery

Dorsalis pollicis artery

Subtendinous bursa of extensor carpi radialis brevis

Radial artery in snuff box

Extensor carpi radialis brevis

Abductor pollicis longus

Dorsal carpal branch

Extensor pollicis longus

Extensor pollicis brevis

Extensor carpi radialis longus

B

Lateral Views

6.78 Lateral aspect of wrist and hand

A. Anatomical snuff box—I. **B.** Anatomical snuff box—II.
In **A**:
- The depression at the base of the thumb, the "anatomical snuff box," retains its name from an archaic habit.
- Note the superficial veins, including the cephalic vein of forearm and/or its tributaries, and cutaneous nerves crossing the snuff box.

In **B**:
- Three long tendons of the thumb form the boundaries of the snuff box; the extensor pollicis longus forms the medial boundary and the abductor pollicis longus and extensor pollicis brevis the lateral boundary.
- The radial artery crosses the floor of the snuff box and travels between the two heads of the 1st dorsal interosseous.
- The adductor pollicis and 1st dorsal interosseous are supplied by the ulnar nerve.

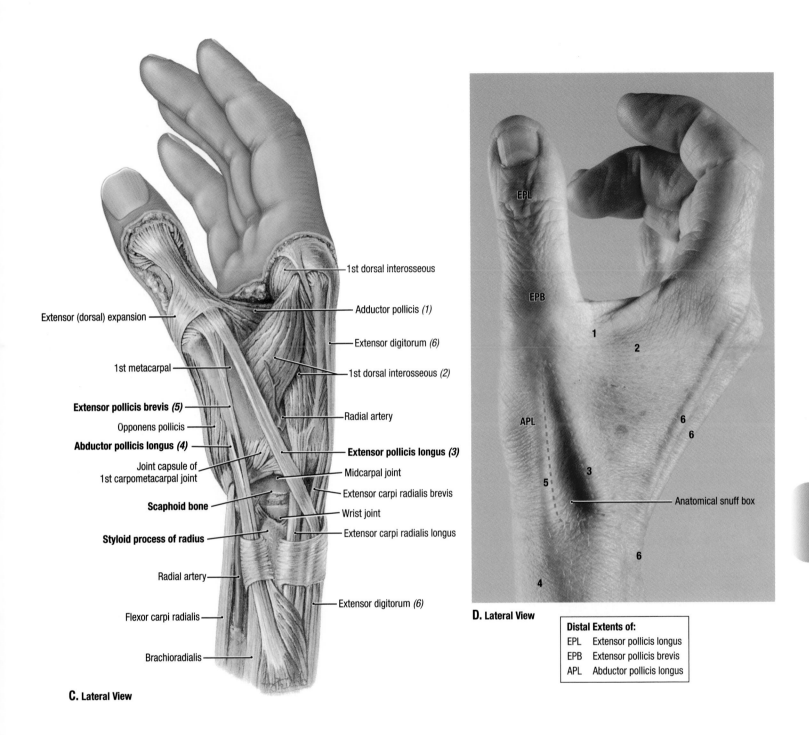

C. Lateral View

1st dorsal interosseous

Adductor pollicis *(1)*

Extensor digitorum *(6)*

1st dorsal interosseous *(2)*

Radial artery

Extensor pollicis longus *(3)*

Midcarpal joint

Extensor carpi radialis brevis

Wrist joint

Extensor carpi radialis longus

Extensor digitorum *(6)*

Extensor (dorsal) expansion

1st metacarpal

Extensor pollicis brevis *(5)*

Opponens pollicis

Abductor pollicis longus *(4)*

Joint capsule of 1st carpometacarpal joint

Scaphoid bone

Styloid process of radius

Radial artery

Flexor carpi radialis

Brachioradialis

D. Lateral View

EPL

EPB

APL

Anatomical snuff box

Distal Extents of:	
EPL	Extensor pollicis longus
EPB	Extensor pollicis brevis
APL	Abductor pollicis longus

6.78   **Lateral aspect of wrist and hand *(continued)***

C. Anatomical snuff box—III. **D.** Surface anatomy.

    In **C**: Note the scaphoid bone, the wrist joint proximal to the scaphoid, and the midcarpal joint distal to it.

Fracture of the scaphoid often results from a fall on the palm with the hand abducted. The fracture occurs across the narrow part ("waist") of the scaphoid. Pain occurs primarily on the lateral side of the wrist, especially during dorsiflexion and abduction of the hand. Initial radiographs of the wrist may not reveal a fracture, but radiographs taken 10–14 days later reveal a fracture because bone resorption has occurred. Owing to the poor blood supply to the proximal part of the scaphoid, union of the fractured parts may take several months. Avascular necrosis of the proximal fragment of the scaphoid (pathological death of bone resulting from poor blood supply) may occur and produce degenerative joint disease of the wrist.

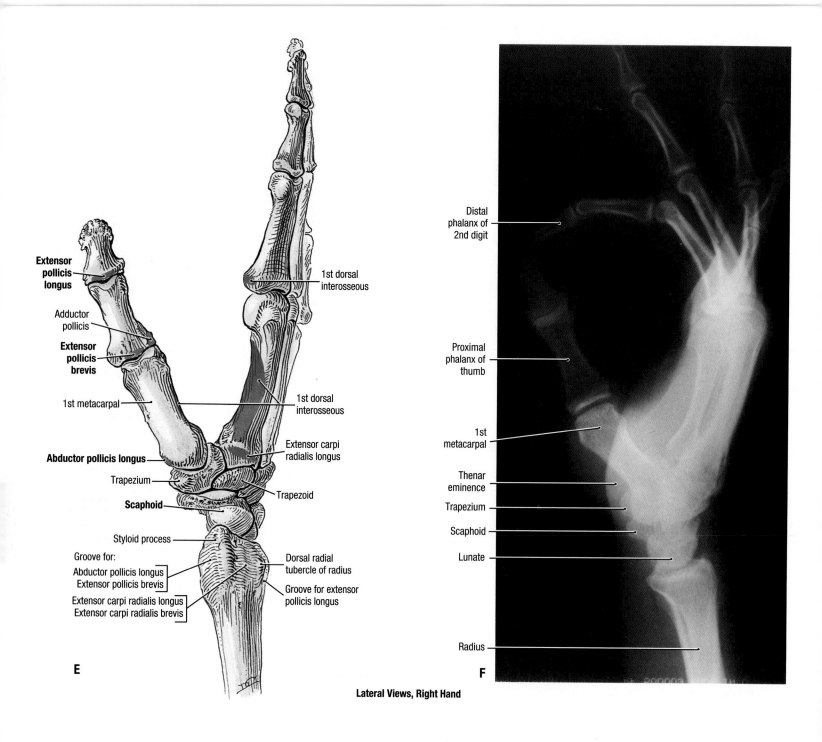

Extensor pollicis longus

Adductor pollicis

Extensor pollicis brevis

1st metacarpal

Abductor pollicis longus

Trapezium

Scaphoid

Styloid process

Groove for:
Abductor pollicis longus
Extensor pollicis brevis

Extensor carpi radialis longus
Extensor carpi radialis brevis

1st dorsal interosseous

1st dorsal interosseous

Extensor carpi radialis longus

Trapezoid

Dorsal radial tubercle of radius

Groove for extensor pollicis longus

E

Distal phalanx of 2nd digit

Proximal phalanx of thumb

1st metacarpal

Thenar eminence

Trapezium

Scaphoid

Lunate

Radius

F

Lateral Views, Right Hand

6.78   Lateral aspect of wrist and hand *(continued)*

E. Bony hand showing muscle attachments. **F.** Radiograph.

• The anatomical snuff box is limited proximally by the styloid process of the radius and distally by the base of the 1st metacarpal; aspects of the two lateral bones of the carpus (scaphoid and trapezium) form the floor of the snuff box.

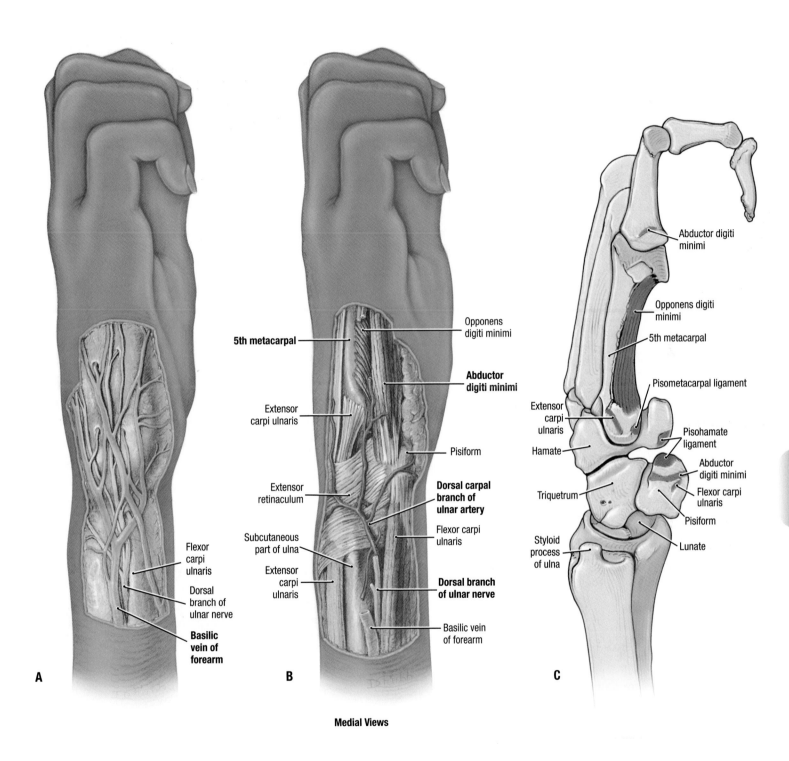

A. Superficial dissection. **B.** Deep dissection. **C.** Bony hand showing sites of muscular and ligamentous attachments. The extensor carpi ulnaris is inserted directly into the base of the fifth metacarpal, but the flexor carpi ulnaris inserts indirectly to the base of the fifth metacarpal and the hook of the hamate through the pisiform and pisohamate and pisometacarpal ligaments.

6.79 **Medial aspect of wrist and hand**

Medial Views

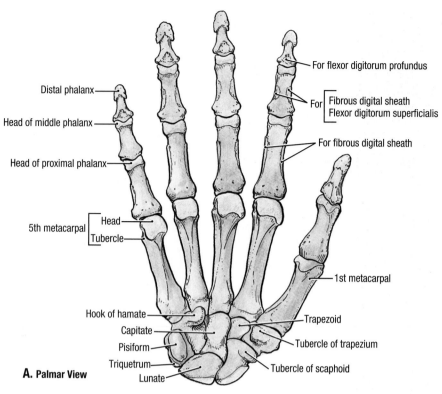

A. Palmar View

Distal phalanx
Head of middle phalanx
Head of proximal phalanx
5th metacarpal { Head, Tubercle }
Hook of hamate
Capitate
Pisiform
Triquetrum
Lunate

For flexor digitorum profundus
For { Fibrous digital sheath / Flexor digitorum superficialis }
For fibrous digital sheath
1st metacarpal
Trapezoid
Tubercle of trapezium
Tubercle of scaphoid

6.80 Bones of hand

A. Palmar view. **B.** Dorsal view.

The eight carpal bones form two rows: in the distal row, the hamate, capitate, trapezoid, and trapezium; the trapezium forming a saddle-shaped joint with the 1st metacarpal; in the proximal row, the scaphoid, lunate, and pisiform; the pisiform is superimposed on the triquetrum.

Severe crushing injuries of the hand may produce multiple metacarpal fractures, resulting in instability of the hand. Similar injuries of the distal phalanges are common (e.g., when a finger is caught in a car door).

A fracture of a distal phalanx is usually comminuted, and a painful hematoma (collection of blood) develops. Fractures of the proximal and middle phalanges are usually the result of crushing or hypertension injuries.

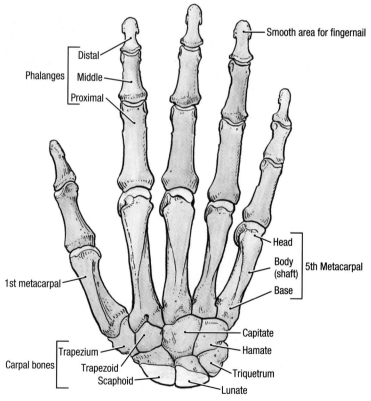

Smooth area for fingernail
Phalanges { Distal / Middle / Proximal }
1st metacarpal
5th Metacarpal { Head / Body (shaft) / Base }
Carpal bones { Trapezium / Trapezoid / Scaphoid }
Capitate
Hamate
Triquetrum
Lunate

B. Dorsal View

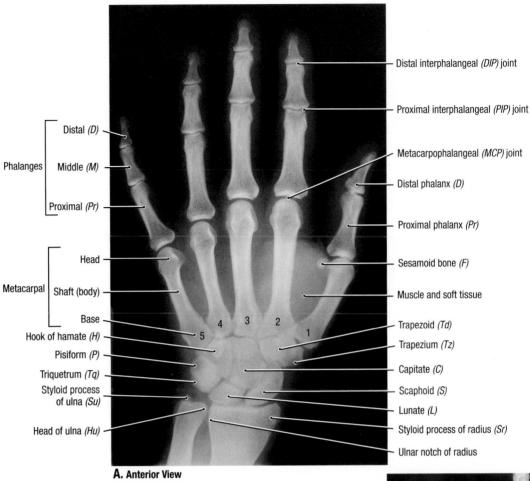

A. Anterior View

Distal interphalangeal (DIP) joint

Proximal interphalangeal (PIP) joint

Metacarpophalangeal (MCP) joint

Distal phalanx (D)

Proximal phalanx (Pr)

Sesamoid bone (F)

Muscle and soft tissue

Trapezoid (Td)

Trapezium (Tz)

Capitate (C)

Scaphoid (S)

Lunate (L)

Styloid process of radius (Sr)

Ulnar notch of radius

Phalanges — Distal (D), Middle (M), Proximal (Pr)

Metacarpal — Head, Shaft (body), Base

Hook of hamate (H)

Pisiform (P)

Triquetrum (Tq)

Styloid process of ulna (Su)

Head of ulna (Hu)

6.81 **Imaging of bones of wrist and hand**

A. Radiograph. **B.** Three-dimensional computer-generated image of wrist and hand (letters correspond to structures labeled in **A**).

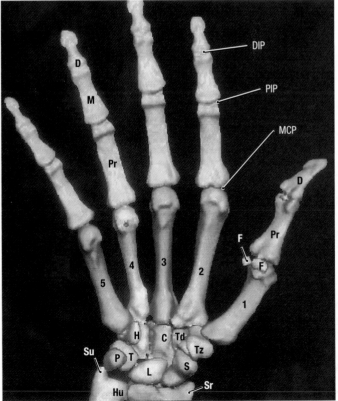

B. Anterior View

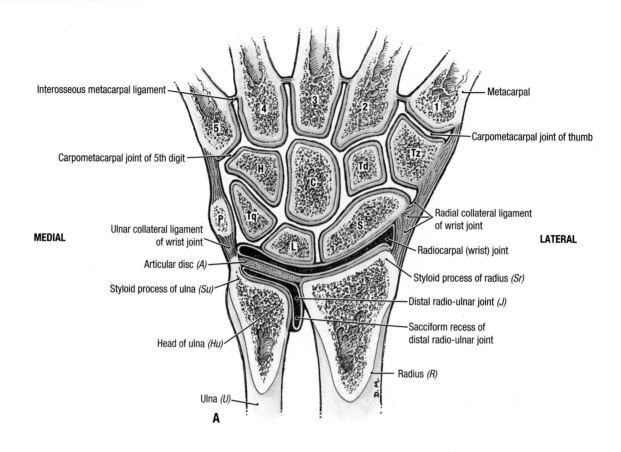

Interosseous metacarpal ligament

Carpometacarpal joint of 5th digit

MEDIAL

Ulnar collateral ligament of wrist joint

Articular disc *(A)*

Styloid process of ulna *(Su)*

Head of ulna *(Hu)*

Ulna *(U)*

A

Metacarpal

Carpometacarpal joint of thumb

Radial collateral ligament of wrist joint

LATERAL

Radiocarpal (wrist) joint

Styloid process of radius *(Sr)*

Distal radio-ulnar joint *(J)*

Sacciform recess of distal radio-ulnar joint

Radius *(R)*

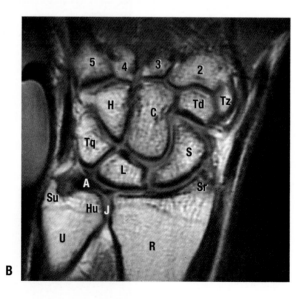

B

6.82   Coronal section of wrist

A. Schematic illustration. **B.** Coronal MRI. *A*, articular disc; *J*, distal radio-ulnar joint (letters correspond to structures labeled in **A** and Figure 6.81A).

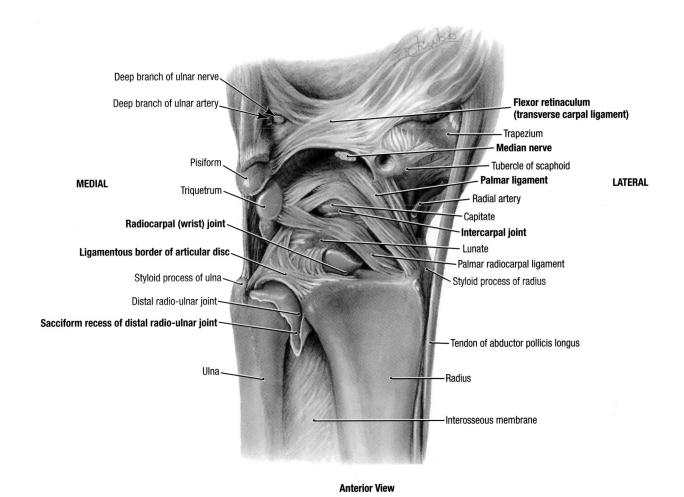

Deep branch of ulnar nerve

Deep branch of ulnar artery

Flexor retinaculum
(transverse carpal ligament)

Trapezium

Median nerve

Pisiform

Tubercle of scaphoid

Palmar ligament

MEDIAL

Triquetrum

Radial artery

Capitate

Radiocarpal (wrist) joint

Intercarpal joint

Lunate

Ligamentous border of articular disc

Palmar radiocarpal ligament

Styloid process of ulna

Styloid process of radius

Distal radio-ulnar joint

Sacciform recess of distal radio-ulnar joint

Tendon of abductor pollicis longus

Ulna

Radius

Interosseous membrane

LATERAL

Anterior View

| 6.83 | **Ligaments of distal radio-ulnar, radiocarpal, and intercarpal joints** |

The hand is forcibly extended. Observe the palmar radiocarpal ligament passing from the radius to the two rows of carpal bones; they are strong and directed, so that the hand moves with the radius during supination.

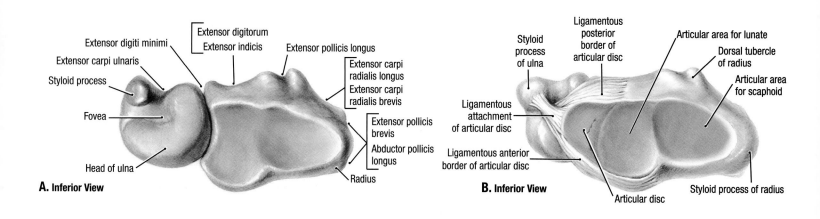

A. Inferior View

Extensor digiti minimi
Extensor carpi ulnaris
Styloid process
Fovea
Head of ulna
Extensor digitorum
Extensor indicis
Extensor pollicis longus
Extensor carpi radialis longus
Extensor carpi radialis brevis
Extensor pollicis brevis
Abductor pollicis longus
Radius

B. Inferior View

Styloid process of ulna
Ligamentous posterior border of articular disc
Ligamentous attachment of articular disc
Ligamentous anterior border of articular disc
Articular disc
Articular area for lunate
Dorsal tubercle of radius
Articular area for scaphoid
Styloid process of radius

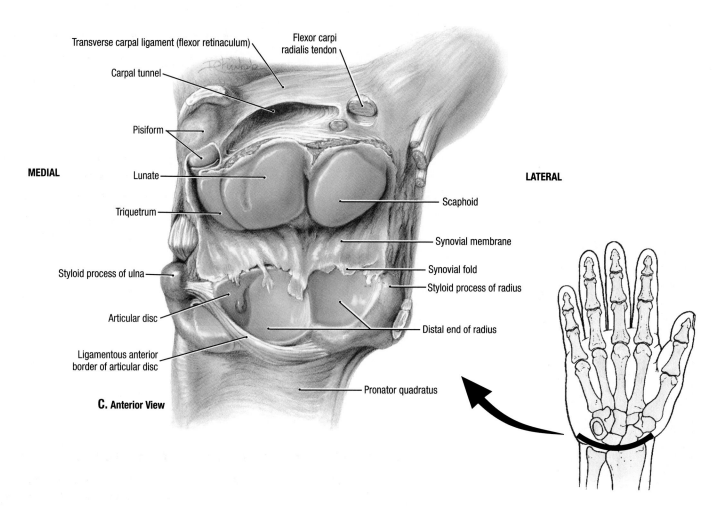

Transverse carpal ligament (flexor retinaculum)
Carpal tunnel
Pisiform
Lunate
Triquetrum
Styloid process of ulna
Articular disc
Ligamentous anterior border of articular disc
Flexor carpi radialis tendon
MEDIAL
Scaphoid
LATERAL
Synovial membrane
Synovial fold
Styloid process of radius
Distal end of radius
Pronator quadratus

C. Anterior View

6.84   Radiocarpal (wrist) joint

A. Distal ends of radius and ulna showing grooves for tendons on the posterior aspects. **B.** Articular disc. The articular disc unites the distal ends of the radius and ulna; it is fibrocartilaginous at the triangular area between the head of the ulna and the lunate bone, but ligamentous and pliable elsewhere. The cartilaginous part commonly has a fissure or perforation, as shown here. **C.** Articular surface of the radiocarpal joint, which is opened anteriorly. The lunate articulates with the radius and articular disc; only during adduction of the wrist does the triquetrum come into articulation with the disc. The perforation in the disc and the associated roughened surface of the lunate are a common occurrence.

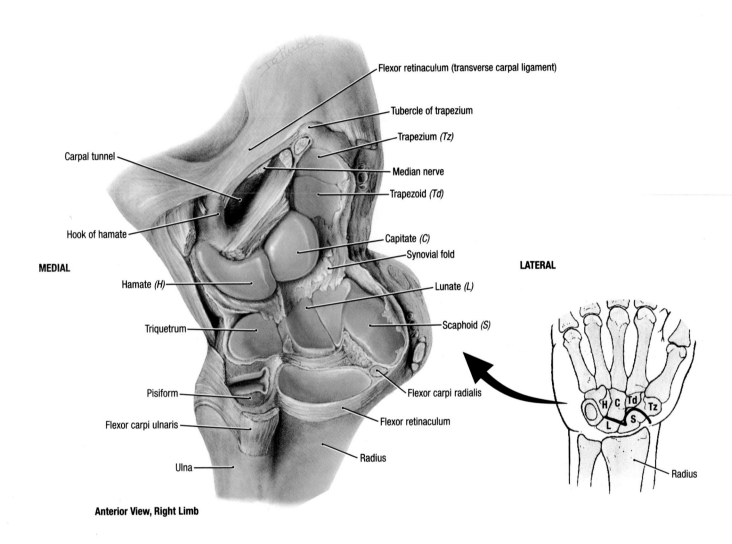

Flexor retinaculum (transverse carpal ligament)

Tubercle of trapezium

Trapezium *(Tz)*

Median nerve

Trapezoid *(Td)*

Capitate *(C)*

Synovial fold

Lunate *(L)*

Scaphoid *(S)*

Flexor carpi radialis

Flexor retinaculum

Radius

Carpal tunnel

Hook of hamate

MEDIAL

Hamate *(H)*

Triquetrum

Pisiform

Flexor carpi ulnaris

Ulna

LATERAL

Radius

Anterior View, Right Limb

| **6.85** | **Articular surfaces of midcarpal (transverse carpal) joint, opened anteriorly** |

- The flexor retinaculum (transverse carpal ligament) is cut; the proximal part of the ligament, which spans from the pisiform to the scaphoid, is relatively weak; the distal part, which passes from the hook of the hamate to the tubercle of the trapezium, is strong.
- Observe the sinuous surfaces of the opposed bones: the trapezium and trapezoid together form a concave, oval surface for

the scaphoid, and the capitate and hamate together form a convex surface for the scaphoid, lunate, and triquetrum.

Anterior dislocation of the lunate is a serious injury that usually results from a fall on the dorsiflexed wrist. The lunate is pushed to the palmar surface of the wrist and may compress the median nerve and lead to carpal tunnel syndrome. Because of poor blood supply, avascular necrosis of the lunate may occur.

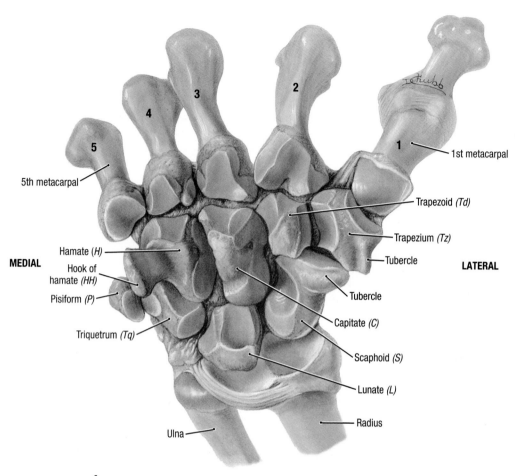

A. Anterior View, Right Limb

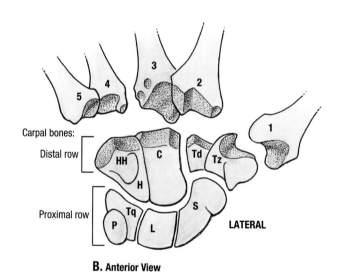

B. Anterior View

6.86 **Carpal bones and bases of metacarpals**

A. Open intercarpal and carpometacarpal joints. The dorsal ligaments remain intact, and all the joints have been hyperextended, permitting study of articular facets. **B.** Diagram of the articular surfaces of the carpometacarpal joints (*letters* refer to structures labeled in **A**).

- The capitate articulates with three metacarpals (2nd, 3rd, and 4th).
- The 2nd metacarpal articulates with three carpals (trapezium, trapezoid, and capitate).
- The 2nd and 3rd carpometacarpal joints are practically immobile; the 1st is saddle-shaped, and the 4th and 5th are hinge-shaped synovial joints.

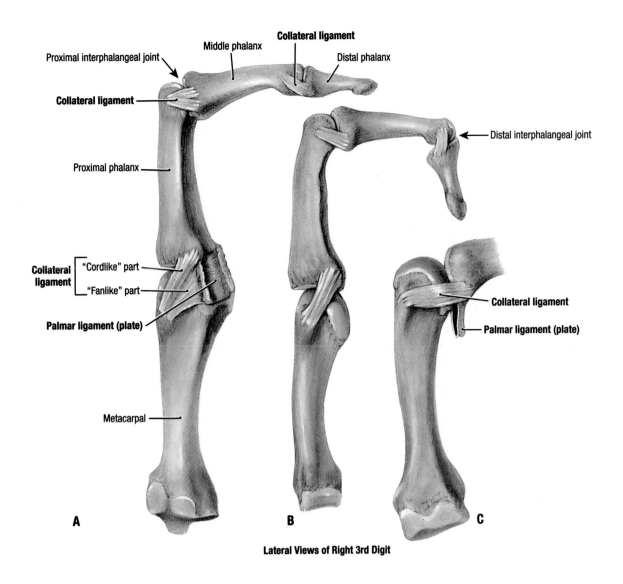

Lateral Views of Right 3rd Digit

6.87   **Collateral ligaments of metacarpophalangeal and interphalangeal joints of third digit**

A. Extended metacarpophalangeal and distal interphalangeal joints. **B.** Flexed interphalangeal joints. **C.** Flexed metacarpophalangeal joint.

- A fibrocartilaginous plate, the palmar ligament, hangs from the base of the proximal phalanx; is fixed to the head of the metacarpal by the weaker, fanlike part of the collateral ligament (**A**); and moves like a visor across the metacarpal head (**C**).
- The extremely strong, cordlike parts of the collateral ligaments of this joint (**A** and **B**) are eccentrically attached to the metacarpal heads; they are slack during extension and taut during flexion (**C**), so the fingers cannot be spread (abducted) unless the hand is open; the interphalangeal joints have similar ligaments.

Skier's thumb refers to the rupture or chronic laxity of the collateral ligament of the 1st metacarpophalangeal joint. The injury results from hyperextension of the joint, which occurs when the thumb is held by the ski pole while the rest of the hand hits the ground or enters the snow.

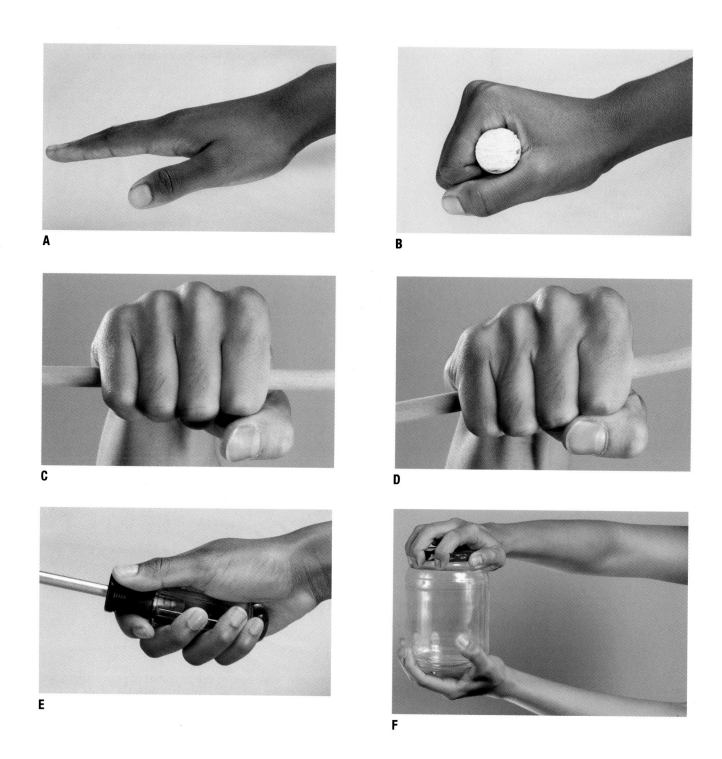

6.88   **Grasp, pinch, and movements of the thumb**

A. The extended hand. **B.** Cylindrical (power) grasp. When grasping an object, the metacarpophalangeal and interphalangeal joints are flexed, but the radiocarpal joints are extended. Without wrist extension the grip is weak and insecure. **C.** Loose cylindri-cal grasp. **D.** Firm cylindrical (power) grasp. The heads of the 4th and 5th metacarpals have moved in a palmar direction. **E.** Centralized (power) grasp. **F.** Disc (power) grasp.

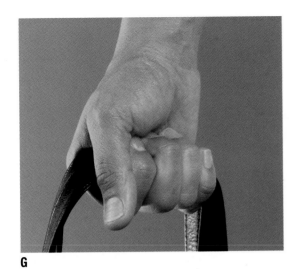

G

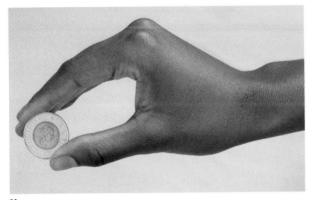

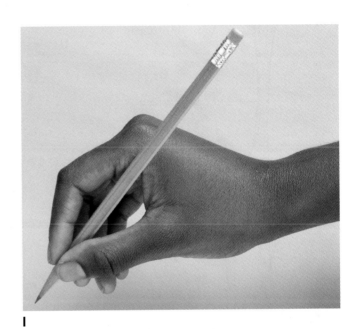

I

H

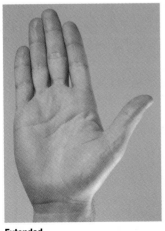
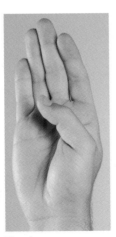
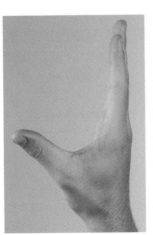
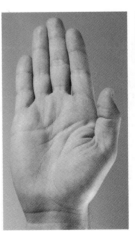
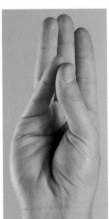

| Extended | Flexed | Abducted | Adducted | Opposed to little finger |

J

6.88   **Grasp, pinch, and movements of the thumb** *(continued)*

G. Hook grasp. This grasp involves primarily the long flexors of the fingers, which are flexed to a varying degree depending on the size of the object. **H.** Fingertip pinch. **I.** Tripod (three-jaw chuck) pinch. **J.** Positions of the thumb.

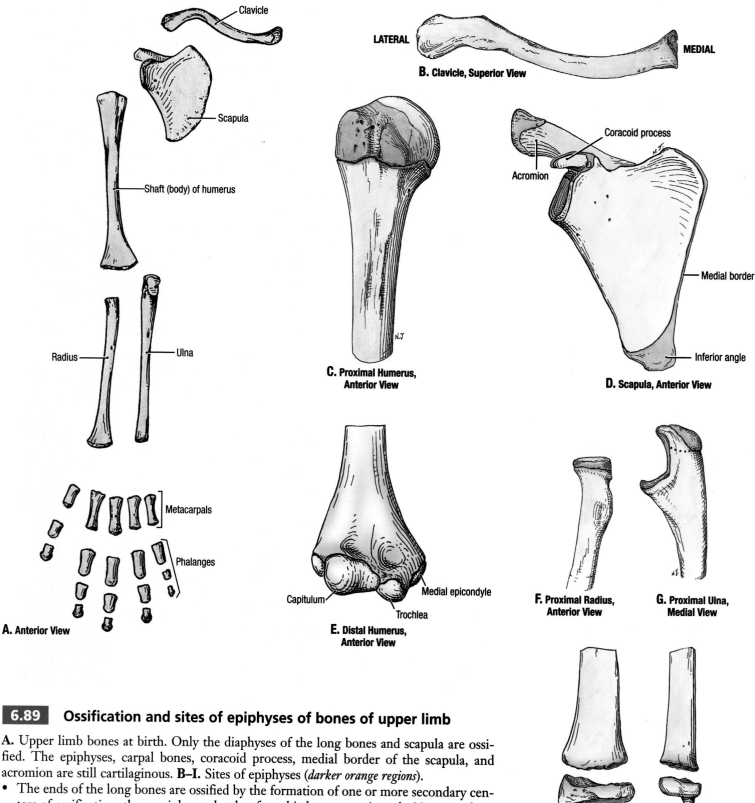

A. Anterior View

Clavicle

Scapula

Shaft (body) of humerus

Radius

Ulna

Metacarpals

Phalanges

B. Clavicle, Superior View

LATERAL

MEDIAL

C. Proximal Humerus, Anterior View

D. Scapula, Anterior View

Coracoid process

Acromion

Medial border

Inferior angle

E. Distal Humerus, Anterior View

Capitulum

Trochlea

Medial epicondyle

F. Proximal Radius, Anterior View

G. Proximal Ulna, Medial View

H. Distal Radius, Anterior View

I. Distal Ulna, Anterior View

6.89 **Ossification and sites of epiphyses of bones of upper limb**

A. Upper limb bones at birth. Only the diaphyses of the long bones and scapula are ossified. The epiphyses, carpal bones, coracoid process, medial border of the scapula, and acromion are still cartilaginous. **B–I.** Sites of epiphyses (*darker orange regions*).

- The ends of the long bones are ossified by the formation of one or more secondary centers of ossification; these epiphyses develop from birth to approximately 20 years of age in the clavicle, humerus, radius, ulna, metacarpals, and phalanges.

Without knowledge of bone growth and the appearance of bones in radiographic and other diagnostic images at various ages, a displaced epiphysial plate could be mistaken for a fracture, and separation of an epiphysis could be interpreted as a displaced piece of fractured bone. Knowledge of the patient's age and the location of epiphyses can prevent these errors.

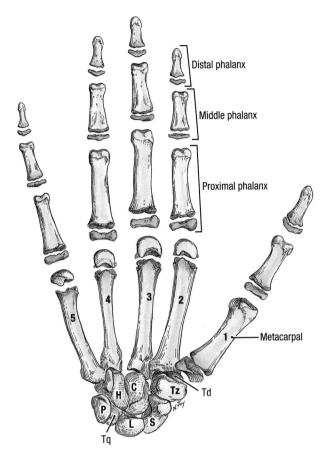

J. Anterior View (Right Hand)

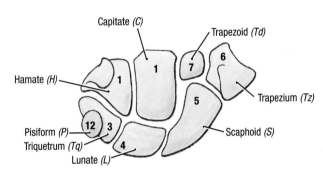

Capitate (C)
Trapezoid (Td)
Hamate (H)
Trapezium (Tz)
Pisiform (P)
Scaphoid (S)
Triquetrum (Tq)
Lunate (L)

Numbers: approximate age of ossification of carpal bones in years

K. Anterior View

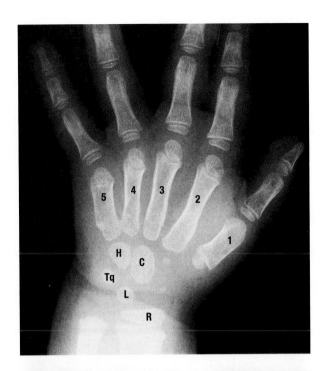

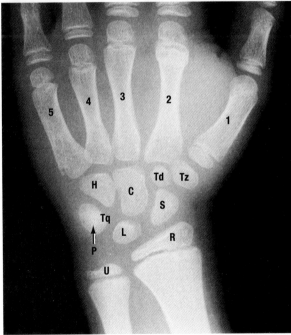

L. Anteroposterior View, Right Hand
Epiphyses in radiographs appear as radiolucent lines

6.89 **Ossification and sites of epiphyses of bones of upper limb (continued)**

J. Sequence of ossification of carpal bones. **K.** Ossification of bones of hand. Note the phalanges have a single proximal epiphysis and metacarpals 2, 3, 4, and 5 have single distal epiphyses. The 1st metacarpal behaves as a phalanx by having proximal epiphysis. Short-lived epiphyses may appear at the other ends of metacarpals 1 and/or 2. There are individual and gender differences in sequence and timing of ossification. **L.** Radiographs of stages of ossification of wrist and hand. *Top,* a 2½-year-old child; the lunate is ossifying, and the distal radial epiphysis *(R)* is present *(C,* capitate; *H,* hamate; *Tq,* triquetrum; *L,* lunate). *Bottom,* an 11-year-old child. All carpal bones are ossified *(S,* scaphoid; *Td,* trapezoid; *Tz,* trapezium; *arrowhead,* pisiform), and the distal epiphysis of the ulna *(U)* has ossified.

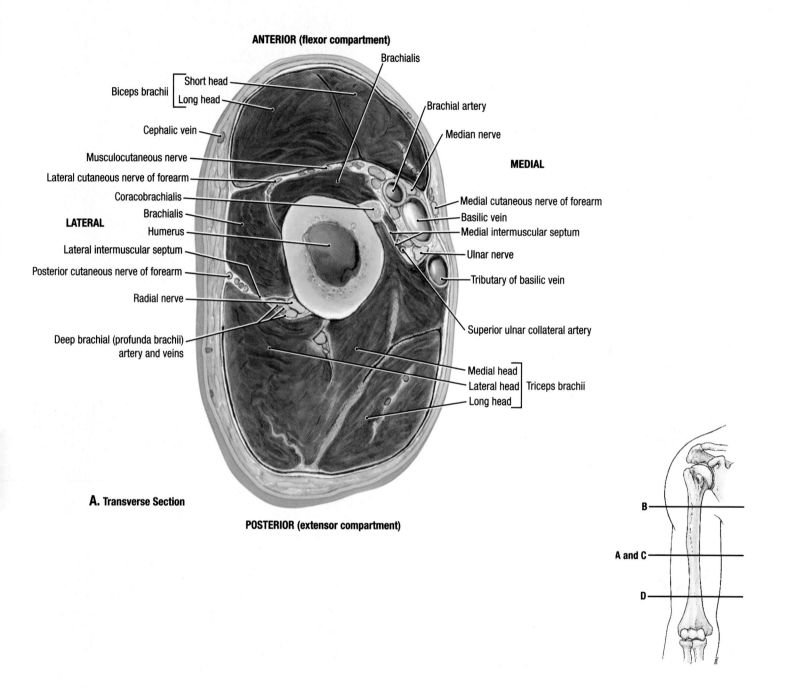

ANTERIOR (flexor compartment)

Brachialis

Biceps brachii [Short head
Long head]

Cephalic vein

Brachial artery

Median nerve

MEDIAL

Musculocutaneous nerve

Lateral cutaneous nerve of forearm

Coracobrachialis

LATERAL

Brachialis

Humerus

Lateral intermuscular septum

Posterior cutaneous nerve of forearm

Radial nerve

Deep brachial (profunda brachii) artery and veins

Medial cutaneous nerve of forearm

Basilic vein

Medial intermuscular septum

Ulnar nerve

Tributary of basilic vein

Superior ulnar collateral artery

Medial head
Lateral head] Triceps brachii
Long head

A. Transverse Section

POSTERIOR (extensor compartment)

B

A and C

D

6.90 **Transverse section and transverse (axial) MRIs of the arm**

A. Transverse section through arm.

- The body (shaft) of the humerus is nearly circular, and its cortex is thickest at this level.
- Three heads (lateral, medial, and long) of the triceps muscle occupy the posterior compartment of the arm.
- The radial nerve and deep artery and veins of arm lie in contact with the radial groove of the humerus.

- The musculocutaneous nerve lies in the plane between the biceps and brachialis muscles.
- The median nerve crosses to the medial side of the brachial artery and veins, the ulnar nerve passes posteriorly onto the medial side of the triceps muscle, and the basilic vein (appearing here as two vessels) has pierced the deep fascia.

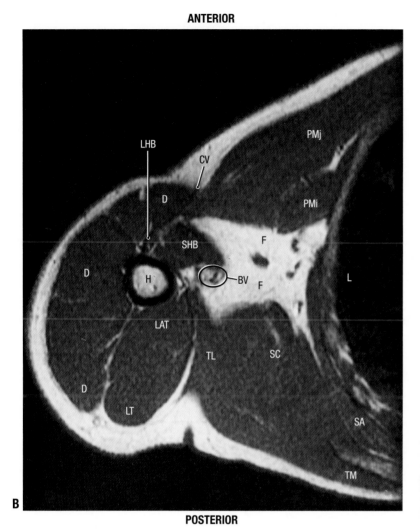

Key for B, E, and D:

BB	Biceps brachii	LT	Long head of triceps brachii
BC	Brachialis	MI	Medial intermuscular septum
BR	Brachioradialis	MT	Medial head of triceps brachii
BS	Basilic vein	PMi	Pectoralis minor
BV	Brachial vessels and nerves	PMj	Pectoralis major
CV	Cephalic vein	SA	Serratus anterior
D	Deltoid	SC	Subscapularis
F	Fat in axilla	SHB	Short head of biceps brachii
H	Humerus	T	Deltoid tuberosity
L	Lung	TL	Teres major and latissimus dorsi
LAT	Lateral head of triceps brachii		
LHB	Long head of biceps brachii	TM	Teres minor
LI	Lateral intermuscular septum	TR	Triceps brachii

6.90   **Transverse section and transverse (axial) MRIs of the arm (continued)**

B. Transverse MRI through the proximal arm. **C.** Transverse MRI though the middle of the arm. **D.** Transverse MRI through the distal arm.

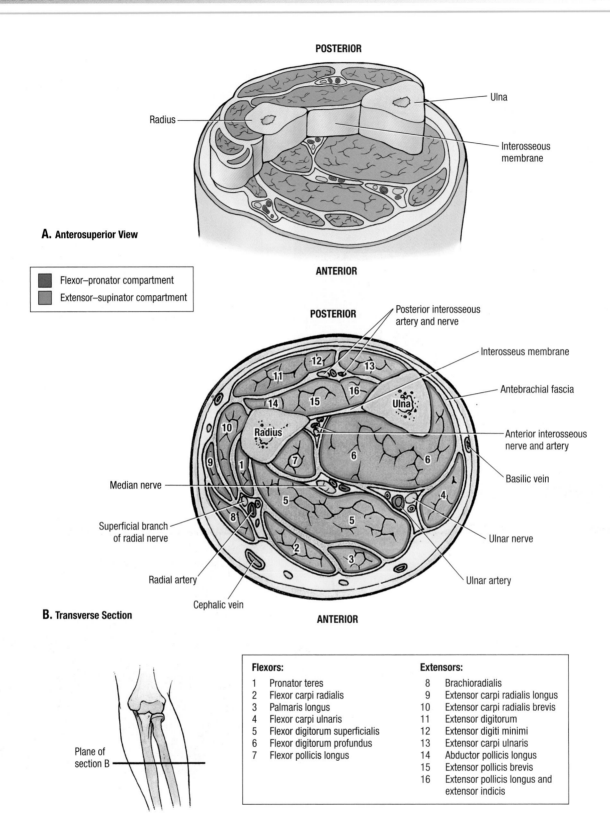

POSTERIOR

Ulna

Radius

Interosseous
membrane

A. Anterosuperior View

ANTERIOR

☐ Flexor–pronator compartment
☐ Extensor–supinator compartment

POSTERIOR

Posterior interosseous
artery and nerve

Interosseus membrane

Antebrachial fascia

Anterior interosseous
nerve and artery

Basilic vein

Median nerve

Superficial branch
of radial nerve

Ulnar nerve

Radial artery

Ulnar artery

Cephalic vein

B. Transverse Section

ANTERIOR

Plane of
section B

Flexors:		Extensors:	
1	Pronator teres	8	Brachioradialis
2	Flexor carpi radialis	9	Extensor carpi radialis longus
3	Palmaris longus	10	Extensor carpi radialis brevis
4	Flexor carpi ulnaris	11	Extensor digitorum
5	Flexor digitorum superficialis	12	Extensor digiti minimi
6	Flexor digitorum profundus	13	Extensor carpi ulnaris
7	Flexor pollicis longus	14	Abductor pollicis longus
		15	Extensor pollicis brevis
		16	Extensor pollicis longus and extensor indicis

6.91   **Transverse sections and transverse (axial) MRIs of forearm**

A. Stepped transverse sections of the anterior and posterior compartments. **B.** Contents of the anterior and posterior compartments.

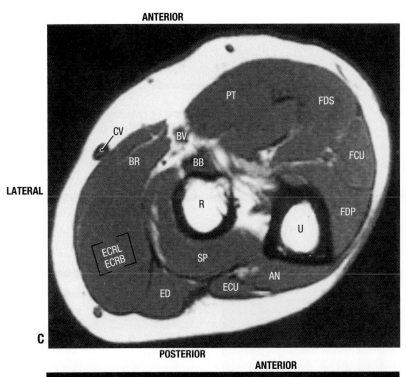

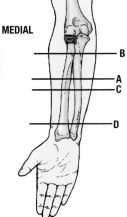

Key for C, D, and E:

AN	Anconeus
APL	Abductor pollicis longus
AV	Anterior interosseous vessels and nerve
BB	Biceps brachii
BR	Brachioradialis
BV	Brachial vessels
CV	Cephalic vein
ECRB	Extensor carpi radialis brevis
ECRL	Extensor carpi radialis longus
ECU	Extensor carpi ulnaris
ED	Extensor digitorum
EPB	Extensor pollicis brevis
EPL	Extensor pollicis longus
FCR	Flexor carpi radialis
FCU	Flexor carpi ulnaris
FDP	Flexor digitorum profundus
FDS	Flexor digitorum superficialis
FPL	Flexor pollicis longus
INT	Interosseous membrane
PQ	Pronator quadratus
PT	Pronator teres
R	Radius
RV	Radial vessels
SP	Supinator
U	Ulnar
UN	Ulnar vessels and nerve

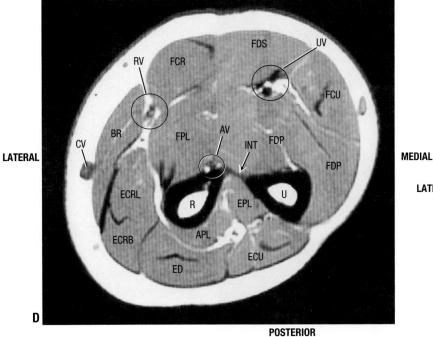

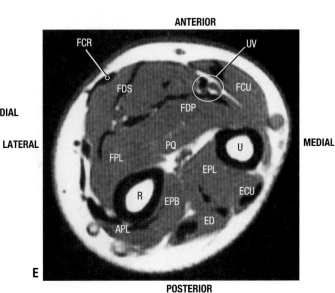

6.91 **Transverse section and transverse (axial) MRIs of forearm** *(continued)*

C. Transverse MRI through the proximal forearm. **D.** Transverse MRI through the middle forearm. **E.** Transverse MRI through the distal forearm.

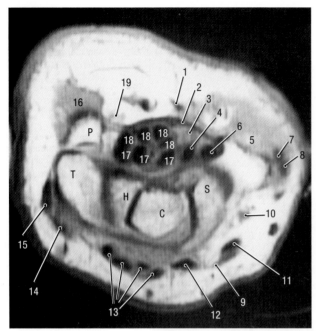

A. Transverse MRI

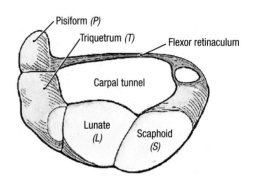

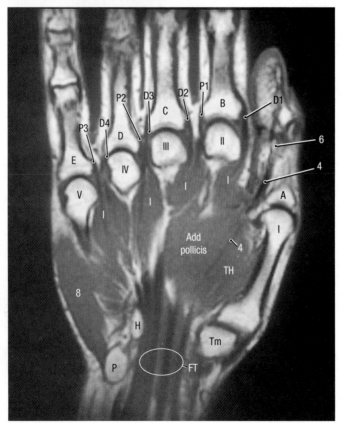

B. Coronal MRI

6.92   **Transverse (axial) section and MRIs through carpal tunnel**

A. Transverse MRI through the proximal carpal tunnel (*numbers* and *letters* in MRIs refer to structures in **D**). **B.** Coronal MRI of wrist and hand showing the course of the long flexor tendons in the carpal tunnel (*numbers* and *letters* in MRIs refer to structures in **D**). *FT,* long flexor tendons in carpal tunnel; *TH,* thenar muscles; *P,* pisiform; *H,* hook of hamate; *Tm,* trapezium; *I,* interossei, *A–E,* proximal phalanges.

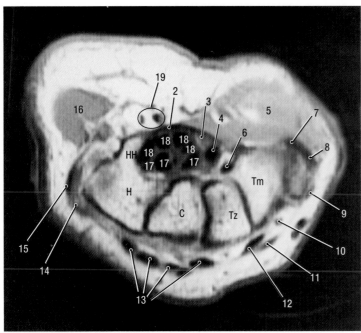

C. Transverse MRI

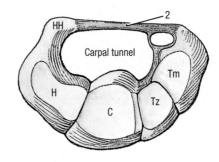

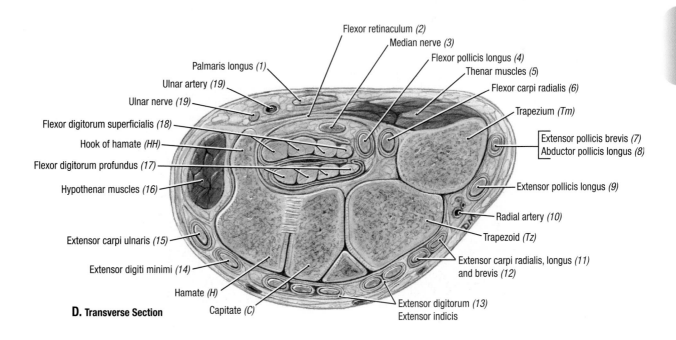

Flexor retinaculum *(2)*

Median nerve *(3)*

Flexor pollicis longus *(4)*

Palmaris longus *(1)*

Thenar muscles *(5)*

Ulnar artery *(19)*

Flexor carpi radialis *(6)*

Ulnar nerve *(19)*

Trapezium *(Tm)*

Flexor digitorum superficialis *(18)*

Extensor pollicis brevis *(7)*
Abductor pollicis longus *(8)*

Hook of hamate *(HH)*

Flexor digitorum profundus *(17)*

Extensor pollicis longus *(9)*

Hypothenar muscles *(16)*

Radial artery *(10)*

Extensor carpi ulnaris *(15)*

Trapezoid *(Tz)*

Extensor carpi radialis, longus *(11)*
and brevis *(12)*

Extensor digiti minimi *(14)*

Hamate *(H)*

Extensor digitorum *(13)*
Extensor indicis

Capitate *(C)*

D. Transverse Section

6.92 **Transverse (axial) section and MRIs through carpal tunnel *(continued)***

C. Transverse MRI through the distal carpal tunnel *(numbers* and *letters* in MRIs refer to
structures in **D**). **D.** Transverse section of carpal tunnel through the distal row of carpal
bones.

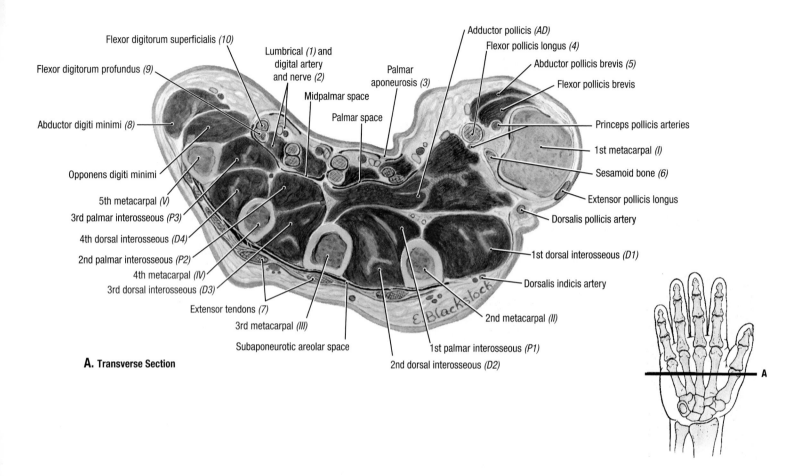

Flexor digitorum superficialis *(10)*
Lumbrical *(1)* and digital artery and nerve *(2)*
Flexor digitorum profundus *(9)*
Midpalmar space
Palmar aponeurosis *(3)*
Palmar space
Adductor pollicis *(AD)*
Flexor pollicis longus *(4)*
Abductor pollicis brevis *(5)*
Flexor pollicis brevis
Abductor digiti minimi *(8)*
Princeps pollicis arteries
Opponens digiti minimi
1st metacarpal *(I)*
Sesamoid bone *(6)*
5th metacarpal *(V)*
3rd palmar interosseous *(P3)*
4th dorsal interosseous *(D4)*
2nd palmar interosseous *(P2)*
Extensor pollicis longus
Dorsalis pollicis artery
1st dorsal interosseous *(D1)*
4th metacarpal *(IV)*
3rd dorsal interosseous *(D3)*
Dorsalis indicis artery
Extensor tendons *(7)*
3rd metacarpal *(III)*
2nd metacarpal *(II)*
Subaponeurotic areolar space
1st palmar interosseous *(P1)*
2nd dorsal interosseous *(D2)*

A. Transverse Section

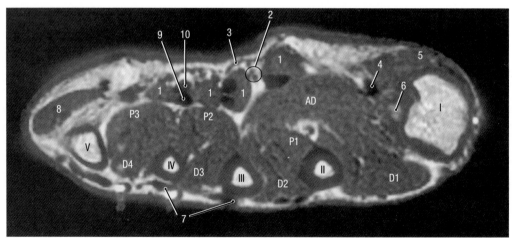

B. Transverse MRI

6.93   **Transverse section and MRI through palm (metacarpals) at level of adductor pollicis**

CHAPTER 7

HEAD

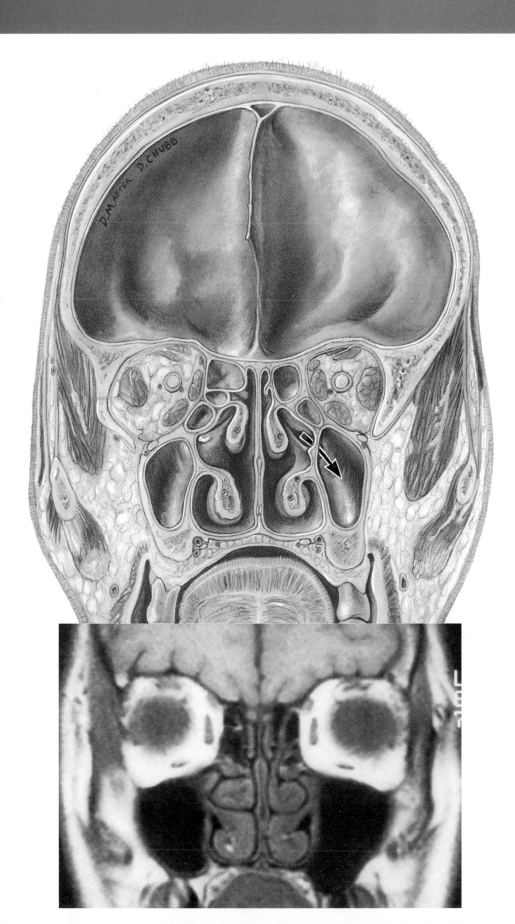

- Cranium **608**
- Face and Scalp **626**
- Circulation and Innervation of Cranial Cavity **632**
- Meninges and Meningeal Spaces **636**
- Cranial Base and Cranial Nerves **640**
- Blood Supply of Brain **646**
- Orbit and Eyeball **650**
- Parotid Region **662**
- Temporal Region and Infratemporal Fossa **664**
- Temporomandibular Joint **672**
- Tongue **676**
- Palate **682**
- Teeth **685**
- Nose, Paranasal Sinuses, and Pterygopalatine Fossa **690**
- Ear **703**
- Lymphatic Drainage of Head **716**
- Autonomic Innervation of Head **717**
- Imaging of Head **718**
- Neuroanatomy: Overview and Ventricular System **722**
- Telencephalon (Cerebrum) and Diencephalon **725**
- Brainstem and Cerebellum **734**
- Imaging of Brain **740**

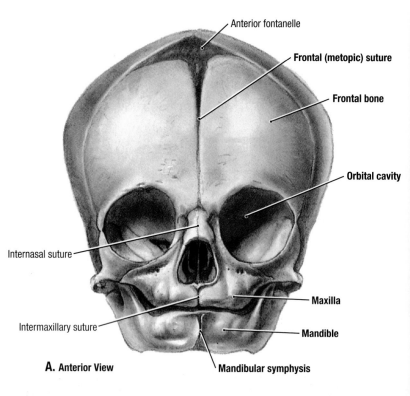

Anterior fontanelle
Frontal (metopic) suture
Frontal bone
Orbital cavity
Internasal suture
Maxilla
Intermaxillary suture
Mandible
A. Anterior View
Mandibular symphysis

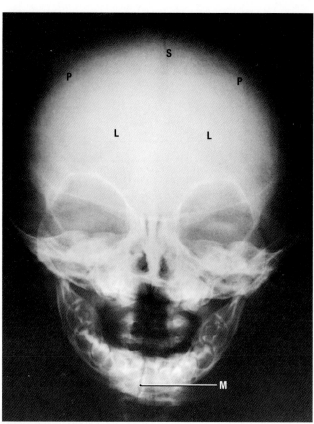

B. Anteroposterior View

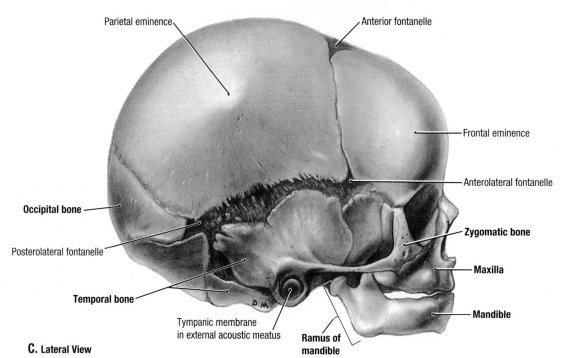

Parietal eminence
Anterior fontanelle
Frontal eminence
Anterolateral fontanelle
Occipital bone
Zygomatic bone
Posterolateral fontanelle
Maxilla
Temporal bone
Mandible
Tympanic membrane
in external acoustic meatus
Ramus of
mandible
C. Lateral View

7.1   Cranium at birth and in early childhood

A. Cranium at birth, anterior aspect. **B.** Radiograph of 6½-month-old child. **C.** Cranium at birth, lateral aspect.
Compared with the adult skull (Figs. 7.2–7.4):
• The maxilla and mandible are proportionately small.

• The mandibular symphysis, which closes during the second year, and the frontal suture, which closes during the sixth year, are still open (unfused).
• The orbital cavities are proportionately large, but the face is small; the facial skeleton forming only one eighth of the whole cranium, while in the adult, it forms one third.

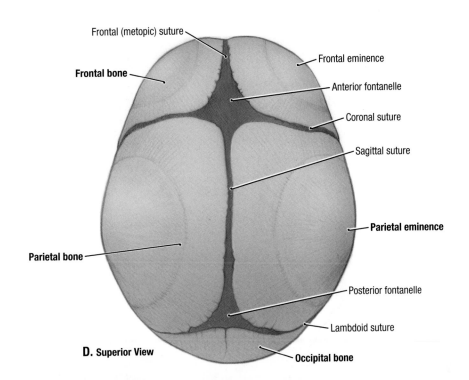

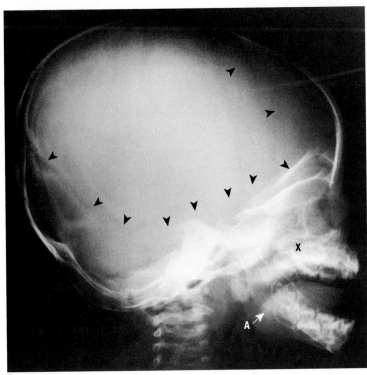

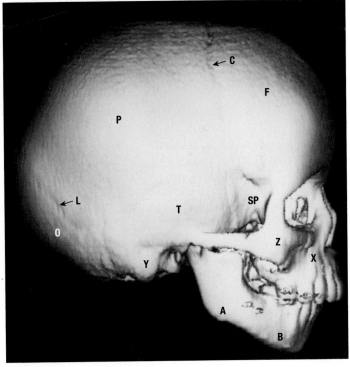

Key for B, E and F

A   Angle of mandible
B   Body of mandible
C   Coronal suture
F   Frontal bone
L   Lambdoid suture
M   Mandibular symphysis
O   Occipital bone
P   Parietal eminence
S   Sagittal suture
SP   Sphenoid
T   Temporal bone
X   Maxilla
Y   Mastoid process
Z   Zygomatic bone

Arrowheads = Membranous outline of parietal bone

Frontal (metopic) suture
Frontal bone
Frontal eminence
Anterior fontanelle
Coronal suture
Sagittal suture
Parietal eminence
Parietal bone
Posterior fontanelle
Lambdoid suture
Occipital bone

D. Superior View

E. Lateral View

F. Lateral View

7.1   Cranium at birth and in early childhood (continued)

D. Cranium at birth, superior aspect. **E.** Radiograph of 6½-month-old child. **F.** Three-dimensional computer-generated images of 3-year-old child's cranium.

- The parietal eminence is a rounded cone. Ossification, which starts at the eminences, has not yet reached the ultimate four angles of the parietal bone; accordingly, these regions are membranous, and the membrane is blended with the pericranium externally and the dura mater internally to form the fontanelles. The fontanelles are usually closed by the second year; there is no mastoid process until the second year.

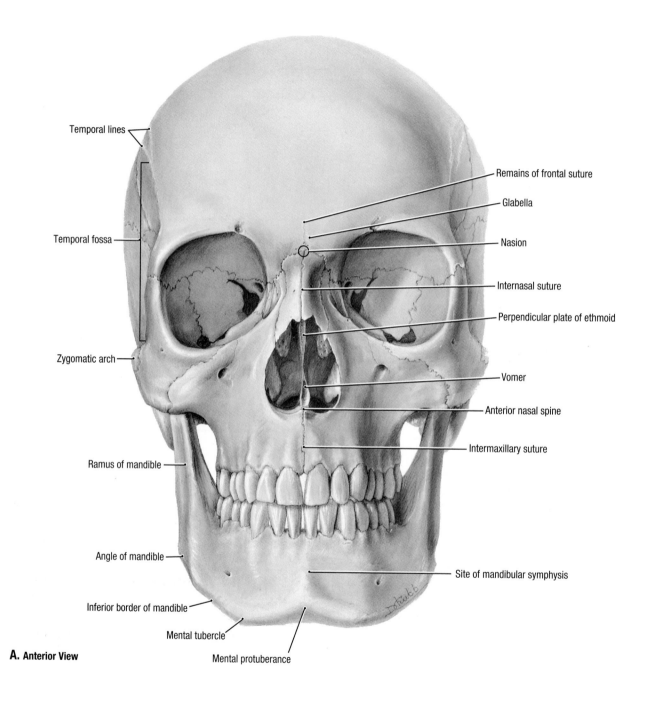

Temporal lines

Temporal fossa

Zygomatic arch

Ramus of mandible

Angle of mandible

Inferior border of mandible

Mental tubercle

A. Anterior View

Mental protuberance

Remains of frontal suture

Glabella

Nasion

Internasal suture

Perpendicular plate of ethmoid

Vomer

Anterior nasal spine

Intermaxillary suture

Site of mandibular symphysis

7.2   **Cranium, facial (frontal) aspect**

A. Formations of the bony cranium. **B.** Bones of cranium and their features. The individual bones forming the cranium are color coded. For the orbital cavity, see also Figure 7.31A.

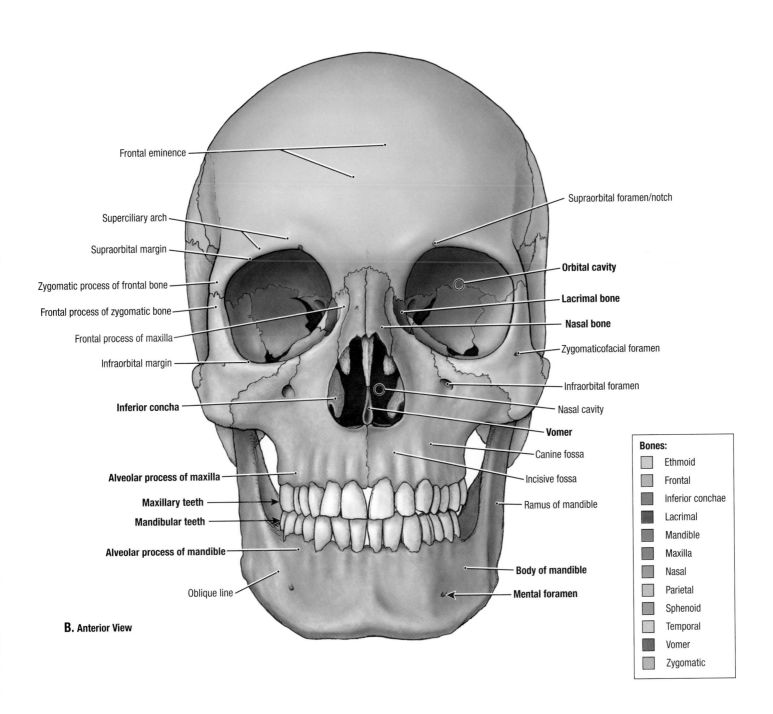

Frontal eminence

Superciliary arch

Supraorbital margin

Zygomatic process of frontal bone

Frontal process of zygomatic bone

Frontal process of maxilla

Infraorbital margin

Inferior concha

Alveolar process of maxilla

Maxillary teeth

Mandibular teeth

Alveolar process of mandible

Oblique line

B. Anterior View

Supraorbital foramen/notch

Orbital cavity

Lacrimal bone

Nasal bone

Zygomaticofacial foramen

Infraorbital foramen

Nasal cavity

Vomer

Canine fossa

Incisive fossa

Ramus of mandible

Body of mandible

Mental foramen

Bones:

- Ethmoid
- Frontal
- Inferior conchae
- Lacrimal
- Mandible
- Maxilla
- Nasal
- Parietal
- Sphenoid
- Temporal
- Vomer
- Zygomatic

7.2   Cranium, facial (frontal) aspect *(continued)*

Extraction of teeth causes the alveolar bone to resorb in the affected regions(s). Following complete loss or extraction of maxillary teeth, the sockets begin to fill in with bone, and the alveolar process begins to resorb. Similarly, extraction of mandibular teeth causes the bone to resorb. Gradually, the mental foramen lies near the superior border of the body of the mandible. In some cases, the mental foramina disappear, exposing the mental nerves to injury.

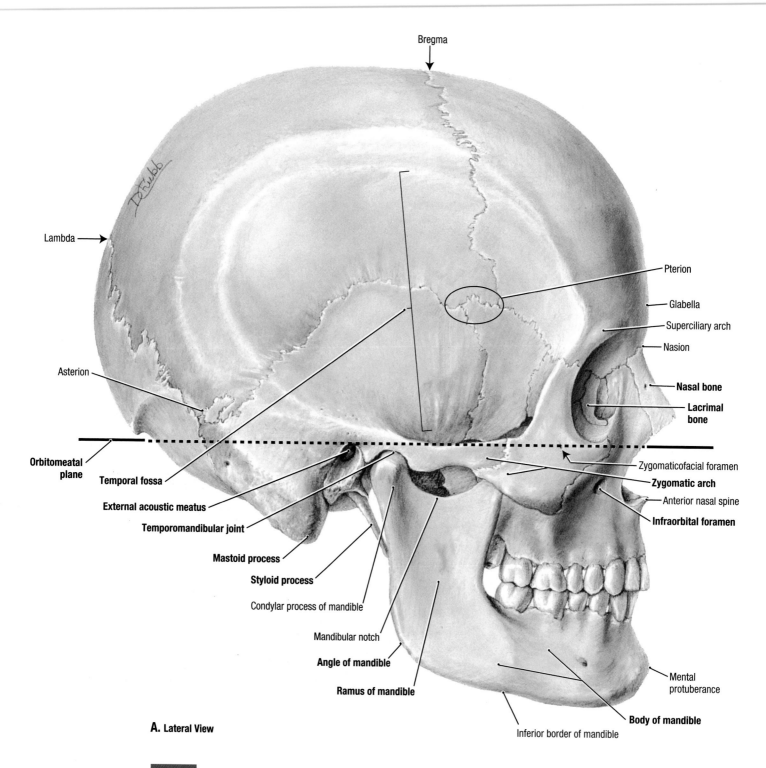

Bregma

Lambda

Asterion

Orbitomeatal
plane

Temporal fossa

External acoustic meatus

Temporomandibular joint

Mastoid process

Styloid process

Condylar process of mandible

Mandibular notch

Angle of mandible

Ramus of mandible

Pterion

Glabella

Superciliary arch

Nasion

Nasal bone

**Lacrimal
bone**

Zygomaticofacial foramen

Zygomatic arch

Anterior nasal spine

Infraorbital foramen

Mental
protuberance

Body of mandible

Inferior border of mandible

A. Lateral View

7.3 Cranium, lateral aspect

A. Bony cranium. **B.** Cranium with bones color coded. The cranium is in the anatomical position when the orbitomeatal plane is horizontal.

The convexity of the neurocranium (braincase) distributes and thereby minimizes the effects of a blow to it. However, hard blows to the head in thin areas of the cranium (e.g., in the temporal fossa) are likely to produce depressed fractures, in which a fragment of bone is depressed inward, compressing and/or injuring the brain. In comminuted fractures, the bone is broken into several pieces. Linear fractures, the most frequent type, usually occur at the point of impact, but fracture lines often radiate away from it in two or more directions.

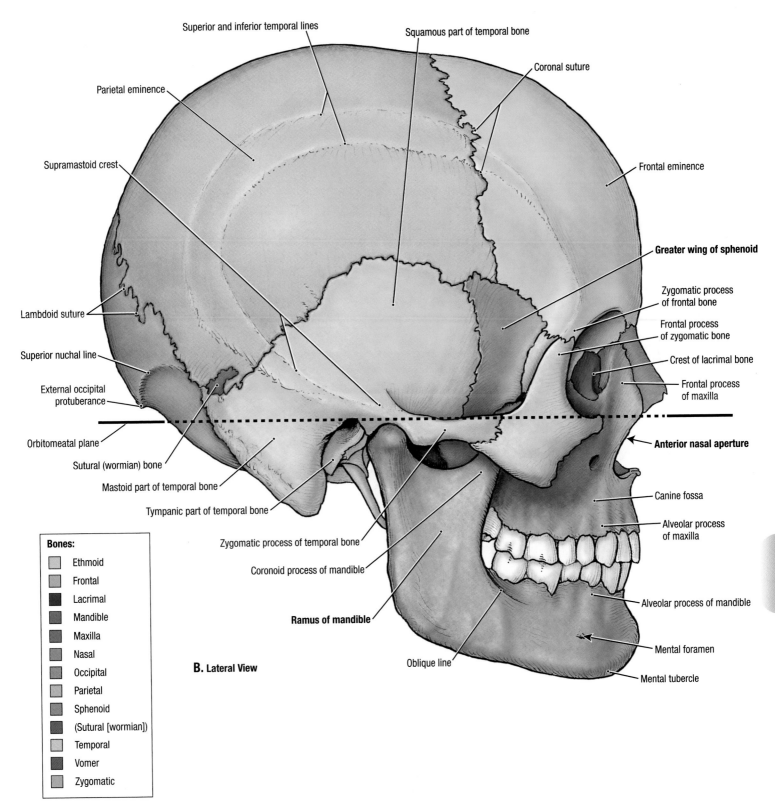

Superior and inferior temporal lines

Squamous part of temporal bone

Coronal suture

Parietal eminence

Frontal eminence

Supramastoid crest

Greater wing of sphenoid

Zygomatic process of frontal bone

Frontal process of zygomatic bone

Crest of lacrimal bone

Lambdoid suture

Frontal process of maxilla

Superior nuchal line

External occipital protuberance

Anterior nasal aperture

Orbitomeatal plane

Canine fossa

Sutural (wormian) bone

Alveolar process of maxilla

Mastoid part of temporal bone

Tympanic part of temporal bone

Zygomatic process of temporal bone

Coronoid process of mandible

Alveolar process of mandible

Ramus of mandible

Mental foramen

Oblique line

Mental tubercle

B. Lateral View

Bones:

- Ethmoid
- Frontal
- Lacrimal
- Mandible
- Maxilla
- Nasal
- Occipital
- Parietal
- Sphenoid
- (Sutural [wormian])
- Temporal
- Vomer
- Zygomatic

7.3 **Cranium, lateral aspect** *(continued)*

If the area of the neurocranium is thick at the site of impact, the bone usually bends inward without fracturing; however, a fracture may occur some distance from the site of direct trauma where the calvaria is thinner. In a contrecoup (counterblow) fracture, the fracture occurs on the opposite side of the cranium rather than at the point of impact.

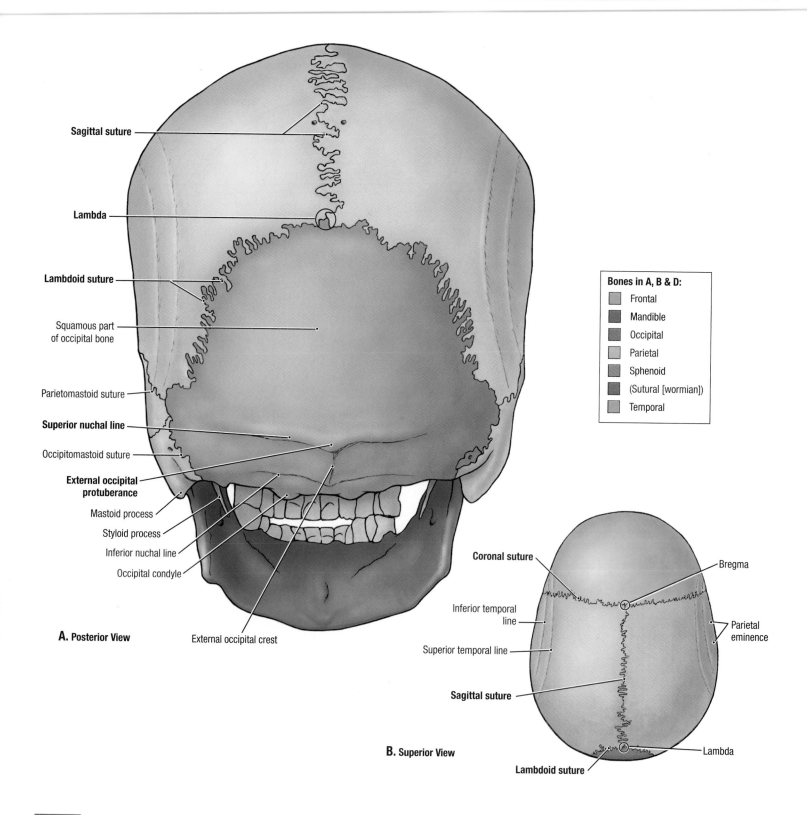

Bones in A, B & D:
- Frontal
- Mandible
- Occipital
- Parietal
- Sphenoid
- (Sutural [wormian])
- Temporal

A. Posterior View

B. Superior View

7.4   **Cranium, occipital aspect, calvaria, and anterior part of posterior cranial fossa**

A. Posterior aspect. **B.** Superior aspect.

   A. The lambda, near the center of this convex surface, is located at the junction of the superior and lambdoid sutures. **B.** The roof of the neurocranium, or calvaria (skullcap), is formed primarily by the paired parietal bones, the frontal bone, and the occipital bone.

Premature closure of the coronal suture results in a high, tower-like cranium, called oxycephaly or turricephaly. Premature closure of sutures usually does not affect brain development. When premature closure occurs on one side only, the cranium is asymmetrical, a condition known as plagiocephaly.

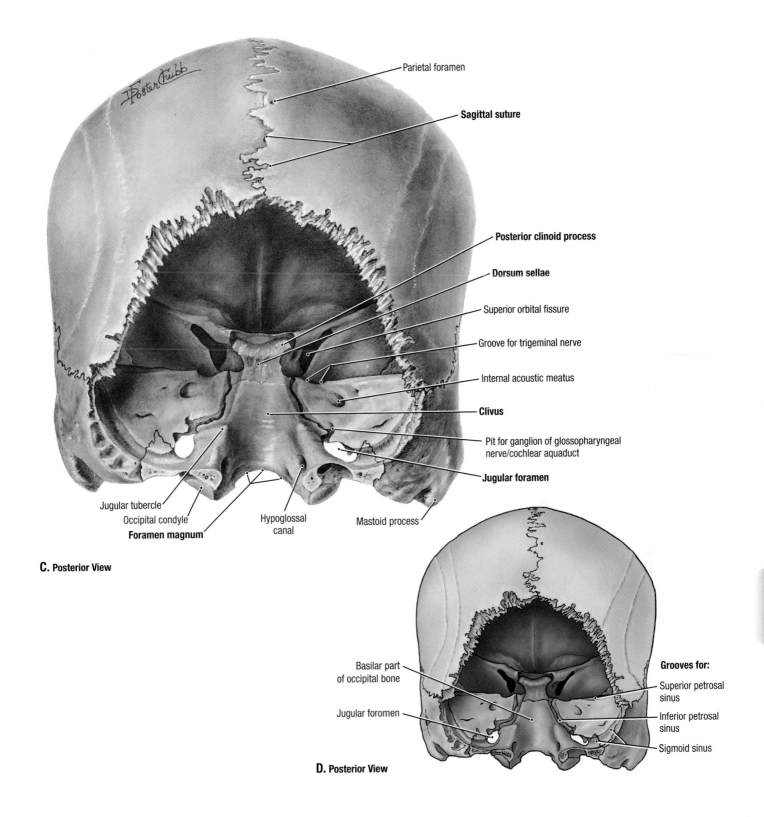

C. Posterior View

- Parietal foramen
- **Sagittal suture**
- **Posterior clinoid process**
- **Dorsum sellae**
- Superior orbital fissure
- Groove for trigeminal nerve
- Internal acoustic meatus
- **Clivus**
- Pit for ganglion of glossopharyngeal nerve/cochlear aquaduct
- **Jugular foramen**
- Mastoid process

Jugular tubercle
Occipital condyle
Foramen magnum
Hypoglossal canal

D. Posterior View

Basilar part of occipital bone
Jugular foromen

Grooves for:
- Superior petrosal sinus
- Inferior petrosal sinus
- Sigmoid sinus

7.4   **Cranium, occipital aspect, calvaria, and anterior part of posterior cranial fossa (continued)**

C and D. Cranium after removal of squamous part of occipital bone.
- The dorsum sellae projects from the body of the sphenoid; the posterior clinoid processes form its superolateral corners.
- The clivus is the slope descending from the dorsum sellae to the foramen magnum.

- The grooves for the sigmoid sinus and inferior petrosal sinus lead inferiorly to the jugular foramen.

Premature closure of the sagittal suture, in which the anterior fontanelle is small or absent, results in a long, narrow, wedge-shaped cranium, a condition called scaphocephaly.

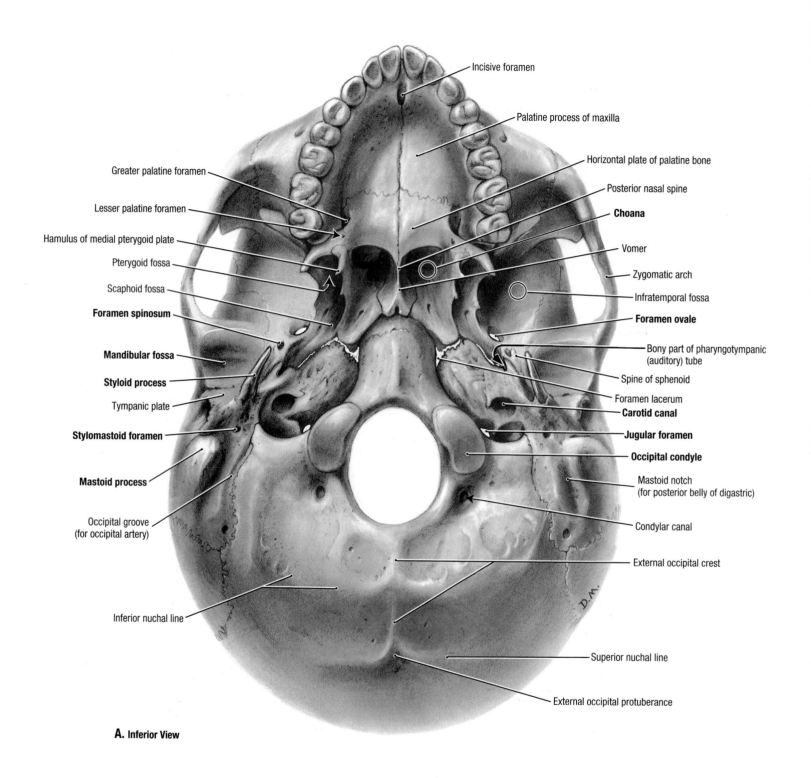

Incisive foramen

Palatine process of maxilla

Greater palatine foramen

Lesser palatine foramen

Hamulus of medial pterygoid plate

Pterygoid fossa

Scaphoid fossa

Foramen spinosum

Mandibular fossa

Styloid process

Tympanic plate

Stylomastoid foramen

Mastoid process

Occipital groove
(for occipital artery)

Inferior nuchal line

Horizontal plate of palatine bone

Posterior nasal spine

Choana

Vomer

Zygomatic arch

Infratemporal fossa

Foramen ovale

Bony part of pharyngotympanic
(auditory) tube

Spine of sphenoid

Foramen lacerum

Carotid canal

Jugular foramen

Occipital condyle

Mastoid notch
(for posterior belly of digastric)

Condylar canal

External occipital crest

Superior nuchal line

External occipital protuberance

A. Inferior View

7.5 **Cranium, inferior aspect**

A. Bony cranium. **B.** Diagram of cranium with bones color coded.

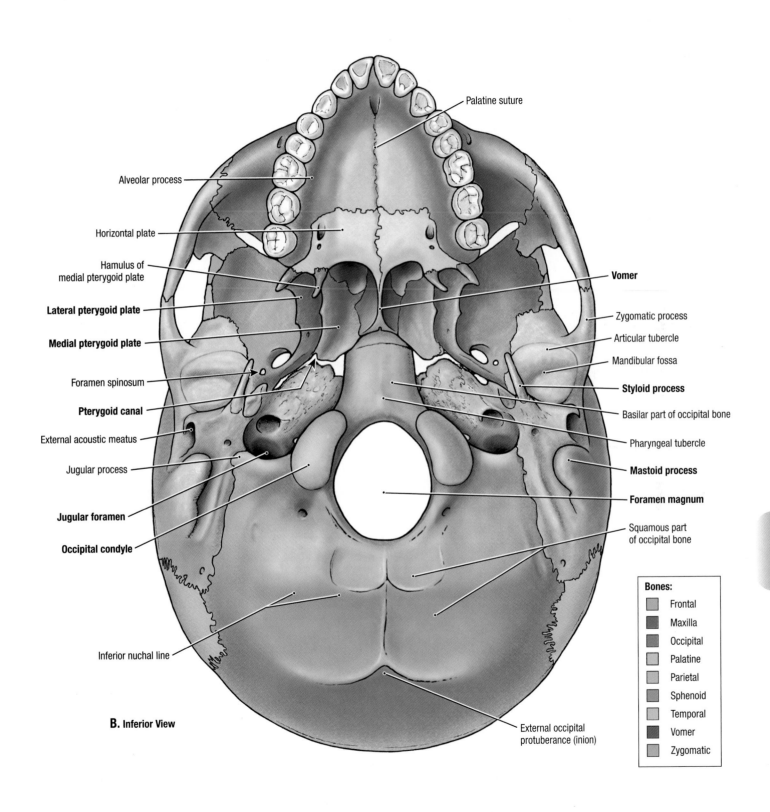

Palatine suture

Alveolar process

Horizontal plate

Hamulus of
medial pterygoid plate

Lateral pterygoid plate

Medial pterygoid plate

Foramen spinosum

Pterygoid canal

External acoustic meatus

Jugular process

Jugular foramen

Occipital condyle

Inferior nuchal line

B. Inferior View

Vomer

Zygomatic process

Articular tubercle

Mandibular fossa

Styloid process

Basilar part of occipital bone

Pharyngeal tubercle

Mastoid process

Foramen magnum

Squamous part
of occipital bone

External occipital
protuberance (inion)

Bones:

Frontal

Maxilla

Occipital

Palatine

Parietal

Sphenoid

Temporal

Vomer

Zygomatic

7.5   **Cranium, inferior aspect (continued)**

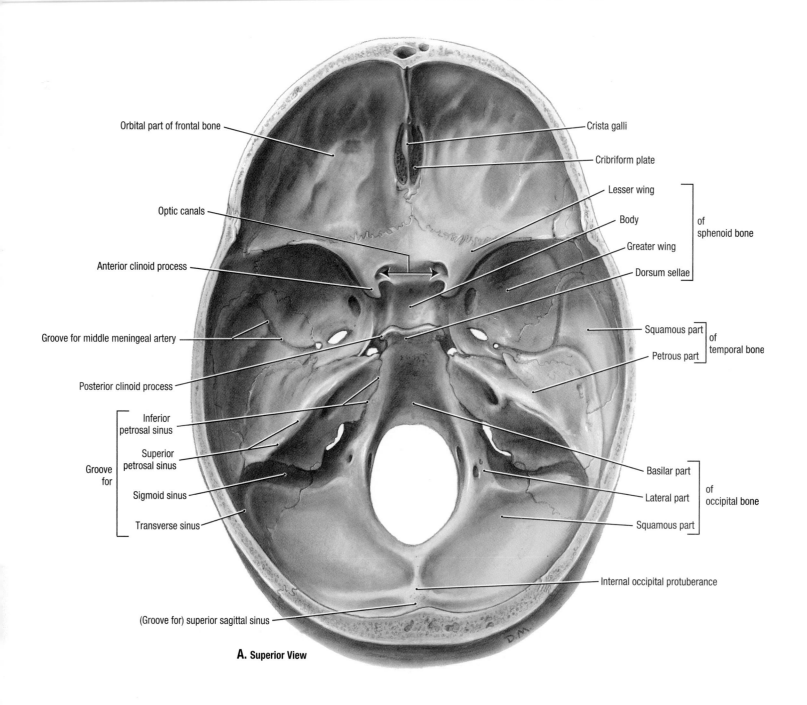

Orbital part of frontal bone

Optic canals

Anterior clinoid process

Groove for middle meningeal artery

Posterior clinoid process

Groove for:

Inferior petrosal sinus

Superior petrosal sinus

Sigmoid sinus

Transverse sinus

(Groove for) superior sagittal sinus

Crista galli

Cribriform plate

Lesser wing

Body — of sphenoid bone

Greater wing

Dorsum sellae

Squamous part — of temporal bone

Petrous part

Basilar part — of occipital bone

Lateral part

Squamous part

Internal occipital protuberance

A. Superior View

7.6   Interior of the cranial base

A. Bony cranial base. **B.** Diagrammatic cranial base with bones color coded.

In **A:**

- Three bones contribute to the anterior cranial fossa: the orbital part of the frontal bone, the cribriform plate of the ethmoid, and the lesser wing of the sphenoid.
- The four parts of the occipital bone are the basilar, right and left lateral, and squamous.
- Fractures in the floor of the anterior cranial fossa may involve the cribriform plate of the ethmoid, resulting in leakage of CSF through the nose (CSF rhinorrhea). CSF rhinorrhea may be a primary indication of a cranial base fracture which increases the risk of meningitis, because an infection could spread to the meninges from the ear or nose.

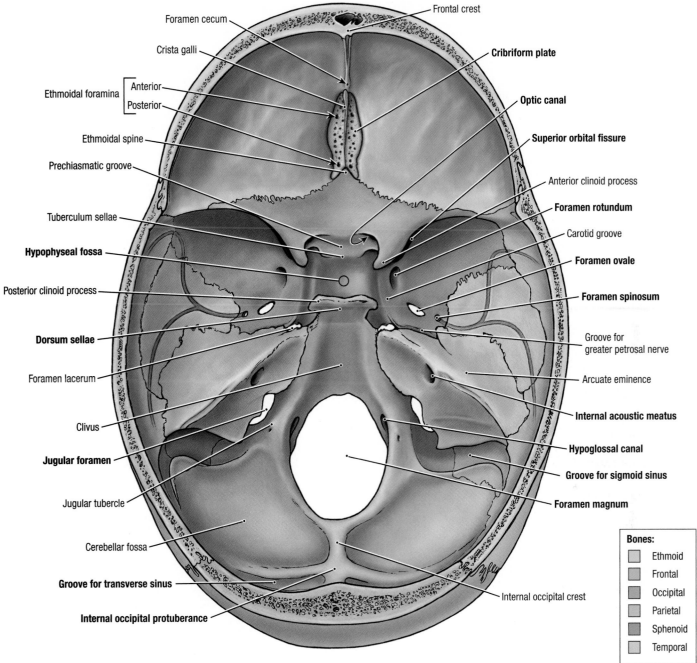

Foramen cecum

Crista galli

Ethmoidal foramina [Anterior / Posterior]

Ethmoidal spine

Prechiasmatic groove

Tuberculum sellae

Hypophyseal fossa

Posterior clinoid process

Dorsum sellae

Foramen lacerum

Clivus

Jugular foramen

Jugular tubercle

Cerebellar fossa

Groove for transverse sinus

Internal occipital protuberance

Frontal crest

Cribriform plate

Optic canal

Superior orbital fissure

Anterior clinoid process

Foramen rotundum

Carotid groove

Foramen ovale

Foramen spinosum

Groove for greater petrosal nerve

Arcuate eminence

Internal acoustic meatus

Hypoglossal canal

Groove for sigmoid sinus

Foramen magnum

Internal occipital crest

Bones:
- Ethmoid
- Frontal
- Occipital
- Parietal
- Sphenoid
- Temporal

B. Superior View

7.6   Interior of the cranial base *(continued)*

In **B,** note the following midline features:

- In the anterior cranial fossa, the frontal crest and crista galli for anterior attachment of the falx cerebri have between them the foramen cecum, which, during development, transmits a vein connecting the superior sagittal sinus with the veins of the frontal sinus and root of the nose.
- In the middle cranial fossa, the tuberculum sellae, hypophyseal fossa, dorsum sellae, and posterior clinoid processes constitute the sella turcica (L. Turkish saddle).
- In the posterior cranial fossa, note the clivus, foramen magnum, internal occipital crest for attachment of the falx cerebelli, and the internal occipital protuberance, from which the grooves for the transverse sinuses course laterally.

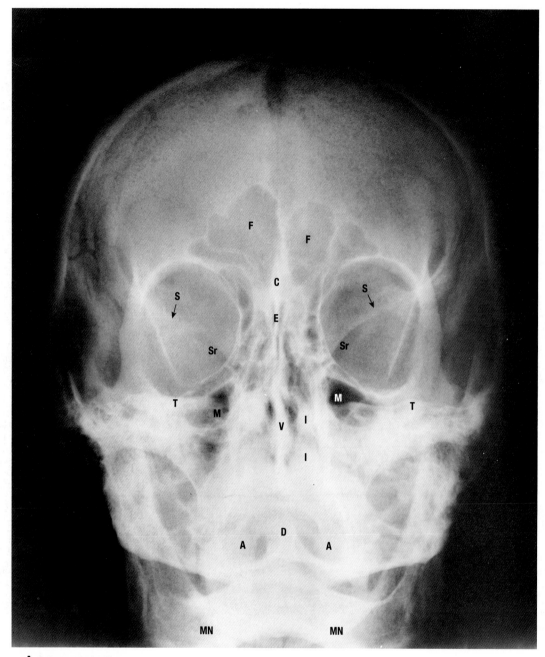

A. Anteroposterior View

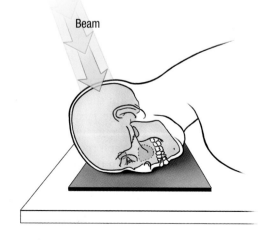

Beam

7.7   Radiographs of the cranium

A. Posteroanterior (Caldwell) radiograph. This view places the orbits centrally in the head and is used to examine the orbits and paranasal sinuses. Observe in **A**:

- The labeled features include the superior orbital fissure *(Sr)*, lesser wing of the sphenoid *(S)*, superior surface of the petrous part of the temporal bone *(T)*, crista galli *(C)*, frontal sinus *(F)*, mandible *(MN)*, and maxillary sinus *(M)*.
- The nasal septum is formed by the perpendicular plate of the ethmoid *(E)* and the vomer *(V)*; note the inferior and middle conchae *(I)* of the lateral wall of the nose.
- Superimposed on the facial skeleton are the dens *(D)* and lateral masses of the atlas *(A)*.

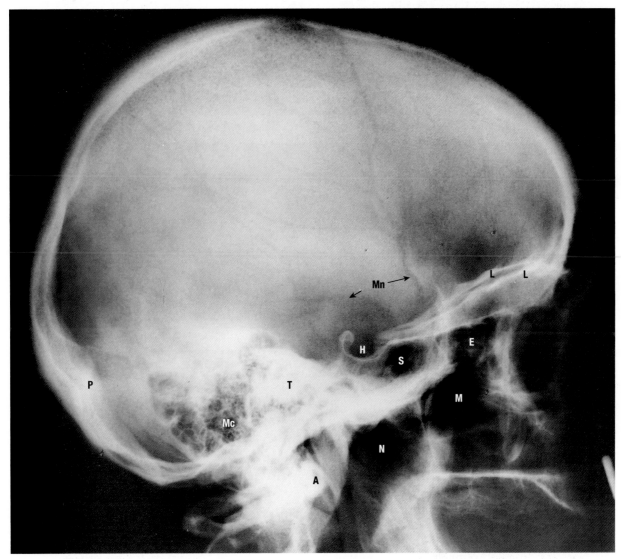

B. Lateral View

7.7 Radiographs of the cranium *(continued)*

B. Lateral radiograph of the cranium. Most of the relatively thin bone of the facial skeleton (viscerocranium) is radiolucent (appears black).

- The labeled features include the ethmoidal cells (*E*), sphenoidal (*S*) and maxillary (*M*) sinuses, the hypophyseal fossa (*H*) for the pituitary gland, the petrous part of the temporal bone (*T*), mastoid cells (*Mc*), grooves for the branches of the middle meningeal vessels (*Mn*), arch of the atlas (*A*), internal occipital protuberance (*P*), and the nasopharynx (*N*).
- The right and left orbital plates of the frontal bone are not superimposed; thus, the floor of the anterior cranial fossa appears as two lines (*L*).

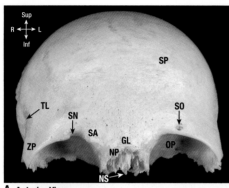

A. Anterior View

B. Inferior View

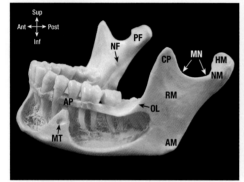

C. Lateral View

D. Posteromedial View

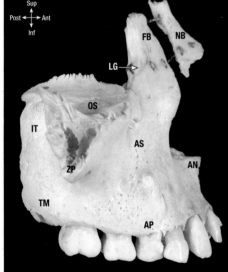

E. Lateral View

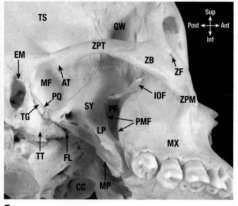

F. Inferolateral View

Key

Frontal Bone

EN	Ethmoidal notch
FL	Fossa for lacrimal gland
FS	Opening of frontal sinus
GL	Glabella
NP	Nasal part
NS	Nasal spine
OP	Orbital part
RE	Root of ethmoid cells
SA	Superciliary arch
SM	Sphenoidal margin
SN	Supra-orbital notch
SO	Supra-orbital foramen
SP	Squamous part
SU	Supra-orbital margin
TL	Temporal line
TS	Temporal surface
ZP	Zygomatic process

Mandible

AM	Angle of mandible
AP	Alveolar part
CP	Coronoid process
HM	Head of mandible
LI	Lingula
ML	Mylohyoid groove
MN	Mandibular notch
MS	Superior and inferior mental spines
MT	Mental foramen
NF	Mandibular foramen
NM	Neck of mandible
PF	Pterygoid fovea
RM	Ramus of mandible
SL	Sublingual fossa
SM	Submandibular fossa

Pterygopalatine fossa

PF	Pterygopalatine fossa
MF	Mandibular fossa
AT	Articular tubercle
ZPT	Zygomatic process of temporal bone
CC	Carotid canal
FL	Foramen lacerum
ZF	Zygomaticofacial foramen
PQ	Petrosquamous fissure
TG	Tegmen tympani
TT	Temporal bone (tympanic part)
ZB	Zygomatic bone
MX	Maxilla
IOF	Inferior orbital fissure
PMF	Pterygomaxillary fissure
ZPM	Zygomatic process of maxilla
EM	External acoustic meatus
GW	Greater wing of sphenoid
LP	Lateral pterygoid plate
MP	Medial pterygoid plate
SY	Stylomastoid foramen

Maxilla and nasal bone

AN	Anterior nasal spine
AP	Alveolar part
AS	Anterior surface of maxilla
FP	Frontal process of maxilla
IT	Infratemporal surface of maxilla
LG	Lacrimal groove
NB	Nasal bone
OS	Orbital surface
TM	Tuberosity
ZP	Zygomatic process

7.8   **Superficial bones of facial skeleton**

A and **B.** Frontal bone. **C** and **D.** Mandible. **E.** Maxilla. **F.** Infratemporal fossa.

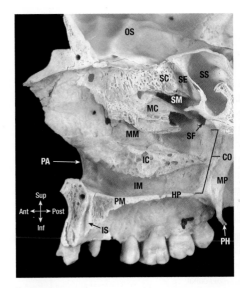

A. Medial View

C. Anterior View

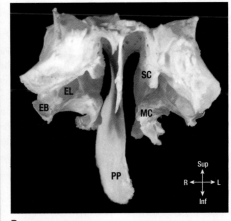

B. Anterior View

D. Posterior View

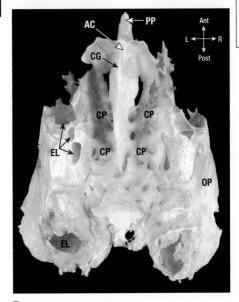

E. Superior View

Key

Lateral Wall of Nose

CO	Choana (posterior nasal aperture)
HP	Horizontal plate of palatine bone
IC	Inferior nasal concha
IS	Incisive canal
IM	Inferior nasal meatus
MC	Middle nasal concha
MM	Middle nasal meatus
PH	Pterygoid hamulus
PM	Palatine process of maxilla
OS	Orbital surface of frontal bone
PA	Piriform aperture
PM	Palatine process of maxilla
SC	Superior nasal concha
SE	Spheno-ethmoidal recess
SF	Sphenopalatine foramen
SM	Superior nasal meatus
SS	Sphenoidal sinus

Palatine Bone

HP	Horizontal plate
NC	Nasal crest
OP	Orbital process
PP	Perpendicular plate
PY	Pyramidal process

Ethmoid Bone

AC	Ala of crista galli
CG	Crista galli
CP	Cribriform plate
EB	Ethmoidal bulla
EL	Ethmoidal labyrinth (ethmoidal cells)
MC	Middle nasal concha
OP	Orbital plate
PP	Perpendicular plate
SC	Superior nasal concha

7.9   **Deep bones of facial skeleton**

A. Lateral wall of nose. **B.** Palatine bone. **C–E.** Ethmoid bone.

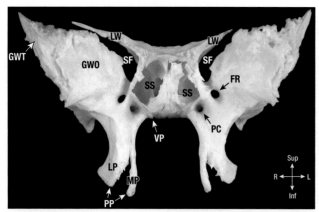

A. Anterior View

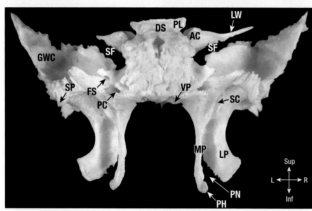

B. Posterior View

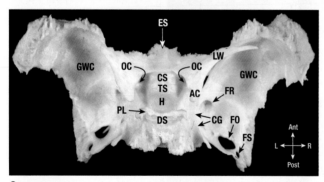

C. Superior View

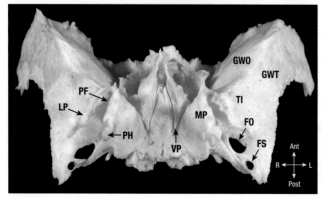

D. Inferior View

Key

AC	Anterior clinoid process
CG	Carotid sulcus
CS	Prechiasmatic sulcus
DS	Dorsum sellae
ES	Ethmoidal spine
FO	Foramen ovale
FR	Foramen rotundum
FS	Foramen spinosum
GWC	Greater wing (cerebral surface)
GWO	Greater wing (orbital surface)
GWT	Greater wing (temporal surface)
H	Hypophysial fossa
LP	Lateral pterygoid plate
LW	Lesser wing
MP	Medial pterygoid plate
OC	Optic canal
PC	Pterygoid canal
PF	Pterygoid fossa
PH	Pterygoid hamulus
PL	Posterior clinoid process
PN	Pterygoid notch
PP	Pterygoid process
SC	Scaphoid fossa
SF	Superior orbital fissure
SP	Spine of sphenoid bone
SS	Sphenoidal sinus (in body of sphenoid)
TI	Greater wing of sphenoid (Infratemporal surface)
TS	Tuberculum sellae
VP	Vaginal process

7.10   Sphenoid bone

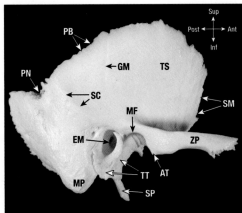

A. Lateral View

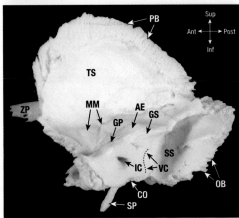

B. Medial View

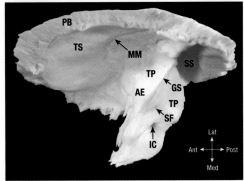

C. Superior View

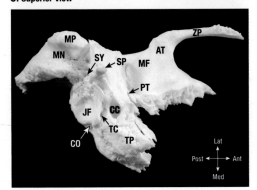

D. Inferior View

Key

AE	Arcuate eminence
AT	Articular tubercle
CC	Carotid canal
CO	Cochlear canaliculus
EM	External acoustic meatus
GM	Groove for middle temporal artery
GP	Hiatus for greater petrosal nerve
GS	Groove for superior petrosal sinus
IC	Internal acoustic meatus
JF	Jugular fossa
MF	Mandibular fossa
MM	Groove for middle meningeal artery
MN	Mastoid notch
MP	Mastoid process
OB	Occipital border
PB	Parietal border
PN	Parietal notch
PT	Petrotympanic fissure
SC	Supramastoid crest
SF	Subarcuate fossa
SM	Sphenoid margin
SP	Styloid process
SS	Groove for sigmoid sinus
SY	Stylomastoid foramen
TC	Tympanic canaliculus
TP	Temporal bone (petrous part)
TS	Temporal bone (squamous part)
TT	Temporal bone (tympanic part)
VC	Vestibular canaliculus
ZP	Zygomatic process

7.11   Temporal bone

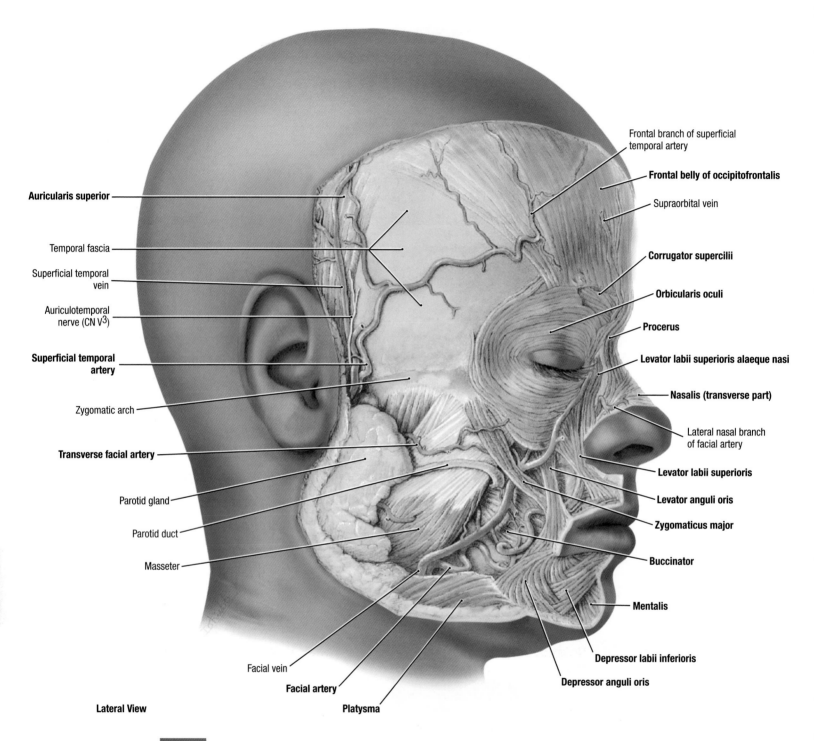

Auricularis superior

Temporal fascia

Superficial temporal vein

Auriculotemporal nerve (CN V³)

Superficial temporal artery

Zygomatic arch

Transverse facial artery

Parotid gland

Parotid duct

Masseter

Facial vein

Facial artery

Lateral View

Platysma

Frontal branch of superficial temporal artery

Frontal belly of occipitofrontalis

Supraorbital vein

Corrugator supercilii

Orbicularis oculi

Procerus

Levator labii superioris alaeque nasi

Nasalis (transverse part)

Lateral nasal branch of facial artery

Levator labii superioris

Levator anguli oris

Zygomaticus major

Buccinator

Mentalis

Depressor labii inferioris

Depressor anguli oris

7.12   Muscles of facial expression and arteries of the face

- The muscles of facial expression are the superficial sphincters and dilators of the openings of the head; all are supplied by the facial nerve (CN VII). The masseter and temporalis (the latter covered here by temporal fascia) are muscles of mastication that are innervated by the trigeminal nerve (CN V).

- The pulses of the superficial temporal and facial arteries can be used for taking the pulse. For example, anesthesiologists at the head of the operating table often take the temporal pulse anterior to the auricle as the artery crosses the zygomatic arch to supply the scalp. The facial pulse can be palpated where the facial artery crosses the inferior border of the mandible immediately anterior to the masseter.

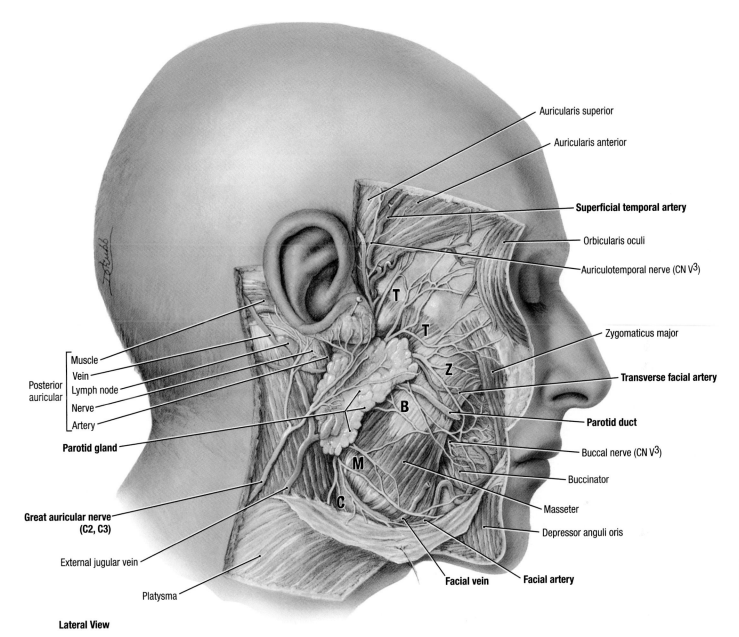

Auricularis superior

Auricularis anterior

Superficial temporal artery

Orbicularis oculi

Auriculotemporal nerve (CN V³)

Zygomaticus major

Transverse facial artery

Parotid duct

Buccal nerve (CN V³)

Buccinator

Masseter

Depressor anguli oris

Facial artery

Facial vein

Posterior auricular
— Muscle
— Vein
— Lymph node
— Nerve
— Artery

Parotid gland

Great auricular nerve (C2, C3)

External jugular vein

Platysma

Lateral View

7.13 Relationships of the branches of the facial nerve and vessels to the parotid gland and duct

- The parotid duct extends across the masseter muscle just inferior to the zygomatic arch; the duct turns medially to pierce the buccinator.
- The facial nerve (CN VII) innervates the muscles of facial expression; it forms a plexus within the parotid gland, the branches of which radiate over the face, anastomosing with each other and the branches of the trigeminal nerve. After emerging from the stylomastoid foramen, the main stem of the facial nerve has posterior auricular, digastric, and stylohyoid branches; the parotid plexus gives rise to temporal (T), zygomatic (Z), buccal (B), marginal mandibular (M), cervical (C), and posterior auricular branches.
- During parotidectomy (surgical excision of the parotid gland), identification, dissection, and preservation of the branches of the facial nerve are critical.
- The parotid gland may become infected by infectious agents that pass through the bloodstream, as occurs in mumps, an acute communicable viral disease. Infection of the gland causes inflammation (parotiditis) and swelling of the gland. Severe pain occurs because the parotid sheath, innervated by the great auricular nerve, limits swelling.

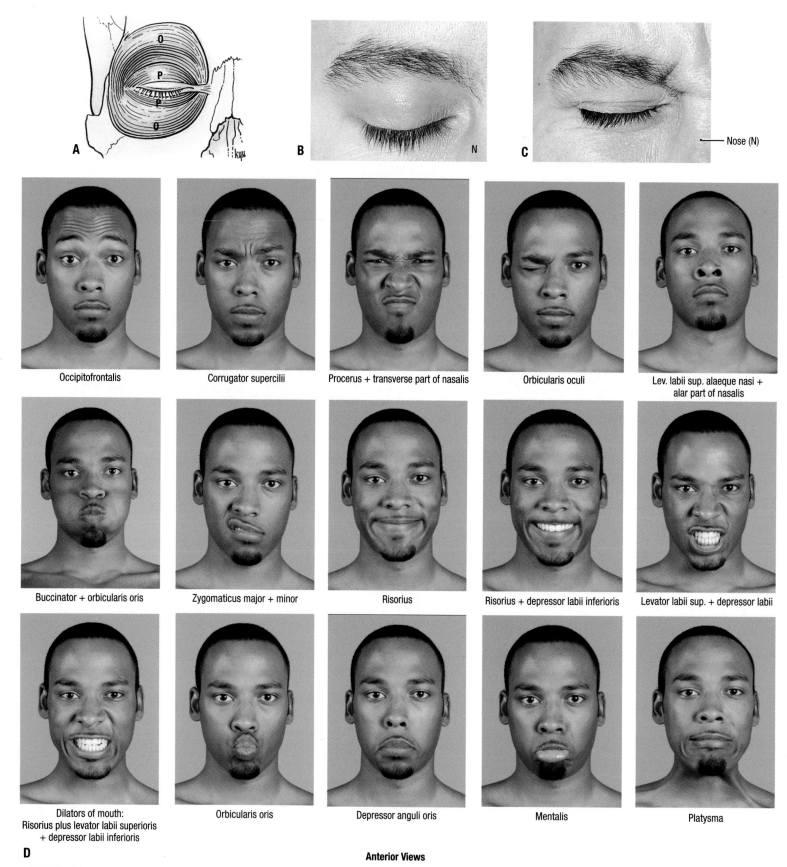

A

B   N

C   — Nose (N)

Occipitofrontalis

Corrugator supercilii

Procerus + transverse part of nasalis

Orbicularis oculi

Lev. labii sup. alaeque nasi + alar part of nasalis

Buccinator + orbicularis oris

Zygomaticus major + minor

Risorius

Risorius + depressor labii inferioris

Levator labii sup. + depressor labii

Dilators of mouth:
Risorius plus levator labii superioris + depressor labii inferioris

Orbicularis oris

Depressor anguli oris

Mentalis

Platysma

D

Anterior Views

7.14 Muscles of facial expression

A. Orbicularis oculi: palpebral (P) and orbital (O) parts. The lacrimal portion (not shown) passes posterior to the lacrimal sac and helps spread of lacrimal secretions. **B.** Gentle closure of eyelid—palpebral part. **C.** Tight closure of eyelid—orbital part. **D.** Actions of selected muscles of facial expression.

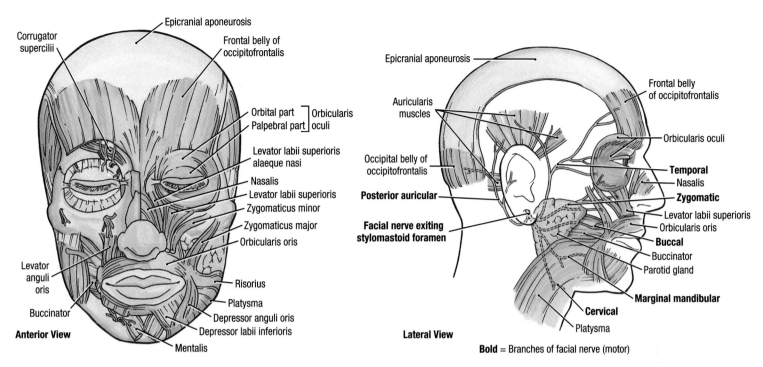

Corrugator supercilii
Epicranial aponeurosis
Frontal belly of occipitofrontalis
Orbital part | Orbicularis
Palpebral part | oculi
Levator labii superioris alaeque nasi
Nasalis
Levator labii superioris
Zygomaticus minor
Zygomaticus major
Orbicularis oris
Levator anguli oris
Risorius
Buccinator
Platysma
Depressor anguli oris
Depressor labii inferioris
Mentalis

Anterior View

Epicranial aponeurosis
Auricularis muscles
Occipital belly of occipitofrontalis
Frontal belly of occipitofrontalis
Orbicularis oculi
Temporal
Nasalis
Zygomatic
Levator labii superioris
Orbicularis oris
Buccal
Buccinator
Parotid gland
Posterior auricular
Facial nerve exiting stylomastoid foramen
Marginal mandibular
Cervical
Platysma

Lateral View

Bold = Branches of facial nerve (motor)

TABLE 7.1 MAIN MUSCLES OF FACIAL EXPRESSION[a]

Muscle	Origin	Insertion	Action
Frontal belly of occipitofrontalis	Epicranial aponeurosis	Skin of forehead	Elevates eyebrows and forehead
Orbicularis oculi	Medial orbital margin, medial palpebral ligament, and lacrimal bone	Skin around margin of orbit; tarsal plate	Closes eyelids
Nasalis	Superior part of canine ridge of maxilla	Nasal cartilages	Flares nostrils
Orbicularis oris	Some fibers arise near median plane of maxilla superiorly and mandible inferiorly; other fibers arise from deep surface of skin	Mucous membrane of lips	Compresses and protrudes lips (e.g., purses them during whistling, sucking, and kissing)
Levator labii superioris	Frontal process of maxilla and infraorbital region	Skin of upper lip and alar cartilage of nose	Elevates lip, dilates nostril, and raises angle of mouth
Platysma	Superficial fascia of deltoid and pectoral regions	Mandible, skin of cheek, angle of mouth, and orbicularis oris	Depresses mandible and tenses skin of lower face and neck
Mentalis	Incisive fossa of mandible	Skin of chin	Protrudes lower lip
Buccinator	Mandible, pterygomandibular raphe, and alveolar processes of maxilla and mandible	Angle of mouth	Presses cheek against molar teeth to keep food between teeth; expels air from oral cavity as occurs when playing a wind instrument

[a]All of these muscles are supplied by the facial nerve (CN VII).

Injury to the facial nerve (CN VII) or its branches produces paralysis of some or all of the facial muscles on the affected side (Bell palsy). The affected area sags, and facial expression is distorted. The loss of tonus of the orbicularis oculi causes the inferior lid to evert (fall away from the surface of the eyeball). As a result, the lacrimal fluid is not spread over the cornea, preventing adequate lubrication, hydration, and flushing of the cornea. This makes the cornea vulnerable to ulceration. If the injury weakens or paralyzes the buccinator and orbicularis oris, food will accumulate in the oral vestibule during chewing, usually requiring continual removal with a finger. When the sphincters or dilators of the mouth are affected, displacement of the mouth (drooping of the corner) is produced by gravity and contraction of unopposed contralateral facial muscles, resulting in food and saliva dribbling out of the side of the mouth. Weakened lip muscles affect speech. Affected people cannot whistle or blow a wind instrument effectively. They frequently dab their eyes and mouth with a handkerchief to wipe the fluid (tears and saliva) that runs from the drooping lid and mouth.

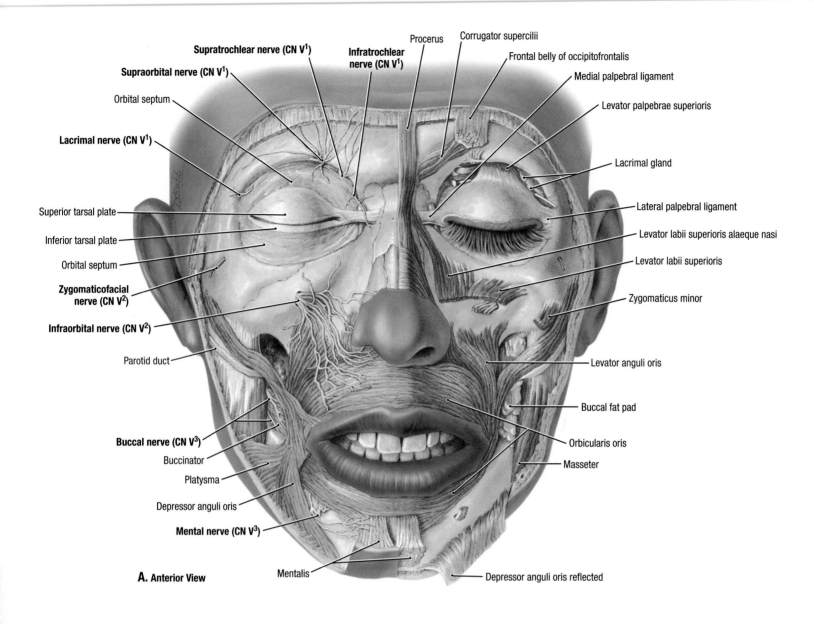

Supratrochlear nerve (CN V¹)
Supraorbital nerve (CN V¹)
Orbital septum
Lacrimal nerve (CN V¹)
Superior tarsal plate
Inferior tarsal plate
Orbital septum
Zygomaticofacial nerve (CN V²)
Infraorbital nerve (CN V²)
Parotid duct
Buccal nerve (CN V³)
Buccinator
Platysma
Depressor anguli oris
Mental nerve (CN V³)
Mentalis
A. Anterior View

Procerus
Corrugator supercilii
Infratrochlear nerve (CN V¹)
Frontal belly of occipitofrontalis
Medial palpebral ligament
Levator palpebrae superioris
Lacrimal gland
Lateral palpebral ligament
Levator labii superioris alaeque nasi
Levator labii superioris
Zygomaticus minor
Levator anguli oris
Buccal fat pad
Orbicularis oris
Masseter
Depressor anguli oris reflected

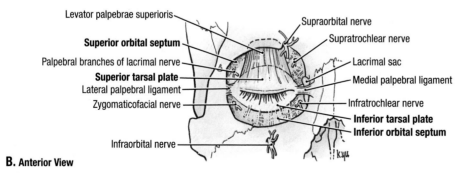

Levator palpebrae superioris
Superior orbital septum
Palpebral branches of lacrimal nerve
Superior tarsal plate
Lateral palpebral ligament
Zygomaticofacial nerve
Infraorbital nerve
B. Anterior View

Supraorbital nerve
Supratrochlear nerve
Lacrimal sac
Medial palpebral ligament
Infratrochlear nerve
Inferior tarsal plate
Inferior orbital septum

7.15   Cutaneous branches of trigeminal nerve, muscles of facial expression, and eyelid

A. Dissection of face. B. Orbital septum and eyelid.
Because the face does not have a distinct layer of deep fascia and the subcutaneous tissue is loose between the attachments of facial muscles, facial lacerations tend to gap (part widely). Consequently, the skin must be sutured carefully to prevent scarring. The looseness of the subcutaneous tissue also enables fluid and blood to accumulate in the loose connective tissue after bruising of the face.

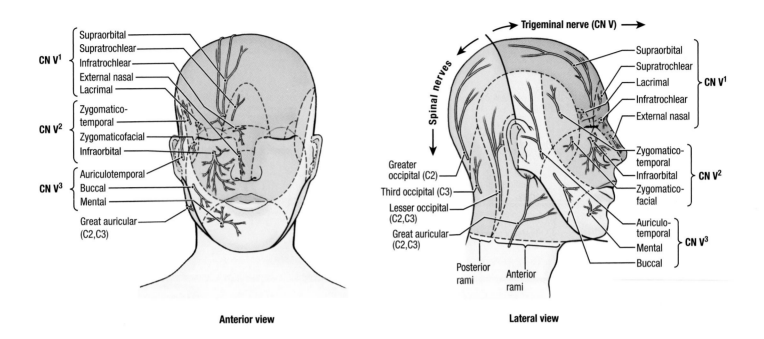

Anterior view

Lateral view

TABLE 7.2 NERVES OF FACE AND SCALP

Nerve	Origin	Course	Distribution
Frontal	Ophthalmic nerve (CN V¹)	Crosses orbit on superior aspect of levator palpebrae superioris; divides into supraorbital and supratrochlear branches	Skin of forehead, scalp, superior eyelid, and nose; conjunctiva of superior lid and mucosa of frontal sinus
Supraorbital	Continuation of frontal nerve (CN V¹)	Emerges through supraorbital notch, or foramen, and and breaks up into small branches	Mucous membrane of frontal sinus and conjunctiva (lining) of superior eyelid; skin of forehead as far as vertex
Supratrochlear	Frontal nerve (CN V¹)	Continues anteromedially along roof of orbit, passing lateral to trochlea	Skin in middle of forehead to hairline
Infratrochlear	Nasociliary nerve (CN V¹)	Follows medial wall of orbit passing inferior to trochlea to superior eyelid	Skin and conjunctiva (lining) of superior eye lid
Lacrimal	Ophthalmic nerve (CN V¹)	Passes through palpebral fascia of superior eyelid near lateral angle (canthus) of eye	Lacrimal gland and small area of skin and conjunctiva of lateral part of superior eyelid
External nasal	Anterior ethmoidal nerve (CN V¹)	Runs in nasal cavity and emerges on face between nasal bone and lateral nasal cartilage	Skin on dorsum of nose, including tip of nose
Zygomatic	Maxillary nerve (CN V²)	Arises in floor of orbit, divides into zygomaticofacial and zygomaticotemporal nerves, which traverse foramina of same name	Skin over zygomatic arch and anterior temporal region; carries postsynaptic parasympathetic fibers from pterygopalatine ganglion to lacrimal nerve
Infraorbital	Terminal branch of maxillary nerve (CN V²)	Runs in floor of orbit and emerges at infraorbital foramen	Skin of cheek, inferior lid, lateral side of nose and inferior septum and superior lip, upper premolar incisors and canine teeth; mucosa of maxillary sinus and superior lip
Auriculotemporal	Mandibular nerve (CN V³)	From posterior division of CN V³, it passes between neck of mandible and external acoustic meatus to accompany superficial temporal artery	Skin anterior to ear and posterior temporal region, tragus and part of helix of auricle, and roof of external acoustic meatus and upper tympanic membrane
Buccal	Mandibular nerve (CN V³)	From the anterior division of CN V³ in infratemporal fossa, it passes anteriorly to reach cheek	Skin and mucosa of cheek, buccal gingiva adjacent to 2nd and 3rd molar teeth
Mental	Terminal branch of inferior alveolar nerve (CN V³)	Emerges from mandibular canal at mental foramen	Skin of chin and inferior lip and mucosa of lower lip

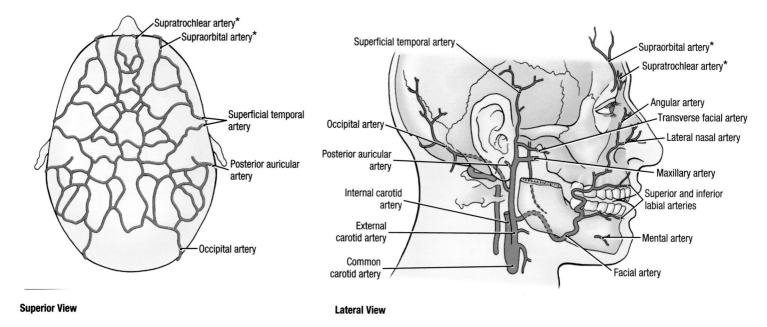

Superior View

Lateral View

*Source= internal carotid artery (ophthalmic artery); all other labeled arteries are from external carotid

TABLE 7.3 ARTERIES OF FACE AND SCALP

Artery	Origin	Course	Distribution
Facial	External carotid artery	Ascends deep to submandibular gland, winds around inferior border of mandible and enters face	Muscles of facial expression and face
Inferior labial	Facial artery near angle of mouth	Runs medially in lower lip	Lower lip and chin
Superior labial		Runs medially in upper lip	Upper lip and ala (side) and septum of nose
Lateral nasal	Facial artery as it ascends alongside nose	Passes to ala of nose	Skin on ala and dorsum of nose
Angular	Terminal branch of facial artery	Passes to medial angle (canthus) of eye	Superior part of cheek and lower eyelid
Occipital	External carotid artery	Passes medial to posterior belly of digastric and mastoid process; accompanies occipital nerve in occipital region	Scalp of back of head, as far as vertex
Posterior auricular		Passes posteriorly, deep to parotid, along styloid process between mastoid and ear	Scalp posterior to auricle and auricle
Superficial temporal	Smaller terminal branch of external carotid artery	Ascends anterior to ear to temporal region and ends in scalp	Facial muscles and skin of frontal and temporal regions
Transverse facial	Superficial temporal artery within parotid gland	Crosses face superficial to masseter and inferior to zygomatic arch	Parotid gland and duct, muscles and skin of face
Mental	Terminal branch of inferior alveolar artery	Emerges from mental foramen and passes to chin	Facial muscles and skin of chin
*Supraorbital	Terminal branch of ophthalmic artery, a branch of internal carotid artery	Passes superiorly from supraorbital foramen	Muscles and skin of forehead and scalp
*Supratrochlear		Passes superiorly from supratrochlear notch	Muscles and skin of scalp

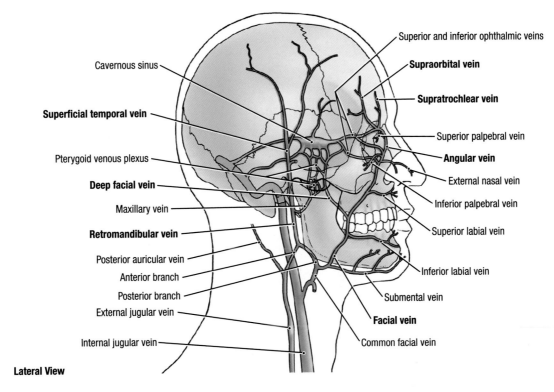

Lateral View

TABLE 7.4 VEINS OF FACE

Vein	Origin	Course	Termination	Area Drained
Supratrochlear	Begins from a venous plexus on the forehead and scalp, through which it communicates with the frontal branch of the superficial temporal vein, its contralateral partner, and the supraorbital vein	Descends near the midline of the forehead to the root of the nose where it joins the supraorbital vein	Angular vein at the root of the nose	Anterior part of scalp and forehead
Supraorbital	Begins in the forehead by anastomosing with a frontal tributary of the superficial temporal vein	Passes medially superior to the orbit and joins the supratrochlear vein; a branch passes through the supraorbital notch and joins with the superior ophthalmic vein		
Angular	Begins at root of nose by union of supratrochlear and supraorbital veins	Descends obliquely along the root and side of the nose to the inferior margin of the orbit	Becomes the facial vein at the inferior margin of the orbit	In addition to above, drains upper and lower lids and conjunctiva; may receive drainage from cavernous sinus
Facial	Continuation of angular vein past inferior margin of orbit	Descends along lateral border of the nose, receiving external nasal and inferior palpebral veins, then obliquely across face to mandible; receives anterior division of retromandibular vein, after which it is sometimes called the common facial vein	Internal jugular vein opposite or inferior to the level of the hyoid bone	Anterior scalp and forehead, eyelids, external nose, and anterior cheek, lips, chin, and submandibular gland
Deep facial	Pterygoid venous plexus	Runs anteriorly on maxilla above buccinator and deep to masseter, emerging medial to anterior border of masseter onto face	Enters posterior aspect of facial vein	Infratemporal fossa (most areas supplied by maxillary artery)
Superficial temporal	Begins from a widespread plexus of veins on the side of the scalp and along the zygomatic arch	Its frontal and parietal tributaries unite anterior to the auricle; it crosses the temporal root of the zygomatic arch to pass from the temporal region and enters the substance of the parotid gland	Joins the maxillary vein posterior to the neck of the mandible to form the retromandibular vein	Side of the scalp, superficial aspect of the temporal muscle, and external ear
Retromandibular	Formed anterior to the ear by the union of the superficial temporal and maxillary veins	Runs posterior and deep to the ramus of the mandible through the substance of the parotid gland; communicates at its inferior end with the facial vein	*Anterior branch* unites with facial vein to form common facial vein; *posterior branch* unites with the posterior auricular vein to form the external jugular vein	Parotid gland and masseter muscle

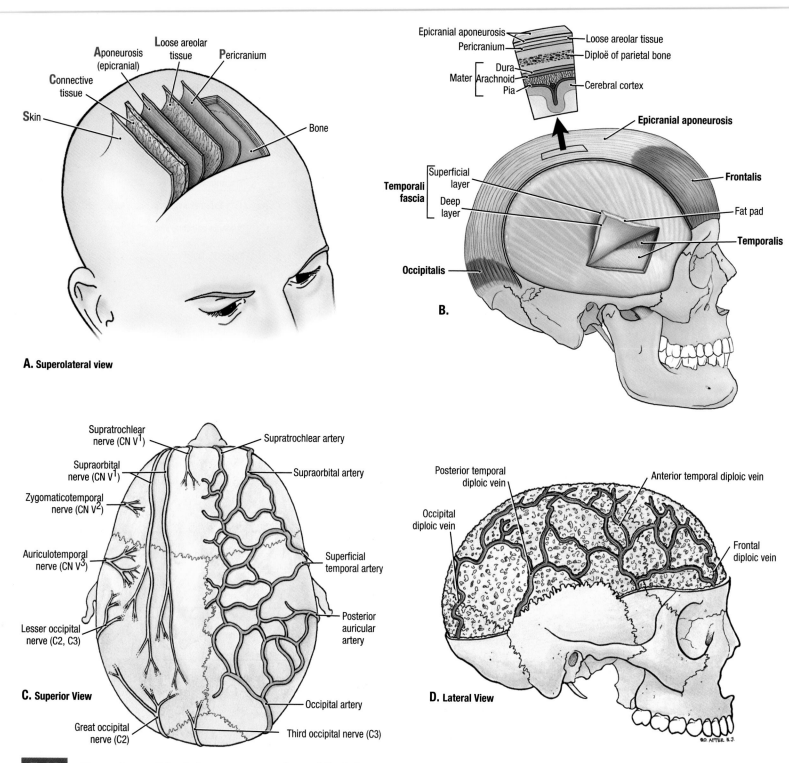

A. Superolateral view

B.

C. Superior View

D. Lateral View

7.16   Branches of facial nerve, muscles of facial expression, and scalp

A. Layers of scalp. **B.** Occipitofrontalis and temporal muscles and fascia. **C.** Sensory nerves and arteries of the scalp. **D.** Diploic veins. The outer layer of the compact bone of the cranium has been filed away, exposing the channels for the diploic veins in the cancellous bone that composes the diploë.

The loose areolar tissue layer is the danger area of the scalp because pus or blood spreads easily in it. Infection in this layer can pass into the cranial cavity through emissary veins, which pass through parietal foramina in the calvaria and reach intracranial structures such as the meninges. An infection cannot pass into the neck because the occipital belly of the occipitofrontalis attaches to the occipital bone and mastoid parts of the temporal bones. Neither can a scalp infection spread laterally beyond the zygomatic arches because the epicranial aponeurosis is continuous with the temporalis fascia that attaches to these arches. An infection or fluid (e.g., pus or blood) can enter the eyelids and the root of the nose because the frontal belly of the occipitofrontalis inserts into the skin and dense subcutaneous tissue and does not attach to the bone. Ecchymoses, or purple patches, develop as a result of extravasation of blood into the subcutaneous tissue and skin of the eyelids and surrounding regions.

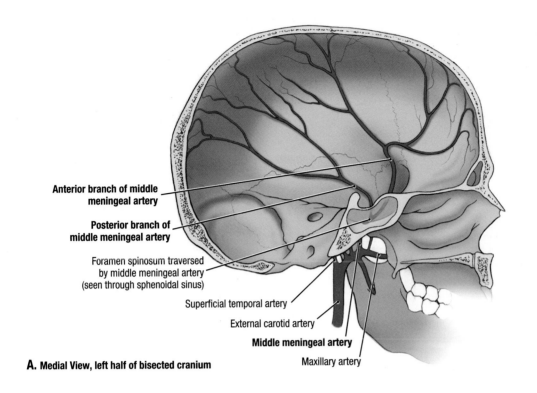

Anterior branch of middle
meningeal artery

Posterior branch of
middle meningeal artery

Foramen spinosum traversed
by middle meningeal artery
(seen through sphenoidal sinus)

Superficial temporal artery

External carotid artery

Middle meningeal artery

Maxillary artery

A. Medial View, left half of bisected cranium

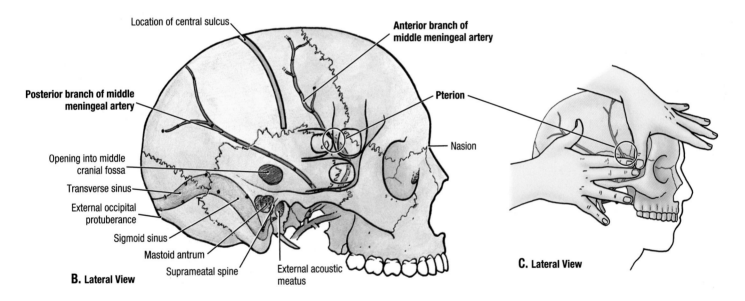

Location of central sulcus

Anterior branch of
middle meningeal artery

Posterior branch of middle
meningeal artery

Pterion

Nasion

Opening into middle
cranial fossa

Transverse sinus

External occipital
protuberance

Sigmoid sinus

Mastoid antrum

Suprameatal spine

External acoustic
meatus

B. Lateral View

C. Lateral View

| 7.17 | **Middle meningeal artery and pterion** |

A. Course of the middle meningeal artery in the cranium. **B.** Surface projections of internal features of the neurocranium. **C.** Locating the pterion. The pterion is located two fingers breadth superior to the zygomatic arch and one thumb breadth posterior to the frontal process of the zygomatic bone (approximately 4 cm superior to the midpoint of the zygomatic arch); the anterior branch of the middle meningeal artery crosses the pterion.

A hard blow to the side of the head may fracture the thin bones forming the pterion, rupturing the anterior branch of the middle meningeal artery crossing the pterion. The resulting extradural (epidural) hematoma exerts pressure on the underlying cerebral cortex. Untreated middle meningeal artery hemorrhage may cause death in a few hours.

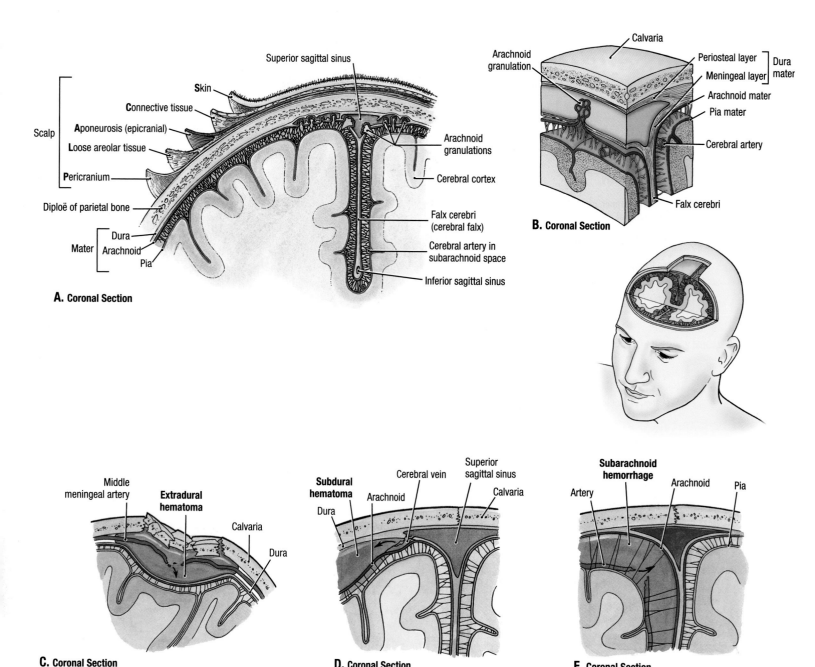

A. Coronal Section
- Superior sagittal sinus
- Skin
- Connective tissue
- Aponeurosis (epicranial)
- Loose areolar tissue
- Pericranium
- Scalp
- Diploë of parietal bone
- Mater — Dura, Arachnoid, Pia
- Arachnoid granulations
- Cerebral cortex
- Falx cerebri (cerebral falx)
- Cerebral artery in subarachnoid space
- Inferior sagittal sinus

B. Coronal Section
- Calvaria
- Arachnoid granulation
- Periosteal layer / Meningeal layer — Dura mater
- Arachnoid mater
- Pia mater
- Cerebral artery
- Falx cerebri

C. Coronal Section
- Middle meningeal artery
- Extradural hematoma
- Calvaria
- Dura

D. Coronal Section
- Subdural hematoma
- Dura
- Arachnoid
- Cerebral vein
- Superior sagittal sinus
- Calvaria

E. Coronal Section
- Subarachnoid hemorrhage
- Artery
- Arachnoid
- Pia

7.18 **Layers of the scalp and meninges**

A. Scalp, cranium, and meninges. **B.** Meninges and their relationship to the calvaria. The three meningeal spaces include the extradural (epidural) space between the cranial bones and dura, which is a potential space normally (it becomes a real space pathologically if blood accumulates in it); the similarly potential subdural space between the dura and arachnoid; and the subarachnoid space, the normal realized space between the arachnoid and pia, which contains cerebrospinal fluid (CSF). **C.** Extradural (epidural) hematomas result from bleeding from a torn middle meningeal artery. **D.** Subdural hematomas commonly result from tearing of a cerebral vein as it enters the superior sagittal sinus. E. Subarachnoid hemorrhage results from bleeding within the subarachnoid space, e.g., from rupture of an aneurysm.

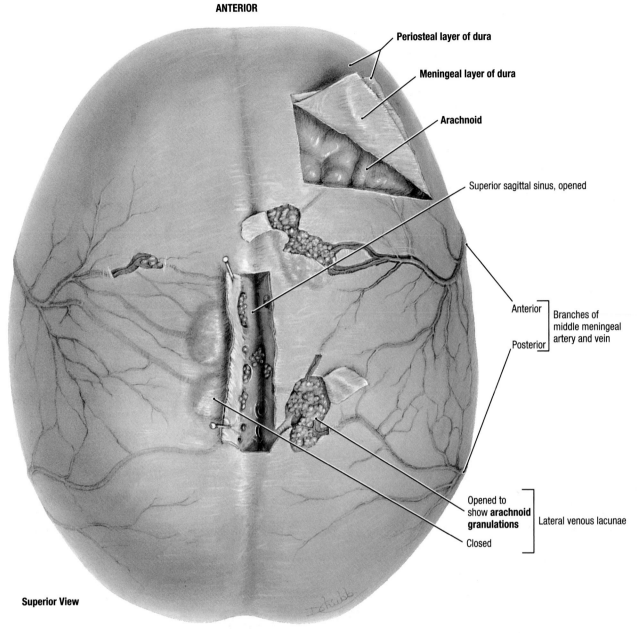

ANTERIOR

Periosteal layer of dura

Meningeal layer of dura

Arachnoid

Superior sagittal sinus, opened

Anterior ⎤ Branches of
            ⎥ middle meningeal
Posterior ⎦ artery and vein

Opened to
show **arachnoid
granulations** ⎤
                ⎥ Lateral venous lacunae
Closed ⎦

Superior View

POSTERIOR

7.19 Dura mater and arachnoid granulations

- The calvaria is removed. In the median plane, the thick roof of the superior sagittal sinus is partly pinned aside, and laterally, the thin roofs of two lateral lacunae are reflected.
- The middle meningeal artery lies in a venous channel (middle meningeal vein), which enlarges superiorly into a lateral lacunae. Other channels drain the lateral lacunae into the superior sagittal sinus.
- Arachnoid granulations in the lacunae are responsible for absorption of CSF from the subarachnoid space into the venous system.
- The dura is sensitive to pain, especially where it is related to the dural venous sinuses and meningeal arteries. Although the causes of headache are numerous, distention of the scalp or meningeal vessels (or both) is believed to be one cause of headache. Many headaches appear to be dural in origin, such as the headache occurring after a lumbar spinal puncture for removal of CSF. These headaches are thought to result from stimulation of sensory nerve endings in the dura.

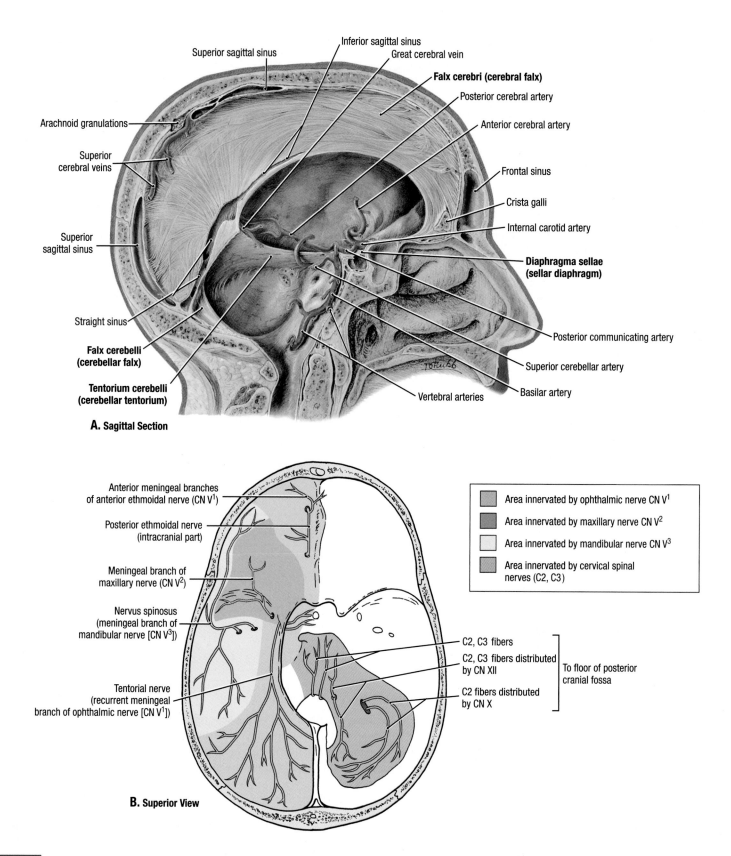

Superior sagittal sinus

Inferior sagittal sinus
Great cerebral vein

Falx cerebri (cerebral falx)

Posterior cerebral artery

Anterior cerebral artery

Arachnoid granulations

Superior cerebral veins

Frontal sinus

Crista galli

Internal carotid artery

Superior sagittal sinus

Diaphragma sellae (sellar diaphragm)

Straight sinus

Posterior communicating artery

Falx cerebelli (cerebellar falx)

Superior cerebellar artery

Basilar artery

Tentorium cerebelli (cerebellar tentorium)

Vertebral arteries

A. Sagittal Section

Anterior meningeal branches of anterior ethmoidal nerve (CN V¹)

Posterior ethmoidal nerve (intracranial part)

Meningeal branch of maxillary nerve (CN V²)

Nervus spinosus (meningeal branch of mandibular nerve [CN V³])

Tentorial nerve (recurrent meningeal branch of ophthalmic nerve [CN V¹])

	Area innervated by ophthalmic nerve CN V¹
	Area innervated by maxillary nerve CN V²
	Area innervated by mandibular nerve CN V³
	Area innervated by cervical spinal nerves (C2, C3)

C2, C3 fibers

C2, C3 fibers distributed by CN XII

C2 fibers distributed by CN X

To floor of posterior cranial fossa

B. Superior View

7.20 **Dura mater**

A. Reflections of the dura mater. **B.** Innervation of the dura of the cranial base. The dura of the cranial base is innervated by branches of the trigeminal nerve and sensory fibers of cervical spinal nerves (C2, C3) passing directly from those nerves or via meningeal branches of the vagus (CN X) and hypoglossal (CN XII) nerves.

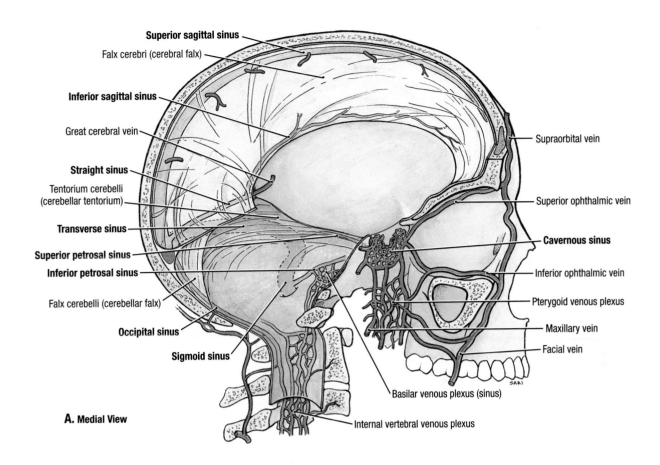

Superior sagittal sinus
Falx cerebri (cerebral falx)
Inferior sagittal sinus
Great cerebral vein
Straight sinus
Tentorium cerebelli (cerebellar tentorium)
Transverse sinus
Superior petrosal sinus
Inferior petrosal sinus
Falx cerebelli (cerebellar falx)
Occipital sinus
Sigmoid sinus
Supraorbital vein
Superior ophthalmic vein
Cavernous sinus
Inferior ophthalmic vein
Pterygoid venous plexus
Maxillary vein
Facial vein
Basilar venous plexus (sinus)
Internal vertebral venous plexus

A. Medial View

7.21   Venous sinuses of the dura mater

A. Schematic of left half of cranial cavity and right facial skeleton. **B.** Venous sinuses of the cranial base.

- The superior sagittal sinus is at the superior border of the falx cerebri, and the inferior sagittal sinus is in its free border. The great cerebral vein joins the inferior sagittal sinus to form the straight sinus.

- The superior sagittal sinus usually becomes the right transverse sinus, right sigmoid sinus, and right internal jugular vein; the straight sinus similarly drains through the left transverse sinus, left sigmoid sinus, and left internal jugular vein.

- The cavernous sinus communicates with the veins of the face through the ophthalmic veins and pterygoid plexus of veins and with the sigmoid sinus through the superior and inferior petrosal sinuses.

- The basilar and occipital sinuses communicate through the foramen magnum with the internal vertebral venous plexuses. Because these venous channels are valveless, compression of the thorax, abdomen, or pelvis, as occurs during heavy coughing and straining, may force venous blood from these regions into the internal vertebral venous system and from it into the dural venous sinuses. As a result, pus in abscesses and tumor cells in these regions may spread to the vertebrae and brain.

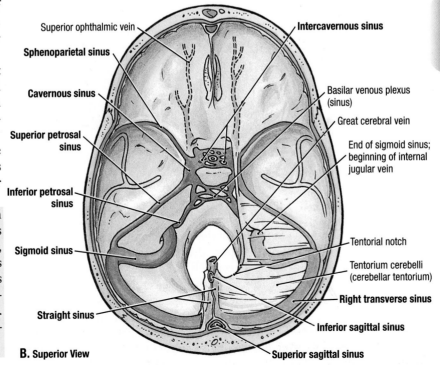

Superior ophthalmic vein
Sphenoparietal sinus
Cavernous sinus
Superior petrosal sinus
Inferior petrosal sinus
Sigmoid sinus
Straight sinus
Intercavernous sinus
Basilar venous plexus (sinus)
Great cerebral vein
End of sigmoid sinus; beginning of internal jugular vein
Tentorial notch
Tentorium cerebelli (cerebellar tentorium)
Right transverse sinus
Inferior sagittal sinus
Superior sagittal sinus

B. Superior View

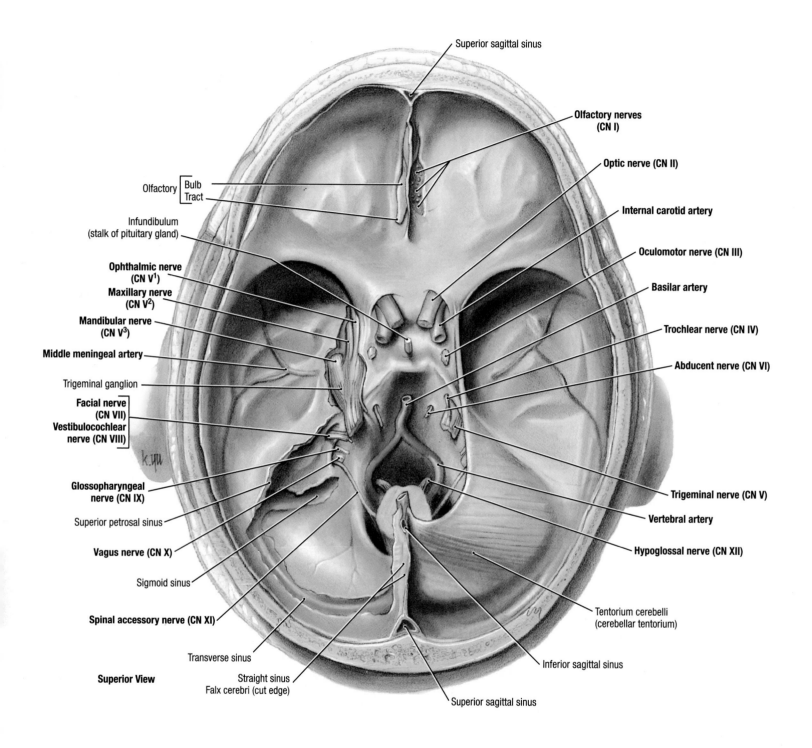

Superior sagittal sinus

Olfactory nerves (CN I)

Optic nerve (CN II)

Olfactory {Bulb Tract

Internal carotid artery

Infundibulum (stalk of pituitary gland)

Oculomotor nerve (CN III)

Ophthalmic nerve (CN V¹)

Basilar artery

Maxillary nerve (CN V²)

Mandibular nerve (CN V³)

Trochlear nerve (CN IV)

Middle meningeal artery

Abducent nerve (CN VI)

Trigeminal ganglion

Facial nerve (CN VII)

Vestibulocochlear nerve (CN VIII)

Trigeminal nerve (CN V)

Glossopharyngeal nerve (CN IX)

Vertebral artery

Superior petrosal sinus

Hypoglossal nerve (CN XII)

Vagus nerve (CN X)

Sigmoid sinus

Spinal accessory nerve (CN XI)

Tentorium cerebelli (cerebellar tentorium)

Transverse sinus

Inferior sagittal sinus

Superior View

Straight sinus
Falx cerebri (cut edge)

Superior sagittal sinus

7.22 **Nerves and vessels of the interior of the base of the cranium**

- On the left of the specimen, the dura mater forming the roof of the trigeminal cave is cut away to expose the trigeminal nerve and its three branches and the sigmoid sinus. The tentorium cerebelli is removed to reveal the transverse and superior petrosal sinuses.
- The frontal lobes of the cerebrum are located in the anterior cranial fossa, the temporal lobes in the middle cranial fossa, and the brainstem and cerebellum in the posterior cranial fossa; the occipital lobes rest on the tentorium cerebelli.
- The sites wherre the 12 cranial nerves and the internal carotid, vertebral, basilar, and middle meningeal arteries penetrate the dura mater are shown.

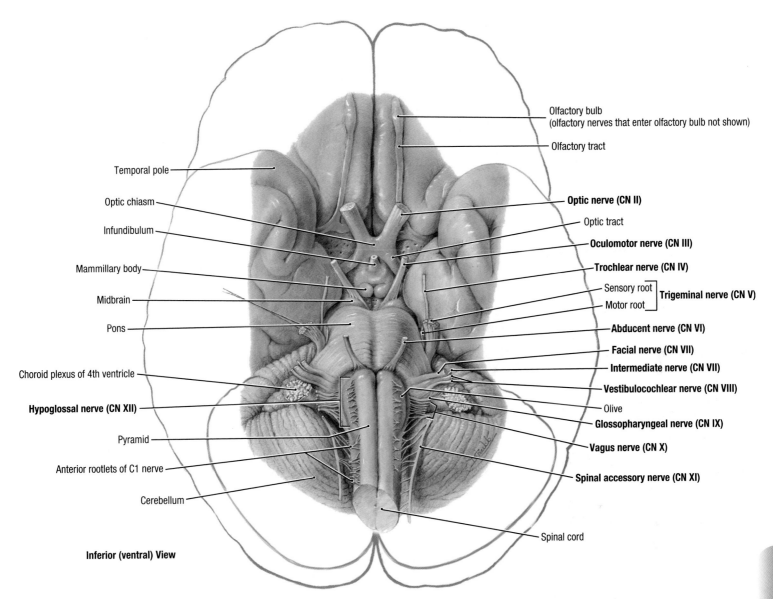

Olfactory bulb
(olfactory nerves that enter olfactory bulb not shown)

Olfactory tract

Temporal pole

Optic chiasm

Infundibulum

Mammillary body

Midbrain

Pons

Choroid plexus of 4th ventricle

Hypoglossal nerve (CN XII)

Pyramid

Anterior rootlets of C1 nerve

Cerebellum

Inferior (ventral) View

Optic nerve (CN II)

Optic tract

Oculomotor nerve (CN III)

Trochlear nerve (CN IV)

Sensory root ⎤
                ⎥ **Trigeminal nerve (CN V)**
Motor root ⎦

Abducent nerve (CN VI)

Facial nerve (CN VII)

Intermediate nerve (CN VII)

Vestibulocochlear nerve (CN VIII)

Olive

Glossopharyngeal nerve (CN IX)

Vagus nerve (CN X)

Spinal accessory nerve (CN XI)

Spinal cord

7.23   **Base of brain and superficial origins of cranial nerves**

Foramina of skull and their associated cranial nerve(s) are listed below.

OPENINGS BY WHICH CRANIAL NERVES EXIT CRANIAL CAVITY

Foramina/Apertures	Cranial nerve
Anterior cranial fossa	
Cribriform foramina in cribriform plate	Axons of olfactory cells in olfactory epithelium form olfactory nerves (CN I)
Middle cranial fossa	
Optic canal	Optic nerve (CN II)
Superior orbital fissure	Opthalmic nerve (CN V^1), oculomotor nerve (CN III), trochlear nerve (CN IV), abducent nerve (CN VI) and branches of opthalmic nerve (CN V^1)
Foramen rotundum	Maxillary nerve (CN V^2)
Foramen ovale	Mandibular nerve (CN V^3)
Posterior cranial fossa	
Foramen magnum	Spinal accessory nerve (CN XI)
Jugular foramen	Glossopharyngeal nerve (CN IX), vagus nerve (CN X), and spinal accessory nerve (CN XI)
Hypoglossal canal	Hypoglossal nerve (CN XII)

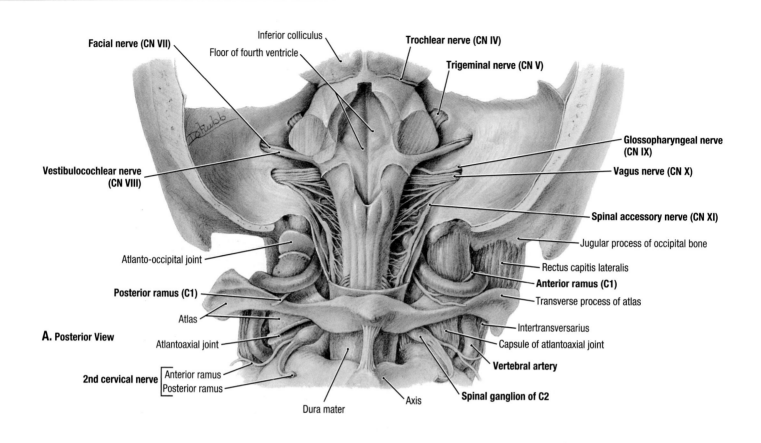

Facial nerve (CN VII)
Floor of fourth ventricle
Inferior colliculus
Trochlear nerve (CN IV)
Trigeminal nerve (CN V)
Glossopharyngeal nerve (CN IX)
Vagus nerve (CN X)
Vestibulocochlear nerve (CN VIII)
Spinal accessory nerve (CN XI)
Jugular process of occipital bone
Atlanto-occipital joint
Rectus capitis lateralis
Anterior ramus (C1)
Posterior ramus (C1)
Transverse process of atlas
Atlas
Intertransversarius
A. Posterior View
Atlantoaxial joint
Capsule of atlantoaxial joint
Vertebral artery
2nd cervical nerve {Anterior ramus / Posterior ramus}
Spinal ganglion of C2
Dura mater
Axis

7.24 Posterior exposures of cranial nerves

A and **B.** Squamous part of occipital bone has been removed posterior to foramen magnum to reveal posterior cranial fossa. **A.** Brainstem in situ. **B.** Right side, with brainstem removed. The trochlear nerves (CN IV) arise from the dorsal aspect of the midbrain, just inferior to the inferior colliculi.

- The sensory and motor roots of the trigeminal nerves (CN V) pass anterolaterally to enter the mouth of the trigeminal cave.
- The facial (CN VII) and vestibulocochlear (CN VIII) nerves course laterally to enter the internal acoustic meatus.
- The glossopharyngeal nerve (CN IX) pierces the dura mater separately but passes with the vagus (CN X) and spinal accessory (CN XI) nerves through the jugular foramen.

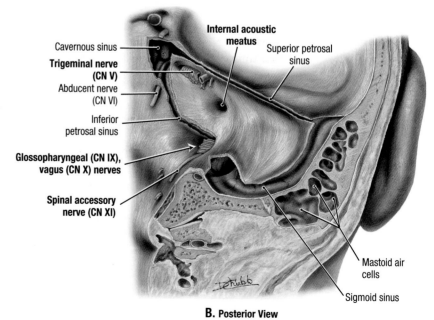

Cavernous sinus
Internal acoustic meatus
Superior petrosal sinus
Trigeminal nerve (CN V)
Abducent nerve (CN VI)
Inferior petrosal sinus
Glossopharyngeal (CN IX), vagus (CN X) nerves
Spinal accessory nerve (CN XI)
Mastoid air cells
Sigmoid sinus

B. Posterior View

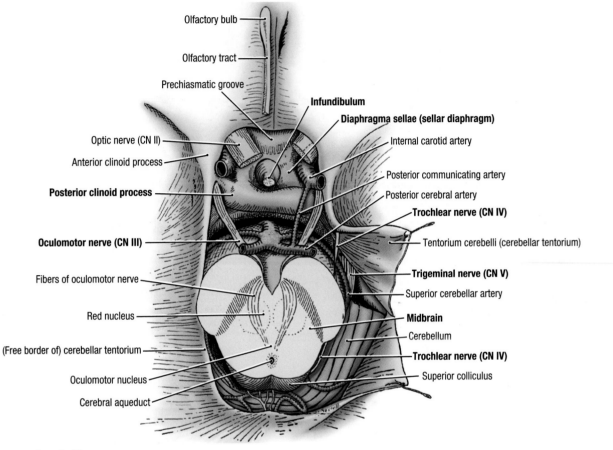

Olfactory bulb

Olfactory tract

Prechiasmatic groove

Infundibulum

Diaphragma sellae (sellar diaphragm)

Optic nerve (CN II)

Internal carotid artery

Anterior clinoid process

Posterior communicating artery

Posterior clinoid process

Posterior cerebral artery

Trochlear nerve (CN IV)

Oculomotor nerve (CN III)

Tentorium cerebelli (cerebellar tentorium)

Fibers of oculomotor nerve

Trigeminal nerve (CN V)

Superior cerebellar artery

Red nucleus

Midbrain

Cerebellum

(Free border of) cerebellar tentorium

Trochlear nerve (CN IV)

Oculomotor nucleus

Superior colliculus

Cerebral aqueduct

Superior View

7.25   Tentorial notch

- The brain has been removed by cutting through the midbrain, revealing the tentorial notch through which the brainstem extends from the posterior into the middle cranial fossa.
- On the right side of the specimen, the tentorium cerebelli is divided and reflected. The trochlear nerve (CN IV) passes around the midbrain under the free edge of the tentorium cerebelli; the roots of the trigeminal nerve (CN V) enter the mouth of the trigeminal cave.
- There is a circular opening in the diaphragma sellae for the infundibulum, the stalk of the pituitary gland.
- The oculomotor nerve (CN III) passes laterally around the posterior clinoid process and then passes between the posterior cerebral and superior cerebellar arteries.
- The tentorial notch is the opening in the tentorium cerebelli for the brainstem, which is slightly larger than is necessary to accommodate the midbrain. Hence, space-occupying lesions, such as tumors in the supratentorial compartment, produce increased intracranial pressure that may cause part of the adjacent temporal lobe of the brain to herniate through the tentorial notch. During tentorial herniation, the temporal lobe may be lacerated by the tough tentorium cerebelli, and the oculomotor nerve (CN III) may be stretched, compressed, or both. Oculomotor lesions may produce paralysis of the extrinsic eye muscles supplied by CN III.

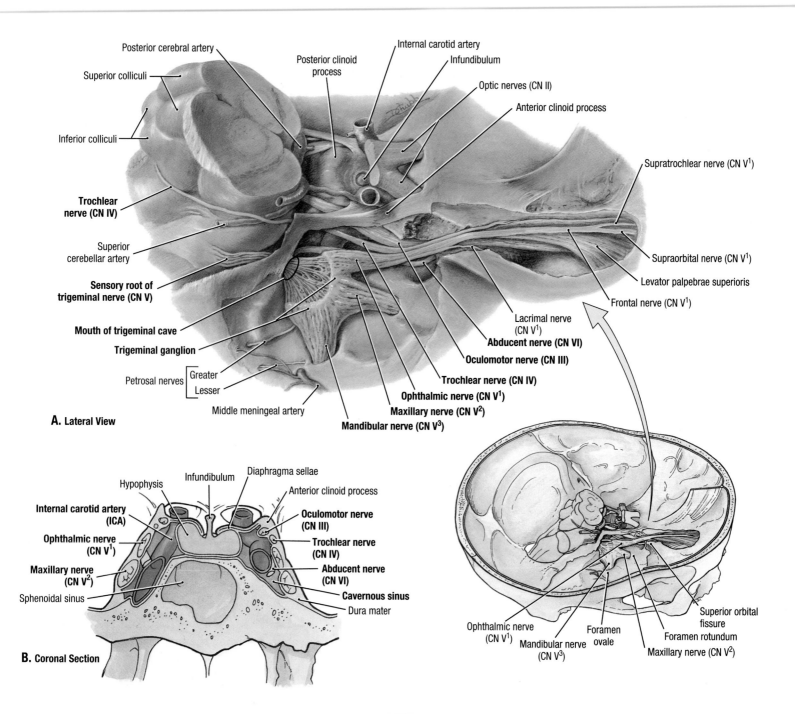

Posterior cerebral artery

Superior colliculi

Inferior colliculi

Posterior clinoid
process

Internal carotid artery

Infundibulum

Optic nerves (CN II)

Anterior clinoid process

Supratrochlear nerve (CN V¹)

**Trochlear
nerve (CN IV)**

Superior
cerebellar artery

**Sensory root of
trigeminal nerve (CN V)**

Mouth of trigeminal cave

Trigeminal ganglion

Petrosal nerves { Greater / Lesser }

Middle meningeal artery

Supraorbital nerve (CN V¹)

Levator palpebrae superioris

Frontal nerve (CN V¹)

Lacrimal nerve
(CN V¹)

Abducent nerve (CN VI)

Oculomotor nerve (CN III)

Trochlear nerve (CN IV)

Ophthalmic nerve (CN V¹)

Maxillary nerve (CN V²)

Mandibular nerve (CN V³)

A. Lateral View

Hypophysis

Infundibulum

Diaphragma sellae

Anterior clinoid process

**Internal carotid artery
(ICA)**

**Ophthalmic nerve
(CN V¹)**

**Maxillary nerve
(CN V²)**

Sphenoidal sinus

**Oculomotor nerve
(CN III)**

**Trochlear nerve
(CN IV)**

**Abducent nerve
(CN VI)**

Cavernous sinus

Dura mater

B. Coronal Section

Ophthalmic nerve
(CN V¹)

Mandibular nerve
(CN V³)

Foramen
ovale

Superior orbital
fissure

Foramen rotundum

Maxillary nerve (CN V²)

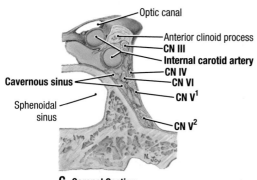

Optic canal

Anterior clinoid process

CN III

Internal carotid artery

CN IV

CN VI

CN V¹

Cavernous sinus

Sphenoidal
sinus

CN V²

C. Coronal Section

7.26 **Nerves and vessels of middle cranial fossa—I**

A. Superficial dissection. The tentorium cerebelli is cut away . The dura
mater is largely removed from the middle cranial fossa. The roof of the
orbit is partly removed. **B** and **C.** Coronal sections through the cavernous sinus.

In fractures of the cranial base, the internal carotid artery may be
torn, producing an arteriovenous fistula within the cavernous sinus.
Arterial blood rushes into the sinus, enlarging it and forcing retrograde
blood flow into its venous tributaries, especially the ophthalmic veins.
As a result, the eyeball protrudes (exophthalmos) and the conjunctiva
becomes engorged (chemosis). Because CN III, CN IV, CN VI, CN
V1, and CN V2 lie in or close to the lateral wall of the cavernous sinus,
these nerves may also be affected.

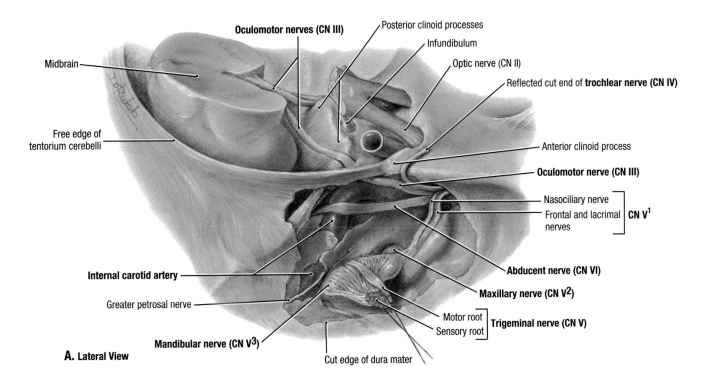

A. Lateral View

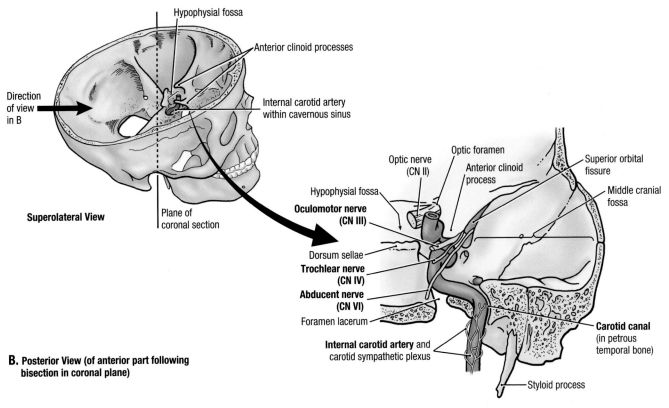

Superolateral View

B. Posterior View (of anterior part following bisection in coronal plane)

7.27 **Nerves and vessels of middle cranial fossa—II**

A. Deep dissection. The roots of the trigeminal nerve are divided, withdrawn from the mouth of the trigeminal cave, and turned anteriorly. The trochlear nerve is reflected anteriorly. **B.** Course of the internal carotid artery.

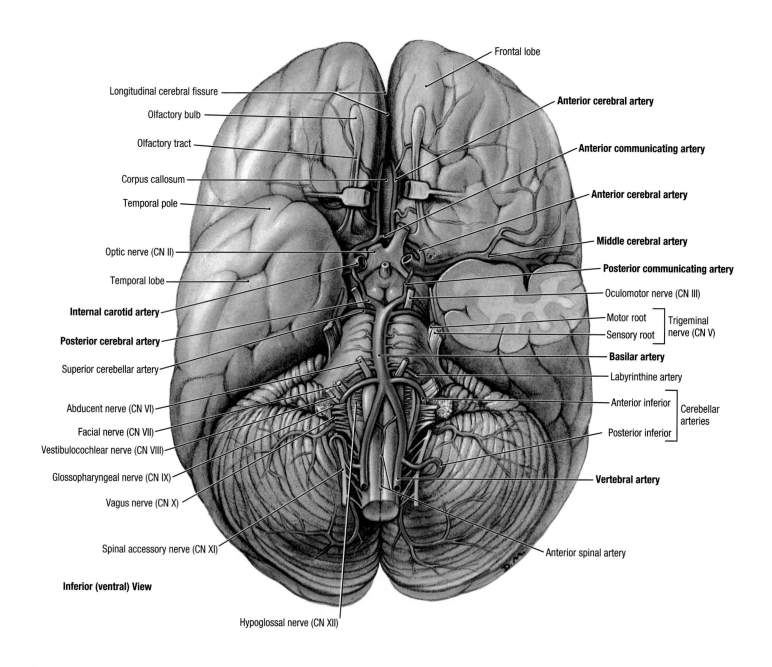

Longitudinal cerebral fissure

Olfactory bulb

Olfactory tract

Corpus callosum

Temporal pole

Optic nerve (CN II)

Temporal lobe

Internal carotid artery

Posterior cerebral artery

Superior cerebellar artery

Abducent nerve (CN VI)

Facial nerve (CN VII)

Vestibulocochlear nerve (CN VIII)

Glossopharyngeal nerve (CN IX)

Vagus nerve (CN X)

Spinal accessory nerve (CN XI)

Inferior (ventral) View

Hypoglossal nerve (CN XII)

Frontal lobe

Anterior cerebral artery

Anterior communicating artery

Anterior cerebral artery

Middle cerebral artery

Posterior communicating artery

Oculomotor nerve (CN III)

Motor root | Trigeminal
Sensory root | nerve (CN V)

Basilar artery

Labyrinthine artery

Anterior inferior | Cerebellar
Posterior inferior | arteries

Vertebral artery

Anterior spinal artery

7.28   Base of brain and cerebral arterial circle

The left temporal pole is removed to enable visualization of the middle cerebral artery in the lateral fissure. The frontal lobes are separated to expose the anterior cerebral arteries and corpus callosum.

An ischemic stroke denotes the sudden development of neurological deficits that are consequences of impaired cerebral blood flow. The most common causes of strokes are spontaneous cerebrovascular accidents such as cerebral embolism, cerebral thrombosis, cerebral hemorrhage, and subarachnoid hemorrhage (Rowland, 2000). The cerebral arterial circle is an important means of collateral circulation in the event of gradual obstruction of one of the major arteries forming the circle. Sudden occlusion, even if only partial, results in neurological deficits. In elderly persons, the anastomoses are often inadequate when a large artery (e.g., internal carotid) is occluded, even if the occlusion is gradual. In such cases function is impaired at least to some degree.

Hemorrhagic stroke follows the rupture of an artery or a saccular aneurysm, a saclike dilation on a weak part of the arterial wall. The most common type of saccular aneurysm is a berry aneurysm, occurring in the vessels of or near the cerebral arterial circle. In time, especially in people with hypertension (high blood pressure), the weak part of the arterial wall expands and may rupture, allowing blood to enter the subarachnoid space.

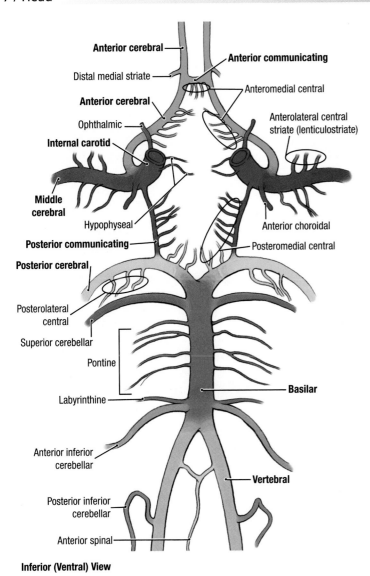

Inferior (Ventral) View

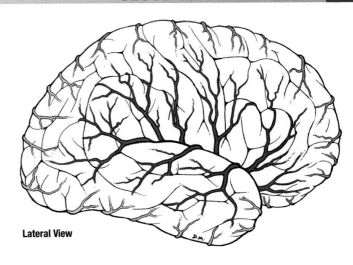

Lateral View

Blood is supplied to the cerebral hemispheres by the anterior (*green*), middle (*purple*), and posterior (*yellow*) cerebral arteries.

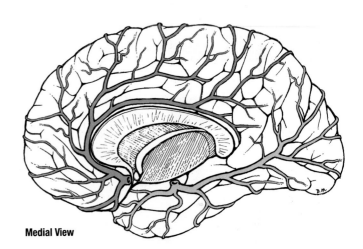

Medial View

TABLE 7.5 ARTERIAL SUPPLY TO BRAIN

Artery	Origin	Distribution
Vertebral	Subclavian artery	Cranial meninges and cerebellum
Posterior inferior cerebellar	Vertebral artery	Posteroinferior aspect of cerebellum
Basilar	Formed by junction of vertebral arteries	Brainstem, cerebellum, and cerebrum
Pontine		Numerous branches to brainstem
Anterior inferior cerebellar	Basilar artery	Inferior aspect of cerebellum
Superior cerebellar		Superior aspect of cerebellum
Internal carotid	Common carotid artery at superior border of thyroid cartilage	Gives branches in cavernous sinus and provides supply to brain
Anterior cerebral	Internal carotid artery	Cerebral hemispheres, except for occipital lobes
Middle cerebral	Continuation of the internal carotid artery distal to anterior cerebral artery	Most of lateral surface of cerebral hemispheres
Posterior cerebral	Terminal branch of basilar artery	Inferior aspect of cerebral hemisphere and occipital lobe
Anterior communicating	Anterior cerebral artery	Cerebral arterial circle
Posterior communicating	Internal carotid artery	

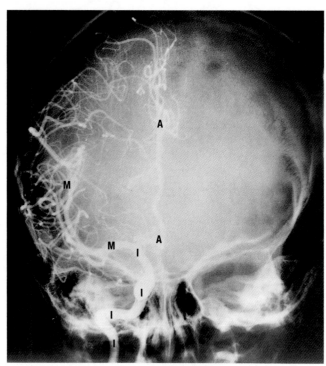

A. Posteroanterior View

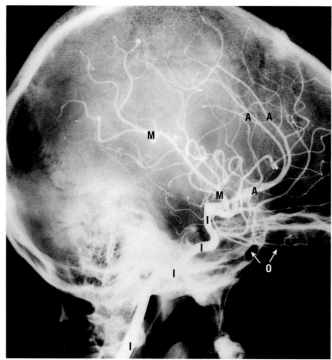

B. Lateral View

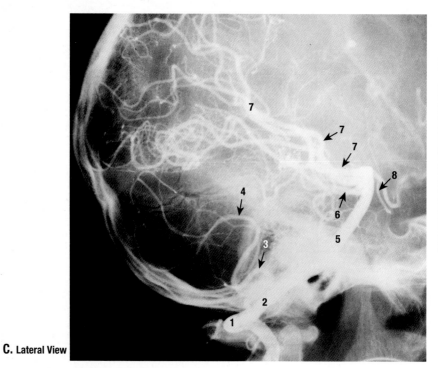

C. Lateral View

A	Anterior cerebral artery
M	Middle cerebral artery
I	Internal carotid artery
0	Ophthalmic artery
1	Vertebral artery on posterior arch of atlas
2	Vertebral artery entering skull through foramen magnum
3	Posterior inferior cerebellar artery
4	Anterior inferior cerebellar artery
5	Basilar artery
6	Superior cerebellar artery
7	Posterior cerebellar artery
8	Posterior communicating artery

7.29 **Arteriograms**

A and **B.** Carotid arteriogram. The four letter Is indicate the parts of the internal carotid artery: cervical, before entering the cranium; petrous, within the temporal bone; cavernous, within the sinus; and cerebral, within the cranial subarachnoid space. **C.** Vertebral arteriogram. Transient ischemic attacks (TIAs) refer to neurological symptoms resulting from ischemia (deficient blood supply) of the brain. The symptoms of a TIA may be ambiguous: staggering, dizziness, light-headedness, fainting, and paresthesias (e.g., tingling in a limb). Most TIAs last a few minutes, but some persist longer. Individuals with TIAs are at increased risk for myocardial infarction and ischemic stroke (Brust, 2000).

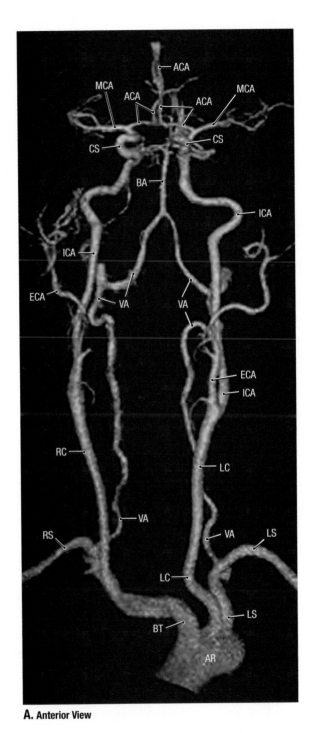

A. Anterior View

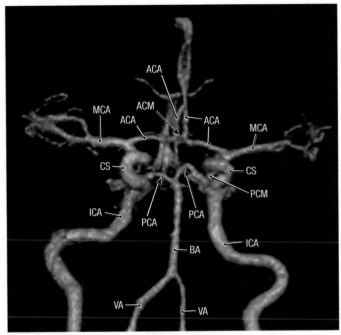

B. Anterior View

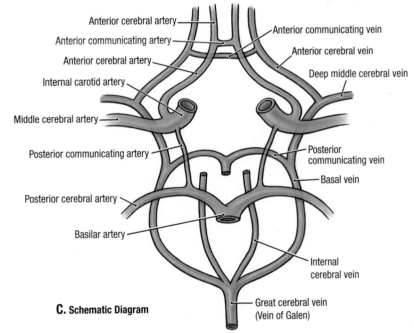

C. Schematic Diagram

ACM	Anterior communicating artery	BT	Brachiocephalic trunk	LC	Left common carotid artery	PCM	Posterior communicating artery
ACA	Anterior cerebral artery	CS	Carotid siphon	LS	Left subclavian artery	RC	Right common carotid artery
AR	Arch of aorta	ECA	External carotid artery	MCA	Middle cerebral artery	RS	Right subclavian artery
BA	Basilar artery	ICA	Internal carotid artery	PCA	Posterior cerebral artery	VA	Vertebral artery

7.30   **Blood supply of head and neck**

A. CT angiogram of arteries of head and neck. **B.** CT angiogram of cerebral arterial circle (circle of Willis). **C.** Schematic diagram of cerebral arterial circle and veins of cerebral base.

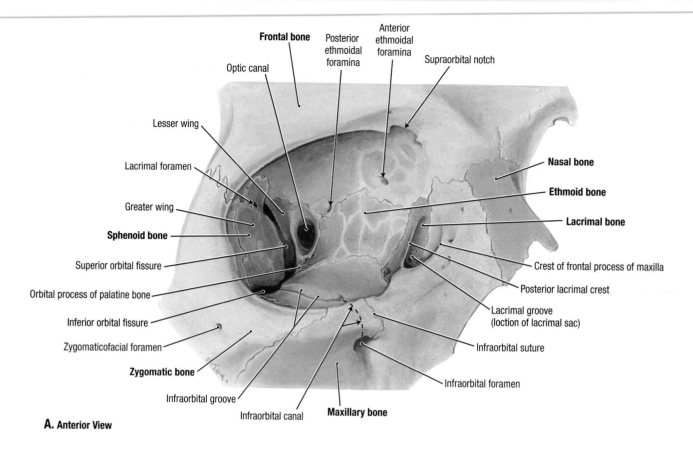

Frontal bone
Posterior ethmoidal foramina
Anterior ethmoidal foramina
Supraorbital notch
Optic canal
Lesser wing
Lacrimal foramen
Nasal bone
Greater wing
Ethmoid bone
Sphenoid bone
Lacrimal bone
Superior orbital fissure
Crest of frontal process of maxilla
Orbital process of palatine bone
Posterior lacrimal crest
Inferior orbital fissure
Lacrimal groove (loction of lacrimal sac)
Zygomaticofacial foramen
Infraorbital suture
Zygomatic bone
Infraorbital foramen
Infraorbital groove
Infraorbital canal
Maxillary bone

A. Anterior View

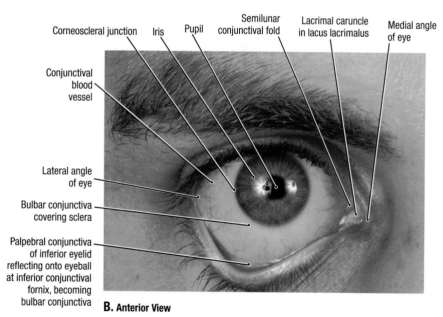

Corneoscleral junction
Iris
Pupil
Semilunar conjunctival fold
Lacrimal caruncle in lacus lacrimalus
Medial angle of eye
Conjunctival blood vessel
Lateral angle of eye
Bulbar conjunctiva covering sclera
Palpebral conjunctiva of inferior eyelid reflecting onto eyeball at inferior conjunctival fornix, becoming bulbar conjunctiva

B. Anterior View

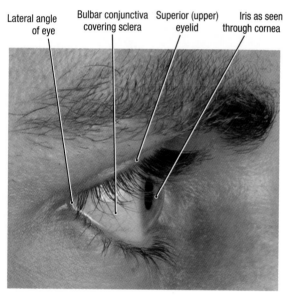

Lateral angle of eye
Bulbar conjunctiva covering sclera
Superior (upper) eyelid
Iris as seen through cornea

C. Lateral View

7.31 **Orbital cavity and surface anatomy of the eye**

A. Bones and features of the orbital cavity. **B** and **C.** Surface anatomy of the eye. In **B,** the inferior eyelid is everted to demonstrate the palpebral conjunctiva. When powerful blows impact directly on the bony rim of the orbit, the resulting fractures usually occur at the sutures between the bones forming the orbital margin. Fractures of the medial wall may involve the ethmoidal and sphenoidal sinuses, whereas fractures in the inferior wall may in-volve the maxillary sinus. Although the superior wall is stronger than the medial and inferior walls, it is thin enough to be translucent and may be readily penetrated. Thus, a sharp object may pass through it into the frontal lobe of the brain. Orbital fractures often result in intraorbital bleeding, which exerts pressure on the eyeball, causing exophthalmos (protrusion of the eyeball).

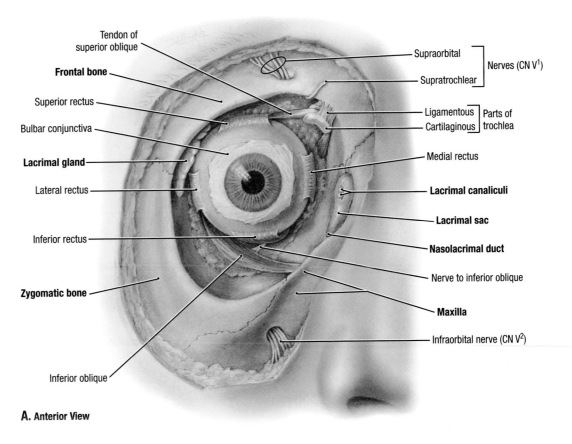

Tendon of superior oblique
Frontal bone
Superior rectus
Bulbar conjunctiva
Lacrimal gland
Lateral rectus
Inferior rectus
Zygomatic bone
Inferior oblique

Supraorbital
Supratrochlear
Nerves (CN V^1)
Ligamentous
Cartilaginous
Parts of trochlea
Medial rectus
Lacrimal canaliculi
Lacrimal sac
Nasolacrimal duct
Nerve to inferior oblique
Maxilla
Infraorbital nerve (CN V^2)

A. Anterior View

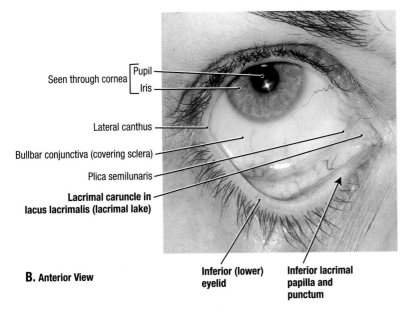

Seen through cornea
Pupil
Iris
Lateral canthus
Bullbar conjunctiva (covering sclera)
Plica semilunaris
Lacrimal caruncle in lacus lacrimalis (lacrimal lake)
Inferior (lower) eyelid
Inferior lacrimal papilla and punctum

B. Anterior View

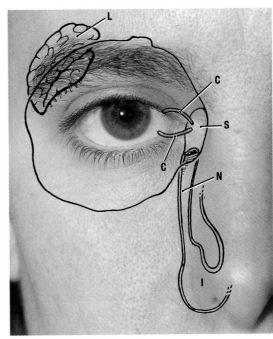

C. Anterior View

7.32   Eye and lacrimal apparatus

A. Anterior dissection of orbital cavity. The eyelids, orbital septum, levator palpebrae superioris, and some fat are removed. **B.** Surface features, with the inferior eyelid everted. **C.** Surface projection of lacrimal apparatus. Tears, secreted by the lacrimal gland (*L*) in the superolateral angle of the bony orbit, pass across the eyeball and enter the lacus lacrimalis (lacrimal lake) at the medial angle of the eye; from here they drain through the lacrimal puncta and lacrimal canaliculi (*C*) to the lacrimal sac (*S*). The lacrimal sac drains into the nasolacrimal duct (*N*), which empties into the inferior meatus (*I*) of the nose.

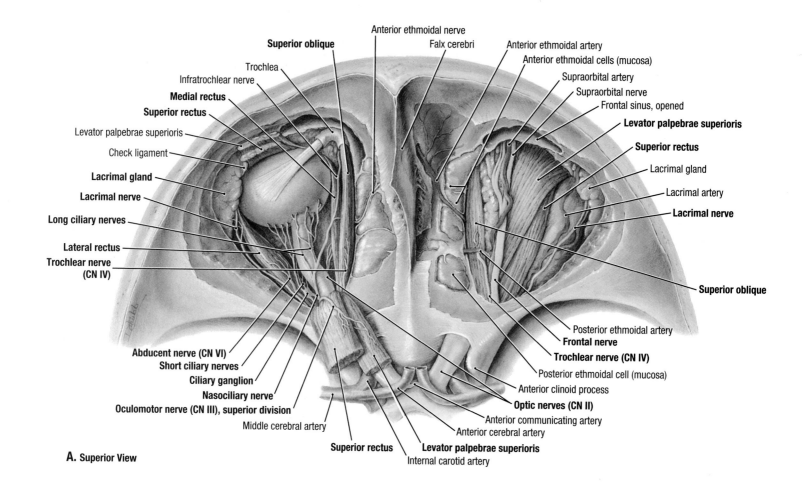

A. Superior View

7.33 **Orbital cavity, superior approach**

A. Superficial dissection.
On the right side of figure **A:**
- The orbital plate of the frontal bone is removed.
- The levator palpebrae superioris muscle lies superficial to the superior rectus muscle.
- The trochlear, frontal, and lacrimal nerves lie immediately inferior to the roof of the orbital cavity.

On the left side of figure **A:**
- The levator palpebrae and superior rectus muscles are reflected.
- The superior division of the oculomotor nerve (CN III) supplies the superior rectus and levator palpebrae muscles.
- The trochlear nerve (CN IV) lies on the medial side of the superior oblique muscle, and the abducent nerve (CN VI) on the medial side of the lateral rectus muscle.
- The lacrimal nerve runs superior to the lateral rectus muscle supplying sensory fibers to the conjunctiva and skin of the superior eyelid; it receives a communicating branch of the zygomaticotemporal nerve carrying secretory motor fibers from the pterygopalatine ganglion to the lacrimal gland.
- The parasympathetic ciliary ganglion, placed between the lateral rectus muscle and the optic nerve (CN II), gives rise to many short ciliary nerves; the nasociliary nerve gives rise to two long ciliary nerves that anastomose with each other and the short ciliary nerves.

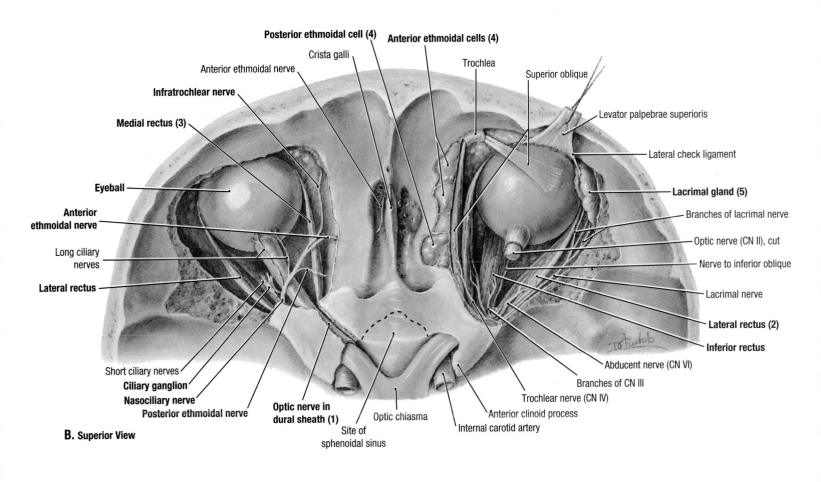

Posterior ethmoidal cell (4)
Crista galli
Anterior ethmoidal cells (4)
Anterior ethmoidal nerve
Trochlea
Superior oblique
Infratrochlear nerve
Levator palpebrae superioris
Medial rectus (3)
Lateral check ligament
Eyeball
Lacrimal gland (5)
Anterior ethmoidal nerve
Branches of lacrimal nerve
Long ciliary nerves
Optic nerve (CN II), cut
Nerve to inferior oblique
Lateral rectus
Lacrimal nerve
Lateral rectus (2)
Inferior rectus
Short ciliary nerves
Abducent nerve (CN VI)
Ciliary ganglion
Branches of CN III
Nasociliary nerve
Trochlear nerve (CN IV)
Posterior ethmoidal nerve
Optic nerve in dural sheath (1)
Optic chiasma
Anterior clinoid process
Internal carotid artery
Site of sphenoidal sinus

B. Superior View

7.33   Orbital cavity, superior approach *(continued)*

B. Deep dissection before *(right side)* and after *(left side)* section of the optic nerve (CN II).
C. Transverse (axial) MRI of orbital cavity. (The *numbers* refer to structures labeled in **B**).
Observe on the right side of figure **B**:

- The eyeball occupies the anterior half of the orbital cavity.
- Nerves supplying the four recti (superior, medial, inferior, lateral) enter their ocular surfaces (the superior rectus is not shown).

Observe on the left of figure **B**:

- The parasympathetic ciliary ganglion lies posteriorly between the lateral rectus muscle and the sheath of the optic nerve.
- The nasociliary nerve (CN V^1) sends a branch to the ciliary ganglion and crosses the optic nerve (CN II), where it gives off two long ciliary nerves (sensory to the eyeball and cornea) and the posterior ethmoidal nerve (to the sphenoidal sinus and posterior ethmoidal cells). The nasociliary nerve then divides into the anterior ethmoidal and infratrochlear nerves.

Because of the closeness of the optic nerve to the sphenoidal sinus and posterior ethmoidal cell, a malignant tumor in these sinuses may erode the thin bony walls of the orbit and compress the optic nerve and orbital contents. Tumors in the orbit produce exophthalmos. A tumor in the middle cranial fossa may enter the orbital cavity through the superior orbital fissure.

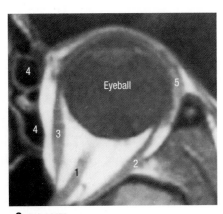

C. Axial MRI

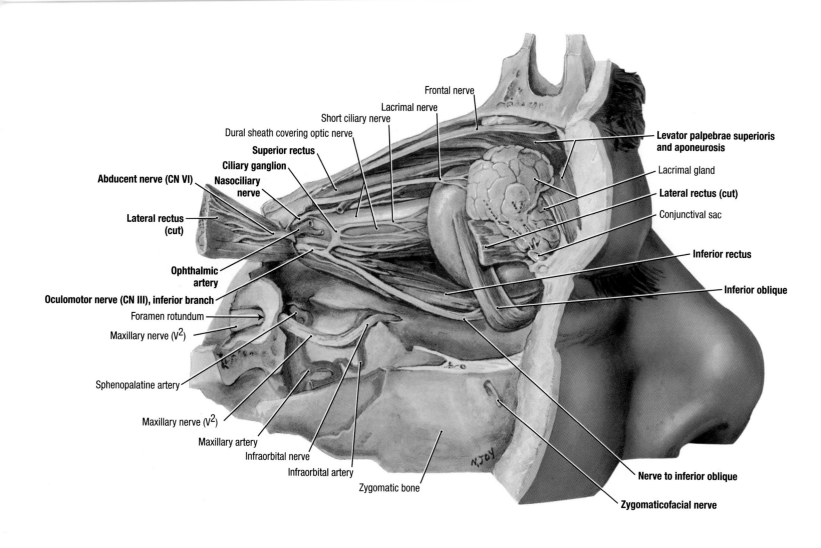

Frontal nerve

Lacrimal nerve

Short ciliary nerve

Dural sheath covering optic nerve

Superior rectus

Ciliary ganglion

Abducent nerve (CN VI)

Nasociliary nerve

Lateral rectus (cut)

Ophthalmic artery

Oculomotor nerve (CN III), inferior branch

Foramen rotundum

Maxillary nerve (V^2)

Sphenopalatine artery

Maxillary nerve (V^2)

Maxillary artery

Infraorbital nerve

Infraorbital artery

Zygomatic bone

Levator palpebrae superioris and aponeurosis

Lacrimal gland

Lateral rectus (cut)

Conjunctival sac

Inferior rectus

Inferior oblique

Nerve to inferior oblique

Zygomaticofacial nerve

7.34 Lateral aspect of the orbit and structure of the eyelid

- The ciliary ganglion receives sensory fibers from the nasociliary branches of VI, postsynaptic sympathetic fibers from the continuation of the internal carotid plexus extending along the ophthalmic artery, and presynaptic parasympathetic fibers from the inferior branch of the oculomotor nerve; only the latter synapse in the ganglion.
- Complete oculomotor nerve palsy affects most of the ocular muscles, the levator palpebrae superioris, and the sphincter pupillae. The superior eyelid droops (ptosis) and cannot be raised voluntarily because of the unopposed activity of the orbicularis oculi (supplied by the facial nerve). The pupil is also fully dilated and nonreactive because of the unopposed dilator pupillae. The pupil is fully abducted and depressed ("down and out") because of the unopposed activity of the lateral rectus and superior oblique, respectively.
- A lesion of the abducent nerve results in loss of lateral gaze to the ipsilateral side because of paralysis of the lateral rectus muscle. On forward gaze, the eye is diverted medially because of the lack of normal resting tone in the lateral rectus, resulting in diplopia (double vision). Horner syndrome results from interruption of a cervical sympathetic trunk and is manifest by the absence of sympathetically stimulated functions on the ipsilateral side of the head. The syndrome includes the following signs: constriction of the pupil (miosis), drooping of the superior eyelid (ptosis), redness and increased temperature of the skin (vasodilatation), and absence of sweating (anhydrosis).

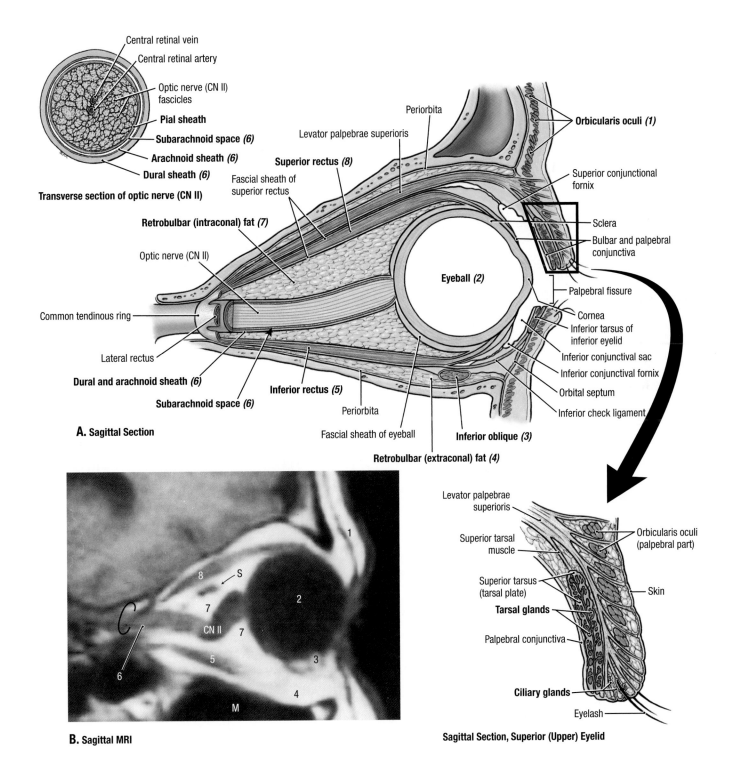

Transverse section of optic nerve (CN II)

- Central retinal vein
- Central retinal artery
- Optic nerve (CN II) fascicles
- **Pial sheath**
- **Subarachnoid space (6)**
- **Arachnoid sheath (6)**
- **Dural sheath (6)**

A. Sagittal Section

- Periorbita
- Levator palpebrae superioris
- **Superior rectus (8)**
- Fascial sheath of superior rectus
- **Retrobulbar (intraconal) fat (7)**
- Optic nerve (CN II)
- Common tendinous ring
- Lateral rectus
- **Dural and arachnoid sheath (6)**
- **Subarachnoid space (6)**
- Periorbita
- Fascial sheath of eyeball
- **Inferior rectus (5)**
- **Inferior oblique (3)**
- **Retrobulbar (extraconal) fat (4)**
- Eyeball (2)
- **Orbicularis oculi (1)**
- Superior conjunctional fornix
- Sclera
- Bulbar and palpebral conjunctiva
- Palpebral fissure
- Cornea
- Inferior tarsus of inferior eyelid
- Inferior conjunctival sac
- Inferior conjunctival fornix
- Orbital septum
- Inferior check ligament

B. Sagittal MRI

Sagittal Section, Superior (Upper) Eyelid

- Levator palpebrae superioris
- Superior tarsal muscle
- Superior tarsus (tarsal plate)
- **Tarsal glands**
- Palpebral conjunctiva
- **Ciliary glands**
- Orbicularis oculi (palpebral part)
- Skin
- Eyelash

7.35   Lateral aspect of the orbit and structure of the eyelid

A. Schematic sagittal and cross-section through optic nerve.
B. Sagittal MRI. The *numbers* refer to structures labeled in **A**; *S,* superior ophthalmic vein; *M,* maxillary sinus; *circled,* optic foramen.

- Foreign objects, such as sand or metal filings, produce corneal abrasions that cause sudden, stabbing eye pain and tears. Opening and closing the eyelids is also painful. Corneal lacerations are caused by sharp objects such as fingernails or the corner of a page of a book.

- Any of the glands in the eyelid may become inflamed and swollen from infection or obstruction of their ducts. If the ducts of the ciliary glands are obstructed, a painful red suppurative (pus-producing) swelling, a sty (hordeolum), develops on the eyelid. Obstruction of a tarsal gland produces inflammation, a tarsal chalazion, that protrudes toward the eyeball and rubs against it as the eyelids blink.

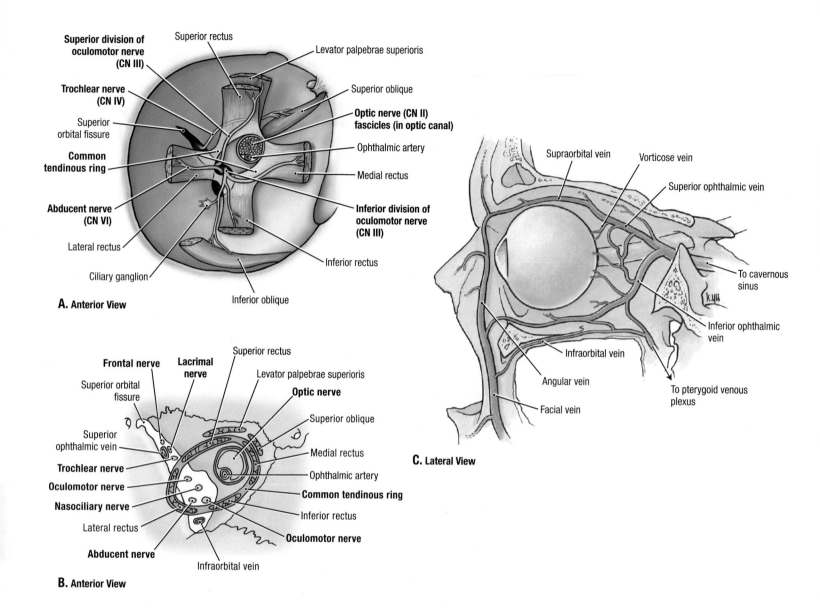

Superior division of oculomotor nerve (CN III)

Superior rectus

Levator palpebrae superioris

Trochlear nerve (CN IV)

Superior oblique

Superior orbital fissure

Optic nerve (CN II) fascicles (in optic canal)

Common tendinous ring

Ophthalmic artery

Medial rectus

Abducent nerve (CN VI)

Inferior division of oculomotor nerve (CN III)

Lateral rectus

Inferior rectus

Ciliary ganglion

Inferior oblique

A. Anterior View

Superior rectus

Frontal nerve

Lacrimal nerve

Levator palpebrae superioris

Superior orbital fissure

Optic nerve

Superior oblique

Superior ophthalmic vein

Medial rectus

Trochlear nerve

Ophthalmic artery

Oculomotor nerve

Common tendinous ring

Nasociliary nerve

Inferior rectus

Lateral rectus

Oculomotor nerve

Abducent nerve

Infraorbital vein

B. Anterior View

Supraorbital vein

Vorticose vein

Superior ophthalmic vein

To cavernous sinus

Inferior ophthalmic vein

Infraorbital vein

Angular vein

To pterygoid venous plexus

Facial vein

C. Lateral View

7.36 Nerves and veins of the orbit

A and **B.** Nerves of orbit in relation to the orbital fissures and the common tendinous ring. The common tendinous ring is formed by the origin of the four recti and encircles the dural sheath of the optic nerve, CN VI, and the superior and inferior branches of CN III; the nasociliary nerve (CN V^1) also passes through this cuff. **C.** Ophthalmic veins. The superior and inferior ophthalmic veins receive the vorticose veins from the eyeball and drain into the cavernous sinus posteriorly and the pterygoid plexus inferiorly. They communicate with the facial and supraorbital veins anteriorly.

- The facial veins make clinically important connections with the cavernous sinus through the superior ophthalmic veins. Cavernous sinus thrombosis usually results from infections in the orbit, nasal sinuses, and superior part of the face (the danger triangle). In persons with thrombophlebitis of the facial vein, pieces of an infected thrombus may extend into the cavernous sinus, producing thrombophlebitis of the cavernous sinus. The infection usually involves only one sinus initially but may spread to the opposite side through the intercavernous sinuses.

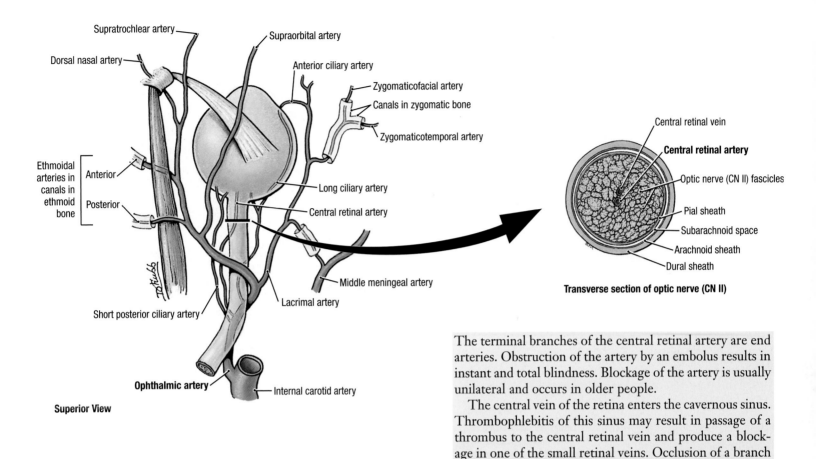

Transverse section of optic nerve (CN II)

The terminal branches of the central retinal artery are end arteries. Obstruction of the artery by an embolus results in instant and total blindness. Blockage of the artery is usually unilateral and occurs in older people.

The central vein of the retina enters the cavernous sinus. Thrombophlebitis of this sinus may result in passage of a thrombus to the central retinal vein and produce a blockage in one of the small retinal veins. Occlusion of a branch of the central vein of the retina usually results in slow, painless loss of vision.

TABLE 7.6 ARTERIES OF ORBIT

Artery	Origin	Courseand Distribution
Ophthalmic	Internal carotid artery	Traverses optic foramen to reach orbital cavity
Central retinal		Runs in dural sheath of optic nerve, entering nerve near eyeball; appears at center of optic disc; supplies optic retina (except cones and rods)
Supraorbital		Passes superiorly and posteriorly from supraorbital foramen to supply forehead and scalp
Supratrochlear		Passes from supraorbital margin to forehead and scalp
Lacrimal		Passes along superior border of lateral rectus muscle to supply lacrimal gland, conjunctiva, and eyelids
Dorsal nasal	Ophthalmic artery	Courses along dorsal aspect of nose and supplies its surface
Short posterior ciliary		Pierces sclera at periphery of optic nerve to supply choroid, which, in turn, supplies cones and rods of optic retina
Long posterior ciliary		Pierces sclera to supply ciliary body and iris
Posterior ethmoidal		Passes through posterior ethmoidal foramen to posterior ethmoidal cells
Anterior ethmoidal		Passes through anterior ethmoidal foramen to anterior cranial fossa; supplies anterior and middle ethmoidal cells, frontal sinus, nasal cavity, and skin on dorsum of nose
Anterior ciliary	Muscular branches of ophthalmic artery	Pierces sclera at attachments of rectus muscles and forms network in iris and ciliary body
Infraorbital	Third part of maxillary artery	Passes along infraorbital groove and exits through infraorbital foramen to face

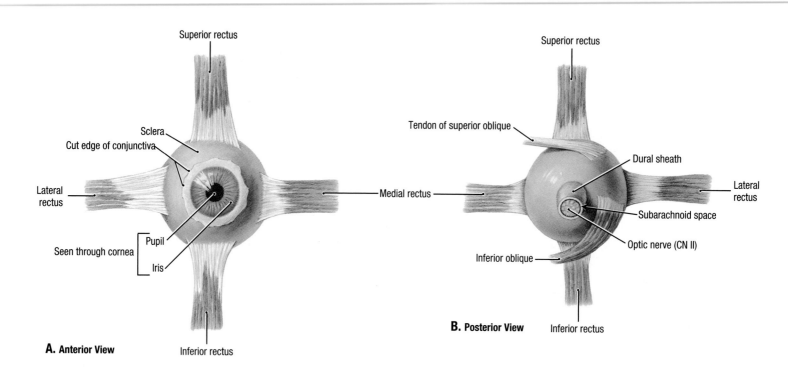

A. Anterior View

Superior rectus

Sclera

Cut edge of conjunctiva

Lateral rectus

Pupil

Seen through cornea

Iris

Inferior rectus

B. Posterior View

Superior rectus

Tendon of superior oblique

Dural sheath

Lateral rectus

Medial rectus

Subarachnoid space

Optic nerve (CN II)

Inferior oblique

Inferior rectus

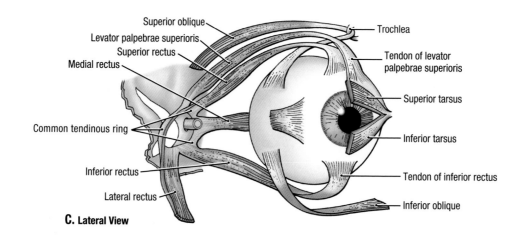

C. Lateral View

Superior oblique

Levator palpebrae superioris

Superior rectus

Medial rectus

Common tendinous ring

Inferior rectus

Lateral rectus

Trochlea

Tendon of levator palpebrae superioris

Superior tarsus

Inferior tarsus

Tendon of inferior rectus

Inferior oblique

TABLE 7.7 MUSCLES OF ORBIT

Muscle	Origin	Insertion	Innervation	Main Action
Levator palpebrae superioris	Lesser wing of sphenoid bone, superior and anterior to optic canal	Tarsal plate and skin of superior (upper) eyelid	Oculomotor nerve (CN III); deep layer (superior tarsal muscle) is supplied by sympathetic fibers	Elevates superior (upper) eyelid
Superior rectus	Common tendinous ring	Sclera just posterior to cornea	Oculomotor nerve (CN III)	Elevates, adducts, and rotates eyeball medially
Inferior rectus				Depresses, adducts, and rotates eyeball laterally
Lateral rectus			Abducent nerve (CN VI)	Abducts eyeball
Medial rectus			Oculomotor nerve (CN III)	Adducts eyeball
Superior oblique	Body of sphenoid bone	Its tendon passes through the trochlea (fibrous ring), changes its direction, and inserts into sclera deep to superior rectus muscle	Trochlear nerve (CN IV)	Abducts, depresses, and medially rotates eyeball
Inferior oblique	Anterior part of floor of orbit	Sclera deep to lateral rectus muscle	Oculomotor nerve (CN III)	Abducts, elevates, and laterally rotates eyeball

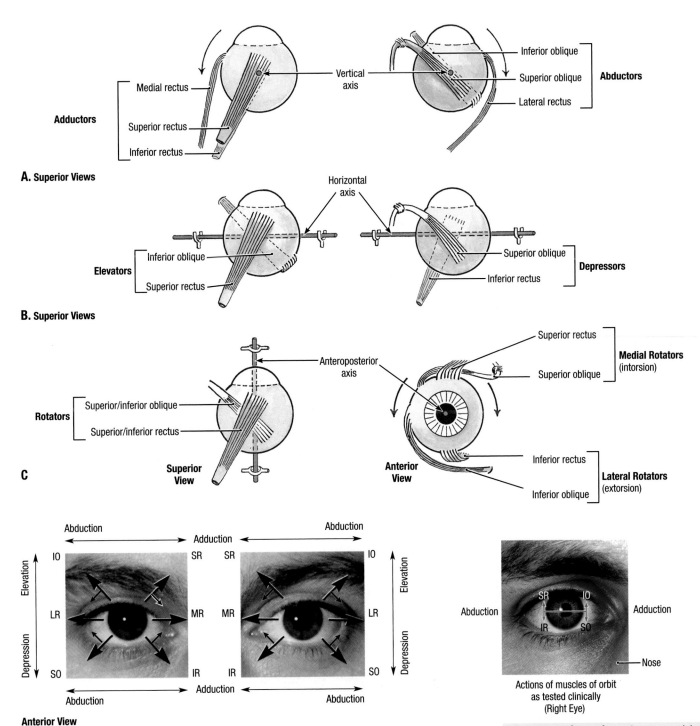

A. Superior Views

B. Superior Views

C

Anterior View

Actions of muscles of orbit
as tested clinically
(Right Eye)

TABLE 7.8 ACTIONS OF MUSCLES OF THE ORBIT STARTING FROM PRIMARY POSITION[a]

Muscle	Main Action		
	Vertical Axis (A)	**Horizontal Axis (B)**	**Anteroposterior Axis (C)**
Superior rectus (SR)	Elevates	Adducts	Rotates medially (intorsion)
Inferior rectus (IR)	Depresses	Adducts	Rotates laterally (extorsion)
Superior oblique (SO)	Depresses	Abducts	Rotates medially (intorsion)
Inferior oblique (IO)	Elevates	Abducts	Rotates laterally (extorsion)
Medial rectus (MR)	N/A	Adducts	N/A
Lateral rectus (LR)	N/A	Abducts	N/A

[a] Primary position, gaze directed anteriorly.

Movement from the primary position always involves more than one muscle acting synergistically. When testing muscles, it is desirable to test actions produced by one muscle acting independently. Because the axes of the orbits diverge and do not correspond to the axis of gaze in the primary position, responsibility for elevation and depression changes with abduction and adduction. When the eye is adducted, the oblique muscles are solely responsible; when the eye is abducted, the rectus muscles are solely responsible.

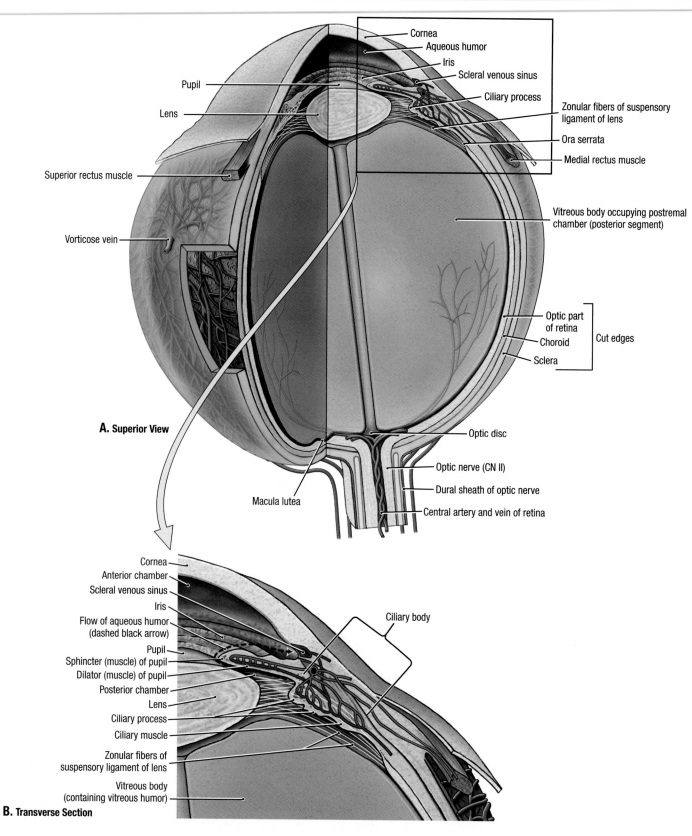

A. Superior View

- Cornea
- Aqueous humor
- Iris
- Scleral venous sinus
- Ciliary process
- Zonular fibers of suspensory ligament of lens
- Ora serrata
- Medial rectus muscle
- Pupil
- Lens
- Superior rectus muscle
- Vorticose vein
- Vitreous body occupying postremal chamber (posterior segment)
- Optic part of retina
- Choroid
- Sclera
- Cut edges
- Optic disc
- Optic nerve (CN II)
- Dural sheath of optic nerve
- Central artery and vein of retina
- Macula lutea

B. Transverse Section

- Cornea
- Anterior chamber
- Scleral venous sinus
- Iris
- Flow of aqueous humor (dashed black arrow)
- Pupil
- Sphincter (muscle) of pupil
- Dilator (muscle) of pupil
- Posterior chamber
- Lens
- Ciliary process
- Ciliary muscle
- Zonular fibers of suspensory ligament of lens
- Vitreous body (containing vitreous humor)
- Ciliary body

7.37   Illustration of a dissected eyeball

A. Parts of the eyeball. **B.** Ciliary region. The aqueous humor is produced by the ciliary processes and provides nutrients for the avascular cornea and lens; the aqueous humor drains into the scleral venous sinus (also called the *sinus venosus sclerae* or *canal of Schlemm*). If drainage of the aqueous humor is reduced significantly, pressure builds up in the chambers of the eye (glaucoma). Blindness can result from compression of the inner layer of the retina and retinal arteries if aqueous humor production is not reduced to maintain normal intraocular pressure.

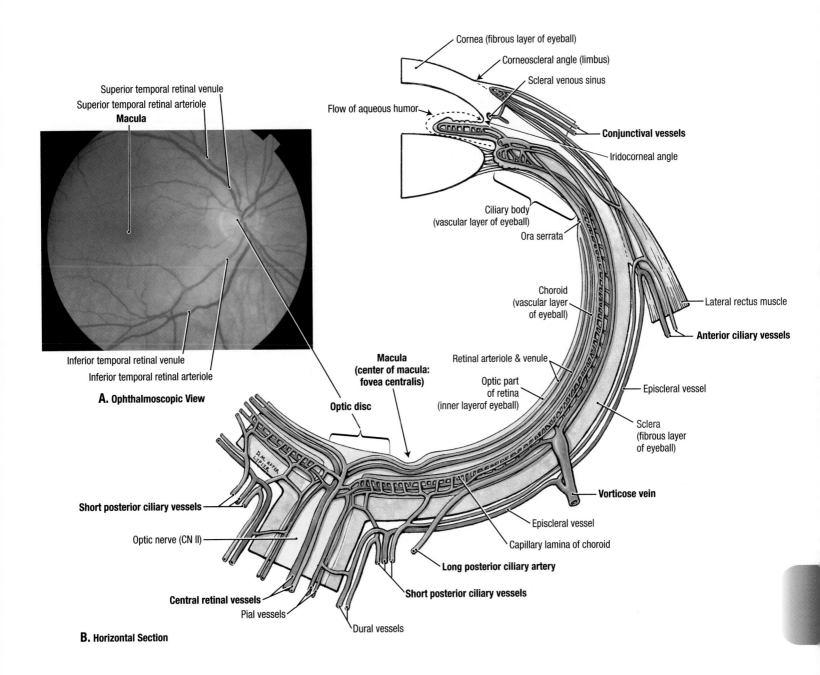

Superior temporal retinal venule
Superior temporal retinal arteriole
Macula

Flow of aqueous humor

Cornea (fibrous layer of eyeball)
Corneoscleral angle (limbus)
Scleral venous sinus

Conjunctival vessels
Iridocorneal angle

Ciliary body
(vascular layer of eyeball)
Ora serrata

Choroid
(vascular layer
of eyeball)

Lateral rectus muscle
Anterior ciliary vessels

Inferior temporal retinal venule
Inferior temporal retinal arteriole

A. Ophthalmoscopic View

**Macula
(center of macula:
fovea centralis)**

Optic disc

Retinal arteriole & venule
Optic part
of retina
(inner layer of eyeball)

Episcleral vessel

Sclera
(fibrous layer
of eyeball)

Short posterior ciliary vessels

Optic nerve (CN II)

Episcleral vessel

Capillary lamina of choroid

Vorticose vein

Central retinal vessels
Pial vessels
Dural vessels

Long posterior ciliary artery
Short posterior ciliary vessels

B. Horizontal Section

7.38   Ocular fundus and blood supply to the eyeball

A. Right ocular fundus, ophthalmoscopic view. Retinal venules (wider) and retinal arterioles (narrower) radiate from the center of the oval optic disc, formed in relation to the entry of the optic nerve into the eyeball. The round, dark area lateral to the disc is the macula; branches of vessels extend to this area, but do not reach its center, the fovea centralis, a depressed spot that is the area of most acute vision. It is avascular but, like the rest of the outermost (cones and rods) layer of the retina, is nourished by the adjacent choriocapillaris. An increase in CSF pressure slows venous return from the retina, causing edema of the retina (fluid accumulation). The edema is viewed during ophthalmoscopy as swelling of the optic disc, a condition called papilledema. **B.** Blood supply to eyeball. The eyeball has three layers: (a) the external, fibrous layer is the sclera and cornea; (b) the middle, vascular layer is the choroid, ciliary body, and iris; and (c) the internal, neural layer or retina consists of a pigment cell layer and a neural layer. The central artery of the retina, a branch of the ophthalmic artery, is an end artery. Of the eight posterior ciliary arteries, six are short posterior ciliary arteries and supply the choroid, which in turn nourishes the outer, nonvascular layer of the retina. Two long posterior ciliary arteries, one on each side of the eyeball, run between the sclera and choroid to anastomose with the anterior ciliary arteries, which are derived from muscular branches. The choroid is drained by posterior ciliary veins, and four to five vorticose veins drain into the ophthalmic veins.

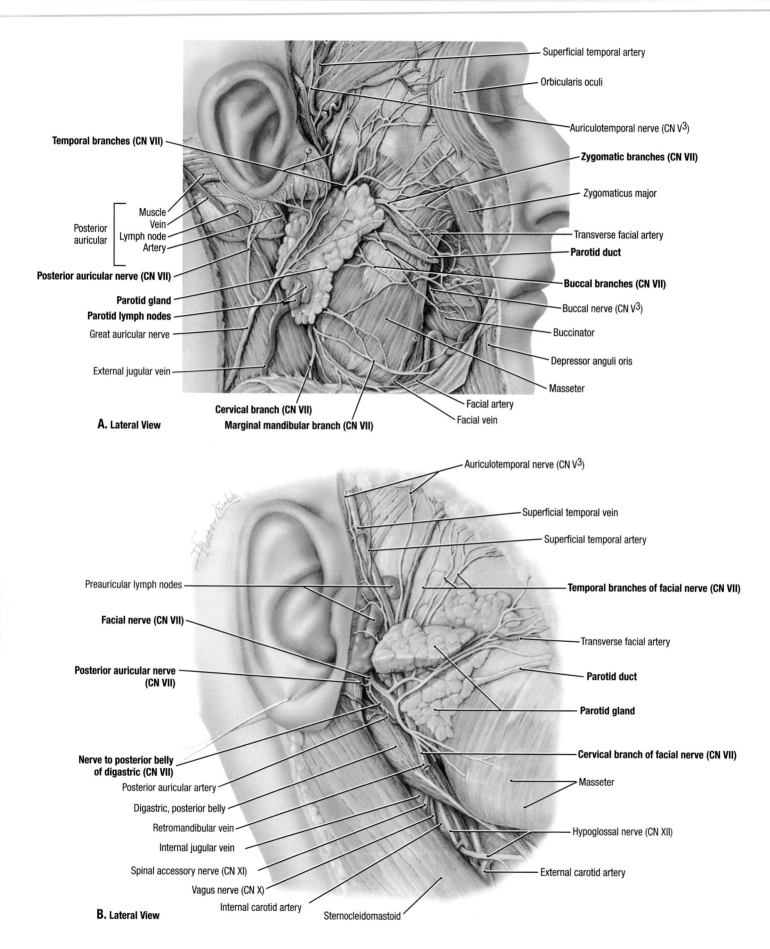

A. Lateral View

Superficial temporal artery

Orbicularis oculi

Auriculotemporal nerve (CN V^3)

Zygomatic branches (CN VII)

Zygomaticus major

Transverse facial artery

Parotid duct

Buccal branches (CN VII)

Buccal nerve (CN V^3)

Buccinator

Depressor anguli oris

Masseter

Facial artery

Facial vein

Temporal branches (CN VII)

Muscle
Vein
Lymph node
Artery
Posterior
auricular

Posterior auricular nerve (CN VII)

Parotid gland
Parotid lymph nodes
Great auricular nerve

External jugular vein

Cervical branch (CN VII)
Marginal mandibular branch (CN VII)

B. Lateral View

Auriculotemporal nerve (CN V^3)

Superficial temporal vein

Superficial temporal artery

Temporal branches of facial nerve (CN VII)

Transverse facial artery

Parotid duct

Parotid gland

Cervical branch of facial nerve (CN VII)

Masseter

Hypoglossal nerve (CN XII)

External carotid artery

Preauricular lymph nodes

Facial nerve (CN VII)

Posterior auricular nerve (CN VII)

Nerve to posterior belly of digastric (CN VII)
Posterior auricular artery
Digastric, posterior belly
Retromandibular vein
Internal jugular vein
Spinal accessory nerve (CN XI)
Vagus nerve (CN X)
Internal carotid artery
Sternocleidomastoid

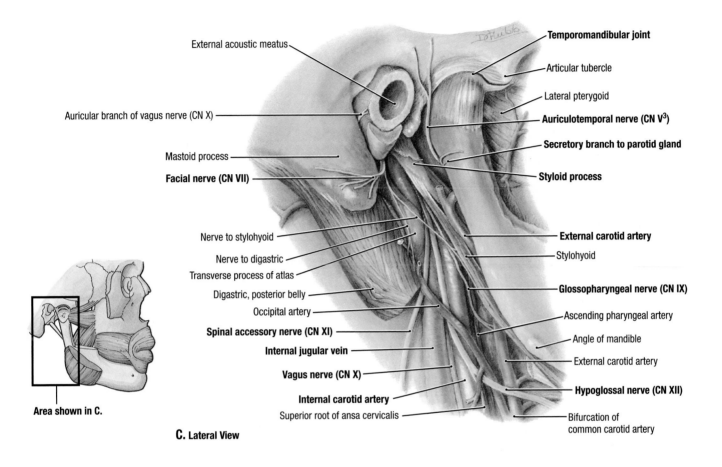

External acoustic meatus

Temporomandibular joint

Articular tubercle

Lateral pterygoid

Auricular branch of vagus nerve (CN X)

Auriculotemporal nerve (CN V³)

Secretory branch to parotid gland

Mastoid process

Facial nerve (CN VII)

Styloid process

Nerve to stylohyoid

External carotid artery

Nerve to digastric

Stylohyoid

Transverse process of atlas

Digastric, posterior belly

Glossopharyngeal nerve (CN IX)

Occipital artery

Ascending pharyngeal artery

Spinal accessory nerve (CN XI)

Angle of mandible

Internal jugular vein

External carotid artery

Vagus nerve (CN X)

Hypoglossal nerve (CN XII)

Internal carotid artery

Superior root of ansa cervicalis

Bifurcation of
common carotid artery

Area shown in C.

C. Lateral View

7.39   Parotid region

A. Superficial dissection. **B.** Deep dissection with part of the gland removed. The facial nerve (CN VII) supplies motor innervation to the muscles of facial expression; it forms a plexus within the parotid gland and the branches of which radiate over the face, anastomosing with each other and the branches of the trigeminal nerve. During parotidectomy (surgical excision of the parotid gland), identification, dissection, and preservation of the facial nerve are critical. **C.** Deep dissection following removal of the parotid gland. The facial nerve, posterior belly of the digastric muscle, and its nerve are retracted; the external carotid artery, stylohyoid muscle, and the nerve to the stylohyoid remain in situ. The internal jugular vein, internal carotid artery, and glossopharyngeal (CN IX), vagus (CN X), accessory (CN XI), and hypoglossal (CN XII) nerves cross anterior to the transverse process of the atlas and deep to the styloid process.

Care must be taken during surgical procedures involving the temporomandibular joint to preserve the branches of the facial nerve that overlie the joint and the articular branches of the auriculotemporal nerve that enter the joint.

Trauma, such as a fractured mandible, may injure the hypoglossal nerve (CN XII), resulting in paralysis and eventual atrophy of one side of the tongue. The tongue deviates to the paralyzed side during protrusion.

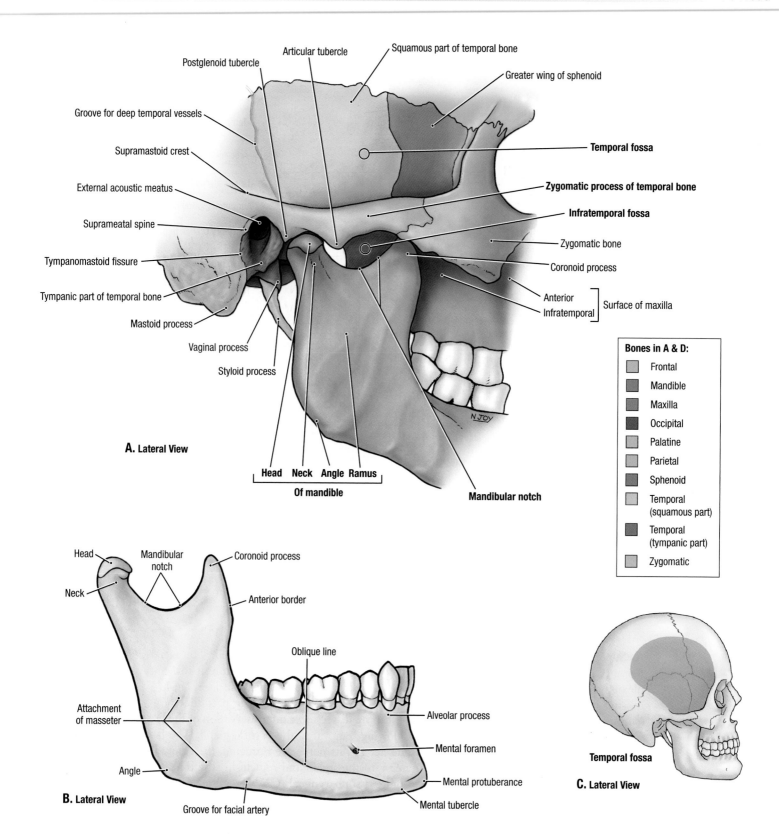

A. Lateral View

Postglenoid tubercle

Articular tubercle

Squamous part of temporal bone

Greater wing of sphenoid

Groove for deep temporal vessels

Supramastoid crest

External acoustic meatus

Suprameatal spine

Tympanomastoid fissure

Tympanic part of temporal bone

Mastoid process

Vaginal process

Styloid process

Temporal fossa

Zygomatic process of temporal bone

Infratemporal fossa

Zygomatic bone

Coronoid process

Anterior

Infratemporal

} Surface of maxilla

Head Neck Angle Ramus

Of mandible

Mandibular notch

Bones in A & D:

Frontal

Mandible

Maxilla

Occipital

Palatine

Parietal

Sphenoid

Temporal (squamous part)

Temporal (tympanic part)

Zygomatic

B. Lateral View

Head

Mandibular notch

Neck

Coronoid process

Anterior border

Oblique line

Attachment of masseter

Alveolar process

Mental foramen

Angle

Mental protuberance

Mental tubercle

Groove for facial artery

Temporal fossa

C. Lateral View

7.40   **Temporal and infratemporal fossa and mandible**

A. Bones and bony features. Note that superficially the zygomatic process of the temporal bone is the boundary between the temporal fossa superiorly and the infratemporal fossa inferiorly. **B.** External surface of the mandible. **C.** Temporal fossa (gray area).

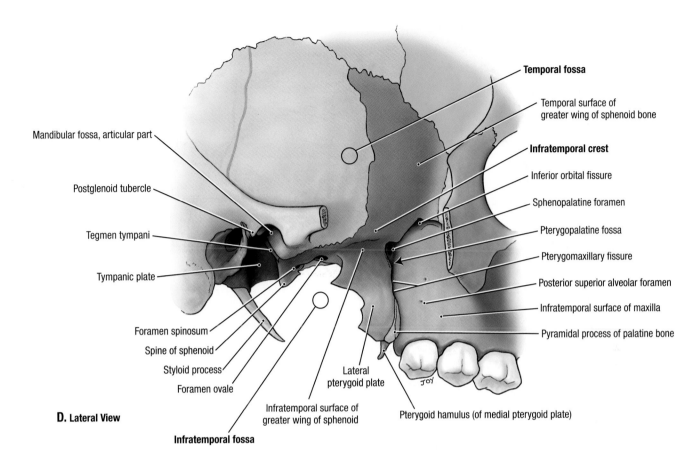

Temporal fossa
Temporal surface of greater wing of sphenoid bone
Mandibular fossa, articular part
Infratemporal crest
Inferior orbital fissure
Postglenoid tubercle
Sphenopalatine foramen
Pterygopalatine fossa
Tegmen tympani
Pterygomaxillary fissure
Posterior superior alveolar foramen
Tympanic plate
Infratemporal surface of maxilla
Pyramidal process of palatine bone
Foramen spinosum
Spine of sphenoid
Styloid process
Lateral pterygoid plate
Foramen ovale
D. Lateral View
Infratemporal surface of greater wing of sphenoid
Pterygoid hamulus (of medial pterygoid plate)
Infratemporal fossa

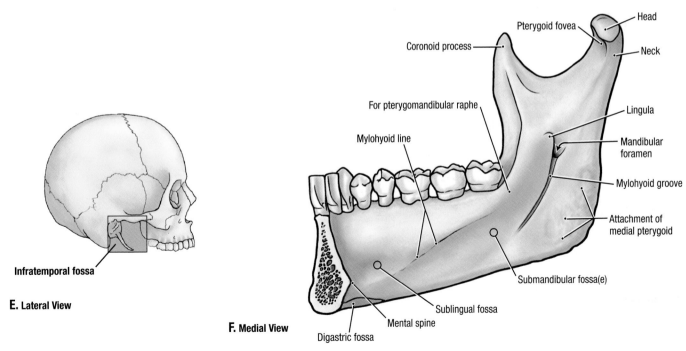

Pterygoid fovea
Head
Coronoid process
Neck
For pterygomandibular raphe
Lingula
Mylohyoid line
Mandibular foramen
Mylohyoid groove
Attachment of medial pterygoid
Infratemporal fossa
Submandibular fossa(e)
E. Lateral View
Sublingual fossa
F. Medial View
Mental spine
Digastric fossa

7.40   **Temporal and infratemporal fossa and mandible** *(continued)*

D. Bones and bony features of the infratemporal fossa. The mandible and part of the zygomatic arch have been removed. Deeply, the infratemporal crest separates the temporal and infratemporal fossae. **E.** Infratemporal fossa (gray area). **F.** Internal surface of the mandible.

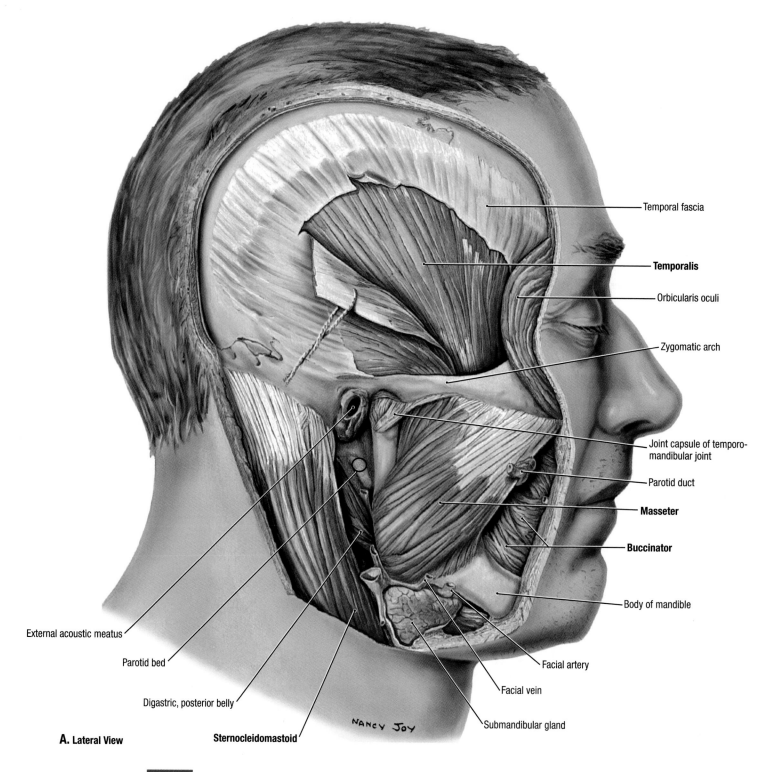

Temporal fascia

Temporalis

Orbicularis oculi

Zygomatic arch

Joint capsule of temporo-
mandibular joint

Parotid duct

Masseter

Buccinator

Body of mandible

Facial artery

Facial vein

Submandibular gland

External acoustic meatus

Parotid bed

Digastric, posterior belly

Sternocleidomastoid

NANCY JOY

A. Lateral View

7.41   Temporalis and masseter

A. Superficial dissection.
- The temporalis and masseter muscles are supplied by the trigeminal nerve (CN V), and both elevate the mandible. The buccinator muscle, supplied by the facial nerve (CN VII), functions during chewing to keep food between the teeth but does not act on the mandible.
- The sternocleidomastoid muscle, supplied by the spinal accessory nerve (CN XI), is the chief flexor of the head and neck; it forms the lateral part of the posterior boundary of the parotid region/parotid bed.

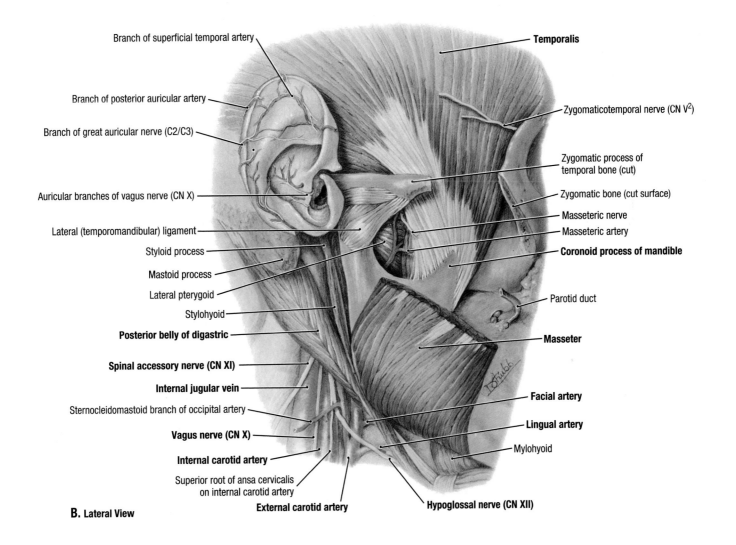

Branch of superficial temporal artery

Branch of posterior auricular artery

Branch of great auricular nerve (C2/C3)

Auricular branches of vagus nerve (CN X)

Lateral (temporomandibular) ligament

Styloid process

Mastoid process

Lateral pterygoid

Stylohyoid

Posterior belly of digastric

Spinal accessory nerve (CN XI)

Internal jugular vein

Sternocleidomastoid branch of occipital artery

Vagus nerve (CN X)

Internal carotid artery

Superior root of ansa cervicalis
on internal carotid artery

External carotid artery

B. Lateral View

Temporalis

Zygomaticotemporal nerve (CN V²)

Zygomatic process of
temporal bone (cut)

Zygomatic bone (cut surface)

Masseteric nerve

Masseteric artery

Coronoid process of mandible

Parotid duct

Masseter

Facial artery

Lingual artery

Mylohyoid

Hypoglossal nerve (CN XII)

| **7.41** | **Temporalis and masseter** *(continued)* |

B. Deep dissection.
- Parts of the zygomatic arch and the masseter muscle have been removed to expose the attachment of the temporalis muscle to the coronoid process of the mandible.
- The carotid sheath surrounding the internal jugular vein, internal carotid artery, and the vagus nerve (CN X) has been removed. The external carotid artery and its lingual, facial, and occipital branches, and the spinal accessory (CN XI) and hypoglossal (CN XII) nerves pass deep to the posterior belly of the digastric muscle.

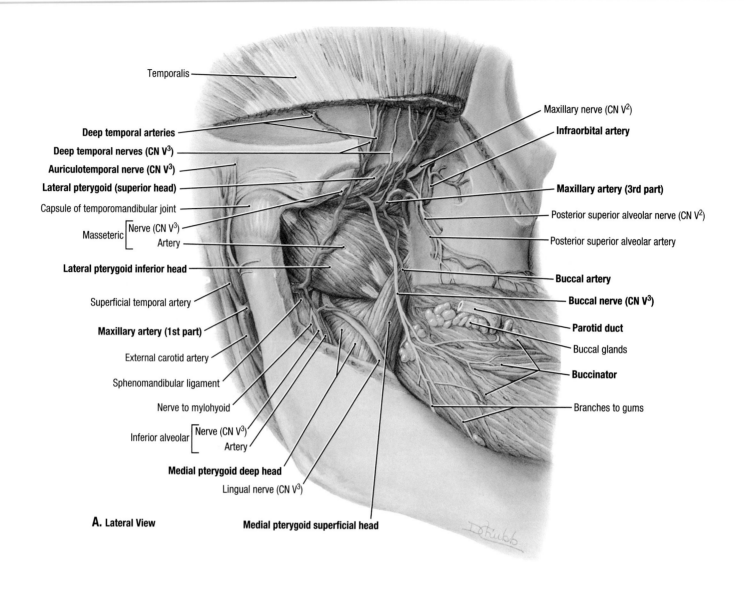

Temporalis

Deep temporal arteries

Deep temporal nerves (CN V³)

Auriculotemporal nerve (CN V³)

Lateral pterygoid (superior head)

Capsule of temporomandibular joint

Masseteric ⎡ Nerve (CN V³)
         ⎣ Artery

Lateral pterygoid inferior head

Superficial temporal artery

Maxillary artery (1st part)

External carotid artery

Sphenomandibular ligament

Nerve to mylohyoid

Inferior alveolar ⎡ Nerve (CN V³)
              ⎣ Artery

Medial pterygoid deep head

Lingual nerve (CN V³)

Maxillary nerve (CN V²)

Infraorbital artery

Maxillary artery (3rd part)

Posterior superior alveolar nerve (CN V²)

Posterior superior alveolar artery

Buccal artery

Buccal nerve (CN V³)

Parotid duct

Buccal glands

Buccinator

Branches to gums

A. Lateral View   **Medial pterygoid superficial head**

7.42   Infratemporal region

A. Superficial dissection.

- The maxillary artery, the larger of two terminal branches of the external carotid, is divided into three parts relative to the lateral pterygoid muscle.
- The buccinator is pierced by the parotid duct, the ducts of the buccal glands, and sensory branches of the buccal nerve.
- The lateral pterygoid muscle arises by two heads (parts), one head from the roof, and the other head from the medial wall of the infratemporal fossa; both heads insert in relation to the temporomandibular joint—the superior head attaching primarily to the articular disc of the joint and the inferior head primarily to the anterior aspect of the neck of the mandible (pterygoid fovea).
- Because of the close relationship of the facial and auriculotemporal nerves to the temporomandibular joint (TMJ), care must be taken during surgical procedures to preserve both the branches of the facial nerve overlying it and the articular branches of the auriculotemporal nerve that enter the posterior part of the joint. Injury to articular branches of the auriculotemporal nerve supplying the TMJ—associated with traumatic dislocation and rupture of the joint capsule and lateral ligament—leads to laxity and instability of the TMJ.

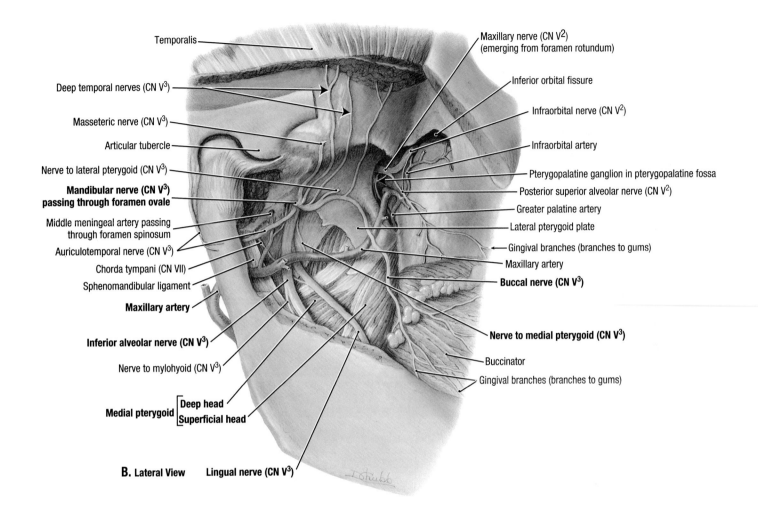

Temporalis

Maxillary nerve (CN V²) (emerging from foramen rotundum)

Deep temporal nerves (CN V³)

Inferior orbital fissure

Masseteric nerve (CN V³)

Infraorbital nerve (CN V²)

Articular tubercle

Infraorbital artery

Nerve to lateral pterygoid (CN V³)

Pterygopalatine ganglion in pterygopalatine fossa

Mandibular nerve (CN V³) passing through foramen ovale

Posterior superior alveolar nerve (CN V²)

Greater palatine artery

Middle meningeal artery passing through foramen spinosum

Lateral pterygoid plate

Auriculotemporal nerve (CN V³)

Gingival branches (branches to gums)

Chorda tympani (CN VII)

Maxillary artery

Sphenomandibular ligament

Buccal nerve (CN V³)

Maxillary artery

Inferior alveolar nerve (CN V³)

Nerve to medial pterygoid (CN V³)

Nerve to mylohyoid (CN V³)

Buccinator

Gingival branches (branches to gums)

Medial pterygoid [**Deep head** / **Superficial head**]

B. Lateral View   Lingual nerve (CN V³)

7.42   Infratemporal region (continued)

B. Deeper dissection.

- The lateral pterygoid muscle and most of the branches of the maxillary artery have been removed to expose the mandibular nerve (CN V³) entering the infratemporal fossa through the foramen ovale and the middle meningeal artery passing through the foramen spinosum.
- The deep head of the medial pterygoid muscle arises from the medial surface of the lateral pterygoid plate and the pyramidal process of the palatine bone. It has a small, superficial head that arises from the tuberosity of the maxilla.
- The inferior alveolar and lingual nerves descend on the medial pterygoid muscle. The inferior alveolar nerve gives off the nerve to mylohyoid and nerve to anterior belly of the digastric muscle, and the lingual nerve receives the chorda tympani, which carries secretory parasympathetic fibers and fibers of taste.
- Motor nerves arising from CN V³ supply the four muscles of mastication: the masseter, temporalis, and lateral and medial pterygoids. The buccal nerve from the mandibular nerve is sensory; the buccal branch of the facial nerve is the motor supply to the buccinator muscle.
- To perform a mandibular nerve block, an anesthetic agent is injected near the mandibular nerve where it enters the infratemporal fossa. This block usually anesthetizes the auriculotemporal, inferior alveolar, lingual, and buccal branches of the mandibular nerve.

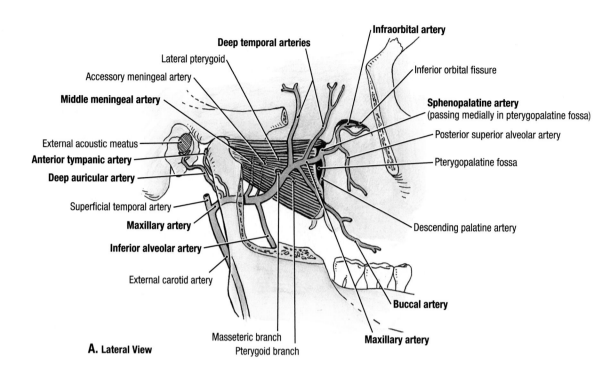

A. Lateral View

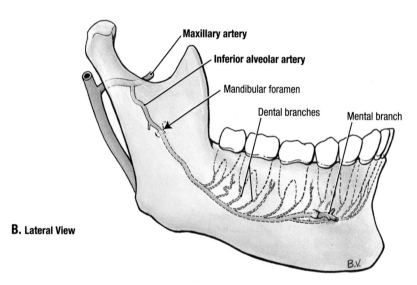

B. Lateral View

7.43 **Branches of maxillary artery**

A. Infratemporal region. **B.** Mandible.

- The maxillary artery arises at the neck of the mandible and is divided into three parts by the lateral pterygoid; it can pass medial or lateral to the lateral pterygoid.
- The branches of the first or retromandibular part pass through foramina or canals: the deep auricular to the external acoustic meatus, the anterior tympanic to the tympanic cavity, the middle and accessory meningeal to the cranial cavity, and the inferior alveolar to the mandible and teeth.
- The branches of the second part (directly related to the lateral pterygoid) supply muscles via the masseteric, deep temporal, pterygoid, and buccal branches.
- The branches of the third (pterygopalatine) part (posterior superior alveolar, infraorbital, descending palatine, and sphenopalatine arteries) arise immediately proximal to and within the pterygopalatine fossa.

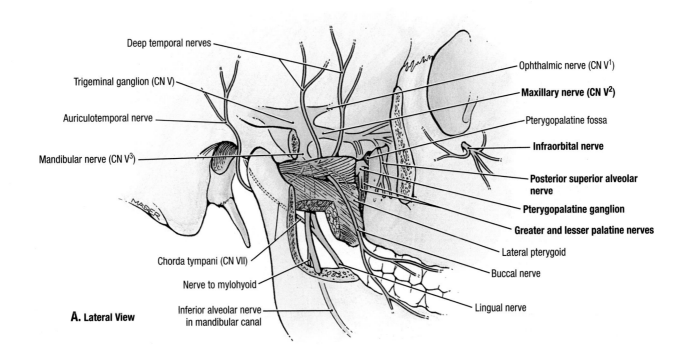

Deep temporal nerves

Trigeminal ganglion (CN V)

Auriculotemporal nerve

Mandibular nerve (CN V³)

Ophthalmic nerve (CN V¹)

Maxillary nerve (CN V²)

Pterygopalatine fossa

Infraorbital nerve

Posterior superior alveolar nerve

Pterygopalatine ganglion

Greater and lesser palatine nerves

Lateral pterygoid

Buccal nerve

Lingual nerve

Chorda tympani (CN VII)

Nerve to mylohyoid

Inferior alveolar nerve in mandibular canal

A. Lateral View

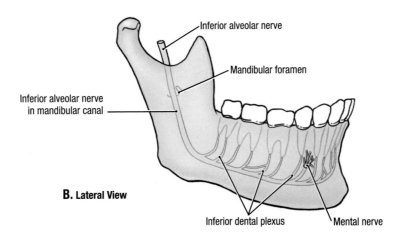

Inferior alveolar nerve

Mandibular foramen

Inferior alveolar nerve in mandibular canal

Inferior dental plexus

Mental nerve

B. Lateral View

7.44   **Branches of maxillary and mandibular nerves**

A. Infratemporal region and pterygopalatine fossa. Branches of the maxillary (CN V²) and mandibular (CN V³) nerves accompany branches from the three parts of the maxillary artery. **B.** Mandible and inferior alveolar nerve.

An alveolar nerve block—commonly used by dentists when repairing mandibular teeth—anesthetizes the inferior alveolar nerve, a branch of CN V³. The anesthetic agent is injected around the mandibular foramen, the opening into the mandibular canal on the medial aspect of the ramus of the mandible. This canal gives passage to the inferior alveolar nerve, artery, and vein. When this nerve block is successful, all mandibular teeth are anesthetized to the median plane. The skin and mucous membrane of the lower lip, the labial alveolar mucosa and gingiva, and the skin of the chin are also anesthetized because they are supplied by the mental branch of this nerve.

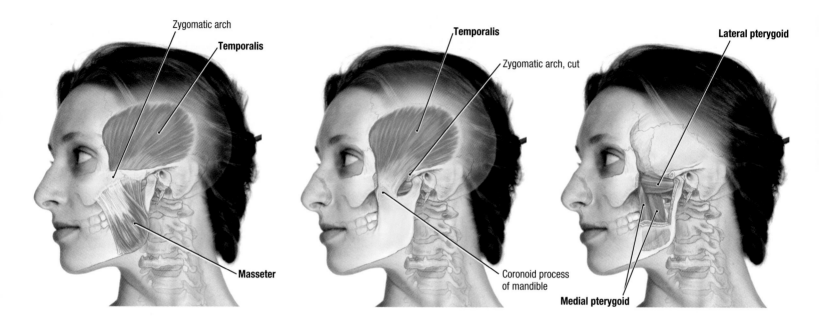

Lateral Views

TABLE 7.9 MUSCLES OF MASTICATION (ACTING ON TEMPOROMANDIBULAR JOINT)

Muscle	Origin	Insertion	Innervation	Main Action
Temporalis	Floor of temporal fossa and deep surface of temporal fascia	Tip and medial surface of coronoid process and anterior border of ramus of mandible	Deep temporal branches of mandibular nerve (CN V³)	Elevates mandible, closing jaws; posterior fibers retrude mandible after protrusion
Masseter	Inferior border and medial surface of zygomatic arch	Lateral surface of ramus of mandible and coronoid process	Mandibular nerve (CN V³) through masseteric nerve that enters deep surface of the muscle	Elevates and protrudes mandible, thus closing jaws; deep fibers retrude it
Lateral pterygoid	*Superior head:* infratemporal surface and infratemporal crest of greater wing of sphenoid bone *Inferior head:* lateral surface of lateral pterygoid plate	Neck of mandible, articular disc, and capsule of temporo-mandibular joint	Mandibular nerve (CN V³) through lateral pterygoid nerve which enters its deep surface	*Acting bilaterally,* protrude mandible and depress chin; *Acting unilaterally* alternately, they produce side-to-side movements of mandible
Medial pterygoid	*Deep head:* medial surface of lateral pterygoid plate and pyramidal process of palatine bone *Superficial head:* tuberosity of maxilla	Medial surface of ramus of mandible, inferior to mandibular foramen	Mandibular nerve (CN V³) through medial pterygoid nerve	Helps elevate mandible, closing jaws; *acting bilaterally* protrude mandible; *acting unilaterally,* protrudes side of jaw; acting alternately, they produce a grinding motion

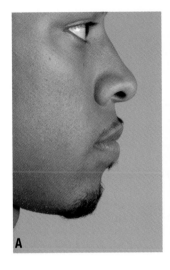
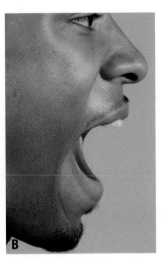
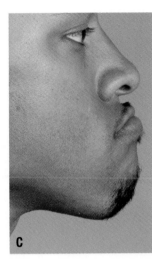
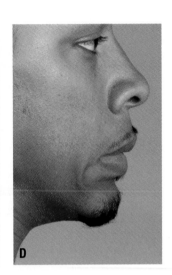

Lateral Views

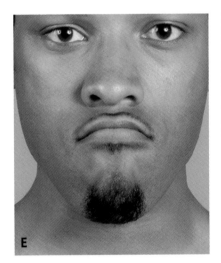
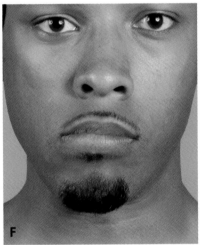
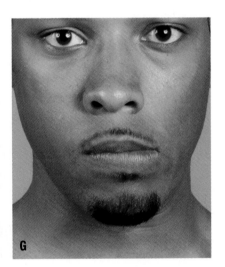

Anterior Views

TABLE 7.10 MOVEMENTS OF THE TEMPOROMANDIBULAR JOINT

Movements	Muscles
Elevation (close mouth) (A)	Temporalis, masseter, and medial pterygoid
Depression (open mouth) (B)	Lateral pterygoid; suprahyoid and infrahyoid muscles; gravity
Protrusion (protrude chin) (C and E)	Lateral pterygoid, masseter, and medial pterygoid
Retrusion (retrude chin) (D)	Temporalis (posterior oblique and near horizontal fibers) and masseter
Lateral movements (grinding and chewing) (F and G)	Temporalis of same side, pterygoids of opposite side, and masseter

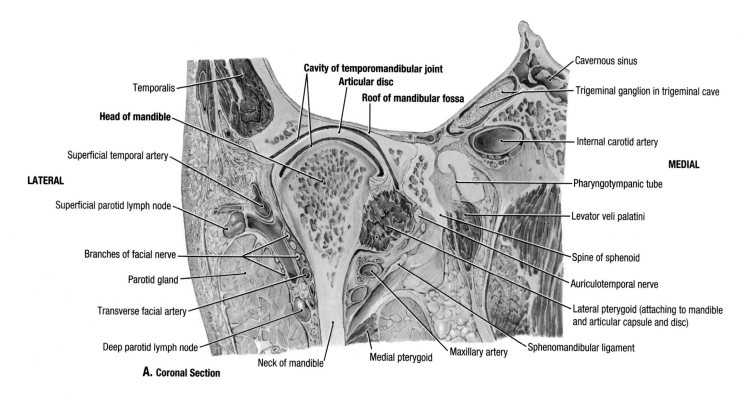

Temporalis

Cavity of temporomandibular joint
Articular disc

Roof of mandibular fossa

Cavernous sinus

Trigeminal ganglion in trigeminal cave

Head of mandible

Superficial temporal artery

LATERAL

Internal carotid artery

MEDIAL

Superficial parotid lymph node

Pharyngotympanic tube

Levator veli palatini

Branches of facial nerve

Parotid gland

Spine of sphenoid

Auriculotemporal nerve

Transverse facial artery

Lateral pterygoid (attaching to mandible
and articular capsule and disc)

Deep parotid lymph node

Neck of mandible

Medial pterygoid

Maxillary artery

Sphenomandibular ligament

A. Coronal Section

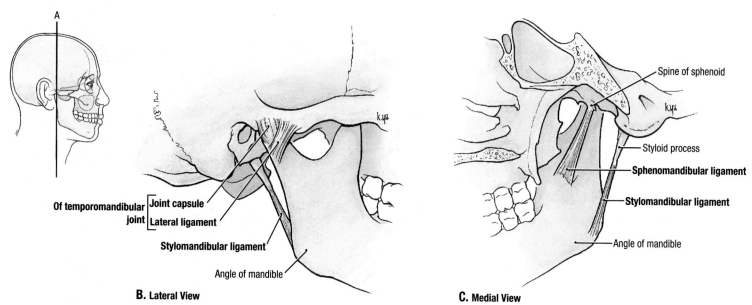

Of temporomandibular joint | **Joint capsule**
Lateral ligament

Stylomandibular ligament

Angle of mandible

B. Lateral View

Spine of sphenoid

Styloid process

Sphenomandibular ligament

Stylomandibular ligament

Angle of mandible

C. Medial View

7.45 Temporomandibular joint

A. Coronal section. **B.** Temporomandibular joint and stylomandibular ligament. The joint capsule of the temporomandibular joint attaches to the margins of the mandibular fossa and articular tubercle of the temporal bone and around the neck of the mandible; the lateral (temporomandibular) ligament strengthens the lateral aspect of the joint. **C.** Stylomandibular and sphenomandibular ligaments. The strong sphenomandibular ligament descends from near the spine of the sphenoid to the lingula of the mandible and is the "swinging hinge" by which the mandible is suspended; the weaker stylomandibular ligament is a thickened part of the parotid sheath that joins the styloid process to the angle of the mandible.

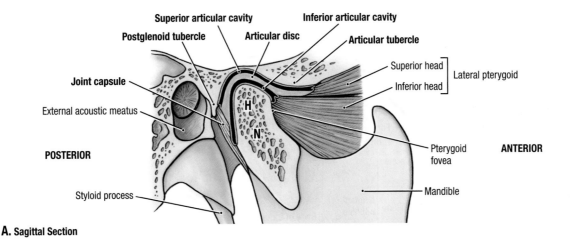

A. Sagittal Section

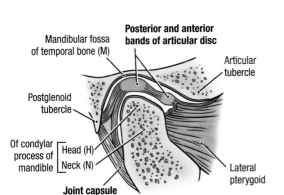

B. Closed Mouth, Sagittal Section

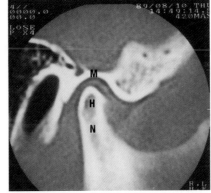

Sagittal CT

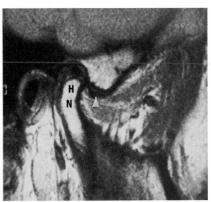

Sagittal MRI

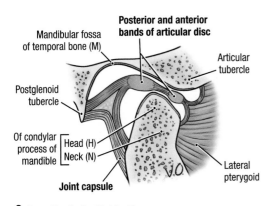

C. Open Mouth, Sagittal Section

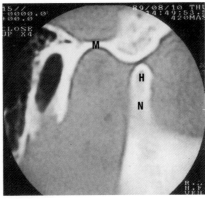

Sagittal CT

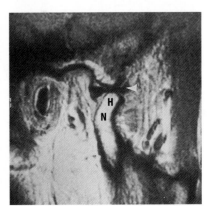

Sagittal MRI

7.46   **Sectional anatomy of temporomandibular joint (TMJ)**

A. TMJ and related structures, sagittal section. **B.** Sagittal orientation figure, CT, and MRI—mouth closed. **C.** Sagittal orientation figure, CT, and MRI—mouth opened widely. The articular disc divides the articular cavity into superior and inferior compartments, each lined by a separate synovial membrane.

During yawning or taking large bites, excessive contraction of the lateral pterygoids can cause the head of the mandible to dislocate (pass anterior to the articular tubercle). In this position, the mouth remains wide open, and the person cannot close it without manual distraction.

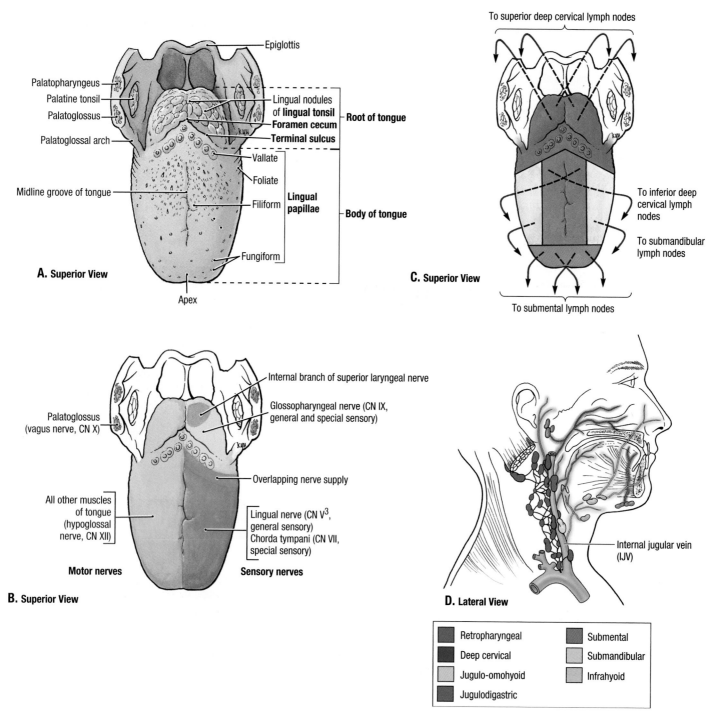

A. **Superior View**

- Epiglottis
- Palatopharyngeus
- Palatine tonsil
- Palatoglossus
- Palatoglossal arch
- Lingual nodules of **lingual tonsil**
- **Foramen cecum**
- **Terminal sulcus** — **Root of tongue**
- Vallate
- Foliate
- Midline groove of tongue
- Filiform — **Lingual papillae**
- Fungiform — **Body of tongue**
- Apex

B. **Superior View**

- Internal branch of superior laryngeal nerve
- Glossopharyngeal nerve (CN IX, general and special sensory)
- Palatoglossus (vagus nerve, CN X)
- Overlapping nerve supply
- All other muscles of tongue (hypoglossal nerve, CN XII)
- Lingual nerve (CN V^3, general sensory)
- Chorda tympani (CN VII, special sensory)
- **Motor nerves**
- **Sensory nerves**

C. **Superior View**

- To superior deep cervical lymph nodes
- To inferior deep cervical lymph nodes
- To submandibular lymph nodes
- To submental lymph nodes

D. **Lateral View**

- Internal jugular vein (IJV)

Retropharyngeal		Submental
Deep cervical		Submandibular
Jugulo-omohyoid		Infrahyoid
Jugulodigastric		

7.47   Tongue

A. Features of dorsum of the tongue. The foramen cecum is the upper end of the primitive thyroglossal duct; the arms of the V-shaped terminal sulcus diverge from the foramen, demarcating the posterior third of the tongue from the anterior two thirds. **B.** General sensory, special sensory (taste), and motor innervation of tongue. **C.** Lymphatic drainage of dorsum of tongue. **D.** Lymphatic drainage of tongue, mouth, nasal cavity, and nose.

Malignant tumors in the posterior part of the tongue metastasize to the superior deep cervical lymph nodes on both sides. In contrast, tumors in the apex and anterolateral parts usually do not metastasize to the inferior deep cervical nodes until late in the disease. Because the deep nodes are closely related to the internal jugular vein (IJV), metastases from the carcinoma may spread to the submental and submandibular regions and along the IJV into the neck.

One may touch the anterior part of the tongue without feeling discomfort; however, when the posterior part is touched, one usually gags. CN IX and CN X are responsible for the muscular contraction of each side of the pharynx. Glossopharyngeal branches (CN IX) provide the afferent limb of the gag reflex.

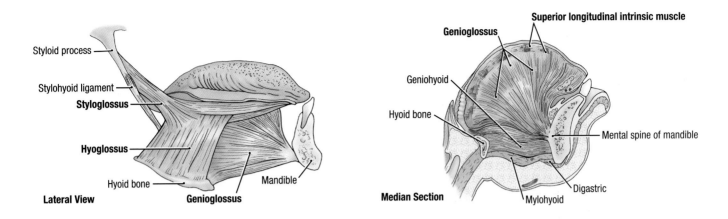

Styloid process

Stylohyoid ligament

Styloglossus

Hyoglossus

Hyoid bone

Lateral View

Mandible

Genioglossus

Genioglossus

Superior longitudinal intrinsic muscle

Geniohyoid

Hyoid bone

Mental spine of mandible

Digastric

Mylohyoid

Median Section

TABLE 7.11 MUSCLES OF TONGUE

Extrinsic Muscles

Muscle	Origin	Insertion	Innervation	Main Action
Genioglossus	Superior part of mental spine of mandible	Dorsum of tongue and body of hyoid bone	Hypoglossal nerve (CN XII)	Depresses tongue; its posterior part pulls tongue anteriorly for protrusion[a]
Hyoglossus	Body and greater horn of hyoid bone	Side and inferior aspect of tongue		Depresses and retracts tongue
Styloglossus	Styloid process of temporal bone and stylohyoid ligament	Side and inferior aspect of tongue		Retracts tongue and draws it up to create a trough for swallowing
Palatoglossus	Palatine aponeurosis of soft palate	Side of tongue	CN X and pharyngeal plexus	Elevates posterior part of tongue

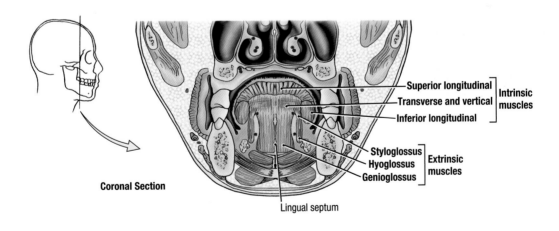

Coronal Section

Superior longitudinal

Transverse and vertical

Intrinsic muscles

Inferior longitudinal

Styloglossus

Hyoglossus

Genioglossus

Extrinsic muscles

Lingual septum

Intrinsic Muscles

Muscle	Origin	Insertion	Innervation	Main Action
Superior longitudinal	Submucous fibrous layer and lingual septum	Margins and mucous membrane of tongue	Hypoglossal nerve (CN XII)	Curls tip and sides of tongue superiorly and shortens tongue
Inferior longitudinal	Root of tongue and body of hyoid bone	Apex of tongue		Curls tip of tongue inferiorly and shortens tongue
Transverse	Lingual septum	Fibrous tissue at margins of tongue		Narrows and elongates the tongue[a]
Vertical	Superior surface of borders of tongue	Inferior surface of borders of tongue		Flattens and broadens the tongue[a]

[a]Acts simultaneously to protrude tongue.

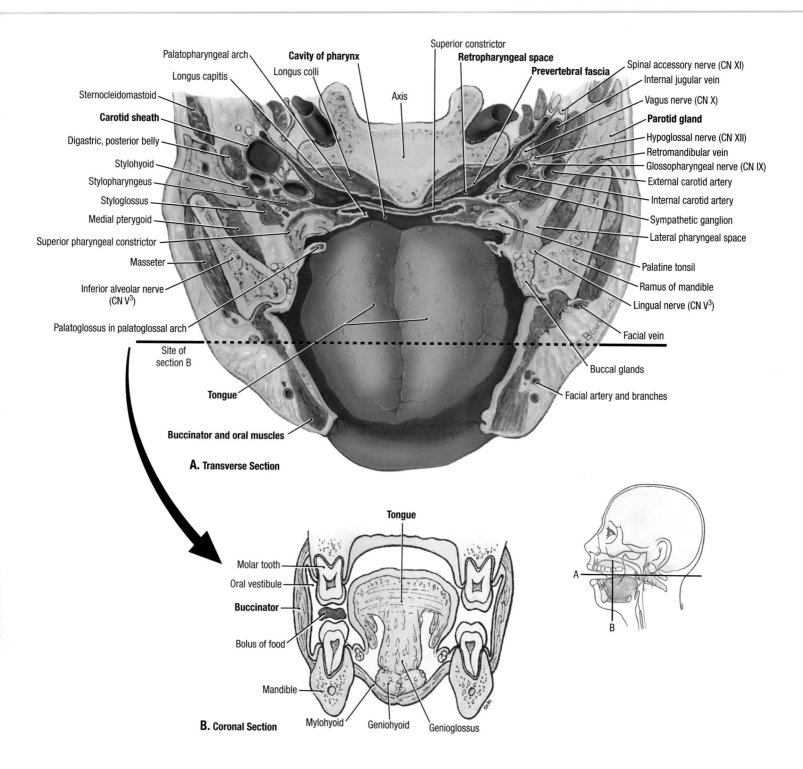

Palatopharyngeal arch
Longus capitis
Sternocleidomastoid
Carotid sheath
Digastric, posterior belly
Stylohyoid
Stylopharyngeus
Styloglossus
Medial pterygoid
Superior pharyngeal constrictor
Masseter
Inferior alveolar nerve (CN V³)
Palatoglossus in palatoglossal arch

Cavity of pharynx
Longus colli
Axis
Superior constrictor
Retropharyngeal space
Prevertebral fascia

Spinal accessory nerve (CN XI)
Internal jugular vein
Vagus nerve (CN X)
Parotid gland
Hypoglossal nerve (CN XII)
Retromandibular vein
Glossopharyngeal nerve (CN IX)
External carotid artery
Internal carotid artery
Sympathetic ganglion
Lateral pharyngeal space
Palatine tonsil
Ramus of mandible
Lingual nerve (CN V³)
Facial vein
Buccal glands
Facial artery and branches

Site of section B
Tongue
Buccinator and oral muscles

A. Transverse Section

Tongue
Molar tooth
Oral vestibule
Buccinator
Bolus of food
Mandible
Mylohyoid   Geniohyoid   Genioglossus

B. Coronal Section

A   B

7.48   Sections through mouth

A. The viscerocranium has been sectioned at the C1 vertebral level, the plane of section passing through the oral fissure anteriorly. The retropharyngeal space (opened up in this specimen) allows the pharynx to contract and relax during swallowing; the retropharyngeal space is closed laterally at the carotid sheath and limited posteriorly by the prevertebral fascia. The beds of the parotid glands are also demonstrated. **B.** Schematic coronal section demonstrating how the tongue and buccinator (or, anteriorly, the orbicularis oris) work together to retain food between the teeth when chewing. The buccinator and superior part of the orbicularis oris are innervated by the buccal branch of the facial nerve (CN VII).

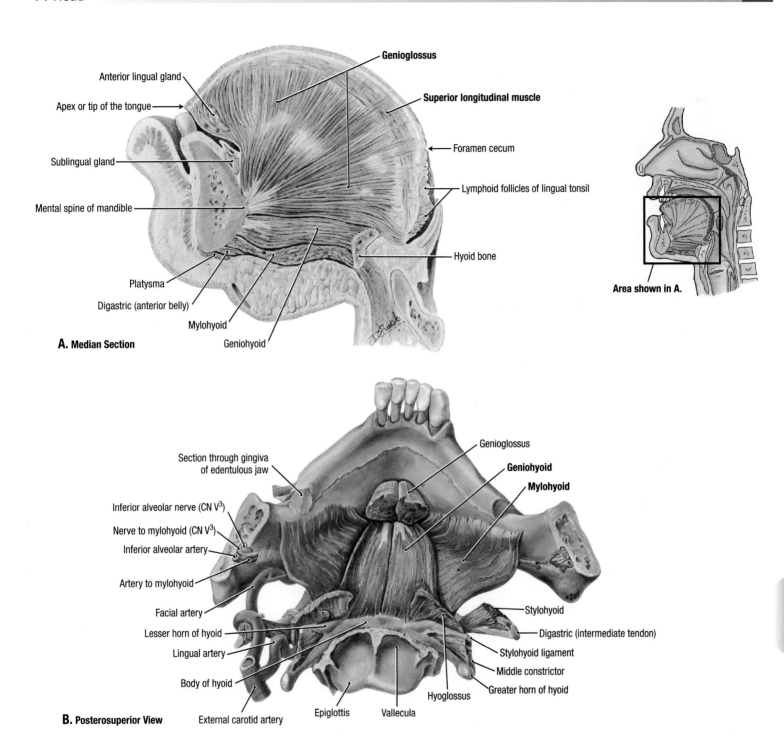

A. Median Section

- Anterior lingual gland
- Apex or tip of the tongue
- Sublingual gland
- Mental spine of mandible
- Platysma
- Digastric (anterior belly)
- Mylohyoid
- Geniohyoid
- **Genioglossus**
- **Superior longitudinal muscle**
- Foramen cecum
- Lymphoid follicles of lingual tonsil
- Hyoid bone

Area shown in A.

B. Posterosuperior View

- Section through gingiva of edentulous jaw
- Inferior alveolar nerve (CN V³)
- Nerve to mylohyoid (CN V³)
- Inferior alveolar artery
- Artery to mylohyoid
- Facial artery
- Lesser horn of hyoid
- Lingual artery
- Body of hyoid
- External carotid artery
- Epiglottis
- Vallecula
- Genioglossus
- **Geniohyoid**
- **Mylohyoid**
- Stylohyoid
- Digastric (intermediate tendon)
- Stylohyoid ligament
- Middle constrictor
- Greater horn of hyoid
- Hyoglossus

7.49   Tongue and floor of mouth

A. Median section though the tongue and lower jaw. The tongue is composed mainly of muscle; extrinsic muscles alter the position of the tongue, and intrinsic muscles alter its shape. The genioglossus is the extrinsic muscle apparent in this plane, and the superior longitudinal muscle is the intrinsic muscle. **B.** Muscles of the floor of the mouth viewed posterosuperiorly. The mylohyoid muscle extends between the two mylohyoid lines of the mandible. It has a thick, free posterior border and becomes thinner anteriorly.

When the genioglossus is paralyzed, the tongue mass has a tendency to shift posteriorly, obstructing the airway and presenting the risk of suffocation. Total relaxation of the genioglossus muscles occurs during general anesthesia; therefore, the tongue of an anesthetized patient must be prevented from relapsing by inserting an airway.

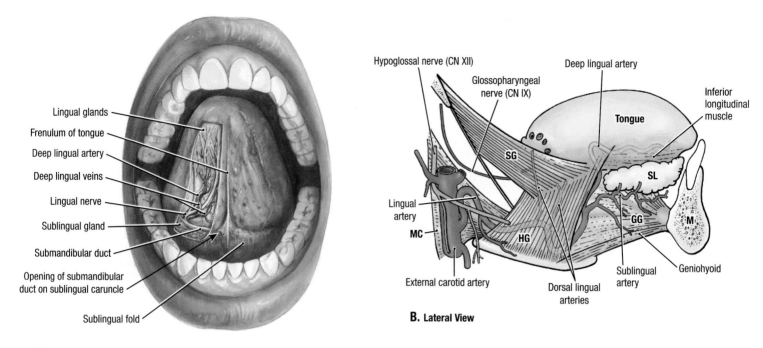

A. Anterior View

Lingual glands
Frenulum of tongue
Deep lingual artery
Deep lingual veins
Lingual nerve
Sublingual gland
Submandibular duct
Opening of submandibular duct on sublingual caruncle
Sublingual fold

B. Lateral View

Hypoglossal nerve (CN XII)
Glossopharyngeal nerve (CN IX)
Deep lingual artery
Inferior longitudinal muscle
Tongue
SG
SL
Lingual artery
MC
GG
M
HG
External carotid artery
Dorsal lingual arteries
Sublingual artery
Geniohyoid

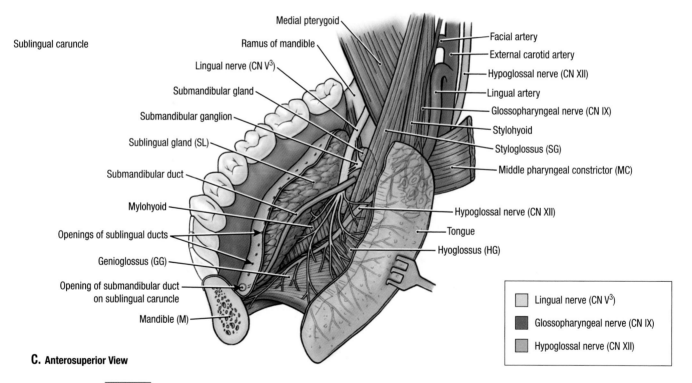

C. Anterosuperior View

Sublingual caruncle
Medial pterygoid
Ramus of mandible
Lingual nerve (CN V³)
Submandibular gland
Submandibular ganglion
Sublingual gland (SL)
Submandibular duct
Mylohyoid
Openings of sublingual ducts
Genioglossus (GG)
Opening of submandibular duct on sublingual caruncle
Mandible (M)

Facial artery
External carotid artery
Hypoglossal nerve (CN XII)
Lingual artery
Glossopharyngeal nerve (CN IX)
Stylohyoid
Styloglossus (SG)
Middle pharyngeal constrictor (MC)
Hypoglossal nerve (CN XII)
Tongue
Hyoglossus (HG)

Lingual nerve (CN V³)
Glossopharyngeal nerve (CN IX)
Hypoglossal nerve (CN XII)

7.50   Arteries and nerves of the tongue

A. Inferior surface of the tongue and floor of the mouth. The thin sublingual mucosa has been removed on the left side. **B.** Course and distribution of the lingual artery. **C.** Dissection of right side of floor of mouth. Letters in parentheses refer to **B**.

The parotid and submandibular salivary glands may be examined radiographically after the injection of a contrast medium into their ducts. This special type of radiograph (sialogram) demonstrates the salivary ducts and some secretory units. Because of the small size and number of sublingual ducts of the sublingual glands, one cannot usually inject contrast medium into them.

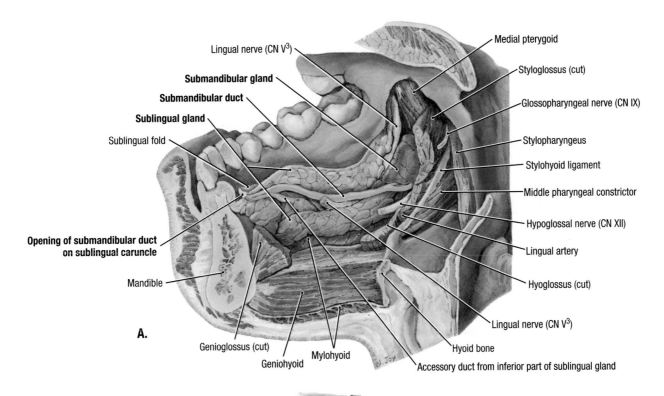

Lingual nerve (CN V³)

Submandibular gland

Submandibular duct

Sublingual gland

Sublingual fold

Opening of submandibular duct on sublingual caruncle

Mandible

Medial pterygoid

Styloglossus (cut)

Glossopharyngeal nerve (CN IX)

Stylopharyngeus

Stylohyoid ligament

Middle pharyngeal constrictor

Hypoglossal nerve (CN XII)

Lingual artery

Hyoglossus (cut)

Lingual nerve (CN V³)

Hyoid bone

Accessory duct from inferior part of sublingual gland

A.

Genioglossus (cut)

Geniohyoid   Mylohyoid

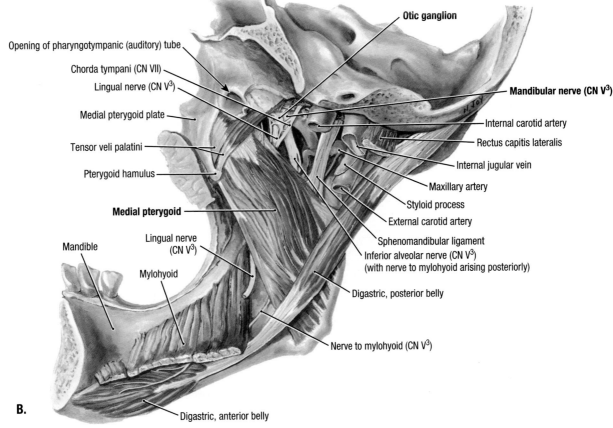

Opening of pharyngotympanic (auditory) tube

Chorda tympani (CN VII)

Lingual nerve (CN V³)

Medial pterygoid plate

Tensor veli palatini

Pterygoid hamulus

Medial pterygoid

Mandible

Lingual nerve (CN V³)

Mylohyoid

Otic ganglion

Mandibular nerve (CN V³)

Internal carotid artery

Rectus capitis lateralis

Internal jugular vein

Maxillary artery

Styloid process

External carotid artery

Sphenomandibular ligament

Inferior alveolar nerve (CN V³)
(with nerve to mylohyoid arising posteriorly)

Digastric, posterior belly

Nerve to mylohyoid (CN V³)

B.

Digastric, anterior belly

Medial Views

7.51   Muscles, glands, and vessels of floor of mouth and medial aspect of mandible

A. Sublingual and submandibular glands. The tongue has been excised. **B.** Structures related to the medial surface of the mandible. The otic ganglion lies medial to the mandibular nerve

(CN V³) and between the foramen ovale superiorly and the medial pterygoid muscle inferiorly.

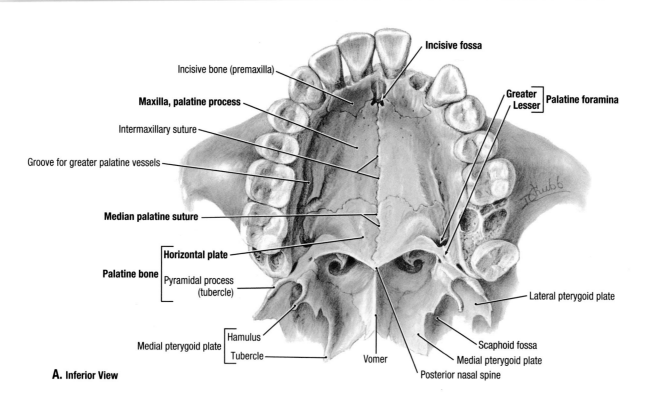

Incisive fossa

Incisive bone (premaxilla)

Maxilla, palatine process

Intermaxillary suture

Groove for greater palatine vessels

Greater
Lesser **Palatine foramina**

Median palatine suture

Palatine bone { **Horizontal plate**

Pyramidal process
(tubercle)

Lateral pterygoid plate

Medial pterygoid plate { Hamulus
                         Tubercle

Scaphoid fossa

Medial pterygoid plate

Vomer

Posterior nasal spine

A. Inferior View

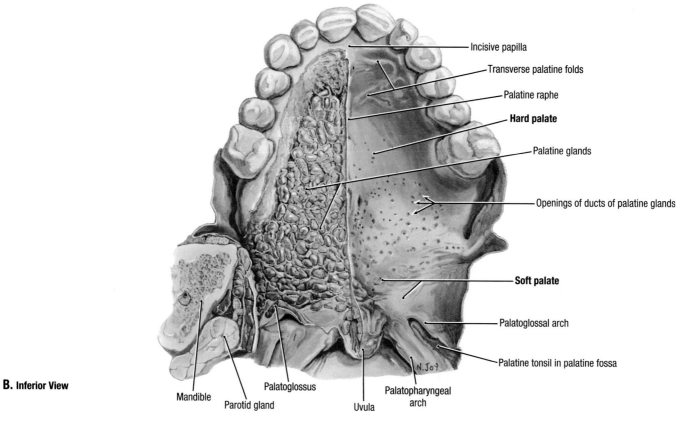

Incisive papilla

Transverse palatine folds

Palatine raphe

Hard palate

Palatine glands

Openings of ducts of palatine glands

Soft palate

Palatoglossal arch

Palatine tonsil in palatine fossa

Mandible

Parotid gland

Palatoglossus

Uvula

Palatopharyngeal
arch

B. Inferior View

7.52   **Palate**

A. Bones of the hard palate. The palatine aponeurosis, which forms the fibrous "skeleton" of the soft palate, stretches between the hamuli of the medial pterygoid plates. **B.** Mucous membrane and glands of palate.

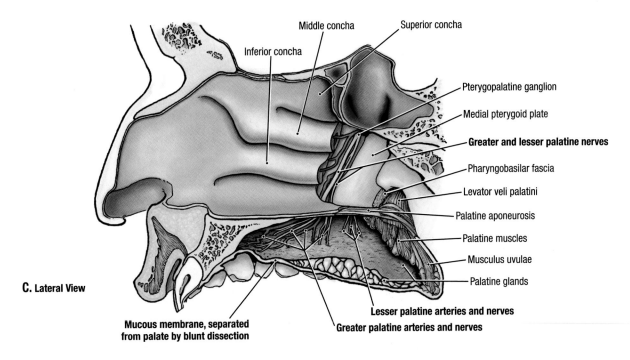

Middle concha
Superior concha
Inferior concha
Pterygopalatine ganglion
Medial pterygoid plate
Greater and lesser palatine nerves
Pharyngobasilar fascia
Levator veli palatini
Palatine aponeurosis
Palatine muscles
Musculus uvulae
Palatine glands

C. Lateral View

Mucous membrane, separated
from palate by blunt dissection

Lesser palatine arteries and nerves
Greater palatine arteries and nerves

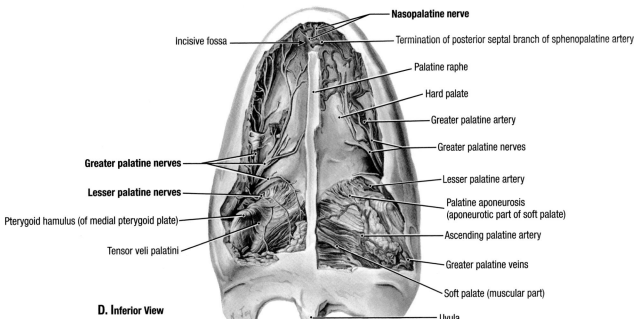

Incisive fossa
Nasopalatine nerve
Termination of posterior septal branch of sphenopalatine artery
Palatine raphe
Hard palate
Greater palatine artery
Greater palatine nerves
Greater palatine nerves
Lesser palatine artery
Lesser palatine nerves
Palatine aponeurosis
(aponeurotic part of soft palate)
Pterygoid hamulus (of medial pterygoid plate)
Ascending palatine artery
Tensor veli palatini
Greater palatine veins
Soft palate (muscular part)

D. Inferior View

Uvula

7.52 **Palate (continued)**

C. Nerves and vessels of palatine canal. The lateral wall of the nasal cavity is shown. The posterior ends of the middle and inferior conchae are excised along with the mucoperiosteum; the thin, perpendicular plate of the palatine bone is removed to expose the palatine nerves and arteries. **D.** Dissection of an edentulous palate. The greater palatine nerve supplies the gingivae and hard palate, the nasopalatine nerve the incisive region, and the lesser palatine nerves the soft palate. The nasopalatine nerves can be anesthetized by injecting anesthetic into the mouth of the incisive fossa in the hard palate. The anesthetized tissues are the palatal mucosa, the lingual gingivae, the six anterior maxillary teeth, and associated alveolar bone. The greater palatine nerve can be anesthetized by injecting anesthetic into the greater palatine foramen. The nerve emerges between the second and third maxillary molar teeth. This nerve block anesthetizes the palatal mucosa and lingual gingivae posterior to the maxillary canine teeth, and the underlying bone of the palate.

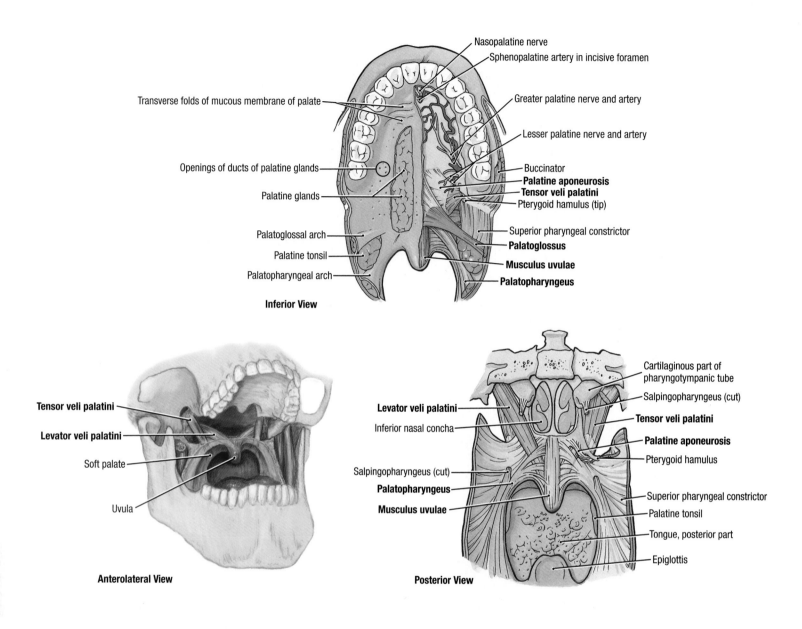

Inferior View

Anterolateral View

Posterior View

TABLE 7.12 MUSCLES OF SOFT PALATE

Muscle	Superior Attachment	Inferior Attachment	Innervation	Main Action(s)
Levator veli palatini	Cartilage of pharyngotympanic tube and petrous part of temporal bone		Pharyngeal branch of vagus nerve through pharyngeal plexus	Elevates soft palate during swallowing and yawning
Tensor veli palatini	Scaphoid fossa of medial pterygoid plate, spine of sphenoid bone, and cartilage of pharyngotympanic tube	Palatine aponeurosis	Medial pterygoid nerve (CN V³) through otic ganglion	Tenses soft palate and opens mouth of pharyngotympanic tube during swallowing and yawning
Palatoglossus	Palatine aponeurosis	Side of tongue	Pharyngeal branch of vagus nerve (CN X) via pharyngeal plexus	Elevates posterior part of tongue and draws soft palate onto tongue
Palatopharyngeus	Hard palate and palatine aponeurosis	Lateral wall of pharynx		Tenses soft palate and pulls walls of pharynx superiorly, anteriorly, and medially during swallowing
Musculus uvulae	Posterior nasal spine and palatine aponeurosis	Mucosa of uvula		Shortens uvula and pulls it superiorly

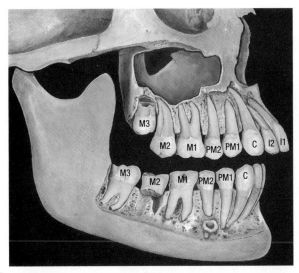

A. Lateral View

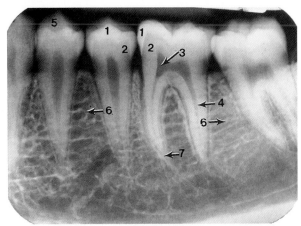

B. Lateral Radiograph

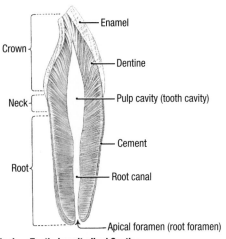

Incisor Tooth, Longitudinal Section

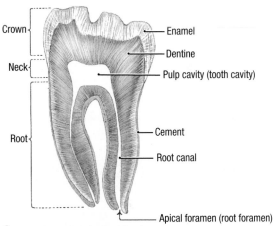

C. Molar Tooth, Longitudinal Section

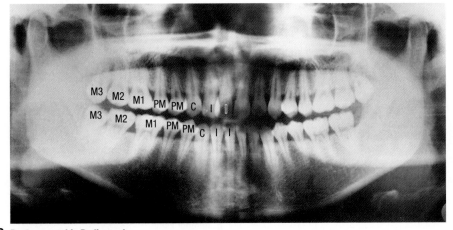

D. Pantomographic Radiograph

7.53   **Permanent teeth—I**

A. Teeth in situ with roots exposed. Incisors *(I1, I2)*, canine *(C1)*, premolars *(PM1, PM2)*, and molars *(M1, M2, M3)*. The roots of the 2nd lower molar have been removed. **B.** Lateral radiograph. *(1)* enamel, *(2)* dentin, *(3)* pulp chamber, *(4)* pulp canal, *(5)* buccal cusp, *(6)* alveolar bone, and *(7)* root apex. **C.** Longitudinal sections of an incisor and a molar tooth. **D.** Pantomographic radiograph of mandible and maxilla. The left lower third molar is not present.

Decay of the hard tissues of a tooth results in the formation of dental caries (cavities). Invasion of the pulp of the tooth by a carious lesion (cavity) results in infection and irritation of the tissues in the pulp cavity. This condition causes an inflammatory process (pulpitis). Because the pulp cavity is a rigid space, the swollen pulpal tissues cause pain (toothache).

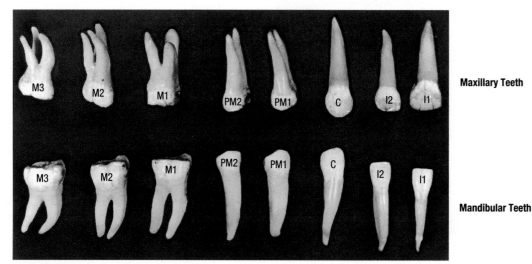

A. Vestibular View

Maxillary Teeth

Mandibular Teeth

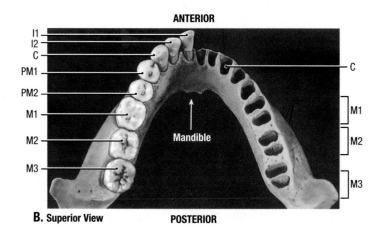

B. Superior View

C. Superior View

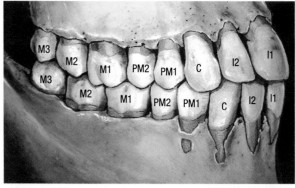

D. Anterolateral View

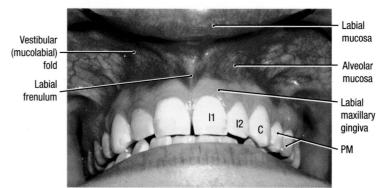

E. Anterior View

7.54 **Permanent teeth—II**

A. Removed teeth, displaying roots. There are 32 permanent teeth; 8 are on each side of each dental arch on the top (maxillary teeth) and bottom (mandibular teeth): 2 incisors *(I1–2)*, 1 canine *(C)*, 2 premolars *(PM1–2)*, and 3 molars *(M1–3)*. **B.** Permanent mandibular teeth and their sockets. **C.** Permanent maxillary teeth and their sockets. **D.** Teeth in occlusion. **E.** Vestibule and gingivae of the maxilla

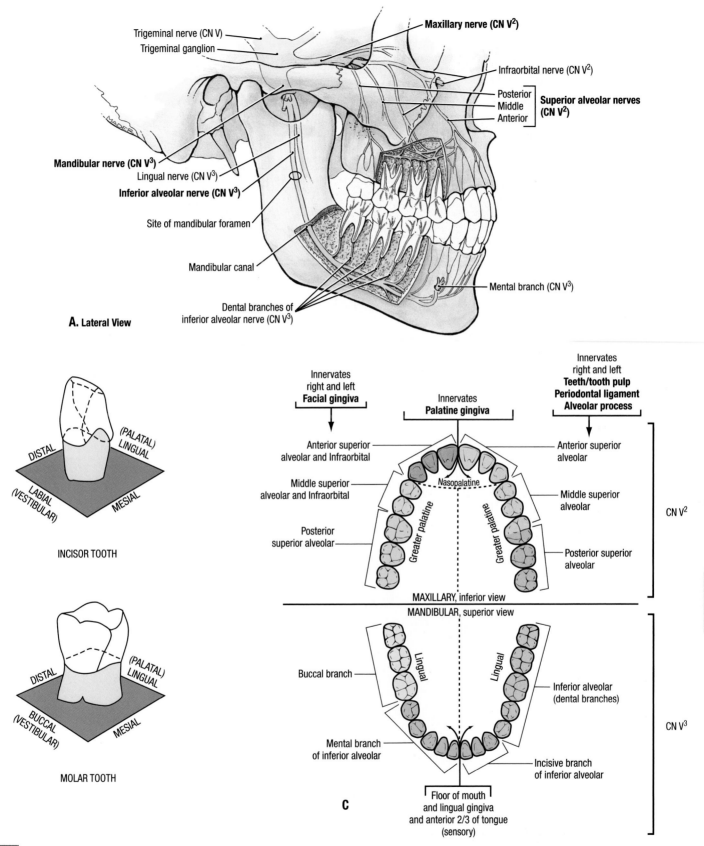

7.55   **Innervation of teeth**

A. Superior and inferior alveolar nerves. **B.** Surfaces of an incisor and molar tooth. **C.** Innervation of the mouth and teeth.

Improper oral hygiene results in food deposits in tooth and gingival crevices, which may cause inflammation of the gingivae (gingivitis). If untreated, the disease spreads to other supporting structures (including the alveolar bone), producing periodontitis. Periodontitis results in inflammation of the gingivae and may result in absorption of alveolar bone and gingival recession. Gingival recession exposes the sensitive cement of the teeth.

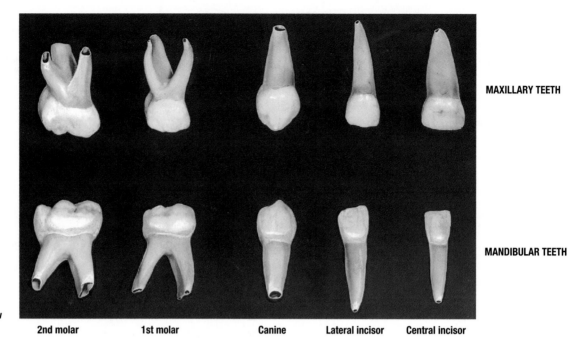

A. Vestibular View

| 2nd molar | 1st molar | Canine | Lateral incisor | Central incisor |

MAXILLARY TEETH

MANDIBULAR TEETH

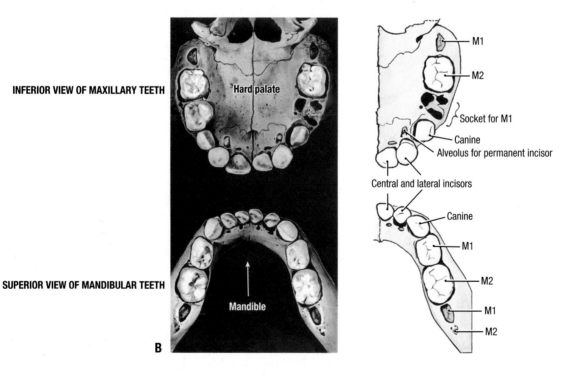

INFERIOR VIEW OF MAXILLARY TEETH

Hard palate

M1

M2

Socket for M1

Canine

Alveolus for permanent incisor

Central and lateral incisors

Canine

M1

M2

M1

M2

SUPERIOR VIEW OF MANDIBULAR TEETH

Mandible

B

7.56 Primary teeth

A. Removed teeth. There are 20 primary (deciduous) teeth, 5 in each half of the mandible and 5 in each maxilla. They are named central incisor, lateral incisor, canine, 1st molar *(M1)*, and 2nd molar *(M2)*. Primary teeth differ from permanent teeth in that the primary teeth are smaller and whiter; the molars also have more bulbous crowns and more divergent roots. **B.** Teeth in situ, younger than 2 years of age. Permanent teeth are colored orange; the crowns of the unerupted 1st and 2nd permanent molars are partly visible.

TABLE 7.13 PRIMARY AND SECONDARY DENTITION

Deciduous Teeth	Medial Incisor	Lateral Incisor	Canine	First Molar	Second Molar
Eruption (months)[a]	6–8	8–10	16–20	12–16	20–24
Shedding (years)	6–7	7–8	10–12	9–11	10–12

[a]In some normal infants, the first teeth (medial incisors) may not erupt until 12 to 13 months of age

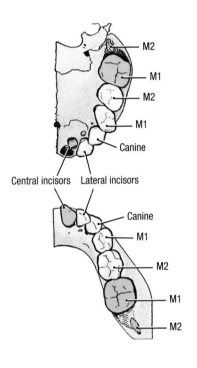

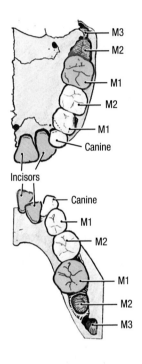

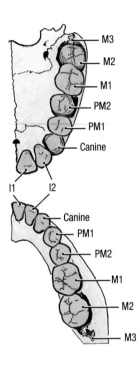

Age: 6–7 years

The 1st molars (6-year molars) have fully erupted, the primary central incisor has been shed, the lower central incisor is almost fully erupted, and the upper central incisor is descending into the vacated socket.

Age: 8 years

All of the permanent incisors have erupted; however, the lower lateral incisor is only partially erupted.

Age: 12 years

The primary teeth have been replaced by 20 permanent teeth, and the 1st and 2nd molars (12-year molars) have erupted; the canines, 2nd premolars, and 2nd molars (especially those in the upper jaw) have not erupted fully, nor have their bony sockets closed around them. By age 12, 28 permanent teeth are in evidence; the last 4 teeth, the 3rd molars, may erupt any time after this, or never.

Permanent Teeth	Medial Incisor	Lateral Incisor	Canine	First Premolar	Second Premolar	First Molar	Second Molar	Third Molar
Eruption (years)	7–8	8–9	10–12	10–11	11–12	6–7	12	13–25

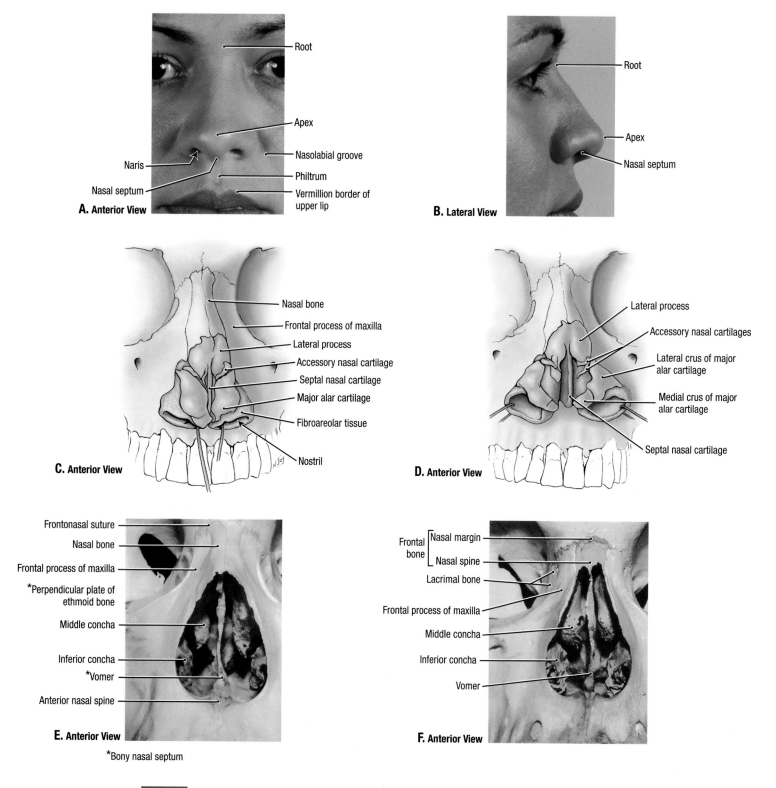

A. Anterior View
- Root
- Apex
- Nasolabial groove
- Naris
- Philtrum
- Nasal septum
- Vermillion border of upper lip

B. Lateral View
- Root
- Apex
- Nasal septum

C. Anterior View
- Nasal bone
- Frontal process of maxilla
- Lateral process
- Accessory nasal cartilage
- Septal nasal cartilage
- Major alar cartilage
- Fibroareolar tissue
- Nostril

D. Anterior View
- Lateral process
- Accessory nasal cartilages
- Lateral crus of major alar cartilage
- Medial crus of major alar cartilage
- Septal nasal cartilage

E. Anterior View
- Frontonasal suture
- Nasal bone
- Frontal process of maxilla
- *Perpendicular plate of ethmoid bone
- Middle concha
- Inferior concha
- *Vomer
- Anterior nasal spine

*Bony nasal septum

F. Anterior View
- Frontal bone { Nasal margin, Nasal spine }
- Lacrimal bone
- Frontal process of maxilla
- Middle concha
- Inferior concha
- Vomer

7.57   Surface anatomy, cartilages, and bones of nose

A. Surface features of anterior aspect of nose. **B.** Surface features of lateral aspect of nose. **C.** Nasal cartilages, with the septum pulled inferiorly. **D.** Nasal cartilages, separated and retracted laterally. **E.** Lower conchae and bony septum seen through the piriform aperture. The margin of the piriform aperture is sharp and formed by the maxillae and nasal bones. **F.** Nasal bones removed. The areas of the frontal processes of the maxillae *(yellow)* and of the frontal bone *(blue)* that articulate with the nasal bones can be seen.

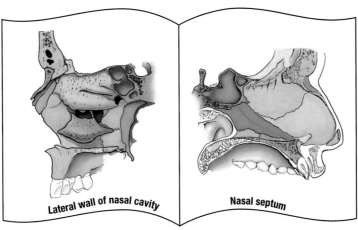

Lateral wall of nasal cavity   Nasal septum

Right Nasal Cavity

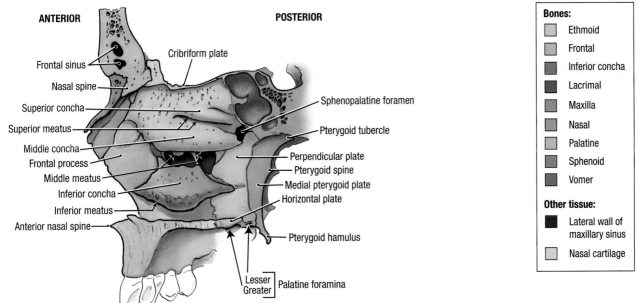

ANTERIOR   POSTERIOR

Frontal sinus
Nasal spine
Superior concha
Superior meatus
Middle concha
Frontal process
Middle meatus
Inferior concha
Inferior meatus
Anterior nasal spine

Cribriform plate

Sphenopalatine foramen
Pterygoid tubercle
Perpendicular plate
Pterygoid spine
Medial pterygoid plate
Horizontal plate

Pterygoid hamulus

Lesser Greater Palatine foramina

A. Medial View of Lateral Wall

Bones:
- Ethmoid
- Frontal
- Inferior concha
- Lacrimal
- Maxilla
- Nasal
- Palatine
- Sphenoid
- Vomer

Other tissue:
- Lateral wall of maxillary sinus
- Nasal cartilage

7.58   **Bones of the lateral wall and septum of the nose**

A. Lateral wall of nose. The superior and middle conchae are parts of the ethmoid bone, whereas the inferior concha is itself a bone. **B.** Nasal septum.

Deformity of the external nose usually is present with a fracture, particularly when a lateral force is applied by someone's elbow, for example. When the injury results from a direct blow (e.g., from a hockey stick), the cribriform plate of the ethmoid bone may fracture, resulting in CSF rhinorrhea.

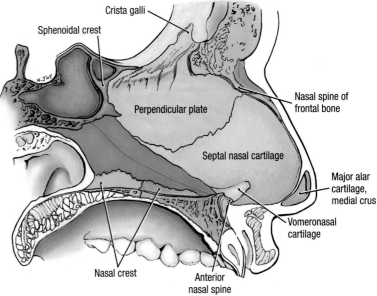

Crista galli
Sphenoidal crest

Nasal spine of frontal bone

Perpendicular plate

Septal nasal cartilage

Major alar cartilage, medial crus

Vomeronasal cartilage

Nasal crest   Anterior nasal spine

B. Lateral View of Nasal Septum

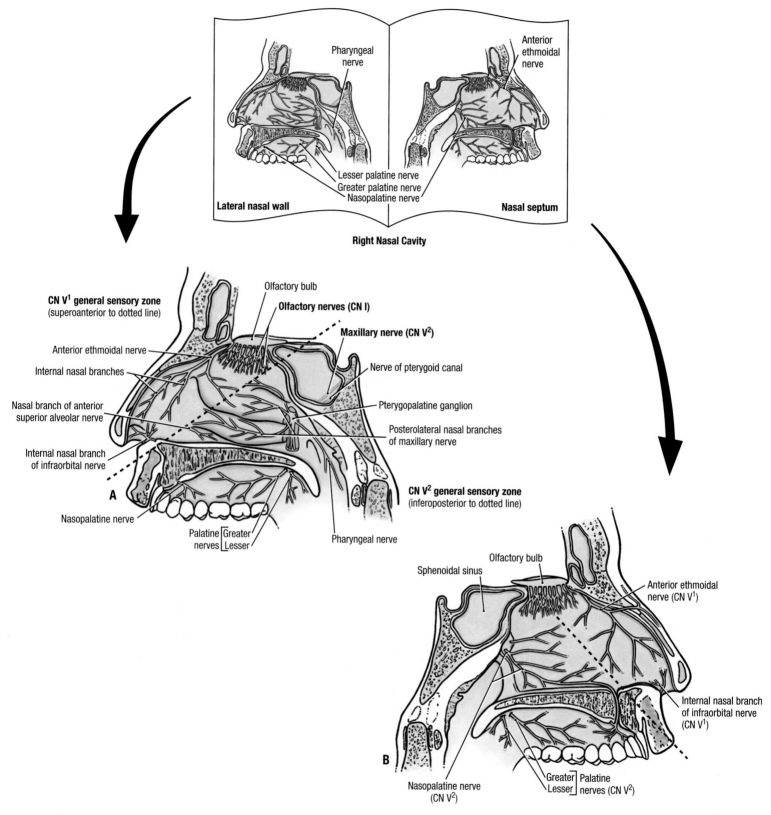

7.59   Innervation of lateral wall and septum of the nose

A. Lateral wall of nose. *Dotted diagonal lines* demarcate CN V¹ and CN V² general sensory zones. The olfactory neuroepithelium is in the superior part of the lateral and septal walls of the nasal cavity. The central processes of the olfactory neurosensory cells of each side form approximately 20 bundles that together form an olfactory nerve (CN I). **B.** Nasal septum. The nasopalatine nerve from the pterygopalatine ganglion supplies the posteroinferior septum, and the anterior ethmoidal nerve (branch of V¹) supplies the anterosuperior septum.

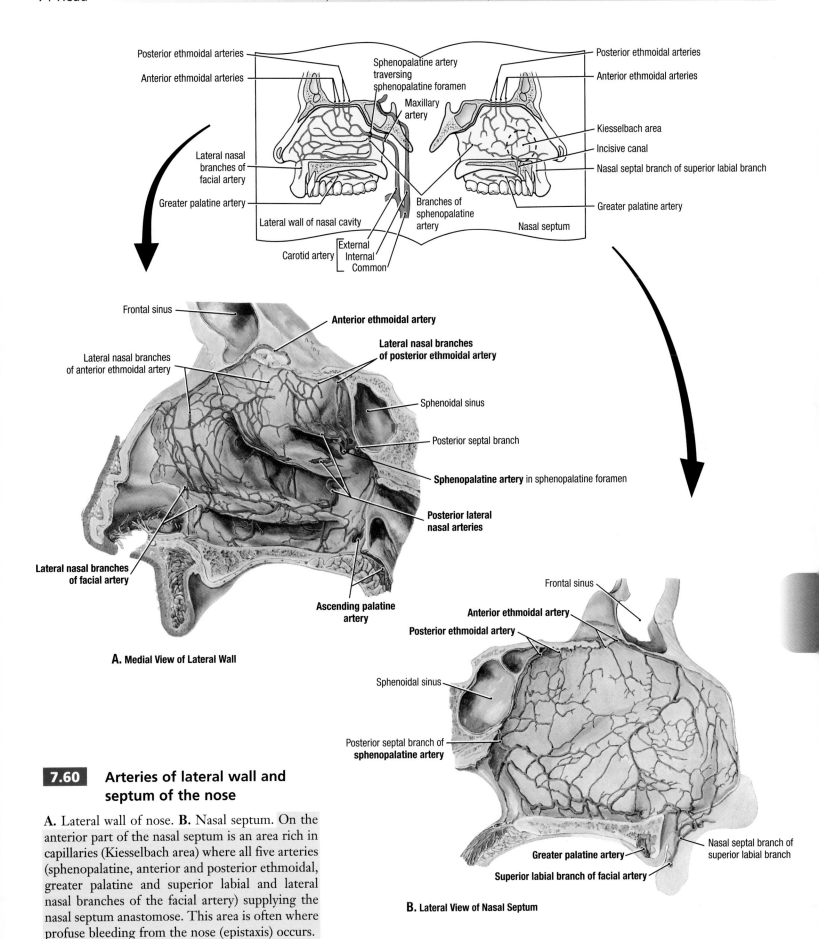

Posterior ethmoidal arteries

Anterior ethmoidal arteries

Sphenopalatine artery traversing sphenopalatine foramen

Maxillary artery

Posterior ethmoidal arteries

Anterior ethmoidal arteries

Kiesselbach area

Incisive canal

Nasal septal branch of superior labial branch

Lateral nasal branches of facial artery

Greater palatine artery

Lateral wall of nasal cavity

Branches of sphenopalatine artery

Greater palatine artery

Nasal septum

Carotid artery

External
Internal
Common

A. Medial View of Lateral Wall

Frontal sinus

Lateral nasal branches of anterior ethmoidal artery

Lateral nasal branches of facial artery

Anterior ethmoidal artery

Lateral nasal branches of posterior ethmoidal artery

Sphenoidal sinus

Posterior septal branch

Sphenopalatine artery in sphenopalatine foramen

Posterior lateral nasal arteries

Ascending palatine artery

B. Lateral View of Nasal Septum

Frontal sinus

Anterior ethmoidal artery

Posterior ethmoidal artery

Sphenoidal sinus

Posterior septal branch of **sphenopalatine artery**

Greater palatine artery

Superior labial branch of facial artery

Nasal septal branch of superior labial branch

7.60 Arteries of lateral wall and septum of the nose

A. Lateral wall of nose. **B.** Nasal septum. On the anterior part of the nasal septum is an area rich in capillaries (Kiesselbach area) where all five arteries (sphenopalatine, anterior and posterior ethmoidal, greater palatine and superior labial and lateral nasal branches of the facial artery) supplying the nasal septum anastomose. This area is often where profuse bleeding from the nose (epistaxis) occurs.

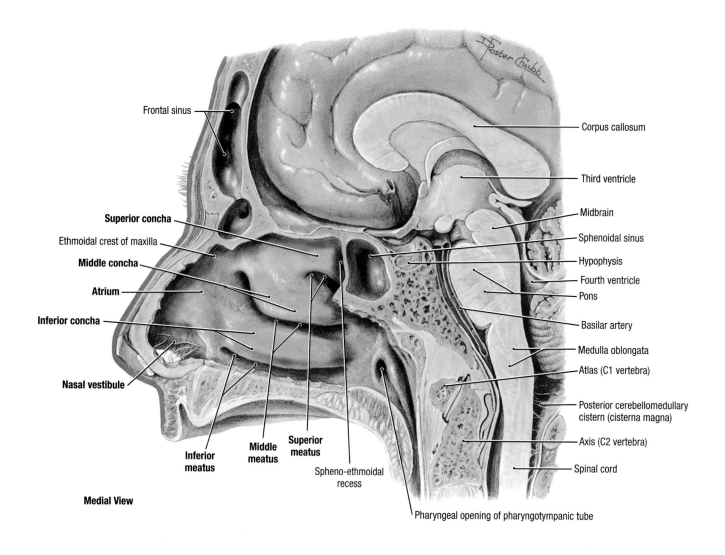

Frontal sinus

Corpus callosum

Third ventricle

Midbrain

Superior concha

Ethmoidal crest of maxilla

Sphenoidal sinus

Middle concha

Hypophysis

Fourth ventricle

Atrium

Pons

Inferior concha

Basilar artery

Medulla oblongata

Atlas (C1 vertebra)

Nasal vestibule

Posterior cerebellomedullary cistern (cisterna magna)

Axis (C2 vertebra)

Spinal cord

Superior meatus

Middle meatus

Inferior meatus

Spheno-ethmoidal recess

Medial View

Pharyngeal opening of pharyngotympanic tube

7.61 **Right half of hemisected head demonstrating upper respiratory tract**

- The vestibule is superior to the nostril and anterior to the inferior meatus; hairs grow from its skin-lined surface. The atrium is superior to the vestibule and anterior to the middle meatus.
- The inferior and middle conchae curve inferiorly and medially from the lateral wall, dividing it into three nearly equal parts and covering the inferior and middle meatuses, respectively. The middle concha ends inferior to the sphenoidal sinus, and the inferior concha ends inferior to the middle concha, just anterior to the orifice of the auditory tube. The superior concha is small and anterior to the sphenoidal sinus.
- The roof comprises an anterior sloping part corresponding to the bridge of the nose; an intermediate horizontal part; a perpendicular part anterior to the sphenoidal sinus; and a curved part, inferior to the sinus, that is continuous with the roof of the nasopharynx.

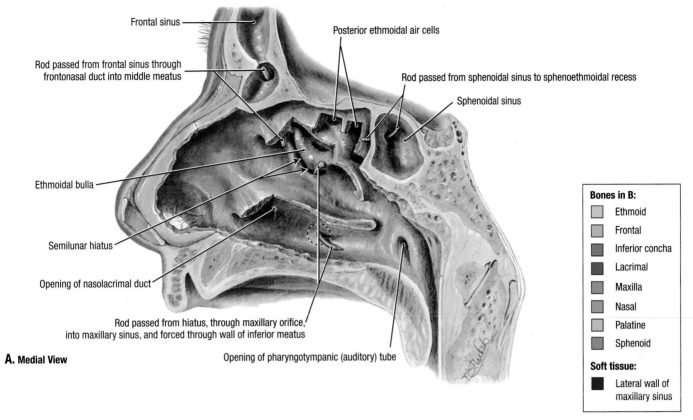

Frontal sinus

Rod passed from frontal sinus through
frontonasal duct into middle meatus

Posterior ethmoidal air cells

Rod passed from sphenoidal sinus to sphenoethmoidal recess

Sphenoidal sinus

Ethmoidal bulla

Semilunar hiatus

Opening of nasolacrimal duct

Rod passed from hiatus, through maxillary orifice,
into maxillary sinus, and forced through wall of inferior meatus

Opening of pharyngotympanic (auditory) tube

A. Medial View

Bones in B:
- Ethmoid
- Frontal
- Inferior concha
- Lacrimal
- Maxilla
- Nasal
- Palatine
- Sphenoid

Soft tissue:
- Lateral wall of maxillary sinus

7.62

Communications through the lateral wall of the nasal cavity

A. Dissection. Parts of the superior, middle, and inferior conchae are cut away to reveal the openings of the air sinuses. **B.** Diagrams of the bones and openings of the lateral wall of nasal cavity following dissection. Note one *arrow* passing from the frontal sinus through the frontonasal duct into the middle meatus and another *arrow* coming from the anteromedial orbit via the nasolacrimal canal.

The nasal mucosa becomes swollen and inflamed (rhinitis) during upper respiratory infections and allergic reactions (e.g., hay fever). Swelling of this mucous membrane occurs readily because of its vascularity and abundant mucosal glands. Infections of the nasal cavities may spread to the anterior cranial fossa through the cribriform plate, nasopharynx and retropharyngeal soft tissues, middle ear through the pharyngotympanic (auditory) tube, paranasal sinuses, lacrimal apparatus, and conjunctiva.

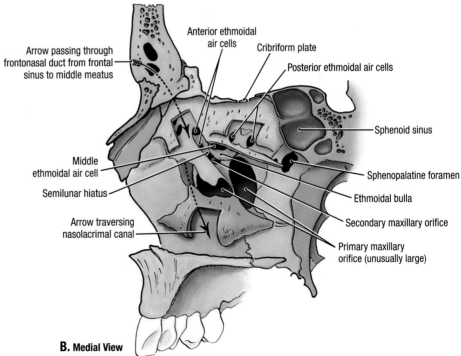

Arrow passing through
frontonasal duct from frontal
sinus to middle meatus

Anterior ethmoidal
air cells

Cribriform plate

Posterior ethmoidal air cells

Sphenoid sinus

Middle
ethmoidal air cell

Semilunar hiatus

Arrow traversing
nasolacrimal canal

Sphenopalatine foramen

Ethmoidal bulla

Secondary maxillary orifice

Primary maxillary
orifice (unusually large)

B. Medial View

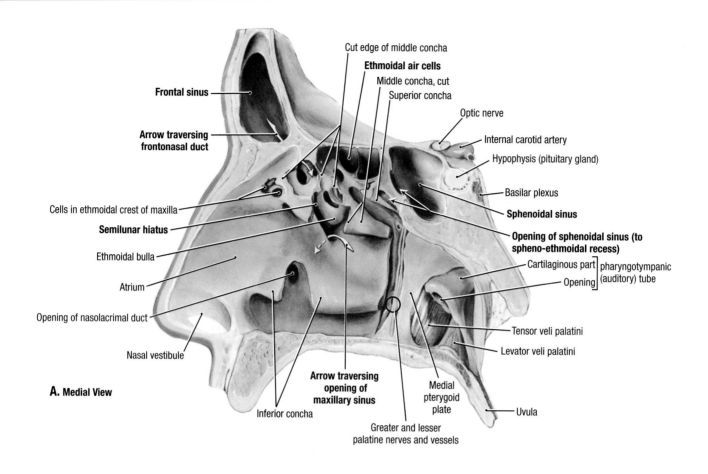

A. Medial View

Cut edge of middle concha
Ethmoidal air cells
Middle concha, cut
Superior concha
Optic nerve
Internal carotid artery
Hypophysis (pituitary gland)
Basilar plexus
Sphenoidal sinus
Opening of sphenoidal sinus (to spheno-ethmoidal recess)
Cartilaginous part ⎤ pharyngotympanic
Opening ⎦ (auditory) tube
Tensor veli palatini
Levator veli palatini
Uvula

Frontal sinus
Arrow traversing frontonasal duct
Cells in ethmoidal crest of maxilla
Semilunar hiatus
Ethmoidal bulla
Atrium
Opening of nasolacrimal duct
Nasal vestibule
Arrow traversing opening of maxillary sinus
Inferior concha
Greater and lesser palatine nerves and vessels
Medial pterygoid plate

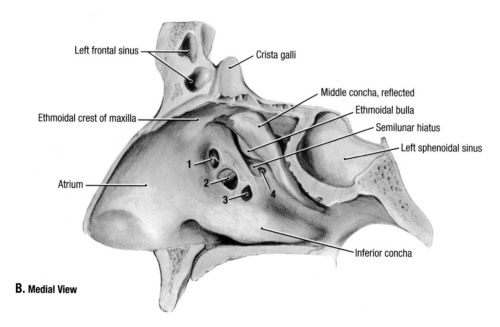

B. Medial View

Left frontal sinus
Crista galli
Middle concha, reflected
Ethmoidal bulla
Semilunar hiatus
Left sphenoidal sinus
Ethmoidal crest of maxilla
Atrium
1
2
3
4
Inferior concha

7.63   Paranasal sinuses, openings, and palatine muscles in the lateral wall of the nasal cavity

A. Dissection. Parts of the middle and inferior conchae and lateral wall of the nasal cavity are cut away to expose the nerves and vessels in the palatine canal and the extrinsic palatine muscles. **B.** Accessory maxillary orifices. In addition to the primary, or normal, ostium (not shown), there are four secondary, or acquired, ostia (numbered 1–4).

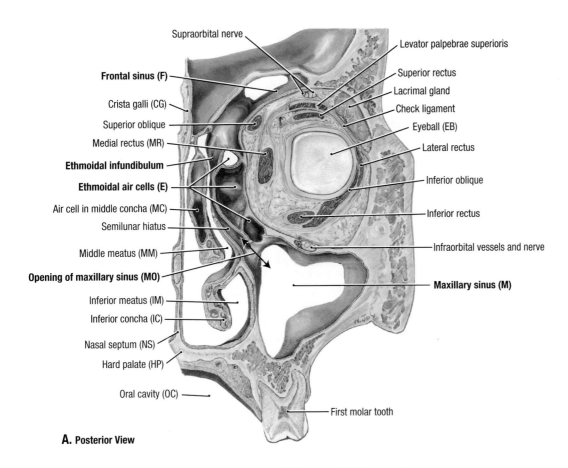

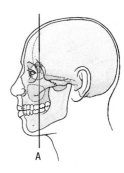

Supraorbital nerve

Levator palpebrae superioris

Frontal sinus (F)

Superior rectus

Crista galli (CG)

Lacrimal gland

Superior oblique

Check ligament

Medial rectus (MR)

Eyeball (EB)

Ethmoidal infundibulum

Lateral rectus

Ethmoidal air cells (E)

Inferior oblique

Air cell in middle concha (MC)

Semilunar hiatus

Inferior rectus

Middle meatus (MM)

Opening of maxillary sinus (MO)

Infraorbital vessels and nerve

Inferior meatus (IM)

Maxillary sinus (M)

Inferior concha (IC)

Nasal septum (NS)

Hard palate (HP)

Oral cavity (OC)

First molar tooth

A. Posterior View

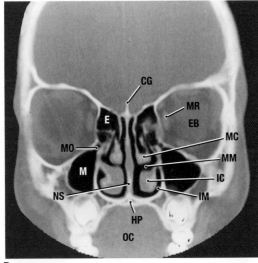

B. Posterior View

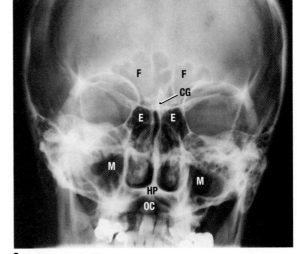

C. Anteroposterior View

7.64   **Paranasal sinuses and nasal cavity**

A. Coronal section of right side of the head. **B.** CT scan. **C.** Radiograph of cranium. Letters in **B** and **C** refer to structures labeled in **A**.

If nasal drainage is blocked, infections of the ethmoidal cells of the ethmoidal sinuses may break through the fragile medial wall of the orbit. Severe infections from this source may cause blindness but could also affect the dural sheath of the optic nerve, causing optic neuritis.

During removal of a maxillary molar tooth, a fracture of a root may occur. If proper retrieval methods are not used, a piece of the root may be driven superiorly into the maxillary sinus.

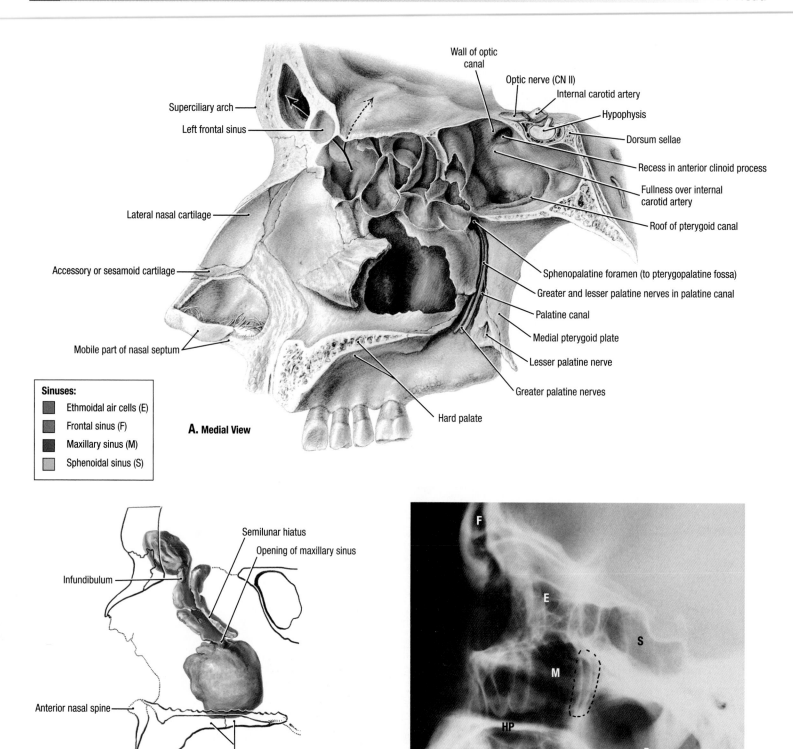

Superciliary arch

Left frontal sinus

Lateral nasal cartilage

Accessory or sesamoid cartilage

Mobile part of nasal septum

Wall of optic canal

Optic nerve (CN II)

Internal carotid artery

Hypophysis

Dorsum sellae

Recess in anterior clinoid process

Fullness over internal carotid artery

Roof of pterygoid canal

Sphenopalatine foramen (to pterygopalatine fossa)

Greater and lesser palatine nerves in palatine canal

Palatine canal

Medial pterygoid plate

Lesser palatine nerve

Greater palatine nerves

Hard palate

Sinuses:
- Ethmoidal air cells (E)
- Frontal sinus (F)
- Maxillary sinus (M)
- Sphenoidal sinus (S)

A. Medial View

Semilunar hiatus

Opening of maxillary sinus

Infundibulum

Anterior nasal spine

Hard palate (HP)

B. Medial View

C. Lateral View

7.65 Paranasal sinuses

A. Opened sinuses, color coded. **B.** Cast of frontal and maxillary sinuses. **C.** Radiograph of cranium. *P*, pharynx; *dotted lines*, pterygopalatine fossa. Letters refer to structures labeled in **B.** The maxillary sinuses are the most commonly infected, probably because their ostia are small and located high on their superomedial walls, a poor location for natural drainage of the sinus. When the mucous membrane of the sinus is congested, the maxillary ostia often are obstructed. The maxillary sinus can be cannulated and drained by passing a canula from the nares through the maxillary ostium into the sinus.

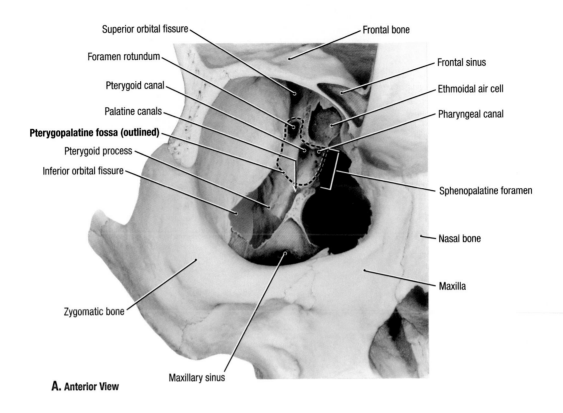

Superior orbital fissure

Foramen rotundum

Pterygoid canal

Palatine canals

Pterygopalatine fossa (outlined)

Pterygoid process

Inferior orbital fissure

Zygomatic bone

Maxillary sinus

Frontal bone

Frontal sinus

Ethmoidal air cell

Pharyngeal canal

Sphenopalatine foramen

Nasal bone

Maxilla

A. Anterior View

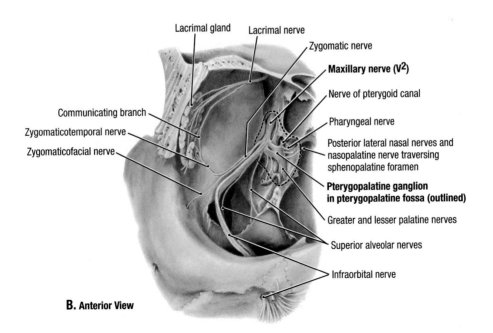

Lacrimal gland   Lacrimal nerve

Zygomatic nerve

Maxillary nerve (V²)

Nerve of pterygoid canal

Communicating branch

Zygomaticotemporal nerve

Zygomaticofacial nerve

Pharyngeal nerve

Posterior lateral nasal nerves and
nasopalatine nerve traversing
sphenopalatine foramen

**Pterygopalatine ganglion
in pterygopalatine fossa (outlined)**

Greater and lesser palatine nerves

Superior alveolar nerves

Infraorbital nerve

B. Anterior View

7.66   **Pterygopalatine fossa, orbital approach**

A. Bones and foramina. **B.** Maxillary nerve. In **A** and **B**, the pterygopalatine fossa has been
exposed through the floor of the orbit and maxillary sinus.

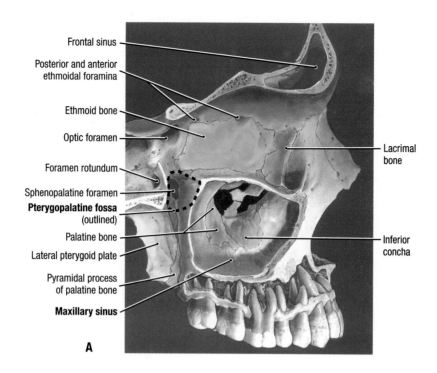

Frontal sinus

Posterior and anterior
ethmoidal foramina

Ethmoid bone

Optic foramen

Foramen rotundum

Sphenopalatine foramen

Pterygopalatine fossa
(outlined)

Palatine bone

Lateral pterygoid plate

Pyramidal process
of palatine bone

Maxillary sinus

Lacrimal
bone

Inferior
concha

A

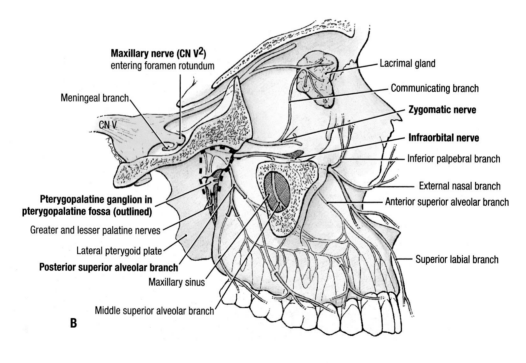

Maxillary nerve (CN V²)
entering foramen rotundum

Meningeal branch

CN V

**Pterygopalatine ganglion in
pterygopalatine fossa (outlined)**

Greater and lesser palatine nerves

Lateral pterygoid plate

Posterior superior alveolar branch

Maxillary sinus

Middle superior alveolar branch

B

Lacrimal gland

Communicating branch

Zygomatic nerve

Infraorbital nerve

Inferior palpebral branch

External nasal branch

Anterior superior alveolar branch

Superior labial branch

Lateral Views

7.67   Nerves of the pterygopalatine fossa

A. Medial half of the right viscerocranium following sagittal sectioning through the maxillary sinus. The inferior concha *(orange)* and palatine bone *(pink)* form part of the medial wall of the maxillary sinus. Note the ethmoid *(yellow)* and lacrimal *(blue)* bones of the medial wall of the orbital cavity and the sphenopalatine foramen opening into the nasal cavity from the pterygopalatine fossa. **B.** Maxillary nerve (CN V²) and branches.

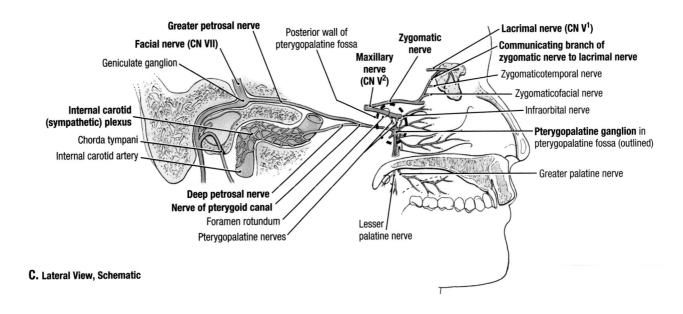

C. Lateral View, Schematic

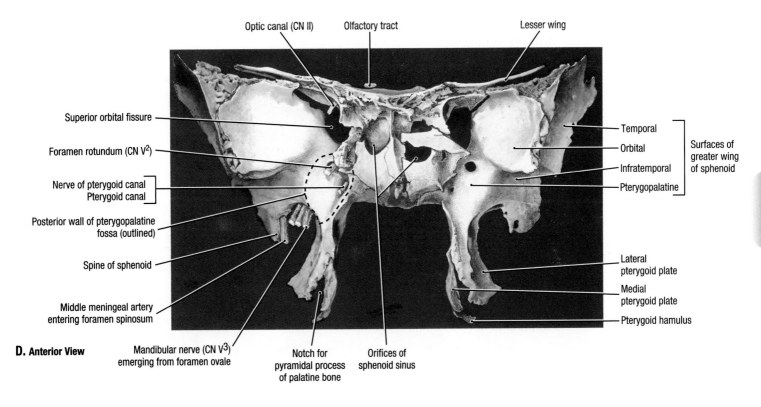

D. Anterior View

7.67   **Nerves of the pterygopalatine fossa** *(continued)*

C. Autonomic innervation of the lacrimal gland and glands of the palatine and nasal mucosa. **D.** Sphenoid bone, anterior surface of the body, pterygoid process, and central parts of the greater and lesser wings.

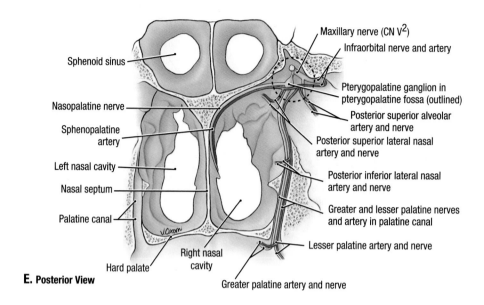

Sphenoid sinus

Nasopalatine nerve

Sphenopalatine artery

Left nasal cavity

Nasal septum

Palatine canal

Hard palate

Right nasal cavity

Maxillary nerve (CN V²)

Infraorbital nerve and artery

Pterygopalatine ganglion in pterygopalatine fossa (outlined)

Posterior superior alveolar artery and nerve

Posterior superior lateral nasal artery and nerve

Posterior inferior lateral nasal artery and nerve

Greater and lesser palatine nerves and artery in palatine canal

Lesser palatine artery and nerve

Greater palatine artery and nerve

E. Posterior View

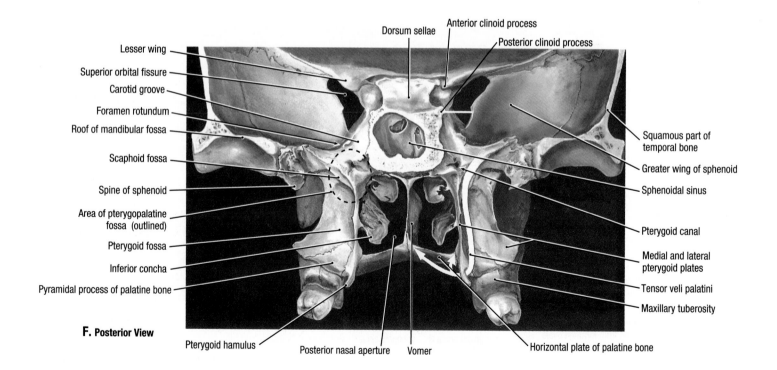

Lesser wing

Superior orbital fissure

Carotid groove

Foramen rotundum

Roof of mandibular fossa

Scaphoid fossa

Spine of sphenoid

Area of pterygopalatine fossa (outlined)

Pterygoid fossa

Inferior concha

Pyramidal process of palatine bone

Dorsum sellae

Anterior clinoid process

Posterior clinoid process

Squamous part of temporal bone

Greater wing of sphenoid

Sphenoidal sinus

Pterygoid canal

Medial and lateral pterygoid plates

Tensor veli palatini

Maxillary tuberosity

Pterygoid hamulus

Posterior nasal aperture

Vomer

Horizontal plate of palatine bone

F. Posterior View

7.67   Nerves of the pterygopalatine fossa (continued)

E. Coronal section through nasal cavities, sphenoidal sinuses, and right pterygopalatine fossa, in the plane of the palatine canal, demonstrating the course of the nasopalatine and greater and lesser palatine nerves. **F.** Anterior part of cranium following coronal sectioning in the plane of the foramen lacerum demonstrating the posterior wall of the pterygopalatine fossa.

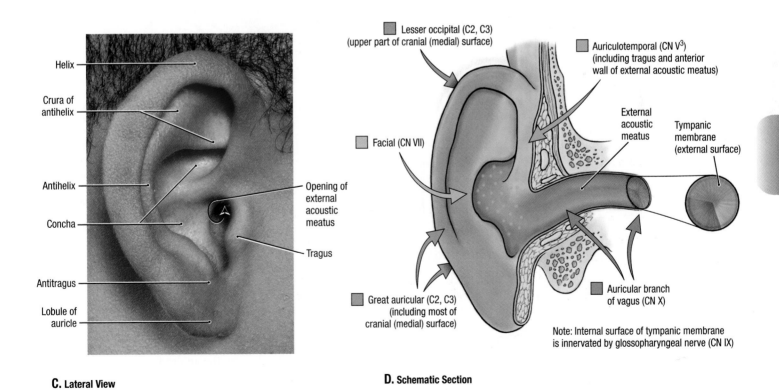

POSTERIOR   Helix   **ANTERIOR**

Scapha

Triangular fossa   Crura of antihelix

Auricular tubercle

Helix   Crus of helix

Antihelix

Concha

Tragus

Antitragus

Intertragic notch

Lobule of auricle
(lobe of ear)

A. Lateral View

Helix

Spine of helix

Crus of helix

Lamina of tragus

Tail of helix

Fissure of tragus

B. Lateral View

Helix

Crura of
antihelix

Antihelix

Opening of
external
acoustic
meatus

Concha

Tragus

Antitragus

Lobule of
auricle

C. Lateral View

☐ Lesser occipital (C2, C3)
(upper part of cranial (medial) surface)

☐ Auriculotemporal (CN V³)
(including tragus and anterior
wall of external acoustic meatus)

☐ Facial (CN VII)

External
acoustic
meatus

Tympanic
membrane
(external surface)

☐ Great auricular (C2, C3)
(including most of
cranial (medial) surface)

☐ Auricular branch
of vagus (CN X)

Note: Internal surface of tympanic membrane
is innervated by glossopharyngeal nerve (CN IX)

D. Schematic Section

7.68 **Auricle**

A. Features of auricle. **B.** Cartilage of auricle. **C.** Surface anatomy of auricle.

A. Superior View

POSTERIOR

LATERAL

Malleus
Incus } Ossicles
Stapes

Auricle

Semicircular canals

Tympanic cavity

Endolymphatic sac

Vestibular aqueduct

External acoustic meatus

Cochlear aqueduct

Lobule of auricle

Internal acoustic meatus

Tympanic membrane

Tensor tympani

Cochlea

Pharyngotympanic (auditory) tube

Bony part

Cartilaginous part

MEDIAL

Levator veli palatini

ANTERIOR

Semicircular duct and canal

Endolymphatic sac

Vestibular aqueduct containing endolymphatic duct

Dura mater

Base of stapes in oval window

Perilymphatic duct (aqueduct of cochlea)

Stapes

Internal ear

Incus

Malleus

Temporal bone

External Ear

External acoustic meatus

Cochlear duct

Tympanic membrane

Secondary tympanic membrane in round window

Tympanic cavity (Middle ear)

Vestibule of bony labyrinth

Pharyngotympanic tube

B. Schematic Anterior View

7.69   **External, middle, and internal ear—I: overviews**

A. Right temporal bone and auricle, sectioned in planes of (1) externa acoustic meatus and (2) pharyngotympanic tube. **B.** Schematic section of petrous temporal bone.

- The external ear comprises the auricle and external acoustic (auditory) meatus.
- The middle ear (tympanum) lies between the tympanic membrane and internal ear. Three ossicles extend from the lateral to the medial walls of the tympanum. Of these, the malleus is attached to the tympanic membrane. The stapes is attached by the anular ligament to the fenestra vestibuli (oval window), and the incus connects to the malleus and stapes. The pharyngotympanic tube, extending from the nasopharynx, opens into the anterior wall of the tympanic cavity.
- The membranous labyrinth comprises a closed system of membranous tubes and bulbs filled with fluid (endolymph) and bathed in surrounding fluid, called *perilymph* (*purple* in **B**); both membranous labyrinth and perilymph are contained within the bony labyrinth.

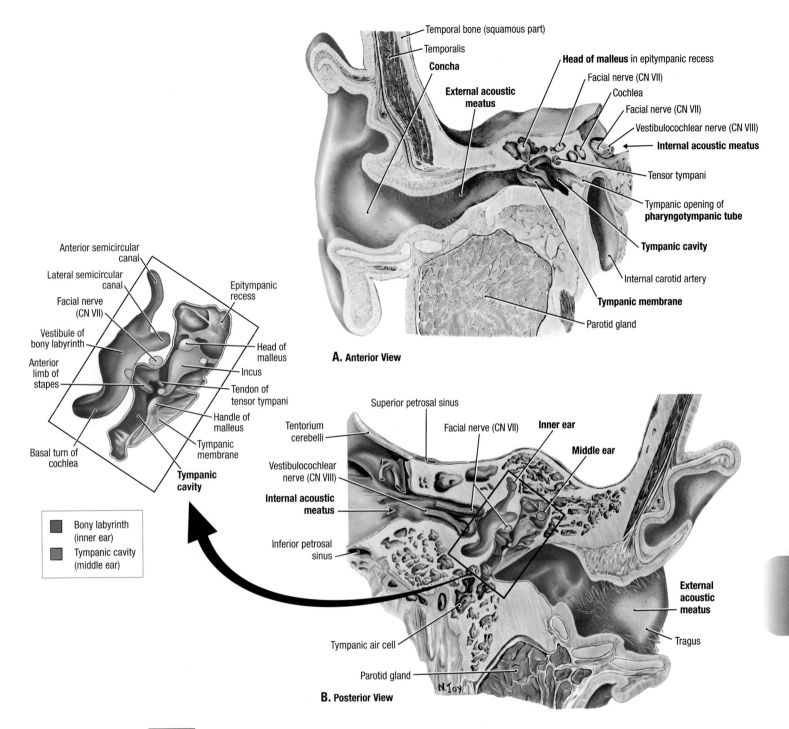

A. Anterior View

Temporal bone (squamous part)
Temporalis
Concha
External acoustic meatus
Head of malleus in epitympanic recess
Facial nerve (CN VII)
Cochlea
Facial nerve (CN VII)
Vestibulocochlear nerve (CN VIII)
Internal acoustic meatus
Tensor tympani
Tympanic opening of **pharyngotympanic tube**
Tympanic cavity
Internal carotid artery
Tympanic membrane
Parotid gland

Anterior semicircular canal
Lateral semicircular canal
Facial nerve (CN VII)
Vestibule of bony labyrinth
Anterior limb of stapes
Basal turn of cochlea
Epitympanic recess
Head of malleus
Incus
Tendon of tensor tympani
Handle of malleus
Tympanic membrane
Tympanic cavity

Bony labyrinth (inner ear)
Tympanic cavity (middle ear)

Superior petrosal sinus
Tentorium cerebelli
Vestibulocochlear nerve (CN VIII)
Internal acoustic meatus
Inferior petrosal sinus
Facial nerve (CN VII)
Inner ear
Middle ear
External acoustic meatus
Tragus
Tympanic air cell
Parotid gland

B. Posterior View

7.70   External, middle, and internal ear—II: coronally sectioned

A. Anterior portion. **B.** Posterior portion. The inset *(outlined by the box)* is an enlargement of the structures of the middle and internal ear as they appear in B.

• The external acoustic meatus is about 3 cm long; half is cartilaginous and half is bony. It is narrowest at the isthmus, near the junction of the cartilaginous and bony parts.

• The external acoustic meatus is innervated by the auriculotemporal branch of the mandibular nerve (CN V³) and the auricular branches of the vagus nerve (CN X); the middle ear is innervated by the glossopharyngeal nerve (CN IX).

• The cartilaginous part of the external acoustic meatus is lined with thick skin; the bony part is lined with thin epithelium that adheres to the periosteum and forms the outermost layer of the tympanic membrane.

POSTERIOR   ANTERIOR

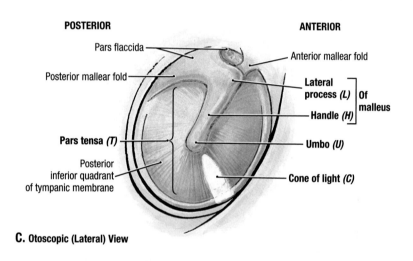

Posterior mallear fold

Pars flaccida

Anterior mallear fold

Lateral process
of malleus

Handle of malleus

Umbo

Cone of light

A. Lateral View

POSTERIOR   ANTERIOR

Lateral ligament of malleus

Lateral process of malleus

Posterior mallear fold

Long limb of incus (I)

Pyramidal
eminence

Stapedius tendon

Posterior limb of stapes (S)

Fossa of round window

Anterior mallear fold

Tensor tympani tendon

Processus
cochleariformis

Handle of malleus

Promontory

Tympanic nerve
(branch of CN IX)

Tympanic cells

B. Lateral View

POSTERIOR   ANTERIOR

Pars flaccida

Posterior mallear fold

Pars tensa (T)

Posterior
inferior quadrant
of tympanic membrane

Anterior mallear fold

Lateral
process (L)   Of
malleus

Handle (H)

Umbo (U)

Cone of light (C)

C. Otoscopic (Lateral) View

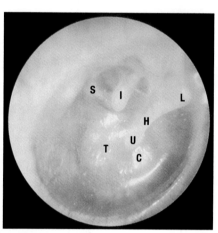

D. Otoscopic (Lateral) View

<table>
<tr><td>**7.71**</td><td>**Tympanic membrane**</td></tr>
</table>

A. External (lateral) surface of tympanic membrane. **B.** Tympanic membrane removed, demonstrating structures that lie medially. **C.** Diagram of otoscopic view of tympanic membrane. **D.** Otoscopic view of tympanic membrane. Letter labels are identified in **C.**

- The oval tympanic membrane is a shallow cone deepest at the central apex, the umbo, where the membrane is attached to the tip of the handle of the malleus. The handle of the malleus is attached to the membrane along its entire length as it extends anterosuperiorly toward the periphery of the membrane.

- Superior to the lateral process of the malleus, the membrane is thin (pars flaccida); the flaccid part lacks the radial and circular fibers present in the remainder of the membrane (pars tensa). The junction between the two parts is marked by anterior and posterior mallear folds.

- The lateral surface of the tympanic membrane is innervated by the auricular branch of the auriculotemporal nerve (CN V^3) and the auricular branch of the vagus nerve (CN X); the medial surface is innervated by tympanic branches of CN IX.

Examination of the external acoustic meatus and tympanic membrane begins by straightening the meatus. In adults, the helix is grasped and pulled posterosuperiorly (up, out, and back). These movements reduce the curvature of the external acoustic meatus, facilitating insertion of the otoscope. The external acoustic meatus is relatively short in infants; therefore, extra care must be taken to prevent damage to the tympanic membrane.

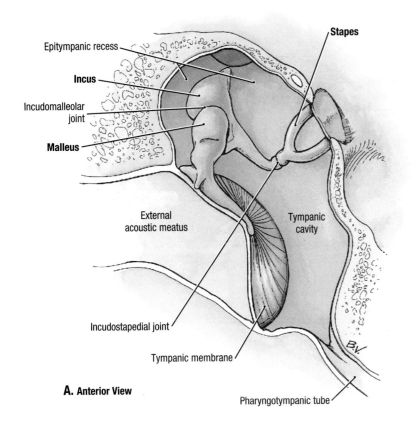

A. Anterior View

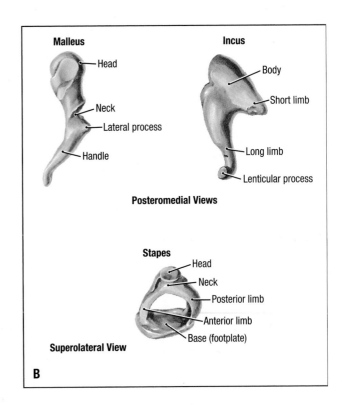

B

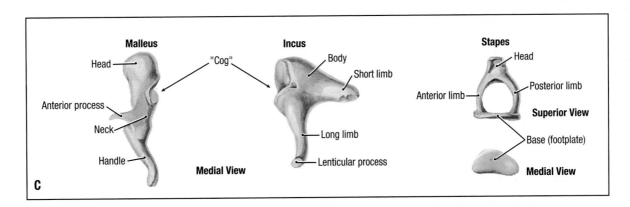

C

7.72   **Ossicles of the middle ear**

A. Ossicles in situ, as revealed by a coronal section of the temporal bone. **B** and **C.** Isolated ossicles.
- The head of the malleus and body and short process of the incus lie in the epitympanic recess, and the handle of the malleus is embedded in the tympanic membrane.
- The saddle-shaped articular surface of the head of the malleus and the reciprocally shaped articular surface of the body of the incus form the incudomalleolar synovial joint.
- A convex articular facet at the end of the long process of the incus articulates with the head of the stapes to compose the incudostapedial synovial joint.

- An earache and bulging red tympanic membrane may indicate pus or fluid in the middle ear, a sign of otitis media. Infection of the middle ear often is secondary to upper respiratory infections. Inflammation and swelling of the mucous membrane lining the tympanic cavity may cause partial or complete blockage of the pharyngotympanic tube. The tympanic membrane becomes red and bulges, and the person may complain of "ear popping." If untreated, otitis media may produce impaired hearing as the result of scarring of the auditory ossicles, limiting the ability of these bones to move in response to sound.

Tegmen tympani
Epitympanic recess
Lesser petrosal nerve
Malleus
Prominence of lateral semicircular canal
Incus
Facial nerve (CN VII) traversing facial canal
Aditus to mastoid antrum
Chorda tympani
Prominence of canal for facial nerve
Tensor tympani
Stapes
LATERAL
Tympanic plexus on **promontory**
MEDIAL
Tympanic membrane
Stapedius tendon
Pyramid
Tympanic nerve

A. Anterior View

Head
Anterior process   **Malleus**
SUPERIOR
Epitympanic recess
Neck of malleus
POSTERIOR
Anterior ligament of malleus
Lateral ligament of malleus
Superior recess of tympanic membrane
ANTERIOR
Tensor tympani
Tympanic opening of pharyngotympanic tube
Chorda tympani
Tubal cells
Anterior recess of tympanic membrane
Facial nerve in its sheath within facial canal
Posterior recess of tympanic membrane
Tendon of tensor tympani
B. Medial View of Lateral Wall
Tympanic cells
Margin of tympanic membrane
Handle of malleus
Tympanic membrane

7.73   Structures of the tympanic cavity

A. Schematic illustration of the tympanic cavity with the anterior wall removed. **B.** Lateral wall of the tympanic cavity. The facial nerve lies within the facial canal surrounded by a tough periosteal tube; the chorda tympani leaves the facial nerve and lies within two crescentic folds of mucous membrane, crossing the neck of the malleus superior to the tendon of tensor tympani.

Perforation of the tympanic membrane (ruptured eardrum) may result from otitis media. Perforation may also result from foreign bodies in the external acoustic meatus, trauma, or excessive pressure. Because the superior half of the tympanic membrane is much more vascular than the inferior half, incisions are made posteroinferiorly through the membrane. This incision also avoids injury to the chorda tympani nerve and auditory ossicles.

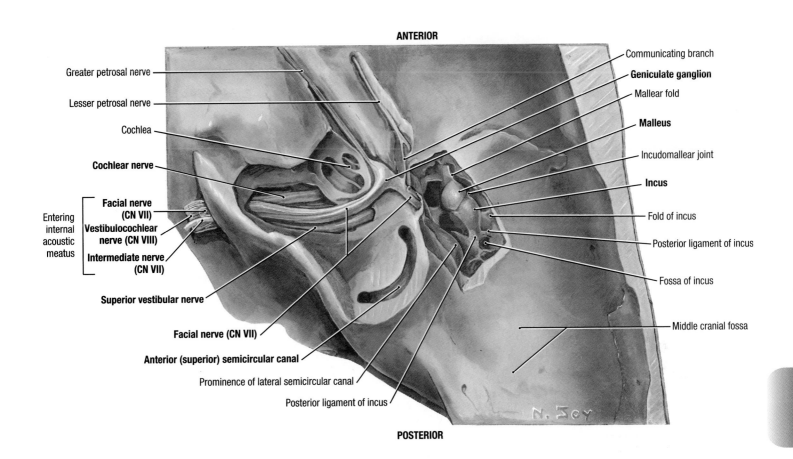

ANTERIOR

Greater petrosal nerve

Lesser petrosal nerve

Cochlea

Cochlear nerve

Entering internal acoustic meatus
- **Facial nerve (CN VII)**
- **Vestibulocochlear nerve (CN VIII)**
- **Intermediate nerve (CN VII)**

Superior vestibular nerve

Facial nerve (CN VII)

Anterior (superior) semicircular canal

Prominence of lateral semicircular canal

Posterior ligament of incus

POSTERIOR

Communicating branch

Geniculate ganglion

Mallear fold

Malleus

Incudomallear joint

Incus

Fold of incus

Posterior ligament of incus

Fossa of incus

Middle cranial fossa

7.74   Middle and inner ear _in situ_

The tegmen tympani has been removed to expose the middle ear, the arcuate eminence has been removed to expose the anterior semicircular canal, and the course of the facial and vestibulocochlear nerves through the internal acoustic meatus and internal ear is demonstrated. At the geniculate ganglion, the facial nerve executes a sharp bend, called the genu, and then curves posteroinferiorly within the bony facial canal; the thin lateral wall of the facial canal separates the facial nerve from the tympanic cavity of the middle ear.

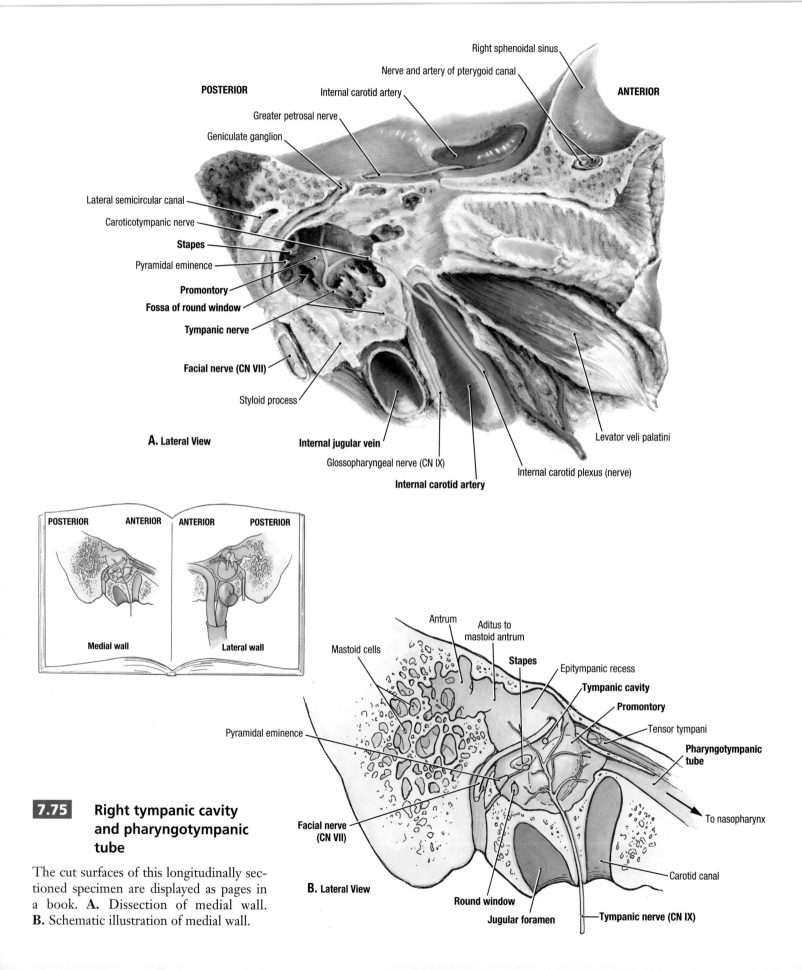

Right sphenoidal sinus

Nerve and artery of pterygoid canal

Internal carotid artery

POSTERIOR

ANTERIOR

Greater petrosal nerve

Geniculate ganglion

Lateral semicircular canal

Caroticotympanic nerve

Stapes

Pyramidal eminence

Promontory

Fossa of round window

Tympanic nerve

Facial nerve (CN VII)

Styloid process

A. Lateral View

Levator veli palatini

Internal jugular vein

Glossopharyngeal nerve (CN IX)

Internal carotid artery

Internal carotid plexus (nerve)

POSTERIOR **ANTERIOR** **ANTERIOR** **POSTERIOR**

Medial wall **Lateral wall**

Antrum

Aditus to mastoid antrum

Mastoid cells

Stapes

Epitympanic recess

Tympanic cavity

Promontory

Tensor tympani

Pyramidal eminence

Pharyngotympanic tube

To nasopharynx

Facial nerve (CN VII)

Carotid canal

B. Lateral View

Round window

Jugular foramen

Tympanic nerve (CN IX)

7.75 **Right tympanic cavity and pharyngotympanic tube**

The cut surfaces of this longitudinally sectioned specimen are displayed as pages in a book. **A.** Dissection of medial wall. **B.** Schematic illustration of medial wall.

ANTERIOR   POSTERIOR

Right sphenoidal sinus

Cavernous sinus

Cartilage of pharyngotympanic tube

Middle meningeal artery

Isthmus of **pharyngotympanic tube**

Lesser petrosal nerve

Tensor tympani

Processus cochleariformis

Head of **malleus**

Chorda tympani

Tympanic membrane

Mastoid process and cells

Levator veli palatini

Pharyngeal opening of pharyngotympanic tube

Internal carotid artery

Internal jugular vein

Facial nerve (CN VII)

C. Medial View

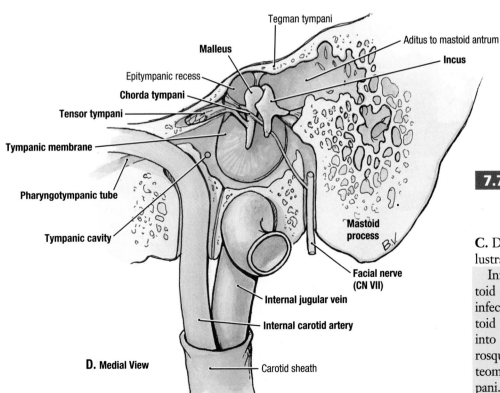

Tegman tympani

Malleus

Epitympanic recess

Chorda tympani

Tensor tympani

Tympanic membrane

Pharyngotympanic tube

Tympanic cavity

Aditus to mastoid antrum

Incus

Mastoid process

Facial nerve (CN VII)

Internal jugular vein

Internal carotid artery

Carotid sheath

D. Medial View

7.75 **Right tympanic cavity and pharyngotympanic tube** *(continued)*

C. Dissection of lateral wall. **D.** Schematic illustration of lateral wall.

Infections of the mastoid antrum and mastoid cells (mastoiditis) result from middle ear infections that cause inflammation of the mastoid process. Infections may spread superiorly into the middle cranial fossa through the petrosquamous fissure in children or may cause osteomyelitis (bone infection) of the tegmen tympani. Since the advent of antibiotics, mastoiditis is uncommon.

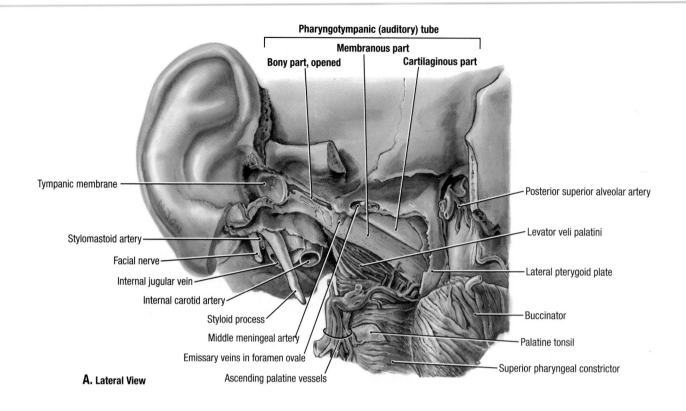

Pharyngotympanic (auditory) tube

Membranous part

Bony part, opened   **Cartilaginous part**

Tympanic membrane

Stylomastoid artery

Facial nerve

Internal jugular vein

Internal carotid artery

Styloid process

Middle meningeal artery

Emissary veins in foramen ovale

Ascending palatine vessels

Posterior superior alveolar artery

Levator veli palatini

Lateral pterygoid plate

Buccinator

Palatine tonsil

Superior pharyngeal constrictor

A. Lateral View

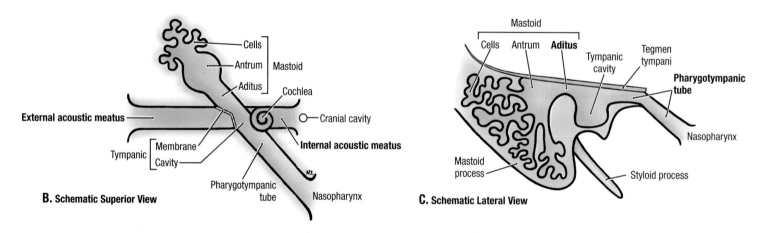

Cells

Antrum] Mastoid

Aditus]

Cochlea

External acoustic meatus

Cranial cavity

[Membrane

Tympanic [Cavity

Internal acoustic meatus

Pharyngotympanic tube

Nasopharynx

B. Schematic Superior View

Mastoid

Cells   Antrum   **Aditus**   Tympanic cavity   Tegmen tympani

Pharygotympanic tube

Nasopharynx

Mastoid process

Styloid process

C. Schematic Lateral View

7.76   Right tympanic cavity and pharyngotympanic tube

A. Dissection demonstrating lateral aspect of pharyngotympanic tube and structures located medially. **B.** Schematic illustration demonstrating relationship between internal and external acoustic meatuses. **C.** Diagram of tegmen tympani. **D.** Spaces of tympanic bone. **E.** Relationship of tympanic cavity to internal carotid artery, sigmoid sinus, and middle cranial fossa.

- The general direction of the pharyngotympanic tube is superior, posterior, and lateral from the nasopharynx to the tympanic cavity.
- The cartilaginous part of the tube rests throughout its length on the levator veli palatini muscle.
- The line of the meatuses and the line of the airway, from nasopharynx to mastoid cells, intersect at the tympanic cavity.
- The tegmen tympani forms the roof of the tympanic cavity and mastoid antrum.
- The internal carotid artery is the primary relationship of the anterior wall, the internal jugular vein is the primary relationship of the floor, and the facial nerve is the primary relationship of the posterior wall.

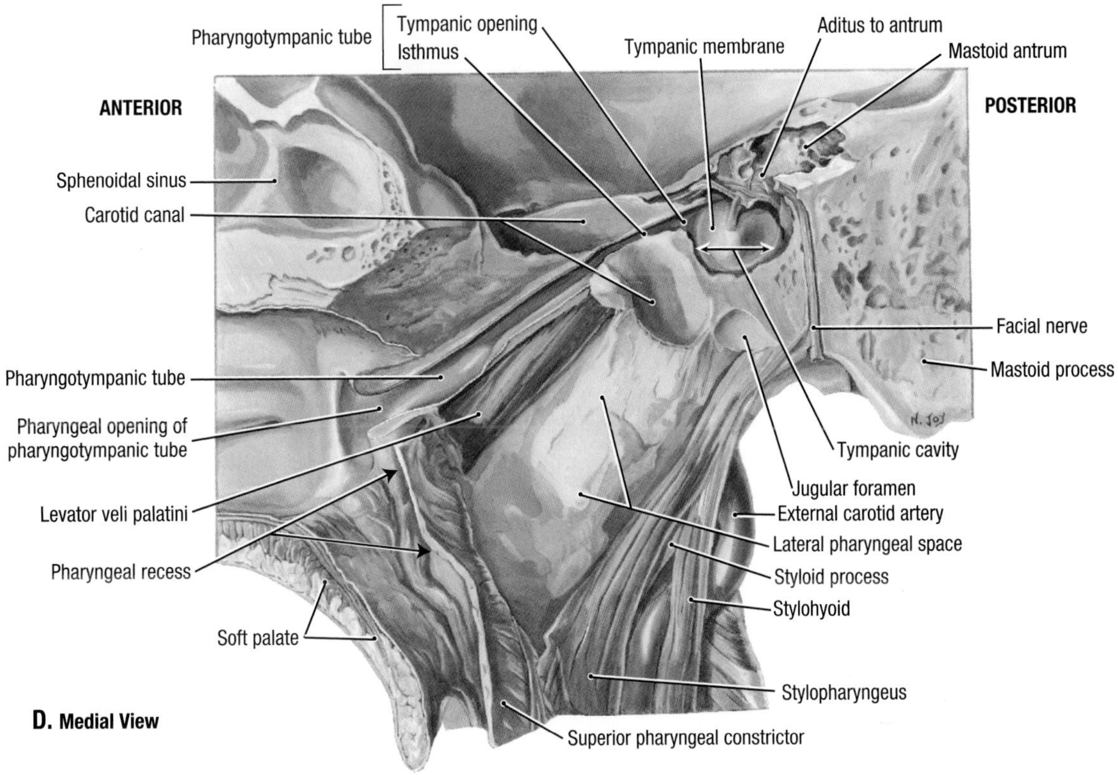

Pharyngotympanic tube
Tympanic opening
Isthmus
Tympanic membrane
Aditus to antrum
Mastoid antrum

ANTERIOR
POSTERIOR

Sphenoidal sinus
Carotid canal

Facial nerve
Mastoid process

Pharyngotympanic tube

Pharyngeal opening of pharyngotympanic tube

Levator veli palatini

Pharyngeal recess

Soft palate

Tympanic cavity

Jugular foramen
External carotid artery
Lateral pharyngeal space
Styloid process
Stylohyoid

Stylopharyngeus

D. Medial View

Superior pharyngeal constrictor

SUPERIOR

Facial nerve (CN VII)
Tegmen tympani
Mastoid antrum

Tendon of tensor tympani

ANTERIOR
POSTERIOR

Tympanic opening of pharyngotympanic (auditory) tube

Internal carotid artery in carotid canal

Superior bulb of internal jugular vein

Sigmoid sinus

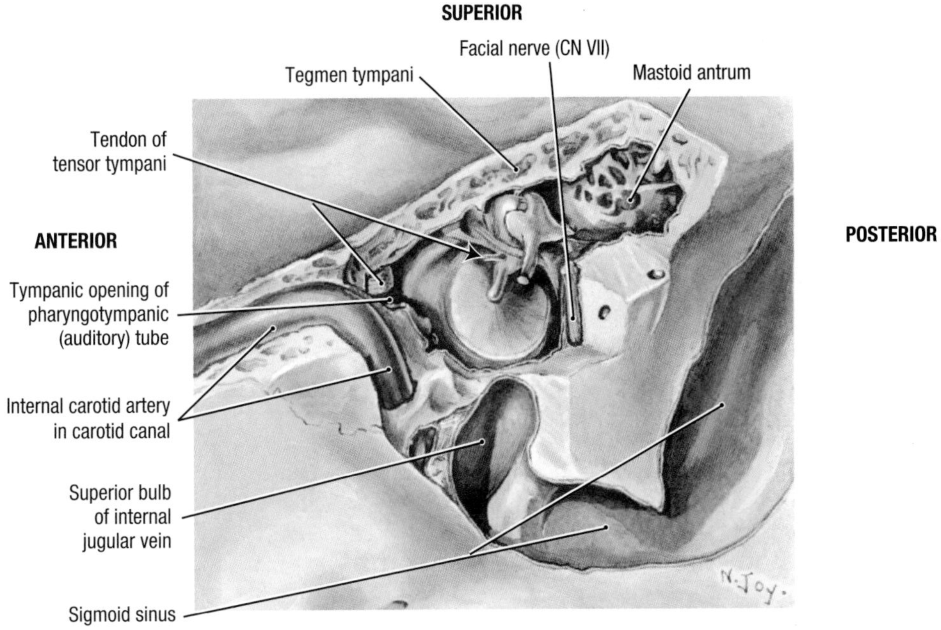

E. Medial View

7.76   **Right tympanic cavity and pharyngotympanic tube** *(continued)*

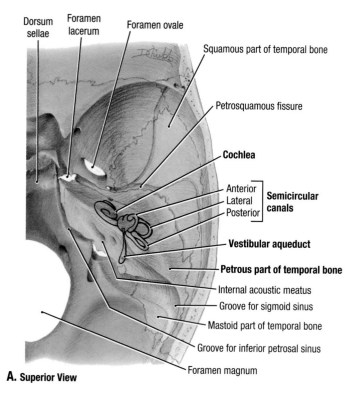

Dorsum sellae
Foramen lacerum
Foramen ovale
Squamous part of temporal bone
Petrosquamous fissure
Cochlea
Anterior
Lateral — **Semicircular canals**
Posterior
Vestibular aqueduct
Petrous part of temporal bone
Internal acoustic meatus
Groove for sigmoid sinus
Mastoid part of temporal bone
Groove for inferior petrosal sinus
Foramen magnum

A. Superior View

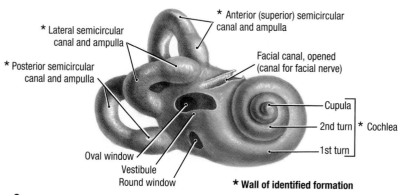

* Lateral semicircular canal and ampulla
* Anterior (superior) semicircular canal and ampulla
* Posterior semicircular canal and ampulla
Facial canal, opened (canal for facial nerve)
Cupula
2nd turn — * Cochlea
1st turn
Oval window
Vestibule
Round window

C. Anterolateral View

* **Wall of identified formation**

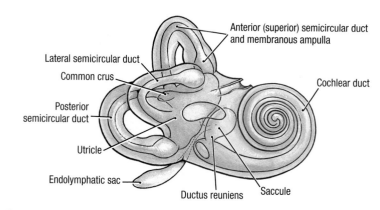

Lateral semicircular duct
Common crus
Posterior semicircular duct
Utricle
Anterior (superior) semicircular duct and membranous ampulla
Cochlear duct
Endolymphatic sac
Ductus reuniens
Saccule

D. Anterolateral View

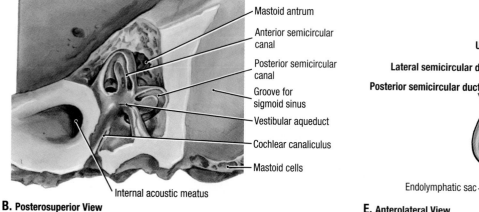

Mastoid antrum
Anterior semicircular canal
Posterior semicircular canal
Groove for sigmoid sinus
Vestibular aqueduct
Cochlear canaliculus
Mastoid cells
Internal acoustic meatus

B. Posterosuperior View

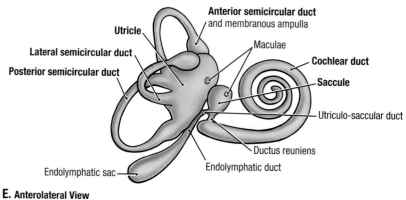

Utricle
Anterior semicircular duct and membranous ampulla
Maculae
Lateral semicircular duct
Posterior semicircular duct
Cochlear duct
Saccule
Utriculo-saccular duct
Ductus reuniens
Endolymphatic sac
Endolymphatic duct

E. Anterolateral View

7.77 Bony and membranous labyrinths

A. Location and orientation of bony labyrinth within petrous temporal bone. **B.** Semicircular canals and aqueducts *in situ*. The tegmen tympani has been excised, and the softer bone surrounding the harder bone of the otic capsule has been drilled away. **C.** Walls of left bony labyrinth (otic capsule). The bony labyrinth is the fluid-filled space contained within this formation. **D.** Membranous labyrinth as it lies within the surrounding bony labyrinth. **E.** Isolated left membranous labyrinth.

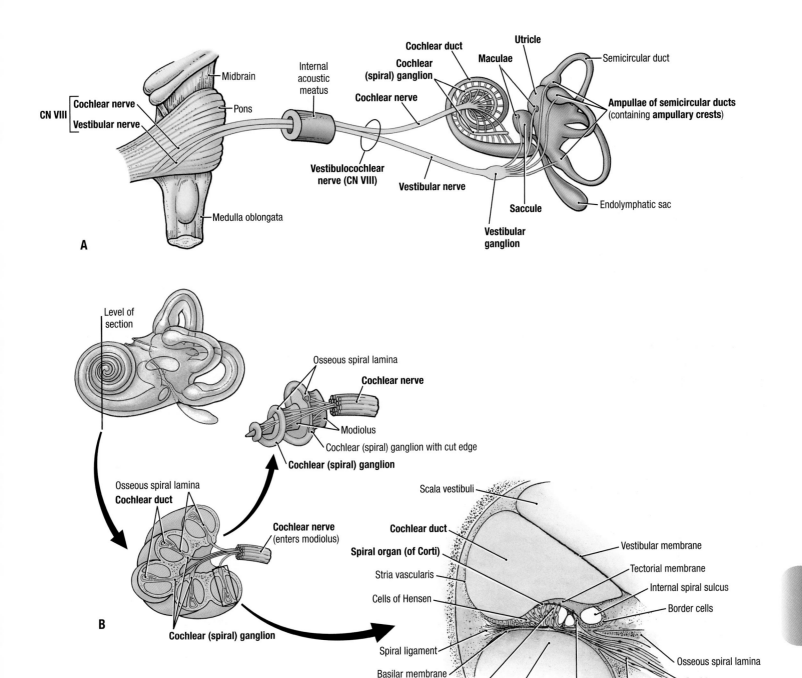

7.78 **Vestibulocochlear nerve and structure of cochlea**

A. Distribution of vestibulocochlear nerve (schematic). **B.** Structure of cochlea. The cochlea has been sectioned along the bony core of the cochlea (modiolus), the axis about which the cochlea winds. An isolated modiolus is shown after the turns of the cochlea are removed, leaving only the spiral lamina winding around it. The *large drawing* shows the details of the *area enclosed in the rectangle*, including a cross-section of the cochlear duct of the membranous labyrinth.

- The maculae of the membranous labyrinth are primarily static organs, which have small dense particles (otoliths) embedded

among the hair cells. Under the influence of gravity, the otoliths cause bending of the hair cells, which stimulate the vestibular nerve and provide awareness of the position of the head in space; the hairs also respond to quick tilting movements and to linear acceleration and deceleration. Motion sickness results mainly from discordance between vestibular and visual stimuli.

- Persistent exposure to excessively loud sound causes degenerative changes in the spiral organ, resulting in high-tone deafness. This type of hearing loss commonly occurs in workers who are exposed to loud noises and do not wear protective earmuffs.

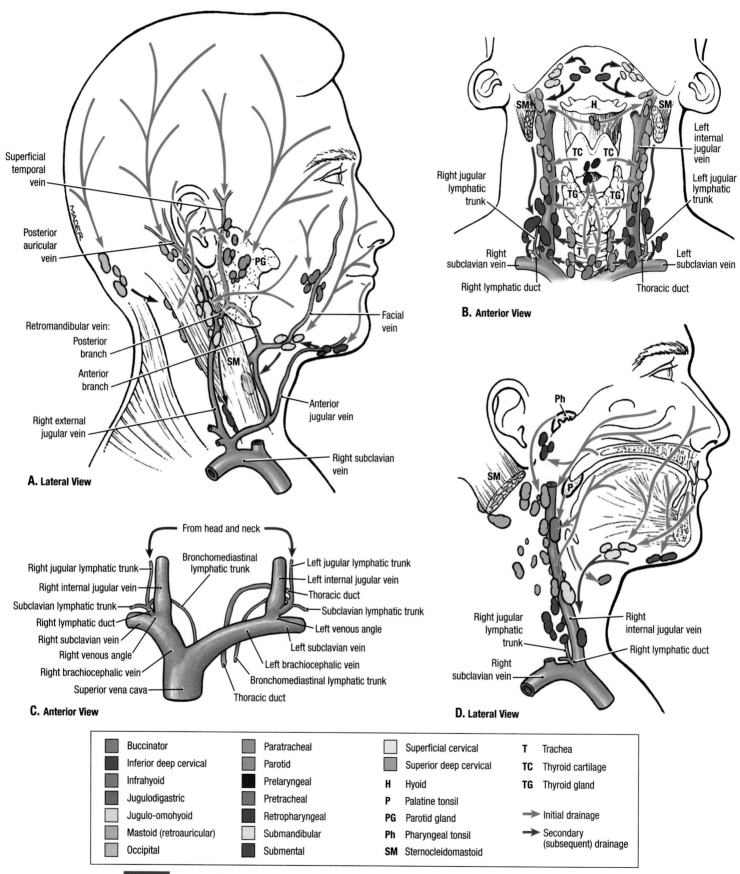

A. Lateral View

B. Anterior View

C. Anterior View

D. Lateral View

Buccinator	Paratracheal	Superficial cervical	T Trachea
Inferior deep cervical	Parotid	Superior deep cervical	TC Thyroid cartilage
Infrahyoid	Prelaryngeal	H Hyoid	TG Thyroid gland
Jugulodigastric	Pretracheal	P Palatine tonsil	
Jugulo-omohyoid	Retropharyngeal	PG Parotid gland	→ Initial drainage
Mastoid (retroauricular)	Submandibular	Ph Pharyngeal tonsil	→ Secondary (subsequent) drainage
Occipital	Submental	SM Sternocleidomastoid	

7.79 **Lymphatic and venous drainage of the head and neck**

A. Superficial drainage. **B.** Drainage of the trachea, thyroid gland, larynx, and floor of mouth. **C.** Termination of right and left jugular lymphatic trunks. **D.** Deep drainage.

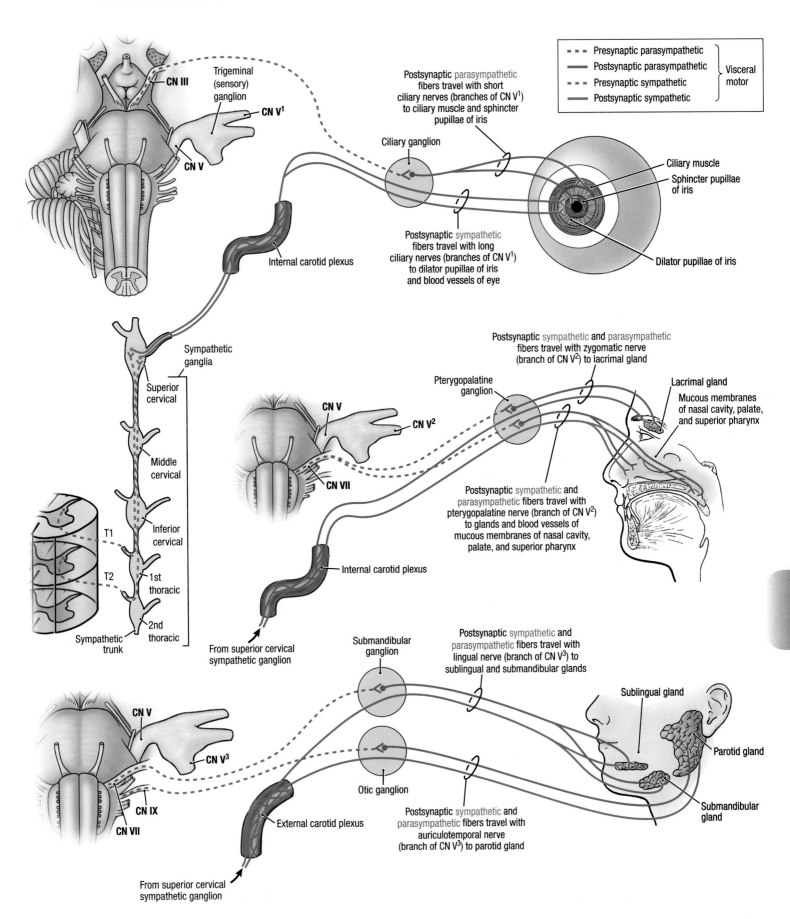

7.80 **Autonomic innervation of the head**

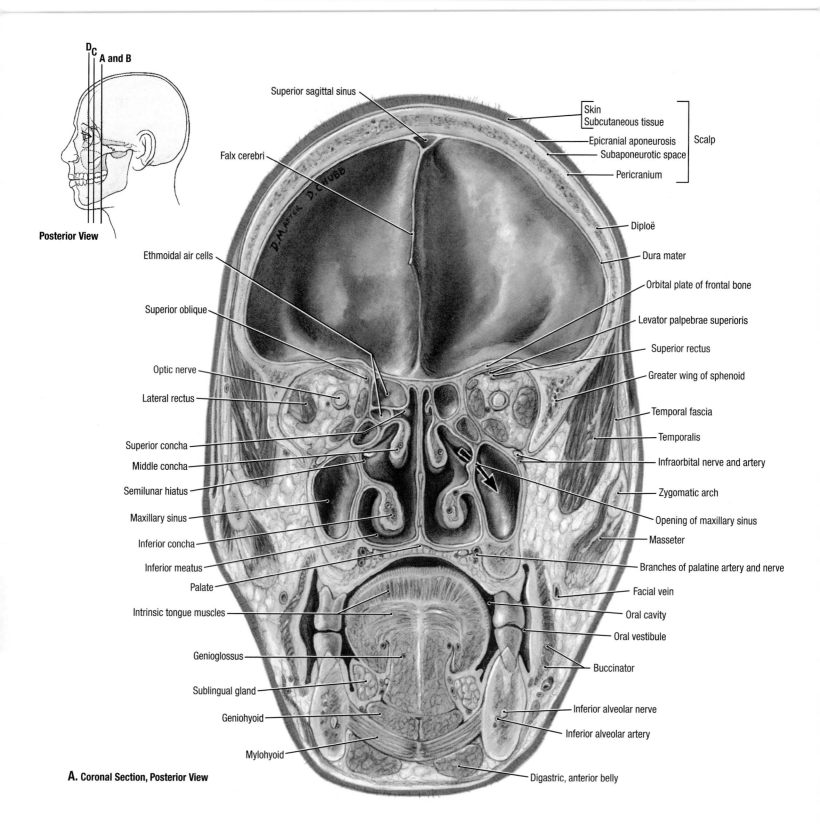

Posterior View

Superior sagittal sinus

Falx cerebri

Ethmoidal air cells

Superior oblique

Optic nerve

Lateral rectus

Superior concha

Middle concha

Semilunar hiatus

Maxillary sinus

Inferior concha

Inferior meatus

Palate

Intrinsic tongue muscles

Genioglossus

Sublingual gland

Geniohyoid

Mylohyoid

A. Coronal Section, Posterior View

Skin
Subcutaneous tissue
Epicranial aponeurosis
Subaponeurotic space   Scalp
Pericranium

Diploë

Dura mater

Orbital plate of frontal bone

Levator palpebrae superioris

Superior rectus

Greater wing of sphenoid

Temporal fascia

Temporalis

Infraorbital nerve and artery

Zygomatic arch

Opening of maxillary sinus

Masseter

Branches of palatine artery and nerve

Facial vein

Oral cavity

Oral vestibule

Buccinator

Inferior alveolar nerve

Inferior alveolar artery

Digastric, anterior belly

7.81 **Coronal section and MRI imaging of nasopharynx and oral cavity**

A. Coronal section. **B–D.** Coronal MRIs.

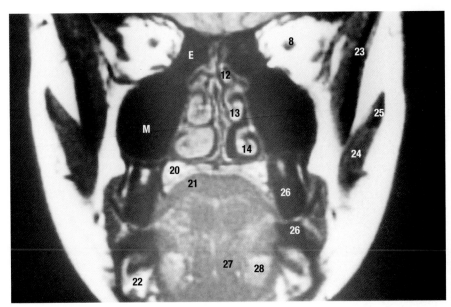

B

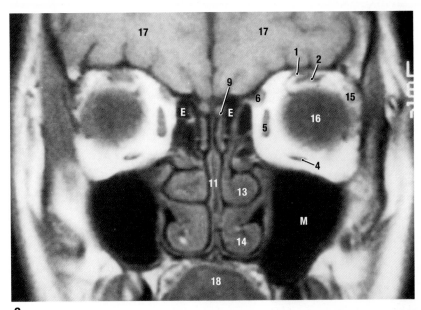

C

1	Levator palpebrae superioris
2	Superior rectus
3	Lateral rectus
4	Inferior rectus
5	Medial rectus
6	Superior oblique
7	Inferior oblique
8	Optic nerve
9	Olfactory bulb
10	Crista galli
11	Nasal septum
12	Superior concha
13	Middle concha
14	Inferior concha
15	Lacrimal gland
16	Eyeball
17	Frontal lobe
18	Tongue
19	Infraorbital vessels and nerve
20	Hard palate
21	Intrinsic muscles of tongue
22	Mandible
23	Temporalis
24	Masseter
25	Zygomatic arch
26	Molar teeth
27	Genioglossus
28	Sublingual gland
M	Maxillary sinus
E	Ethmoidal air cell

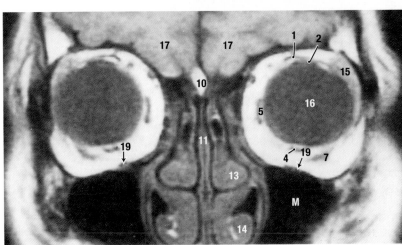

Posterior Views

D

7.81 Coronal section and MRI imaging of nasopharynx and oral cavity *(continued)*

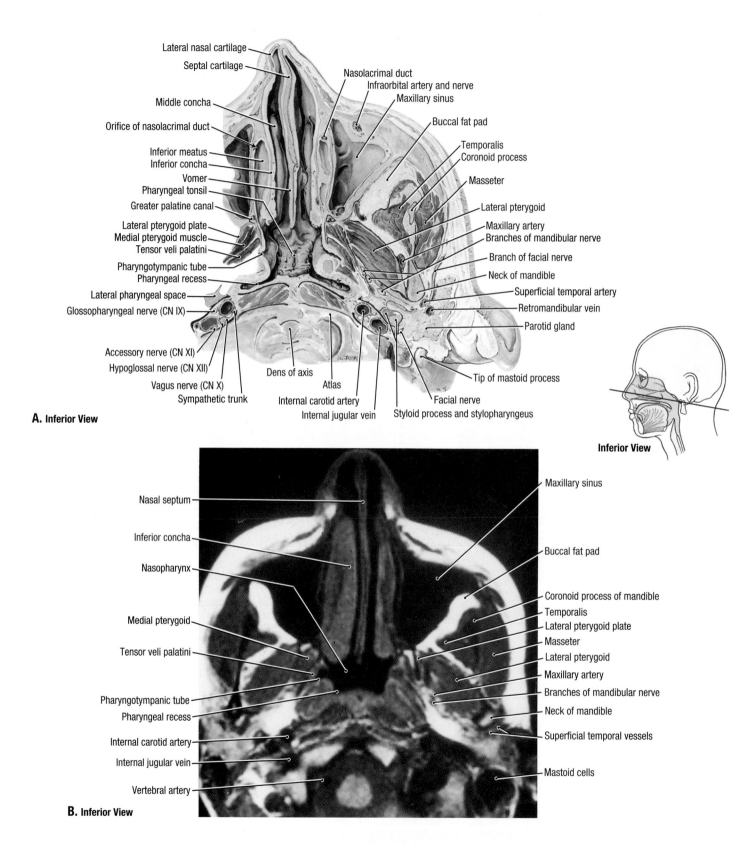

Lateral nasal cartilage

Septal cartilage

Nasolacrimal duct

Infraorbital artery and nerve

Maxillary sinus

Middle concha

Orifice of nasolacrimal duct

Buccal fat pad

Temporalis

Coronoid process

Inferior meatus

Inferior concha

Masseter

Vomer

Pharyngeal tonsil

Lateral pterygoid

Greater palatine canal

Maxillary artery

Lateral pterygoid plate

Branches of mandibular nerve

Medial pterygoid muscle

Tensor veli palatini

Branch of facial nerve

Pharyngotympanic tube

Neck of mandible

Pharyngeal recess

Lateral pharyngeal space

Superficial temporal artery

Glossopharyngeal nerve (CN IX)

Retromandibular vein

Parotid gland

Accessory nerve (CN XI)

Hypoglossal nerve (CN XII)

Dens of axis

Tip of mastoid process

Vagus nerve (CN X)

Atlas

Sympathetic trunk

Internal carotid artery

Facial nerve

Internal jugular vein

Styloid process and stylopharyngeus

A. Inferior View

Inferior View

Nasal septum

Maxillary sinus

Inferior concha

Buccal fat pad

Nasopharynx

Coronoid process of mandible

Temporalis

Lateral pterygoid plate

Medial pterygoid

Masseter

Tensor veli palatini

Lateral pterygoid

Maxillary artery

Branches of mandibular nerve

Pharyngotympanic tube

Neck of mandible

Pharyngeal recess

Internal carotid artery

Superficial temporal vessels

Internal jugular vein

Mastoid cells

Vertebral artery

B. Inferior View

7.82 **Transverse section and MRI imaging of nasal cavity and naso-pharynx**

A. Transverse section of left side of head. **B.** Transverse (axial) MRI scan.

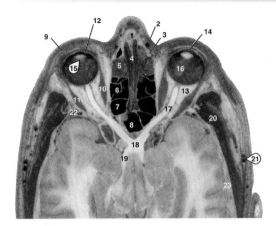

A. Transverse Section

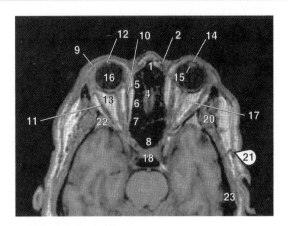

B. Transverse (axial) MRI Scan

Key

1	Nasal bones	7	Posterior ethmoidal air cell	13	Retrobulbar fat	19	Optic tract
2	Angular artery	8	Sphenoid sinus	14	Anterior chamber	20	Temporalis muscle
3	Frontal process of maxilla	9	Orbicularis oculi muscle	15	Lens	21	Superficial temporal vessels
4	Nasal septum	10	Medial rectus muscle	16	Vitreous body	22	Greater wing of sphenoid
5	Anterior ethmoidal cell	11	Lateral rectus muscle	17	Optic nerve	23	Squamous portion of temporal bone
6	Middle ethmoidal cell	12	Cornea	18	Optic chiasm		

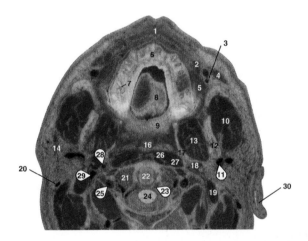

C. Transverse Section

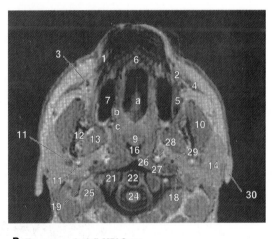

D. Transverse (axial) MRI Scan

Key

1	Orbicularis oris muscle	12	Ramus of mandible	23	Transverse ligament of Atlas
2	Levator anguli oris muscle	13	Lateral pterygoid muscle	24	Spinal cord
3	Facial artery and vein	14	Parotid gland	25	Vertebral artery in foramina transversaria
4	Zygomaticus major muscle	15	Superficial temporal vessels	26	Longus colli muscle
5	Buccinator muscle	16	Region of pharyngeal tubercle	27	Longus capitis muscle
6	Maxilla	17	Sphenoid bone	28	Internal carotid artery
7	Alveolar process of maxilla	18	Stylohyoid ligament and muscle	29	Internal jugular vein
8	Dorsum of the tongue	19	Posterior belly of digastric muscle	30	Interior portion of helix of auricle
9	Soft palate (uvula apparent in radiographs)	20	Occipital artery	a	Hard palate
10	Masseter muscle	21	First cervical vertebrae (Atlas)	b	Palatoglossus muscle
11	Retromandibular vein	22	Dens (Axis)	c	Palatopharyngeus muscle

7.83   MRIs of oropharynx

A and **B.** Transverse (axial) MRIs. **C** and **D.** Coronal MRIs. **E.** Sagittal MRI

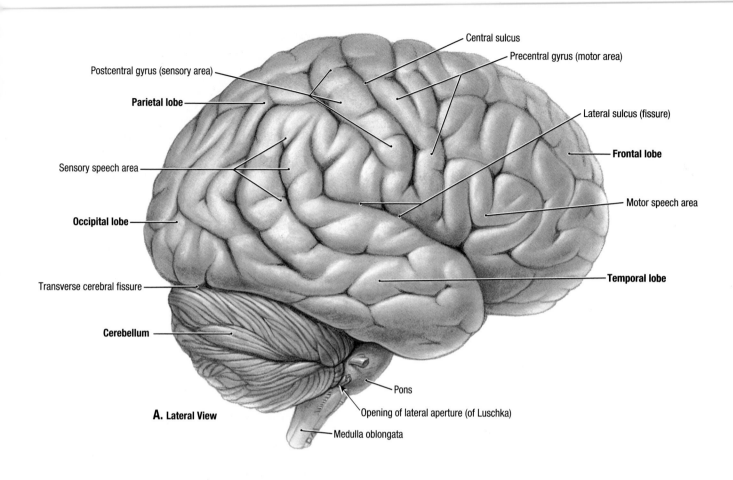

A. **Lateral View**

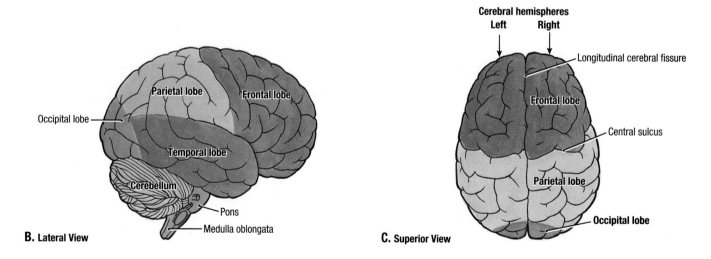

B. **Lateral View**

C. **Superior View**

7.84 **Brain**

A. Cerebrum, cerebellum, and brainstem, lateral aspect. **B.** Lobes of the cerebral hemispheres, lateral aspect. **C.** Lobes of the cerebral hemispheres, superior aspect.

Cerebral contusion (bruising) results from brain trauma in which the pia is stripped from the injured surface of the brain and may be torn, allowing blood to enter the subarachnoid space. The bruising results from the sudden impact of the moving brain against the stationary cranium or from the suddenly moving cranium against the stationary brain. Cerebral contusion may result in an extended loss of consciousness

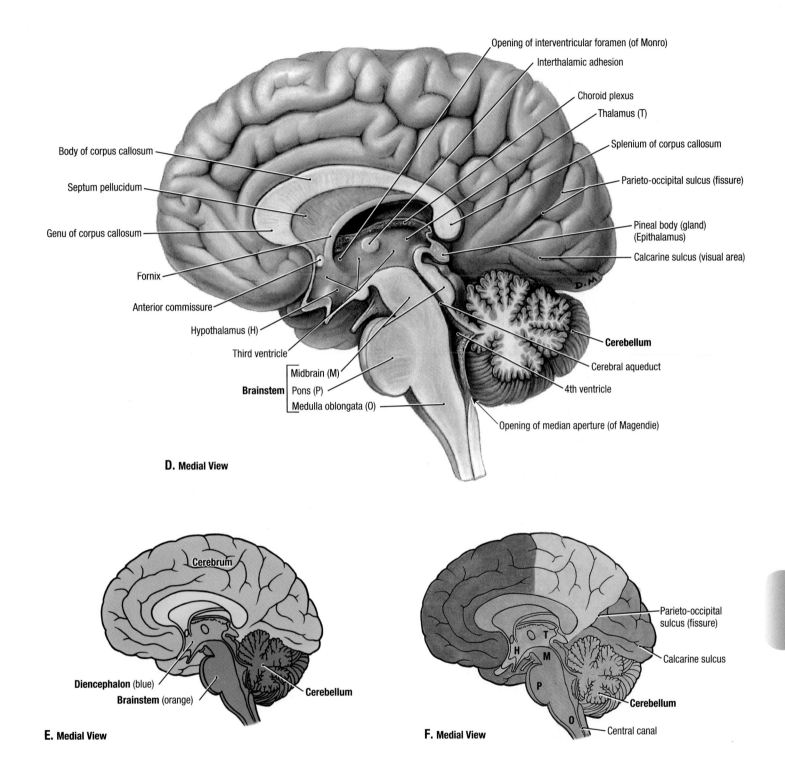

Body of corpus callosum

Septum pellucidum

Genu of corpus callosum

Fornix

Anterior commissure

Hypothalamus (H)

Third ventricle

Midbrain (M)

Brainstem   Pons (P)

Medulla oblongata (O)

D. Medial View

Opening of interventricular foramen (of Monro)

Interthalamic adhesion

Choroid plexus

Thalamus (T)

Splenium of corpus callosum

Parieto-occipital sulcus (fissure)

Pineal body (gland) (Epithalamus)

Calcarine sulcus (visual area)

Cerebellum

Cerebral aqueduct

4th ventricle

Opening of median aperture (of Magendie)

Cerebrum

Diencephalon (blue)

Brainstem (orange)

Cerebellum

E. Medial View

Parieto-occipital sulcus (fissure)

Calcarine sulcus

Cerebellum

Central canal

F. Medial View

7.84   **Brain** *(continued)*

D. Cerebrum, cerebellum, and brainstem, median section. **E.** Parts of the brain, median section. **F.** Lobes of the cerebral hemisphere, median section. See **D** for labeling key.

Cerebral compression may be produced by intracranial collections of blood, obstruction of CSF circulation or absorption, intracranial tumors or abscesses, and brain swelling caused by brain edema, an increase in brain volume resulting from an increase in water and sodium content.

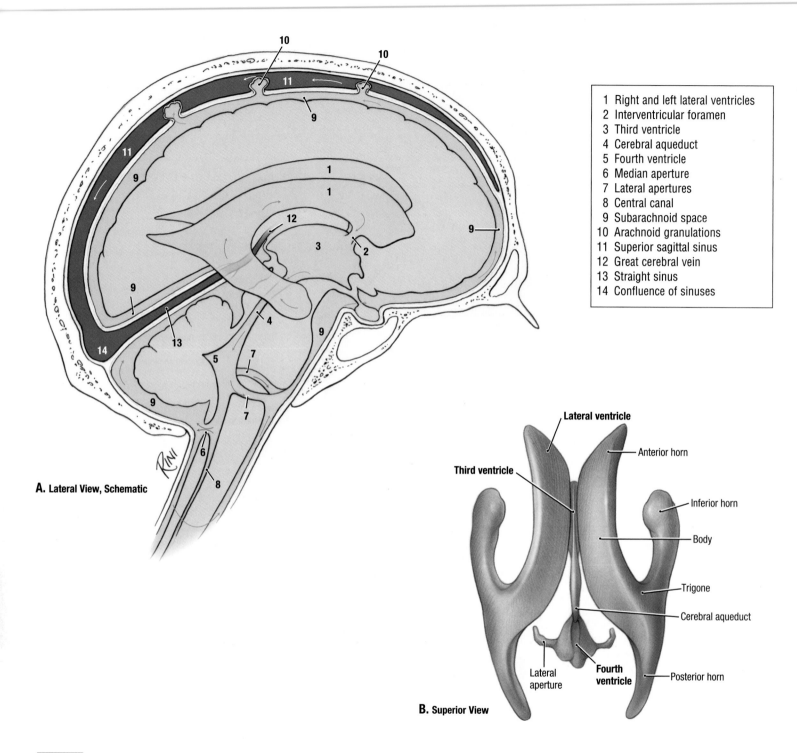

1 Right and left lateral ventricles
2 Interventricular foramen
3 Third ventricle
4 Cerebral aqueduct
5 Fourth ventricle
6 Median aperture
7 Lateral apertures
8 Central canal
9 Subarachnoid space
10 Arachnoid granulations
11 Superior sagittal sinus
12 Great cerebral vein
13 Straight sinus
14 Confluence of sinuses

A. Lateral View, Schematic

Lateral ventricle
Anterior horn
Third ventricle
Inferior horn
Body
Trigone
Cerebral aqueduct
Lateral aperture
Fourth ventricle
Posterior horn

B. Superior View

7.85 Ventricular system

A. Circulation of cerebrospinal fluid (CSF). **B.** Ventricles: lateral, third, and fourth.

- The ventricular system consists of two lateral ventricles located in the cerebral hemispheres, a third ventricle located between the right and left halves of the diencephalon, and a fourth ventricle located in the posterior parts of the pons and medulla.
- CSF secreted by choroid plexus in the ventricles drains via the interventricular foramen from the lateral to the third ventricle, via the cerebral aqueduct from the third to the fourth ventricle,

and via median and lateral apertures into the subarachnoid space. CSF is absorbed by arachnoid granulations into the venous sinuses (especially the superior sagittal sinus).

- Overproduction of CSF, obstruction of its flow, or interference with its absorption results in an excess of CSF in the ventricles and enlargement of the head, a condition known as hydrocephalus. Excess CSF dilates the ventricles; thins the brain; and, in infants, separates the bones of the calvaria because the sutures and fontanelles are still open.

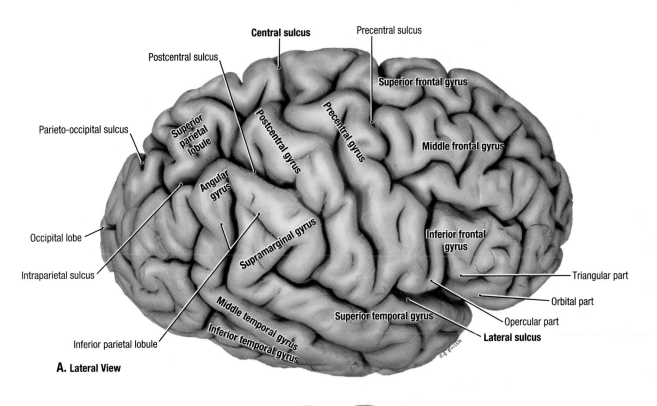

A. Lateral View

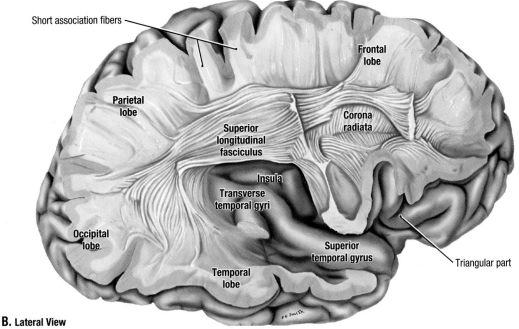

B. Lateral View

7.86   Serial dissections of the lateral aspect of the cerebral hemisphere

The dissections begin from the lateral surface of the cerebral hemisphere (**A**) and proceed sequentially medially (**B–F**).

A. Sulci and gyri of the lateral surface of one cerebral hemisphere. Each gyrus is a fold of cerebral cortex with a core of white matter. The furrows are called *sulci*. The pattern of sulci and gyri formed shortly before birth is recognizable in some adult brains, as shown in this specimen. Usually the expanding cortex acquires secondary foldings, which make identification of this basic pattern more difficult. **B.** Superior longitudinal fasciculus, transverse temporal gyri, and insula. The cortex and short association fiber bundles around the lateral fissure have been removed.

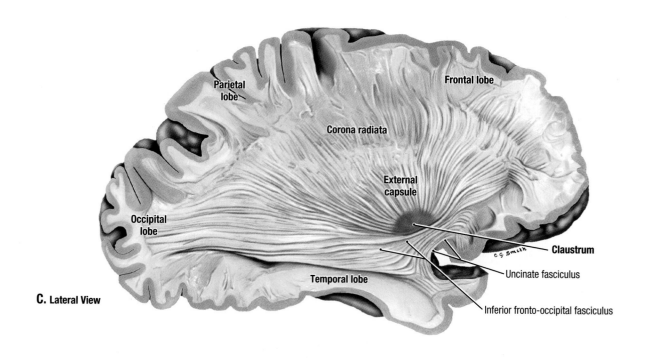

C. Lateral View

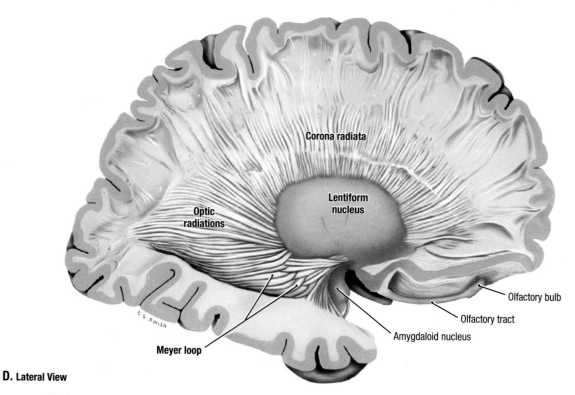

D. Lateral View

7.86   **Serial dissections of the lateral aspect of the cerebral hemisphere (*continued*)**

C. Uncinate and inferior fronto-occipital fasciculi and external capsule. The external capsule consists of projection fibers that pass between the claustrum laterally and the lentiform nucleus medially. **D.** Lentiform nucleus and corona radiata. The inferior longitudinal and uncinate fasciculi, claustrum, and external capsule have been removed. The fibers of the optic radiations convey impulses from the right half of the retina of each eye; the fibers extending closest to the temporal pole (Meyer's loop) carry impulses from the lower portion of each retina.

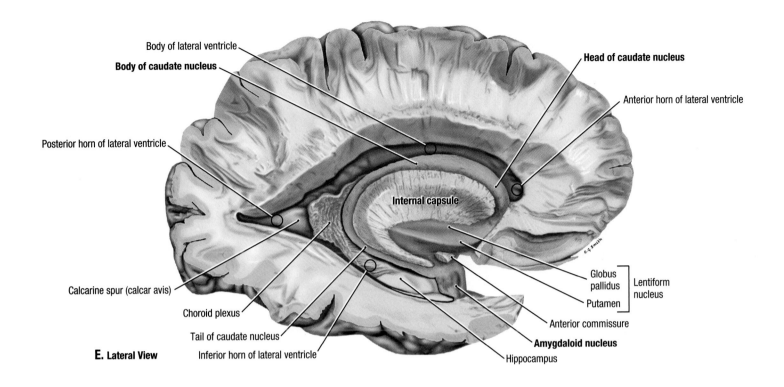

Body of lateral ventricle

Body of caudate nucleus

Posterior horn of lateral ventricle

Head of caudate nucleus

Anterior horn of lateral ventricle

Internal capsule

Calcarine spur (calcar avis)

Globus pallidus

Putamen

Lentiform nucleus

Choroid plexus

Tail of caudate nucleus

Anterior commissure

Amygdaloid nucleus

Inferior horn of lateral ventricle

Hippocampus

E. Lateral View

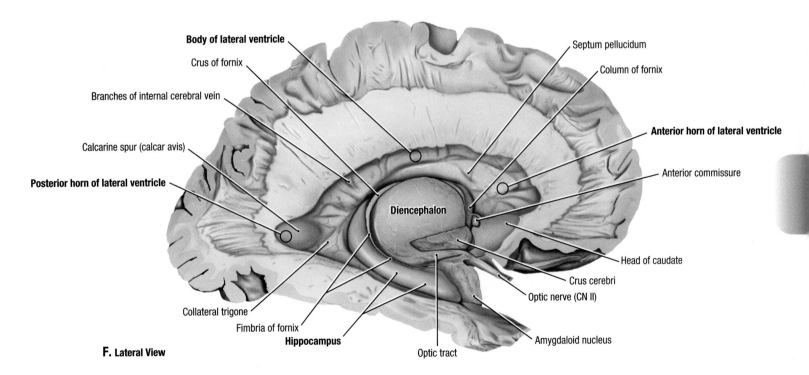

Body of lateral ventricle

Crus of fornix

Branches of internal cerebral vein

Septum pellucidum

Column of fornix

Calcarine spur (calcar avis)

Anterior horn of lateral ventricle

Posterior horn of lateral ventricle

Anterior commissure

Diencephalon

Head of caudate

Crus cerebri

Optic nerve (CN II)

Collateral trigone

Fimbria of fornix

Hippocampus

Optic tract

Amygdaloid nucleus

F. Lateral View

7.86   **Serial dissections of the lateral aspect of the cerebral hemisphere *(continued)***

E. Caudate and amygdaloid nuclei and internal capsule. The lateral wall of the lateral ventricle, the marginal part of the internal capsule, the anterior commissure, and the superior part of the lentiform nucleus have been removed. **F.** Lateral ventricle, hippocampus, and diencephalon. The inferior parts of the lentiform nucleus, internal capsule, and caudate nucleus have been removed.

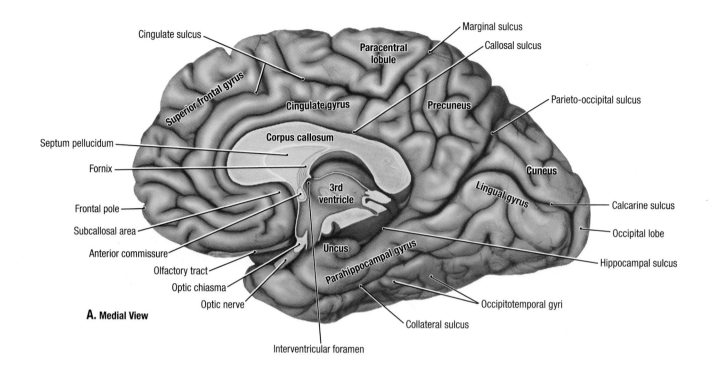

Cingulate sulcus

Paracentral lobule

Marginal sulcus

Callosal sulcus

Superior frontal gyrus

Cingulate gyrus

Precuneus

Parieto-occipital sulcus

Corpus callosum

Septum pellucidum

Fornix

Cuneus

Lingual gyrus

Calcarine sulcus

3rd ventricle

Frontal pole

Subcallosal area

Anterior commissure

Olfactory tract

Optic chiasma

Optic nerve

Uncus

Parahippocampal gyrus

Occipital lobe

Hippocampal sulcus

Occipitotemporal gyri

A. Medial View

Collateral sulcus

Interventricular foramen

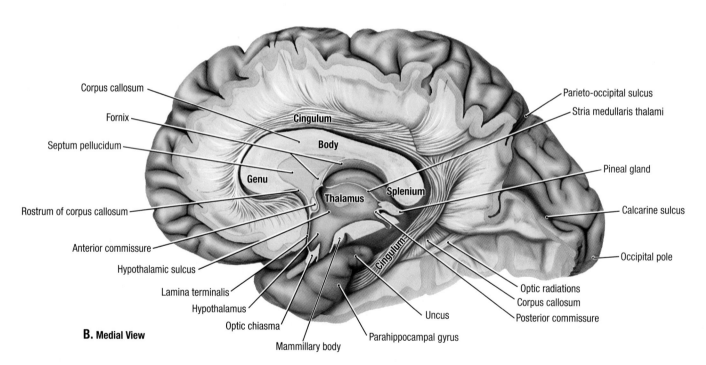

Corpus callosum

Fornix

Septum pellucidum

Cingulum

Body

Parieto-occipital sulcus

Stria medullaris thalami

Genu

Rostrum of corpus callosum

Thalamus

Splenium

Pineal gland

Calcarine sulcus

Anterior commissure

Hypothalamic sulcus

Lamina terminalis

Hypothalamus

Optic chiasma

Cingulum

Occipital pole

Optic radiations

Corpus callosum

Posterior commissure

B. Medial View

Uncus

Parahippocampal gyrus

Mammillary body

7.87   Serial dissections of the medial aspect of cerebral hemisphere

The dissections begin from the medial surface of the cerebral hemisphere (**A**) and proceed sequentially laterally (**B–D**).

A. Sulci and gyri of medial surface of cerebral hemisphere. The corpus callosum consists of the rostrum, genu, body, and splenium; the cingulate and parahippocampal gyri from the limbic lobe. **B.** Cingulum. The cortex and short association fibers were removed from the medial aspect of the hemisphere. The cingulum is a long association fiber bundle that lies in the core of the cingulate and parahippocampal gyri.

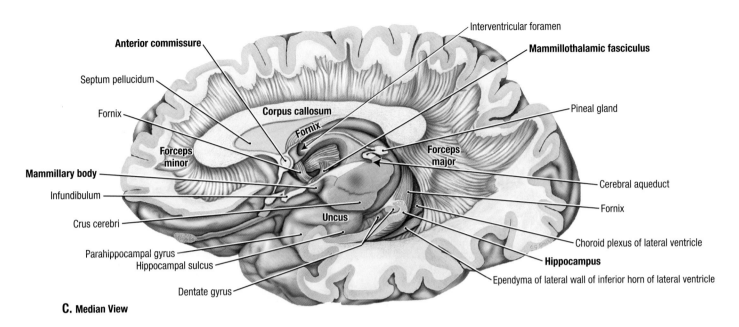

C. Median View

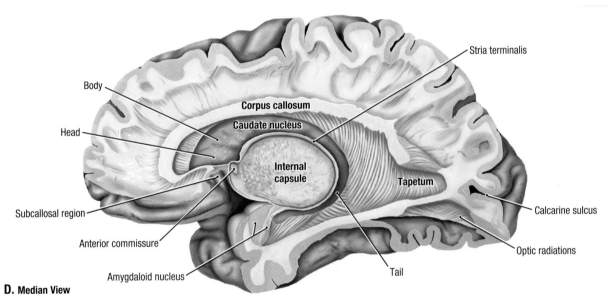

D. Median View

7.87 **Serial dissections of the medial aspect of cerebral hemisphere (continued)**

C. Fornix, mamillothalamic fasciculus, and forceps major and minor. The cingulum and a portion of the wall of the third ventricle have been removed. The fornix begins at the hippocampus and terminates in the mammillary body by passing anterior to the interventricular foramen and posterior to the anterior commissure. The mamillothalamic fasciculus emerges from the mammillary body and terminates in the anterior nucleus of the thalamus. **D.** Caudate nucleus and internal capsule. The diencephalon was removed, along with the ependyma of the lateral ventricle, except where it covers the caudate and amygdaloid nuclei. **E.** Corpus callosum. The body of the corpus callosum connects the two cerebral hemispheres; the minor (frontal) forceps (at the genu of corpus callosum) connects the frontal lobes, and the major (occipital) forceps (at splenium) connects the occipital lobes.

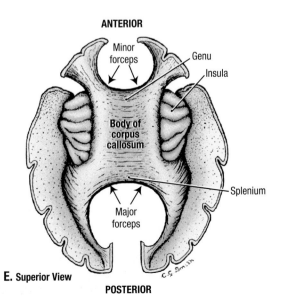

E. Superior View

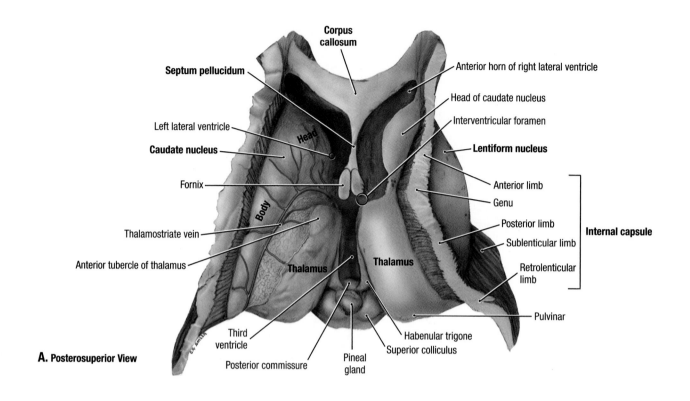

A. Posterosuperior View

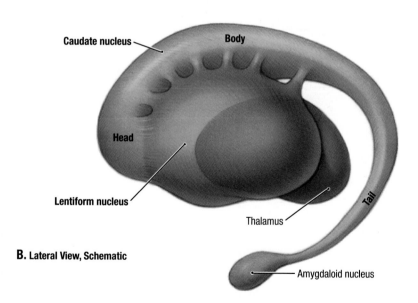

B. Lateral View, Schematic

7.88   **Caudate and lentiform nuclei**

A. Relationship to the lateral ventricles and internal capsule. The dorsal surface of the diencephalon has been exposed by dissecting away the two cerebral hemispheres, except the anterior part of the corpus callosum, the inferior part of the septum pellucidum, the internal capsule, and the caudate and lentiform nuclei. On the right side of the specimen, the thalamus, caudate, and lentiform nuclei have been cut horizontally at the level of the interventricular foramen. The parts of the internal capsule include the anterior, posterior, retrolenticular sublenticular limbs, and genu. **B.** Schematic illustration of nuclei.

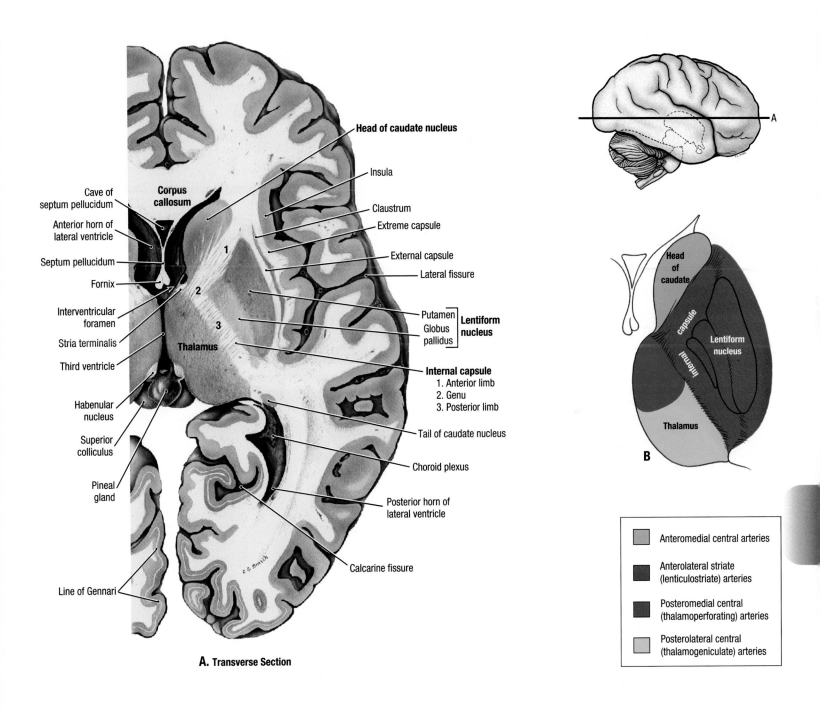

A. **Transverse Section**

Head of caudate nucleus

Insula

Claustrum

Extreme capsule

External capsule

Lateral fissure

Putamen   Lentiform
Globus   nucleus
pallidus

Internal capsule
1. Anterior limb
2. Genu
3. Posterior limb

Tail of caudate nucleus

Choroid plexus

Posterior horn of
lateral ventricle

Calcarine fissure

Cave of
septum pellucidum

Corpus
callosum

Anterior horn of
lateral ventricle

Septum pellucidum

Fornix

Interventricular
foramen

Stria terminalis

Third ventricle

Habenular
nucleus

Superior
colliculus

Pineal
gland

Line of Gennari

1

2

3

Thalamus

Head
of
caudate

Internal capsule

Lentiform
nucleus

Thalamus

B

Anteromedial central arteries

Anterolateral striate
(lenticulostriate) arteries

Posteromedial central
(thalamoperforating) arteries

Posterolateral central
(thalamogeniculate) arteries

7.89   **Axial sections through the thalamus, caudate nucleus, and
lentiform nucleus**

A. Relationships of the internal capsule. **B.** Blood supply of region.

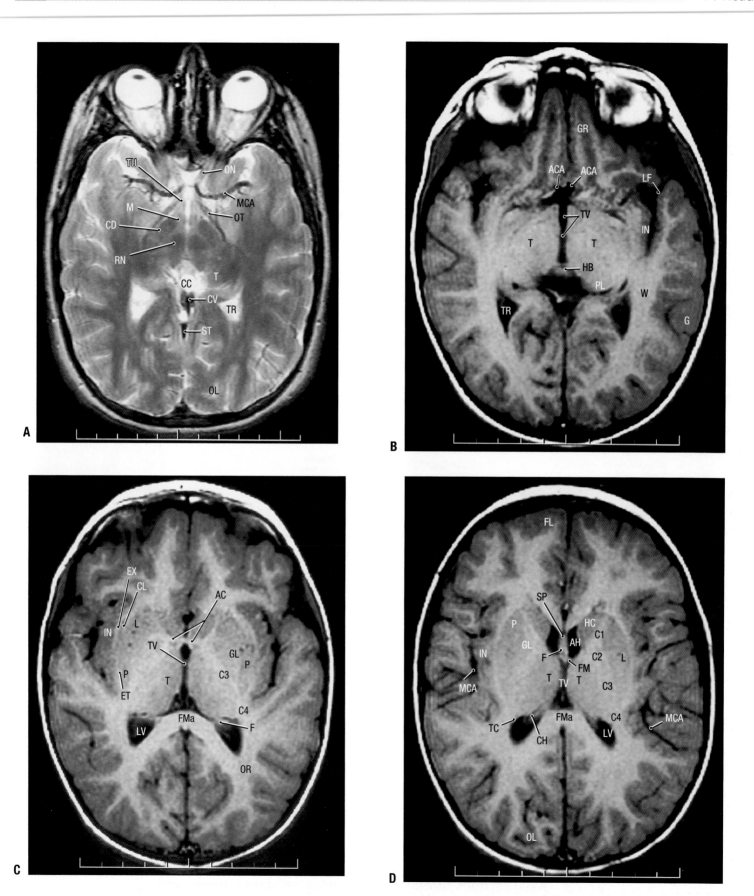

7.90   Axial (transverse) MRIs through the cerebral hemispheres

See orientation drawing for sites of scans **A–F. A** is T2 weighted, and **B–F** are T1 weighted.

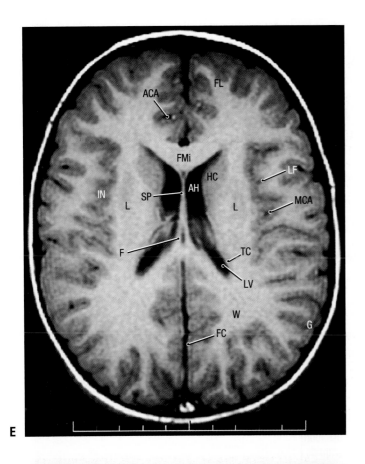

E

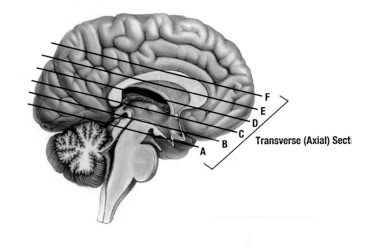

Transverse (Axial) Secti

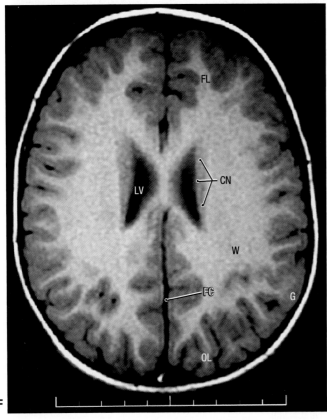

F

AC	Anterior commissure	GL	Globus pallidus
ACA	Anterior cerebral artery	GR	Gyrus rectus
AH	Anterior horn of lateral ventricle	HB	Habenular commissure
C1	Anterior limb of internal capsule	HC	Head of caudate nucleus
		IN	Insular cortex
C2	Genu of internal capsule	L	Lentiform nucleus
C3	Posterior limb of internal capsule	LF	Lateral fissure
		LV	Lateral ventricle
C4	Retrolenticular limb of internal capsule	M	Mammillary body
		MCA	Middle cerebral artery
CC	Collicular cistern	OL	Occipital lobe
CD	Cerebral peduncle	ON	Optic nerve
CH	Choroid plexus	OR	Optic radiations
CL	Claustrum	OT	Optic tract
CN	Caudate nucleus	P	Putamen
CV	Great cerebral vein	PL	Pulvinar
ET	External capsule	RN	Red nucleus
EX	Extreme capsule	SP	Septum pellucidum
F	Fornix	ST	Straight sinus
FC	Falx cerebri	T	Thalamus
FL	Frontal lobe	TC	Tail of caudate nucleus
FM	Interventricular foramen	TR	Trigone of lateral ventricle
FMa	Forceps major	TU	Tuber cinereum
FMi	Forceps minor	TV	Third ventricle
G	Gray matter	W	White matter

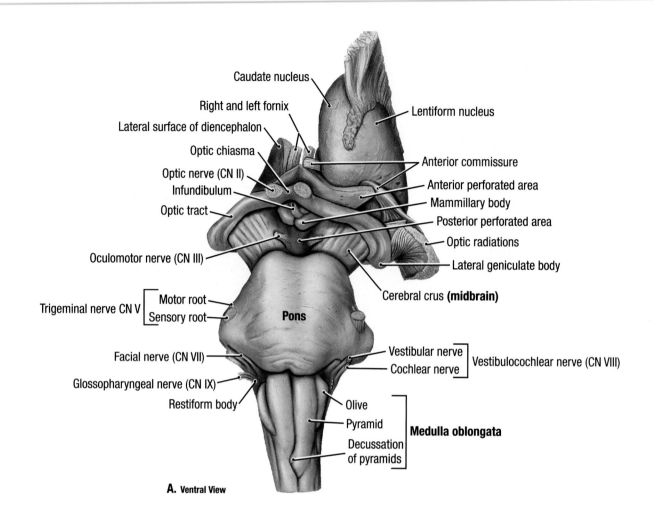

Caudate nucleus

Right and left fornix

Lateral surface of diencephalon

Optic chiasma

Optic nerve (CN II)

Infundibulum

Optic tract

Oculomotor nerve (CN III)

Lentiform nucleus

Anterior commissure

Anterior perforated area

Mammillary body

Posterior perforated area

Optic radiations

Lateral geniculate body

Cerebral crus **(midbrain)**

Trigeminal nerve CN V { Motor root / Sensory root }

Pons

Facial nerve (CN VII)

Glossopharyngeal nerve (CN IX)

Restiform body

Vestibular nerve

Cochlear nerve

Vestibulocochlear nerve (CN VIII)

Olive

Pyramid

Decussation of pyramids

Medulla oblongata

A. Ventral View

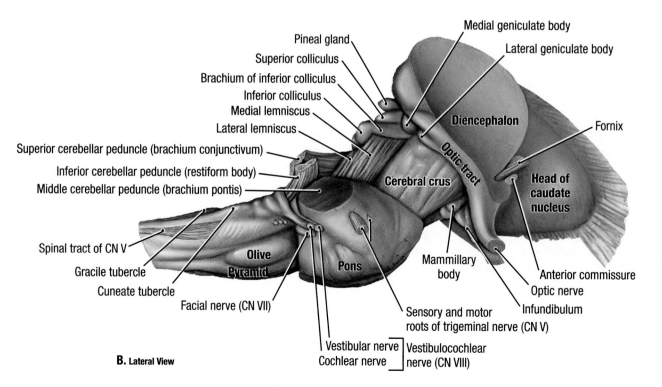

Pineal gland

Superior colliculus

Brachium of inferior colliculus

Inferior colliculus

Medial lemniscus

Lateral lemniscus

Superior cerebellar peduncle (brachium conjunctivum)

Inferior cerebellar peduncle (restiform body)

Middle cerebellar peduncle (brachium pontis)

Medial geniculate body

Lateral geniculate body

Diencephalon

Fornix

Optic tract

Cerebral crus

Head of caudate nucleus

Spinal tract of CN V

Gracile tubercle

Cuneate tubercle

Facial nerve (CN VII)

Olive

Pyramid

Pons

Mammillary body

Anterior commissure

Optic nerve

Infundibulum

Sensory and motor roots of trigeminal nerve (CN V)

Vestibular nerve

Cochlear nerve

Vestibulocochlear nerve (CN VIII)

B. Lateral View

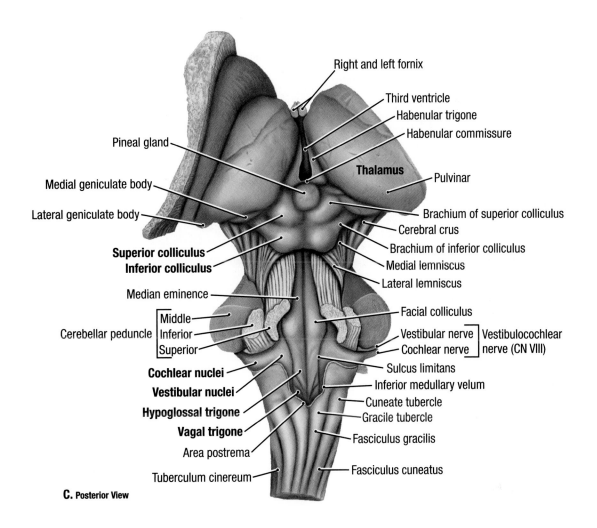

Right and left fornix

Third ventricle

Habenular trigone

Habenular commissure

Pineal gland

Thalamus

Pulvinar

Medial geniculate body

Lateral geniculate body

Brachium of superior colliculus

Cerebral crus

Brachium of inferior colliculus

Superior colliculus

Inferior colliculus

Medial lemniscus

Lateral lemniscus

Median eminence

Facial colliculus

Middle

Inferior

Superior

Cerebellar peduncle

Vestibular nerve

Cochlear nerve

Vestibulocochlear nerve (CN VIII)

Cochlear nuclei

Sulcus limitans

Vestibular nuclei

Inferior medullary velum

Hypoglossal trigone

Cuneate tubercle

Gracile tubercle

Vagal trigone

Fasciculus gracilis

Area postrema

Tuberculum cinereum

Fasciculus cuneatus

C. Posterior View

7.91   **Brainstem**

The brainstem has been exposed by removing the cerebellum, all of the right cerebral hemisphere, and the major portion of the left hemisphere. **A.** Ventral aspect.

- The brainstem consists of the medulla oblongata, pons, and midbrain.
- The pyramid is on the ventral surface of the medulla; the decussation of the pyramids is formed by the decussating (crossing) lateral corticospinal tract.
- The trigeminal nerve (CN V) emerges as sensory and motor roots.
- The crus cerebri are part of the midbrain;
- The oculomotor nerve emerges from the interpeduncular fossa.

B. Lateral aspect.

- The vestibulocochlear nerve (CN VIII) consists of two nerves, the vestibular and cochlear nerves.
- The spinal tract of the trigeminal nerve is exposed where it comes to the surface of the medulla to form the tuber cinereum.
- The three are cerebellar peduncles: superior, middle, and inferior.
- The medial and lateral lemnisci on the lateral aspect of the midbrain

C. Dorsal aspect.

- Ridges are formed by the fasciculus gracilis and cuneatus.
- The gracile and cuneate tubercles are the site of the nucleus cuneatus and nucleus gracilis.
- The diamond-shaped floor of the fourth ventricle; lateral to the sulcus limitans are the vestibular and cochlear nuclei and medially are the hypoglossal and vagal trigones and the facial colliculus.
- The superior and inferior colliculi form the dorsal surface of the midbrain.

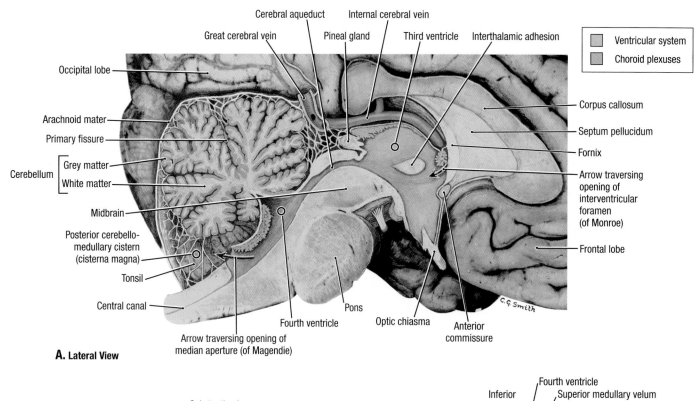

A. Lateral View

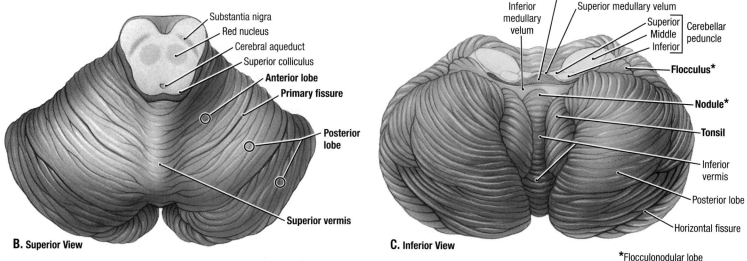

B. Superior View

C. Inferior View

*Flocculonodular lobe

7.92 Cerebellum

A. Median section. The arachnoid mater was removed except where it covered the cerebellum and the occipital lobe. CSF may be obtained, for diagnostic purposes, from the posterior cerebellomedullary cistern, using a procedure known as cisternal puncture. The subarachnoid space or the ventricular system may also be entered for measuring or monitoring CSF pressure, injecting antibiotics, or administering contrast media for radiography. **B.** Superior view of the cerebellum. The right and left cerebellar hemispheres are united by the superior vermis; the anterior and posterior lobes are separated by the primary fissure. **C.** Inferior view of cerebellum. The flocculonodular lobe, the oldest part of the cerebellum, consists of the flocculus and nodule; the cerebellar tonsils typically extend into the foramen magnum.

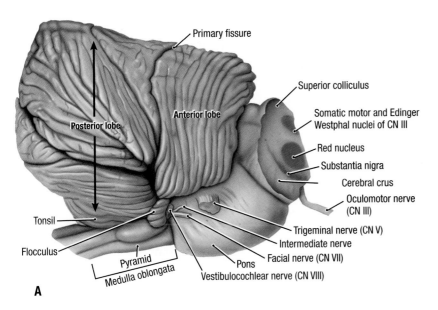

A

Primary fissure

Posterior lobe

Anterior lobe

Superior colliculus

Somatic motor and Edinger
Westphal nuclei of CN III

Red nucleus

Substantia nigra

Cerebral crus

Oculomotor nerve
(CN III)

Tonsil

Flocculus

Pyramid

Medulla oblongata

Pons

Trigeminal nerve (CN V)

Intermediate nerve

Facial nerve (CN VII)

Vestibulocochlear nerve (CN VIII)

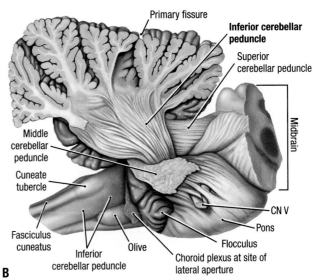

B

Primary fissure

**Inferior cerebellar
peduncle**

Superior
cerebellar peduncle

Middle
cerebellar
peduncle

Cuneate
tubercle

Fasciculus
cuneatus

Inferior
cerebellar peduncle

Olive

Midbrain

CN V

Pons

Flocculus

Choroid plexus at site of
lateral aperture

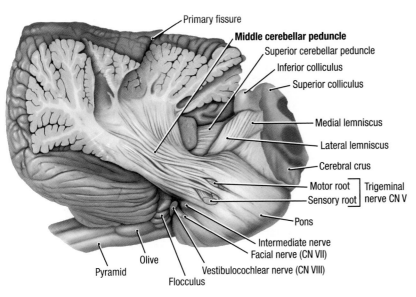

C

Primary fissure

Middle cerebellar peduncle

Superior cerebellar peduncle

Inferior colliculus

Superior colliculus

Medial lemniscus

Lateral lemniscus

Cerebral crus

Motor root ⎤ Trigeminal
Sensory root ⎦ nerve CN V

Pons

Intermediate nerve

Facial nerve (CN VII)

Vestibulocochlear nerve (CN VIII)

Pyramid

Olive

Flocculus

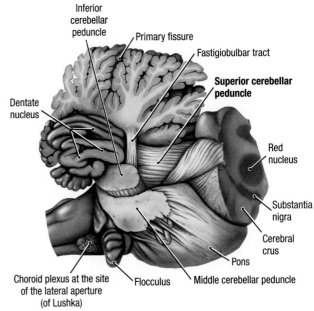

D

Inferior
cerebellar
peduncle

Primary fissure

Fastigiobulbar tract

**Superior cerebellar
peduncle**

Dentate
nucleus

Red
nucleus

Substantia
nigra

Cerebral
crus

Pons

Choroid plexus at the site
of the lateral aperture
(of Lushka)

Flocculus

Middle cerebellar peduncle

Lateral Views

7.93   Serial dissections of the cerebellum

The series begins with the lateral surface of the cerebellar hemispheres (**A**) and proceeds medially in sequence (**B–D**).

A. Cerebellum and brainstem. **B.** Inferior cerebellar peduncle. The fibers of the middle cerebellar peduncle were cut dorsal to the trigeminal nerve and peeled away to expose the fibers of the inferior cerebellar peduncle. **C.** Middle cerebellar peduncle. The fibers of the middle cerebellar peduncle were exposed by peeling away the lateral portion of the lobules of the cerebellar hemisphere. **D.** Superior cerebellar peduncle and dentate nucleus. The fibers of the inferior cerebellar peduncle were cut just dorsal to the previously sectioned middle cerebellar peduncle and peeled away until the gray matter of the dentate nucleus could be seen.

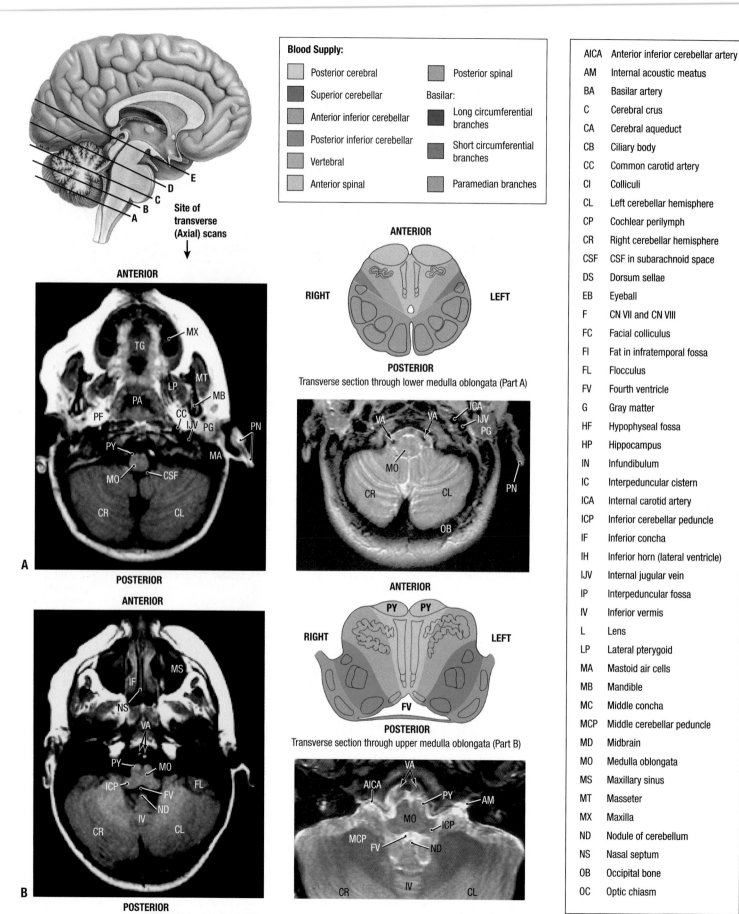

Site of transverse (Axial) scans

Blood Supply:

Posterior cerebral
Superior cerebellar
Anterior inferior cerebellar
Posterior inferior cerebellar
Vertebral
Anterior spinal

Posterior spinal

Basilar:
Long circumferential branches
Short circumferential branches
Paramedian branches

AICA	Anterior inferior cerebellar artery
AM	Internal acoustic meatus
BA	Basilar artery
C	Cerebral crus
CA	Cerebral aqueduct
CB	Ciliary body
CC	Common carotid artery
CI	Colliculi
CL	Left cerebellar hemisphere
CP	Cochlear perilymph
CR	Right cerebellar hemisphere
CSF	CSF in subarachnoid space
DS	Dorsum sellae
EB	Eyeball
F	CN VII and CN VIII
FC	Facial colliculus
FI	Fat in infratemporal fossa
FL	Flocculus
FV	Fourth ventricle
G	Gray matter
HF	Hypophyseal fossa
HP	Hippocampus
IN	Infundibulum
IC	Interpeduncular cistern
ICA	Internal carotid artery
ICP	Inferior cerebellar peduncle
IF	Inferior concha
IH	Inferior horn (lateral ventricle)
IJV	Internal jugular vein
IP	Interpeduncular fossa
IV	Inferior vermis
L	Lens
LP	Lateral pterygoid
MA	Mastoid air cells
MB	Mandible
MC	Middle concha
MCP	Middle cerebellar peduncle
MD	Midbrain
MO	Medulla oblongata
MS	Maxillary sinus
MT	Masseter
MX	Maxilla
ND	Nodule of cerebellum
NS	Nasal septum
OB	Occipital bone
OC	Optic chiasm

Transverse section through lower medulla oblongata (Part A)

Transverse section through upper medulla oblongata (Part B)

7.94 Axial (transverse) MRIs through the brainstem, inferior views

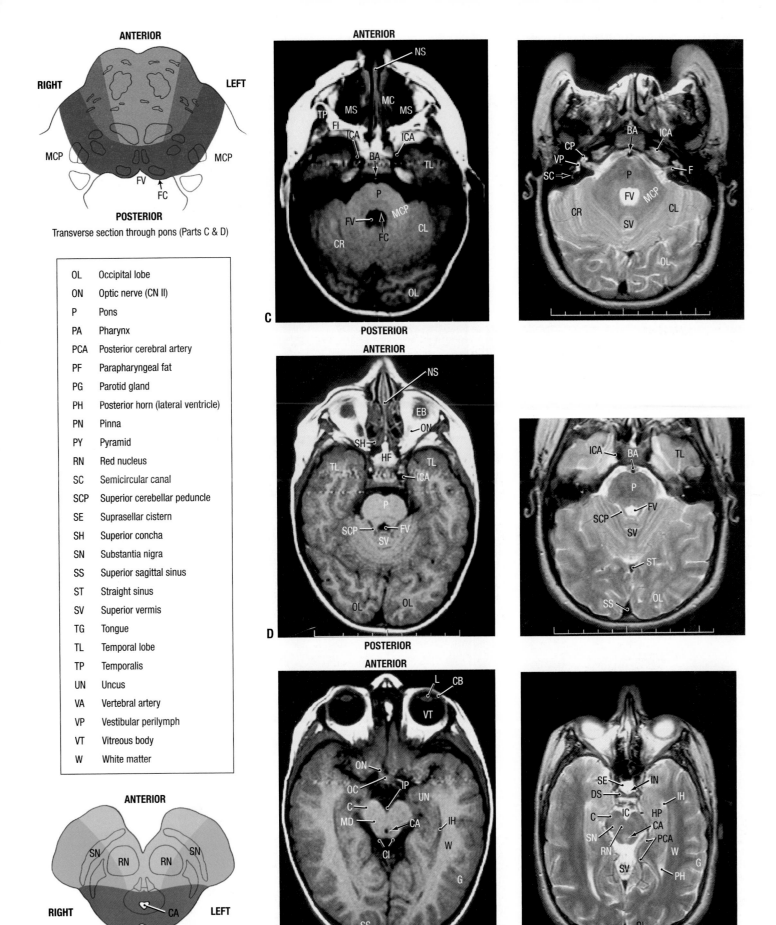

ANTERIOR

RIGHT — LEFT

MCP — MCP

FV

FC

POSTERIOR

Transverse section through pons (Parts C & D)

OL	Occipital lobe
ON	Optic nerve (CN II)
P	Pons
PA	Pharynx
PCA	Posterior cerebral artery
PF	Parapharyngeal fat
PG	Parotid gland
PH	Posterior horn (lateral ventricle)
PN	Pinna
PY	Pyramid
RN	Red nucleus
SC	Semicircular canal
SCP	Superior cerebellar peduncle
SE	Suprasellar cistern
SH	Superior concha
SN	Substantia nigra
SS	Superior sagittal sinus
ST	Straight sinus
SV	Superior vermis
TG	Tongue
TL	Temporal lobe
TP	Temporalis
UN	Uncus
VA	Vertebral artery
VP	Vestibular perilymph
VT	Vitreous body
W	White matter

ANTERIOR

SN — SN
RN — RN

RIGHT — CA — LEFT

POSTERIOR

Transverse section through midbrain (Part E)

7.94   Axial (transverse) MRIs through the brainstem, inferior views *(continued)*

Images on left side of page are T1 weighted, and images on the right side are T2 weighted.

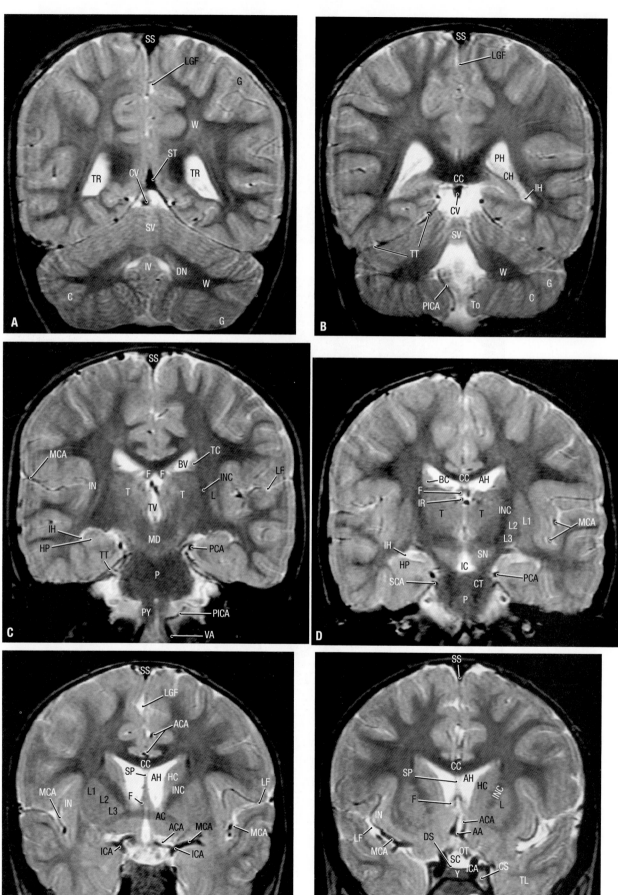

AA Anterior communicating artery
AC Anterior commissure
ACA Anterior cerebral artery
AH Anterior horn of lateral ventricle
BC Body of caudate nucleus
BV Body of lateral ventricle
C Cerebellum
CC Corpus callosum
CH Choroid plexus
CS Cavernous sinus
CT Corticospinal tract
CV Great cerebral vein
DN Dentate nucleus
DS Diaphragma sellae
F Fornix
FV Fourth ventricle
G Gray matter
HC Head of caudate nucleus
HP Hippocampus
IC Interpeduncular cistern
ICA Internal carotid artery
IH Interior horn of lateral ventricle
IN Insular cortex
INC Internal capsule
IR Intervertebral vein
IV Inferior vermis
L Lentiform nucleus
L1 Putamen
L2 External (lateral) segment of
     globus pallidus
L3 Internal (medial) segment of
     globus pallidus
LF Lateral fissure
LGF Longitudinal fissure
MCA Middle cerebral artery
MD Midbrain
OT Optic tract
P Pons
PCA Posterior cerebral artery
PH Posterior horn of lateral ventricle
PICA Posterior inferior cerebellar artery
PY Pyramid
S Carotid siphon
SC Supracellebellar cistern
SCA Superior cerebellar artery
SN Substantia nigra
SP Septum pellucidum
SS Superior sagittal sinus
ST Straight sinus
SV Superior vermis
T Thalamus
TC Tail of caudate nucleus
TL Temporal lobe
To Cerebellar tonsil
TR Trigone of lateral ventricle
TT Tentorium cerebelli
TV Third ventricle
VA Vertebral artery
W White matter
Y Hypophysis

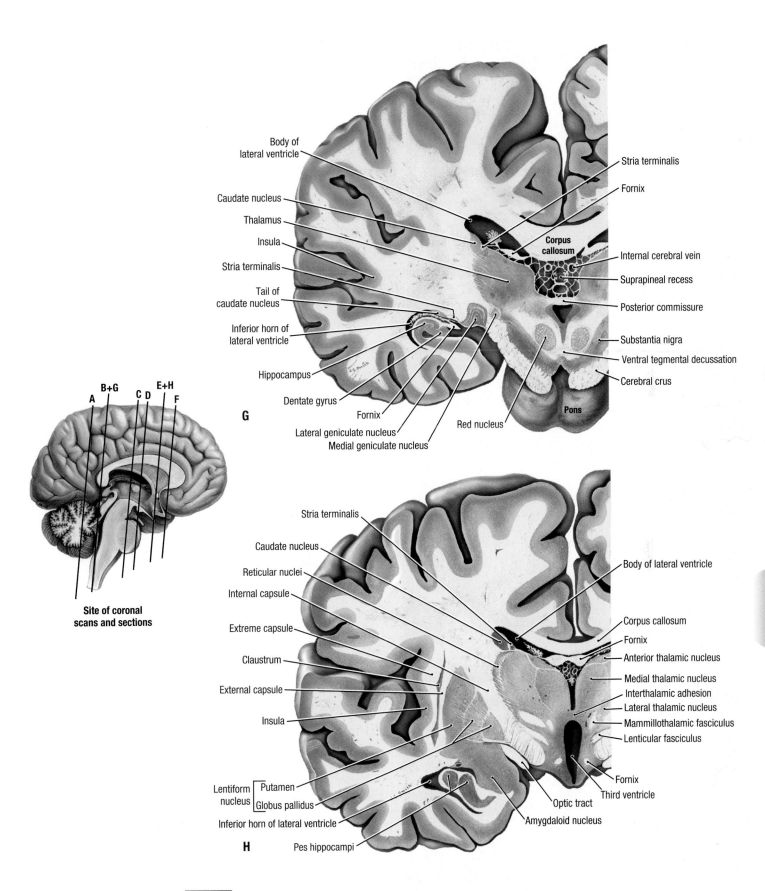

Body of lateral ventricle

Caudate nucleus

Thalamus

Insula

Stria terminalis

Tail of caudate nucleus

Inferior horn of lateral ventricle

Hippocampus

Dentate gyrus

Fornix

Lateral geniculate nucleus

Medial geniculate nucleus

Stria terminalis

Fornix

Corpus callosum

Internal cerebral vein

Suprapineal recess

Posterior commissure

Substantia nigra

Ventral tegmental decussation

Cerebral crus

Red nucleus

Pons

G

A   B+G   C D   E+H   F

Site of coronal scans and sections

Stria terminalis

Caudate nucleus

Reticular nuclei

Internal capsule

Extreme capsule

Claustrum

External capsule

Insula

Lentiform nucleus { Putamen / Globus pallidus }

Inferior horn of lateral ventricle

Body of lateral ventricle

Corpus callosum

Fornix

Anterior thalamic nucleus

Medial thalamic nucleus

Interthalamic adhesion

Lateral thalamic nucleus

Mammillothalamic fasciculus

Lenticular fasciculus

Fornix

Third ventricle

Optic tract

Amygdaloid nucleus

Pes hippocampi

H

7.95   Coronal MRIs (T2 weighted) and sections of brain

A–F. Coronal MRIs. **G–H.** Coronal sections, posterior views.

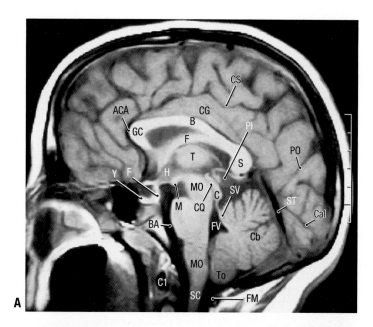

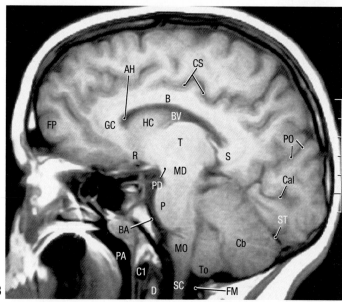

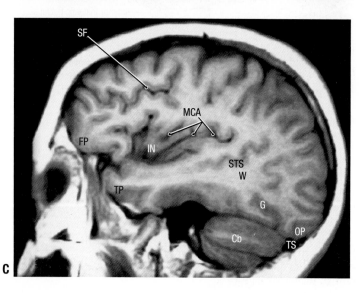

ACA	Anterior cerebral artery
AH	Anterior horn of lateral ventricle
B	Body of corpus callosum
BA	Basilar artery
BV	Body of lateral ventricle
C	Colliculi
C1	Anterior tubercle of atlas
Cal	Calcarine sulcus
Cb	Cerebellum
CG	Cingulate nucleus
CQ	Cerebral aqueduct
CS	Cingulate sulcus
D	Dens (odontoid process)
F	Fornix
FM	Foramen magnum
FP	Frontal pole
FV	Fourth ventricle
G	Cerebral cortex (gray matter)
GC	Genus of corpus callosum
H	Hypothalamus
HC	Head of caudate nucleus
I	Infundibulum
IN	Insular cortex
M	Mammillary body
MCA	Middle cerebral artery
MD	Midbrain
OP	Occipital pole
P	Pons
PA	Pharynx
PD	Cerebral peduncle
PI	Pineal
PO	Parieto-occipital fissure
R	Rostrum of corpus callosum
S	Splenium of corpus callosum
SC	Spinal cord
SF	Superior frontal sulcus
ST	Straight sinus
STS	Superior temporal sulcus
SV	Superior medullary vellum
T	Thalamus
To	Cerebral tonsil
TP	Temporal pole
TS	Transverse sinus
W	White matter
Y	Hypophysis

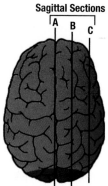

Sagittal Sections

7.96   **Sagittal MRIs (T1 weighted) and median section of brain**

See orientation drawing for sites of scans **A–C.**

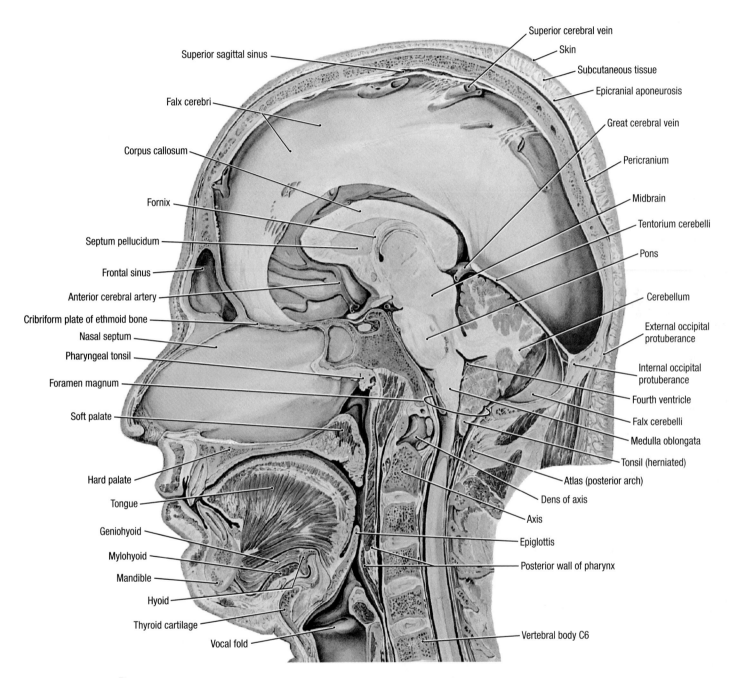

Superior cerebral vein
Skin
Superior sagittal sinus
Subcutaneous tissue
Epicranial aponeurosis
Falx cerebri
Great cerebral vein
Corpus callosum
Pericranium
Fornix
Midbrain
Tentorium cerebelli
Septum pellucidum
Pons
Frontal sinus
Anterior cerebral artery
Cerebellum
Cribriform plate of ethmoid bone
External occipital
protuberance
Nasal septum
Pharyngeal tonsil
Internal occipital
protuberance
Foramen magnum
Fourth ventricle
Soft palate
Falx cerebelli
Medulla oblongata
Hard palate
Tonsil (herniated)
Atlas (posterior arch)
Tongue
Dens of axis
Geniohyoid
Axis
Mylohyoid
Epiglottis
Mandible
Posterior wall of pharynx
Hyoid
Thyroid cartilage
Vocal fold
Vertebral body C6

D. Median Section

7.96 **Sagittal MRIs (T1 weighted) and median section of brain** *(continued)*

Increased intracranial pressure (e.g., due to a tumor) may cause displacement of the cerebellar tonsils through the foramen magnum, resulting in a formial (tonsillar) herniation. Compression of the brainstem, if severe, may result in respiratory and cardiac arrest.

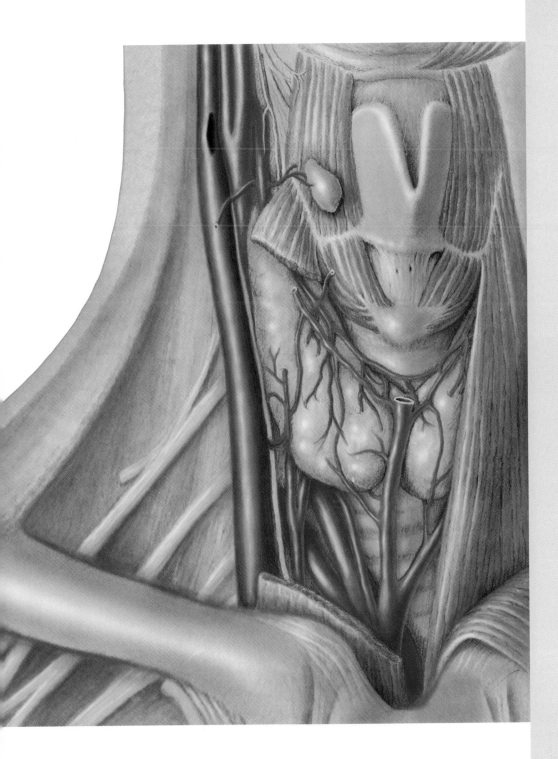

- Subcutaneous Structures and Cervical Fascia **746**
- Skeleton of Neck **750**
- Regions of Neck **752**
  - Lateral Region (Posterior Triangle) of Neck **754**
  - Anterior Region (Anterior Triangle) of Neck **758**
    - Neurovascular Structures of Neck **762**
    - Visceral Compartment of Neck **768**
    - Root and Prevertebral Region of Neck **772**
    - Submandibular Region and Floor of Mouth **778**
  - Posterior Cervical Region **783**
- Pharynx **786**
- Isthmus of Fauces **792**
- Larynx **798**
- Sectional Anatomy and Imaging of Neck **806**

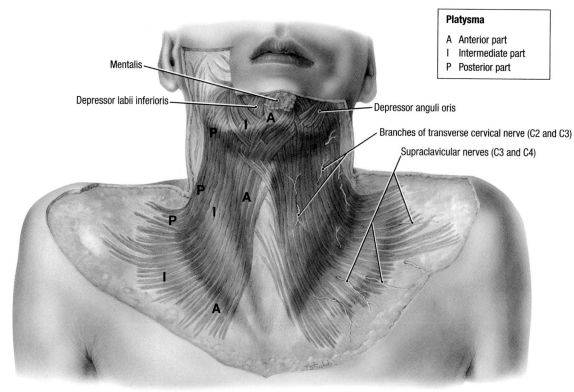

Platysma
A   Anterior part
I   Intermediate part
P   Posterior part

Mentalis

Depressor labii inferioris

Depressor anguli oris

Branches of transverse cervical nerve (C2 and C3)

Supraclavicular nerves (C3 and C4)

A. Anterior View

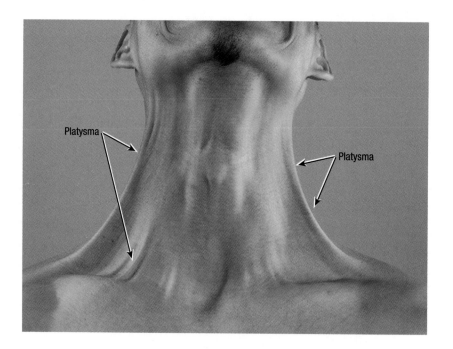

Platysma

Platysma

TABLE 8.1 PLATYSMA

Muscle	Superior Attachment	Inferior Attachment	Innervation	Main Action
Platysma	*Anterior part:* Fibers interlace with contra-lateral muscle *Intermediate part:* Fibers pass deep to depressors anguli oris and labii inferioris to attach to inferior border of mandible *Posterior part:* Skin/subcutaneous tissue of lower face lateral to mouth	Subcutaneous tissue overlying superior parts of pectoralis major and sometimes deltoid muscles	Cervical branch of facial nerve (CN VII)	Draws corner of mouth inferiorly and widens it as in expressions of sadness and fright; draws the skin of the neck superiorly, forming tense vertical and oblique ridges over the anterior neck

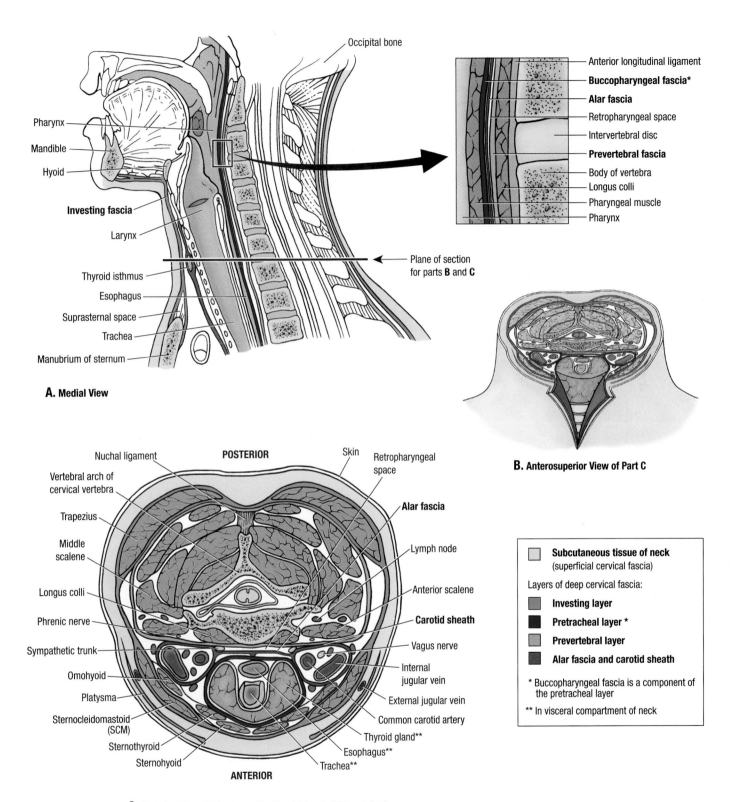

A. Medial View

Occipital bone

Pharynx
Mandible
Hyoid

Investing fascia

Larynx

Thyroid isthmus
Esophagus
Suprasternal space
Trachea
Manubrium of sternum

Plane of section
for parts **B** and **C**

Anterior longitudinal ligament
Buccopharyngeal fascia*
Alar fascia
Retropharyngeal space
Intervertebral disc
Prevertebral fascia
Body of vertebra
Longus colli
Pharyngeal muscle
Pharynx

B. Anterosuperior View of Part C

Nuchal ligament   **POSTERIOR**   Skin   Retropharyngeal space

Vertebral arch of cervical vertebra
Trapezius
Middle scalene
Longus colli
Phrenic nerve
Sympathetic trunk
Omohyoid
Platysma
Sternocleidomastoid (SCM)
Sternothyroid
Sternohyoid

Alar fascia
Lymph node
Anterior scalene
Carotid sheath
Vagus nerve
Internal jugular vein
External jugular vein
Common carotid artery
Thyroid gland**
Esophagus**
Trachea**

ANTERIOR

☐ **Subcutaneous tissue of neck**
(superficial cervical fascia)

Layers of deep cervical fascia:

■ **Investing layer**
■ **Pretracheal layer ***
■ **Prevertebral layer**
■ **Alar fascia and carotid sheath**

* Buccopharyngeal fascia is a component of the pretracheal layer

** In visceral compartment of neck

C. Superior View of Transverse Section (at level of C7 vertebra)

8.1   **Subcutaneous tissue and deep fascia of neck**

Sectional demonstrations of the fasciae of the neck. **A.** Fasciae of the neck are continuous inferiorly and superiorly with thoracic and cranial fasciae. The *inset* illustrates the fascia of the retropharyngeal region. **B.** Relationship of the main layers of deep cervical fascia and the carotid sheath. Midline access to the cervical viscera is possible with minimal disruption of tissues. **C.** The concentric layers of fascia are apparent in this transverse section of neck at the level indicated in **A.**

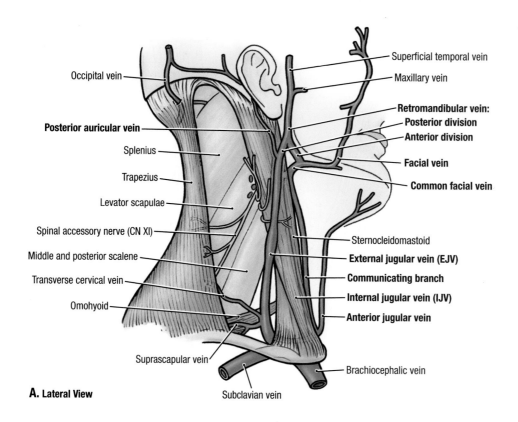

Occipital vein

Posterior auricular vein

Splenius

Trapezius

Levator scapulae

Spinal accessory nerve (CN XI)

Middle and posterior scalene

Transverse cervical vein

Omohyoid

Suprascapular vein

Superficial temporal vein

Maxillary vein

Retromandibular vein:
Posterior division
Anterior division

Facial vein

Common facial vein

Sternocleidomastoid

External jugular vein (EJV)

Communicating branch

Internal jugular vein (IJV)

Anterior jugular vein

Brachiocephalic vein

Subclavian vein

A. Lateral View

8.2   Superficial veins of the neck

A. Schematic illustration of superficial veins of the neck. The superficial temporal and maxillary veins merge to form the retromandibular vein. The posterior division of the retromandibular vein unites with the posterior auricular vein to form the external jugular vein (EJV). The facial vein receives the anterior division of the retromandibular vein, forming the common facial vein that empties into the internal jugular vein. **B.** Surface anatomy of the external jugular vein and the muscles bounding the lateral cervical region (posterior triangle) of the neck.

The EJV may serve as an "internal barometer." When venous pressure is in the normal range, the EJV is usually visible superior to the clavicle for only a short distance. However, when venous pressure rises (e.g., as in heart failure) the vein is prominent throughout its course along the side of the neck. Consequently, routine observation for distention of the EJVs during physical examinations may reveal diagnostic signs of heart failure, obstruction of the superior vena cava, enlarged supraclavicular lymph nodes, or increased intrathoracic pressure.

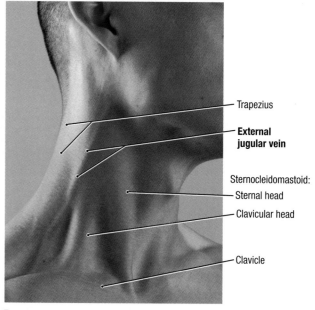

Trapezius

External
jugular vein

Sternocleidomastoid:
Sternal head
Clavicular head

Clavicle

B. Lateral View

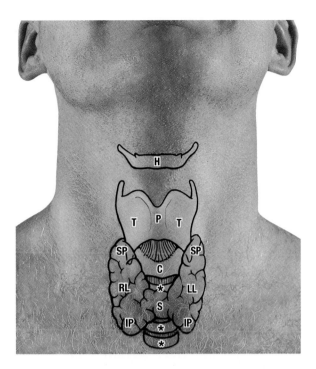

Anterior View

C	Cricoid cartilage	RL	Right lobe of thyroid gland
H	Hyoid	S	Isthmus
IP	Inferior pole of thyroid gland	SP	Superior pole of thyroid gland
LL	Left lobe of thyroid gland	T	Thyroid cartilage
P	Laryngeal prominence	★	Tracheal rings

8.3   Surface anatomy of hyoid and cartilages of anterior neck

The U-shaped hyoid lies superior to the thyroid cartilage at the level of the C4 and C5 vertebrae. The laryngeal prominence is produced by the fused laminae of the thyroid cartilage, which meet in the median plane. The cricoid cartilage can be felt inferior to the laryngeal prominence. It lies at the level of the C6 vertebra. The cartilaginous tracheal rings are palpable in the inferior part of the neck. The 2nd–4th rings cannot be felt because the isthmus of the thyroid, connecting its right and left lobes, covers them. The first tracheal ring is just superior to the isthmus.

Tracheostomy

A transverse incision through the skin of the neck and anterior wall of the trachea (*tracheostomy*) establishes an airway in patients with upper airway obstruction or respiratory failure. The infrahyoid muscles are retracted laterally, and the isthmus of the thyroid gland is either divided or retracted superiorly. An opening is made in the trachea between the 1st and 2nd tracheal rings or through the 2nd through 4th rings. A *tracheostomy tube* is then inserted into the trachea and secured. To avoid complications during a tracheostomy, the following anatomical relationships are important:

- The *inferior thyroid veins* arise from a venous plexus on the thyroid gland and descend anterior to the trachea (see Fig. 8.13).
- A small *thyroid ima artery* is present in approximately 10% of people; it ascends from the brachiocephalic trunk or the arch of the aorta to the isthmus of the thyroid gland (see Fig. 8.15).
- The *left brachiocephalic vein*, jugular venous arch, and pleurae may be encountered, particularly in infants and children.
- The *thymus* covers the inferior part of the trachea in infants and children.
- The trachea is small, mobile, and soft in infants, making it easy to cut through its posterior wall and damage the esophagus.

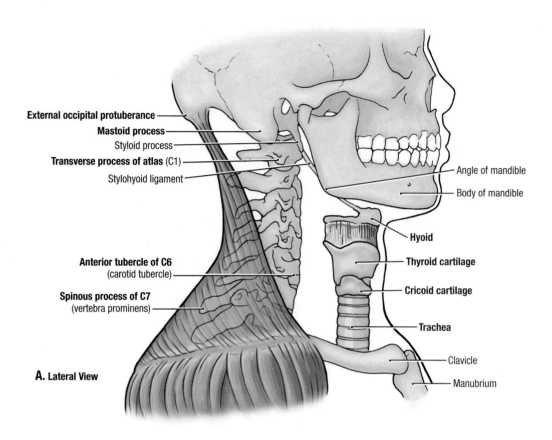

External occipital protuberance
Mastoid process
Styloid process
Transverse process of atlas (C1)
Stylohyoid ligament

Angle of mandible
Body of mandible

Hyoid

Anterior tubercle of C6
(carotid tubercle)

Thyroid cartilage

Spinous process of C7
(vertebra prominens)

Cricoid cartilage

Trachea

Clavicle

Manubrium

A. Lateral View

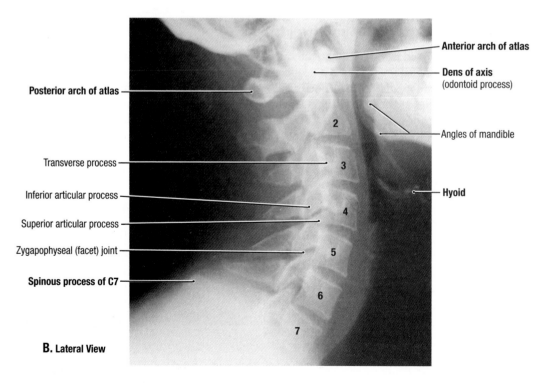

Anterior arch of atlas

Dens of axis
(odontoid process)

Posterior arch of atlas

Angles of mandible

Transverse process

Inferior articular process

Hyoid

Superior articular process

Zygapophyseal (facet) joint

Spinous process of C7

B. Lateral View

8.4   **Bones and cartilages of the neck**

A. Bony and cartilaginous landmarks of the neck. **B.** Radiograph of hyoid bone and cervical vertebrae. Because the upper cervical vertebrae lie posterior to the upper and lower jaws and teeth, they are best seen radiographically in lateral views.

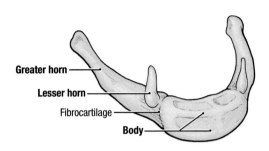

C. Right Anterolateral View of Hyoid

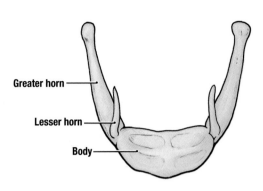

D. Anterosuperior View of Hyoid

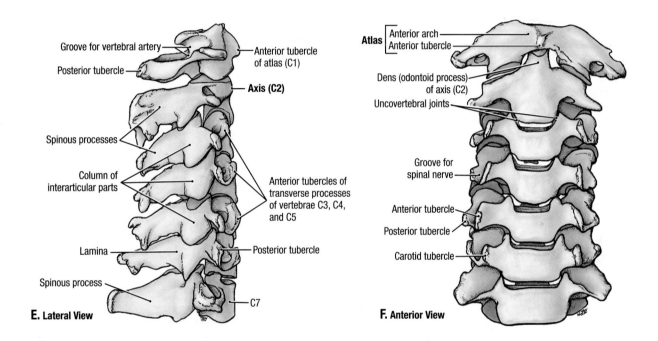

E. Lateral View

F. Anterior View

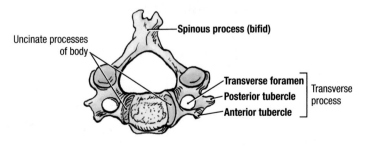

G. Superior View of Typical Cervical Vertebra (e.g., C4)

8.4 **Bones and cartilages of the neck** *(continued)*

C and **D.** Features of hyoid bone. **E** and **F.** Articulated cervical vertebrae. **G.** Features of typical cervical vertebrae.

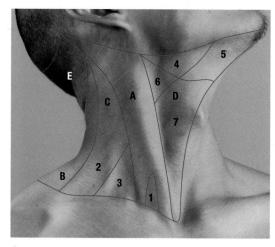

A Anterolateral view

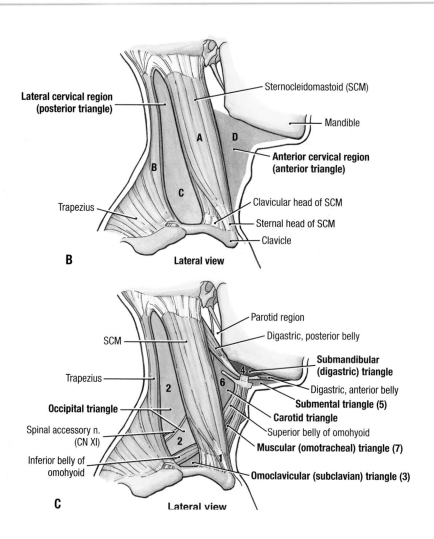

TABLE 8.2 CERVICAL REGIONS AND CONTENTS[a]

Region	Main Contents and Underlying Structures
Sternocleidomastoid region (A)	Sternocleidomastoid (SCM) muscle; superior part of the external jugular vein; greater auricular nerve; transverse cervical nerve
Lesser supraclavicular fossa (1)	Inferior part of internal jugular vein
Posterior cervical region (B)	Trapezius muscle; cutaneous branches of posterior rami of cervical spinal nerves; suboccipital region (E) lies deep to superior part of this region
Lateral cervical region (posterior triangle) (C) Occipital triangle (2)	Part of external jugular vein; posterior branches of cervical plexus of nerves; spinal accessory nerve; trunks of brachial plexus; transverse cervical artery; cervical lymph nodes
Omoclavicular triangle	Subclavian artery (3rd part); part of subclavian vein (variable); suprascapular artery; supraclavicular lymph nodes
Anterior cervical region (anterior triangle) (D) Submandibular (digastric) triangle (4)	Submandibular gland almost fills triangle; submandibular lymph nodes; hypoglossal nerve; mylohyoid nerve; parts of facial artery and vein
Submental triangle (5)	Submental lymph nodes and small veins that unite to form anterior jugular vein
Carotid triangle (6)	Common carotid artery and its branches; internal jugular vein and its tributaries; vagus nerve; external carotid artery and some of its branches; hypoglossal nerve and superior root of ansa cervicalis; spinal accessory nerve; thyroid gland, larynx, and pharynx; deep cervical lymph nodes; branches of cervical plexus
Muscular (omotracheal) triangle (7)	Sternothyroid and sternohyoid muscles; thyroid and parathyroid glands

[a]Letters and numbers in parentheses refer to Figures A and B.

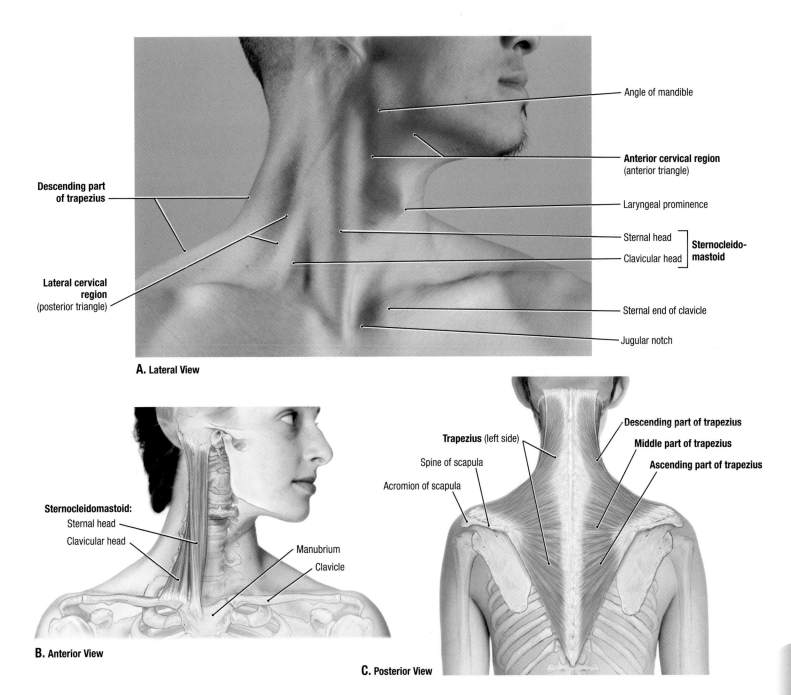

A. Lateral View

B. Anterior View

C. Posterior View

Labels for A (Lateral View):
- Descending part of trapezius
- Lateral cervical region (posterior triangle)
- Angle of mandible
- **Anterior cervical region** (anterior triangle)
- Laryngeal prominence
- Sternal head
- Clavicular head
- **Sternocleido-mastoid**
- Sternal end of clavicle
- Jugular notch

Labels for B (Anterior View):
- Sternocleidomastoid:
  - Sternal head
  - Clavicular head
- Manubrium
- Clavicle

Labels for C (Posterior View):
- **Trapezius** (left side)
- Spine of scapula
- Acromion of scapula
- **Descending part of trapezius**
- **Middle part of trapezius**
- **Ascending part of trapezius**

TABLE 8.3 STERNOCLEIDOMASTOID AND TRAPEZIUS

Muscle	Superior Attachment	Inferior Attachment	Innervation	Main Action
Sternocleidomastoid	Lateral surface of mastoid process of temporal bone; lateral half of superior nuchal line	*Sternal head:* anterior surface of manubrium of sternum *Clavicular head:* superior surface of medial third of clavicle	Spinal accessory nerve (CN XI) [motor] and C2 and C3 nerves (pain and proprioception)	*Unilateral contraction:* laterally flexes neck; rotates neck so face is turned superiorly toward opposite side; *Bilateral contraction:* (1) extends neck at atlanto-occipital joints, (2) flexes cervical vertebrae so that chin approaches manubrium, or (3) extends superior cervical vertebrae while flexing inferior vertebrae, so chin is thrust forward with head kept level; with cervical vertebrae fixed, may elevate manubrium and medial end of clavicles, assisting deep respiration.
Trapezius	Medial third of superior nuchal line, external occipital protuberance, nuchal ligament, spinous processes of C7–T12 vertebrae, lumbar and sacral spinous processes	Lateral third of clavicle, acromion, spine of scapula	Spinal accessory nerve (CN XI) [motor] and C2 and C3 nerves (pain and proprioception)	*Superior fibers* elevate pectoral girdle, maintain level of shoulders against gravity or resistance; *middle fibers* retract scapula; and *inferior fibers* depress shoulders; *superior* and *inferior fibers* work together to rotate scapula upward; *when shoulders are fixed,* bilateral contraction extends neck; unilateral contraction produces lateral flexion to same

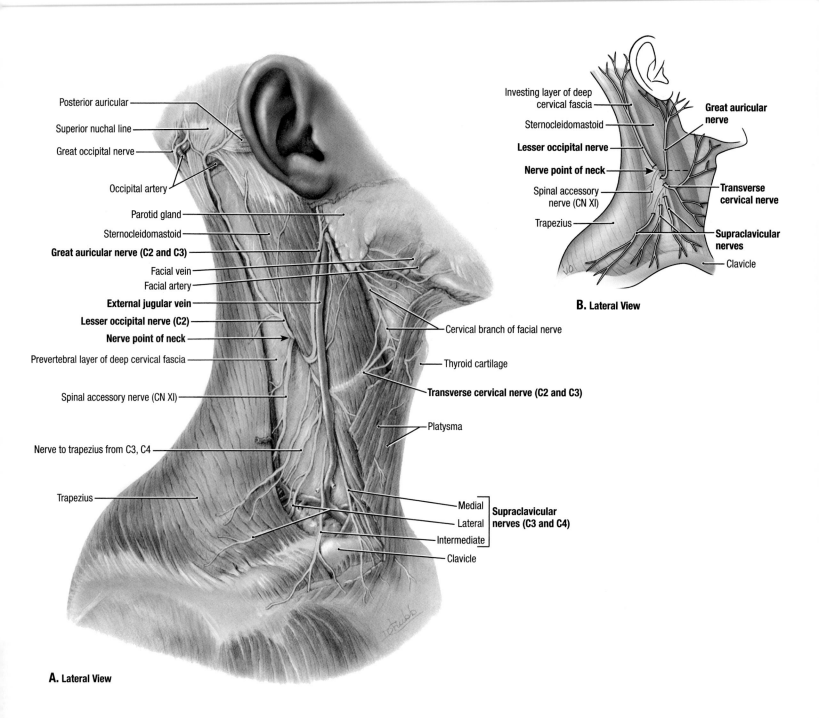

Posterior auricular

Superior nuchal line

Great occipital nerve

Occipital artery

Parotid gland

Sternocleidomastoid

Great auricular nerve (C2 and C3)

Facial vein

Facial artery

External jugular vein

Lesser occipital nerve (C2)

Nerve point of neck

Prevertebral layer of deep cervical fascia

Spinal accessory nerve (CN XI)

Nerve to trapezius from C3, C4

Trapezius

Cervical branch of facial nerve

Thyroid cartilage

Transverse cervical nerve (C2 and C3)

Platysma

Medial
Lateral   **Supraclavicular nerves (C3 and C4)**
Intermediate

Clavicle

A. Lateral View

Investing layer of deep cervical fascia

Sternocleidomastoid

Lesser occipital nerve

Nerve point of neck

Spinal accessory nerve (CN XI)

Trapezius

Great auricular nerve

Transverse cervical nerve

Supraclavicular nerves

Clavicle

B. Lateral View

8.5   Serial dissection of lateral cervical region (posterior triangle of neck)

A. External jugular vein and cutaneous branches of cervical plexus. Subcutaneous fat, the part of the plasma overlying the inferior part of the lateral cervical region, and the investing layer of deep cervical fascia have all been removed. The external jugular vein descends vertically across the sternocleidomastoid and pierces the prevertebral layer of deep cervical fascia superior to the clavicle.

B and **C.** Branches of the cervical plexus
• Branches arising from the nerve loop between the anterior rami of C2 and C3 are the lesser occipital, great auricular, and transverse cervical nerves.

• Branches arising from the loop formed between the anterior rami of C3 and C4 are the supraclavicular nerves, which emerge as a common trunk under cover of the SCM.

Regional anesthesia is often used for surgical procedures in the neck region or upper limb. In a cervical plexus block, an anesthetic agent is injected at several points along the posterior border of the SCM, mainly at its midpoint, the nerve point of the neck.

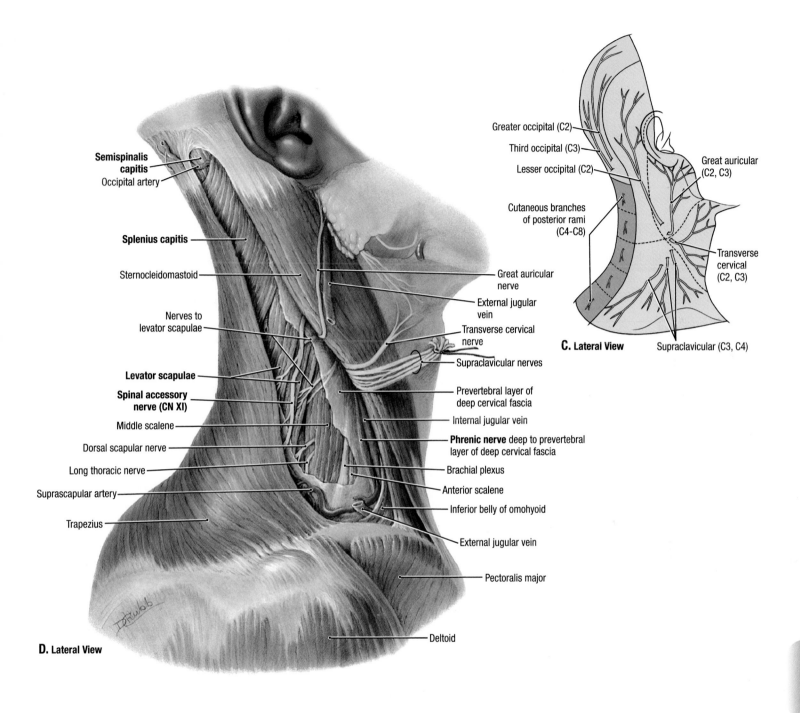

Semispinalis capitis
Occipital artery
Splenius capitis
Sternocleidomastoid
Nerves to levator scapulae
Levator scapulae
Spinal accessory nerve (CN XI)
Middle scalene
Dorsal scapular nerve
Long thoracic nerve
Suprascapular artery
Trapezius

Great auricular nerve
External jugular vein
Transverse cervical nerve
Supraclavicular nerves
Prevertebral layer of deep cervical fascia
Internal jugular vein
Phrenic nerve deep to prevertebral layer of deep cervical fascia
Brachial plexus
Anterior scalene
Inferior belly of omohyoid
External jugular vein
Pectoralis major
Deltoid

D. Lateral View

Greater occipital (C2)
Third occipital (C3)
Lesser occipital (C2)
Cutaneous branches of posterior rami (C4-C8)
Great auricular (C2, C3)
Transverse cervical (C2, C3)
Supraclavicular (C3, C4)

C. Lateral View

| **8.5** | **Serial dissection of lateral cervical region** *(continued)* |

D. Muscles forming the floor of the lateral cervical region. The prevertebral layer of deep cervical fascia has been partially removed, and the motor nerves and most of the floor of the region are exposed.

- The spinal accessory nerve (CN XI) supplies the SCM and trapezius muscles; between them, it courses along the levator scapulae muscle but is separated from it by the prevertebral layer of deep cervical fascia.

- The phrenic nerve (C3, C4, C5) supplies the diaphragm and is located deep to the prevertebral layer of deep cervical fascia on the anterior surface of the anterior scalene muscle.

Severance of a phrenic nerve results in an ipsilateral paralysis of the diaphragm. A phrenic nerve block produces a short period of paralysis of the diaphragm on one side (e.g., for a lung operation). The anesthetic agent is injected around the nerve where it lies on the anterior surface of the anterior scalene muscle.

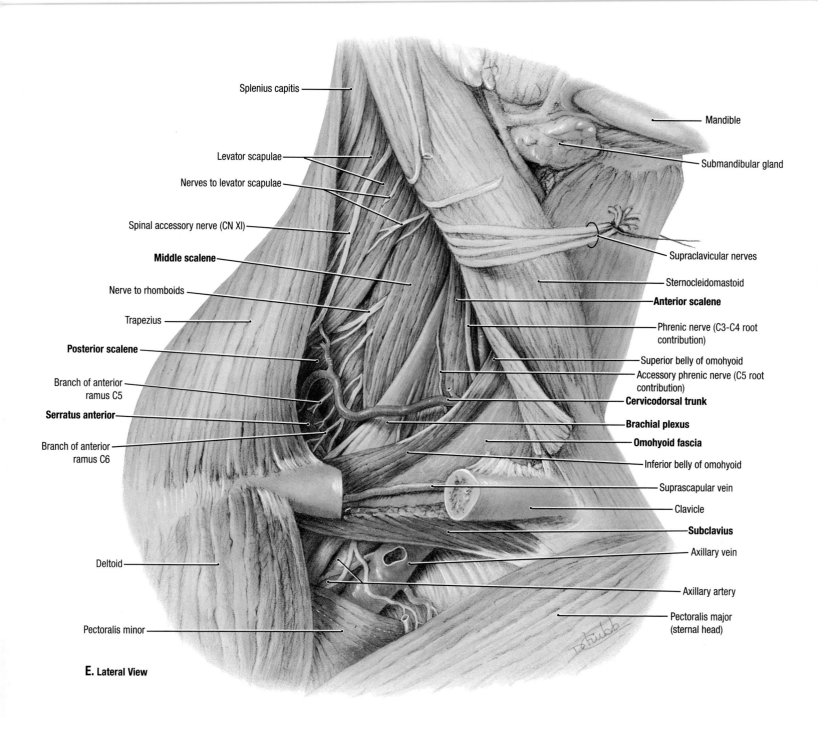

Splenius capitis

Levator scapulae

Nerves to levator scapulae

Spinal accessory nerve (CN XI)

Middle scalene

Nerve to rhomboids

Trapezius

Posterior scalene

Branch of anterior ramus C5

Serratus anterior

Branch of anterior ramus C6

Deltoid

Pectoralis minor

Mandible

Submandibular gland

Supraclavicular nerves

Sternocleidomastoid

Anterior scalene

Phrenic nerve (C3-C4 root contribution)

Superior belly of omohyoid

Accessory phrenic nerve (C5 root contribution)

Cervicodorsal trunk

Brachial plexus

Omohyoid fascia

Inferior belly of omohyoid

Suprascapular vein

Clavicle

Subclavius

Axillary vein

Axillary artery

Pectoralis major (sternal head)

E. Lateral View

8.5   **Serial dissection of lateral cervical region (continued)**

E. Vessels and motor nerves of the lateral cervical region. The clavicular head of the pectoralis major muscle and part of the clavicle have been removed.

The muscles that form the floor of the region are the semispinalis capitis, splenius capitis and levator scapulae superiorly and the anterior middle and posterior scalenes and serratus anterior inferiorly.

• The brachial plexus emerges between the anterior and middle scalene muscles.

A supraclavicular brachial plexus block may be utilized for anesthesia of the upper limb. The anesthetic agent is injected around the supraclavicular part of the brachial plexus. The main injection site is superior to the midpoint of the clavicle.

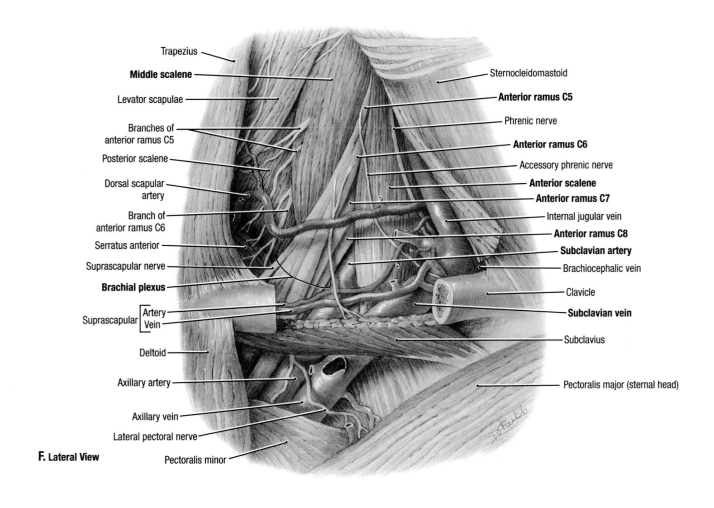

Trapezius

Middle scalene

Levator scapulae

Branches of
anterior ramus C5

Posterior scalene

Dorsal scapular
artery

Branch of
anterior ramus C6

Serratus anterior

Suprascapular nerve

Brachial plexus

Suprascapular { Artery
Vein

Deltoid

Axillary artery

Axillary vein

Lateral pectoral nerve

F. Lateral View

Pectoralis minor

Sternocleidomastoid

Anterior ramus C5

Phrenic nerve

Anterior ramus C6

Accessory phrenic nerve

Anterior scalene

Anterior ramus C7

Internal jugular vein

Anterior ramus C8

Subclavian artery

Brachiocephalic vein

Clavicle

Subclavian vein

Subclavius

Pectoralis major (sternal head)

8.5   Serial dissection of lateral cervical region *(continued)*

F. Structures of the omoclavicular (subclavian) triangle. The omohyoid muscle and fascia have been removed, exposing the brachial plexus and subclavian vessels.

- The anterior rami of C5–T1 form the brachial plexus (the anterior ramus of T1 lies posterior to the subclavian artery).
- The brachial plexus and subclavian artery emerge between the middle and anterior scalene muscles.
- The anterior scalene muscle lies between the subclavian artery and vein.

The right or left subclavian vein is often the site of placement for a central venous catheter, used to insert intravenous tubes ("central venous lines") for the administration of parenteral nutritional fluids or medications, for testing blood chemistry or central venous pressure, or inserting electrode wires for heart pacemaker devices. The relationships of the subclavian vein to the sternocleidomastoid muscle, clavicle, sternoclavicular joint and 1st rib are of clinical importance in line placement, and there is danger of puncture of the pleura or subclavian artery if the procedure is not performed correctly.

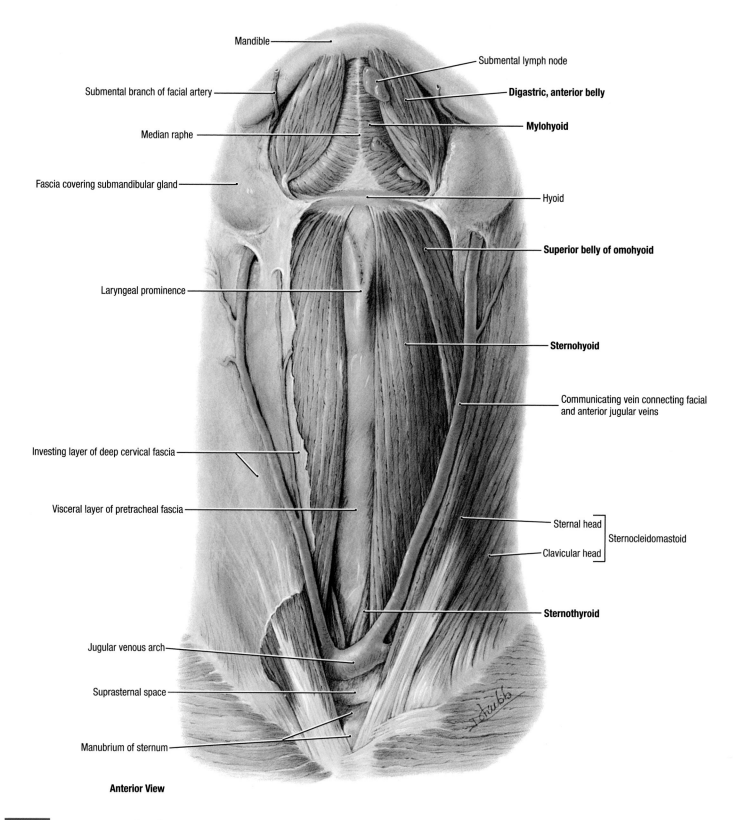

Mandible

Submental lymph node

Submental branch of facial artery

Digastric, anterior belly

Mylohyoid

Median raphe

Fascia covering submandibular gland

Hyoid

Superior belly of omohyoid

Laryngeal prominence

Sternohyoid

Communicating vein connecting facial and anterior jugular veins

Investing layer of deep cervical fascia

Visceral layer of pretracheal fascia

Sternal head

Sternocleidomastoid

Clavicular head

Sternothyroid

Jugular venous arch

Suprasternal space

Manubrium of sternum

Anterior View

8.6 Supra- and infrahyoid muscles

Much of the investing layer of deep cervical fascia has been removed.

- The anterior bellies of the digastric muscles form the sides of the suprahyoid part of the anterior cervical region, or submental triangle (floor of mouth). The hyoid bone forms the triangle's base, and the mylohyoid muscles are its floor.

- The infrahyoid part of the anterior cervical region is shaped like an elongated diamond bounded by the sternohyoid muscle superiorly and sternothyroid muscle inferiorly.

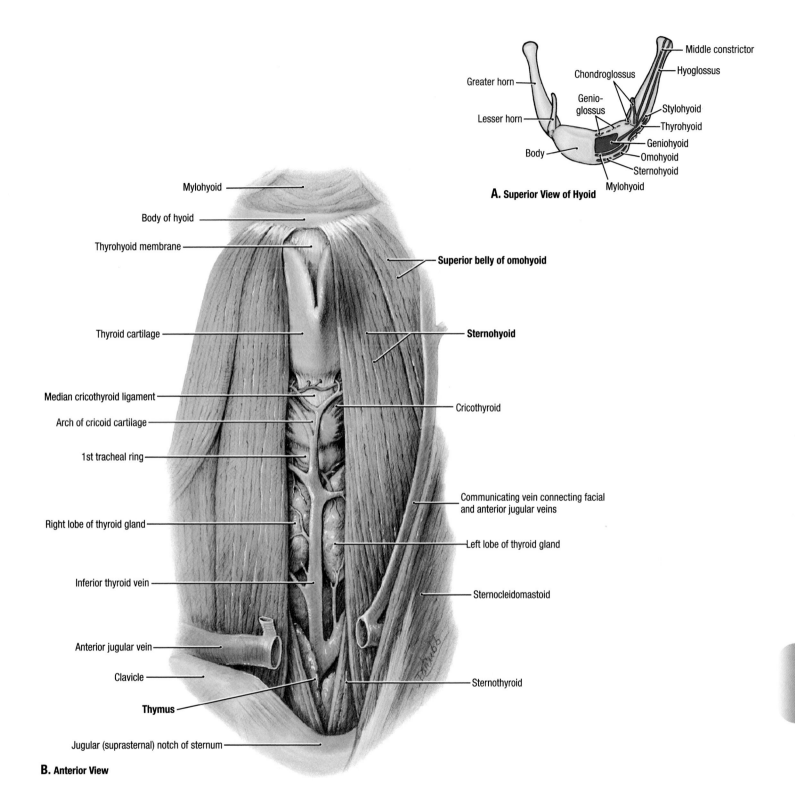

A. Superior View of Hyoid

Greater horn

Lesser horn

Body

Chondroglossus

Genio-glossus

Middle constrictor

Hyoglossus

Stylohyoid

Thyrohyoid

Geniohyoid

Omohyoid

Sternohyoid

Mylohyoid

B. Anterior View

Mylohyoid

Body of hyoid

Thyrohyoid membrane

Thyroid cartilage

Median cricothyroid ligament

Arch of cricoid cartilage

1st tracheal ring

Right lobe of thyroid gland

Inferior thyroid vein

Anterior jugular vein

Clavicle

Thymus

Jugular (suprasternal) notch of sternum

Superior belly of omohyoid

Sternohyoid

Cricothyroid

Communicating vein connecting facial and anterior jugular veins

Left lobe of thyroid gland

Sternocleidomastoid

Sternothyroid

8.7   Infrahyoid region, superficial muscular layer

A. Muscular attachments onto the hyoid bone.
B. The pretracheal fascia, right anterior jugular vein, and jugular venous arch have been removed.
- A persistent thymus projects superiorly from the thorax.
- The two superficial depressors of the larynx ("strap muscles") are the omohyoid (only the superior belly of which is seen here) and sternohyoid.

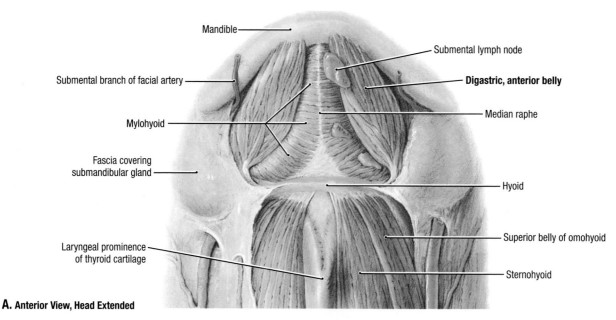

Mandible

Submental lymph node

Submental branch of facial artery

Digastric, anterior belly

Mylohyoid

Median raphe

Fascia covering submandibular gland

Hyoid

Superior belly of omohyoid

Laryngeal prominence of thyroid cartilage

Sternohyoid

A. Anterior View, Head Extended

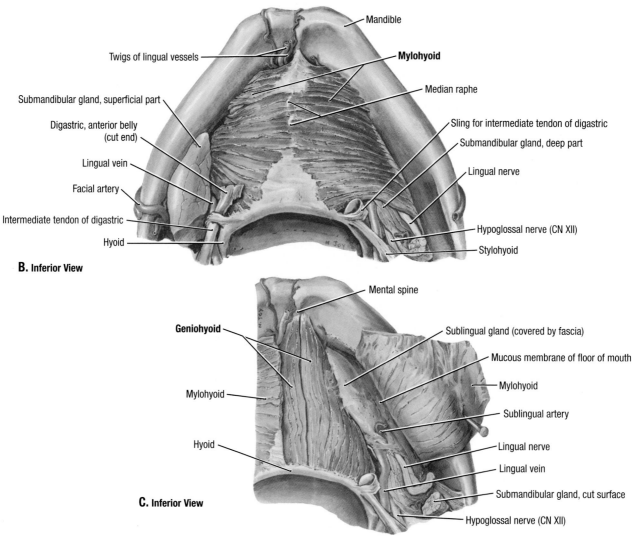

Mandible

Twigs of lingual vessels

Mylohyoid

Submandibular gland, superficial part

Median raphe

Digastric, anterior belly (cut end)

Sling for intermediate tendon of digastric

Submandibular gland, deep part

Lingual vein

Lingual nerve

Facial artery

Intermediate tendon of digastric

Hypoglossal nerve (CN XII)

Hyoid

Stylohyoid

B. Inferior View

Mental spine

Geniohyoid

Sublingual gland (covered by fascia)

Mucous membrane of floor of mouth

Mylohyoid

Mylohyoid

Sublingual artery

Lingual nerve

Hyoid

Lingual vein

Submandibular gland, cut surface

C. Inferior View

Hypoglossal nerve (CN XII)

8.8 **Suprahyoid region (submental triangle)**

A. Superficial layer—anterior belly of digastric. **B.** Intermediate layer—mylohyoid muscles. **C.** Deep layer—geniohyoid muscles.

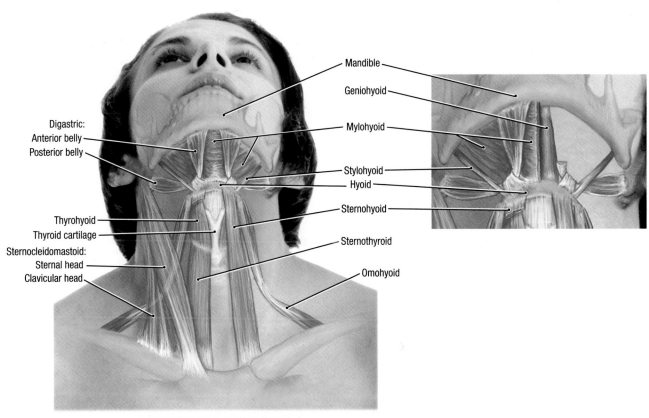

Anterior View, Head and Neck Extended

TABLE 8.4 SUPRAHYOID AND INFRAHYOID MUSCLES

Muscle	Origin	Insertion	Innervation	Main Action
Suprahyoid muscles				
Mylohyoid	Mylohyoid line of mandible	Raphe and body of hyoid bone	Nerve to mylohyoid, a branch of inferior alveolar nerve (CN V^3)	Elevates hyoid bone, floor of mouth and tongue during swallowing and speaking
Digastric	*Anterior belly:* digastric fossa of mandible *Posterior belly:* mastoid notch of temporal bone	Intermediate tendon to body and greater horn of hyoid bone	*Anterior belly:* nerve to mylohyoid, a branch of inferior alveolar nerve (CN V^3) *Posterior belly:* facial nerve (CN VII)	Elevates hyoid bone and steadies it during swallowing and speaking; depresses mandible against resistance
Geniohyoid	Inferior mental spine of mandible	Body of hyoid bone	C1 via the hypoglossal nerve (CN XII)	Pulls hyoid bone anterosuperiorly, shortens floor of mouth, and widens pharynx
Stylohyoid	Styloid process of temporal bone		Cervical branch of facial nerve (CN VII)	Elevates and retracts hyoid bone, thereby elongating floor of mouth
Infrahyoid muscles				
Sternohyoid	Manubrium of sternum and medial end of clavicle	Body of hyoid bone	C1–C3 by a branch of ansa cervicalis	Depresses hyoid bone after it has been elevated during swallowing
Omohyoid	Superior border of scapula near suprascapular notch	Inferior border of hyoid bone		Depresses, retracts, and steadies hyoid bone
Sternothyroid	Posterior surface of manubrium of sternum	Oblique line of thyroid cartilage	C2 and C3 by a branch of ansa cervicalis	Depresses hyoid bone and larynx
Thyrohyoid	Oblique line of thyroid cartilage	Inferior border of body and greater horn of hyoid bone	C1 via hypoglossal nerve (CN XII)	Depresses hyoid bone and elevates larynx

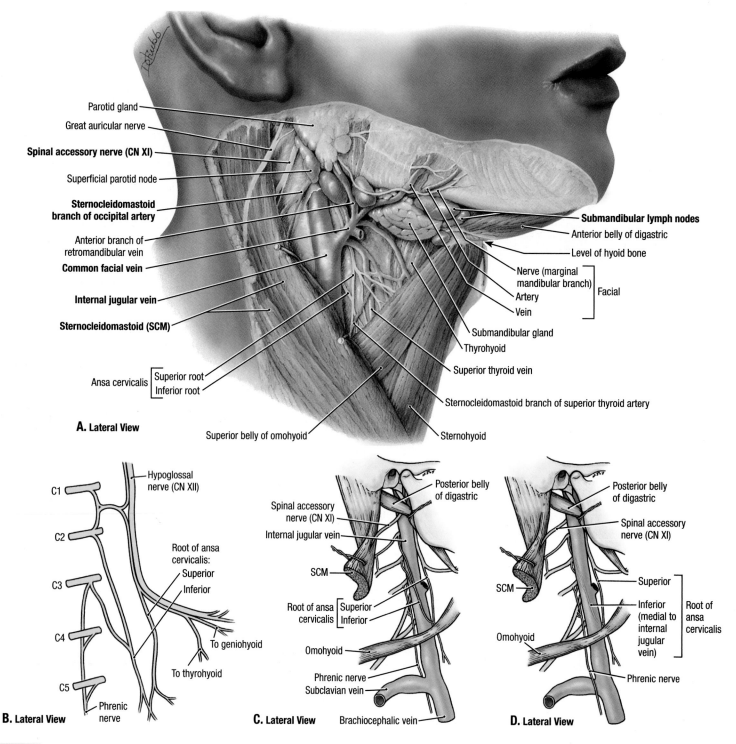

A. Lateral View

Parotid gland
Great auricular nerve
Spinal accessory nerve (CN XI)
Superficial parotid node
Sternocleidomastoid branch of occipital artery
Anterior branch of retromandibular vein
Common facial vein
Internal jugular vein
Sternocleidomastoid (SCM)
Ansa cervicalis — Superior root / Inferior root
Superior belly of omohyoid

Submandibular lymph nodes
Anterior belly of digastric
Level of hyoid bone
Nerve (marginal mandibular branch)
Artery
Vein — Facial
Submandibular gland
Thyrohyoid
Superior thyroid vein
Sternocleidomastoid branch of superior thyroid artery
Sternohyoid

B. Lateral View

C1
C2
C3
C4
C5
Phrenic nerve

Hypoglossal nerve (CN XII)
Root of ansa cervicalis:
Superior
Inferior
To geniohyoid
To thyrohyoid

C. Lateral View

Spinal accessory nerve (CN XI)
Internal jugular vein
SCM
Root of ansa cervicalis — Superior / Inferior
Omohyoid
Phrenic nerve
Subclavian vein
Brachiocephalic vein

Posterior belly of digastric

D. Lateral View

SCM
Omohyoid

Posterior belly of digastric
Spinal accessory nerve (CN XI)
Superior
Inferior (medial to internal jugular vein) — Root of ansa cervicalis
Phrenic nerve

8.9   **Superficial dissection of carotid triangle**

A. The skin, subcutaneous tissue (with platysma), and the investing layer of deep cervical fascia, including the sheaths of the parotid and submandibular glands, have been removed.
- The spinal accessory nerve (XI) enters the deep surface of the sternocleidomastoid muscle and is joined along its anterior border by the sternocleidomastoid branch of the occipital artery.
- The (common) facial vein joins the internal jugular vein near the level of the hyoid bone; here, the facial vein is joined by several other veins.

- The submandibular lymph nodes lie deep to the investing layer of deep cervical fascia in the submandibular triangle; some of the nodes lie deep in the submandibular gland.

B. Diagram of the motor branches of cervical plexus.

C. Typical relationships of ansa cervicalis, spinal accessory nerve (CN XI), and phrenic nerve to the internal jugular and subclavian veins.

D. Atypical relationships.

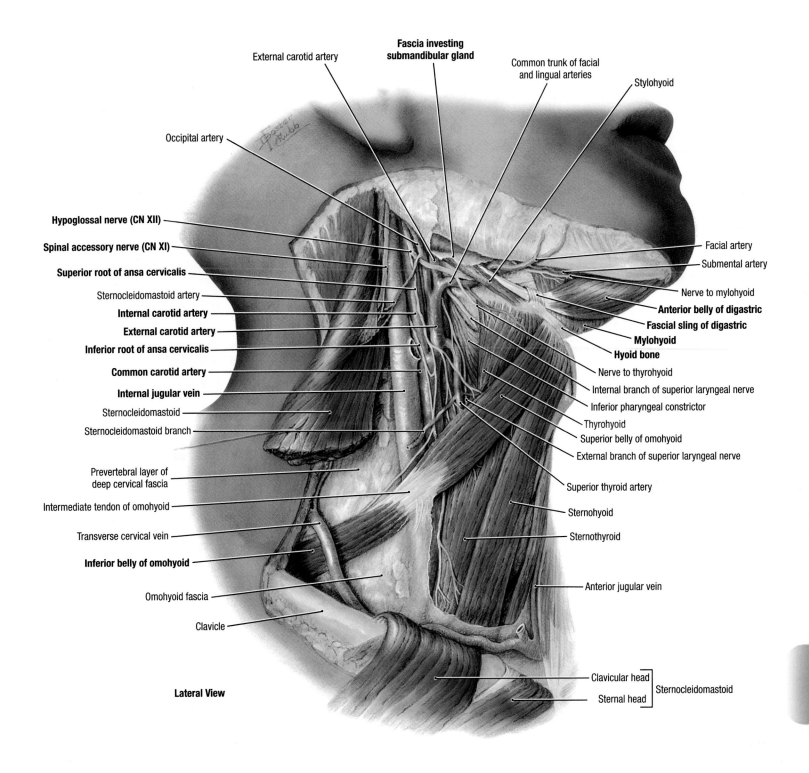

External carotid artery

Fascia investing submandibular gland

Common trunk of facial and lingual arteries

Stylohyoid

Occipital artery

Hypoglossal nerve (CN XII)

Spinal accessory nerve (CN XI)

Superior root of ansa cervicalis

Sternocleidomastoid artery

Internal carotid artery

External carotid artery

Inferior root of ansa cervicalis

Common carotid artery

Internal jugular vein

Sternocleidomastoid

Sternocleidomastoid branch

Prevertebral layer of deep cervical fascia

Intermediate tendon of omohyoid

Transverse cervical vein

Inferior belly of omohyoid

Omohyoid fascia

Clavicle

Lateral View

Facial artery

Submental artery

Nerve to mylohyoid

Anterior belly of digastric

Fascial sling of digastric

Mylohyoid

Hyoid bone

Nerve to thyrohyoid

Internal branch of superior laryngeal nerve

Inferior pharyngeal constrictor

Thyrohyoid

Superior belly of omohyoid

External branch of superior laryngeal nerve

Superior thyroid artery

Sternohyoid

Sternothyroid

Anterior jugular vein

Clavicular head ⎤
                    ⎥ Sternocleidomastoid
Sternal head   ⎦

8.10   Deep dissection of carotid triangle

The sternocleidomastoid muscle has been severed; the inferior portion reflected inferiorly and superior portion posteriorly.

- The tendon of the digastric muscle is connected to the hyoid bone by a fascial sling derived from the muscular part of the pretracheal layer of deep cervical fascia; the tendon of the omohyoid muscle is similarly tethered to the clavicle.
- In this specimen, the facial and lingual arteries arise from a common trunk and pass deep to the stylohyoid and digastric muscles.
- The hypoglossal nerve (CN XII) crosses the internal and external carotid arteries and gives off two branches, the superior root of the ansa cervicalis and the nerve to the thyrohyoid, before passing anteriorly deep to the mylohyoid muscle. In this specimen, the inferior root of the ansa cervicalis lies deep to the internal jugular vein and emerges at its medial aspect.

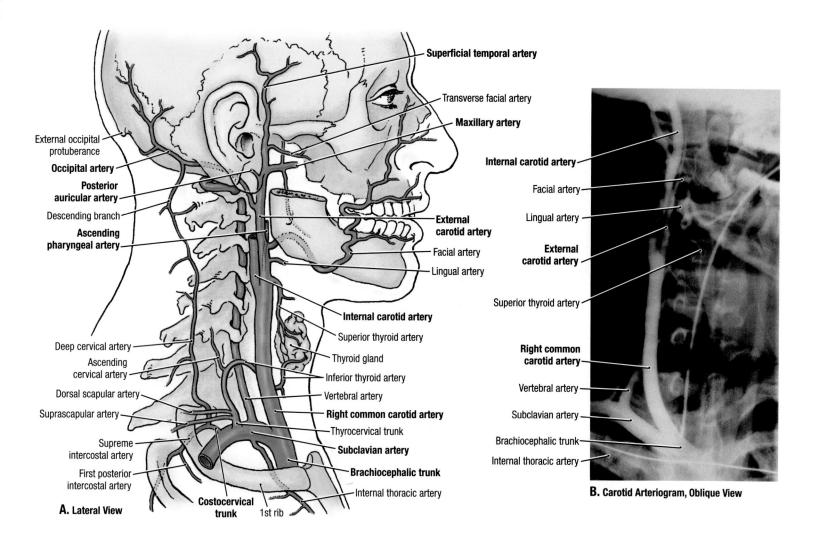

A. Lateral View

External occipital protuberance
Occipital artery
Posterior auricular artery
Descending branch
Ascending pharyngeal artery
Deep cervical artery
Ascending cervical artery
Dorsal scapular artery
Suprascapular artery
Supreme intercostal artery
First posterior intercostal artery
Costocervical trunk
1st rib

Superficial temporal artery
Transverse facial artery
Maxillary artery
External carotid artery
Facial artery
Lingual artery
Internal carotid artery
Superior thyroid artery
Thyroid gland
Inferior thyroid artery
Vertebral artery
Right common carotid artery
Thyrocervical trunk
Subclavian artery
Brachiocephalic trunk
Internal thoracic artery

Internal carotid artery
Facial artery
Lingual artery
External carotid artery
Superior thyroid artery
Right common carotid artery
Vertebral artery
Subclavian artery
Brachiocephalic trunk
Internal thoracic artery

B. Carotid Arteriogram, Oblique View

TABLE 8.5 ARTERIES OF THE NECK

Artery	Origin	Course and Distribution
Right common carotid	Bifurcation of brachiocephalic trunk	Ascends in neck within carotid sheath with the internal jugular vein and vagus nerve (CN X). Terminates at superior border of thyroid cartilage (C4 vertebral level) by dividing into internal and external carotid arteries
Left common carotid	Arch of aorta	
Right and left internal carotid	Right and left common carotid	No branches in the neck. Enters cranium via carotid canal to supply brain and orbits. Proximal part location of carotid sinus, a baroreceptor that reacts to change in arterial blood pressure. The carotid body, a chemoreceptor that monitors oxygen level in blood, is located in bifurcation of common carotid
Right and left external carotid		Supplies most structures external to cranium; the orbit, part of forehead, and scalp are major exceptions (supplied by ophthalmic artery from intracranial internal carotid artery)
Ascending pharyngeal	External carotid	Ascends on pharynx to supply pharynx, prevertebral muscles, middle ear, and cranial meninges
Occipital		Passes posteriorly, medial and parallel to the posterior belly of digastric, ending in the posterior scalp
Posterior auricular		Ascends posteriorly between external acoustic meatus and mastoid process to supply adjacent muscles, parotid gland, facial nerve, auricle, and scalp

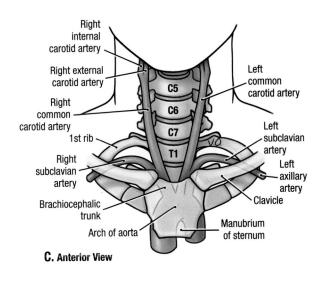

C. Anterior View

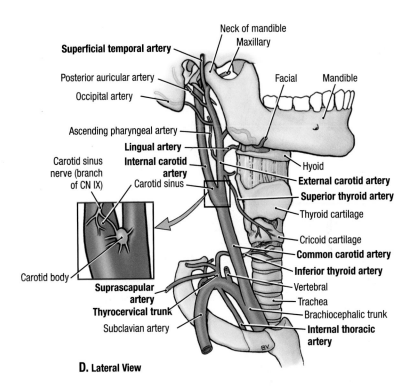

D. Lateral View

TABLE 8.5 ARTERIES OF THE NECK (continued)

Artery	Origin	Course and Distribution
Superior thyroid	External carotid	Runs anteroinferiorly deep to infrahyoid muscles to reach thyroid gland. Supplies thyroid gland, infrahyoid muscles, SCM, and larynx via *superior laryngeal artery*
Lingual		Lies on middle constrictor muscle of pharynx; arches superoanteriorly and passes deep to CN XIII, stylohyoid muscle, and posterior belly of digastric then passes deep to hyoglossus, giving branches to the posterior tongue and bifurcating into *deep lingual* and *sublingual arteries*
Facial		After giving rise to *ascending palatine artery* and a tonsillar branch, it passes superiorly under cover of the angle of the mandible. It then loops anteriorly to supply the submandibular gland and give rise to the *submental artery* to the floor of the mouth before entering the face
Maxillary	Terminal branches of external carotid	Passes posterior to neck of mandible, enters infratemporal fossa then pterygopalatine fossa to supply teeth, nose, ear, and face
Superficial temporal		Ascends anterior to auricle to temporal region and ends in scalp
Vertebral	Subclavian	Passes through the transverse foramina of the transverse processes of vertebrae C1–C6, runs in a groove on the posterior arch of the atlas, and enters the cranial cavity through the foramen magnum
Internal thoracic		No branches in neck; enters thorax
Thyrocervical trunk		Has two branches: the *inferior thyroid artery*, the main visceral artery of the neck; the cervicodorsal trunk sending branches to the lateral cervical region, trapezius, and medial scapular arteries
Costocervical trunk		Trunk passes posterosuperiorly and divides into *superior intercostal* and *deep cervical arteries* to supply the 1st and 2nd intercostal spaces and posterior deep cervical muscles, respectively

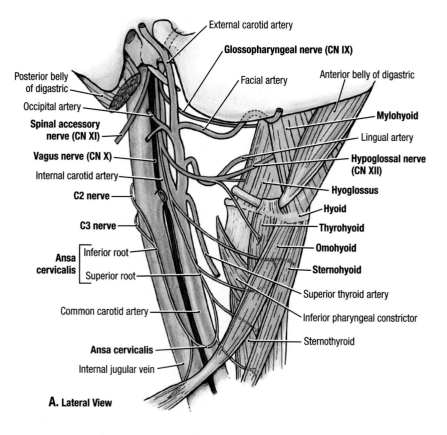

A. Lateral View

Glossopharyngeal—CN IX	Vagus—CN X
Motor: stylopharyngeus, parotid gland **Sensory:** taste: posterior third of tongue; general sensation: pharynx, tonsillar sinus, pharyngotympanic tube, middle ear cavity	**Motor:** palate, pharynx, larynx, trachea, bronchial tree, heart, GI tract to left colic flexure **Sensory:** pharynx, larynx; reflex sensory from tracheo-bronchial tree, lungs, heart, GI tract to left colic flexure
Spinal accessory—CN XI	Hypoglossal—CN XII
Motor: sternocleidomastoid and trapezius	**Motor:** all intrinsic and extrinsic muscles of tongue (excluding palatoglossus— a palatine muscle)

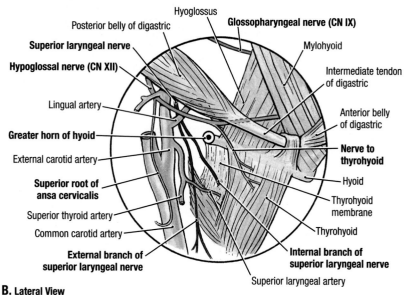

B. Lateral View

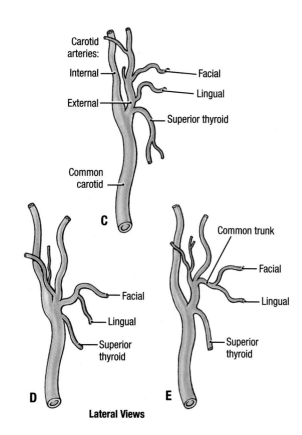

Lateral Views

8.11 **Relationships of nerves and vessels in the carotid triangle of the neck**

A. Ansa cervicalis and the strap muscles. **B.** Hypoglossal nerve (CN XII) and internal and external branches of superior laryngeal nerve (CN X). The tip of the greater hyoid bone, indicated with a *circle* is the reference point for many structures. **C–E.** Variation in the origin of the lingual artery as studied by Dr. Grant in 211 specimens. In 80%, the superior thyroid, lingual, and facial arteries arose separately **(C)**; in 20%, the lingual and facial arteries arose from a common stem inferiorly **(D)** or high on the external carotid artery **(E)**. In one specimen, the superior thyroid and lingual arteries arose from a common stem.

Carotid occlusion, causing stenosis (narrowing) can be relieved by opening the artery at its origin and stripping off the atherosclerotic plaque with the artery's lining (intima). This procedure is called carotid endarterectomy. Because of the relationships of the internal carotid artery, there is a risk of cranial nerve injury during the procedure involving one or more of the following nerves: CN IX, CN X (or its branch, the superior laryngeal nerve), CN XI, or CN XII.

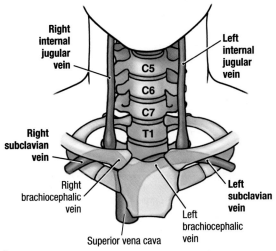

A. Anterior View

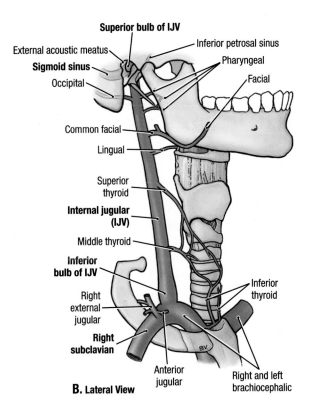

B. Lateral View

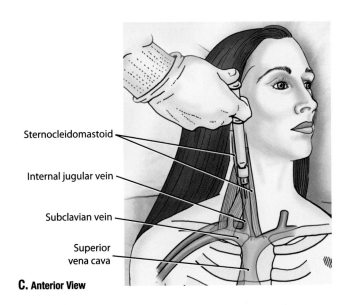

C. Anterior View

8.12   Deep veins of the neck

A. Internal jugular and subclavian veins. **B.** Tributaries of the internal jugular vein (IJV). The IJV begins at the jugular foramen as the continuation of the sigmoid sinus. From a dilated origin, the superior bulb of the IJV, the vein runs inferiorly through the neck in the carotid sheath. Posterior to the sternal end of the clavicle the vein merges perpendicularly with the subclavian vein, forming the "venous angle" that marks the origin of the brachiocephalic vein. The inferior end of the IJV dilates superior to its terminal valve, forming the inferior bulb of the IJV. The valve permits blood to flow toward the heart while preventing backflow into the IJV. **C.** Internal jugular vein puncture. A needle and catheter may be inserted into the IJV for diagnostic or therapeutic purposes. The right internal jugular vein is preferable because it is usually larger and straighter. During this procedure, the clinician palpates the common carotid artery and inserts the needle into the IJV just lateral to it at a 30° angle, aiming at the apex of the triangle between the sternal and clavicular heads of the SCM. The needle is then directed inferolaterally toward the ipsilateral nipple.

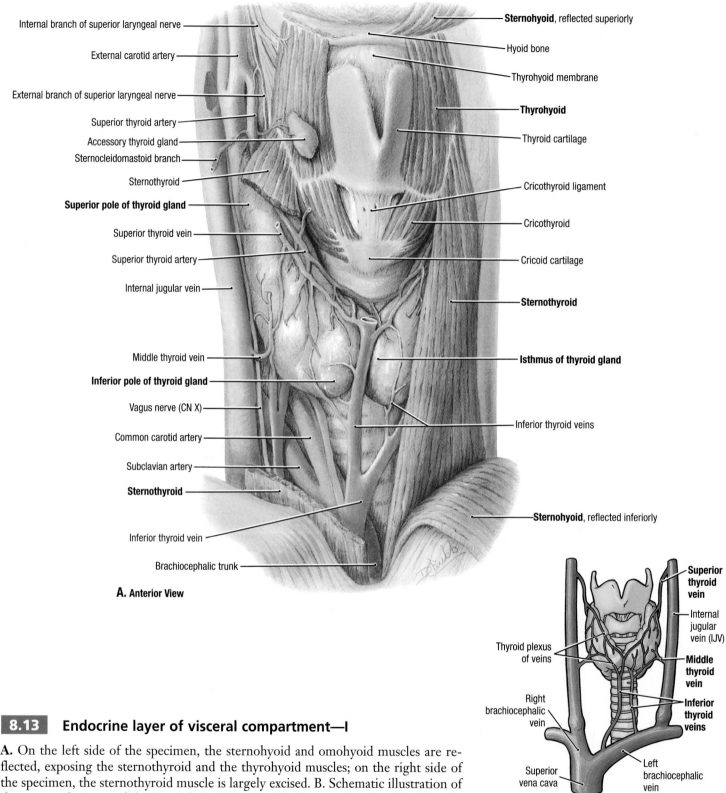

Internal branch of superior laryngeal nerve

External carotid artery

External branch of superior laryngeal nerve

Superior thyroid artery

Accessory thyroid gland

Sternocleidomastoid branch

Sternothyroid

Superior pole of thyroid gland

Superior thyroid vein

Superior thyroid artery

Internal jugular vein

Middle thyroid vein

Inferior pole of thyroid gland

Vagus nerve (CN X)

Common carotid artery

Subclavian artery

Sternothyroid

Inferior thyroid vein

Brachiocephalic trunk

A. Anterior View

Sternohyoid, reflected superiorly

Hyoid bone

Thyrohyoid membrane

Thyrohyoid

Thyroid cartilage

Cricothyroid ligament

Cricothyroid

Cricoid cartilage

Sternothyroid

Isthmus of thyroid gland

Inferior thyroid veins

Sternohyoid, reflected inferiorly

Superior thyroid vein

Internal jugular vein (IJV)

Middle thyroid vein

Inferior thyroid veins

Thyroid plexus of veins

Right brachiocephalic vein

Superior vena cava

Left brachiocephalic vein

B. Anterior View

8.13   Endocrine layer of visceral compartment—I

A. On the left side of the specimen, the sternohyoid and omohyoid muscles are reflected, exposing the sternothyroid and the thyrohyoid muscles; on the right side of the specimen, the sternothyroid muscle is largely excised. B. Schematic illustration of the venous drainage of the thyroid gland. Except for the superior thyroid veins, the thyroid veins are not paired with arteries of corresponding names.

The carotid pulse (neck pulse) is easily felt by palpating the common carotid artery in the side of the neck, where it lies in a groove between the trachea and the infrahyoid muscles. It is usually easily palpated just deep to the anterior border of the SCM at the level of the superior border of the thyroid cartilage. It is routinely checked during cardiopulmonary resuscitation (CPR). Absence of a carotid pulse indicates cardiac arrest.

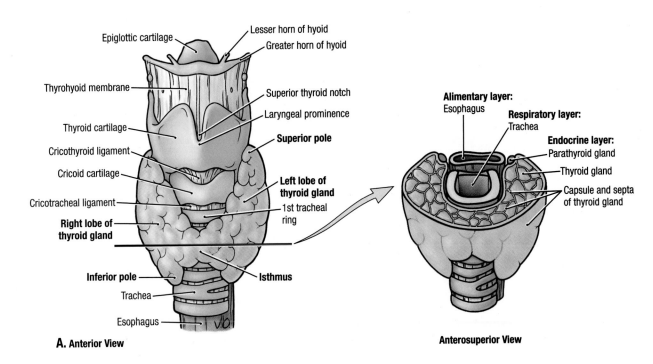

A. Anterior View

Anterosuperior View

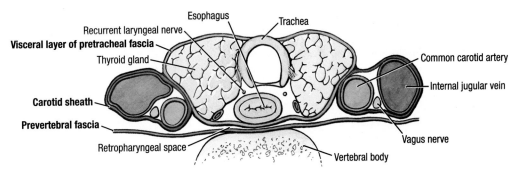

B. Transverse Section, Inferior View

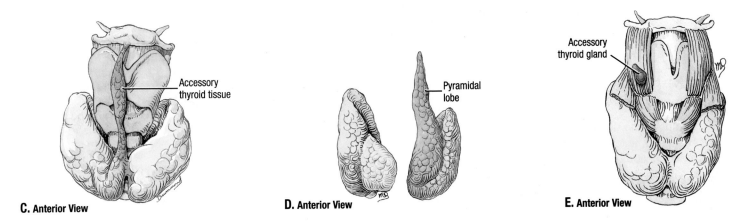

C. Anterior View   D. Anterior View   E. Anterior View

8.14   Endocrine layer of visceral compartment—II

A. Relations of thyroid gland with transverse section showing alimentary, respiratory, and endocrine layers of visceral compartment. **B.** Fascia. **C.** Accessory thyroid tissue along the course of the thyroglossal duct. **D.** Approximately 50% of glands have a pyramidal lobe that extends from near the isthmus to or toward the hyoid bone; the isthmus is occasionally absent, in which case the gland is in two parts. **E.** An accessory thyroid gland can occur between the suprahyoid region and arch of the aorta (see Fig. 8.13A).

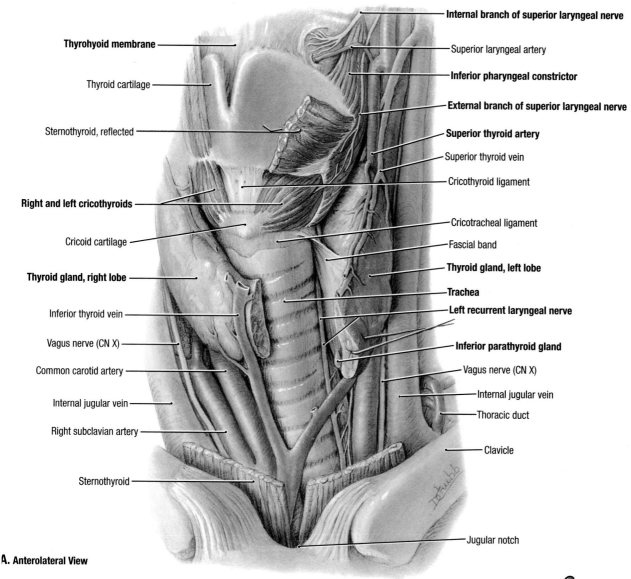

A. Anterolateral View

Internal branch of superior laryngeal nerve

Thyrohyoid membrane

Superior laryngeal artery

Inferior pharyngeal constrictor

Thyroid cartilage

External branch of superior laryngeal nerve

Superior thyroid artery

Sternothyroid, reflected

Superior thyroid vein

Cricothyroid ligament

Right and left cricothyroids

Cricotracheal ligament

Fascial band

Cricoid cartilage

Thyroid gland, left lobe

Thyroid gland, right lobe

Trachea

Left recurrent laryngeal nerve

Inferior thyroid vein

Inferior parathyroid gland

Vagus nerve (CN X)

Vagus nerve (CN X)

Common carotid artery

Internal jugular vein

Internal jugular vein

Thoracic duct

Right subclavian artery

Clavicle

Sternothyroid

Jugular notch

8.15 Respiratory layer of visceral compartment

A. The isthmus of the thyroid gland is divided, and the left lobe is retracted. The left recurrent laryngeal nerve ascends on the lateral aspect of the trachea between the trachea and esophagus. The internal branch of the superior laryngeal nerve runs along the superior border of the inferior pharyngeal constrictor muscle and pierces the thyrohyoid membrane. The external branch of the superior laryngeal nerve lies adjacent to the inferior pharyngeal constrictor muscle and supplies its lower portion; it continues to run along the anterior border of the superior thyroid artery, passing deep to the superior attachment of the sternothyroid muscle, and then supplies the cricothyroid muscle. **B.** Blood supply of the parathyroid glands and courses of the left and right recurrent laryngeal nerves.

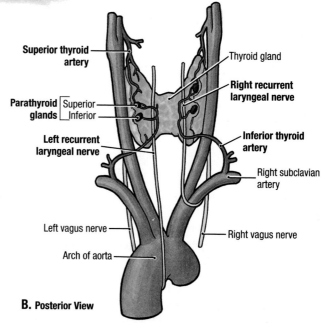

Superior thyroid artery

Thyroid gland

Parathyroid glands { Superior / Inferior }

Right recurrent laryngeal nerve

Left recurrent laryngeal nerve

Inferior thyroid artery

Right subclavian artery

Left vagus nerve

Right vagus nerve

Arch of aorta

B. Posterior View

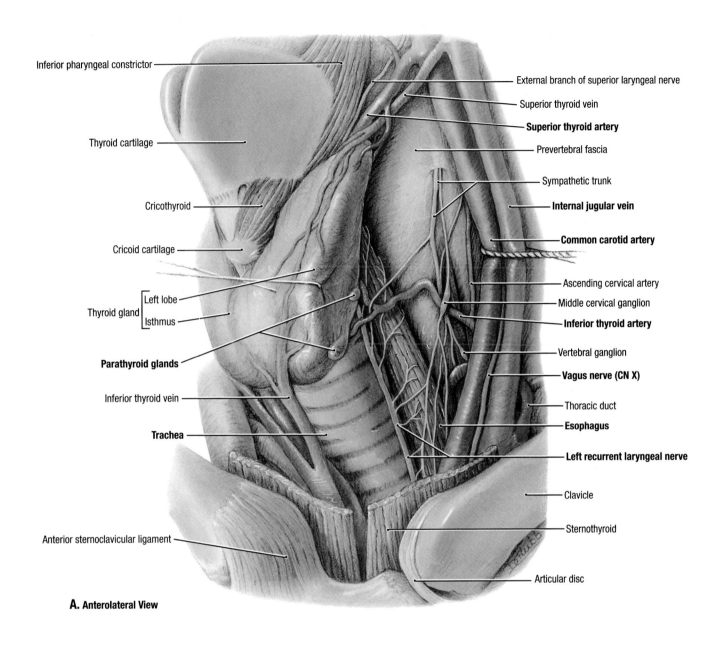

A. Anterolateral View

8.16   Alimentary layer of visceral compartment

A. Dissection of the left side of the root of the neck. The three structures contained in the carotid sheath (internal jugular vein, common carotid artery, and vagus nerve) are retracted. The left recurrent laryngeal nerve ascends on the lateral aspect of the trachea, just anterior to the recess between the trachea and esophagus. **B.** Arterial supply of thyroid gland. The thyroid ima artery is infrequent (10%) and variable in its origin.

During a total thyroidectomy (e.g., excision of a malignant thyroid gland), the parathyroid glands are in danger of being inadvertently damaged or removed. These glands are safe during *subtotal thyroidectomy* because the most posterior part of the thyroid gland usually is preserved. Variability in the position of the parathyroid glands, especially the inferior ones, puts them in danger of being removed during surgery on the thyroid gland. If the parathyroid glands are inadvertently removed during surgery, the patient suffers from *tetany*, a severe convulsive disorder. The generalized convulsive muscle spasms result from a fall in blood calcium levels.

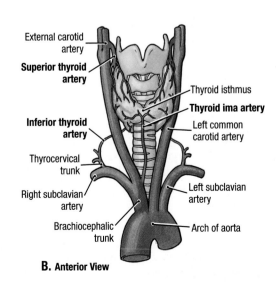

B. Anterior View

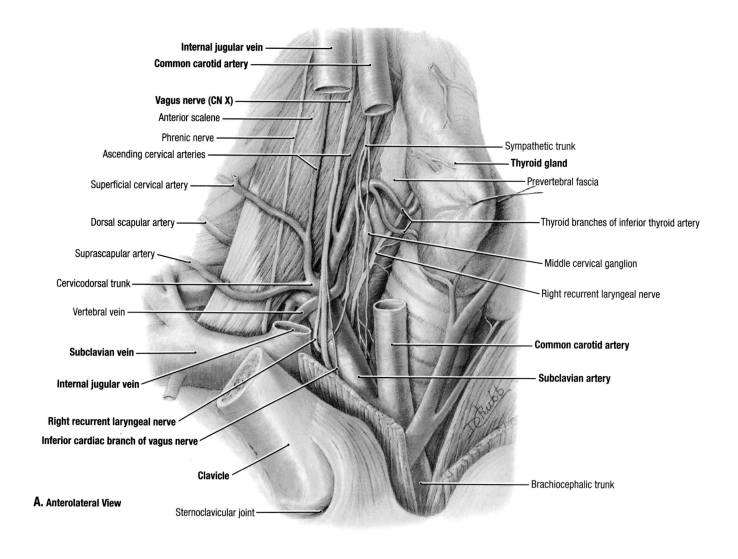

Internal jugular vein
Common carotid artery

Vagus nerve (CN X)
Anterior scalene
Phrenic nerve
Ascending cervical arteries

Superficial cervical artery

Dorsal scapular artery

Suprascapular artery

Cervicodorsal trunk

Vertebral vein

Subclavian vein

Internal jugular vein

Right recurrent laryngeal nerve

Inferior cardiac branch of vagus nerve

Clavicle

A. Anterolateral View

Sternoclavicular joint

Sympathetic trunk
Thyroid gland
Prevertebral fascia
Thyroid branches of inferior thyroid artery

Middle cervical ganglion

Right recurrent laryngeal nerve

Common carotid artery

Subclavian artery

Brachiocephalic trunk

8.17   **Root of the neck**

A. Dissection of the right side of the root of the neck. The clavicle is cut, sections of the common carotid artery and internal jugular vein are removed, and the right lobe of the thyroid gland is retracted. The right vagus nerve crosses the first part of the subclavian artery and gives off an inferior cardiac branch and the right recurrent laryngeal nerve. The right recurrent laryngeal nerve loops inferior to the subclavian artery and passes posterior to the common carotid artery on its way to the posterolateral aspect of the trachea.

- The recurrent laryngeal nerves are vulnerable to injury during thyroidectomy and other surgeries in the anterior cervical region of the neck. Because the terminal branch of this nerve, the inferior laryngeal nerve, innervates the muscles moving the

vocal folds, injury to the nerve results in paralysis of the vocal folds.

- A non-neoplastic and noninflammatory enlargement of the thyroid gland, other than the variable enlargement that may occur during menstruation and pregnancy, is called a goiter. A *goiter* results from a lack of iodine. It is common in certain parts of the world where the soil and water are deficient in iodine and iodized salt is unavailable. The enlarged gland causes a swelling in the neck that may compress the trachea, esophagus, and recurrent laryngeal nerves. When the gland enlarges, it may do so anteriorly, posteriorly, inferiorly, or laterally. It cannot move superiorly because of the superior attachments of the sternothyroid and sternohyoid muscles. Substernal extension of a goiter is also common.

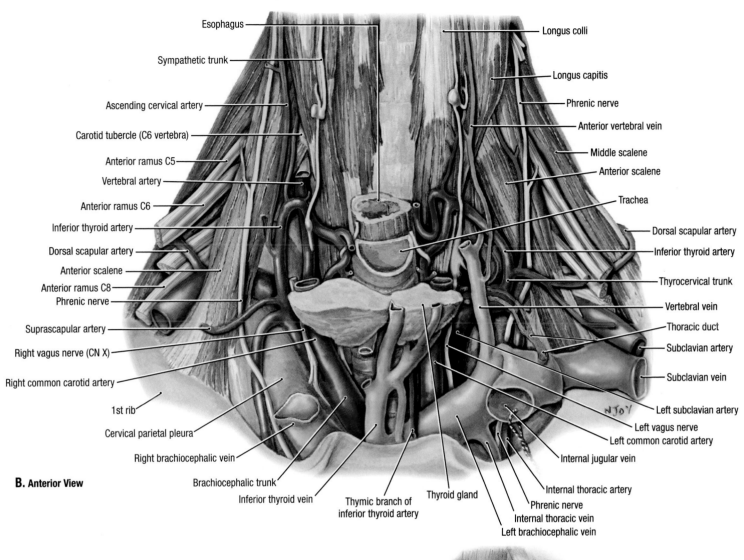

Esophagus

Sympathetic trunk

Ascending cervical artery

Carotid tubercle (C6 vertebra)

Anterior ramus C5

Vertebral artery

Anterior ramus C6

Inferior thyroid artery

Dorsal scapular artery

Anterior scalene

Anterior ramus C8

Phrenic nerve

Suprascapular artery

Right vagus nerve (CN X)

Right common carotid artery

1st rib

Cervical parietal pleura

Right brachiocephalic vein

Longus colli

Longus capitis

Phrenic nerve

Anterior vertebral vein

Middle scalene

Anterior scalene

Trachea

Dorsal scapular artery

Inferior thyroid artery

Thyrocervical trunk

Vertebral vein

Thoracic duct

Subclavian artery

Subclavian vein

Left subclavian artery

Left vagus nerve

Left common carotid artery

Internal jugular vein

Internal thoracic artery

Phrenic nerve

Internal thoracic vein

Left brachiocephalic vein

Thyroid gland

Thymic branch of inferior thyroid artery

Inferior thyroid vein

Brachiocephalic trunk

B. Anterior View

8.17 Root of the neck (continued)

B. Deep anterior dissection. **C.** Dissection of termination of the thoracic duct. The sternocleidomastoid muscle is removed, the sternohyoid muscle is resected, and the omohyoid portion of the pretracheal fascia is partially removed. The thoracic duct arches laterally in the neck, passing posterior to the carotid sheath and anterior to the vertebral artery, thyrocervical trunk, and subclavian arteries; it enters the angle formed by the junction of the left subclavian and internal jugular veins to form the left brachiocephalic vein (the left venous angle).

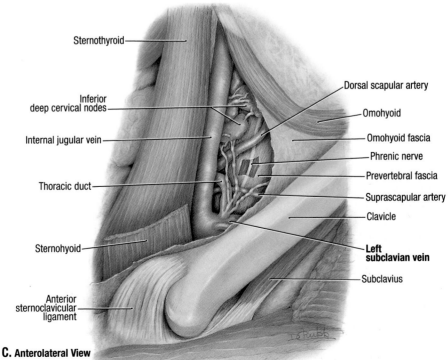

Sternothyroid

Inferior deep cervical nodes

Internal jugular vein

Thoracic duct

Sternohyoid

Anterior sternoclavicular ligament

Dorsal scapular artery

Omohyoid

Omohyoid fascia

Phrenic nerve

Prevertebral fascia

Suprascapular artery

Clavicle

Left subclavian vein

Subclavius

C. Anterolateral View

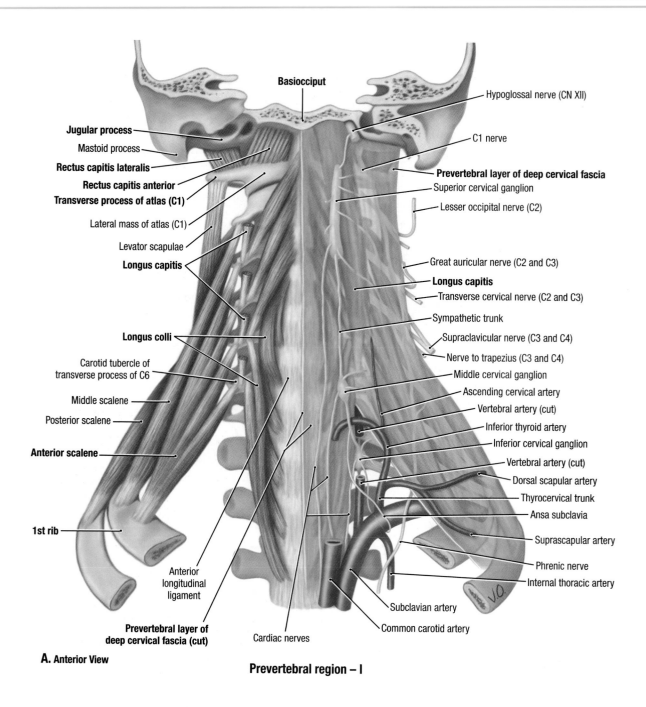

A. Anterior View

Prevertebral region – I

TABLE 8.6 ANTERIOR VERTEBRAL MUSCLES

Muscle	Superior Attachment	Inferior Attachment	Innervation	Main Action
Longus colli	Anterior tubercle of C1 vertebra (atlas); bodies of C1–C3 and transverse processes of C3–C6 vertebrae	Bodies of C5–T3 vertebrae, transverse processes of C3–C5 vertebrae	Anterior rami of C2–C6 spinal nerves	Flexes neck with rotation (torsion) to opposite side if acting unilaterally[a]
Longus capitis	Basilar part of occipital bone (basiocciput)	Anterior tubercles of C3–C6 transverse processes	Anterior rami of C1–C3 spinal nerves	Flexes head[b]
Rectus capitis lateralis	Jugular process of occipital bone	Transverse process of C1 vertebra (atlas)	From loop between C1 and C2 spinal nerves	Flexes head and helps to stabilize it[b]

[a]Flexion of neck, anterior (or lateral) bending of cervical vertebrae C2–C7.
[b]Flexion of head, anterior (or lateral) bending of head relative to vertebral column at atlanto-occipital joints.

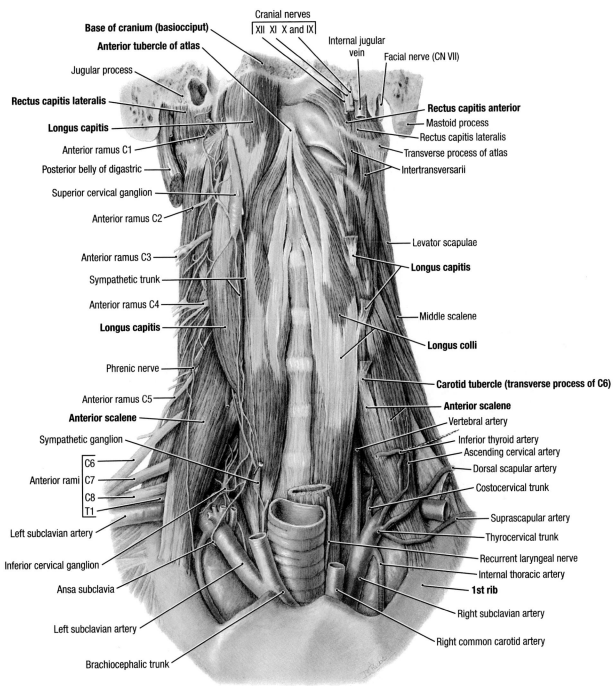

Cranial nerves
XII XI X and IX

Base of cranium (basiocciput)
Anterior tubercle of atlas
Jugular process
Rectus capitis lateralis
Longus capitis
Anterior ramus C1
Posterior belly of digastric
Superior cervical ganglion
Anterior ramus C2
Anterior ramus C3
Sympathetic trunk
Anterior ramus C4
Longus capitis
Phrenic nerve
Anterior ramus C5
Anterior scalene
Sympathetic ganglion
Anterior rami { C6 C7 C8 T1 }
Left subclavian artery
Inferior cervical ganglion
Ansa subclavia
Left subclavian artery
Brachiocephalic trunk

Internal jugular vein
Facial nerve (CN VII)
Rectus capitis anterior
Mastoid process
Rectus capitis lateralis
Transverse process of atlas
Intertransversarii
Levator scapulae
Longus capitis
Middle scalene
Longus colli
Carotid tubercle (transverse process of C6)
Anterior scalene
Vertebral artery
Inferior thyroid artery
Ascending cervical artery
Dorsal scapular artery
Costocervical trunk
Suprascapular artery
Thyrocervical trunk
Recurrent laryngeal nerve
Internal thoracic artery
1st rib
Right subclavian artery
Right common carotid artery

B. Anterior View

Prevertebral region – II

TABLE 8.6 ANTERIOR VERTEBRAL MUSCLES (continued)

Muscle	Superior Attachment	Inferior Attachment	Innervation	Main Action
Rectus capitis anterior	Base of cranium, just anterior to occipital condyle	Anterior surface of lateral mass of atlas (C1 vertebra)	Branches from loop between C1 and C2 spinal nerves	Flexes head[b]
Anterior scalene	Transverse processes of C4–C6 vertebrae	1st rib	Cervical spinal nerves C4–C6	

[a]Flexion of neck, anterior (or lateral) bending of cervical vertebrae C2–C7.
[b]Flexion of head, anterior (or lateral) bending of head relative to vertebral column at atlanto-occipital joints.

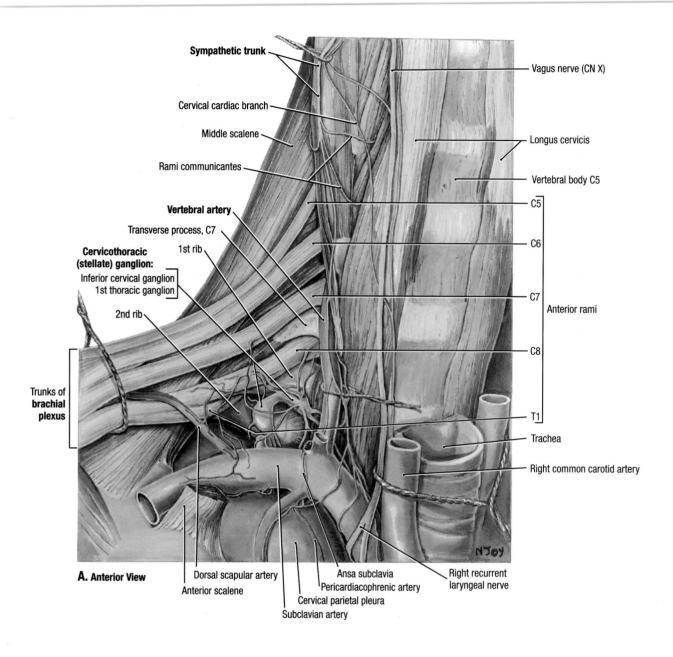

Sympathetic trunk

Cervical cardiac branch

Middle scalene

Rami communicantes

Vertebral artery

Transverse process, C7

Cervicothoracic (stellate) ganglion:

1st rib

Inferior cervical ganglion
1st thoracic ganglion

2nd rib

Trunks of **brachial plexus**

Vagus nerve (CN X)

Longus cervicis

Vertebral body C5

C5

C6

C7

Anterior rami

C8

T1

Trachea

Right common carotid artery

A. Anterior View

Dorsal scapular artery

Anterior scalene

Ansa subclavia

Pericardiacophrenic artery

Cervical parietal pleura

Subclavian artery

Right recurrent laryngeal nerve

8.18 Brachial plexus and sympathetic trunk in the root of the neck

A. Dissection of right side of specimen. The pleura has been depressed, the vertebral artery retracted medially, and the brachial plexus retracted superiorly to reveal the cervicothoracic (stellate) ganglion (the combined inferior cervical and 1st thoracic ganglia). Anesthetic injected around the cervicothoracic (stellate) ganglion blocks transmission of stimuli through the cervical and superior thoracic ganglia. This ganglion block may relieve vascular spasms involving the brain and upper limb. It is also useful when deciding if surgical resection of the ganglion would be beneficial to a person with excess vasoconstriction of the ipsilateral limb. **B.** Relation of brachial plexus and subclavian artery to anterior and middle scalene muscles.

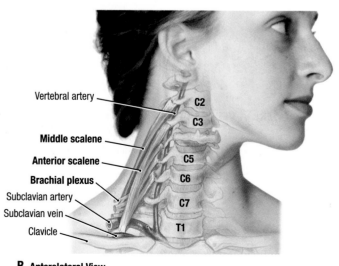

Vertebral artery

Middle scalene

Anterior scalene

Brachial plexus

Subclavian artery

Subclavian vein

Clavicle

C2

C3

C5

C6

C7

T1

B. Anterolateral View

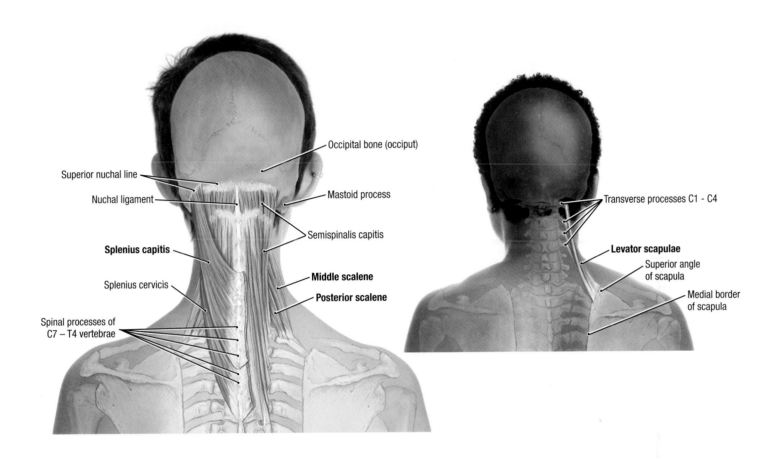

Occipital bone (occiput)

Superior nuchal line

Nuchal ligament

Mastoid process

Semispinalis capitis

Splenius capitis

Splenius cervicis

Middle scalene

Posterior scalene

Spinal processes of
C7 – T4 vertebrae

Transverse processes C1 - C4

Levator scapulae

Superior angle
of scapula

Medial border
of scapula

TABLE 8.7 LATERAL VERTEBRAL MUSCLES

Muscle	Superior Attachment	Inferior Attachment	Innervation	Main Action
Splenius capitis	Inferior half of nuchal ligament and spinous processes of C7 and superior 3–4 thoracic vertebrae	Lateral aspect of mastoid process and lateral third of superior nuchal line	Posterior rami of middle cervical spinal nerves	Laterally flexes and rotates head and neck to same side; acting bilaterally, extend head and neck[a]
Levator scapulae	Posterior tubercles of transverse processes of C1–C4 vertebrae	Superior part of medial border of scapula	Dorsal scapular nerve (C5) and cervical spinal nerves C3 and C4	Elevates scapula and tilts its glenoid cavity inferiorly by rotating scapula
Middle scalene	Posterior tubercles of transverse processes of C2–C7 vertebrae	Superior surface of 1st rib posterior to groove for subclavian artery	Anterior rami of cervical spinal nerves	Flexes neck laterally; elevates 1st rib during forced inspiration[b]
Posterior scalene		External border of 2nd rib	Anterior rami of cervical spinal nerves C4 to C8	Flexes neck laterally; elevates 2nd rib during forced inspiration[b]

[a]Rotation of head occurs at atlantoaxial joints.
[b]Flexion of neck anterior (or lateral) bending of cervical vertebrae C2–C7.

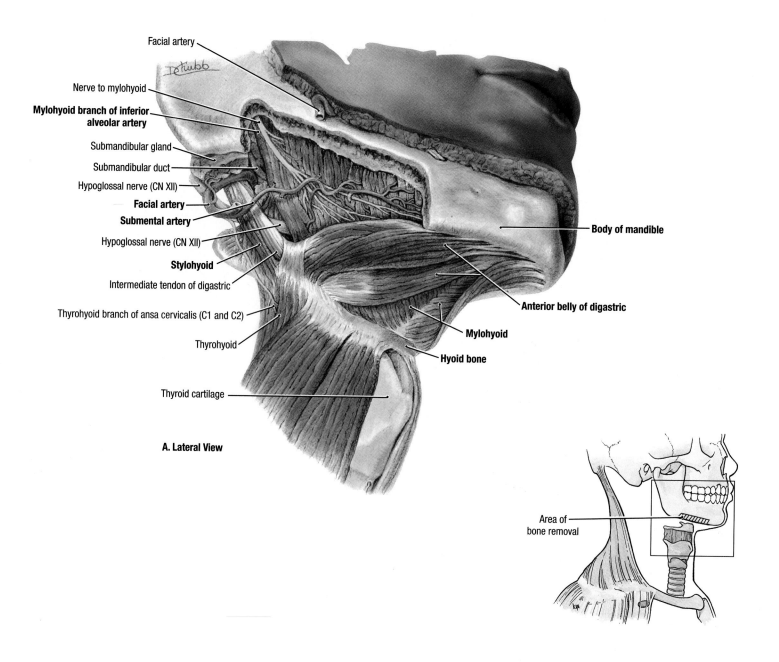

Facial artery

Nerve to mylohyoid

Mylohyoid branch of inferior alveolar artery

Submandibular gland

Submandibular duct

Hypoglossal nerve (CN XII)

Facial artery

Submental artery

Hypoglossal nerve (CN XII)

Stylohyoid

Intermediate tendon of digastric

Thyrohyoid branch of ansa cervicalis (C1 and C2)

Thyrohyoid

Thyroid cartilage

Body of mandible

Anterior belly of digastric

Mylohyoid

Hyoid bone

A. Lateral View

Area of bone removal

8.19   **Serial dissection of submandibular region and floor of mouth—I**

Mylohyoid and digastric muscles. **A.** Structures overlying the mandible and a portion of the body of the mandible have been removed.

- The stylohyoid and posterior belly and intermediate tendon of the digastric muscle form the posterior border of the submandibular triangle; the facial artery passes superficial to these muscles.
- The anterior belly of the digastric muscle forms the anterior border of the submandibular triangle. In this specimen, the anterior belly has an additional origin from the hyoid bone; the mylohyoid muscle forms the medial wall of the triangle and has a thick, free posterior border.
- The nerve to mylohyoid, which supplies the mylohyoid muscle and anterior belly of the digastric muscle, is accompanied by the mylohyoid branch of the inferior alveolar artery posteriorly and the submental artery from the facial artery anteriorly.

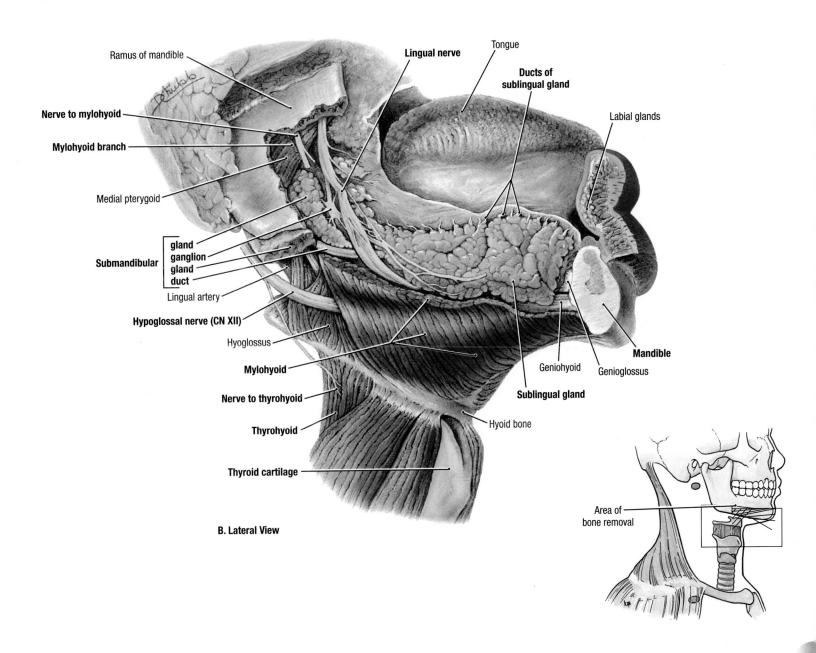

B. Lateral View

8.19   **Serial dissection of submandibular region and floor of mouth—II**

B. Sublingual and submandibular glands. The body and adjacent portion of the ramus of the mandible have been removed.
- The sublingual salivary gland lies posterior to the mandible and is in contact with the deep part of the submandibular gland posteriorly.
- Numerous fine ducts pass from the superior border of the sublingual gland to open on the sublingual fold of the overlying mucosa.
- The lingual nerve lies between the sublingual gland and the deep part of the submandibular gland; the submandibular ganglion is suspended from this nerve.
- Spinal nerve C1 fibers, conveyed by the hypoglossal nerve (CN XII), pass to the thyrohyoid muscle before the hypoglossal nerve passes deep to the mylohyoid muscle.

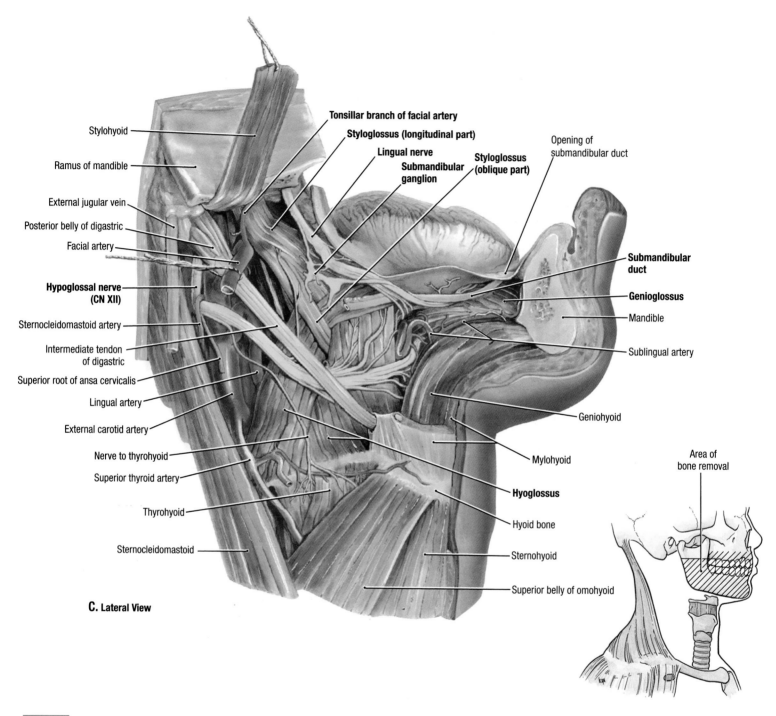

Stylohyoid

Ramus of mandible

External jugular vein

Posterior belly of digastric

Facial artery

Hypoglossal nerve (CN XII)

Sternocleidomastoid artery

Intermediate tendon of digastric

Superior root of ansa cervicalis

Lingual artery

External carotid artery

Nerve to thyrohyoid

Superior thyroid artery

Thyrohyoid

Sternocleidomastoid

Tonsillar branch of facial artery

Styloglossus (longitudinal part)

Lingual nerve

Submandibular ganglion

Styloglossus (oblique part)

Opening of submandibular duct

Submandibular duct

Genioglossus

Mandible

Sublingual artery

Geniohyoid

Mylohyoid

Area of bone removal

Hyoglossus

Hyoid bone

Sternohyoid

Superior belly of omohyoid

C. Lateral View

8.19 **Serial dissection of submandibular region and floor of mouth—III**

C. Hyoglossus muscle, lingual and hypoglossal nerves (CN XII). All of the right half of the mandible, except the superior part of the ramus, has been removed. The stylohyoid muscle is reflected superiorly, and the posterior belly of the digastric muscle is left in situ.

- The hyoglossus muscle ascends from the greater horn and body of the hyoid bone to the side of the tongue.
- The styloglossus muscle is crossed by the tonsillar branch of the facial artery posterosuperiorly, and its oblique part interdigitates with bundles of the hyoglossus muscle inferiorly.

- The hypoglossal nerve supplies all of the muscles of the tongue, both extrinsic and intrinsic, except the palatoglossus (a palatine muscle, innervated by CN X).
- The submandibular duct runs anteriorly in contact with the hyoglossus and genioglossus muscles to its opening on the side of the frenulum of the tongue.
- The lingual nerve is in contact with the mandible posteriorly, looping inferior to the submandibular duct and ending in the tongue. The submandibular ganglion is suspended from the lingual nerve; twigs leave the nerve to supply the mucous membrane.

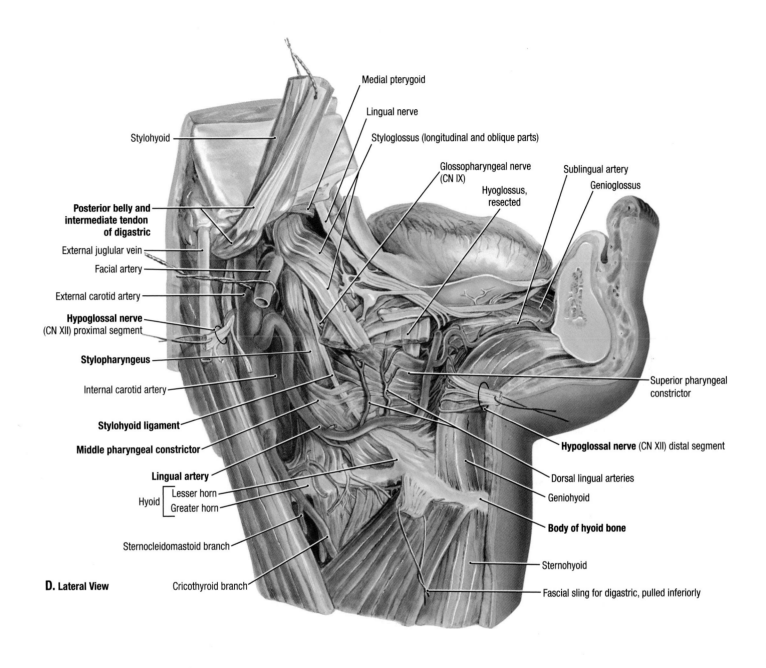

Medial pterygoid

Lingual nerve

Styloglossus (longitudinal and oblique parts)

Stylohyoid

Glossopharyngeal nerve (CN IX)

Sublingual artery

Genioglossus

Hyoglossus, resected

Posterior belly and intermediate tendon of digastric

External juglular vein

Facial artery

External carotid artery

Hypoglossal nerve (CN XII) proximal segment

Stylopharyngeus

Internal carotid artery

Superior pharyngeal constrictor

Stylohyoid ligament

Middle pharyngeal constrictor

Hypoglossal nerve (CN XII) distal segment

Lingual artery

Dorsal lingual arteries

Geniohyoid

Hyoid — Lesser horn / Greater horn

Body of hyoid bone

Sternocleidomastoid branch

Sternohyoid

D. Lateral View

Cricothyroid branch

Fascial sling for digastric, pulled inferiorly

8.19   **Serial dissection of submandibular region and floor of mouth—IV**

D. Genioglossus and geniohyoid muscles. The stylohyoid, posterior belly and intermediate tendon of the digastric muscle are reflected superiorly, the hypoglossal nerve is divided, and the hyoglossus muscle is mostly removed.

- The lingual artery passes deep to the hyoglossus muscle (resected here), close to the greater horn of the hyoid, and then passes lateral to the middle pharyngeal constrictor muscle, stylohyoid ligament, and genioglossus muscle and turns into the tongue as the deep lingual arteries.

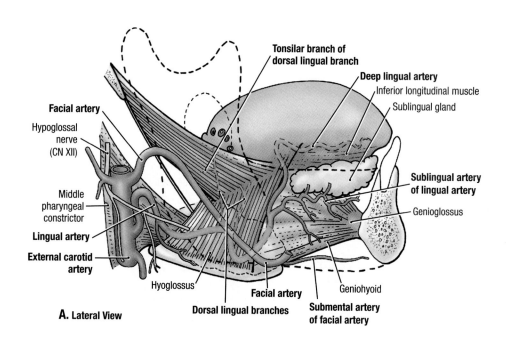

A. Lateral View

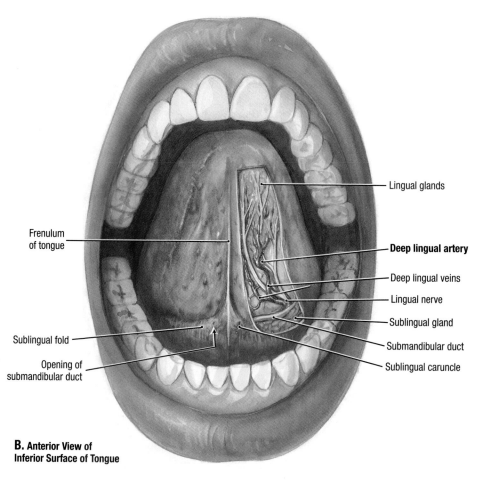

**B. Anterior View of
Inferior Surface of Tongue**

8.20 **Lingual and facial arteries in submandibular region and floor of mouth**

A. Course of the lingual artery. **B.** Inferior surface of the tongue and floor of the mouth.

In **A**:

• The dorsal lingual arteries supply the root of the tongue and palatine tonsil, the deep lingual artery supplies the body of the tongue, and the sublingual branch supplies the floor of the mouth.

In **B**:

• The inferior (sublingual) surface of the tongue is covered by a mucous membrane through which the underlying deep lingual veins can be seen.

• The sublingual caruncle, a papilla on each side of the frenulum, marks the location of the opening of the submandibular duct.

Posterior Views

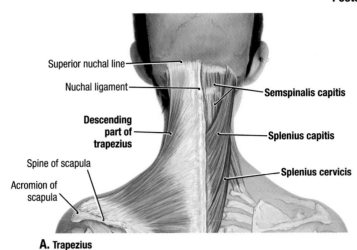

Superior nuchal line
Nuchal ligament
Descending part of trapezius
Spine of scapula
Acromion of scapula
Semspinalis capitis
Splenius capitis
Splenius cervicis

A. Trapezius

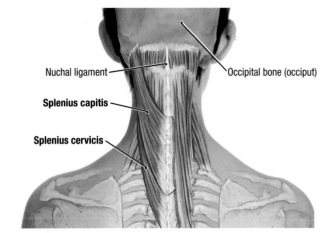

Nuchal ligament
Splenius capitis
Splenius cervicis
Occipital bone (occiput)

B. Splenius

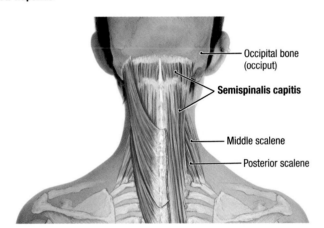

Occipital bone (occiput)
Semispinalis capitis
Middle scalene
Posterior scalene

C. Semispinalis

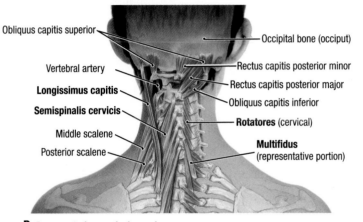

Obliquus capitis superior
Vertebral artery
Longissimus capitis
Semispinalis cervicis
Middle scalene
Posterior scalene
Occipital bone (occiput)
Rectus capitis posterior minor
Rectus capitis posterior major
Obliquus capitis inferior
Rotatores (cervical)
Multifidus (representative portion)

D. Deep posterior cervical muscles

TABLE 8.8 MUSCLES OF POSTERIOR CERVICAL REGION

Muscle	Superior Attachment	Inferior Attachment	Innervation	Main Action
Extrinsic muscle of back (superior axioappendicular muscle)				
Descending part of trapezius	Medial third of superior nuchal line; external occipital protuberance; nuchal ligament	Lateral third of clavicle and lateral aspect of acromion of scapula	Spinal accessory nerve (CN XI)	Elevates scapulae and works with other parts of muscle to retract scapulae; with shoulder fixed, contributes to extension of head, side bending (lateral flexion) of neck
Intrinsic muscles of back—superficial layer				
Splenius	Nuchal ligament and spinous processes of C7 toT3–T4 vertebrae	*Splenius capitis:* fibers run superolaterally to mastoid process of temporal bone and lateral third of superior nuchal line of occipital bone *Splenius cervicis:* Tubercles of transverse processes of C1–C4 vertebrae	Posterior rami of spinal nerves	*Acting unilaterally:* laterally flex and rotate head to side of active muscle *Acting bilaterally:* extend head and neck
Intrinsic muscles of back—intermediate layer				
Longissimus	Transverse processes of T1–T5 vertebrae	*Longissimus capitis:* posterior mastoid process *Longissimus cervicis:* transverse processes of C2–C6	Posterior rami of spinal nerves	Extends vertebral column; longissimus capitis turns face ipsilaterally
Intrinsic muscles of back—deep layer				
Semispinalis	Transverse processes of C4-T5 vertebrae	*Semispinalis capitis:* Superior nuchal line of occipital bone *Semispinalis cervicis:* Spinous processes of cervical vertebrae		*Acting unilaterally:* contribute to contralateral rotation; *Acting bilaterally:* extend head and neck
Multifidus of cervical region	Transverse processes of T1–T3 Articular processes of C4–C7 vertebrae	Spinous processes 2–4 segments inferior to attachment	Posterior rami of spinal nerves	Stabilizes vertebrae during local movements of vertebral column
Rotatores	Transverse processes	Junction of lamina and transverse process, or spinous process of vertebra immediately (brevis) or two segments (longus) superior to origin		Stabilize, assist with local extension and rotatory movements; may function as proprioceptive organs

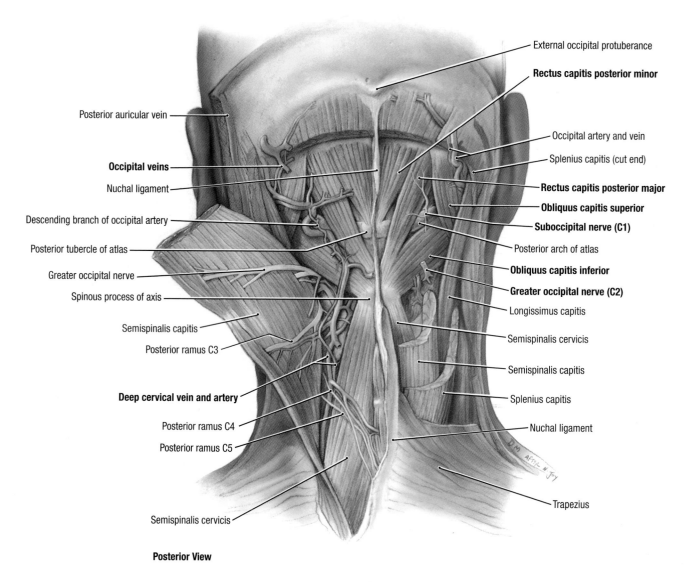

External occipital protuberance

Rectus capitis posterior minor

Posterior auricular vein

Occipital artery and vein

Splenius capitis (cut end)

Occipital veins

Rectus capitis posterior major

Nuchal ligament

Obliquus capitis superior

Descending branch of occipital artery

Suboccipital nerve (C1)

Posterior tubercle of atlas

Posterior arch of atlas

Greater occipital nerve

Obliquus capitis inferior

Spinous process of axis

Greater occipital nerve (C2)

Longissimus capitis

Semispinalis capitis

Semispinalis cervicis

Posterior ramus C3

Semispinalis capitis

Deep cervical vein and artery

Splenius capitis

Posterior ramus C4

Nuchal ligament

Posterior ramus C5

Trapezius

Semispinalis cervicis

Posterior View

8.21   Suboccipital region

A. Dissection. B. Schematic illustration.

- The suboccipital triangle is bounded by three muscles: obliquus capitis inferior and superior, and rectus capitis posterior major.
- The suboccipital nerve (posterior ramus of C1) emerges through the suboccipital triangle to innervate the muscles forming the triangle.

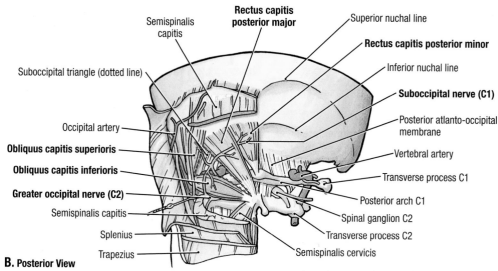

Semispinalis capitis

Rectus capitis posterior major

Superior nuchal line

Rectus capitis posterior minor

Suboccipital triangle (dotted line)

Inferior nuchal line

Suboccipital nerve (C1)

Occipital artery

Posterior atlanto-occipital membrane

Obliquus capitis superioris

Obliquus capitis inferioris

Vertebral artery

Greater occipital nerve (C2)

Transverse process C1

Semispinalis capitis

Posterior arch C1

Splenius

Spinal ganglion C2

Trapezius

Transverse process C2

Semispinalis cervicis

B. Posterior View

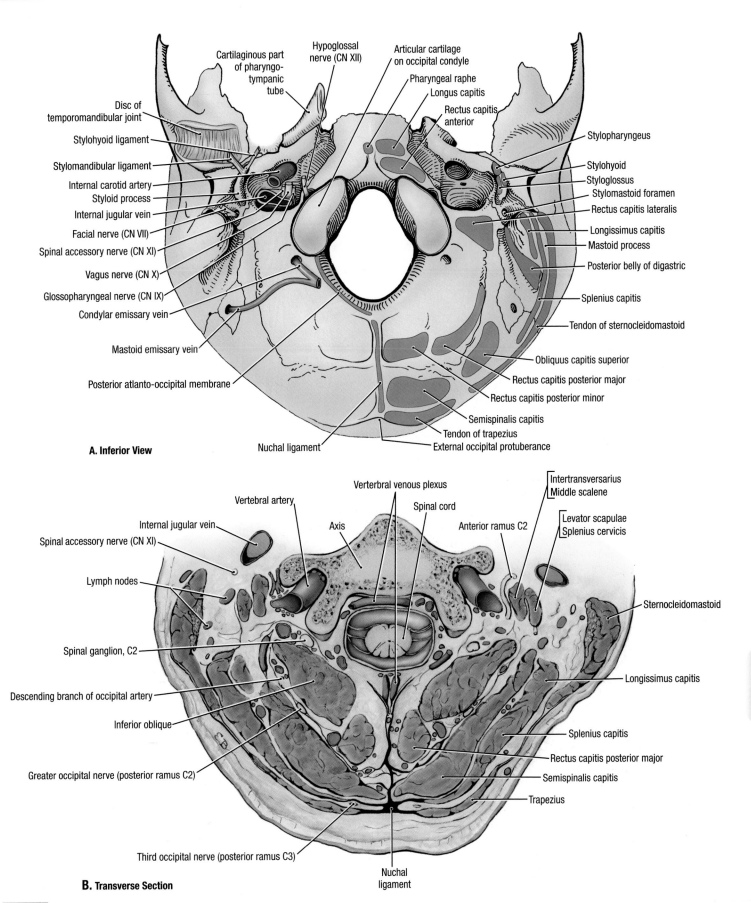

A. Inferior View

Cartilaginous part of pharyngo-tympanic tube

Disc of temporomandibular joint

Stylohyoid ligament

Stylomandibular ligament

Internal carotid artery

Styloid process

Internal jugular vein

Facial nerve (CN VII)

Spinal accessory nerve (CN XI)

Vagus nerve (CN X)

Glossopharyngeal nerve (CN IX)

Condylar emissary vein

Mastoid emissary vein

Posterior atlanto-occipital membrane

Hypoglossal nerve (CN XII)

Articular cartilage on occipital condyle

Pharyngeal raphe

Longus capitis

Rectus capitis anterior

Stylopharyngeus

Stylohyoid

Styloglossus

Stylomastoid foramen

Rectus capitis lateralis

Longissimus capitis

Mastoid process

Posterior belly of digastric

Splenius capitis

Tendon of sternocleidomastoid

Obliquus capitis superior

Rectus capitis posterior major

Rectus capitis posterior minor

Semispinalis capitis

Tendon of trapezius

External occipital protuberance

Nuchal ligament

B. Transverse Section

Verterbral venous plexus

Vertebral artery

Internal jugular vein

Spinal accessory nerve (CN XI)

Lymph nodes

Spinal ganglion, C2

Descending branch of occipital artery

Inferior oblique

Greater occipital nerve (posterior ramus C2)

Axis

Spinal cord

Anterior ramus C2

Intertransversarius
Middle scalene

Levator scapulae
Splenius cervicis

Sternocleidomastoid

Longissimus capitis

Splenius capitis

Rectus capitis posterior major

Semispinalis capitis

Trapezius

Third occipital nerve (posterior ramus C3)

Nuchal ligament

8.22   Posterior cervical region—base of skull and transverse section

A. Muscular attachments to and neurovascular relationships at the base of the skull. **B.** Transverse section through the axis (C2).

Structures exiting via jugular foramen

| CN X | CN IX | CN XI | Jugular bulb |

Hypoglossal nerve (CN XII)

Basiocciput

Pharyngobasilar fascia

Internal carotid artery

Stylohyoid

Posterior belly of digastric

Glossopharyngeal nerve (CN IX)

Stylopharyngeus

Superior pharyngeal constrictor

Ascending pharyngeal artery

Submandibular gland

Carotid arteries — External / Internal / Common

Inferior pharyngeal constrictor

Left lobe of thyroid gland

Left recurrent laryngeal nerve

Parathyroid glands — Superior / Inferior

Esophagus

A. Posterior View

M. Sewell.

Internal jugular vein

Styloid process

Facial nerve (CN VII)

Parotid gland

Posterior belly of digastric (cut)

Stylopharyngeus

Superior cervical ganglion

Pharyngeal / Superior laryngeal — Branches of CN X

Hypoglossal nerve (CN XII)

Spinal accessory nerve (CN XI)

Middle pharyngeal constrictor

Sternocleidomastoid

Internal jugular vein

Vagus nerve (CN X)

Common carotid artery

Sympathetic trunk

Right lobe of thyroid gland

Sheath of thyroid gland

Parathyroid gland

Inferior thyroid artery

Right recurrent laryngeal nerve

Paratracheal lymph nodes

8.23   **External pharynx—I**

A. Illustration of a dissection similar to **B.** The sympathetic trunk (including the superior cervical ganglion), which normally lies posterior to the internal carotid artery, has been retracted medially.

• The pharyngobasilar fascia, between the superior pharyngeal constrictor muscle and the base of the skull, attaches the phar-

ynx to the occipital bone and forms the wall of the noncollapsible pharyngeal recesses.

• As they exit the jugular foramen, CN IX lies anterior to CN X, and CN XI; CN XII, exiting the hypoglossal canal, lies medially.

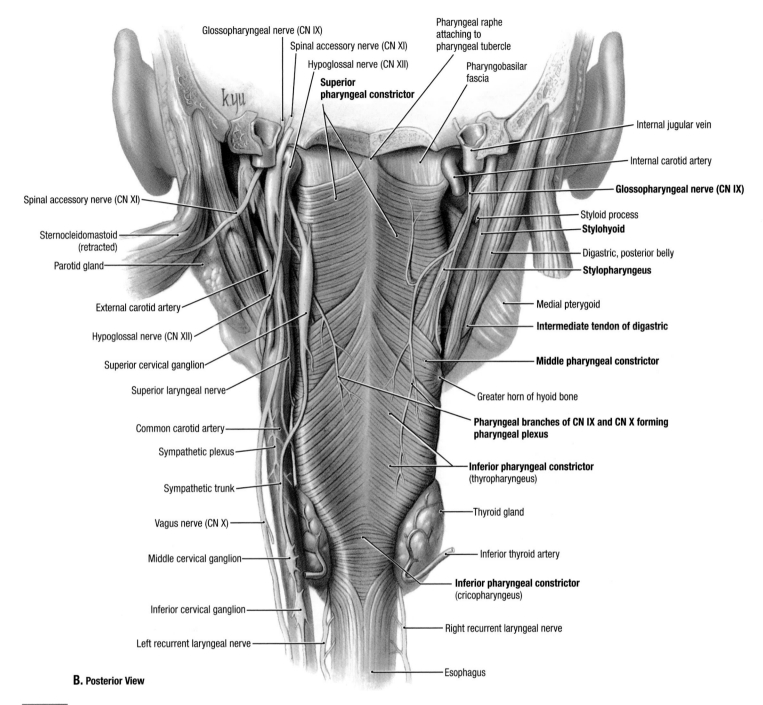

Glossopharyngeal nerve (CN IX)

Spinal accessory nerve (CN XI)

Hypoglossal nerve (CN XII)

Superior pharyngeal constrictor

Pharyngeal raphe attaching to pharyngeal tubercle

Pharyngobasilar fascia

Internal jugular vein

Internal carotid artery

Glossopharyngeal nerve (CN IX)

Styloid process

Stylohyoid

Digastric, posterior belly

Stylopharyngeus

Medial pterygoid

Intermediate tendon of digastric

Middle pharyngeal constrictor

Greater horn of hyoid bone

Pharyngeal branches of CN IX and CN X forming pharyngeal plexus

Inferior pharyngeal constrictor (thyropharyngeus)

Thyroid gland

Inferior thyroid artery

Inferior pharyngeal constrictor (cricopharyngeus)

Right recurrent laryngeal nerve

Esophagus

Spinal accessory nerve (CN XI)

Sternocleidomastoid (retracted)

Parotid gland

External carotid artery

Hypoglossal nerve (CN XII)

Superior cervical ganglion

Superior laryngeal nerve

Common carotid artery

Sympathetic plexus

Sympathetic trunk

Vagus nerve (CN X)

Middle cervical ganglion

Inferior cervical ganglion

Left recurrent laryngeal nerve

B. Posterior View

8.23   External pharynx—II

B. Dissection. A large wedge of occipital bone (including the foramen magnum) and the articulated cervical vertebrae have been separated from the remainder (anterior portion) of the head and cervical viscera at the retropharyngeal space and removed.

- The pharynx is a unique portion of the alimentary tract, having a circular layer of muscle externally and a longitudinal layer internally.
- The circular layer of the pharynx consists of the three pharyngeal constrictor muscles (superior, middle, and inferior), which overlap one another.
- On the right side of the specimen, the stylopharyngeus muscle and glossopharyngeal nerve (IX) pass from the medial side of the

styloid process anteromedially through the interval between the superior and middle pharyngeal constrictor muscles to become part of the internal longitudinal layer. The stylohyoid muscle passes from the lateral side of the styloid process anterolaterally and splits on its way to the hyoid bone to accommodate passage of the intermediate tendon of the digastric.

- Pharyngeal branches of the glossopharyngeal nerve (CN IX) and the vagus nerve (CN X) form the pharyngeal plexus, which provides most of the pharyngeal innervation. The glossopharyngeal nerve supplies the sensory component, while the vagus supplies motor innervation.

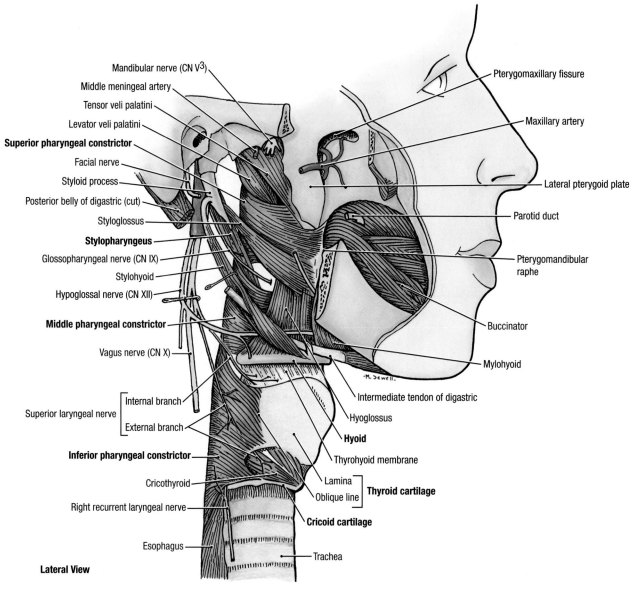

Lateral View

TABLE 8.9 MUSCLES OF PHARYNX

Muscle	Origin	Insertion	Innervation	Main Action(s)
Superior pharyngeal constrictor	Pterygoid hamulus, pterygo-mandibular raphe, posterior end of mylohyoid line of mandible, and side of tongue	Pharyngeal raphe	Pharyngeal and superior laryngeal branches of vagus (CN X) through pharyngeal plexus	Constrict wall of pharynx during swallowing
Middle pharyngeal constrictor	Stylohyoid ligament and superior (greater) and inferior (lesser) horns of hyoid bone			
Inferior pharyngeal constrictor				
Thyropharyngeus	Oblique line of thyroid cartilage			
Cricopharyngeus (see Fig. 8.20B)	Side of cricoid cartilage	Contralateral side of cricoid cartilage	Pharyngeal and superior laryngeal branches of vagus (CN X) through pharyngeal plexus + external laryngeal plexus	Serves as superior esophageal sphincter
Palatopharyngeus (see Fig. 8.21B)	Hard palate and palatine aponeurosis	Posterior border of lamina of thyroid cartilage and side of pharynx and esophagus	Pharyngeal and superior laryngeal branches of vagus (CN X) through pharyngeal plexus	Elevate pharynx and larynx during swallowing and speaking
Salpingopharyngeus (see Fig. 8.21B)	Cartilaginous part of pharyngotympanic tube	Blends with palatopharyngeus		
Stylopharyngeus	Styloid process of temporal bone	Posterior and superior borders of thyroid cartilage with palatopharyngeus	Glossopharyngeal nerve (CN IX)	

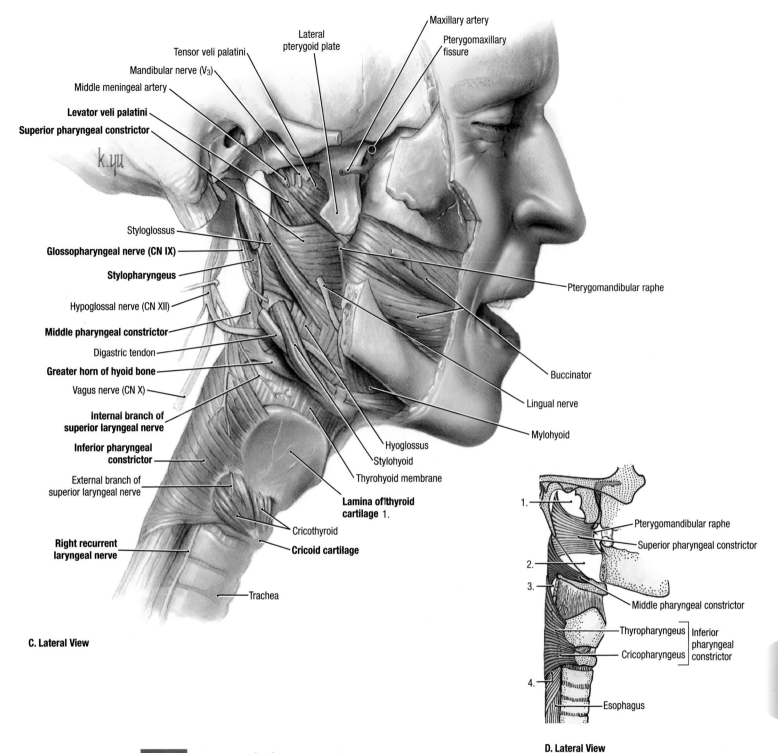

Maxillary artery

Lateral
pterygoid plate

Pterygomaxillary
fissure

Tensor veli palatini

Mandibular nerve (V₃)

Middle meningeal artery

Levator veli palatini

Superior pharyngeal constrictor

Styloglossus

Glossopharyngeal nerve (CN IX)

Stylopharyngeus

Hypoglossal nerve (CN XII)

Middle pharyngeal constrictor

Digastric tendon

Greater horn of hyoid bone

Vagus nerve (CN X)

**Internal branch of
superior laryngeal nerve**

**Inferior pharyngeal
constrictor**

External branch of
superior laryngeal nerve

**Right recurrent
laryngeal nerve**

Trachea

Cricothyroid

Cricoid cartilage

**Lamina of thyroid
cartilage** 1.

Thyrohyoid membrane

Stylohyoid

Hyoglossus

Mylohyoid

Lingual nerve

Buccinator

Pterygomandibular raphe

C. Lateral View

Pterygomandibular raphe

Superior pharyngeal constrictor

Middle pharyngeal constrictor

Thyropharyngeus ⎤ Inferior
　　　　　　　 ⎬ pharyngeal
Cricopharyngeus ⎦ constrictor

Esophagus

D. Lateral View

8.23　**External pharynx—III**

C and **D.** Observe that there are gaps in the pharyngeal musculature (1–4 in **D**) allowing the entry of structures:

1. Superior to the superior constrictor muscle: levator veli palatini muscle and pharyngo-tympanic (auditory) tube (see Fig. 8.24B)
2. Between the superior and middle constrictors: stylopharyngeus muscle, CN IX, and stylohyoid ligament
3. Between the middle and inferior constrictors: internal branch of superior laryngeal nerve and superior laryngeal artery and nerve (not shown)
4. Inferior to the inferior constrictor muscle: recurrent laryngeal nerve

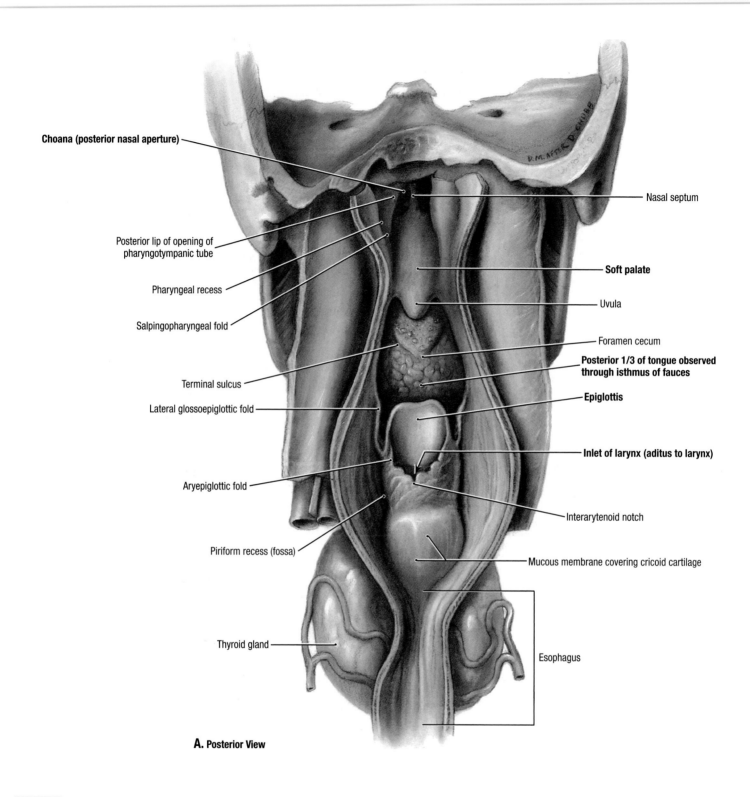

Choana (posterior nasal aperture)

Posterior lip of opening of pharyngotympanic tube

Pharyngeal recess

Salpingopharyngeal fold

Terminal sulcus

Lateral glossoepiglottic fold

Aryepiglottic fold

Piriform recess (fossa)

Thyroid gland

Nasal septum

Soft palate

Uvula

Foramen cecum

Posterior 1/3 of tongue observed through isthmus of fauces

Epiglottis

Inlet of larynx (aditus to larynx)

Interarytenoid notch

Mucous membrane covering cricoid cartilage

Esophagus

A. Posterior View

8.24   Internal pharynx—I

A. Dissection. The posterior wall of the pharynx has been split in the midline and the halves retracted laterally to reveal the internal aspect of the anterior wall of the pharynx, occupied by communications that define three parts of the pharynx: (1) the nasal part (nasopharynx), superior to the level of the soft palate, communicates anteriorly through the choanae with the nasal cavities; (2) the oral part (oropharynx), between the soft palate and the epiglottis, communicates anteriorly through the isthmus of the fauces with the oral cavity; and (3) the laryngeal part (laryngopharynx), posterior to the larynx, communicates with the vestibule of the larynx through the inlet of (aditus to) the larynx. The pharynx extends from the cranial base to the inferior border of the cricoid cartilage. Inferiorly, it is narrowed by the encircling cricopharyngeus.

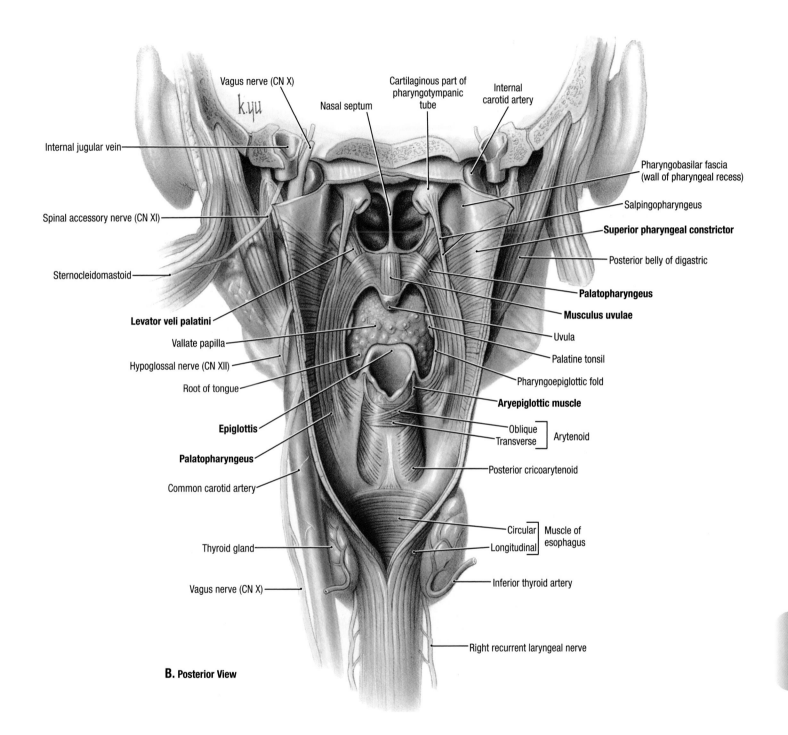

Vagus nerve (CN X)

k.yu

Nasal septum

Cartilaginous part of pharyngotympanic tube

Internal carotid artery

Internal jugular vein

Spinal accessory nerve (CN XI)

Sternocleidomastoid

Levator veli palatini

Vallate papilla

Hypoglossal nerve (CN XII)

Root of tongue

Epiglottis

Palatopharyngeus

Common carotid artery

Thyroid gland

Vagus nerve (CN X)

Pharyngobasilar fascia (wall of pharyngeal recess)

Salpingopharyngeus

Superior pharyngeal constrictor

Posterior belly of digastric

Palatopharyngeus

Musculus uvulae

Uvula

Palatine tonsil

Pharyngoepiglottic fold

Aryepiglottic muscle

Oblique
Transverse } Arytenoid

Posterior cricoarytenoid

Circular
Longitudinal } Muscle of esophagus

Inferior thyroid artery

Right recurrent laryngeal nerve

B. Posterior View

8.24   Internal pharynx—II

B. Illustration. The posterior wall of the pharynx has been split in the midline and reflected laterally as in **A**; then, the mucous membrane was removed to expose the underlying musculature. The muscles of the soft palate, pharynx, and larynx work together during swallowing, elevating the soft palate, narrowing the pharyngeal isthmus (passageway between the nasal and oral parts of the pharynx) and laryngeal inlet, retracting the epiglottis, and closing the glottis, to keep food and drink out of the nasopharynx and larynx as they pass from oral cavity to esophagus. At other times, as when blowing one's nose, the palatopharyngeus muscles, partially encircling the opening to the oral cavity, constrict this opening and depress the soft palate, working with placement and expansion of the posterior tongue to direct expired air through the nasal cavity.

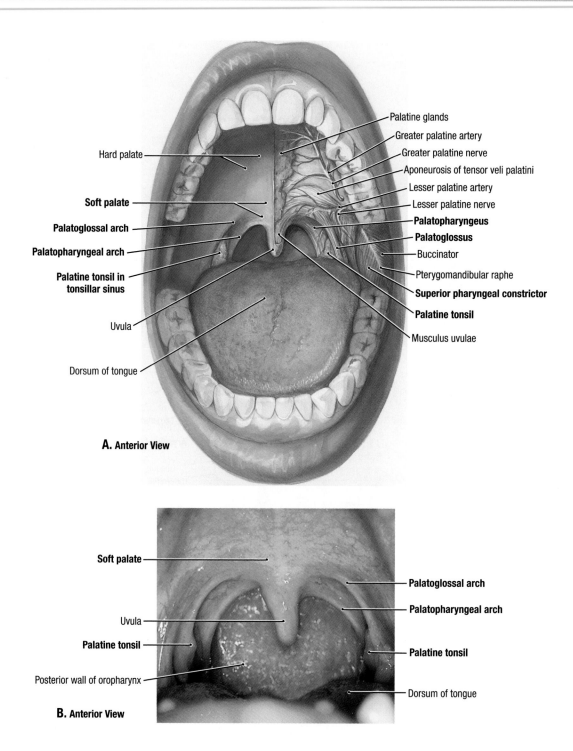

Palatine glands
Greater palatine artery
Greater palatine nerve
Aponeurosis of tensor veli palatini
Lesser palatine artery
Lesser palatine nerve
Palatopharyngeus
Palatoglossus
Buccinator
Pterygomandibular raphe
Superior pharyngeal constrictor
Palatine tonsil
Musculus uvulae

Hard palate
Soft palate
Palatoglossal arch
Palatopharyngeal arch
Palatine tonsil in tonsillar sinus
Uvula
Dorsum of tongue

A. Anterior View

Soft palate
Uvula
Palatine tonsil
Posterior wall of oropharynx

Palatoglossal arch
Palatopharyngeal arch
Palatine tonsil
Dorsum of tongue

B. Anterior View

8.25 **Surface anatomy of isthmus of the fauces (oropharyngeal isthmus)**

A. Oral cavity and isthmus demonstrating the sinus (bed) of the tonsils. **B.** Tonsillar sinuses with palatine tonsils in situ, and oropharynx.

- The fauces (throat), the passage from the mouth to the pharynx, is bounded superiorly by the soft palate, inferiorly by the root (base) of the tongue, and laterally by the palatoglossal and palatopharyngeal arches.
- The palatine tonsils are located between the palatoglossal and palatopharyngeal arches, formed by mucosa overlying the similarly named muscles; the arches form the boundaries, and the superior pharyngeal constrictor the floor, of the tonsillar sinuses.

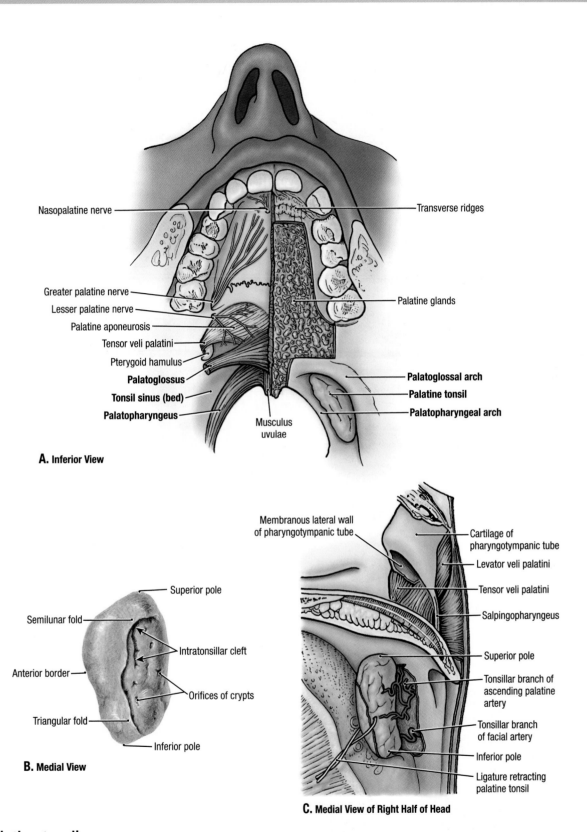

A. Inferior View

B. Medial View

C. Medial View of Right Half of Head

8.26   **Palatine tonsil**

A. Left side: Palatine tonsil in situ and glands of palatine mucosa. Right side: Palatine mucosa and tonsils removed demonstrating palatine nerves and muscles. **B.** Isolated palatine tonsil. **C.** Tonsillectomy. The procedure involves removal of the tonsil and the fascial sheet covering the tonsillar sinus. Because of the rich blood supply of the tonsil, bleeding commonly arises from the large external palatine vein or less commonly from the tonsillar artery or other arterial twigs. The glossopharyngeal nerve accompanies the tonsillar artery on the lateral wall of the pharynx and is vulnerable to injury because this wall is thin. The internal carotid artery is especially vulnerable when it is tortuous, as it lies directly lateral to the tonsil.

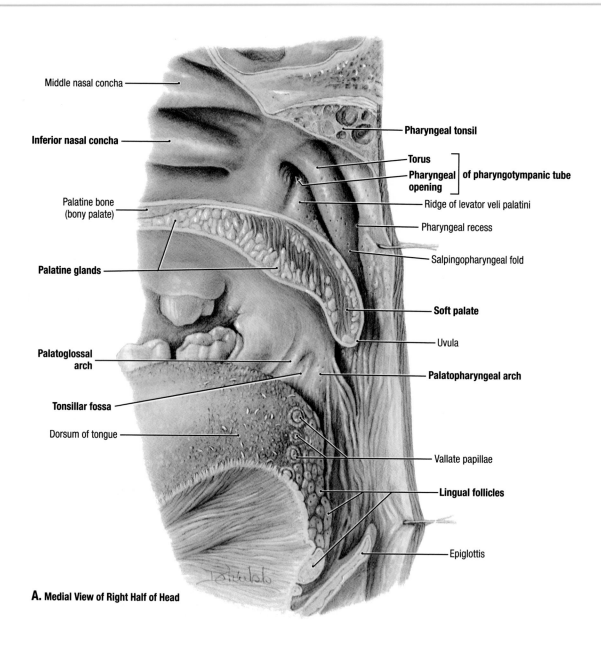

Middle nasal concha

Inferior nasal concha

Palatine bone
(bony palate)

Palatine glands

Palatoglossal
arch

Tonsillar fossa

Dorsum of tongue

Pharyngeal tonsil

Torus
Pharyngeal } **of pharyngotympanic tube**
opening

Ridge of levator veli palatini

Pharyngeal recess

Salpingopharyngeal fold

Soft palate

Uvula

Palatopharyngeal arch

Vallate papillae

Lingual follicles

Epiglottis

A. Medial View of Right Half of Head

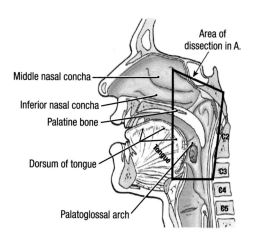

Area of
dissection in A.

Middle nasal concha

Inferior nasal concha

Palatine bone

Dorsum of tongue

Palatoglossal arch

C2

C3

C4

C5

**8.27   Serial dissection of isthmus of fauces and lateral wall of
nasopharynx —I**

- The pharyngeal opening of the pharyngotympanic tube is located approximately 1 cm
  posterior to the inferior concha.
- The numerous pinpoint orifices of the ducts of the mucous glands can be seen in the
  mucosa of the torus.
- The pharyngeal tonsil lies in the mucous membrane of the roof and posterior wall of
  the nasopharynx.
- The palatine glands lie in the soft palate.
- The palatine tonsil lies in the tonsillar sinus between the palatoglossal and palatopharyngeal arches.
- Each lingual follicle has the duct of a mucous gland opening onto its surface; collectively, the follicles are known as the lingual tonsil.

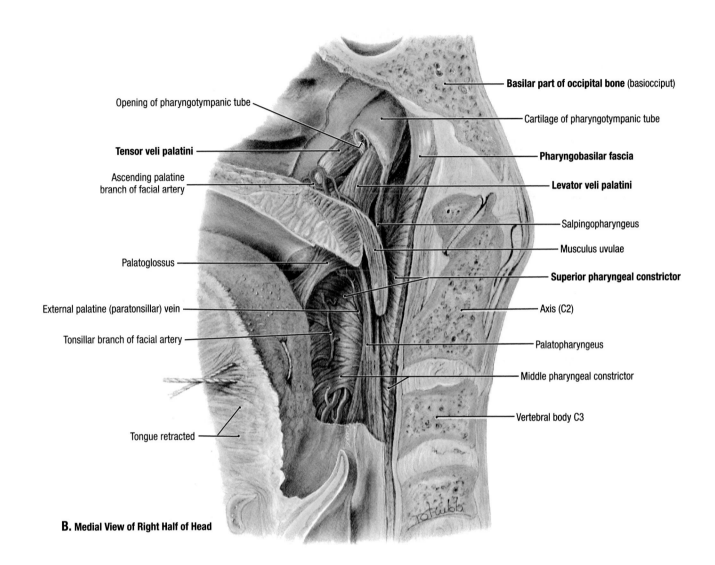

Opening of pharyngotympanic tube

Tensor veli palatini

Ascending palatine branch of facial artery

Palatoglossus

External palatine (paratonsillar) vein

Tonsillar branch of facial artery

Tongue retracted

Basilar part of occipital bone (basiocciput)

Cartilage of pharyngotympanic tube

Pharyngobasilar fascia

Levator veli palatini

Salpingopharyngeus

Musculus uvulae

Superior pharyngeal constrictor

Axis (C2)

Palatopharyngeus

Middle pharyngeal constrictor

Vertebral body C3

B. Medial View of Right Half of Head

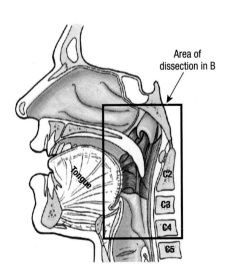

Area of dissection in B

8.27   **Serial dissection of isthmus of fauces and lateral wall of nasopharynx—II**

Muscles underlying tonsillar sinus and wall of nasopharynx. The palatine and pharyngeal tonsils and mucous membrane have been removed. The pharyngobasilar fascia, which attaches the pharynx to the basilar part of the occipital bone was also removed, except at the superior, arched border of the superior pharyngeal constrictor.

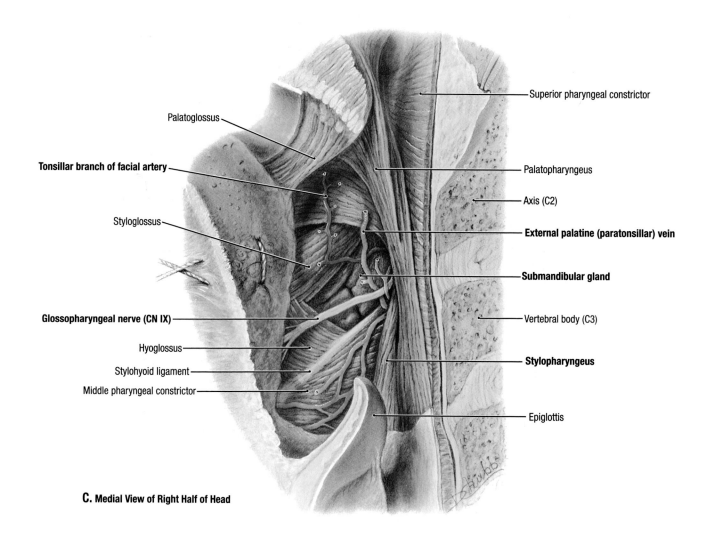

Palatoglossus

Tonsillar branch of facial artery

Styloglossus

Glossopharyngeal nerve (CN IX)

Hyoglossus

Stylohyoid ligament

Middle pharyngeal constrictor

Superior pharyngeal constrictor

Palatopharyngeus

Axis (C2)

External palatine (paratonsillar) vein

Submandibular gland

Vertebral body (C3)

Stylopharyngeus

Epiglottis

C. Medial View of Right Half of Head

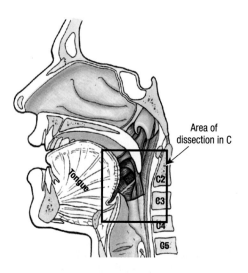

Area of dissection in C

8.27 Serial dissection of isthmus of the fauces and lateral wall of nasopharynx—III

Neurovascular structures of tonsillar sinus and longitudinal muscles of the pharynx.
- In this deeper dissection, the tongue was pulled anteriorly, and the inferior part of the origin of the superior pharyngeal constrictor muscle was cut away.
- The glossopharyngeal nerve passes to the posterior one third of the tongue and lies anterior to the stylopharyngeus muscle.
- The tonsillar branch of the facial artery sends a branch (cut short here) to accompany the glossopharyngeal nerve to the tongue; the submandibular gland is seen lateral to the artery and external palatine (paratonsillar) vein.

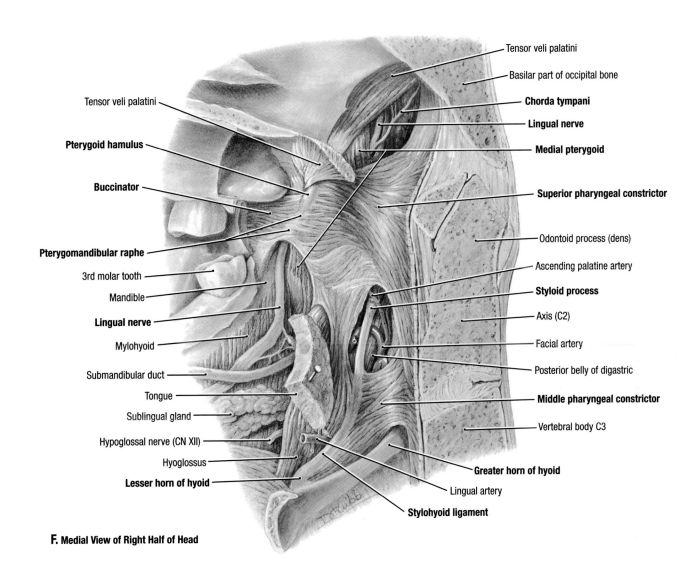

Tensor veli palatini
Basilar part of occipital bone
Chorda tympani
Lingual nerve
Medial pterygoid
Superior pharyngeal constrictor
Odontoid process (dens)
Ascending palatine artery
Styloid process
Axis (C2)
Facial artery
Posterior belly of digastric
Middle pharyngeal constrictor
Vertebral body C3
Greater horn of hyoid
Lingual artery

Tensor veli palatini
Pterygoid hamulus
Buccinator
Pterygomandibular raphe
3rd molar tooth
Mandible
Lingual nerve
Mylohyoid
Submandibular duct
Tongue
Sublingual gland
Hypoglossal nerve (CN XII)
Hyoglossus
Lesser horn of hyoid
Stylohyoid ligament

F. Medial View of Right Half of Head

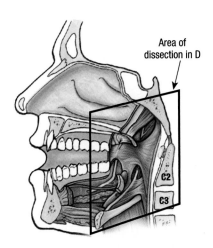

Area of dissection in D

8.27 **Serial dissection of isthmus of the fauces lateral wall of nasopharynx—IV**

- The superior pharyngeal constrictor muscle arises from (a) the pterygomandibular raphe, which unites it to the buccinator muscle; (b) the bones at each end of the raphe, the hamulus of the medial pterygoid plate superiorly and the mandible inferiorly; and (c) the root (posterior part) of the tongue.
- The middle pharyngeal constrictor muscle arises from the angle formed by the greater and lesser horns of the hyoid bone and from the stylohyoid ligament; in this specimen, the styloid process is long and, therefore, a lateral relation of the tonsil.
- The lingual nerve is joined by the chorda tympani, disappears at the posterior border of the medial pterygoid muscle, and reappears at the anterior border to follow the mandible.

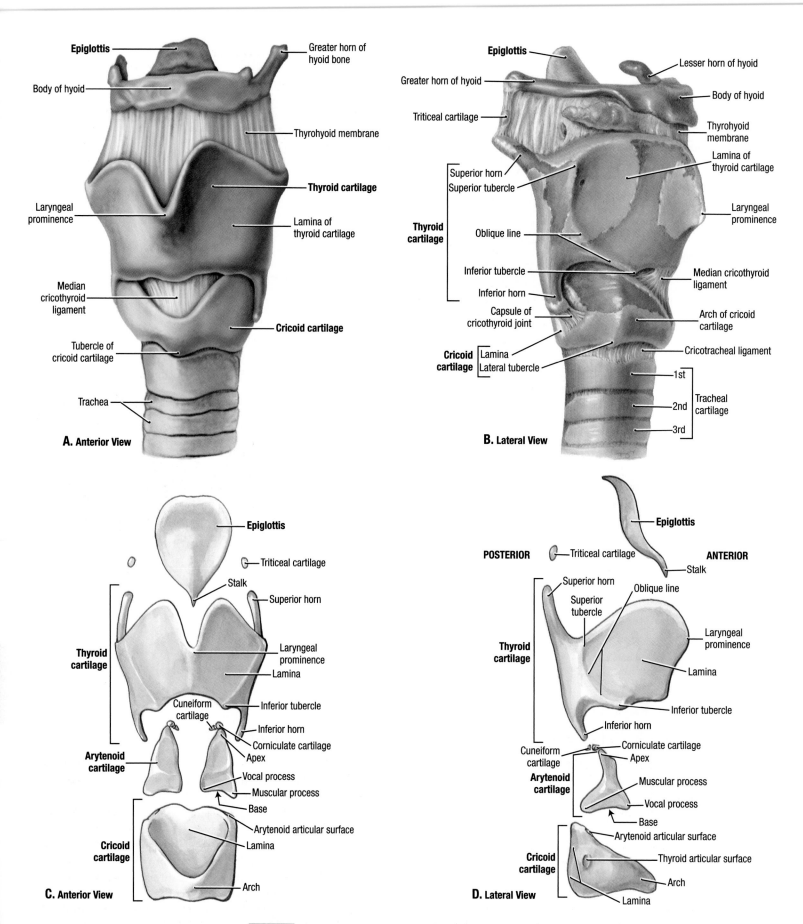

A. Anterior View

Epiglottis
Greater horn of hyoid bone
Body of hyoid
Thyrohyoid membrane
Thyroid cartilage
Laryngeal prominence
Lamina of thyroid cartilage
Median cricothyroid ligament
Cricoid cartilage
Tubercle of cricoid cartilage
Trachea

B. Lateral View

Epiglottis
Lesser horn of hyoid
Greater horn of hyoid
Body of hyoid
Triticeal cartilage
Thyrohyoid membrane
Superior horn
Superior tubercle
Lamina of thyroid cartilage
Thyroid cartilage
Oblique line
Laryngeal prominence
Inferior tubercle
Median cricothyroid ligament
Inferior horn
Capsule of cricothyroid joint
Arch of cricoid cartilage
Cricoid cartilage Lamina Lateral tubercle
Cricotracheal ligament
1st
2nd   Tracheal cartilage
3rd

C. Anterior View

Epiglottis
Triticeal cartilage
Stalk
Superior horn
Thyroid cartilage
Laryngeal prominence
Lamina
Cuneiform cartilage
Inferior tubercle
Inferior horn
Corniculate cartilage
Apex
Arytenoid cartilage
Vocal process
Muscular process
Base
Arytenoid articular surface
Cricoid cartilage
Lamina
Arch

D. Lateral View

Epiglottis
POSTERIOR
Triticeal cartilage
ANTERIOR
Stalk
Superior horn
Oblique line
Superior tubercle
Thyroid cartilage
Laryngeal prominence
Lamina
Inferior tubercle
Inferior horn
Cuneiform cartilage
Corniculate cartilage
Apex
Arytenoid cartilage
Muscular process
Vocal process
Base
Arytenoid articular surface
Thyroid articular surface
Cricoid cartilage
Arch
Lamina

8.28   **Cartilages of the laryngeal skeleton**

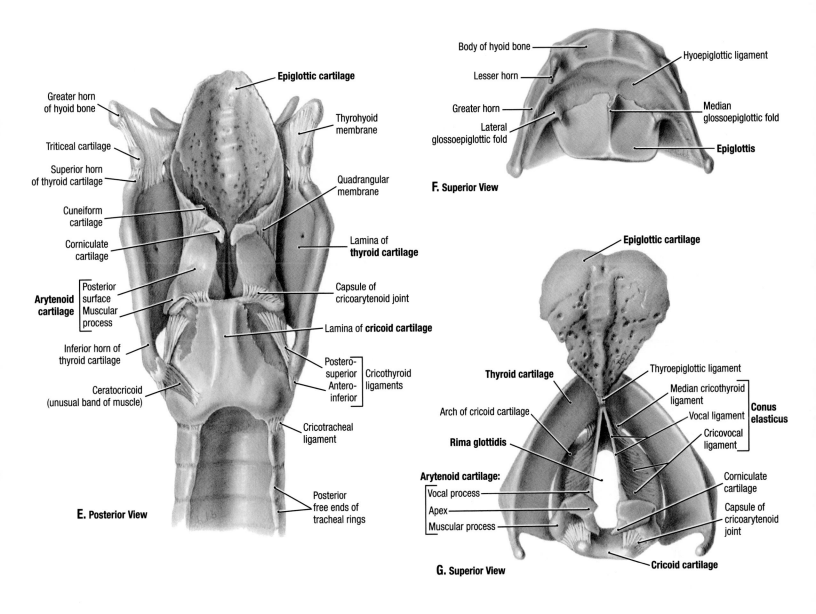

E. Posterior View

Epiglottic cartilage

Greater horn of hyoid bone

Thyrohyoid membrane

Triticeal cartilage

Superior horn of thyroid cartilage

Cuneiform cartilage

Corniculate cartilage

Quadrangular membrane

Lamina of **thyroid cartilage**

Arytenoid cartilage — Posterior surface / Muscular process

Capsule of cricoarytenoid joint

Lamina of **cricoid cartilage**

Inferior horn of thyroid cartilage

Postero-superior / Antero-inferior — Cricothyroid ligaments

Ceratocricoid (unusual band of muscle)

Cricotracheal ligament

Posterior free ends of tracheal rings

F. Superior View

Body of hyoid bone

Lesser horn

Greater horn

Lateral glossoepiglottic fold

Hyoepiglottic ligament

Median glossoepiglottic fold

Epiglottis

G. Superior View

Epiglottic cartilage

Thyroid cartilage

Arch of cricoid cartilage

Rima glottidis

Arytenoid cartilage: Vocal process / Apex / Muscular process

Thyroepiglottic ligament

Median cricothyroid ligament

Vocal ligament

Cricovocal ligament

Conus elasticus

Corniculate cartilage

Capsule of cricoarytenoid joint

Cricoid cartilage

8.28   **Cartilages of the laryngeal skeleton (continued)**

A, B, and **E.** Articulated laryngeal skeleton. **C** and **D.** Cartilages disarticulated and separated. **F.** Epiglottis and hyoepiglottic ligament. **G.** Conus elasticus and rima glottidis.

- The larynx extends vertically from the tip of the epiglottis to the inferior border of the cricoid cartilage. The hyoid bone is generally not regarded as part of the larynx.
- The cricoid cartilage is the only cartilage that totally encircles the airway.
- The rima glottidis is the aperture between the vocal folds. During normal respiration, it is narrow and wedge shaped; during forced respiration, it is wide. Variations in the tension

and length of the vocal folds, in the width of the rima glottidis, and in the intensity of the expiratory effort produce changes in the pitch of the voice.

- Laryngeal fractures may result from blows received in sports such as kickboxing and hockey or from compression by a shoulder strap during an automobile accident. Laryngeal fractures produce submucous hemorrhage and edema, respiratory obstruction, hoarseness, and sometimes a temporary inability to speak. The thyroid, cricoid, and most of the arytenoid cartilages often ossify as age advances, commencing at approximately 25 years of age in the thyroid cartilage.

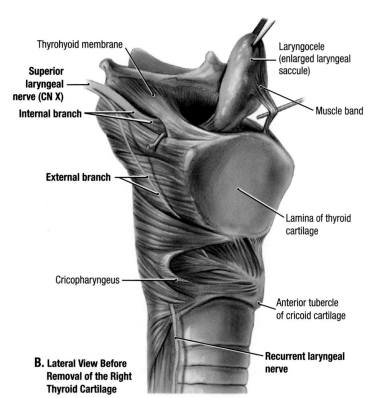

Greater horn of hyoid bone

Thyrohyoid membrane

Epiglottis

Internal branch | **Superior laryngeal nerve**
External branch | **(CN X)**

Median raphe of pharynx

Thyropharyngeus

Inferior pharyngeal constrictor

Cricopharyngeus

Sheath of thyroid gland

Right lobe of thyroid gland

Parathyroid glands { Superior / Inferior

Parathyroid glands

Inferior thyroid artery

Esophagus

Right recurrent laryngeal nerve (CN X)

Submucous coat of esophagus

Paratracheal lymph nodes

A. Posterior View

Incision to open posterior wall of larynx and trachea (Fig. 8.30A)

Thyrohyoid membrane

Laryngocele (enlarged laryngeal saccule)

Superior laryngeal nerve (CN X)

Internal branch

Muscle band

External branch

Lamina of thyroid cartilage

Cricopharyngeus

Anterior tubercle of cricoid cartilage

B. Lateral View Before Removal of the Right Thyroid Cartilage

Recurrent laryngeal nerve

8.29   External larynx and laryngeal nerves

A. Posterior aspect.
- The internal branch of the superior laryngeal nerve innervates the mucous membrane superior to the vocal folds, and the external laryngeal branch supplies the inferior pharyngeal constrictor and cricothyroid muscles.
- The recurrent laryngeal nerve supplies the esophagus, trachea, and inferior pharyngeal constrictor muscle. It supplies sensory innervation inferior to the vocal folds and motor innervation to the intrinsic muscles of the larynx, except the cricothyroid.

B. Laryngocele. A laryngocele (enlarged laryngeal saccule) projects through the thyrohyoid membrane and communicates with the larynx through the ventricle. This air sac can form a bulge in the neck, especially on coughing. The inferior laryngeal nerves are vulnerable to injury during operations in the anterior triangles of the neck. Injury of the nerve results in paralysis of the vocal fold. The voice is initially poor because the paralyzed fold cannot adduct to meet the normal vocal fold. In a bilateral paralysis, the voice is almost absent. Injury to the external branch of the superior laryngeal nerve results in a voice that is monotonous in character because the cricothyroid muscle is unable to vary the tension of the vocal fold. Hoarseness is the most common symptom of serious disorders of the larynx.

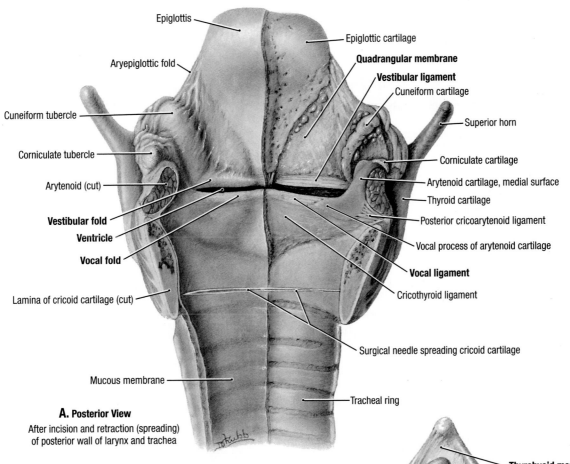

Epiglottis

Aryepiglottic fold

Cuneiform tubercle

Corniculate tubercle

Arytenoid (cut)

Vestibular fold

Ventricle

Vocal fold

Lamina of cricoid cartilage (cut)

Mucous membrane

Epiglottic cartilage

Quadrangular membrane

Vestibular ligament

Cuneiform cartilage

Superior horn

Corniculate cartilage

Arytenoid cartilage, medial surface

Thyroid cartilage

Posterior cricoarytenoid ligament

Vocal process of arytenoid cartilage

Vocal ligament

Cricothyroid ligament

Surgical needle spreading cricoid cartilage

Tracheal ring

A. Posterior View
After incision and retraction (spreading)
of posterior wall of larynx and trachea

8.30   Internal larynx

A. The posterior wall of the larynx was split in the median plane (see Figure 8.29A), and the two sides held apart. On the left side of the specimen, the mucous membrane, which is the innermost coat of the larynx, is intact; on the right side of the specimen, the mucous and submucous coats were peeled off, and the next coat, consisting of cartilages, ligaments, and fibroelastic membrane, was uncovered. **B.** Interior of the larynx superior to the vocal folds. The larynx was sectioned near the median plane to reveal the interior of its left side. Inferior to this level, the right side of the intact larynx was dissected. The thyrohyoid membrane is intact; there is no laryngocele.

- The three compartments of the larynx are (a) the superior compartment of the vestibule, superior to the level of the vestibular folds (false cords); (b) the middle, between the levels of the vestibular and vocal folds; and (c) the inferior, or infraglottic, cavity, inferior to the level of the vocal folds.
- The quadrangular membrane underlies the aryepiglottic fold superiorly and is thickened inferiorly to form the vestibular ligament. The cricothyroid ligament (conus elasticus) begins inferiorly as the strong median cricothyroid ligament and is thickened superiorly as the vocal ligament. The lateral recess between the vocal and vestibular ligaments, lined with mucous membrane, is the ventricle.

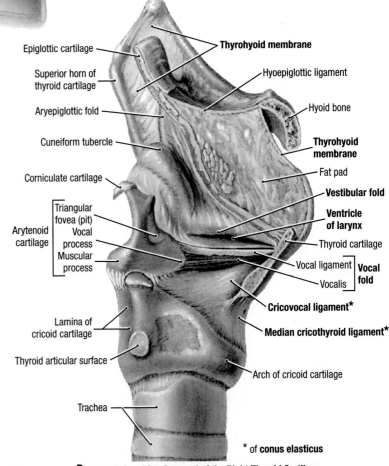

Epiglottic cartilage

Superior horn of
thyroid cartilage

Aryepiglottic fold

Cuneiform tubercle

Corniculate cartilage

Arytenoid
cartilage

Triangular
fovea (pit)
Vocal
process
Muscular
process

Lamina of
cricoid cartilage

Thyroid articular surface

Trachea

Thyrohyoid membrane

Hyoepiglottic ligament

Hyoid bone

**Thyrohyoid
membrane**

Fat pad

Vestibular fold

**Ventricle
of larynx**

Thyroid cartilage

Vocal ligament ⎫ **Vocal**
Vocalis   ⎬ **fold**

Cricovocal ligament*

Median cricothyroid ligament*

Arch of cricoid cartilage

* of **conus elasticus**

B. Lateral View After Removal of the Right Thyroid Cartilage

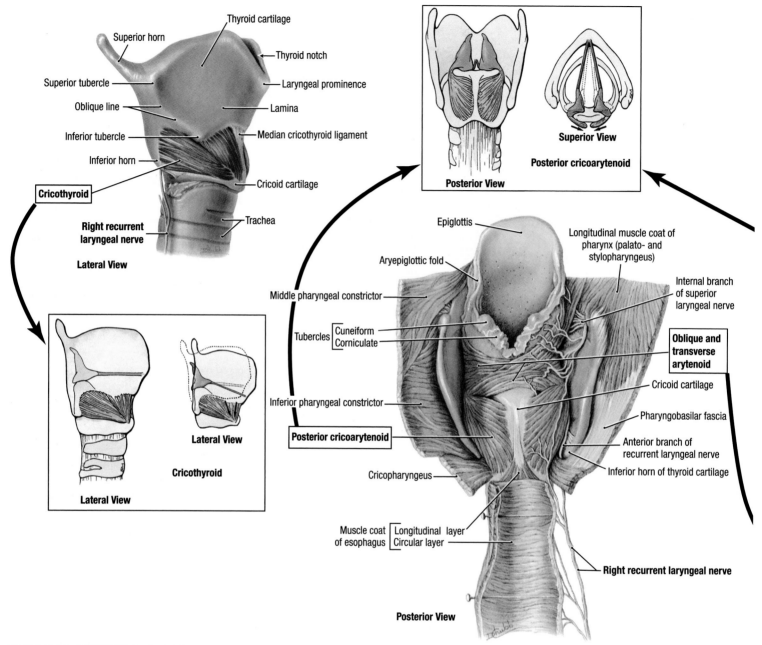

Cricothyroid

Superior horn — Thyroid cartilage — Thyroid notch

Superior tubercle — Laryngeal prominence

Oblique line — Lamina

Inferior tubercle — Median cricothyroid ligament

Inferior horn —

Cricoid cartilage

Right recurrent laryngeal nerve — Trachea

Lateral View

Lateral View

Lateral View

Cricothyroid

Posterior View — **Posterior cricoarytenoid**

Superior View — **Posterior cricoarytenoid**

Epiglottis — Longitudinal muscle coat of pharynx (palato- and stylopharyngeus)

Aryepiglottic fold — Internal branch of superior laryngeal nerve

Middle pharyngeal constrictor —

Tubercles [Cuneiform / Corniculate] — **Oblique and transverse arytenoid**

Cricoid cartilage

Inferior pharyngeal constrictor — Pharyngobasilar fascia

Posterior cricoarytenoid — Anterior branch of recurrent laryngeal nerve

Inferior horn of thyroid cartilage

Cricopharyngeus —

Muscle coat of esophagus [Longitudinal layer / Circular layer]

Right recurrent laryngeal nerve

Posterior View

TABLE 8.10 MUSCLES OF LARYNX

Muscle	Origin	Insertion	Innervation	Main Action(s)
Cricothyroid	Anterolateral part of cricoid cartilage	Inferior margin and inferior horn of thyroid cartilage	External branch of superior laryngeal nerve (CN X)	Tenses vocal fold
Posterior cricoarytenoid	Posterior surface of laminae of cricoid cartilage	Muscular process of arytenoid cartilage	Recurrent laryngeal nerve (CN X)	Abducts vocal fold
Lateral cricoarytenoid	Arch of cricoid cartilage			Adducts vocal fold
Thyroarytenoid[a]	Posterior surface of thyroid cartilage			Relaxes vocal fold
Transverse and oblique arytenoids[b]	One arytenoid cartilage	Opposite arytenoid cartilage		Close inlet of larynx by approximating arytenoid cartilages
Vocalis[c]	Angle between laminae of thyroid cartilage	Vocal ligament, between origin and vocal process of arytenoid cartilage		Alters vocal fold during phonation

[a]Superior fibers of the thyroarytenoid muscle pass into the aryepiglottic fold, and some of them reach the epiglottic cartilage. These fibers constitute the thyroepiglottic muscle, which widens the inlet of the larynx.
[b]Some fibers of the oblique arytenoid muscle continue as the aryepiglottic muscle.
[c]This slender muscular slip is derived from inferior deeper fibers of the thyroarytenoid muscle.

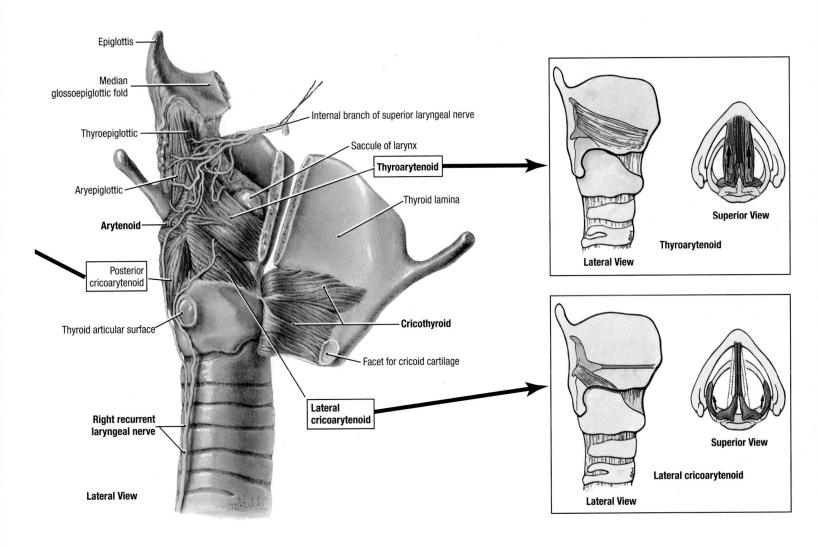

Epiglottis

Median
glossoepiglottic fold

Thyroepiglottic

Aryepiglottic

Arytenoid

Posterior
cricoarytenoid

Thyroid articular surface

**Right recurrent
laryngeal nerve**

Lateral View

Internal branch of superior laryngeal nerve

Saccule of larynx

Thyroarytenoid

Thyroid lamina

Cricothyroid

Facet for cricoid cartilage

**Lateral
cricoarytenoid**

Thyroarytenoid

Superior View

Lateral View

Lateral cricoarytenoid

Superior View

Lateral View

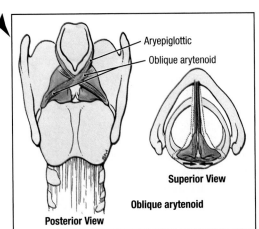

Aryepiglottic

Oblique arytenoid

Superior View

Oblique arytenoid

Posterior View

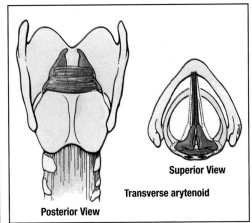

Superior View

Transverse arytenoid

Posterior View

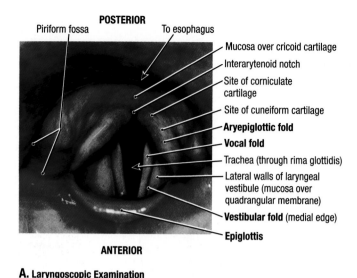

A. Laryngoscopic Examination

Labels (clockwise from top): POSTERIOR · Piriform fossa · To esophagus · Mucosa over cricoid cartilage · Interarytenoid notch · Site of corniculate cartilage · Site of cuneiform cartilage · **Aryepiglottic fold** · **Vocal fold** · Trachea (through rima glottidis) · Lateral walls of laryngeal vestibule (mucosa over quadrangular membrane) · **Vestibular fold** (medial edge) · **Epiglottis** · ANTERIOR

B. Superior View

Labels: POSTERIOR · Rima glottidis · **Corniculate tubercle** · **Cuneiform tubercle** · Piriform fossa · **Aryepiglottic fold** · Greater horn of hyoid · **Epiglottis** · Epiglottic tubercle · **Vestibular fold** · Ventricle of larynx · **Vocal fold** · ANTERIOR

C. Coronal MRI

Labels: Pre-epiglottic fat · Tongue · 1 · 2 · 3 · 4 · 5

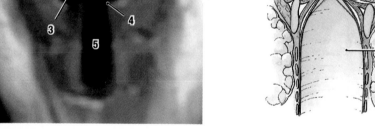

D. Posterior View

Labels: Aryepiglottic fold · Vestibule (1) · Vestibular fold (2) · Ventricle (3) · Vocal fold (4) (conus elasticus) · Trachea (5)

8.31 Laryngoscopic examination and MRI imaging of larynx

A. Laryngoscopic examination.
Laryngoscopy is the procedure used to examine the interior of the larynx. The larynx may be examined visually by indirect laryngoscopy using a laryngeal mirror or it may be viewed by direct laryngoscopy using a tubular and endoscopic instrument, a laryngoscope. The vestibular and vocal folds can be observed.

B. Vocal folds and rima glottidis.
The inlet, or aditus, to the larynx is bounded anteriorly by the epiglottis; posteriorly by the arytenoid cartilages, the corniculate cartilages that cap them, and the interarytenoid fold that unites them; and on each side by the aryepiglottic fold, which contains the superior end of the cuneiform cartilage.
C. Coronal MRI. **D.** Coronal section. Numbers in parentheses on diagram refer to numbered structures on MRI.

A foreign object, such as a piece of steak, may accidentally aspirate through the laryngeal inlet into the vestibule of the larynx, where it becomes trapped superior to the vestibular folds. When a foreign object enters the vestibule, the laryngeal muscles go into spasm, tensing the vocal folds. The rima glottidis closes and no air enters the trachea. Asphyxiation occurs, and the person will die in approximately 5 minutes from lack of oxygen if the obstruction is not removed. Emergency therapy must be given to open the airway. The procedure used depends on the condition of the patient, the facilities available, and the experience of the person giving first aid. Because the lungs still contain air, sudden compression of the abdomen (Heimlich maneuver) causes the diaphragm to elevate and compress the lungs, expelling air from the trachea into the larynx. This maneuver may dislodge the food or other material from the larynx.

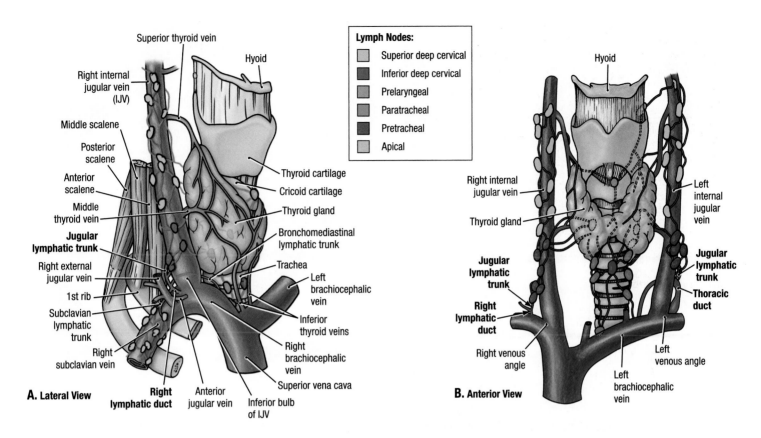

8.32   **Lymphatic drainage of thyroid gland, larynx, and trachea**

Radical neck dissections are performed when cancer invades the lymphatics. During the procedure, the deep cervical lymph nodes and the tissues around them are removed as completely as possible. Although major arteries, the brachial plexus, CN X, and the phrenic nerve are preserved, most cutaneous branches of the cervical plexus are removed. The aim of the dissection is to remove all tissue that contains lymph nodes in one piece.

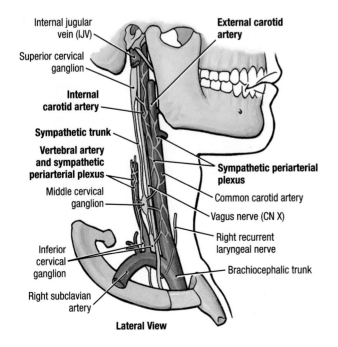

8.33   **Sympathetic trunk and sympathetic periarterial plexus**

A lesion of a sympathetic trunk in the neck results in a sympathetic disturbance called Horner syndrome, which is characterized by

- Pupillary constriction resulting from paralysis of the dilator pupillae muscle
- Ptosis (drooping of the superior eyelid), resulting from paralysis of the smooth (tarsal) muscle intermingled with striated muscle of the levator palpebrae superioris
- Sinking in of the eyeball (enophthalmos), possibly caused by paralysis of smooth (orbitalis) muscle in the floor of the orbit
- Vasodilation and absence of sweating on the face and neck (anhydrosis), caused by a lack of sympathetic (vasoconstrictive) nerve supply to the blood vessels and sweat glands

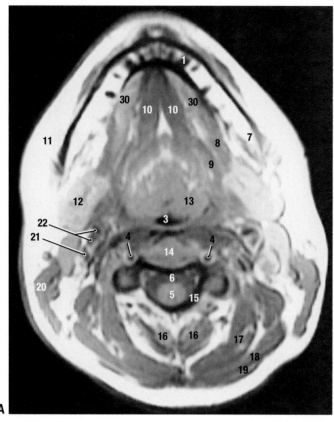

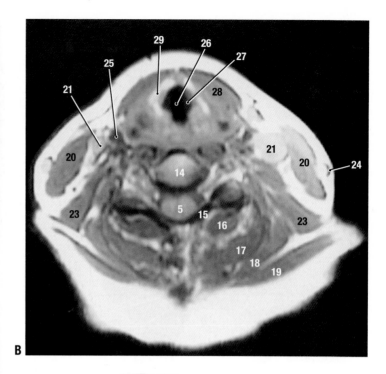

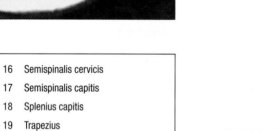

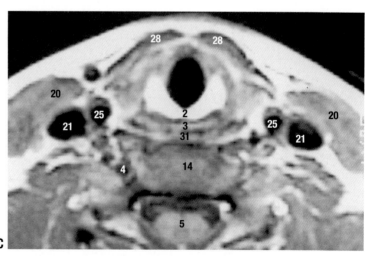

Inferior Views

1	Tooth	16	Semispinalis cervicis
2	Cricoid cartilage	17	Semispinalis capitis
3	Pharynx	18	Splenius capitis
4	Vertebral artery	19	Trapezius
5	Spinal cord	20	Sternocleidomastoid
6	Cerebrospinal fluid in	21	Internal jugular vein
	subarachnoid space	22	Bifurcation of common carotid artery
7	Body of mandible	23	Levator scapulae
8	Mylohyoid	24	External jugular vein
9	Hyoglossus	25	Common carotid artery
10	Genioglossus	26	Rima glottidis
11	Buccal fat pad	27	Vocal fold
12	Submandibular gland	28	Strap muscles
13	Intrinsic muscles of tongue	29	Thyroid cartilage
14	Vertebral body	30	Sublingual gland
15	Lamina of vertebra	31	Inferior pharyngeal constrictor

8.34   **Transverse MRIs of neck**

The orientation figure indicates the vertebral level of the MRI sections.

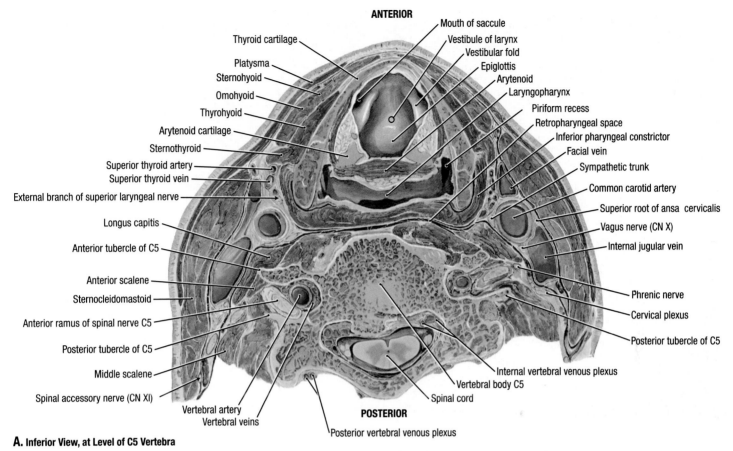

ANTERIOR

Mouth of saccule

Thyroid cartilage

Vestibule of larynx

Vestibular fold

Platysma

Epiglottis

Sternohyoid

Arytenoid

Omohyoid

Laryngopharynx

Thyrohyoid

Piriform recess

Arytenoid cartilage

Retropharyngeal space

Sternothyroid

Inferior pharyngeal constrictor

Superior thyroid artery

Facial vein

Superior thyroid vein

Sympathetic trunk

External branch of superior laryngeal nerve

Common carotid artery

Longus capitis

Superior root of ansa cervicalis

Anterior tubercle of C5

Vagus nerve (CN X)

Internal jugular vein

Anterior scalene

Sternocleidomastoid

Anterior ramus of spinal nerve C5

Phrenic nerve

Posterior tubercle of C5

Cervical plexus

Middle scalene

Posterior tubercle of C5

Spinal accessory nerve (CN XI)

Vertebral artery

Internal vertebral venous plexus

Vertebral veins

Vertebral body C5

Spinal cord

POSTERIOR

Posterior vertebral venous plexus

A. Inferior View, at Level of C5 Vertebra

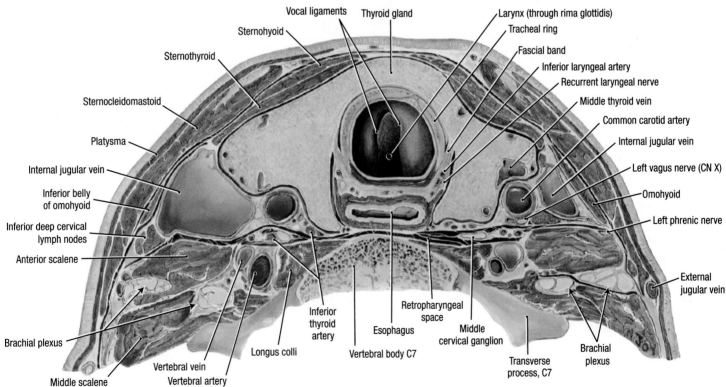

Vocal ligaments

Thyroid gland

Larynx (through rima glottidis)

Sternohyoid

Tracheal ring

Sternothyroid

Fascial band

Inferior laryngeal artery

Sternocleidomastoid

Recurrent laryngeal nerve

Middle thyroid vein

Platysma

Common carotid artery

Internal jugular vein

Internal jugular vein

Left vagus nerve (CN X)

Inferior belly of omohyoid

Omohyoid

Inferior deep cervical lymph nodes

Left phrenic nerve

Anterior scalene

External jugular vein

Brachial plexus

Inferior thyroid artery

Retropharyngeal space

Middle cervical ganglion

Brachial plexus

Middle scalene

Vertebral vein

Longus colli

Esophagus

Vertebral body C7

Transverse process, C7

Vertebral artery

B. Inferior View, at Level of C7 Vertebra

8.35   **Transverse anatomical sections of neck**

Level of C7 Vertebra

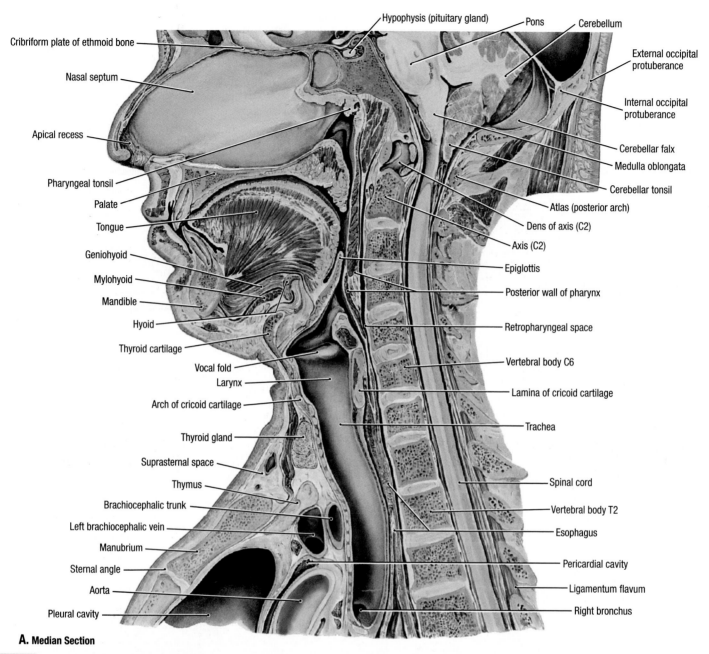

Hypophysis (pituitary gland)

Pons

Cerebellum

Cribriform plate of ethmoid bone

External occipital protuberance

Nasal septum

Internal occipital protuberance

Apical recess

Cerebellar falx

Medulla oblongata

Pharyngeal tonsil

Cerebellar tonsil

Palate

Atlas (posterior arch)

Tongue

Dens of axis (C2)

Geniohyoid

Axis (C2)

Mylohyoid

Epiglottis

Mandible

Posterior wall of pharynx

Hyoid

Retropharyngeal space

Thyroid cartilage

Vertebral body C6

Vocal fold

Lamina of cricoid cartilage

Larynx

Arch of cricoid cartilage

Trachea

Thyroid gland

Suprasternal space

Spinal cord

Thymus

Vertebral body T2

Brachiocephalic trunk

Esophagus

Left brachiocephalic vein

Manubrium

Pericardial cavity

Sternal angle

Aorta

Ligamentum flavum

Pleural cavity

Right bronchus

A. Median Section

8.36   Median section and MRI scan of head and neck

A. Median anatomical section.

Swallowing. (1) The bolus of food is squeezed to the back of the mouth by pushing the tongue against the palate. (2) The nasopharynx is sealed off, and the larynx is elevated, enlarging the pharynx to receive food. (3) The pharyngeal sphincters contract sequentially, squeezing food into the esophagus. The epiglottis deflects the bolus from but does not close the inlet to the larynx and trachea. (4) The bolus of food moves down the esophagus by peristaltic contractions.

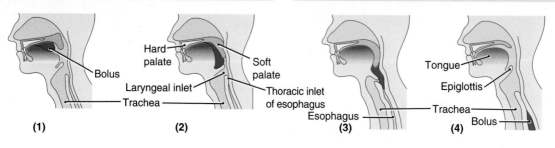

Bolus

Hard palate

Soft palate

Laryngeal inlet

Thoracic inlet of esophagus

Trachea

Esophagus

Tongue

Epiglottis

Trachea

Bolus

(1)   (2)   (3)   (4)

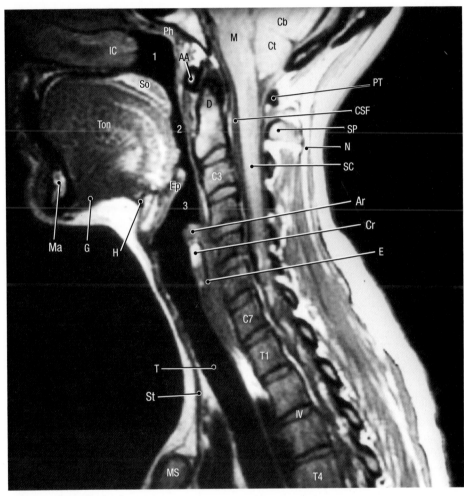

B. Median MRI Scan

1	Nasopharynx
2	Oropharynx
3	Laryngopharynx
AA	Anterior arch of C1
Ar	Arytenoid cartilage
C3-T4	Vertebral bodies
Cb	Cerebellum
Cr	Cricoid cartilage
CSF	Cerebrospinal fluid in subarachnoid space
Ct	Tonsil of cerebellum
D	Dens
E	Esophagus
Ep	Epiglottis
G	Genioglossus
H	Hyoid
IC	Inferior concha
IV	Intervertebral disc
M	Medulla oblongata
Ma	Mandible
MS	Manubrium of sternum
N	Nuchal ligament
Ph	Pharyngeal tonsil (adenoid)
PT	Posterior tubercle of C1
SC	Spinal cord
So	Soft palate
SP	Spinous process
St	Strap muscles
T	Trachea
Ton	Tongue

8.36 Median section and MRI scan of head and neck *(continued)*

8.37 Doppler US color flow study of carotid artery

Ultrasonography is a useful diagnostic imaging technique for studying soft tissues of the neck. Ultrasound provides images of many abnormal conditions noninvasively, at relatively low cost, and with minimal discomfort. Ultrasound is useful for distinguishing solid from cystic masses, for example, which may be difficult to determine during physical examination. Vascular imaging of arteries and veins of the neck is possible using intravascular ultrasonography. The images are produced by placing the transducer over the blood vessel. Doppler ultrasound techniques help evaluate blood flow through a vessel (e.g., for detecting stenosis [narrowing] of a carotid artery).

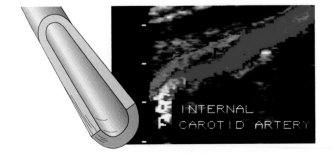

INTERNAL CAROTID ARTERY

CHAPTER 9

CRANIAL NERVES

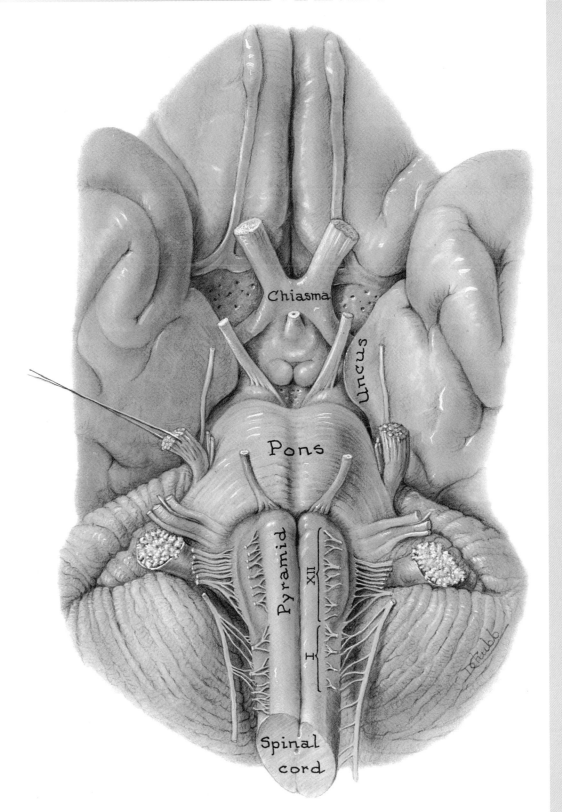

Chiasma

Uncus

Pons

Pyramid

XII

II

Spinal
cord

- Overview of Cranial
  Nerves 812
- Cranial Nerve Nuclei 816
- Cranial Nerve I: Olfactory 818
- Cranial Nerve II: Optic 819
- Cranial Nerves III, IV, and VI:
  Oculomotor, Trochlear, and
  Abducent 821
- Cranial Nerve V:
  Trigeminal 824
- Cranial Nerve VII: Facial 830
- Cranial Nerve VIII:
  Vestibulocochlear 832
- Cranial Nerve IX:
  Glossopharyngeal 834
- Cranial Nerve X: Vagus 836
- Cranial Nerve XI: Spinal
  Accessory 838
- Cranial Nerve XII:
  Hypoglossal 839
- Summary of Autonomic
  Ganglia of Head 840
- Summary of Cranial Nerve
  Lesions 841
- Sectional Imaging of Cranial
  Nerves 842

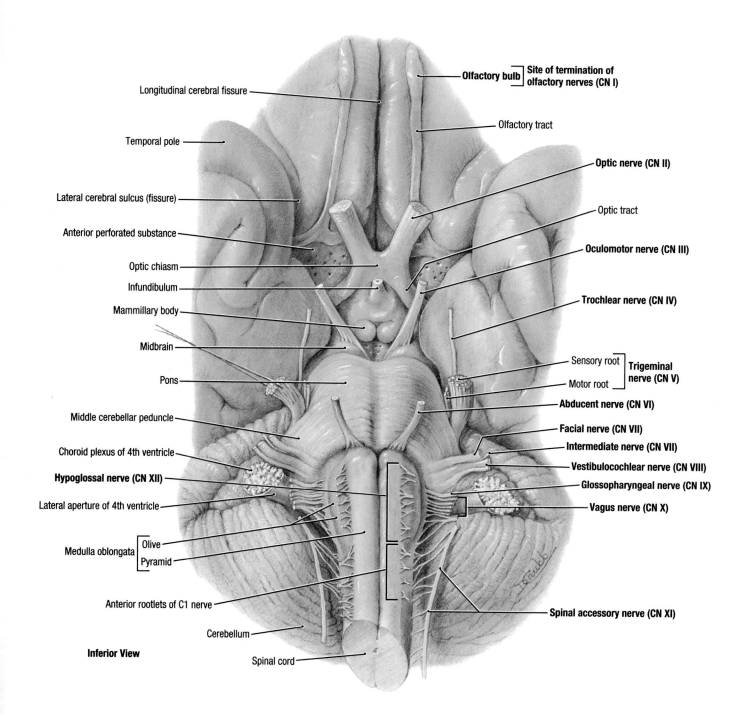

Longitudinal cerebral fissure

Temporal pole

Lateral cerebral sulcus (fissure)

Anterior perforated substance

Optic chiasm

Infundibulum

Mammillary body

Midbrain

Pons

Middle cerebellar peduncle

Choroid plexus of 4th ventricle

Hypoglossal nerve (CN XII)

Lateral aperture of 4th ventricle

Medulla oblongata [Olive / Pyramid]

Anterior rootlets of C1 nerve

Cerebellum

Inferior View

Spinal cord

Olfactory bulb] **Site of termination of olfactory nerves (CN I)**

Olfactory tract

Optic nerve (CN II)

Optic tract

Oculomotor nerve (CN III)

Trochlear nerve (CN IV)

Sensory root] **Trigeminal nerve (CN V)**
Motor root

Abducent nerve (CN VI)

Facial nerve (CN VII)

Intermediate nerve (CN VII)

Vestibulocochlear nerve (CN VIII)

Glossopharyngeal nerve (CN IX)

Vagus nerve (CN X)

Spinal accessory nerve (CN XI)

9.1 **Cranial nerves in relation to the base of the brain**

Cranial nerves are nerves that exit from the cranial cavity through openings in the cranium. There are 12 pairs of cranial nerves that are named and numbered in rostrocaudal sequence of their superficial origins from the brain, brainstem, and superior spinal cord. The olfactory nerves (CN I, not shown) end in the olfactory bulb. The entire origin of the spinal accessory nerve (CN XI) from the spinal cord is not included here; it extends inferiorly as far as the C6 spinal cord segment.

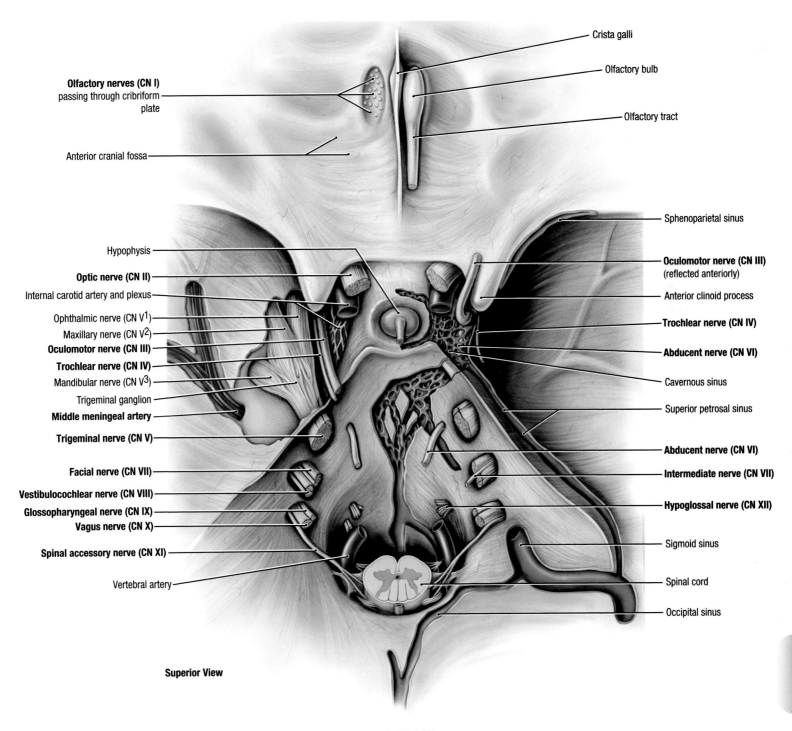

ANTERIOR

Crista galli

Olfactory bulb

Olfactory nerves (CN I) passing through cribriform plate

Olfactory tract

Anterior cranial fossa

Sphenoparietal sinus

Hypophysis

Oculomotor nerve (CN III) (reflected anteriorly)

Optic nerve (CN II)

Anterior clinoid process

Internal carotid artery and plexus

Ophthalmic nerve (CN V^1)

Trochlear nerve (CN IV)

Maxillary nerve (CN V^2)

Abducent nerve (CN VI)

Oculomotor nerve (CN III)

Trochlear nerve (CN IV)

Cavernous sinus

Mandibular nerve (CN V^3)

Trigeminal ganglion

Superior petrosal sinus

Middle meningeal artery

Trigeminal nerve (CN V)

Abducent nerve (CN VI)

Facial nerve (CN VII)

Intermediate nerve (CN VII)

Vestibulocochlear nerve (CN VIII)

Hypoglossal nerve (CN XII)

Glossopharyngeal nerve (CN IX)

Vagus nerve (CN X)

Sigmoid sinus

Spinal accessory nerve (CN XI)

Vertebral artery

Spinal cord

Occipital sinus

Superior View

POSTERIOR

9.2 **Cranial nerves in relation to the internal aspect of the cranial base**

The venous sinuses have been opened on the right side. The ophthalmic division of the trigeminal nerve (CN V^1), and the trochlear (CN IV) and oculomotor (CN III) nerves have been dissected from the lateral wall of the cavernous sinus.

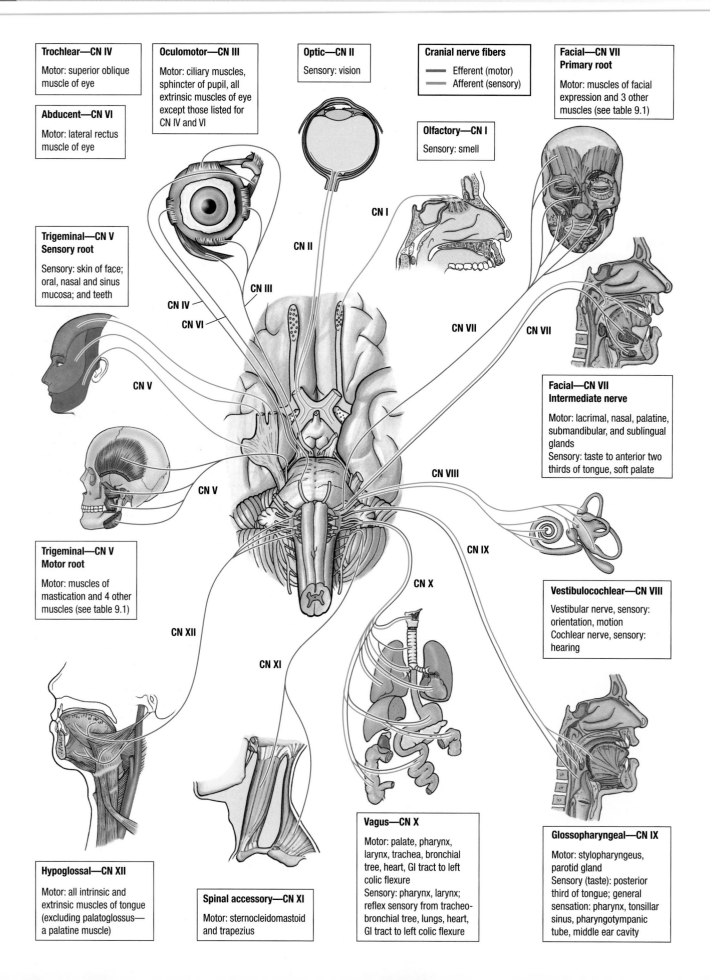

Trochlear—CN IV

Motor: superior oblique muscle of eye

Abducent—CN VI

Motor: lateral rectus muscle of eye

Oculomotor—CN III

Motor: ciliary muscles, sphincter of pupil, all extrinsic muscles of eye except those listed for CN IV and VI

Optic—CN II

Sensory: vision

Cranial nerve fibers

▬▬▬ Efferent (motor)
▬▬▬ Afferent (sensory)

Facial—CN VII
Primary root

Motor: muscles of facial expression and 3 other muscles (see table 9.1)

Olfactory—CN I

Sensory: smell

Trigeminal—CN V
Sensory root

Sensory: skin of face; oral, nasal and sinus mucosa; and teeth

Facial—CN VII
Intermediate nerve

Motor: lacrimal, nasal, palatine, submandibular, and sublingual glands
Sensory: taste to anterior two thirds of tongue, soft palate

Vestibulocochlear—CN VIII

Vestibular nerve, sensory: orientation, motion
Cochlear nerve, sensory: hearing

Trigeminal—CN V
Motor root

Motor: muscles of mastication and 4 other muscles (see table 9.1)

Hypoglossal—CN XII

Motor: all intrinsic and extrinsic muscles of tongue (excluding palatoglossus—a palatine muscle)

Spinal accessory—CN XI

Motor: sternocleidomastoid and trapezius

Vagus—CN X

Motor: palate, pharynx, larynx, trachea, bronchial tree, heart, GI tract to left colic flexure
Sensory: pharynx, larynx; reflex sensory from tracheo-bronchial tree, lungs, heart, GI tract to left colic flexure

Glossopharyngeal—CN IX

Motor: stylopharyngeus, parotid gland
Sensory (taste): posterior third of tongue; general sensation: pharynx, tonsillar sinus, pharyngotympanic tube, middle ear cavity

CN I
CN II
CN III
CN IV
CN VI
CN V
CN V
CN VII
CN VII
CN VIII
CN IX
CN X
CN XI
CN XII

TABLE 9.1 SUMMARY OF CRANIAL NERVES

Nerve	Components	Location of Nerve Cell Bodies	Cranial Exit	Main Action
Olfactory (CN I)	Special sensory	Olfactory epithelium (olfactory cells)	Foramina in cribriform plate of ethmoid bone	Smell from nasal mucosa of roof of each nasal cavity, superior sides of nasal septum and superior concha
Optic (CN II)	Special sensory	Retina (ganglion cells)	Optic canal	Vision from retina
Oculomotor (CN III)	Somatic motor	Midbrain	Superior orbital fissure	Motor to superior, inferior, and medial rectus, inferior oblique, and levator palpebrae superioris muscle that raise upper eyelid and rotates eyeball superiorly, inferiorly, and medially
	Visceral motor (parasympathetic)	Presynaptic: midbrain; Postsynaptic: ciliary ganglion		Secretomotor to sphincter pupillae and ciliary muscles that constrict pupil and accommodate lens of eye
Trochlear (CN IV)	Somatic motor	Midbrain		Motor to superior oblique that assists in rotating eye inferolaterally
Trigeminal (CN V) Ophthalmic division (CN V^1)	General sensory	Trigeminal ganglion		Sensation from cornea, skin of forehead, scalp, eyelids, nose, and mucosa of nasal cavity and paranasal sinuses
Maxillary division (CN V^2)	General sensory	Trigeminal ganglion	Foramen rotundum	Sensation from skin of face over maxilla including upper lip, maxillary teeth, mucosa of nose, maxillary sinuses, and palate
Mandibular division (CN V^3)	Branchial motor	Pons	Foramen ovale	Motor to muscles of mastication, mylohyoid, anterior belly of digastric, tensor veli palatini, and tensor tympani
	General sensory	Trigeminal ganglion		Sensation from the skin over mandible, including lower lip and side of head, mandibular teeth, temporomandibular joint, and mucosa of mouth and anterior two thirds of the tongue
Abducent (CN VI)	Somatic motor	Pons	Superior orbital fissure	Motor to lateral rectus that rotates eye laterally
Facial (CN VII)	Branchial motor	Pons	Internal acoustic meatus, facial canal, and stylomastoid foramen	Motor to muscles of facial expression and scalp; also supplies stapedius of middle ear, stylohyoid, and posterior belly of digastric
	Special sensory	Geniculate ganglion		Taste from anterior two thirds of tongue, floor of mouth, and palate
	General sensory			Sensation from skin of external acoustic meatus
	Visceral motor (parasympathetic)	Presynaptic: pons; Postsynaptic: pterygopalatine ganglion and submandibular ganglion		Secretomotor to submandibular and sublingual salivary glands, lacrimal gland, and glands of nose and palate
Vestibulocochlear (CN VIII) Vestibular	Special sensory	Vestibular ganglion	Internal acoustic meatus	Vestibular sensation from semicircular ducts, utricle, and saccule related to position and movement of head
Cochlear	Special sensory	Spiral ganglion		Hearing from spiral organ
Glossopharyngeal (CN IX)	Branchial motor	Medulla	Jugular foramen	Motor to stylopharyngeus that assists with swallowing
	Visceral motor (parasympathetic)	Presynaptic: medulla; Postsynaptic: otic ganglion		Secretomotor to parotid gland
	Visceral sensory	Inferior ganglion		Visceral sensation from parotid gland, carotid body and sinus, pharynx, and middle ear
	Special sensory	Superior ganglion		Taste from posterior third of tongue
	General sensory	Inferior ganglion		Cutaneous sensation from external ear
Vagus (CN X)	Branchial motor	Medulla		Motor to constrictor muscles of pharynx, intrinsic muscles of larynx, muscles of palate (except tensor veli palatine), and striated muscle in superior two thirds of esophagus
	Visceral motor (parasympathetic)	Presynaptic: medulla; Postsynaptic: neurons in, on, or near viscera		Motor to smooth muscle of trachea, bronchi, and digestive tract, moderates cardiac pacemaker and vasoconstrictor of coronary arteries
	Special sensory	Inferior ganglion		Visceral sensation from base of tongue, pharynx, larynx, trachea, bronchi, heart, esophagus, stomach, and intestine
	General sensory	Superior ganglion		Sensation from auricle, external acoustic meatus, and dura mater of posterior cranial fossa
	Somatic motor	Medulla		Motor to striated muscles of soft palate, pharynx, and larynx
Spinal accessory nerve (CN XI)	Somatic motor	Cervical spinal cord		Motor to sternocleidomastoid and trapezius
Hypoglossal (CN XII)	Somatic motor	Medulla	Hypoglossal canal	Motor to muscles of tongue (except palatoglossus)

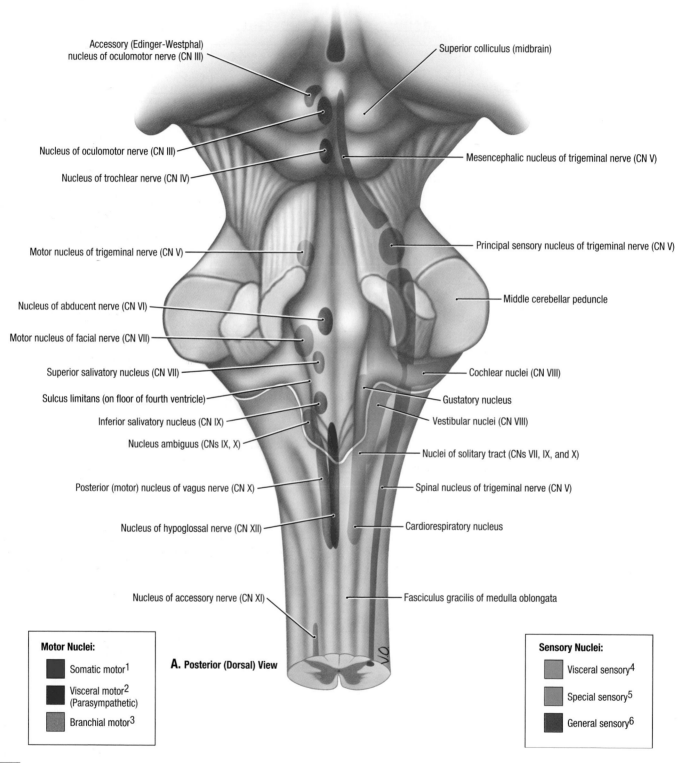

Accessory (Edinger-Westphal) nucleus of oculomotor nerve (CN III)

Superior colliculus (midbrain)

Nucleus of oculomotor nerve (CN III)

Nucleus of trochlear nerve (CN IV)

Mesencephalic nucleus of trigeminal nerve (CN V)

Motor nucleus of trigeminal nerve (CN V)

Principal sensory nucleus of trigeminal nerve (CN V)

Middle cerebellar peduncle

Nucleus of abducent nerve (CN VI)

Motor nucleus of facial nerve (CN VII)

Superior salivatory nucleus (CN VII)

Cochlear nuclei (CN VIII)

Sulcus limitans (on floor of fourth ventricle)

Gustatory nucleus

Inferior salivatory nucleus (CN IX)

Vestibular nuclei (CN VIII)

Nucleus ambiguus (CNs IX, X)

Nuclei of solitary tract (CNs VII, IX, and X)

Posterior (motor) nucleus of vagus nerve (CN X)

Spinal nucleus of trigeminal nerve (CN V)

Nucleus of hypoglossal nerve (CN XII)

Cardiorespiratory nucleus

Nucleus of accessory nerve (CN XI)

Fasciculus gracilis of medulla oblongata

Motor Nuclei:

Somatic motor[1]

Visceral motor[2] (Parasympathetic)

Branchial motor[3]

A. Posterior (Dorsal) View

Sensory Nuclei:

Visceral sensory[4]

Special sensory[5]

General sensory[6]

9.3   Cranial nerve nuclei

The fibers of the cranial nerves are connected to nuclei (groups of nerve cell bodies in the central nervous system), in which afferent (sensory) fibers terminate and from which efferent (motor) fibers originate. Nuclei of common functional types (motor, sensory, parasympathetic, and special sensory nuclei) have a generally columnar placement within the brainstem, with the sulcus limitans demarcating motor and sensory columns.

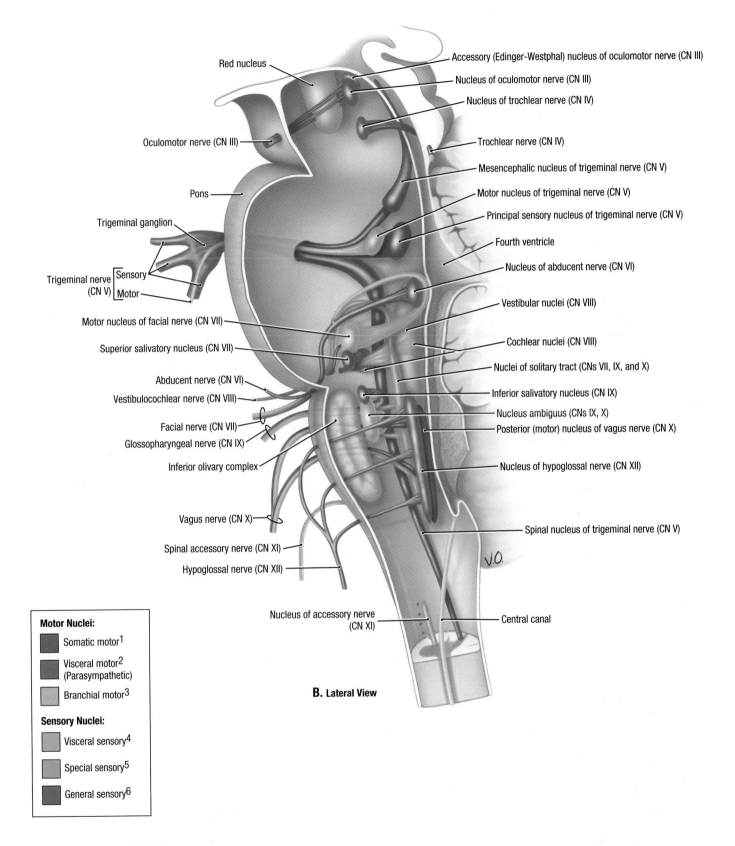

Red nucleus

Accessory (Edinger-Westphal) nucleus of oculomotor nerve (CN III)

Nucleus of oculomotor nerve (CN III)

Nucleus of trochlear nerve (CN IV)

Oculomotor nerve (CN III)

Trochlear nerve (CN IV)

Mesencephalic nucleus of trigeminal nerve (CN V)

Pons

Motor nucleus of trigeminal nerve (CN V)

Principal sensory nucleus of trigeminal nerve (CN V)

Trigeminal ganglion

Fourth ventricle

Trigeminal nerve (CN V) [Sensory / Motor]

Nucleus of abducent nerve (CN VI)

Vestibular nuclei (CN VIII)

Motor nucleus of facial nerve (CN VII)

Cochlear nuclei (CN VIII)

Superior salivatory nucleus (CN VII)

Nuclei of solitary tract (CNs VII, IX, and X)

Abducent nerve (CN VI)

Inferior salivatory nucleus (CN IX)

Vestibulocochlear nerve (CN VIII)

Nucleus ambiguus (CNs IX, X)

Facial nerve (CN VII)

Posterior (motor) nucleus of vagus nerve (CN X)

Glossopharyngeal nerve (CN IX)

Inferior olivary complex

Nucleus of hypoglossal nerve (CN XII)

Vagus nerve (CN X)

Spinal nucleus of trigeminal nerve (CN V)

Spinal accessory nerve (CN XI)

Hypoglossal nerve (CN XII)

V.O.

Nucleus of accessory nerve (CN XI)

Central canal

B. Lateral View

Motor Nuclei:

■ Somatic motor[1]

■ Visceral motor[2] (Parasympathetic)

■ Branchial motor[3]

Sensory Nuclei:

■ Visceral sensory[4]

■ Special sensory[5]

■ General sensory[6]

9.3   Cranial nerve nuclei (continued)

[1]General somatic efferent (GSE); [2]General visceral efferent (GVE); [3]Special visceral efferent (SVE); [4]Special/General visceral afferent (SVA/GVA); [5]Special somatic afferent; [6]General somatic afferent (GSA).

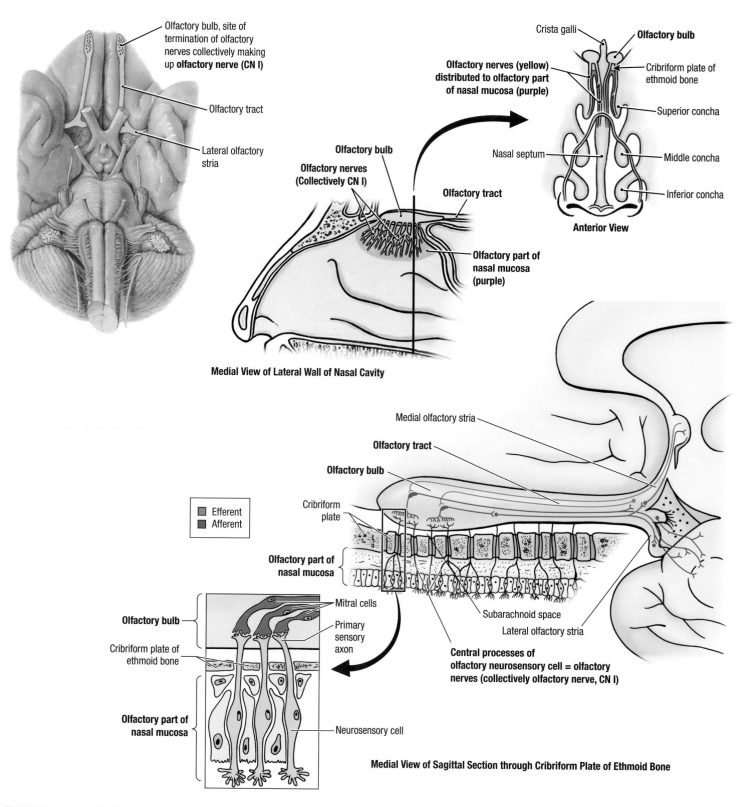

Olfactory bulb, site of termination of olfactory nerves collectively making up **olfactory nerve (CN I)**

Olfactory tract

Lateral olfactory stria

Crista galli

Olfactory bulb

Cribriform plate of ethmoid bone

Superior concha

Olfactory nerves (yellow) distributed to olfactory part of nasal mucosa (purple)

Nasal septum

Middle concha

Inferior concha

Anterior View

Olfactory bulb

Olfactory nerves (Collectively CN I)

Olfactory tract

Olfactory part of nasal mucosa (purple)

Medial View of Lateral Wall of Nasal Cavity

Medial olfactory stria

Olfactory tract

Olfactory bulb

Cribriform plate

Efferent
Afferent

Olfactory part of nasal mucosa

Subarachnoid space

Lateral olfactory stria

Central processes of olfactory neurosensory cell = olfactory nerves (collectively olfactory nerve, CN I)

Mitral cells

Olfactory bulb

Primary sensory axon

Cribriform plate of ethmoid bone

Olfactory part of nasal mucosa

Neurosensory cell

Medial View of Sagittal Section through Cribriform Plate of Ethmoid Bone

TABLE 9.2 OLFACTORY NERVE (CN I)

Nerve	Functional Components	Cells of Origin/ Termination	Cranial Exit	Distribution and Functions
Olfactory	Special sensory	Olfactory epithelium (olfactory cells/olfactory bulb)	Foramina in cribriform plate of ethmoid bone	Smell from nasal mucosa of roof and superior sides of nasal septum and superior concha of each nasal cavity

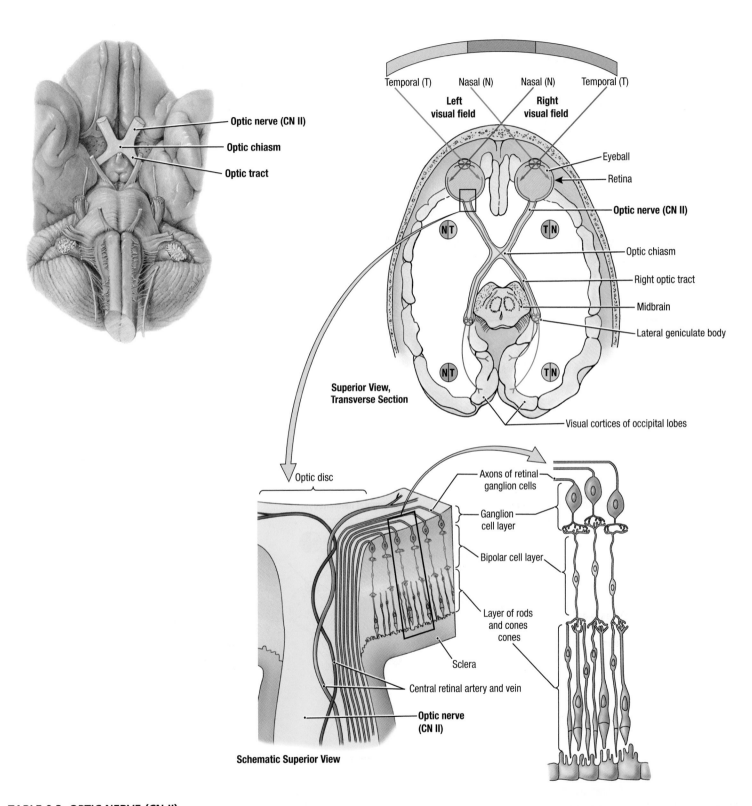

Superior View,
Transverse Section

Schematic Superior View

TABLE 9.3 OPTIC NERVE (CN II)

Nerve	Functional Components	Cells of Origin/ Termination	Cranial Exit	Distribution and Functions
Optic	Special sensory	Retina (ganglion cells)/ lateral geniculate body (nucleus)	Optic canal	Vision from retina

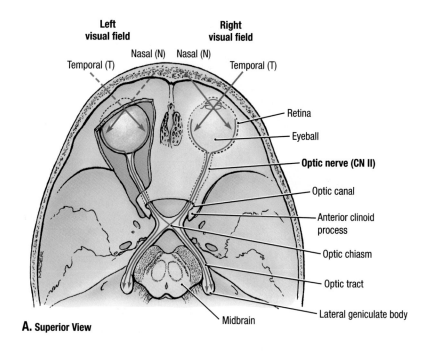

A. Superior View

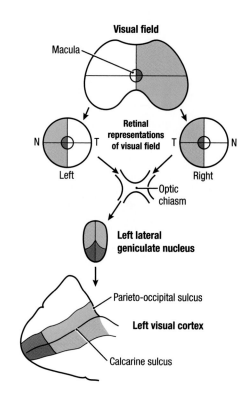

B

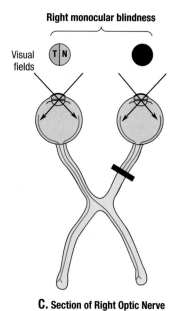

C. Section of Right Optic Nerve

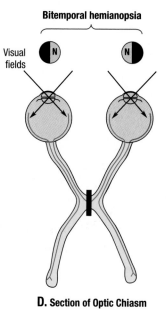

D. Section of Optic Chiasm

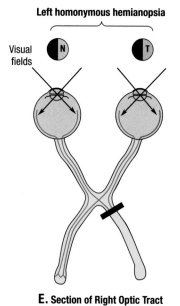

E. Section of Right Optic Tract

9.4 **Visual pathway**

A. The visual pathway in situ. B. Visual field representation on retinae, lateral geniculate nucleus, and visual cortex. C–E. Schematic illustrations of lesions of the visual pathway.

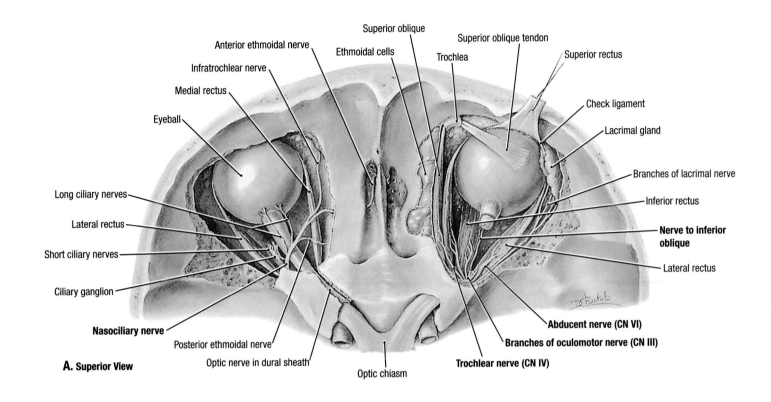

A. Superior View

Superior oblique

Anterior ethmoidal nerve

Ethmoidal cells

Infratrochlear nerve

Medial rectus

Eyeball

Long ciliary nerves

Lateral rectus

Short ciliary nerves

Ciliary ganglion

Nasociliary nerve

Posterior ethmoidal nerve

Optic nerve in dural sheath

Optic chiasm

Superior oblique tendon

Trochlea

Superior rectus

Check ligament

Lacrimal gland

Branches of lacrimal nerve

Inferior rectus

Nerve to inferior oblique

Lateral rectus

Abducent nerve (CN VI)

Branches of oculomotor nerve (CN III)

Trochlear nerve (CN IV)

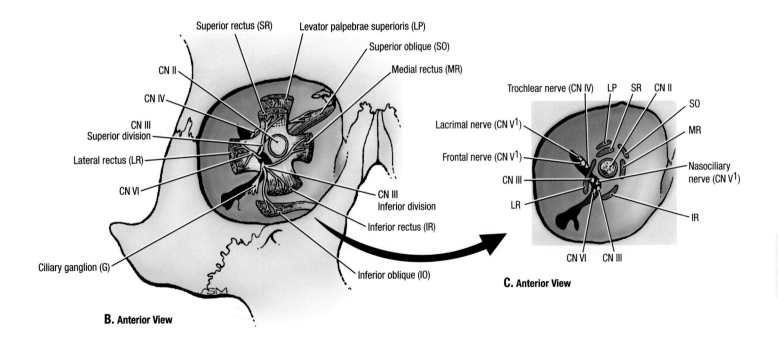

B. Anterior View

Superior rectus (SR)

Levator palpebrae superioris (LP)

Superior oblique (SO)

Medial rectus (MR)

CN II

CN IV

CN III
Superior division

Lateral rectus (LR)

CN VI

Ciliary ganglion (G)

CN III
Inferior division

Inferior rectus (IR)

Inferior oblique (IO)

C. Anterior View

Trochlear nerve (CN IV)   LP   SR   CN II

Lacrimal nerve (CN V¹)

Frontal nerve (CN V¹)

CN III

LR

SO

MR

Nasociliary nerve (CN V¹)

IR

CN VI   CN III

9.5   Overview of muscles and nerves of orbit

A. Orbital cavities, dissected from a superior approach. **B.** Structures of apex of orbit.
C. Relationship of muscle attachments and nerves at apex of orbit.

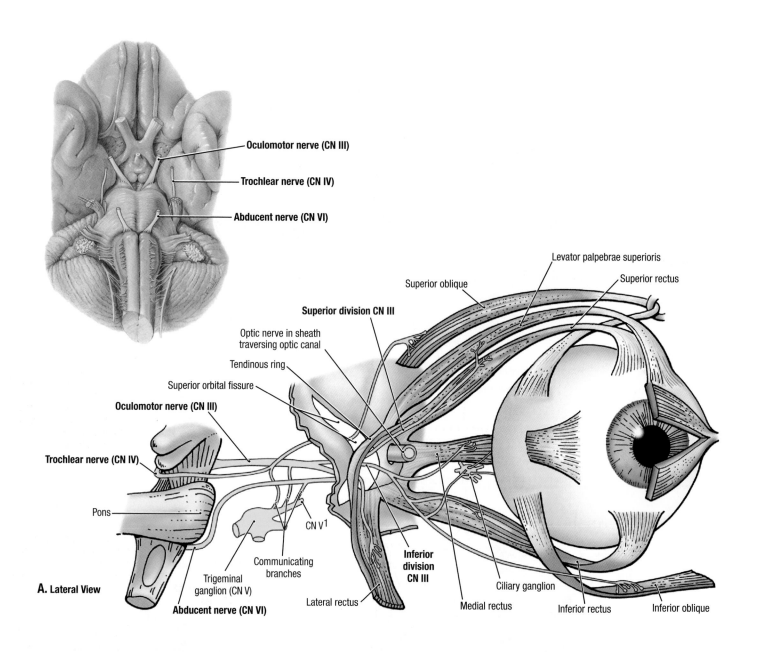

Oculomotor nerve (CN III)

Trochlear nerve (CN IV)

Abducent nerve (CN VI)

Levator palpebrae superioris

Superior oblique

Superior rectus

Superior division CN III

Optic nerve in sheath traversing optic canal

Tendinous ring

Superior orbital fissure

Oculomotor nerve (CN III)

Trochlear nerve (CN IV)

Pons

CN V¹

Inferior division CN III

Communicating branches

Ciliary ganglion

Trigeminal ganglion (CN V)

Medial rectus

Inferior rectus

Inferior oblique

A. Lateral View

Abducent nerve (CN VI)

Lateral rectus

TABLE 9.4 OCULOMOTOR (CN III), TROCHLEAR (CN IV), AND ABDUCENT (CN VI) NERVES[a]

Nerve	Functional Components	Cells of Origin/ Termination	Cranial Exit	Distribution and Functions
Oculomotor	Somatic motor	Oculomotor nucleus	Superior orbital fissure	Motor to superior, inferior, and medial recti, inferior oblique, and levator palpebrae superioris muscles; raises upper eyelid; rotates eyeball superiorly, inferiorly, and medially
	Visceral motor (parasympathetic)	Presynaptic: midbrain (Edinger-Westphal nucleus); Postsynaptic: ciliary ganglion		Motor to sphincter pupillae and ciliary muscle that constrict pupil and accommodate lens of eyeball
Trochlear	Somatic motor	Trochlear nucleus		Motor to superior oblique that assists in rotating eyeball inferolaterally
Abducent	Somatic motor	Abducent nucleus		Motor to lateral rectus that rotates eyeball laterally

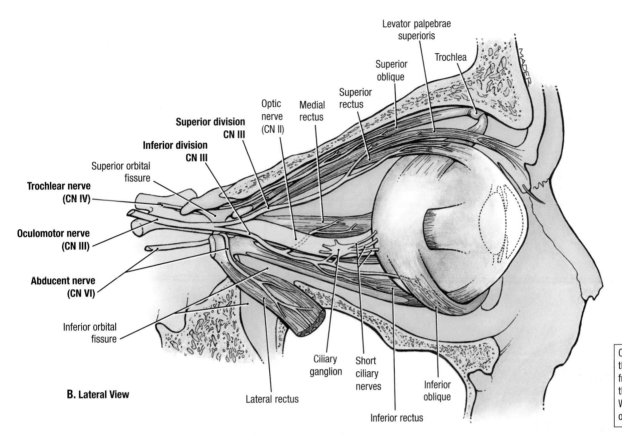

Levator palpebrae superioris

Trochlea

Superior oblique

Superior rectus

Optic nerve (CN II)

Medial rectus

Superior division CN III

Inferior division CN III

Superior orbital fissure

Trochlear nerve (CN IV)

Oculomotor nerve (CN III)

Abducent nerve (CN VI)

Inferior orbital fissure

B. Lateral View

Lateral rectus

Ciliary ganglion

Short ciliary nerves

Inferior oblique

Inferior rectus

CN II contains parasympathetic fibers originating from nerve cell bodies of the accessory (Edinger-Westphal) nucleus of the oculomotor nerve

↓

Fibers synapse in the ciliary ganglion, consisting of post-synaptic parasympathetic nerve cell bodies associated with CN V^1

↓

Short ciliary nerves (CN V^1) carry post-synaptic parasympathetic fibers to the ciliary and constrictor pupillae muscles.

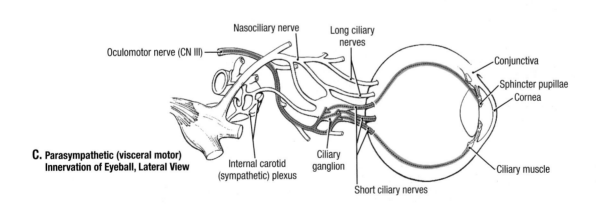

Nasociliary nerve

Long ciliary nerves

Oculomotor nerve (CN III)

Conjunctiva

Sphincter pupillae

Cornea

C. Parasympathetic (visceral motor) Innervation of Eyeball, Lateral View

Internal carotid (sympathetic) plexus

Ciliary ganglion

Short ciliary nerves

Ciliary muscle

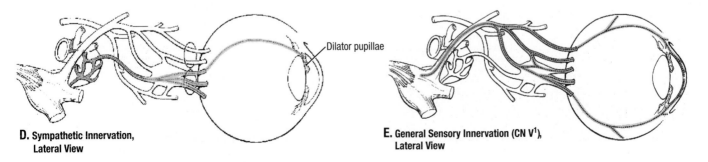

Dilator pupillae

D. Sympathetic Innervation, Lateral View

E. General Sensory Innervation (CN V^1), Lateral View

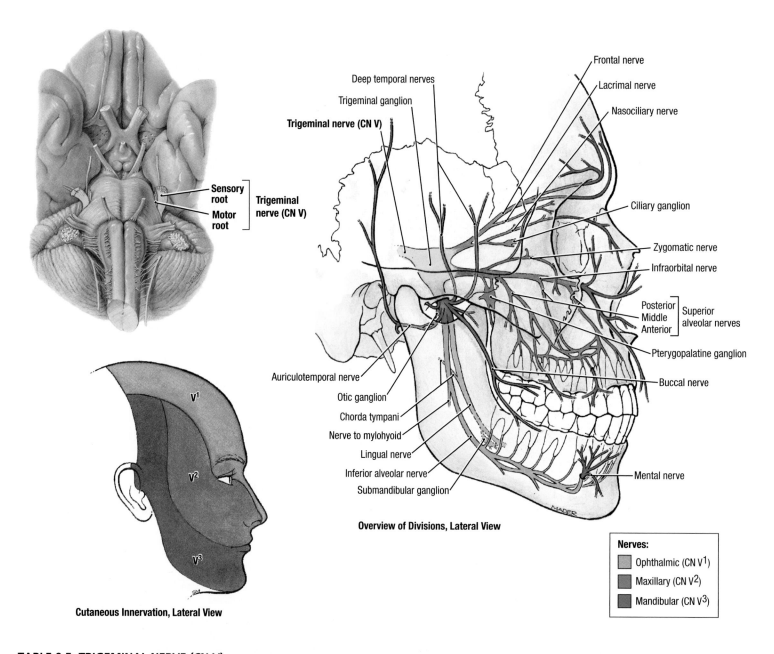

Cutaneous Innervation, Lateral View

Overview of Divisions, Lateral View

Nerves:
- ☐ Ophthalmic (CN V¹)
- ☐ Maxillary (CN V²)
- ☐ Mandibular (CN V³)

TABLE 9.5 TRIGEMINAL NERVE (CN V)

Nerve	Functional Components	Cells of Origin/ Termination	Cranial Exit	Distribution and Functions
Ophthalmic division (CN V¹)	General sensory	Trigeminal ganglion/spinal, principal and mesencephalic nucleus of CN V	Superior orbital fissure	Sensation from cornea, skin of forehead, scalp, eyelids, nose, and mucosa of nasal cavity and paranasal sinuses
Maxillary division (CN V²)			Foramen rotundum	Sensation from skin of face over maxilla including upper lip, maxillary teeth, mucosa of nose, maxillary sinuses, and palate
Mandibular division (CN V³)			Foramen ovale	Sensation from the skin over mandible, including lower lip and side of head, mandibular teeth, temporomandibular joint, and mucosa of mouth and anterior two thirds of tongue
	Branchial motor	Trigeminal motor nucleus		Motor to muscles of mastication, mylohyoid, anterior belly of digastric, tensor veli palatini, and tensor tympani

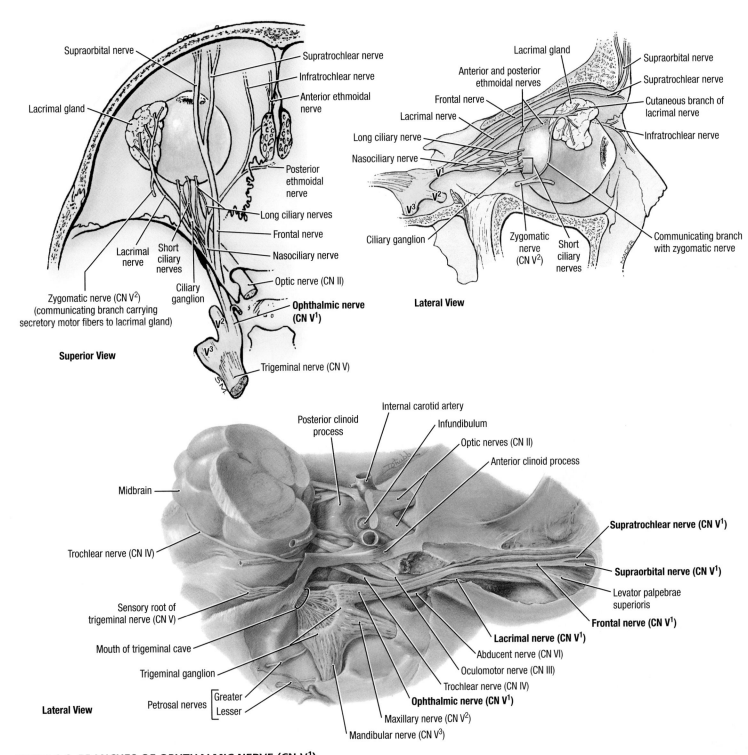

Superior View

Lateral View

Lateral View

TABLE 9.6 BRANCHES OF OPHTHALMIC NERVE (CN V¹)

Function	Branches

The ophthalmic nerve is a sensory nerve passing through the superior orbital fissure that supplies the eyeball and conjunctiva, lacrimal gland and sac, nasal mucosa, frontal sinus, external nose, upper eyelid, forehead, scalp, and central dura mater of anterior cranial fossa	Lacrimal nerve
	
	Frontal nerve
	   Supraorbital nerve
	   Supratrochlear nerve
	
	Nasociliary nerve
	   Short ciliary nerves
	   Long ciliary nerves
	   Infratrochlear nerve
	   Anterior and posterior ethmoidal nerves

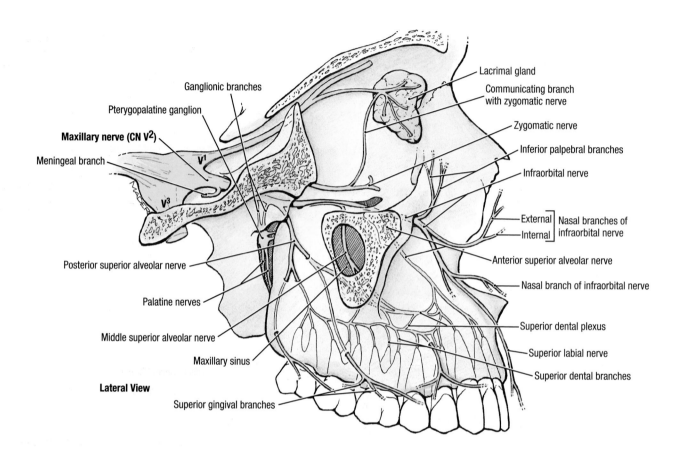

Ganglionic branches

Lacrimal gland

Communicating branch with zygomatic nerve

Pterygopalatine ganglion

Maxillary nerve (CN V²)

Zygomatic nerve

Inferior palpebral branches

V^1

Meningeal branch

Infraorbital nerve

V^3

External | Nasal branches of
Internal | infraorbital nerve

Anterior superior alveolar nerve

Posterior superior alveolar nerve

Nasal branch of infraorbital nerve

Palatine nerves

Superior dental plexus

Middle superior alveolar nerve

Superior labial nerve

Maxillary sinus

Superior dental branches

Lateral View

Superior gingival branches

TABLE 9.7 BRANCHES OF MAXILLARY NERVE (CN V²)

Function	Branches

The maxillary nerve is a sensory nerve passing through the foramen rotundum that supplies sensation to the face, upper teeth and gums, mucous membrane of the nasal cavity, palate and roof of the pharynx, maxillary, ethmoidal, and sphenoidal sinuses, and secretory fibers from the pterygopalatine ganglion, which pass with the zygomatic and lacrimal nerves to the lacrimal gland	Meningeal branch
	
	Zygomatic nerve
	   Zygomaticofacial nerve
	   Zygomaticotemporal nerve
	
	Posterior superior alveolar nerves
	
	Infraorbital nerve
	   Anterior and middle superior alveolar
	     nerves
	   Superior labial branches
	   Inferior palpebral branches
	   External and internal nasal branches
	
	Greater palatine nerve
	   Posterior inferior lateral nasal branches
	
	Lesser palatine nerve
	   Posterior superior lateral nasal branches
	
	Nasopalatine nerve
	
	Pharyngeal nerve

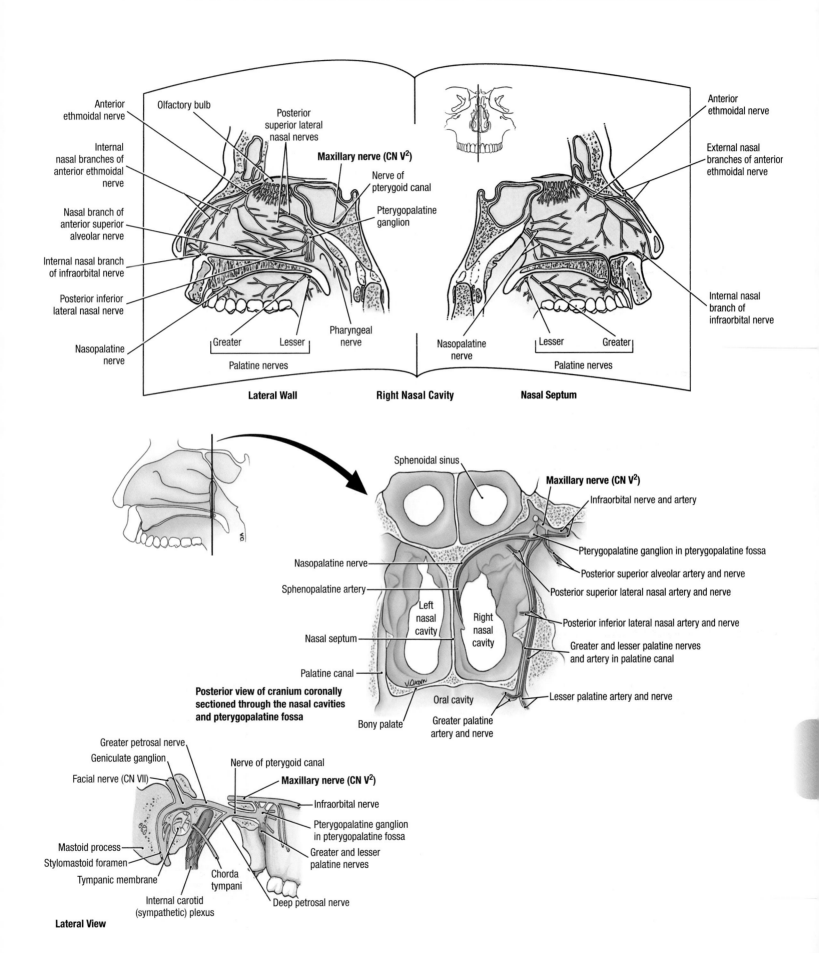

Lateral Wall   **Right Nasal Cavity**   **Nasal Septum**

Posterior view of cranium coronally sectioned through the nasal cavities and pterygopalatine fossa

Lateral View

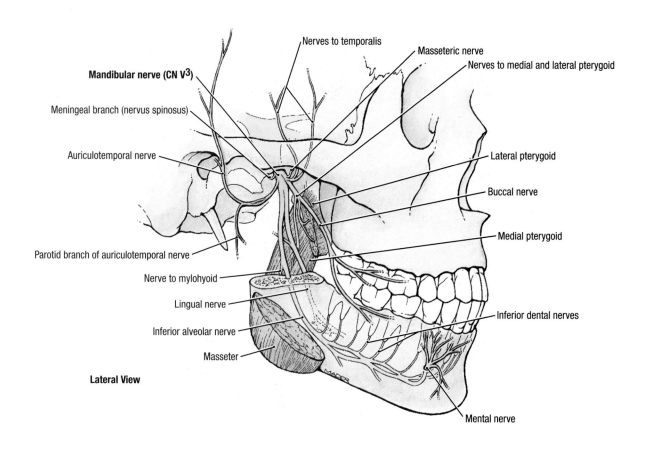

Nerves to temporalis

Masseteric nerve

Nerves to medial and lateral pterygoid

Mandibular nerve (CN V³)

Meningeal branch (nervus spinosus)

Auriculotemporal nerve

Lateral pterygoid

Buccal nerve

Medial pterygoid

Parotid branch of auriculotemporal nerve

Nerve to mylohyoid

Lingual nerve

Inferior alveolar nerve

Inferior dental nerves

Masseter

Lateral View

Mental nerve

TABLE 9.8 BRANCHES OF MANDIBULAR NERVE (CN V³)

Function	Branches

The mandibular nerve is a sensory and motor nerve passing through the foramen ovale. General sensory branches supply the lower teeth, gums, lip, auricle, external acoustic meatus, outer surface of tympanic membrane, cheek, anterior two thirds of tongue, and floor of mouth. CN V³ also conveys secretory fibers from the otic ganglion to the parotid gland. Taste from the anterior two thirds of the tongue and presynaptic secretomotor fibers to the submandibular ganglion are conveyed to the nerve by the chorda tympani. Postsynaptic fibers from the submandibular ganglion pass to the submandibular and sublingual glands	Meningeal branch
	 Buccal nerve
	 Auriculotemporal nerve
	    Inferior alveolar nerve
	    Inferior dental nerves
	    Mental nerve
	    Incisive nerve
	 Lingual nerve

Motor branches supply the muscles of mastication and other muscles derived from the first branchial arches	Masseter Temporalis Medial and lateral pterygoids Tensor veli palatini Mylohyoid Anterior belly of digastric Tensor tympani

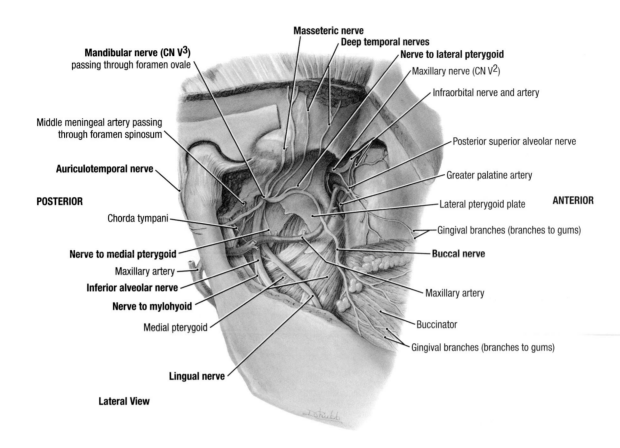

Masseteric nerve

Deep temporal nerves

Mandibular nerve (CN V³)
passing through foramen ovale

Nerve to lateral pterygoid

Maxillary nerve (CN V²)

Infraorbital nerve and artery

Middle meningeal artery passing
through foramen spinosum

Posterior superior alveolar nerve

Auriculotemporal nerve

Greater palatine artery

POSTERIOR

Lateral pterygoid plate

ANTERIOR

Chorda tympani

Gingival branches (branches to gums)

Nerve to medial pterygoid

Buccal nerve

Maxillary artery

Maxillary artery

Inferior alveolar nerve

Nerve to mylohyoid

Buccinator

Medial pterygoid

Gingival branches (branches to gums)

Lingual nerve

Lateral View

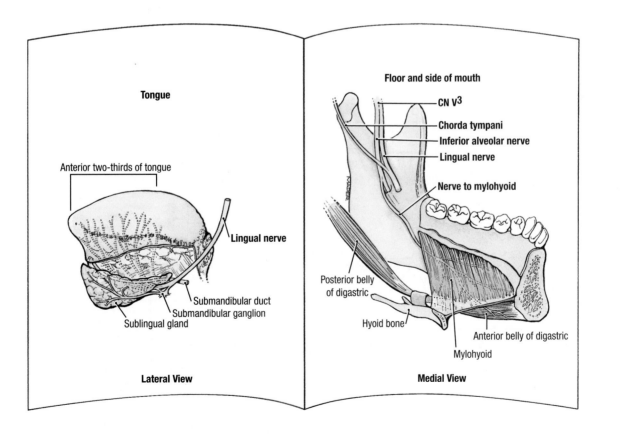

Tongue

Floor and side of mouth

CN V³

Anterior two-thirds of tongue

Chorda tympani

Inferior alveolar nerve

Lingual nerve

Nerve to mylohyoid

Lingual nerve

Posterior belly
of digastric

Submandibular duct
Submandibular ganglion

Hyoid bone

Sublingual gland

Anterior belly of digastric

Mylohyoid

Lateral View

Medial View

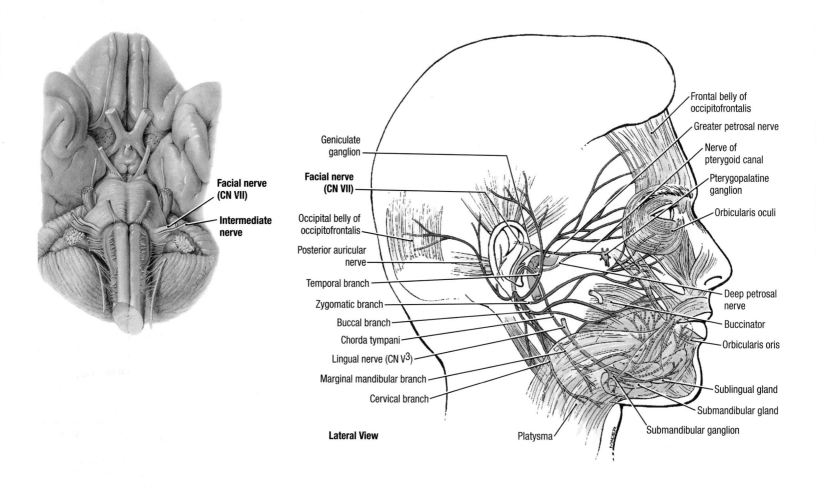

Lateral View

TABLE 9.9 FACIAL NERVE (CN VII), INCLUDING MOTOR ROOT AND INTERMEDIATE NERVE[a]

Nerve	Functional Components	Cells of Origin/ Termination	Cranial Exit	Distribution and Functions
Temporal, zygomatic, buccal, mandibular, cervical, and posterior auricular nerves, nerve to posterior belly of digastric, nerve to stylohyoid, nerve to stapedius	Branchial motor	Facial motor nucleus	Stylomastoid foramen	Motor to muscles of facial expression and scalp; also supplies stapedius of middle ear, stylohyoid, and posterior belly of digastric
Intermediate nerve through chorda tympani	Special sensory	Geniculate ganglion/ solitary nucleus	Internal acoustic meatus/ facial canal/petro-tympanic fissure	Taste from anterior two thirds of tongue, floor of mouth, and palate
Intermediate nerve	General sensory	Geniculate ganglion/spinal trigeminal nucleus	Internal acoustic meatus	Sensation from skin of external acoustic meatus
Intermediate nerve through greater petrosal nerve	Visceral sensory	Solitary nucleus	Internal acoustic meatus/ facial canal/foramen for greater petrosal nerve	Visceral sensation from mucous membranes of nasopharynx and palate
Greater petrosal nerve Chorda tympani	Visceral motor (parasympathetic)	Presynaptic: superior salivatory nucleus; Postsynaptic: pterygopalatine ganglion (greater petrosal nerve) and submandibular ganglion (chorda tympani)	Internal acoustic meatus/ facial canal/foramen for greater petrosal nerve, (greater petrosal nerve) petrotympanic fissure (chorda tympani)	Secretomotor to lacrimal gland and glands of the nose and palate (greater petrosal nerve); submandibular and sublingual salivary glands (chorda tympani)

[a] See also Table 9.15.

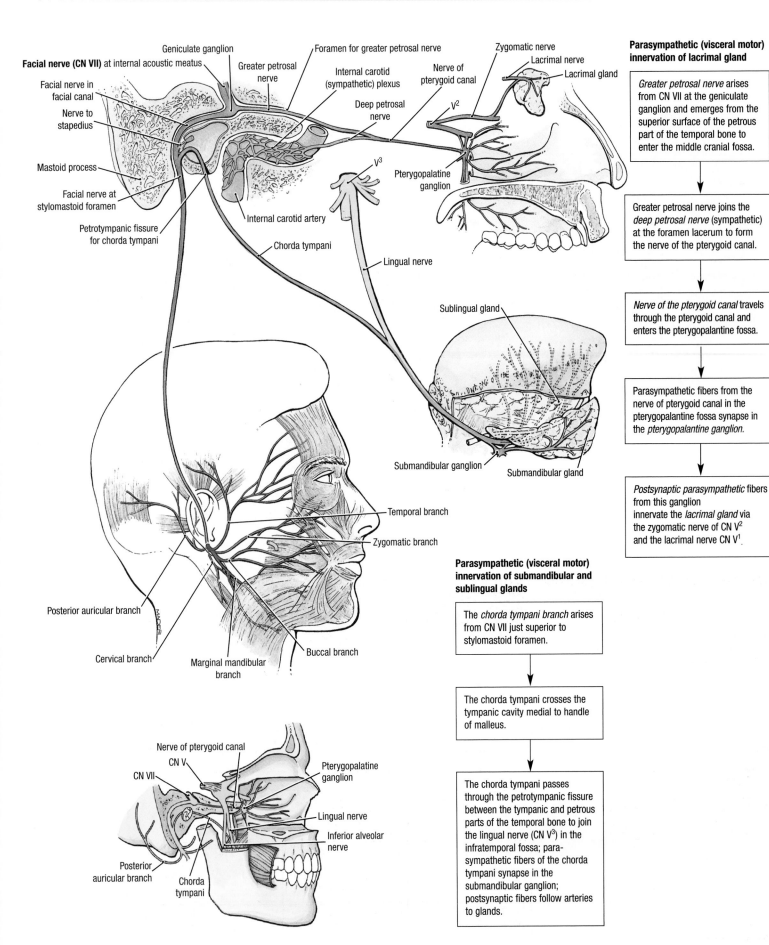

Facial nerve (CN VII) at internal acoustic meatus

Geniculate ganglion

Greater petrosal nerve

Foramen for greater petrosal nerve

Internal carotid (sympathetic) plexus

Zygomatic nerve

Lacrimal nerve

Lacrimal gland

Nerve of pterygoid canal

Deep petrosal nerve

V²

Facial nerve in facial canal

Nerve to stapedius

Internal carotid artery

V³

Pterygopalatine ganglion

Mastoid process

Facial nerve at stylomastoid foramen

Petrotympanic fissure for chorda tympani

Chorda tympani

Lingual nerve

Sublingual gland

Temporal branch

Zygomatic branch

Posterior auricular branch

Cervical branch

Marginal mandibular branch

Buccal branch

Submandibular ganglion

Submandibular gland

Nerve of pterygoid canal

CN V

CN VII

Pterygopalatine ganglion

Lingual nerve

Inferior alveolar nerve

Posterior auricular branch

Chorda tympani

Parasympathetic (visceral motor) innervation of lacrimal gland

Greater petrosal nerve arises from CN VII at the geniculate ganglion and emerges from the superior surface of the petrous part of the temporal bone to enter the middle cranial fossa.

Greater petrosal nerve joins the *deep petrosal nerve* (sympathetic) at the foramen lacerum to form the nerve of the pterygoid canal.

Nerve of the pterygoid canal travels through the pterygoid canal and enters the pterygopalatine fossa.

Parasympathetic fibers from the nerve of pterygoid canal in the pterygopalantine fossa synapse in the *pterygopalantine ganglion.*

Postsynaptic parasympathetic fibers from this ganglion innervate the *lacrimal gland* via the zygomatic nerve of CN V² and the lacrimal nerve CN V¹.

Parasympathetic (visceral motor) innervation of submandibular and sublingual glands

The *chorda tympani branch* arises from CN VII just superior to stylomastoid foramen.

The chorda tympani crosses the tympanic cavity medial to handle of malleus.

The chorda tympani passes through the petrotympanic fissure between the tympanic and petrous parts of the temporal bone to join the lingual nerve (CN V³) in the infratemporal fossa; para-sympathetic fibers of the chorda tympani synapse in the submandibular ganglion; postsynaptic fibers follow arteries to glands.

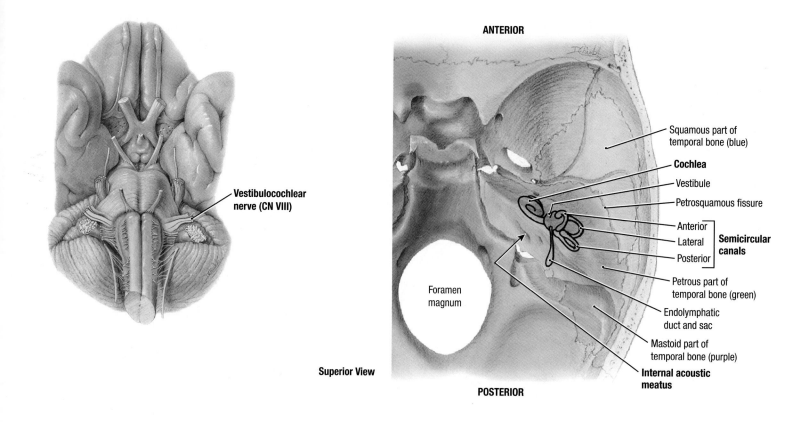

Vestibulocochlear
nerve (CN VIII)

ANTERIOR

Squamous part of
temporal bone (blue)

Cochlea

Vestibule

Petrosquamous fissure

Anterior
Lateral   **Semicircular
canals**
Posterior

Petrous part of
temporal bone (green)

Endolymphatic
duct and sac

Mastoid part of
temporal bone (purple)

**Internal acoustic
meatus**

Foramen
magnum

Superior View

POSTERIOR

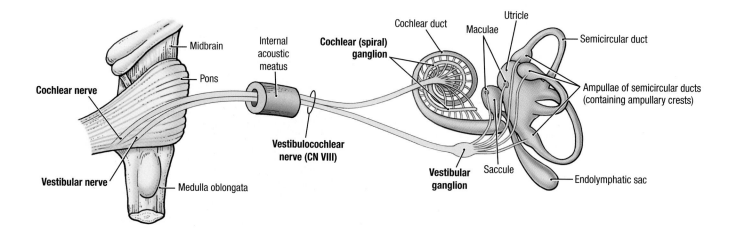

Midbrain

Internal
acoustic
meatus

**Cochlear (spiral)
ganglion**

Cochlear duct

Maculae

Utricle

Semicircular duct

Pons

Cochlear nerve

Vestibular nerve

Medulla oblongata

**Vestibulocochlear
nerve (CN VIII)**

**Vestibular
ganglion**

Saccule

Ampullae of semicircular ducts
(containing ampullary crests)

Endolymphatic sac

TABLE 9.10 VESTIBULOCOCHLEAR NERVE (CN VIII)

Part of Vestibuloccochlear Nerve	Functional Components	Cells of Origin/ Termination	Cranial Exit	Distribution and Functions
Vestibular nerve	Special sensory	Vestibular ganglion/ vestibular nuclei	Internal acoustic meatus	Vestibular sensation from semicircular ducts, utricle, and saccule related to position and movement of head
Cochlear nerve	Special sensory	Spiral ganglion/cochlear nuclei	Internal acoustic meatus	Hearing from spiral organ

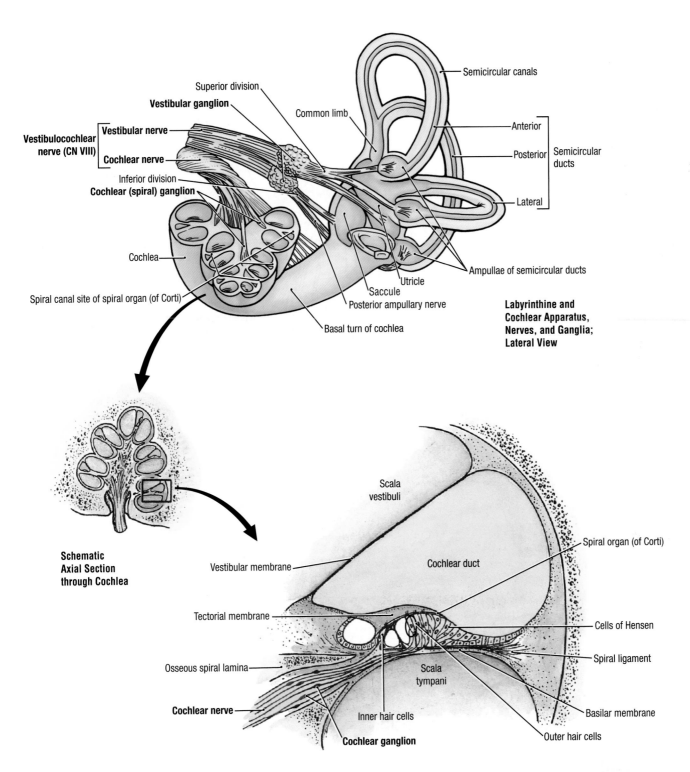

Labyrinthine and Cochlear Apparatus, Nerves, and Ganglia; Lateral View

Schematic Axial Section through Cochlea

Observe in the lower diagram:
- The cochlear duct is a spiral tube fixed to the internal and external walls of the cochlear canal by the spiral ligament.
- The triangular cochlear duct lies between the osseous spiral lamina and the external wall of the cochlear canal.
- The roof of the cochlear duct is formed by the vestibular membrane and the floor by the basilar membrane and osseous spiral lamina.

- The receptor of auditory stimuli is the spiral organ (of Corti), situated on the basilar membrane; it is overlaid by the gelatinous tectorial membrane.
- The spiral organ contains hair cells that respond to vibrations induced in the endolymph by sound waves.
- The fibers of the cochlear nerve are axons of neurons in the spiral ganglion; the peripheral processes enter the spiral organ (of Corti).

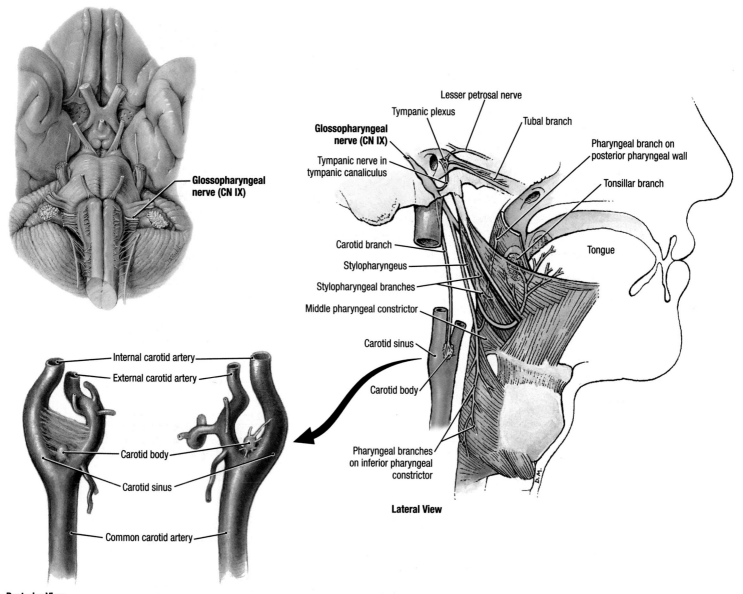

Lesser petrosal nerve

Tympanic plexus

Tubal branch

Glossopharyngeal nerve (CN IX)

Pharyngeal branch on posterior pharyngeal wall

Tympanic nerve in tympanic canaliculus

Tonsillar branch

Carotid branch

Tongue

Stylopharyngeus

Stylopharyngeal branches

Middle pharyngeal constrictor

Carotid sinus

Carotid body

Pharyngeal branches on inferior pharyngeal constrictor

Lateral View

Internal carotid artery

External carotid artery

Carotid body

Carotid sinus

Common carotid artery

Posterior View

Glossopharyngeal nerve (CN IX)

TABLE 9.11 GLOSSOPHARYNGEAL NERVE (CN IX)[a]

Nerve Functions	Functional Components	Cells of Origin/ Termination	Cranial Exit	Distribution and Functions
Glossopharyngeal	Branchial motor	Nucleus ambiguus		Motor to stylopharyngeus that assists with swallowing
	Visceral motor (parasympathetic)	Presynaptic: inferior salivatory nucleus; postsynaptic: otic ganglion	Jugular foramen	Secretomotor to parotid gland
	Visceral sensory	Solitary nucleus, spinal trigeminal nucleus/ inferior ganglion		Visceral sensation from parotid gland, carotid body, carotid sinus, pharynx, and middle ear
	Special sensory	Solitary nucleus/inferior ganglion		Taste from posterior third of tongue
	General sensory	Spinal trigeminal nucleus/ superior ganglion		Cutaneous sensation from external ear

[a] See also Table 9.15.

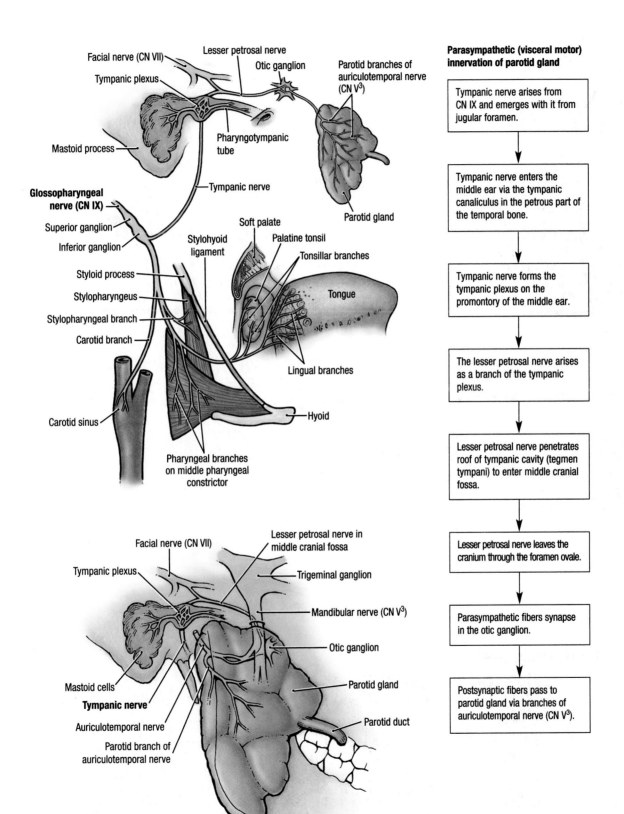

Facial nerve (CN VII)

Lesser petrosal nerve

Otic ganglion

Parotid branches of auriculotemporal nerve (CN V³)

Tympanic plexus

Mastoid process

Pharyngotympanic tube

Tympanic nerve

Parotid gland

Glossopharyngeal nerve (CN IX)

Superior ganglion

Inferior ganglion

Stylohyoid ligament

Soft palate

Palatine tonsil

Tonsillar branches

Styloid process

Stylopharyngeus

Tongue

Stylopharyngeal branch

Carotid branch

Lingual branches

Carotid sinus

Hyoid

Pharyngeal branches on middle pharyngeal constrictor

Facial nerve (CN VII)

Lesser petrosal nerve in middle cranial fossa

Tympanic plexus

Trigeminal ganglion

Mandibular nerve (CN V³)

Otic ganglion

Mastoid cells

Parotid gland

Tympanic nerve

Auriculotemporal nerve

Parotid duct

Parotid branch of auriculotemporal nerve

Lateral View

Parasympathetic (visceral motor) innervation of parotid gland

Tympanic nerve arises from CN IX and emerges with it from jugular foramen.

Tympanic nerve enters the middle ear via the tympanic canaliculus in the petrous part of the temporal bone.

Tympanic nerve forms the tympanic plexus on the promontory of the middle ear.

The lesser petrosal nerve arises as a branch of the tympanic plexus.

Lesser petrosal nerve penetrates roof of tympanic cavity (tegmen tympani) to enter middle cranial fossa.

Lesser petrosal nerve leaves the cranium through the foramen ovale.

Parasympathetic fibers synapse in the otic ganglion.

Postsynaptic fibers pass to parotid gland via branches of auriculotemporal nerve (CN V³).

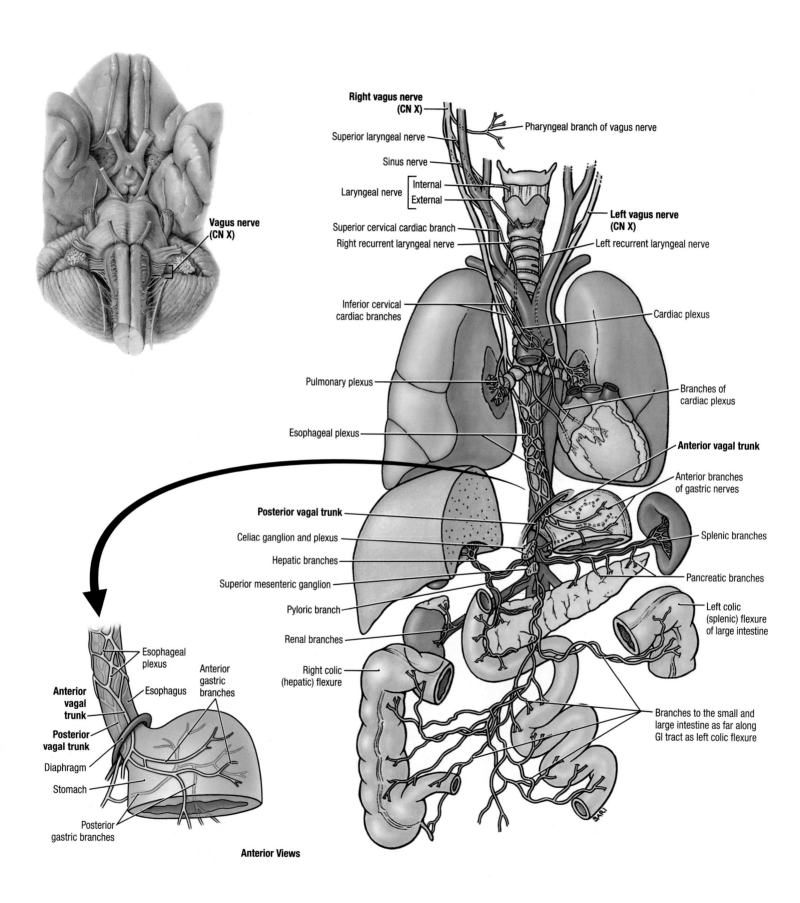

Vagus nerve
(CN X)

Right vagus nerve
(CN X)

Pharyngeal branch of vagus nerve

Superior laryngeal nerve

Sinus nerve

Laryngeal nerve { Internal / External }

Left vagus nerve
(CN X)

Superior cervical cardiac branch

Right recurrent laryngeal nerve

Left recurrent laryngeal nerve

Inferior cervical
cardiac branches

Cardiac plexus

Pulmonary plexus

Branches of
cardiac plexus

Esophageal plexus

Anterior vagal trunk

Anterior branches
of gastric nerves

Posterior vagal trunk

Celiac ganglion and plexus

Splenic branches

Hepatic branches

Pancreatic branches

Superior mesenteric ganglion

Pyloric branch

Left colic
(splenic) flexure
of large intestine

Renal branches

Right colic
(hepatic) flexure

Branches to the small and
large intestine as far along
GI tract as left colic flexure

Esophageal
plexus

Anterior
gastric
branches

Esophagus

Anterior
vagal
trunk

Posterior
vagal trunk

Diaphragm

Stomach

Posterior
gastric branches

Anterior Views

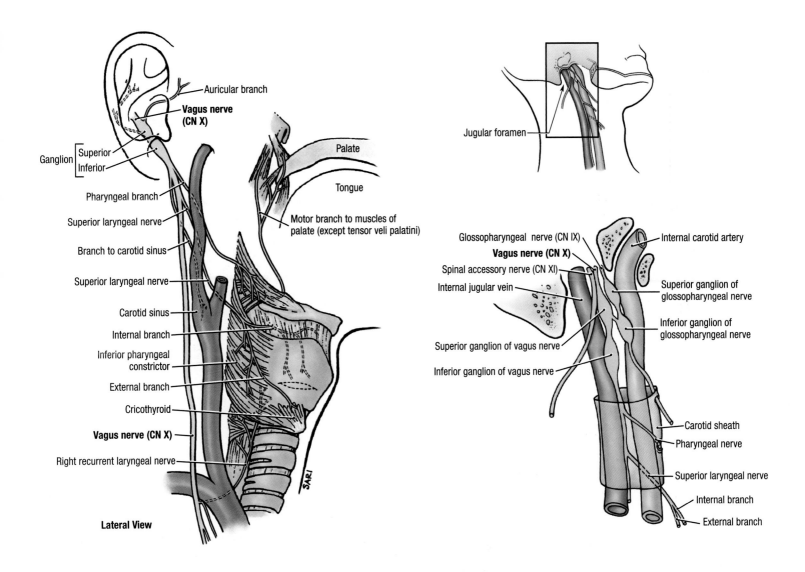

Lateral View

TABLE 9.12 VAGUS NERVE (CN X)

Nerve Functions	Functional Components	Cells of Origin/ Termination	Cranial Exit	Distribution and Functions
Vagus	Branchial motor	Nucleus ambiguus	Jugular foramen	Motor to constrictor muscles of pharynx, intrinsic muscles of larynx, muscles of palate (except tensor veli palatini), and striated muscle in superior two thirds of esophagus
	Visceral motor (parasympathetic)	Presynaptic: dorsal vagal nucleus; Postsynaptic: neurons in, on, or near viscera		Motor to smooth muscle of trachea, bronchi, and digestive tract; moderates cardiac pacemaker and vasoconstrictor of coronary arteries
	Visceral sensory	Solitary nucleus, spinal trigeminal nucleus/ inferior ganglion		Visceral sensation from base of tongue, pharynx, larynx, trachea, bronchi, heart, esophagus, stomach, and intestine
	Special sensory	Solitary nucleus/inferior ganglion		Taste from epiglottis and palate
	General sensory	Spinal trigeminal nucleus/ superior or inferior ganglion		Sensation from auricle, external acoustic meatus, and dura mater of posterior cranial fossa

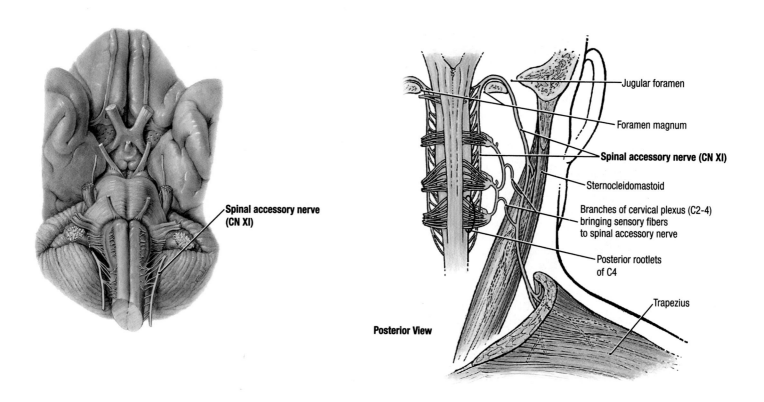

Spinal accessory nerve
(CN XI)

Posterior View

Jugular foramen

Foramen magnum

Spinal accessory nerve (CN XI)

Sternocleidomastoid

Branches of cervical plexus (C2-4)
bringing sensory fibers
to spinal accessory nerve

Posterior rootlets
of C4

Trapezius

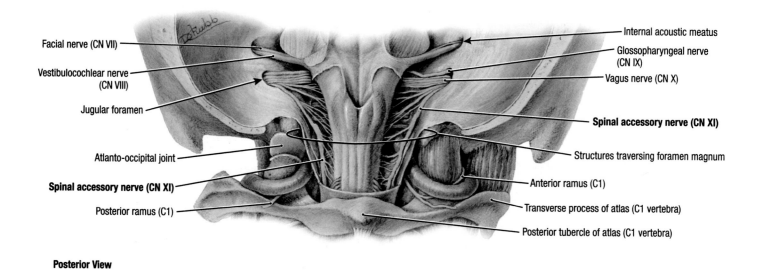

Facial nerve (CN VII)

Vestibulocochlear nerve
(CN VIII)

Jugular foramen

Atlanto-occipital joint

Spinal accessory nerve (CN XI)

Posterior ramus (C1)

Internal acoustic meatus

Glossopharyngeal nerve
(CN IX)

Vagus nerve (CN X)

Spinal accessory nerve (CN XI)

Structures traversing foramen magnum

Anterior ramus (C1)

Transverse process of atlas (C1 vertebra)

Posterior tubercle of atlas (C1 vertebra)

Posterior View

TABLE 9.13   SPINAL ACCESSORY NERVE (CN XI)

Nerve	Functional Components	Cells of Origin/ Termination	Cranial Exit	Distribution and Functions
Spinal accessory	Somatic motor	Accessory nucleus of spinal cord	Jugular foramen	Motor to sternocleidomastoid and trapezius

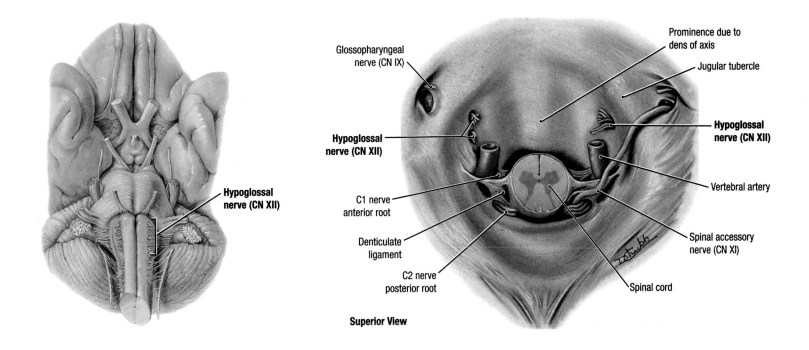

Glossopharyngeal nerve (CN IX)

Prominence due to dens of axis

Jugular tubercle

Hypoglossal nerve (CN XII)

Hypoglossal nerve (CN XII)

Vertebral artery

C1 nerve anterior root

Denticulate ligament

C2 nerve posterior root

Spinal accessory nerve (CN XI)

Spinal cord

Superior View

Hypoglossal nerve (CN XII)

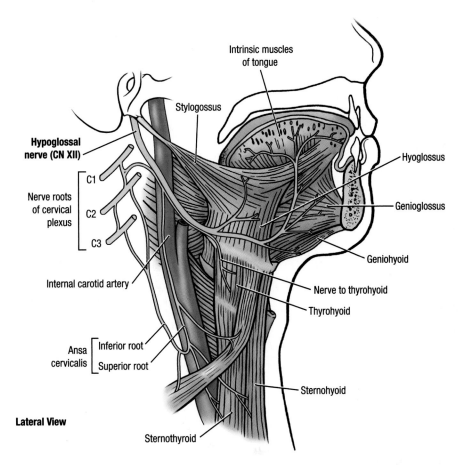

Intrinsic muscles of tongue

Stylogossus

Hypoglossal nerve (CN XII)

C1

C2

Nerve roots of cervical plexus

C3

Internal carotid artery

Hyoglossus

Genioglossus

Geniohyoid

Nerve to thyrohyoid

Thyrohyoid

Ansa cervicalis

Inferior root

Superior root

Sternohyoid

Lateral View

Sternothyroid

TABLE 9.14 HYPOGLOSSAL NERVE (CN XII)

Nerve	Functional Components	Cells of Origin/ Termination	Cranial Exit	Distribution and Functions
Hypoglossal	Somatic motor	Hypoglossal nucleus	Hypoglossal canal	Motor to muscles of tongue (except palatoglossus)

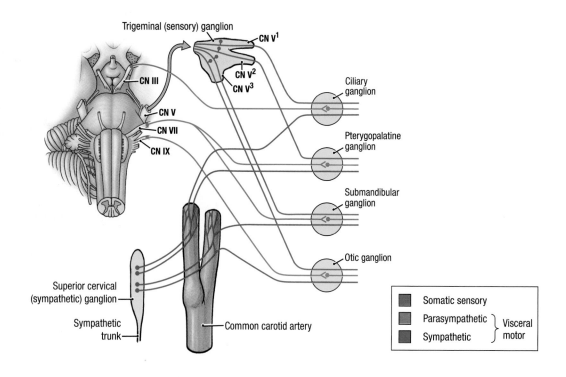

TABLE 9.15 AUTONOMIC GANGLIA OF THE HEAD

Ganglion	Location	Parasympathetic Root (Nucleus of Origin) [a]	Sympathetic Root	Main Distribution
Ciliary	Between optic nerve and lateral rectus, close to apex of orbit	Inferior branch of oculomotor nerve (CN III) (Edinger-Westphal nucleus)	Branch from internal carotid plexus in cavernous sinus	Parasympathetic postsynaptic fibers from ciliary ganglion pass to ciliary muscle and sphincter pupillae of iris; sympathetic postsynaptic fibers from superior cervical ganglion pass to dilator pupillae and blood vessels of eye
Pterygopalatine	In pterygopalatine fossa, where it is attached by pterygopalatine branches of maxillary nerve; located just anterior to opening of pterygoid canal and inferior to CN V²	Greater petrosal nerve from facial nerve (CN VII) (superior salivatory nucleus)	Deep petrosal nerve, a branch of internal carotid plexus that is continuation of postsynaptic fibers of cervical sympathetic trunk; fibers from superior cervical ganglion pass through pterygopalatine ganglion and enter branches of CN V²	Parasympathetic postsynaptic fibers from pterygopalatine ganglion innervate lacrimal gland through zygomatic branch of CN V²; sympathetic postsynaptic fibers from superior cervical ganglion accompany branches of pterygopalatine nerve that are distributed to the nasal cavity, palate, and superior parts of the pharynx
Otic	Between tensor veli palatini and mandibular nerve; lies inferior to foramen ovale	Tympanic nerve from glossopharyngeal nerve (CN IX); tympanic nerve continues from tympanic plexus as lesser petrosal nerve (inferior salivatory nucleus)	Fibers from superior cervical ganglion travel via plexus on middle meningeal artery	Parasympathetic postsynaptic fibers from otic ganglion are distributed to parotid gland through auriculotemporal nerve (branch of CN V³); sympathetic postsynaptic fibers from superior cervical ganglion pass to parotid gland and supply its blood vessels
Submandibular	Suspended from lingual nerve by two short roots; lies on surface of hyoglossus muscle inferior to submandibular duct	Parasympathetic fibers join facial nerve (CN VII) and leave it in its chorda tympani branch, which unites with lingual nerve (superior salivatory nucleus)	Sympathetic fibers from superior cervical ganglion travel via the plexus on facial artery	Postsynaptic parasympathetic fibers from submandibular ganglion are distributed to the sublingual and submandibular glands; sympathetic fibers from superior cervical ganglion supply sublingual and submandibular glands

[a] For location of nuclei, see Figure 9.3.

TABLE 9.16 SUMMARY OF CRANIAL NERVE LESIONS

Nerve	Lesion Type and/or Site	Abnormal Findings
CN I	Fracture of cribriform plate	Anosmia (loss of smell); cerebrospinal fluid (CSF) rhinorrhea (leakage of CSF through nose)
CN II	Direct trauma to orbit or eyeball; fracture involving optic canal	Loss of pupillary constriction
	Pressure on optic pathway; laceration or intracerebral clot in temporal, parietal, or occipital lobes of brain	Visual field defects
	Increased CSF pressure	Swelling of optic disc (papilledema)
CN III	Pressure from herniating uncus on nerve; fracture involving cavernous sinus; aneurysms	Dilated pupil, ptosis, eye rotates inferiorly and laterally (down and out), pupillary reflex on the side of the lesion will be lost
CN IV	Stretching of nerve during its course around brainstem; fracture of orbit	Inability to rotate adducted eye inferiorly
CN V	Injury to terminal branches (particularly CN V^2) in roof of maxillary sinus; pathologic processes (tumors, aneurysms, infections) affecting trigeminal nerve	Loss of pain and touch sensations/paresthesia on face; loss of corneal reflex (blinking when cornea touched); paralysis of muscles of mastication; deviation of mandible to side of lesion when mouth is opened
CN VI	Base of brain or fracture involving cavernous sinus or orbit	Inability to rotate eye laterally; diplopia on lateral gaze
CN VII	Laceration or contusion in parotid region	Paralysis of facial muscles; eye remains open; angle of mouth droops; forehead does not wrinkle
	Fracture of temporal bone	As above, plus associated involvement of cochlear nerve and chorda tympani; dry cornea and loss of taste on anterior two thirds of tongue
	Intracranial hematoma ("stroke")	Weakness (paralysis) of lower facial muscles contralateral to the lesion, upper facial muscles are not affected because they are bilaterally innervated
CN VIII	Tumor of nerve	Progressive unilateral hearing loss; tinnitus (noises in ear); vertigo (loss of balance)
CN IX[a]	Brainstem lesion or deep laceration of neck	Loss of taste on posterior third of tongue; loss of sensation on affected side of soft palate; loss of gag reflex on affected side
CN X	Brainstem lesion or deep laceration of neck	Sagging of soft palate; deviation of uvula to unaffected side; hoarseness owing to paralysis of vocal fold; difficulty in swallowing and speaking
CN XI	Laceration of neck	Paralysis of sternocleidomastoid and superior fibers of trapezius; drooping of shoulder
CN XII	Neck laceration; basal skull fractures	Protruded tongue deviates toward affected side; moderate dysarthria (disturbance of articulation)

[a] Isolated lesions of CN IX are uncommon; usually, CN IX, X, and XI are involved together as they pass through the jugular foramen.

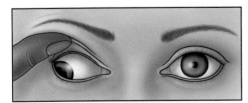

Right eye: Downward and outward gaze, dilated pupil, eyelid manually elevated due to ptosis   Left

Right oculomotor (CN III) nerve palsy

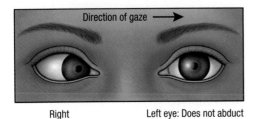

Direction of gaze →

Right   Left eye: Does not abduct

Left abducent (CN VI) nerve palsy

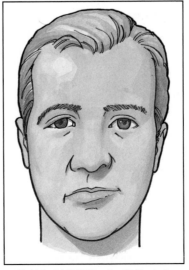

Right facial (CN VII) palsy (Bell palsy)

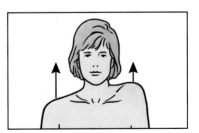

Right CN XI lesion

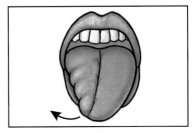

Right CN XII lesion

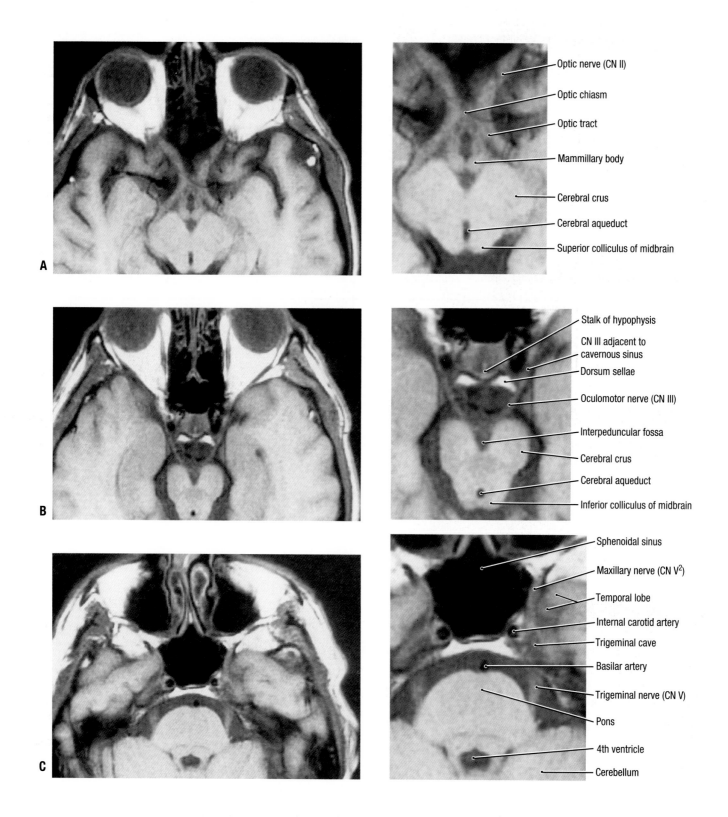

9.6   Transverse MRIs through head, showing cranial nerves

A. Optic nerve (CN II). **B.** Oculomotor nerve (CN III). **C.** Trigeminal nerve (CN V).

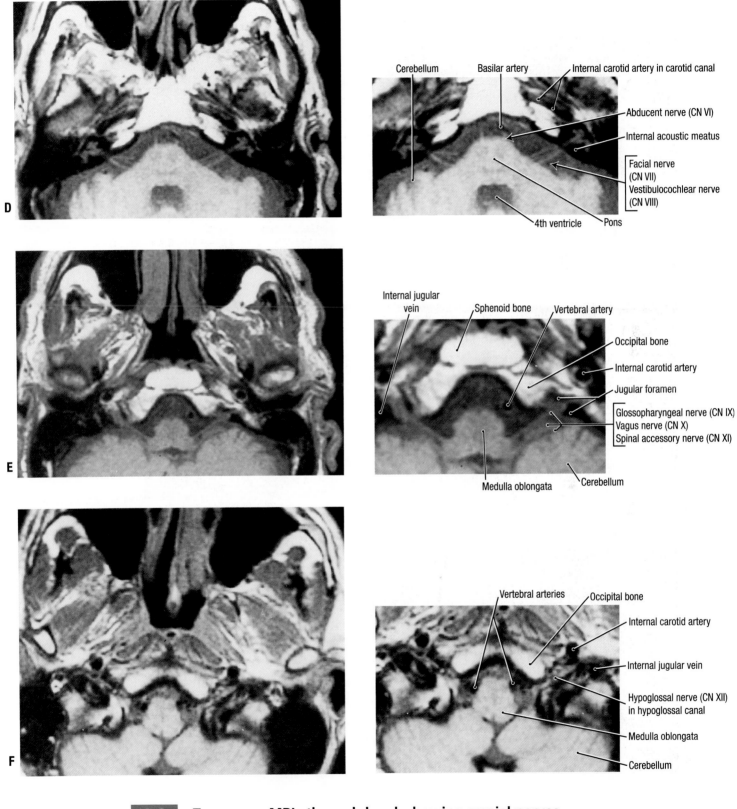

9.6   **Transverse MRIs through head, showing cranial nerves** *(continued)*

D. Abducent (CN VI), facial (CN VII), and vestibulocochlear (CN VIII) nerves.
E. Glossopharyngeal (CN IX), vagus (CN X), and spinal accessory (CN XI) nerves.
F. Hypoglossal nerve (CN XII).

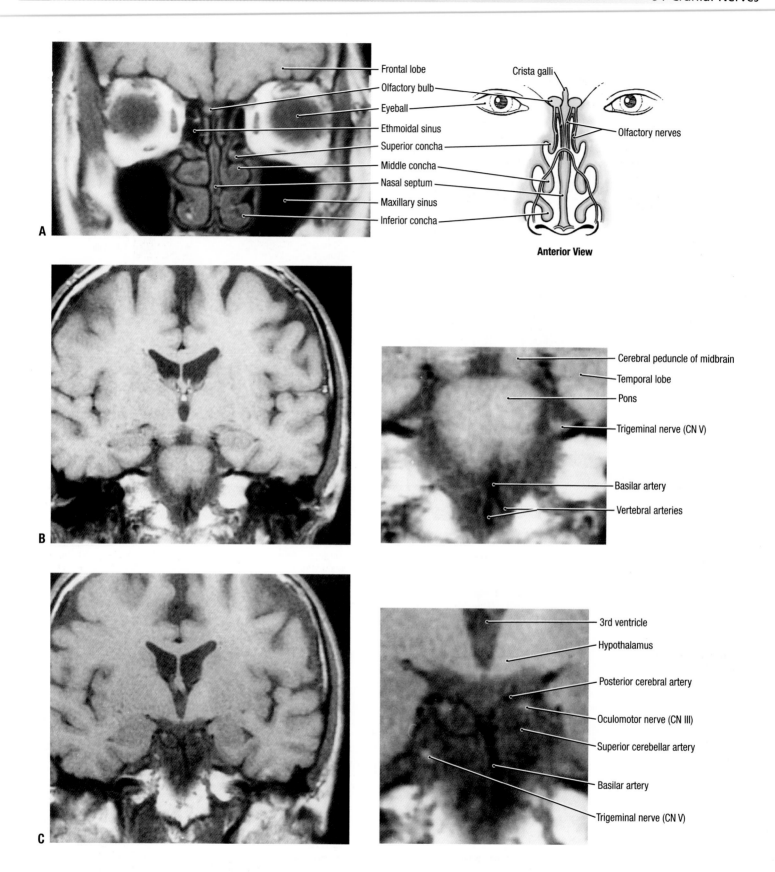

9.7   **Coronal MRIs through head, showing cranial nerves**

A. Olfactory bulb. **B.** Trigeminal (CN V) nerve. **C.** Oculomotor (CN III) and trigeminal (CN V) nerves.

INDEX

Note: Page numbers followed by t denote tables.

Abdomen
    autonomic innervation, 178, 179t
    contents, 119
    magnetic resonance imaging,
        186–189, 191
    ultrasound, 190–191
    vagus nerves in, 181
    viscera, 96, 97, 162, 163
Abdominal wall
    anterior, 102–103, 152, 157
    anterolateral
        arteries, 101
        muscles, 104, 104t
        nerves, 101
        posterior aspect, 118
        structure, 105
        superficial dissection, 100
        surface anatomy, 98–99
    layers, 105
    posterior, 121, 162, 163, 172t
    subperitoneal fat, 164
Acetabular region, 396
Acetabulum, 196–199, 372, 380,
    396–398
Acromion, 511, 518, 519, 527, 529,
    533, 535–537, 598
Amnion, 239
Ampulla, 714
    ductus deferens, 216, 217, 220
    hepatopancreatic, 156
    phrenic, 132
    rectum, 208, 232
Anal column, 209, 211
Anastomosis
    genicular, 417
    knee, 416–417
    portal-systemic, 227
    transverse, 490
    upper limb, 486, 487
Anatomical snuff box, 580, 584, 585
Angiogram
    abdomen, 191
    aorta, 55, 70, 191
    head and neck, 649
    pelvis, 277
    thorax, 41, 92–93
Angle
    acromial, 519, 531
    of clitoris, 272
    costal, 13
    of eye, 650
    inferolateral, 313
    infrasternal, 10
    of mandible, 609, 610, 612, 664
    Q-, 407
    of scapula
        inferior, 11, 511, 518, 522, 523,
            535
        superior, 511, 518, 523, 529,
            536
    sternal, 12, 300, 499, 808
    subpubic, 196, 198, 199
    venous, 76, 716
Ankle, 354
    articular surfaces, 455

coronal section, 456
ligaments, 449, 452, 454
magnetic resonance imaging, 456,
    457
medial aspect, 438, 439
posterior aspect, 450
posteromedial aspect, 451
radiograph, 453, 454
synovial sheaths and tendons, 430,
    431
transverse section, 457
Ankle region, 354
Ansa cervicalis, 762, 763, 766, 807
Antihelix, 703
Antrum
    mastoid, 713
    pyloric, 129, 132, 186, 189
Anulus fibrosus, 304–308
Anus, 161, 252, 271–274, 276–281
Aorta, 20, 29, 50, 57–59, 65, 73, 78,
    83, 117, 120, 124, 130,
    133, 137, 142, 144,
    152–154, 157, 164, 165,
    186, 188, 189, 215, 339,
    808
    abdominal, 74, 85, 123, 163, 175,
        191, 213
    ascending, 27, 41, 46, 49, 51, 59,
        67, 70
        3-D volume reconstruction and
            CT angiogram, 92–93
        magnetic resonance imaging,
            88–91
    bifurcation, 188
    branches, 174
    descending, 65, 67, 70, 71, 81, 351
        3-D volume reconstruction and
            CT angiogram, 92–93
        computed tomography, 6
        magnetic resonance imaging,
            88–91
    dorsal, 67
    thoracic, 68, 69, 74–76, 82, 85
        descending, 119
    ultrasound, 190, 191
Aperture
    anterior nasal, 613
    lateral, 722, 724
    median, 723, 724
Aponeurosis
    bicipital, 522, 523, 525, 538, 539,
        549
    epicranial, 330, 634, 743
    external oblique, 100, 102,
        105–109, 111, 112, 372
    flexor carpi ulnaris with ante-
        brachial fascia, 542
    gastrocnemius, 472
    internal oblique, 105, 107–109,
        112
    levator palpebrae superior, 654
    palatine, 682, 684
    palmar, 554, 560–563, 566, 571,
        606
    palmar carpal, 493

plantar, 443–445, 456
transversus abdominis, 109, 170,
    322, 324
triceps, 527
Appendices epiploicae, 144, 145
Appendix, 97, 128, 136, 139, 140,
    160, 208, 232
    blood supply, 139
    of epididymis, 116
    omental, 136, 140
    of testis, 116
Aqueduct
    cerebral, 523, 723, 724, 729, 738,
        739, 742
    vestibular, 714
Aqueous humor, 660, 661
Arachnoid granulations, 636–638,
    724
Arachnoid mater, 334, 335, 338–340,
    634, 636
Arch
    aortic, 25–27, 29, 39, 46, 47, 49,
        52, 61, 68, 69, 72, 74, 75,
        78, 81, 84, 85, 486
        branches, 70
        double, 71
        magnetic resonance imaging,
            90, 91
        relationship to recurrent laryn-
            geal nerve, 67
        variations, 70, 71
    carpal
        dorsal, 487, 573, 573t, 576
        palmar, 487, 570
    iliopectineal, 373
    longitudinal
        lateral, 466
        medial, 466
    neural, 290
    palatoglossal, 792–794
    palatopharyngeal, 792–794
    palmar
        deep, 486, 487, 550, 551,
            570–573, 573t, 584
        superficial, 486, 487, 550, 551,
            561, 566, 572, 573, 573t
    pancreaticoduodenal
        anterior, 135
        posterior, 135, 153
    plantar, 362, 440
        deep, 446
    pubic, 196, 198, 199
    superciliary, 611, 612
    transverse, 466
    venous
        deep palmar, 488
        dorsal, 363–365, 490
        dorsal digital, 490
        plantar, 363
        superficial palmar, 488
    vertebral, 16, 289
    zygomatic, 610, 612, 615, 666, 719
Areola, 4
Arm, 476, 477
    anterior aspect, 522, 523

compartments, 521, 600
lateral aspect, 524
magnetic resonance imaging, 601
medial aspect, 525
muscles, 519
posterior aspect, 526
Arteriogram
    axillary, 504
    brachial, 551
    carotid, 648
    celiac, 131
    coronary, 54
    hand, 572
    inferior mesenteric, 143
    popliteal, 440
    renal, 167
    superior mesenteric, 141
    vertebral, 648
Arteriole, inferior temporal retinal,
    661
Artery
    acetabular, 401
    alveolar
        inferior, 670, 778
        posterior superior, 712
    anal, inferior, 261, 269
    angular, 632, 632t, 721
    appendicular, 139, 140
    arcuate, 362, 425, 427, 427t
    auricular
        deep, 670
        posterior, 632, 632t, 662, 764,
            764t, 765
    axillary, 8, 22, 486, 487, 503, 508,
        509
    basilar, 298, 341, 638, 640, 646,
        647, 647t, 648, 649, 738,
        739, 742
    brachial, 486, 487, 502, 539–541,
        549–551
        deep, 504, 505t, 510, 521, 527,
            600
    brachiocephalic, 66, 67
    bronchial, 35, 69, 75
    buccal, 668, 670
    calcaneal, medial, 457
    carotid
        common, 71, 738, 739, 763,
            771, 772, 806, 807
            left, 46–49, 66, 67, 70, 71, 74,
                81, 82, 88–91, 773
            right, 26, 48, 66, 67, 70, 71,
                74, 88–90, 486, 764, 764t,
                765, 773
        external, 662, 663, 667, 681,
            713, 763, 764, 764t, 765
        internal, 350, 638, 640,
            644–647, 647t, 648, 649,
            662, 663, 667, 681,
            710–713, 720, 721,
            738–740, 763, 764, 764t,
            765, 785, 809
    celiac, 78, 82, 130, 186, 188, 189
    central
        anteromedial, 731

Artery—*continued*
  posterolateral, 731
  posteromedial, 731
  of retina, 657, 657t, 660, 661
  cerebellar
    anterior inferior, 647, 647t, 648
    posterior, 648
    posterior inferior, 647, 647t, 648, 740
    superior, 341, 638, 647, 647t, 648, 740
  cerebral
    anterior, 638, 646, 647, 647t, 648, 649, 732, 733, 740, 742, 743
    middle, 646, 647, 647t, 648, 649, 732, 733, 740, 742
    posterior, 341, 638, 646, 647, 647t, 649, 738–740
  cervical
    ascending, 341, 772, 773
    deep, 75, 331, 341, 784
    superficial, 486, 772
  ciliary
    anterior, 657t, 661
    long posterior, 657t, 661
    short posterior, 657t, 661
  circumflex femoral
    lateral, 277, 362, 373, 382, 400, 401
    medial, 277, 362, 373, 382, 400, 401
  circumflex humeral
    anterior, 486, 504, 505t, 509
    posterior, 486, 504, 505t, 509, 510, 527, 528, 534, 536
  circumflex iliac
    deep, 101, 108, 109, 111, 112, 118, 224, 242, 362, 372
    superficial, 101, 362, 370, 372
  circumflex scapular, 487, 502, 504, 505t, 509, 510, 528
  colic
    left, 142, 143, 145
    middle, 122, 126, 127, 134, 135, 140–142, 144, 145
      accessory, 127
    right, 127, 134, 140, 141, 145
  collateral
    medial, 486, 487
    middle, 550
    radial, 486, 487, 550
  communicating
    anterior, 646, 647, 647t, 649, 738–740
    posterior, 638, 646, 647, 647t, 648, 649
  coronary, 53, 59, 75
    3-D volume reconstruction and CT angiogram, 92–93
    anterior interventricular branch, 49
    branches, 52
    circumflex branch, 50
    left, 46, 52, 54, 55, 63, 92–93
    magnetic resonance imaging, 88–89
    right, 46, 47, 49, 50, 52, 54, 55, 59, 63, 92–93
    single, 55
  cremasteric, 101, 108, 109, 112, 117
  cystic, 130, 154, 155, 158
  deep
    of arm, 486, 487, 502, 509, 528, 550

  of clitoris, 241
  of thigh, 275, 362, 372, 373, 382, 400
  digital
    common palmar, 487, 561, 566, 569, 570, 572, 573t
    dorsal, 362, 425, 487, 569, 573, 576
    plantar, 362, 443, 446
    proper palmar, 487, 561, 563, 569, 570, 572, 573t
  dorsal
    of clitoris, 241, 254, 272, 274
    of foot, 362, 425–427, 427t, 431, 440, 441t
    of penis, 116, 254, 264, 267
  ductus deferens, 117, 216, 224, 225, 225t, 226
  epigastric
    inferior, 101, 103, 108, 109, 111, 112, 118, 136, 144, 208, 215, 218, 219, 224, 226, 232, 242, 362
    superficial, 101, 102, 370
    superior, 101, 103
  esophageal, 65
  ethmoidal
    anterior, 657t, 693
    posterior, 657t, 693
  facial, 626, 627, 632, 632t, 662, 666, 667, 693, 721, 762–765, 765t, 766, 778, 780, 782, 796
    groove, 664
    transverse, 626, 627, 632, 632t, 662
  femoral, 101, 109, 117, 118, 213, 222, 241, 250, 275, 277, 362, 370–373, 382, 399, 400, 440, 470
  fibular, 362, 424, 427, 436, 437, 440, 441t
  gastric
    left, 75, 122, 126, 127, 129–131, 133–135, 154, 155, 162
    posterior, 130, 135
    right, 127, 129–131, 135, 154, 155
    short, 129–131, 135
  gastro-omental
    left, 124–127, 129–131, 135
    right, 124, 126, 127, 129–131, 134, 135
  gastroduodenal, 130, 131, 133–135, 153–155, 174
  genicular
    descending, 362, 416
    inferior lateral, 362, 404, 416, 417
    inferior medial, 362, 404, 416, 417
    lateral superior, 409
    medial inferior, 408, 435, 440
    medial superior, 408, 440
    middle, 416
    superior lateral, 362, 404, 416, 417
    superior medial, 362, 404, 416, 417
  gluteal
    inferior, 212, 224, 225, 225t, 226, 242, 250, 277, 362, 393t
    superior, 212, 224, 225, 225t, 226, 242, 277, 351, 362, 393t

  gonadal, 165
  hepatic, 124, 131, 147, 149–151, 154, 186
    aberrant, 153, 155
    accessory, 154
    common, 123, 126, 127, 130, 131, 135, 153–155, 174, 186
    proper, 122, 123, 130, 131, 133–135, 154, 155, 158, 174
    variations, 158
  ileal, 141, 145
  ileocolic, 134, 139–141, 144, 145
  iliac
    common, 117, 142, 163, 165, 175, 188, 213, 215, 216, 224, 225, 225t, 226, 240–242, 277, 362
    external, 101, 109, 111, 163, 175, 202, 212, 213, 215, 216, 218, 224, 225, 225t, 226, 240–242, 277, 362, 400
    internal, 163, 165, 175, 202, 212, 213, 215, 216, 224, 225, 225t, 226, 240–242, 243t, 277, 351, 362
  iliolumbar, 224, 225, 225t, 242, 243t
  indicis
    dorsalis, 576, 577, 584, 606
    radialis, 561, 566, 570, 573, 573t, 577
  infraorbital, 657t, 668, 670, 719, 720
  intercostal, 341
    anterior, 20, 22, 23
    posterior, 17, 20, 75, 80–83, 101, 339, 341
    supreme, 72, 75, 81
  interosseous
    anterior, 486, 487, 550, 550t, 551, 557, 573, 576, 602
    common, 486, 487, 550, 550t, 551
    posterior, 338–340, 487, 550, 550t, 551, 573, 577, 602, 634, 636
    posterior recurrent, 577
    recurrent, 487, 543, 550, 550t
  interventricular, 66
    anterior, 46, 47, 52
    posterior, 47
  jejunal, 135, 141, 145
  labial
    anterior, 241
    inferior, 632, 632t
    posterior, 241
    superior, 632, 632t
  lacrimal, 657t
  laryngeal, inferior, 807
  of ligament of head of femur, 401
  lingual, 667, 680, 681, 763–765, 765t, 766, 781, 782
  lumbar, 175, 341
  malleolar
    lateral, 362, 425, 427
    medial, 362, 425, 427
  marginal, 140–143
    left, 46
    right, 46, 55
  maxillary, 384, 668–670, 681, 720, 764, 765, 765t

  medullary
    anterior segmental, 341
    posterior segmental, 341, 342
  meningeal, middle, 618, 635, 637, 640, 670, 712
  mental, 632, 632t
  mesenteric
    inferior, 122, 133, 142–145, 163, 174, 175, 213, 215, 241
    superior, 78, 82, 120, 122, 126, 127, 133–135, 140–142, 145, 153–156, 162, 163, 174, 175, 187–191
  metacarpal
    dorsal, 569, 573, 576
    palmar, 487, 570, 572, 573
  metatarsal
    dorsal, 362, 425
    perforating branches, 425
    plantar, 362, 444, 446
  musculophrenic, 101
  nasal
    dorsal, 657t
    lateral, 632, 632t
    posterior lateral, 693
  obturator, 118, 212, 224, 225, 225t, 242, 243t, 250, 277, 362, 396, 399, 401
    anomalous, 226
  occipital, 330, 331, 333, 632, 632t, 721, 762–764, 764t, 765, 785
  ophthalmic, 648, 654, 657, 657t
  ovarian, 233–235, 241, 243t
  palatine
    ascending, 693, 712
    greater, 683, 693
    lesser, 683
  pancreatic
    dorsal, 135
    greater, 134, 135
    inferior, 135
  pancreaticoduodenal
    anterior inferior, 134, 135
    anterior superior, 134, 135, 145
    posterior inferior, 134, 135, 153
    posterior superior, 134, 135, 153
    superior, 130
  perforating, 362, 372, 393t, 427, 446, 576
  pericardiacophrenic, 80
  perineal, 202, 241
  phrenic
    inferior, 75, 163, 175
    left inferior, 165
    superior, 75
  plantar
    deep, 362, 427, 427t, 446
    lateral, 362, 438, 440, 441t, 443, 446, 456
    medial, 362, 438, 440, 441t, 443, 444, 446, 456
  pollicis
    dorsalis, 572, 573, 576, 577
    princeps, 561, 572, 573, 573t, 606
  pontine, 647, 647t
  popliteal, 362, 402, 404, 416, 419, 420, 437, 440, 441t
  pudendal
    external, 102, 241, 269, 362, 370
    internal, 212, 213, 218, 222, 224, 225, 225t, 226, 241, 242, 243t, 250, 274, 277, 393t

pulmonary, 27, 29, 34, 35, 68
　3-D volume reconstruction and
　　CT angiogram, 41, 92–93
　left, 26, 27, 33, 41, 46, 47, 49,
　　52, 67, 68, 88–90
　relationship to bronchi, 41
　right, 33, 41, 46, 47, 68, 88–89,
　　91
radial, 486, 487, 540, 550, 550t,
　551, 554, 558, 559, 561,
　566, 570–573, 576, 577,
　584, 585, 591, 602, 604,
　605
　dorsal branch, 582
　dorsal carpal branch, 576
　palmar branch, 572
　palmar carpal branch, 570
　recurrent, 486, 487, 540, 550,
　　550t, 551
　superficial palmar branch, 566,
　　570
radicular
　anterior, 341, 342
　posterior, 341, 342
rectal
　inferior, 202, 213, 241
　middle, 212, 213, 224, 225,
　　225t, 226, 241, 242, 243t
　superior, 142, 143, 213, 241
renal, 164, 166, 167
　accessory, 164
　left, 165, 174, 175, 188
　right, 153, 174, 187–189
　of round ligament, 110
sacral
　lateral, 212, 224, 225, 225t, 241,
　　242, 243t, 277, 341
　median, 175, 241
　middle, 277
saphenous, 382
scapular, dorsal, 486, 487, 529,
　772, 773
scrotal, posterior, 261
sigmoid, 142, 143, 145
sphenopalatine, 670, 693
spinal
　anterior, 341, 342
　posterior, 341, 342
splenic, 122, 123, 125–127, 130,
　131, 133–135, 154, 155,
　164, 174, 187–189
striate, anterolateral, 731
stylomastoid, 712
subclavian, 8, 23, 71, 72, 80, 511,
　529, 757, 772, 773
　left, 46, 47, 49, 66–68, 70, 71,
　　74, 81, 88–89, 91, 773
　right, 25, 26, 66–68, 70, 71, 74,
　　84, 88–89, 486
subcostal, 75, 101, 163
submental, 763, 778
subscapular, 486, 487, 504, 505t,
　509
sulcal, 342
supraduodenal, 130, 134
supraorbital, 632, 632t, 657t
suprarenal, 165, 167, 175
suprascapular, 486, 487, 504, 505t,
　528, 529, 531, 537, 772,
　773
supratrochlear, 632, 632t,
　657t
tarsal
　lateral, 362, 425, 427, 427t
　medial, 362, 427

temporal
　deep, 668, 670
　superficial, 626, 627, 632, 632t,
　　662, 720, 721, 764, 765,
　　765t
testicular, 113, 116, 117, 145, 152,
　153, 162, 163, 215, 216,
　225t, 226, 264
thoracic, 175
　internal, 8, 20, 22, 23, 48, 66,
　　67, 70, 72–74, 80, 81,
　　88–89, 486, 504, 505t, 529,
　　764, 765, 765t, 773
　lateral, 8, 486, 502, 504, 505t,
　　509
　superior, 509
　supreme, 504, 505t
thoraco-acromial, 486, 500, 504,
　505t, 508, 531
thoracodorsal, 487, 502, 504, 505t
thyroid
　inferior, 75, 770–773, 807
　superficial, 770, 771
　superior, 762–765, 765t, 766,
　　807
thyroid ima, 749, 771
tibial
　anterior, 362, 424, 425, 427,
　　437, 440, 441t, 457, 472
　anterior recurrent, 362, 417,
　　425
　posterior, 362, 436–438, 440,
　　441t, 443, 446, 451, 457,
　　458, 472
tympanic, anterior, 670
ulnar, 486, 487, 540, 550, 550t,
　551, 555, 556, 558, 559,
　566, 567, 570, 572, 573,
　602, 604, 605
　anterior recurrent, 550, 550t
　deep branch, 567, 570, 572, 591
　deep palmar branch, 572
　dorsal carpal branch, 487, 566,
　　573, 576, 587
　posterior recurrent, 542, 543,
　　550, 550t
　superficial, 541
　superior collateral, 486, 487,
　　504, 505t, 525, 539, 550
ulnar collateral, 521, 600
　inferior, 486, 487, 504, 505t,
　　525, 539, 540, 550, 551
ulnar recurrent, 551
　anterior, 486, 487
　posterior, 486, 487
umbilical, 118, 144, 225, 225t, 241,
　242, 243t
uterine, 212, 234, 235, 240–242,
　243t
vaginal, 234, 235, 241, 242, 243t
vertebral, 74, 88–89, 297–299, 333,
　335, 338, 341, 350, 352,
　486, 529, 638, 640, 642,
　646, 647, 647t, 648, 720,
　721, 738–740, 764, 765,
　765t, 773, 785, 806, 807
vesical, 277
　inferior, 216, 226
　superior, 224, 225, 225t, 226,
　　241, 242, 243t
　of vestibule of vagina, 241
Asterion, 612
Atlas, 294–297, 350, 621, 720, 721,
　743, 751, 808
　anterior arch, 296, 297, 350, 750,

　810
　anterior tubercle, 742
　posterior arch, 296, 297, 318, 331,
　　350, 750
Atrioventricular bundle, 55, 61, 64
Atrium, 694
　left, 29, 47, 53, 58, 60, 64
　　3-D volume reconstruction and
　　　CT angiogram, 41, 92–93
　　interior, 57
　　magnetic resonance imaging,
　　　88–91
　　radiograph, 27
　right, 26, 27, 29, 46, 47, 49, 50, 53,
　　57, 60, 64, 84
　　3-D volume reconstruction and
　　　CT angiogram, 92–93
　　computed tomography, 6
　　interior, 56
　　magnetic resonance imaging,
　　　88–91
Auricle, 721
　of ear, 703, 704
　left, 27, 46, 47, 49, 58, 60, 90
　right, 46, 49, 60
Auscultation
　of heart, 44
　triangle of, 512, 514
Autonomic nervous system, 177, 346
Axilla, 497, 525
　anterior wall, 500
　contents, 502
　medial wall, 509
　posterior wall, 509, 510
　structures, 508
　veins, 501
　walls, 502
Axis, 294–297, 333, 743, 751, 785, 808

Back
　cutaneous nerves, 514
　muscles, 321–329
　　cervical, 783, 783t
　　deep, 123, 171, 186, 189, 323,
　　　325, 329t
　　intermediate, 322, 329t
　　magnetic resonance imaging,
　　　88–89
　　superficial, 321, 329t, 513t
　　transverse section, 324
　surface anatomy, 320, 512
Band
　central, 569, 583
　fascial, 807
　lateral, 569, 583
　spiral, 561
Bare area, 120, 122, 146, 147
Barium enema, 138
Barium swallow, 132
Basioccipital bone, 297
Bile duct, 122–124, 133, 134, 147,
　149–159
Bladder, 96, 97, 118, 120–122, 128,
　136, 165, 205, 208–210,
　215, 276–283, 311, 470
　female, 232, 233, 250
　male, 216–222
　trigone, 217, 221, 234
　uvula, 221
Body
　anococcygeal, 208, 232, 261, 262,
　　273, 275
　ciliary, 661, 738, 739
　erectile, 255, 266
　geniculate

　lateral, 734, 735
　medial, 734, 735
　mamillary, 639, 728, 729, 732–734,
　　742
　perineal, 210, 253, 261–263, 273,
　　276, 277
　pineal, 723, 742
　restiform, 734
　vertebral, 14–16, 72, 78, 88–90, 123,
　　288, 289, 301, 302, 310,
　　337, 743, 806–808, 810
　vitreous, 660, 721, 738, 739
Brain
　arterial supply, 647, 647t
　coronal sections, 741
　lobes, 722
　　frontal, 719, 722, 725, 726, 732,
　　　733
　　occipital, 722, 725, 726, 728,
　　　732, 733, 738, 739
　　parietal, 722, 725, 726
　　temporal, 722, 725, 726,
　　　738–740
　magnetic resonance imaging,
　　732–733, 738–740, 742
　median section, 743
　overview, 722–724
Brainstem, 722, 723, 734–735
Breast
　anatomy, 4, 5
　anterior view, 5
　arterial supply, 8
　axillary process (tail), 4
　bed of, 7
　imaging of, 6
　lymphatic drainage, 9
　sagittal view, 5
　suspensory ligaments, 4–6
Bregma, 614
Bronchial tree, innervation, 84
Bronchogram, of tracheobronchial
　tree, 39–40
Bronchopulmonary segments, 36–37
Bronchus, 33, 71, 80, 81
　anterior basal segmental, 40
　anterior medial basal segmental, 40
　anterior segmental, 40, 41
　apical segmental, 39, 41
　apicoposterior segmental, 39, 40
　inferior lobar
　　left, 38, 39, 41, 74
　　right, 39, 41
　intermediate, 38–40, 74
　intrapulmonary, 69
　left, 33, 36–38
　lingular segmental
　　inferior, 41
　　superior, 41
　lower lobar, right, 38
　main
　　left, 28, 33, 35, 38, 41, 69, 74,
　　　84
　　right, 28, 33, 34, 38, 69, 74, 84,
　　　91
　middle lobar, 41
　　left, 38
　　right, 39
　relationship to pulmonary arteries,
　　41
　right, 33, 36–38, 808
　segmental, 36–38, 40, 41
　superior lobar
　　left, 38, 39, 41, 74
　　right, 38, 39, 41, 74
　superior segmental, 40

Bulb
of duodenum, 189
of internal jugular vein, 767
olfactory, 639, 719, 726, 818, 844
of penis, 209, 216, 217, 262, 266–268, 276, 277, 279
of vestibule, 272, 274
Bulla, ethmoidal, 695
Bundle, atrioventricular, 55, 61, 64
Bundle branch
left, 64
right, 64
Bursa
anserine, 415t
calcaneal, 438, 454, 457
gastrocnemius, medial semitendinous, 415, 415t
iliopectineal, 373
infrapatellar
deep, 415t, 421
subcutaneous, 415t, 421
obturator internus, 395, 399
olecranon, 544, 549
omental, 120, 121, 123–127, 162
popliteus, 415, 415t
prepatellar, subcutaneous, 410, 415t, 421
retromammary, 5
semimembranosus, 415, 415t
subacromial, 531, 534, 536, 537
subdeltoid, 503
subtendinous, 503, 532, 534, 537, 544, 574, 584
suprapatellar, 414, 415t, 420, 421

Calcaneus, 354, 430, 431, 437, 439, 442, 444, 448, 450, 452–454, 456, 458, 459, 461, 464–466
Calcarine spur, 727
Calices, renal, 165–167
Calvaria, 615, 636
Canal
adductor, 373
anal, 208, 210–212, 214, 232, 261, 268, 275
carotid, 616, 625, 645, 713
central, 723, 724
cervical, 238
condylar, 615
femoral, 371
gastric, 129
hypoglossal, 615, 619, 639
infraorbital, 650
inguinal, 103, 217
dissection, 112
structures forming, 108t
nasolacrimal, 695
obturator, 372
optic, 618, 619, 624, 639, 650
palatine, greater, 720
pterygoid, 617, 624, 702
nerve of, 701, 831
pudendal, 219, 261
pyloric, 124, 129
sacral, 197, 198, 202, 313, 316, 317
semicircular, 704, 709, 714, 738, 739, 832
vertebral, 296, 303
Canaliculus
bile, 151
cochlear, 625
lacrimal, 651
tympanic, 625
vestibular, 625

Canine teeth, 685, 688, 689t
Canthus, lateral, 651
Capillaries, lymphatic, 77
Capitate, 552, 574, 588, 589, 591, 593, 594, 599, 604, 605
Capitulum, 518, 544, 547, 549, 552, 598
Capsule
external, 726, 731–733, 741
extreme, 731–733, 741
internal, 727, 729–733, 740, 741
joint, 12
acromioclavicular, 535
glenohumeral (shoulder), 532, 533
hip, 390, 391, 398
knee, 410, 420, 421
temporomandibular, 674, 675
zygapophysial, 304, 305
renal, 171
synovial, 548
Caput medusae, 161
Cardiac cycle, 62
Carina, 38
Carpal bones, 476–479, 588, 589, 594, 599
Carpal tunnel, 493, 592, 593, 604, 605
Carpal tunnel syndrome, 567
Cartilage
articular, 410, 785
arytenoid, 798, 799, 807, 810
auricular, 703, 704
costal, 3, 10, 12, 22, 24, 48, 102, 103, 123, 124, 186, 499
cricoid, 749, 750, 788–790, 798, 799, 806, 808, 810
epiglottic, 799
nasal, 690
alar, 690, 691
septal, 690, 691
thyroid, 716, 743, 749, 750, 779, 788, 789, 798, 799, 806–808
triradiate, 397
vomeronasal, 691
Caruncle
hymenal, 253
lacrimal, 650, 651
sublingual, 782
Cauda equina, 334, 337, 351
Cave, trigeminal, 644
Cavity
abdominal, posterior, 144, 145
amniotic, 238
articular, 674, 675
glenoid, 533–535, 537
nasal, 28, 611, 691–693, 695–697
oral, 128, 697, 718–720, 792
orbital, 608, 611, 650–653
pericardial, 29, 53, 808
peritoneal, 121, 122
pleural, 28, 29, 72, 808
of temporomandibular joint, 674
tympanic, 705, 708, 710–713
Cecum, 96, 97, 122, 128, 136, 138–140, 144, 145, 160
Celiac arteriogram, 131
Cells
ethmoidal air, 621, 653, 695–698, 719, 721
hair, cochlear, 715
mastoid, 621, 711, 738, 739
Cerebellum, 639, 722, 723, 736–740, 742, 743, 808, 810

tonsil of, 736, 740, 808, 810
Cerebral hemispheres, 722, 723
Cerebrospinal fluid, 286, 352, 724, 738, 739, 806, 810
Cervical regions
anterior, 752, 752t, 753
lateral, 752, 752t, 753, 754–757
posterior, 783, 785
Cervix, 208, 232, 250
Chamber
anterior, 660, 721
posterior, 660
Chiasm, optic, 639, 721, 728, 734, 738, 739, 819, 820
Choana, 616, 790
Cholangiography, endoscopic retrograde, 156, 159
Chorda tympani, 681, 708, 711, 797, 831
Choroid, 660, 661
Cingulum, 728
Circle, cerebral arterial, 646, 649
Cistern
cerebral, 732, 733
chyle, 74, 76, 83, 117
collicular, 732, 733
interpeduncular, 738–740, 763
lumbar, 337
supracerebellar, 740
suprasellar, 738, 739
Claustrum, 726, 731–733, 741
Clavicle, 2–4, 8, 10–12, 24, 27, 39, 80, 96, 296, 476, 478, 479, 492, 494, 495, 498, 503, 511, 518, 519, 529–532, 535–537, 598, 763, 772
Cleft
gluteal, 261
intergluteal, 320
pudendal, 110
Clitoris, 273
angle of, 272
body, 255, 272
crus, 234, 272, 274, 275
deep artery, 241
dorsal artery, 241, 254, 272, 274
dorsal nerve, 254, 269, 270, 272, 274
frenulum, 271
glans, 253, 269, 271, 272
prepuce, 253, 269, 271, 274
suspensory ligament, 271
Clivus, 615, 619
Coccyx, 194–198, 202, 208–210, 216, 222, 232, 262, 273, 279, 312, 313
overview, 286, 288
tip, 263
Cochlea, 704, 714, 715, 832
Colliculus, 738, 739, 742
facial, 735, 738, 739
inferior, 734, 735
seminal, 221
superior, 730, 731, 734, 735, 816
Colon, 161
ascending, 96, 97, 119, 122, 128, 133, 136, 138, 140, 141, 143–145, 148, 160, 162, 186, 188
barium enema, 138
descending, 96, 97, 119, 122, 128, 133, 136–138, 142–145, 148, 160, 162, 163, 186, 188, 189

haustrum of, 139
sigmoid, 128, 137, 138, 142, 144, 145, 160, 163, 215, 233, 282
transverse, 96, 119, 121, 122, 124–126, 128, 136–138, 140–142, 145, 152, 187, 189
Commissure
anterior, 723, 727–729, 732–734, 740
habenular, 732, 733, 735
posterior, 728, 730, 741
Compartment(s)
adductor, 562
of arm, 521, 600
central, 562
infracolic, 122
of leg, 369
perineal, 254–255, 258, 259
supracolic, 122
thenar, 562
of thigh, 369
Compressor urethrae, 256t, 257, 260
Computed tomography
breast, 6
cervical vertebrae, 296, 350
cranium, 697
intervertebral disc, 305
lumbar vertebrae, 351
sacroiliac joint, 317, 351
Computed tomography angiogram
head and neck, 649
thorax, 41, 92–93
Concha, 705
inferior, 611, 690, 691, 694, 695, 700, 702, 719, 720, 738, 739, 810
inferior nasal, 794
middle, 690, 691, 694, 719, 720, 738, 739
superior, 691, 694, 719, 738, 739
Condyle
femoral, 419
lateral, 380, 381, 418
medial, 380, 381
lateral, 413
medial, 413
occipital, 614–617, 785
tibial
lateral, 380, 381, 418
medial, 380, 381, 418
Conjunctiva
bulbar, 650, 651
palpebral, 650
Conus arteriosus, 57
Conus elasticus, 799
Conus medullaris, 334, 337
Cornea, 660, 661, 721
Corona radiata, 725, 726
Coronary circulation, 55
Corpus callosum, 723, 728–730, 740–743
Cortex
cerebral, 634, 636
insular, 732, 733, 740, 742
renal, 166
visual, 820
Costovertebral articulations, 14
Cranial nerves
abducent (CN VI), 640, 644, 645, 652, 654, 656, 812–814, 815t, 821, 822, 822t, 823, 841, 841t, 843

facial (CN VII), 640–642, 663, 701, 708–713, 720, 734, 738, 739, 762, 812–814, 815t, 830, 831, 841, 841t, 843
  branches, 627, 629, 634, 662
  motor root, 830
glossopharyngeal (CN IX), 335, 640–642, 663, 680, 681, 720, 734, 766, 785–787, 789, 796, 812–814, 815t, 834–835, 841, 843
hypoglossal (CN XII), 335, 640, 641, 662, 663, 667, 680, 681, 720, 763, 766, 779, 780, 785, 786, 812–814, 815t, 839, 841, 841t, 843
lesions, 841, 841t
magnetic resonance imaging, 842–844
nuclei, 816–817
oculomotor (CN III), 640, 641, 643–645, 652, 654, 656, 734, 812–814, 815t, 821, 822, 822t, 823, 841, 841t, 842, 844
olfactory (CN I), 640, 692, 812–814, 815t, 818, 841
optic (CN II), 640, 641, 652, 653, 655–657, 660, 719, 727, 728, 732–734, 738, 739, 812–814, 815t, 819, 820, 841, 842
overview, 812–814
posterior exposures, 642
spinal accessory (CN XI), 333, 334, 511, 529, 642, 662, 663, 667, 720, 755, 762, 763, 766, 785, 807, 812–814, 815t, 838, 841, 841t, 843
summary, 815t
superficial origins, 641
trigeminal (CN V), 631, 631t, 640–643, 812–814, 815t, 824, 841, 842, 844
  cutaneous branches, 630
  groove for, 615
  mandibular division, 824t, 828–829
  maxillary division, 824t, 826–827
  motor root, 645, 646, 734
  ophthalmic division, 824t, 825
  sensory root, 644–646, 734
  spinal tract, 734
trochlear (CN IV), 640–645, 652, 656, 812–814, 815t, 821, 822, 822t, 823, 841
vagus (CN X), 181, 640–642, 662, 663, 667, 720, 766, 771, 772, 785, 807, 812–814, 815t, 836–837, 841, 843
  in abdomen, 181
  auricular branch, 703
  inferior cardiac branch, 772
  left, 25, 42, 48, 49, 65, 67–69, 81, 84, 85, 773, 836
  right, 25, 42, 48, 67, 68, 72, 80, 84, 85, 773, 836
vestibulocochlear (CN VIII), 640–642, 709, 715, 734, 735, 738, 739, 812–814, 815t, 832–833, 841, 843
Cranium
  base, interior, 618–619
  of child, 608–609
  computed tomography, 697
  facial (frontal) aspect, 610–611
  inferior aspect, 616–617
  lateral aspect, 612–613
  posterior view, 614–615
  radiograph, 608, 609, 620–621, 697, 698
  superior view, 614
Crest
  frontal, 619
  iliac, 104, 169, 194–198, 200, 311, 312, 354, 368, 380, 381, 390, 391, 397
  infratemporal, 665
  intertrochanteric, 381, 398
  lacrimal, 613, 650
  medial, 442
  obturator, 396
  occipital
    external, 614, 615
    internal, 619
  pronator, 552
  pubic, 106, 199, 380
  sacral, 312, 313
    median, 194, 195
  supinator, 544
  supramastoid, 613, 625
  supraventricular, 57
  urethral, 221
Crista galli, 618–620, 638, 697, 719
Crural region, 354
Crus
  cerebral, 727, 729, 734, 735, 738, 739, 741
  of clitoris, 234, 272, 274, 275
  of diaphragm, 26, 74, 82, 85, 123, 172, 174, 186, 187, 352
  lateral, 102, 106, 107, 110, 372
  medial, 102, 106, 107, 110
  of penis, 262, 266, 267, 276, 277
Cubital tunnel, 465, 542, 543
Cuboid, 427, 431, 444, 449, 453, 454, 458, 459, 461, 464, 466
Cuneiform, 453, 459, 462
  first, 452, 465
  lateral, 427, 431, 444, 449, 454, 458
  medial, 427, 444, 449, 452, 458, 464
  middle, 427, 431, 444, 452, 454
Cuneus, 728
Cusp
  anterior, 63
  commissural, 63
  left, 60
  posterior, 63
  septal, 63

Decussation, ventral tegmental, 741
Dens, 296, 297, 299, 350, 352, 742, 810
  of atlas, 750
  of axis, 720, 721, 743, 808
Dermatomes, 348
  of abdomen, 99
  across bed of breast, 7
  of lower limb, 360, 361
  map, 348
  of upper limb, 483
Diaphragm, 23–26, 28, 29, 40, 49, 73–76, 78, 80–83, 85, 118–124, 129, 132, 133, 147, 149, 163, 164, 172–174, 186, 189
  central tendon, 24, 29, 73, 174
  crura, 26, 74, 82, 85, 123, 172, 174, 186, 187, 352
  left dome, 27, 48, 90, 125, 188
  lymphatic drainage, 87
  magnetic resonance imaging, 90
  muscular part, 73
  pelvic, 203, 254, 258, 259, 263
  right dome, 27, 39, 48, 90, 96, 97, 125, 188
  sellar, 643
  surface markings, 45
  vertebral attachment, 24, 172
Diaphragma sellae, 638, 740
Diastole, 62
Diencephalon, 723, 725–734
Digestive system, 128
Disc
  articular, 12, 590, 591
    radiocarpal joint, 592
    sternoclavicular joint, 530
    temporomandibular joint, 674, 675, 785
  intervertebral, 286, 297, 300, 352, 810
    computed tomography, 305
    innervation, 304
    ligaments, 306, 307
    lumbar, 145, 324
    movements, 307
  optic, 660, 661
Diverticulum, ileal, 138, 139
Doppler ultrasound, internal carotid artery, 809
Dorsum sellae, 615, 618, 619, 624, 702, 738, 739
Duct
  bile, 122–124, 133, 134, 147, 149–157, 159
  cochlear, 714, 715, 833
  collecting, 167
  cystic, 123, 152–156, 159, 186
  ejaculatory, 216, 217, 220
  hepatic, 154, 155, 159
    accessory, 159
    common, 123, 152–154, 156, 158, 159, 186
    radiograph, 158
    variations, 159
  lactiferous, 4–6
  lymphatic
    overview, 77
    right, 9, 43, 76, 716, 805
  nasolacrimal, 651, 695, 720
  pancreatic
    accessory, 133, 156, 157
    development, 157
    main, 133, 156, 157
  papillary, 167
  parotid, 627, 630, 662, 666, 668
  semicircular, 714, 715
  submandibular, 681, 779, 780
  thoracic, 29, 69, 73–76, 79, 81–83, 117, 119, 123, 339, 716, 773, 805
  vestibular, greater, 272, 274
Ductules
  efferent, 217
  prostatic, 220
Ductus deferens, 113, 116–118, 163, 210, 215–220, 222, 226, 264
  ampulla, 216, 217, 220
Ductus reuniens, 714
Duodenal cap, 132
Duodenum, 96, 120–122, 126, 128, 129, 131, 135, 142, 144, 152–155, 158, 159, 162, 188, 189
  ascending part, 133t, 156
  blood supply, 135
  bulb of, 189
  descending part, 133t, 145, 156, 157, 186
  inferior part, 133t, 145, 156, 186
  parts, 133, 133t
  radiograph, 132
  relationships, 134
  superior part, 133t, 156
Dura mater, 297, 335, 336, 338–340, 634, 636, 637–639

Ear
  auricle of, 703, 704
  external, 704, 705
  inner, 704, 705, 709
  middle, 704, 705, 709
  ossicles, 704, 707
  pharyngotympanic tube, 28, 615, 681, 695, 704, 705, 710–713, 720, 785, 790, 794
  semicircular canals, 704, 709, 714, 738, 739, 832
  tympanic cavity, 705, 708, 710–713
Ejaculatory duct, 216, 217, 220
Eminence
  arcuate, 619, 625
  frontal, 608, 609, 611, 613
  iliopubic, 197, 198, 312, 372, 380
  intercondylar, 418
  parietal, 608, 609, 613, 614
  thenar, 586
Endocardium, 53
Endometrium, 279, 282, 283
Endoscopic retrograde cholangiography and pancreatography, 156, 159
Epicardium, 53
Epicondyle
  lateral, 380, 418, 518, 519, 523, 524, 542, 544, 547, 548, 552, 574
  medial, 380, 491, 518, 519, 521, 523, 527, 538, 539, 542–544, 546, 548, 552, 574, 598, 600
Epididymis, 112, 113, 116, 117, 216, 217, 264
Epiglottis, 28, 743, 790, 791, 798, 799, 804, 807, 808, 810
Epiphyseal sites, upper limb, 598–599
Esophageal varices, 161
Esophagus, 29, 43, 65–67, 69, 71, 72, 74, 76, 80–82, 84, 85, 119, 122, 124, 127, 129, 161, 162, 174, 186, 188, 771, 773, 807, 808, 810
  3-D volume reconstruction and CT angiogram, 92–93
  abdominal, 128
  arterial supply, 75
  computed tomography, 6
  lymphatic drainage, 87
  magnetic resonance imaging, 88–89
  radiograph, 132
  thoracic, 128

Ethmoid bone, 610, 611, 613, 619, 623, 650, 690, 691, 695, 700
Expansion, extensor, 426, 427, 569, 574, 581–583, 585
Eye, surface anatomy, 650, 651
Eyeball, 653, 660, 661, 697, 719, 738, 739
Eyelid, 629, 650, 651, 654–655

Fabella, 420, 467
Facet
  articular, 442
    inferior, 300, 350
    superior, 14, 297, 300, 303, 338
  costal, 300
    superior, 14
    transverse, 14
  patellar, 411
  talar, 458
Falx cerebelli, 638, 639, 743, 808
Falx cerebri, 636, 638, 639, 732, 733, 743
Fascia
  abdominal, parietal, 219
  alar, 747
  antebrachial, 493, 542, 549, 602
  axillary, 492
  brachial, 492, 493, 539
  buccopharyngeal, 747
  cervical, 747
    deep, 492
    prevertebral layer, 763
  clavipectoral, 492, 500
  cribriform, 368
  crural, 368
  dartos, 113
  deep, 368, 369, 424, 436, 438
  deltoid, 493
  dorsal, 562
  endoabdominal, 219
  endopelvic, 248, 251, 279
  endothoracic, 72, 129
  extraperitoneal, 218
  gluteal, 383
  hypothenar, 560, 562, 563
  investing, 105, 171, 747
  lower limb, 368
  lumbar, 171
  obturator, 202–204, 212, 219, 258, 259, 262, 399
  omohyoid, 756, 763
  palmar, 560, 562
  pectineal, 373
  pectoral, 3, 4, 492–494
  pelvic
    diaphragmatic, 258, 259
    parietal, 219
      tendinous arch, 219
    visceral, 219, 220
  penile, 258, 265
  perineal, 258, 259
  pharyngobasilar, 786, 795
  plantar, 443
  popliteal, 405, 408, 409, 436
  pretracheal, 747, 769
  prevertebral, 678, 747, 769, 772, 774
  psoas, 163, 171, 202, 218, 310
  rectal, 259
  rectovesical, 209
  renal, 164, 171
  scrotal, 258
  spermatic, 108, 112, 113, 116, 264
  temporal, 634, 666
  thenar, 560, 562, 563
  thoracolumbar, 169, 171, 321, 324, 326, 512, 514
  umbilical, 251
  upper limb, 492, 493
  vesical, 251, 259
  visceral, 258
Fascia lata, 106, 112, 271, 274, 368, 470
  tensor, 250, 275, 368, 373, 375, 376, 377t, 381, 383, 385, 386t, 399, 470
Fascia transversalis, 101, 103, 105, 109, 111, 112, 118, 171
Fasciculus
  inferior fronto-occipital, 726
  lenticular, 741
  mammillothalamic, 729, 741
  superior longitudinal, 725
  uncinate, 726
Fasciculus cuneatus, 735
Fasciculus gracilis, 735, 816
Fat, 4, 453
  axillary, 536
  breast, 5
  encapsulated cushions, 456
  epidural, 286, 339
  extraperitoneal, 105, 109
  parapharyngeal, 738, 739
  perinephric, 171, 187
  perirenal, 152, 164, 171
  in popliteal fossa, 419–421
  prefemoral, 420
  renal, 123
  retrobulbar, 655, 721
  retroperitoneal, 187
  retropubic, 208, 232, 279
  subendocardial, 53
  subpericardial, 57
  subperitoneal, 164
  suprapatellar, 420
Fat body, ischioanal, 274
Fat pad, 73, 80, 81, 110, 111, 209, 443
  buccal, 630, 720, 806
  infrapatellar, 410, 420, 421
  synovial, 548
Fauces, isthmus of, 792–797
Femoral region, 354
Femur, 104, 200, 201, 275, 354, 355, 380, 381, 404, 418–420, 470, 471
  condyle, 419
    lateral, 380, 381, 418
    medial, 380, 381
  distal, 411
  head, 200, 222, 373, 380, 394, 399, 400, 470
    blood supply, 401
    ligament of, 222, 396, 399, 401
  neck, 250, 311, 381, 395, 400
  shaft, 400
Fetus, radiograph, 239
Fibers
  afferent, visceral, 246, 346
  efferent, visceral, 346
  intercrural, 102, 106, 110
  motor, somatic, 357
  parasympathetic, 230, 346, 717
  sympathetic, 230, 246, 346, 347, 717
Fibula, 354, 355, 380, 381, 420, 423, 429, 433, 436, 442, 448, 450, 453, 454, 472–473
  apex, 420
  head, 383, 406, 407, 419, 425, 433, 442, 472
  neck, 418, 425, 433
Filum terminale, 334, 336, 337
Finger pad, 588
Fissure
  calcarine, 731
  cerebral, 722
  horizontal, 25, 32, 34, 35
  lateral, 731–733, 740
  longitudinal, 740
  lung, 32, 96, 97
  oblique, 25, 32, 34, 35
  orbital
    inferior, 650
    superior, 615, 619, 624, 639, 650, 702
  parieto-occipital, 742
  petrotympanic, 625
Flexure
  left colic (splenic), 119, 122, 138, 187, 352
  right colic (hepatic), 119, 122, 126, 136, 138, 144
Flocculus, 736, 738, 739
Floor of mouth, 679, 681
Fold
  aryepiglottic, 790, 804
  axillary
    anterior, 2, 495, 497, 525
    posterior, 2, 495, 497, 512, 525
  conjunctival, semilunar, 650
  gastric, 132
  gastropancreatic, 126
  glossoepiglottic, lateral, 790
  gluteal, 195
  ileocecal, inferior, 139
  inguinal, 194, 195
  rectal, 213
    inferior transverse, 211
  rectouterine, 208, 232, 233, 280, 281
  sacrogenital, 215
  salpingopharyngeal, 790
  semilunar, 137
  sublingual, 681
  synovial, 454, 548, 549, 592, 593
    infrapatellar, 410
  umbilical
    lateral, 118, 219, 233
    medial, 218, 219, 226
    median, 118, 219
  vascular, of cecum, 139
  vesical, transverse, 233
  vestibular, 801, 804, 807
  vocal, 743, 801, 804, 806, 808
Follicle, 282, 283
  lingual, 794
Fontanelle
  anterior, 608, 609
  anterolateral, 608
  posterior, 609
  posterolateral, 608
Foot, 354
  arches, 466
  arteries, 441t
  dorsum, 426, 427, 427t, 449
  joints, 460t
  lateral aspect, 428, 429
  ligaments, 449, 464, 465
  medial, 439
  muscles, 428, 429, 444–447, 444t–447t
  postnatal development, 469
  radiograph, 453
  sole, 443–447, 464, 465
Foramen
  cribriform, 639
  ethmoidal
    anterior, 619, 650
    posterior, 619, 650
  incisive, 615
  infraorbital, 611, 612, 650
  interventricular, 724, 728–733
  intervertebral, 286, 302, 304, 339
  jugular, 615–617, 619, 639, 710
  lacrimal, 650
  mental, 611, 613, 664
  obturator, 196–199, 311, 312, 380
  omental, 120, 123, 124, 153, 162
  palatine, 682
    greater, 615
    lesser, 615
  parietal, 615
  sacral, 310, 313, 317, 334
    anterior, 200
    posterior, 201
  sciatic
    greater, 200–202, 390, 391
    lesser, 201, 202, 390
  sphenopalatine, 695, 699, 700
  sternal, 16
  stylomastoid, 616, 625, 785
  supraorbital, 611
  transverse, 16
  vertebral, 289, 297, 301
  zygomaticofacial, 611, 612, 650
Foramen cecum, 619, 676, 790
Foramen lacerum, 615, 619
Foramen magnum, 297, 334, 335, 350, 615, 617, 619, 639, 742, 743
Foramen ovale, 616, 619, 624, 639
Foramen rotundum, 619, 624, 639, 699, 702
Foramen spinosum, 616, 617, 619, 624
Foramen transversarium, 296, 297, 350
Forceps major, 729, 732, 733
Forceps minor, 729, 732, 733
Forearm, 476, 477
  arteries, 550, 550t, 551
  bones, 552, 574
  magnetic resonance imaging, 603
  muscles, 552, 553t, 554, 574, 575t, 576, 577
  radiograph, 545
  transverse section, 602
Foregut, 67
Fornix, 208, 232, 723, 727–735, 740–743
Fossa
  acetabular, 311, 398, 401
  axillary, 2
  canine, 611, 613
  cerebellar, 619
  coronoid, 518, 544
  cranial
    anterior, 641
    middle, 641, 644–645
    posterior, 641, 642
  cubital, 525, 538–540
  gallbladder, 154, 155
  glenoid, 503, 511, 536, 537
  hypophyseal, 619, 621, 624, 738, 739
  iliac, 196, 197, 200, 312, 373, 380
  incisive, 611, 682
  infraspinous, 519

infratemporal, 615, 622, 664, 665
inguinal
  lateral, 219
  medial, 118, 219
intercondylar, 381
interpeduncular, 738, 739
intrabulbar, 209
ischioanal, 118, 213, 218, 219, 222, 250, 258, 259, 261, 262, 268, 269, 271, 273–277, 280, 281
jugular, 625
malleolar, 455
mandibular, 615–617, 625, 674, 702
olecranon, 544
oval, 56, 58
pararectal, 215
paravesical, 215, 219, 233
perineal, parietal, 219
popliteal, 402–404, 416
  fat in, 419–421
pterygoid, 615, 624, 702
pterygopalatine, 622, 699, 700–702
radial, 518, 544
scaphoid, 615, 624, 702
subarcuate, 625
subscapular, 518, 523
supinator, 544
supraclavicular, lesser, 752, 752t
supraspinous, 519
supravesical, 118, 208, 209, 219
temporal, 610, 612, 664, 665
tonsillar, 794
triangular, 703
Fossae ovalis, limbus, 56
Fovea, for ligament of head of femur, 311, 394, 398, 400
Frenulum
  of clitoris, 271
  labial, 253
  of tongue, 782
Frontal bone, 608, 609, 611, 613, 614, 617–619, 622, 650, 651, 664, 691, 695, 699
Fundus
  of gallbladder, 96, 119, 156, 159
  ocular, 661
  of stomach, 129, 132
  of uterus, 234, 237, 279, 282
Furrow, posterior median, 320

Galactogram, 6
Gallbladder, 123, 124, 126–128, 132, 146–148, 150, 152, 153, 156, 157, 160, 186
  body, 156, 159
  endoscopic retrograde cholangiography, 159
  folded, 159
  fossa, 154, 155
  fundus, 96, 119, 156, 159
  lymphatic drainage, 185
  mucous membrane, 156
  neck, 156, 159
Ganglion
  abdominopelvic, 176–178, 179t
  aorticorenal, 177
  celiac, 85, 163, 176, 177, 179, 181
  cervical
    middle, 68, 772, 807
    superior, 786
  cervicothoracic, 68, 72, 84, 85, 776
  ciliary, 652, 653, 717, 840, 840t
  cochlear, 715, 832

enteric, 214
geniculate, 709
mesenteric
  inferior, 176, 177, 230
  superior, 176, 177
otic, 681, 717, 840, 840t
parasympathetic, 230, 246
prevertebral, 214
pterygopalatine, 671, 699–701, 717, 831, 840, 840t
spinal, 17, 214, 246, 333, 334, 336, 642, 785
submandibular, 717, 779, 780, 840, 840t
sympathetic, 80–82, 173, 176, 177, 183, 230, 246, 717
  thoracic, 68, 84, 85
trigeminal, 644, 717
vestibular, 832
Gas, in colon, 141, 143
Genital organs, female, 234
Genital system, autonomic stimulation effects, 230t
Genitalia, external
  female, 253
  male, 216
Genu, articularis, 380, 414
Gingiva
  facial, 687
  palatine, 687
Glabella, 610, 612
Gland
  bulbourethral, 216–218, 254, 268
  ciliary, 655
  lacrimal, 630, 651–653, 701, 719, 831
  mammary, 5
  palatine, 682, 794
  parathyroid, 770, 771
    inferior, 770
  parotid, 350, 627, 662, 663, 678, 716, 720, 721, 738, 739, 762
  pineal, 728–731, 734, 735
  prostate, 118, 209, 210, 216–220, 222, 223, 262, 263, 276–279
  seminal, 118, 210, 216–220, 222, 276, 277, 279
  sublingual, 681, 719, 779, 806, 831
  submandibular, 666, 681, 762, 763, 779, 796, 806, 831
  suprarenal, 183, 352
    left, 97, 123, 125, 131, 133, 162, 163, 165, 181, 186
    lymphatic drainage, 182
    right, 97, 122, 123, 131, 133, 162–164, 181, 187
  tarsal, 655
  thyroid, 75, 716, 749, 759, 768–773, 790, 805, 807, 808
  vestibular, greater, 272, 274
Glans penis, 116, 216, 217, 252, 264, 266–268
Globus pallidus, 732, 733, 740, 741
Gluteal region, 196
  arteries, 393t
  ligaments, 390, 391
  muscles, 384, 385, 386t, 388, 389
  nerves, 392t
Gonadal shield, 143
Gonads, descent, 114
Grasping movements, 596, 597
Gray matter, 732, 733, 738–740, 742

Great vessels, 46–47, 66
Groove
  bicipital, 521, 525, 537, 600
  carotid, 619, 702
  costal, 13
  deltopectoral, 525
  facial artery, 664
  fibularis brevis, 433, 450
  fibularis longus, 427, 431, 433, 444, 447, 450
  flexor digitorum longus, 433, 450
  flexor hallucis longus, 433, 436, 444, 445, 450, 452, 455, 464
  greater petrosal nerve, 619
  infraorbital, 650
  intertubercular, 503, 518
  lacrimal, 650
  meniscus
    lateral, 411
    medial, 411
  middle meningeal, 621
  middle meningeal artery, 625
  middle temporal artery, 625
  obturator, 197
  occipital, 615
  petrosal sinus, 618
  prechiasmatic, 619
  radial, 519
  semimembranosus, 433
  sigmoid sinus, 618, 625
  superior petrosal sinus, 625
  superior sagittal sinus, 618
  tibialis posterior, 433, 450, 452
  transverse sinus, 618, 619
  trigeminal nerve, 615
  ulnar nerve, 519
Gubernacular remnant, 116
Gutter, paracolic, 122
Gyrus
  angular, 725
  cingulate, 728
  dentate, 729, 741
  frontal
    inferior, 725
    middle, 725
    superior, 725, 728
  lingual, 728
  occipitotemporal, 728
  parahippocampal, 728, 729
  postcentral, 722, 725
  precentral, 722, 725
  supramarginal, 725
  temporal
    inferior, 725
    middle, 725
    superior, 725
    transverse, 725
Gyrus rectus, 732, 733

Hallux valgus, 463
Hamate, 552, 574, 587, 593, 594, 599, 604, 605
Hamulus, pterygoid, 615, 617, 624, 681, 702, 797
Hand, 476, 477
  anastomoses, 487
  arteries, 572–573, 573t, 576
  bones, 552, 588, 589
  cutaneous innervation, 578, 579
  dorsal venous network, 491, 580
  dorsum, 580–582
  imaging of, 589
  lateral aspect, 584–586
  medial aspect, 587

muscles, 552
radiograph, 586, 589
surface anatomy, 560
Haustra, 136–140
Head
  autonomic ganglia, 840, 840t
  autonomic innervation, 717–718
  blood supply, 649
  lymphatic drainage, 716
  magnetic resonance imaging, 718–721, 809
  median anatomical section, 808
  veins, 716
Heart, 40, 46–47
  3-D volume reconstruction, 46, 47
  apex, 26–28, 46, 58, 59, 96
  auscultation, 44
  circulation, 55
  conduction system, 64, 129
  coronal section, 28
  crux, 52, 64
  diaphragmatic surface, 55
  excised, 60
  fibrous skeleton, 61
  innervation, 84
  left, interior, 58, 59
  lymphatic drainage, 86, 87
  posterior relationships, 65
  right, interior, 56, 57
  sternocostal surface, 25, 49, 55
  surface markings, 44, 45
Helix, 703
Hemivertebra, 318
Hepatocytes, 151
Hernia, inguinal, 115
Hiatus
  aortic, 165, 174
  esophageal, 74, 174
  greater petrosal nerve, 625
  sacral, 313
  semilunar, 695, 696
  urogenital, 254, 263
Hip bone, 194–196, 198, 286, 312, 316, 354, 355, 397
Hippocampus, 727, 729, 738–741
Hook of hamate, 571, 588, 589, 593, 594, 604, 605
Humerus, 476–479, 503, 518, 519, 521, 523, 534, 546–548, 600
  anatomical neck, 533
  capitulum, 523
  distal, 598
  head, 503, 534, 536, 537
  lymph nodes, 9
  proximal, 598
  shaft, 598
  supracondylar process, 541
  surgical neck, 532, 533, 536
Hyoid bone, 681, 716, 743, 749–751, 759, 762, 763, 766, 778, 797, 808, 810
Hypophysis, 740, 742, 808
Hypothalamus, 723, 728, 742
Hysterosalpingogram, 284

Ileocecal region, 139
Ileum, 96, 121, 128, 136, 137, 139, 140, 144, 145
Ilium, 196, 311, 312, 316, 317, 373, 381, 390, 391, 397, 398
  arcuate line, 199
  articular surface, 312
  body, 351
Incisor teeth, 685, 687, 688, 689t

Incisure, angular, 129, 132
Incus, 704, 706, 707, 709, 711
Infratemporal region, 668–669
Infundibulum, 639, 643, 729, 734, 738, 739, 742
  ethmoidal, 697
  pulmonary, 88–89
Inguinal region
  dissection, 112
  embryology, 114
  female, 110–112
  male, 106–109
Insula, 725, 731, 741
Intertendinous connection, 581, 582
Intestines, 136
Iris, 650, 651, 660, 661
Ischium, 196, 202, 222, 275, 312, 381, 391, 397
  body, 197, 312, 397
  ramus, 197, 199, 312, 397
Isthmus
  oropharyngeal, 792–797
  thyroid gland, 768

Jejunum, 96, 121, 128, 132, 134, 136, 137, 140, 144, 145, 162
Joint
  acromioclavicular, 519, 530, 531, 535, 536
  atlanto-occipital, 298, 299, 332t
  atlantoaxial, 297, 299, 332t
  calcaneocuboid, 430, 460t
  carpometacarpal, 571, 585, 590
  costochondral, 10
  costotransverse, 14, 15, 301
  craniovertebral, 298
  cubonavicular, 462
  cuneonavicular, 460t, 462
  elbow, 476, 477
    anastomoses, 487
    articular surfaces, 549
    bones, 544
    lateral aspect, 547
    magnetic resonance imaging, 546
    medial aspect, 546
    posterior aspect, 542, 543
    radiograph, 544, 547
    synovial capsule, 548
  glenohumeral (shoulder), 476, 477, 528, 530
    interior, 534, 535
    ligaments and articular capsule, 532, 533
    magnetic resonance imaging, 537
    radiograph, 536
    ultrasound, 537
  of head of rib, 14, 301
  hip, 250, 354, 390, 391, 394–395
    coronal section, 398
    magnetic resonance imaging, 399
    radiograph, 398
    transverse section, 399
  humeroulnar, 544
  intercarpal, 591
  interchondral, 12
  intermetatarsal, 460t
  interphalangeal, 460t, 552, 580
    distal, 552, 589, 595
    proximal, 552, 580, 589, 595
  manubriosternal, 10, 12, 48
  metacarpophalangeal, 552, 580, 589, 595

  metatarsophalangeal, 460t, 463
  midcarpal, 585, 593
  patellofemoral, 418
  radiocarpal, 590–592
  radioulnar
    distal, 545, 590, 591
    proximal, 544, 545
  sacrococcygeal, 196
  sacroiliac, 196–199, 310, 311
    articular surfaces, 316
    CT scan, 317, 351
    ligaments, 316
  sternoclavicular, 12, 88–89, 530, 772
  sternocostal, 12
  subtalar, 430, 458, 460t
  talocalcaneal, 459
  talocalcaneonavicular, 458, 460t
  tarsal, transverse, 458, 461
  tarsometatarsal, 460t, 462
  temporomandibular, 612, 663, 666
    movements, 673, 673t
    muscles acting on, 672, 672t
    sectional anatomy, 674–675
  tibiofibular
    proximal, 419
    superior, 442
  uncovertebral, 295, 296
  xiphisternal, 10, 12, 48
  zygapophysial, 296, 302, 304–306, 310
Junction
  anorectal, 211
  corneoscleral, 650
  costochondral, 26
  duodenojejunal, 122, 124, 135, 137, 144
  esophagogastric, 129
  gastroesophageal, 189
  ileocecal, 141
  neurocentral, 290
  xiphisternal, 499

Kidney, 145, 171
  anomalies, 168
  calices, 165–167
  cortex, 166
  ectopic pelvic, 168
  exposures, 169–171
  external features, 166
  hilum, 171
  horseshoe, 168
  left, 97, 122–125, 133, 162, 164, 165, 352
  magnetic resonance imaging, 187–189
  medulla, 166
  right, 97, 122–124, 126, 133, 152, 153, 162, 171, 352
  segments, 167
  structure, 166
  ultrasound, 191
Knee, 354
  anastomoses, 416–417
  anterior aspect, 406, 407
  articular surfaces, 411
  bursae, 415t
  cavity, 421
  coronal section, 419
  distended, 414, 415
  joint capsule, 410, 420, 421
  lateral aspect, 409
  ligaments, 411, 412
  magnetic resonance imaging, 419–421

    medial aspect, 408
    radiograph, 418, 420
    sagittal section, 420–421
Kyphosis
  sacral, 287
  thoracic, 287

Labium majus, 110, 208, 232, 253, 269, 280, 281
Labium minus, 208, 232, 253, 269, 273
Labrum
  acetabular, 394, 396, 398
  glenoid, 503, 533–535, 537
Labyrinth
  bony, 714
  membranous, 714
Lacrimal bone, 611–613, 650, 690, 691, 695, 700
Lambda, 612, 614
Lamina
  chorionic, 238
  of vertebra, 289, 296, 297, 301, 303, 310, 806
Large intestine, lymphatic drainage, 185
Laryngocele, 800
Laryngopharynx, 128, 790, 807, 810
Laryngoscopy, 804
Larynx, 28, 128, 807, 808
  external, 800
  inlet, 790, 804
  internal, 801
  lymphatic drainage, 805
  magnetic resonance imaging, 804
  muscles, 802, 802t
Leg, 354
  anterior aspect, 422–425
  arteries, 441t
  bones, 380, 381, 433
  deep vessels, 424, 425
  lateral aspect, 428, 429
  magnetic resonance imaging, 472–473
  muscles, 423t, 424, 428, 429
    deep, 425, 432t, 436, 437
    superficial, 422, 432t, 434, 435
  nerves, 424, 424t, 425
  posterior, 432–437
  proximal, 380, 381
  transverse sections, 472–473
Lemniscus
  lateral, 734, 735
  medial, 734, 735
Lens, 660, 721, 738, 739
Ligament
  acetabular, transverse, 396, 398
  acromioclavicular, 531
    superior, 530, 532
  alar, 299
  anococcygeal, 250
  anular, 543, 545–548, 551
  apical, 297
  arcuate
    lateral, 172, 174
    medial, 172, 174, 175
    median, 74
  bifurcate, 449, 454, 458
  broad, of uterus, 208, 233–237, 240, 282, 283
  calcaneocuboid
    dorsal, 454, 458
    medial, 454
    plantar, 464
  calcaneofibular, 430, 450, 451, 454, 458

  calcaneonavicular
    lateral, 454, 458
    plantar, 447, 452, 458, 464, 465
  calcaneotibial, 450
  carpal, palmar, 493
  collateral
    of digit, 571, 595
    fibular, 405, 409, 411, 412, 414, 419
    radial, 547, 548, 590
    tibial, 405, 408, 411, 412, 419
    ulnar, 546, 548, 549, 590
  commissural
    distal, 561
    proximal, 561
  conoid, 532
  coracoacromial, 523, 530–533, 535
  coracoclavicular, 529, 530, 532
  coracohumeral, 523, 535
  coronal, 408
  coronary, 120, 122, 146–148, 162, 411
  costoclavicular, 12, 530
  costotransverse, 15
    lateral, 15, 18, 327
    posterior, 327
    superior, 15, 17, 301, 327
  of costovertebral articulations, 15
  costoxiphoid, anterior, 12
  cricothyroid, median, 801
  cricovocal, 801
  cruciate
    anterior, 411–413, 419–421
    inferior longitudinal band, 297
    posterior, 411–413, 415, 419–421
    superior longitudinal band, 297
  cruciform, 299
  cuboideonavicular, dorsal, 458
  cubonavicular, plantar, 465
  cuneocuboid, plantar, 465
  cuneonavicular
    dorsal, 449
    plantar, 465
  deltoid, 438, 448–450, 452, 456
  denticulate, 334, 335
  falciform, 118, 119, 121–123, 126, 146–148, 152, 162, 186
  fundiform, of penis, 107
  gastrocolic, 119, 124–127, 129, 144
  gastrophrenic, 119
  gastrosplenic, 119, 123–125, 129, 131, 164
  glenohumeral
    inferior, 533, 534
    middle, 533, 534
    superior, 533, 534
  of head of femur, 222, 396, 399, 401
  of head of fibula, 442
  hepatoduodenal, 119, 126, 129, 154, 162
  hepatogastric, 119, 126, 129, 154
  humeral, transverse, 530, 532, 537
  hyoepiglottic, 799
  iliofemoral, 200, 201, 394–396, 399, 400
  iliolumbar, 200, 201, 314, 315
  of inferior vena cava, 146
  inguinal, 98, 101, 104, 106, 107, 109, 110, 200, 371–373, 400
  interchondral, 12
  interclavicular, 12, 530
  intermetatarsal

dorsal, 449
plantar, 464, 465
interspinous, 295, 297, 305, 308, 324
intra-articular, 12, 15, 301
ischiofemoral, 395
lacunar, 106, 202, 371–373, 399
lateral
of ankle, 451
of bladder, 220, 251
of temporomandibular joint, 674
longitudinal
anterior, 15, 17, 145, 200, 295, 297, 298, 301, 306, 308, 314, 339
posterior, 297, 306–308
medial, of ankle, 451, 452, 457, 458, 465
meniscofemoral, 419
posterior, 412
metacarpal
deep transverse, 571
interosseous, 590
superficial transverse, 561
metatarsal
deep transverse, 446
superficial transverse, 443
nuchal, 295, 328, 331, 333, 785, 810
of ovary, 233, 236, 237
palmar, 568, 571, 583, 591, 595
palpebral
lateral, 630
medial, 630
patellar, 374–376, 380, 383, 406, 408, 409, 411, 420–422, 424, 425
pectineal, 202, 371
perineal, transverse, 267
periodontal, 687
peritoneal, 120
phrenicocolic, 119, 122, 125
phrenicoesophageal, 129
pisohamate, 552, 570, 571, 587
pisometacarpal, 552, 571, 587
plantar, 446, 447
long, 447, 464
popliteal, oblique, 405
pubic, inferior, 202, 208, 232
pubofemoral, 200
puboprostatic, 209, 210, 263
pubovesical, 251
pulmonary, 34, 35
radiate, 15, 17, 301
sternocostal, anterior, 12
radiocarpal, palmar, 571
radioulnar, 551
retinacular, 583
round, 234
artery of, 110
of liver, 118, 119, 123, 146–148, 152, 154
of uterus, 110, 111, 122, 208, 232, 233, 248, 269, 271, 280, 281
sacrococcygeal
anterior, 200, 314
posterior, 201, 315
sacroiliac
anterior, 200, 314, 316
interosseous, 316, 317
posterior, 201, 315, 316, 390
sacrospinous, 200, 202, 222, 314–316, 390, 391

sacrotuberous, 200–202, 212, 262, 263, 273, 314–316, 390, 391
scapular, superior transverse, 517, 529
skin, 561, 567
sphenomandibular, 674, 681
splenorenal, 122–124, 127, 131, 162, 164
sternoclavicular, anterior, 12, 530
sternohyoid, 350
stylohyoid, 681, 721, 785, 797
stylomandibular, 674, 785
supraspinous, 201, 295, 300, 305, 308, 315
suspensory
of axilla, 492
of breast, 4–6
of clitoris, 271
of lens, 660
of ovary, 208, 232, 233, 236, 237, 248
of penis, 112, 116, 264
talocalcanean
interosseous, 448, 449, 454, 456, 458
lateral, 454
talofibular
anterior, 430, 448, 449, 454
posterior, 450, 451, 456, 457
posterior inferior, 450
talonavicular, dorsal, 449, 452, 454
tarsometatarsal
dorsal, 449
plantar, 464, 465
thyrohyoid, 801
tibiocalcanean, 450, 451
tibiofibular
anterior, 442
anterior inferior, 430, 448, 449, 454
interosseous, 456
posterior, 442, 450
posterior inferior, 450, 451
tibiotalar, posterior, 450–452
transverse, 297, 299, 350, 721
inferior, 442
trapezoid, 532
triangular, 122, 125–127, 146–148, 162
umbilical
medial, 208, 218, 219, 224, 225, 225t, 232, 233, 238, 242
median, 218, 219
uterosacral, 251
vestibular, 801
vocal, 807
Ligamentum arteriosum, 41, 46, 47, 49, 51, 67–69, 75, 81, 409
Ligamentum flavum, 297, 304–306, 308, 338, 808
Ligamentum venosum, 147, 154
Line
arcuate, 103, 118, 199, 219, 312
epiphyseal, 419
of Gennari, 731
gluteal
anterior, 381, 390, 397
inferior, 381, 390, 397
posterior, 381, 390, 397
intertrochanteric, 311, 380, 394
nuchal
inferior, 614, 615, 617
superior, 328, 330, 613–615
oblique, 611, 613

anterior, 544, 552
posterior, 544, 574
pain, pelvic, 230, 231
pectinate, 211
pectineal, 381
soleal, 381, 433
spiral, 381
supracondylar
lateral, 381
medial, 381
temporal, 610
inferior, 613, 614
superior, 613, 614
vertical, 433
Linea alba, 2, 98, 102, 103, 105–107, 351
Linea aspera, 381
Linea semilunaris, 98, 497
Lingula, 26, 35, 41
Lips, 128
Liver, 96, 97, 121, 124, 125, 127, 128, 152, 161, 352
anterior surface, 146
caudate lobe, 123, 125–127, 146–148, 150, 151, 151t, 152, 162, 186
computed tomography, 6
flow of blood and bile in, 151
lobes, 119, 123–126, 146–148, 150, 151, 151t, 160, 162
lobules, 151
lymphatic drainage, 185
magnetic resonance imaging, 187–189
posterior relations, 148
quadrate lobe, 126, 147, 154, 155
segments, 150, 151, 151t
superior surface, 146
visceral (posteroinferior) surface, 147
Lobes
of brain, 722
frontal, 719, 722, 725, 726, 732, 733
occipital, 722, 725, 726, 728, 732, 733, 738, 739
parietal, 722, 725, 726
temporal, 722, 725, 726, 738–740
of liver, 119, 123–126, 146–148, 150, 151, 151t, 160, 162
caudate, 123, 125–127, 146–148, 150, 151, 151t, 152, 162, 186
quadrate, 126, 147, 154, 155
of lung, 28, 32
left, 32, 33, 41
inferior, 25, 186, 188, 189
superior, 25
right, 32, 33, 41
inferior, 83, 187–189
middle, 25
superior, 83
Lobule
of auricle, 703
fat, 5
inferior parietal, 725
liver, 151
paracentral, 728
Lordosis
cervical, 287
lumbar, 287
Lower limb
arteries, 362
bones, 354, 355

bony anomalies, 467
cutaneous nerves, 359
dermatomes, 360, 361
fascia, 368
fascial compartments, 369
joints, 354
lymphatic drainage, 366
motor nerves, 356
myotatic (deep tendon) reflexes, 357
myotomes, 357
postnatal development, 468–469
regions, 354
veins
deep, 363
superficial, 364, 365
Lunate, 552, 574, 586–589, 591–594, 599
Lung, 147
apex, 32, 34, 35
cardiac notch, 26, 32, 96
coronal section, 28
costal surface, 25
extent of, 30–31
fissures, 32, 96, 97
innervation, 42
left, 28, 29, 48, 65, 68, 69, 96, 352
apex, 25, 26
bronchi, 33, 36–38
computed tomography, 6
inferior lobe, 25, 186, 188, 189
lobes, 32, 33, 41
magnetic resonance imaging, 88–91
mediastinal surface and hilum, 35
superior lobe, 25
lobes, 28, 32
lymphatic drainage, 43, 87
mediastinal surface, 25, 34–35
right, 28, 29, 65, 68, 69, 352
apex, 39, 96
bronchi, 33, 36–38
computed tomography, 6
inferior lobe, 83, 187–189
lobes, 32, 33, 41
magnetic resonance imaging, 88–91
mediastinal surface and hilum, 34
middle lobe, 25
superior lobe, 83
root, 25, 28, 48, 81
surface markings, 31t, 45
topography, 26
Lymph nodes, 68, 134, 275, 333
aortic arch, 43
apical, 9
appendicular, 185
auricular, posterior, 662
axillary, 9, 503
apical, 489
central, 489
humeral, 489
pectoral, 489
subscapular, 489
bronchopulmonary, 35, 43
celiac, 182, 184, 185
central, 9
cervical
deep, 676
inferior, 43, 716
superior, 716
superficial, 716
colic, 185

Lymph nodes—*continued*
  cubital, 489, 538
  cystic, 185
  diaphragmatic
    inferior, 185
    superior, 86, 185
  epicolic, 185
  gastro-omental, 184
  hepatic, 185
  humeral, 9
  ileocolic, 185
  iliac
    common, 182, 228, 229, 229t,
      244, 245, 245t
    external, 182, 228, 229, 229t,
      244, 245, 245t
    internal, 182, 228, 229, 244, 245
  infraclavicular, 9, 489
  infrahyoid, 676, 716
  inguinal, 107, 117
    deep, 109, 228, 229, 244, 245,
      366
    superficial, 228, 229, 229t, 244,
      245, 245t, 366, 367, 370
  interpectoral, 9
  jugulo-omohyoid, 676, 716
  jugulodigastric, 676, 716
  lumbar, 117, 183, 185, 228, 229,
    244, 245
  mastoid, 716
  mediastinal, posterior, 76
  mesenteric
    inferior, 182, 185, 228, 229, 244,
      245
    superior, 182, 184, 185
  occipital, 716
  overview, 77
  pancreatic, 184
  pancreaticoduodenal, 153, 184
  paracolic, 145, 185
  paraesophageal, 185
  pararectal, 228, 229, 244, 245
  parasternal, 9, 22, 86, 185
  paratracheal, 716
  parotid, 662, 716
  pectoral, 9
  popliteal, 366
  preauricular, 662
  prelaryngeal, 716
  pretracheal, 716
  pulmonary, 43
  retroauricular, 716
  retropharyngeal, 676, 716
  sacral, 228, 229, 229t, 244, 245,
    245t
  splenic, 184
  submandibular, 676, 716, 762
  submental, 676, 716
  subpyloric, 184
  subscapular, 9
  supraclavicular, 9
  suprapyloric, 184
  thoracic, 86, 87
  tracheal, 43
  tracheobronchial, 74
    inferior, 43
    superior, 43
Lymphatic drainage, 131
  breast, 9
  gallbladder, 185
  head and neck, 716
  large intestine, 185
  larynx, 805
  liver, 185
  lower limb, 366

  lung, 43, 87
  overview, 77
  pancreas, 184
  pelvis and perineum
    female, 244–245, 245t
    male, 228–229, 229t
  scrotum, 117
  small intestine, 184
  spleen, 184
  stomach, 184
  suprarenal gland, 182
  testis, 117
  thorax, 86–87
  tongue, 676
  trachea, 805
  upper limb, 489

Macula, 661, 715
Macula lutea, 660
Magnetic resonance imaging
  abdomen, 186–189, 191
  ankle, 456, 457
  arm, 601
  brain, 732–733, 738–740, 742
  cranial nerves, 842–844
  elbow joint, 546
  forearm, 603
  glenohumeral (shoulder) joint, 537
  head, 718–721, 809
  hip joint, 399
  knee, 419–421
  larynx, 804
  leg, 472–473
  nasopharynx and oral cavity,
    718–720
  oropharynx, 721
  patellofemoral joint, 418
  pelvis and perineum, 276–282
  teeth, 806
  thigh, 470–471
  thorax, 88–91
  through carpal tunnel, 604, 605
  through palm, 606
  vertebrae
    cervical, 352
    lumbar, 343
    thoracic, 300, 352
  vertebral artery, 88–89
Malleolus
  lateral, 354, 422, 426, 427, 429,
    430, 433, 448–451,
    453–457
  medial, 354, 422, 426, 427, 433,
    436, 438, 448–452, 454,
    456, 457, 464, 472
Malleus, 704–709, 711
Mammogram, 6
Mandible, 608, 611, 613, 614, 620,
  622, 664, 719, 738, 739,
  743, 779, 808, 810
  body, 609, 611, 612, 666, 778, 806
  head, 664, 674
  inferior border, 610, 612
  internal surface, 665
  medial aspect, 681
  neck, 664, 720
  ramus, 721
Mandibular teeth, 611
Manubrium, 10, 12, 21, 24, 29, 40,
  48, 88–89, 499, 530, 808,
  810
Margin
  costal, 10, 24
  infraorbital, 611
  sphenoid, 625

  supraorbital, 611
Mass
  fatty, 350
  lateral, 297, 350
Mater
  arachnoid, 334, 335, 338–340, 634,
    636
  dura, 297, 335, 336, 338–340, 634,
    636, 637–639
  pia, 339, 573, 634, 636
Maxilla, 608, 609, 611, 613, 617, 622,
  650, 664, 691, 695, 721,
  738, 739
Maxillary teeth, 611
Meatus
  acoustic
    external, 612, 617, 625, 666,
      703–706, 712
    internal, 615, 619, 625, 639,
      705, 712, 738, 739, 832
  inferior, 694, 697, 720
  middle, 694, 697
  superior, 694
Mediastinum, 28
  anterior, 29
  inferior, 29
  left side, 81
  middle, 29
  posterior, 29
    innervation, 84
    lymphatic drainage, 87
    structures, 82–83
  right side, 80
  subdivisions, 29
  superior, 29, 67–69, 72
    innervation, 84
    root of neck, 67
    superficial dissection, 66
  topography, 26
Medulla oblongata, 352, 722, 723,
  734, 738, 739, 743, 808,
  810
Membrane
  areolar, 152, 153
  atlanto-occipital
    anterior, 297, 298
    posterior, 295, 297, 298, 785
  costocoracoid, 492
  intercostal
    external, 20–22
    internal, 17, 18
  interosseous, 369, 425, 442, 449,
    472, 493, 546, 547, 551,
    591, 602
  obturator, 196, 202, 250, 372, 396
  perineal, 202, 209, 210, 217, 218,
    258, 259, 261, 262, 267,
    268, 271, 272, 274,
    280–282
  quadrangular, 801
  synovial, 12, 396, 398, 410, 421, 592
  tectorial, 297–299
  thyrohyoid, 770, 807
  tympanic, 698, 703–706, 708,
    711–713
Meninges, 335, 636
Meniscus
  lateral, 409, 411–413, 419
  medial, 408, 410–413, 419, 420
Mesentery, 120–122, 134, 137, 144,
  148, 157, 162
Mesoappendix, 139
Mesocolon
  sigmoid, 122, 137, 144, 145, 212,
    215, 233

    transverse, 120–122, 125, 126, 144,
      145, 148, 162
Mesoesophagus, 73
Mesosalpinx, 236, 237
Mesotendon, 569
Mesovarium, 236
Metacarpals, 476–479, 552, 574, 582,
  589, 590, 594, 595, 598,
  599, 606
  fifth, 587, 588, 594
  first, 585, 586, 588, 594, 606
Metatarsals, 427, 431, 444, 453, 462,
  464–466
  fifth, 430, 431, 465
  first, 439, 449, 452, 463, 465
  heads, 443, 447
Meyer loop, 726
Midbrain, 639, 643, 723, 734,
  738–740, 742, 743
Molar teeth, 685, 687, 688, 689t, 719
Mons pubis, 253, 269, 271
Mucosa, nasal, 818
Muscle
  abdominal, posterior, 147
  abductor brevis, 447
  abductor digiti minimi, 430, 444,
    444t, 445, 447, 456, 458,
    552, 564, 565t, 566, 567,
    570, 587, 606
  abductor hallucis, 438, 444, 444t,
    445, 447, 451, 452, 456
  abductor pollicis
    brevis, 552, 561, 564, 565t, 566,
      567, 570, 606
    longus, 481, 552, 566, 567, 571,
      574, 575t, 576, 577, 581,
      582, 584–586, 602, 604,
      605
  adductor brevis, 222, 375, 378t,
    380–382, 396, 447, 447t,
    470
  adductor hallucis, 447
    oblique head, 446, 446t
    transverse head, 446, 446t
  adductor longus, 222, 372–375,
    378t, 379–382, 396, 470
  adductor magnus, 375, 378t,
    379–382, 384, 385, 388,
    389, 396, 405, 408, 470
  adductor pollicis, 480, 552, 564,
    565t, 566, 567, 577,
    584–586, 606
    oblique head, 570
    transverse head, 570
  anconeus, 481, 519, 542, 543, 549,
    574, 575t, 576, 577
  ansa subclavia, 72
  aryepiglottic, 791
  arytenoid, 807
    oblique, 802, 802t
    transverse, 802, 802t
  auricular, posterior, 662
  axioappendicular, 499t
  biceps brachii, 480, 491, 510,
    521–525, 538–540, 552,
    600
    attrition of long head, 541
    long head, 22, 502, 503, 508,
      520, 520t, 521–523, 525,
      530, 533, 537, 600
    short head, 22, 499, 502, 503,
      508, 518, 520, 520t,
      521–523, 525, 530, 534,
      600
    third head, 541

biceps femoris, 380, 402, 403, 406, 407, 409, 419, 421, 434, 435, 437, 470
  long head, 381, 383–385, 387t, 388, 389, 396, 470
  short head, 381, 383–385, 387t, 388, 389, 470
brachialis, 480, 499, 502, 510, 518–520, 520t, 521–525, 527, 539, 540, 549, 552, 600
brachioradialis, 481, 518, 522, 524, 526, 527, 539, 540, 542, 546, 549, 552, 554, 556, 559, 571, 574, 575t, 576, 577, 581, 585, 602
buccinator, 626, 629t, 630, 662, 666, 668, 678, 712, 716, 721, 797
bulbospongiosus, 209, 210, 218, 255, 256t, 257, 260, 261, 271, 272
coccygeus, 203, 203t, 204, 210, 212, 254, 263, 273
  nerve to, 206, 207, 207t
compressor urethrae, 254
coracobrachialis, 22, 480, 499, 502, 503, 508, 510, 518, 520, 520t, 521, 522, 525, 541, 600
corpus cavernosum, 216, 255, 261, 266–268, 276–279
corpus spongiosum, 216, 217, 255, 261, 266–268, 278, 279
corrugator supercilii, 626, 630
cremaster, 107, 108, 111–113, 116
cricoarytenoid
  lateral, 802, 802t, 803
  posterior, 802, 802t, 803
cricopharyngeus, 788, 788t
cricothyroid, 759, 770, 802, 802t, 803
dartos, 113
deltoid, 2, 4, 481, 490, 491, 495, 499–503, 508, 517–519, 522, 523, 525–529, 531, 534, 536, 537
  acromial part, 513, 513t, 514, 524
  clavicular part, 513, 513t, 521, 524, 600
  spinal part, 320, 512, 513, 513t, 514, 521, 524, 600
depressor anguli oris, 626, 630, 662, 746
depressor labii inferioris, 626, 746
digastric, 330
  anterior belly, 681, 758, 760, 761, 761t, 762, 763, 778
  fascial sling, 763
  posterior belly, 333, 350, 666, 667, 681, 721, 761, 761t, 785
  nerve to, 662
erector spinae, 123, 171, 320, 323, 324, 328, 329t, 351
extensor carpi radialis
  brevis, 481, 540, 574, 575t, 576, 577, 581, 582, 584, 585, 602, 604, 605
  longus, 481, 518, 524, 527, 540, 542, 549, 552, 574, 575t, 576, 577, 581, 582, 584–586, 602, 604, 605

extensor carpi ulnaris, 481, 543, 552, 574, 575t, 576, 577, 581, 582, 587, 602, 604, 605
extensor digiti minimi, 481, 574, 575t, 576, 577, 581, 582, 602, 604, 605
extensor digitorum, 431, 481, 569, 574, 575t, 576, 577, 580–582, 585, 602, 604, 605
  brevis, 422, 424–428, 430
  longus, 422, 423, 423t, 424, 426, 428–431, 436, 457, 472
extensor hallucis
  brevis, 422, 426–428, 431
  longus, 422, 423, 423t, 424, 426–428, 431, 457, 472
extensor indicis, 481, 574, 575t, 576, 577, 581, 582, 602, 604, 605
extensor pollicis
  brevis, 481, 574, 575t, 576, 577, 580–582, 584–586, 602, 604, 605
  longus, 481, 574, 575t, 576, 577, 580–582, 584–586, 602, 604–606
extensor retinaculum, 368, 458, 576, 577, 581, 582, 587
facial expression, 626, 628–629, 629t, 634
fibularis brevis, 422–425, 427–429, 429t, 430, 431, 433–435, 439, 449, 454, 456, 457, 472
fibularis longus, 422–425, 428, 429, 429t, 430, 431, 434, 435, 439, 447, 454, 456–458, 472
fibularis tertius, 422, 423, 423t, 424, 426, 427, 429–431, 457
flexor carpi
  radialis, 480, 540, 552, 553t, 554, 568, 570, 571, 585, 593, 602, 604, 605
  ulnaris, 480, 543, 549, 552, 553t, 554–556, 559, 566, 570, 571, 574, 587, 593, 602
flexor digiti minimi, 446, 446t, 447
  brevis, 552, 564, 565t, 567, 570
flexor digitorum
  brevis, 438, 444, 444t, 445, 447, 456
  longus, 432t, 433–439, 443, 445, 447, 448, 451, 456–458, 472
  profundus, 480, 543, 552, 553t, 556, 557, 568, 570, 571, 574, 602, 604–606
  superficialis, 480, 518, 543, 552, 553t, 555, 558, 566, 568, 570, 571, 602, 604–606
flexor hallucis
  brevis, 439, 445, 446, 446t, 447, 452
  longus, 432t, 433, 435–439, 443, 445, 447, 448, 456–458, 472
flexor pollicis
  brevis, 552, 561, 564, 565t, 566, 567, 570, 606

longus, 480, 552, 553t, 555–557, 568, 602, 604–606
flexor retinaculum, 434, 436–438, 493, 554, 564, 567, 568, 570, 571, 591–593, 604, 605
frontalis, 634
gastrocnemius, 408, 409, 435
  lateral head, 381, 383–385, 402, 403, 405, 409, 419, 421, 428, 432t, 433–435, 472
  medial head, 381, 384, 385, 402, 403, 405, 419, 420, 422, 432t, 433–435, 472
gemellus, 381
  inferior, 385, 386t, 388, 389, 391
  nerve to, 206, 207, 207t
  superior, 222, 385, 386t, 388, 389, 391, 399
genioglossus, 677, 677t, 678, 679, 681, 719, 780, 781, 806, 810
geniohyoid, 678, 679, 681, 743, 760, 761, 761t, 781, 808
gluteus maximus, 202, 222, 250, 261, 262, 268, 273, 275, 320, 351, 368, 381, 383, 385, 386t, 388, 389, 399, 470, 472, 514
gluteus medius, 202, 320, 351, 381, 384, 385, 386t, 388, 389, 399
gluteus minimus, 351, 380, 381, 386t, 389, 396
gracilis, 372, 373, 375, 378t, 379, 380, 382, 384, 389, 396, 408, 434, 437, 470, 472
hamstring, 384, 385, 387t, 388, 389
hyoglossus, 677, 677t, 681, 766, 780, 806
hypothenar, 480, 604, 605
iliacus, 118, 163, 172, 172t, 173, 212, 218, 250, 317, 373, 375, 376, 377t, 380, 382
iliococcygeus, 203, 203t, 204, 212, 254, 262, 263
iliocostalis, 18, 323, 324, 351
  cervicis, 323
  lumborum, 323, 328
  thoracis, 323, 328
iliopsoas, 351, 372, 373, 375, 376, 377t, 380, 381, 399
infraspinatus, 481, 503, 512, 516, 517, 517t, 519, 526–528, 537
intercostal, 164
  external, 17–21, 21t, 22, 24, 83, 327, 334
  innermost, 17–21, 21t, 83, 334
  internal, 18–21, 21t, 22–24, 72, 83
interosseous
  dorsal, 447, 447t, 480, 564, 565, 565t, 566, 574, 576, 577, 580–582, 584–586, 606
  palmar, 480, 564, 565, 565t, 606
  plantar, 447, 447t
interspinales, 329t, 330
intertransversarius, 324, 326, 328, 329t, 333, 785
ischiocavernosus, 255, 256t, 257, 261, 271, 276, 277
laryngeal, 802, 802t

longus, 480, 552, 553t, 555–557, 568, 602, 604–606
latissimus dorsi, 4, 7, 73, 100, 123, 169–171, 320, 321, 324, 351, 481, 496, 497, 499, 502, 509, 510, 512, 513, 513t, 514, 518, 521–523, 525, 526, 600
levator anguli oris, 626, 630, 721
levator ani, 118, 203, 203t, 204, 205, 208, 209, 211–213, 216, 218, 220, 232, 250, 261, 268, 272, 273, 276–278, 280, 281
  nerve to, 206, 207, 207t, 210
  tendinous arch, 218, 219
levator costarum, 327, 328, 329t
levator labii superioris, 626, 629t, 630
levator labii superioris alaeque nasi, 630
levator palpebrae superioris, 630, 652, 654, 658, 658t, 719
levator prostatae, 263
levator scapulae, 321, 322, 333, 481, 511, 513, 513t, 514, 518, 519, 529, 755, 777, 777t, 806
levator veli palatini, 684, 684t, 712, 713, 789, 791, 795
levatores costarum, 18, 21, 21t
longissimus, 18, 323, 324, 351, 783, 783t
  capitis, 328, 330, 331, 333, 350, 785
  cervicis, 328
  thoracis, 323, 328
longitudinal
  inferior, 677t
  superior, 677, 677t, 679
longus capitis, 332, 333, 350, 721, 773, 774, 774t, 775, 785, 807
longus colli, 69, 80, 350, 721, 773, 774, 774t, 775, 807
lumbrical, 439, 445, 445t, 480, 556, 563–565, 565t, 566, 567, 571, 606
masseter, 630, 662, 666, 667, 672, 672t, 719–721, 738, 739
mastication, 672, 672t
mentalis, 626, 629t, 630, 746
multifidus, 324, 325, 328, 351, 783, 783t
mylohyoid, 678, 679, 681, 743, 758, 760, 761, 761t, 763, 766, 778, 779, 806, 808
  nerve to, 681, 763, 778, 779, 828, 829
nasalis, 626, 629t
oblique
  external, 2, 3, 7, 19, 22, 24, 73, 98, 100–104, 104t, 105–109, 111, 112, 118, 119, 123, 163, 169–171, 188, 320, 324, 351, 496, 497, 514
  inferior, 651, 654, 658, 658t, 659, 659t, 719
    nerve to, 651, 654, 821
  internal, 19, 24, 101, 103, 104, 104t, 105, 107–109, 111, 112, 118, 119, 163, 169–171, 188, 324, 351, 382, 785
  superior, 330, 651, 652, 658, 658t, 659, 659t, 719

Muscle—*continued*
  obliquus capitis
    inferior, 330–333, 350, 784
    superior, 330–333, 350, 784, 785
  obturator externus, 222, 250, 268, 273, 275, 378t, 380, 391, 394, 396, 470
  obturator internus, 118, 202, 203, 203t, 204, 212, 213, 218, 219, 222, 250, 275, 278, 280–282, 385, 386t, 388, 391
    nerve to, 206, 207, 207t, 392t
  occipitalis, 330, 634
  occipitofrontalis, 626, 629t, 630
  omohyoid, 492, 518, 529, 758, 759, 761, 761t, 762, 766
  opponens brevis, 614
  opponens digiti minimi, 552, 565t, 567, 570, 587, 606
  opponens pollicis, 552, 564, 565t, 567, 570, 585
  orbicularis oculi, 626, 628, 629t, 655, 662, 666, 721
  orbicularis oris, 626, 629t, 630, 721
  palatoglossus, 677, 677t, 684, 684t, 721, 792, 793
  palatopharyngeus, 684, 684t, 721, 788, 788t, 791–793
  palmaris
    brevis, 480, 561, 563, 566
    longus, 480, 553t, 554, 559, 566, 570, 602, 604, 605
  papillary, 58
    anterior, 57, 59, 63, 64
    magnetic resonance imaging, 88–89
    posterior, 57, 59, 63
    septal, 57, 63
  pectinate, 56
  pectineus, 222, 250, 275, 372, 373, 375, 378t, 380–382, 396, 399
  pectoralis major, 4, 7, 22, 100, 103, 490, 492, 496, 499, 502, 503, 508–510, 518, 522, 523
    abdominal part, 494–498, 499t
    clavicular head, 2, 3, 494, 495, 497–499, 499t, 500
    magnetic resonance imaging, 88–89
    sternocostal head, 2, 3, 494, 495, 497–499, 499t, 500, 508
  pectoralis minor, 492, 498, 499, 499t, 500–503, 508, 510, 518, 523, 530
  perineal
    deep transverse, 209, 216, 254, 256t, 257, 263
    superficial, 268
    superficial transverse, 255, 256t, 257, 261, 271
  pes anserinus, 379, 408, 437
  pharyngeal, 681, 788, 788t, 797
  piriformis, 202, 203, 203t, 204, 212, 385, 386t, 388–391
    nerve to, 206, 207, 207t
  plantaris, 381, 385, 405, 432t, 433
  platysma, 3, 494, 626, 629t, 630, 746, 746t, 807
  popliteus, 381, 385, 404, 405, 414, 420, 421, 432t, 433, 435–437, 472

  procerus, 626, 629, 630
  pronator quadratus, 480, 552, 553t, 555–557, 571, 592
  pronator teres, 480, 518, 522, 523, 539, 549, 552, 553t, 554, 555, 557, 574, 577, 602
    deep head, 540
    superficial head, 540
    ulnar head, 518, 552
  psoas, 133, 144, 145, 153, 163, 187, 188, 212, 215, 218, 317, 324, 352, 372, 373
  psoas major, 171, 172, 172t, 173, 250, 334, 351, 375, 376, 377t
  psoas minor, 172, 375
  pterygoid
    lateral, 668, 672, 672t, 720, 721, 738, 739
      nerve to, 828, 829
    medial, 672, 672t, 681, 720, 797
      deep head, 668, 669
      nerve to, 669, 828, 829
      superficial head, 668, 669
  pubococcygeus, 202, 203, 203t, 204, 210, 212, 254, 260, 262, 263
  puboprostaticus, 203, 204, 260
  puborectalis, 203, 203t, 204, 209–212, 222, 260, 263, 275–277
  pubovaginalis, 203, 205, 260, 273
  quadratus femoris, 375, 376, 377t, 381, 385, 386t, 390, 396
    nerve to, 206, 207, 207t, 392t
  quadratus lumborum, 153, 163, 171, 172, 172t, 173, 174, 187, 324, 326, 351
  quadratus plantae, 438, 439, 445, 445t, 451, 452, 456
  rectovesicalis, 260
  rectus
    inferior, 651, 653–655, 658, 658t, 659, 659t, 719
    lateral, 652–654, 658, 658t, 659, 659t, 719, 721
    medial, 651–653, 658, 658t, 659, 659t, 660, 697, 719, 721
    superior, 651, 652, 654, 655, 658, 658t, 659, 659t, 660, 719
  rectus abdominis, 2, 19, 22, 24, 98, 102–104, 104t, 118, 119, 123, 136, 187, 189, 209, 218, 219, 222, 279, 351
  rectus capitis anterior, 332, 333, 774, 775, 775t, 785
  rectus capitis lateralis, 333, 350, 681, 774, 774t, 775, 785
  rectus capitis posterior
    major, 330–333, 350, 784, 785
    minor, 330–333, 350, 784, 785
  rectus femoris, 250, 372–376, 377t, 380–383, 395, 396, 399, 406, 407, 470
  rhomboid, 481, 512, 526
  rhomboid major, 321, 322, 513, 513t, 514, 519, 527
  rhomboid minor, 321, 322, 513, 513t, 514, 519, 529
  rotator cuff, 516–517, 517f, 534, 535
  rotatores, 328, 351, 783, 783t
    brevis, 327
    longus, 327

  salpingopharyngeus, 788, 788t
  sartorius, 250, 372–376, 377t, 379–382, 399, 406, 408, 434, 437, 470
  scalene
    anterior, 22–24, 72, 80, 82, 511, 756, 772–774, 774t, 775, 776, 807
    middle, 22, 24, 72, 333, 511, 756, 776, 777, 777t, 785, 807
    posterior, 22, 24, 756, 777, 777t
  scalenus minimus, 72
  semimembranosus, 379, 381, 384, 385, 387t, 388, 389, 396, 402, 403, 405, 408, 420, 421, 433–437, 470
  semispinalis, 18, 325
    capitis, 325, 328, 330–333, 350, 755, 783, 783t, 785, 806
    cervicis, 328, 330, 331, 783, 783t, 806
  semitendinosus, 379, 381, 384, 385, 387t, 388, 389, 396, 402, 403, 408, 419, 420, 434, 435, 437, 470
  serratus anterior, 2–4, 7, 22, 98, 100, 102, 103, 494–499, 499t, 502, 503, 508–511, 518, 526, 527, 529, 756
    nerve to, 510
  serratus posterior
    inferior, 21, 21t, 73, 169, 170, 322, 511
    superior, 21, 21t, 24, 322
  soleus, 381, 385, 402, 405, 422, 428, 432t, 433–437, 439, 472
  spinalis, 323, 351
  spinalis thoracis, 328
  splenius, 329t
    capitis, 323, 328, 331–333, 350, 755, 777, 777t, 783, 783t, 785, 806
    cervicis, 323, 328, 333, 783, 783t, 785
  sternocleidomastoid, 22, 332, 333, 350, 352, 499, 518, 662, 666, 716, 753, 753t, 759, 762, 763, 807
    artery, 763, 785, 806
    clavicular head, 24, 763
    sternal head, 24, 763
  sternohyoid, 22, 23, 350, 758, 759, 761, 761t, 762, 763, 766, 768, 785, 807
  sternothyroid, 22, 23, 758, 759, 761, 761t, 763, 807
  strap, 806, 810
  styloglossus, 350, 677, 677t, 681, 780, 785
  stylohyoid, 713, 721, 761, 761t, 763, 778, 787
  stylopharyngeus, 350, 681, 713, 720, 785, 787, 788, 788t, 789, 796
  subclavius, 22, 492, 498, 499t, 508–510, 756
  subcostales, 17, 21, 21t
  subscapularis, 481, 499, 502, 503, 508–511, 516, 517, 517t, 518, 522, 523, 525, 527, 530, 534, 537
    nerve to, 502

  supinator, 481, 540, 543, 552, 555, 557, 574, 575t, 577
  supraspinatus, 481, 499, 516, 517, 517t, 518, 519, 522, 523, 528, 529, 531, 537
  suspensory, 133
  temporalis, 634, 666, 667, 672, 672t, 719–721, 738, 739
    nerve to, 828, 829
  tensor fascia lata, 250, 275, 368, 373, 375, 376, 377t, 381, 383, 385, 386t, 399, 470
  tensor tympani, 711, 713
  tensor veli palatini, 681, 684, 684t, 702, 720, 795
  teres major, 320, 481, 499, 502, 509–512, 516, 517, 517t, 518, 521–523, 525–528, 534, 600
    nerve to, 502
  teres minor, 481, 503, 516, 517, 517t, 519, 527, 528, 537
  thenar, 480, 604, 605
  thyroarytenoid, 802, 802t, 803
  thyrohyoid, 761, 761t, 762, 763, 766, 768, 779
    nerve to, 763, 766, 779
  thyropharyngeus, 788, 788t
  tibialis anterior, 422, 423, 423t, 424, 426, 428, 431, 439, 447, 449, 452, 454, 457, 464, 472
  tibialis posterior, 432t, 433–439, 447, 448, 451, 452, 456–458, 464, 472
  of tongue, intrinsic, 806
  transverse, 677t
  transversospinalis, 329t
  transversus abdominis, 19, 22–24, 101, 103, 104, 104t, 105, 108, 109, 111, 112, 118, 119, 163, 170–172, 188, 334, 351
  transversus thoracis, 20, 21, 21t, 23, 73
  trapezius, 321, 331–333, 350, 499, 513, 513t, 514, 518, 519, 537, 753, 753t, 785, 806
    ascending part, 320, 321, 512, 514, 529
    descending part, 320, 321, 512, 514, 526, 529, 783, 783t
    transverse part, 320, 321, 512, 514, 529
  triceps brachii, 502, 519, 527, 543, 546, 547, 574
    lateral head, 481, 519, 520, 520t, 521, 523, 524, 526–528, 600
    long head, 481, 509–511, 518–520, 520t, 521–528, 534, 535, 600
    medial head, 481, 499, 510, 519, 520, 520t, 521–523, 525–527, 600
  uvular, 260, 684, 684t, 791
  vastus intermedius, 374–376, 377t, 380–382, 470
  vastus lateralis, 250, 275, 373–376, 377t, 380–383, 406, 409, 470
  vastus medialis, 375, 376, 377t, 380–382, 385, 406–408, 419–421, 434, 470
    nerve to, 373, 382

vertical, 677t
zygomaticus major, 626, 662, 721
zygomaticus minor, 630
Myelogram, 337
Myocardium, 53, 58, 61
Myometrium, 279–283
Myotome, 348, 349

Nail bed, nerve to, 578
Nasal bone, 611–613, 622, 650, 690, 691, 695, 699, 721
Nasion, 610, 612
Nasopharynx, 128, 621, 718–720, 790, 794–797, 810
Navicular, 427, 431, 449, 454, 459, 461, 462, 464–466
  fossa, 267, 444, 452, 453, 458
  tuberosity, 439
Neck
  arteries, 764, 764t–765t, 765
  blood supply, 649
  bones, 750, 751
  cartilage, 749–751
  Doppler ultrasound, 809
  fascia, 747
  lymphatic drainage, 716
  magnetic resonance imaging, 806, 809
  median anatomical section, 808
  regions, 752, 752t
  root of, 67, 772–773
  transverse anatomical sections, 807
  veins, 716
    deep, 767
    superficial, 748
Nephron, 167
Nerve
  abducent, 640, 644, 645, 652, 654, 656, 812–814, 815t, 821, 822, 822t, 823, 841, 841t, 843
  alveolar
    anterior superior, 692, 826, 827
    inferior, 669, 681, 687, 828, 829
    middle superior, 826, 827
    posterior superior, 671, 826, 827
    superior, 687
  anal, inferior, 214, 231, 261, 269, 270
  anococcygeal, 206
  auricular
    great, 627, 662, 754, 762
    posterior, 186, 189, 629, 662
  auriculotemporal, 631t, 662, 663, 668, 828, 829
  axillary, 345, 481, 506, 507t, 509, 510, 527, 528, 534, 536
  buccal, 629, 630, 631t, 662, 668, 669, 828, 829
  calcaneal, medial, 457
  cardiac, 67
    cervical, 68
      inferior, 68, 84
      middle, 68
    cavernous, 231
  cervical, 629, 639
    transverse, 746, 754
  ciliary
    long, 652, 825
    short, 652, 825
  clunial
    inferior, 270, 359, 392t
    medial, 359, 392t
    superior, 359, 392t
  coccygeal, 206, 207, 207t

cochlear, 709, 715, 734, 735, 832–833
cranial. See Cranial nerves
cutaneous
  of abdomen, lateral, 7
  of arm
    inferior lateral, 484, 485t, 527
    medial, 484, 485t, 506, 507t
    posterior, 484, 485t, 509, 510, 525
    superior lateral, 484, 485t, 528
  of forearm
    lateral, 484, 485t, 521, 538, 539, 549, 579, 600
    medial, 484, 485t, 506, 507t, 508, 521, 538, 600
    posterior, 484, 485t, 521, 527, 578, 579, 600
  lateral dorsal, 359
  of lower limb, 359
  pectoral
    anterior, 3
    lateral, 3, 7
  perforating, 207, 207t
  superficial back, 514
  of thigh
    anterior, 372
    lateral, 163, 172, 173, 359, 372
    posterior, 218, 250, 261, 269, 270, 359, 392t, 399
  of upper limb, 484, 485t
dental, inferior, 828, 829
digital
  common palmar, 566, 567, 569
  common plantar, 444
  plantar, 443
  proper palmar, 561, 563, 566, 567, 569
  proper plantar, 444
dorsal
  of clitoris, 254, 269, 270, 272, 274
  of penis, 116, 202, 231, 254, 264, 265, 267
ethmoidal
  anterior, 638, 653, 692, 825
  posterior, 638, 653, 825
facial, 640–642, 663, 701, 708–713, 720, 734, 738, 739, 762, 812–814, 815t, 830, 831, 841, 841t, 843
  branches, 627, 629, 634, 662
  motor root, 830
femoral, 118, 163, 172, 173, 212, 218, 222, 250, 275, 345, 356, 358t, 359, 372, 373, 382, 399
femoral cutaneous, posterior, 206, 207, 207t
fibular
  common, 345, 356, 358t, 402, 403, 409, 424, 424t, 425, 428, 434–437
  deep, 218, 270, 345, 356, 358t, 359, 424, 424t, 425, 426, 431, 457, 472
  superficial, 270, 345, 356, 358t, 359, 424, 424t, 425, 428, 429
frontal, 631t, 656, 825
genitofemoral, 116, 163, 172, 173, 215
  femoral branch, 109, 112, 359

genital branch, 110–112, 359
glossopharyngeal, 335, 640–642, 663, 680, 681, 720, 734, 766, 785–787, 789, 796, 812–814, 815t, 834–835, 841, 843
gluteal
  inferior, 206, 207, 207t, 250, 392t
  superior, 206, 207, 207t, 392t
hypogastric, 230, 231, 249
hypoglossal, 335, 640, 641, 662, 663, 667, 680, 681, 720, 763, 766, 779, 780, 785, 786, 812–814, 815t, 839, 841, 841t, 843
iliohypogastric, 100, 101, 103, 107, 108, 112, 163, 170–173, 359, 382, 496
ilioinguinal, 101–103, 107, 110–112, 116, 163, 172, 173, 264, 359, 382
incisive, 828, 829
infraorbital, 629, 630, 651, 671, 692, 700, 719, 720, 826, 827
infratrochlear, 629, 630, 631t, 653, 825
intercostal, 17, 19, 20, 22, 23, 72, 80–83, 85, 334, 339
  collateral branches, 17, 18
  lateral cutaneous branch, 19, 502, 511
  lateral pectoral cutaneous branch, 494
  posterior, 18
intercostobrachial, 3, 7, 100, 484, 485t, 494, 496, 502, 509, 511
intermediate, 709, 830
interosseous
  anterior, 480, 557, 602
  posterior, 345, 481, 543, 577, 602
labial
  anterior, 270
  posterior, 270
lacrimal, 629, 630, 631t, 652, 656, 701, 825
laryngeal
  recurrent, 67, 807
    left, 42, 49, 67–69, 81, 84, 85, 770, 771
    relationship to aortic arches, 67
    right, 42, 68, 72, 84, 85, 770, 772, 789, 800
  superior, 763, 766, 770, 789, 800, 807
lingual, 669, 680, 681, 779, 780, 797, 828, 829
mandibular, 638, 640, 644, 645, 669, 671, 681, 687, 720, 824t, 828–829
  marginal, 629
masseteric, 828, 829
maxillary, 638, 640, 644, 645, 671, 692, 699–701, 824t, 826–827
median, 345, 480, 484, 485t, 502, 508, 521, 525, 539–541, 549, 555, 556, 558, 559, 567, 570, 571, 579, 591, 593, 600, 602, 604, 605
  lateral root, 508

medial root, 508
  palmar branch, 579
  palmar cutaneous branch, 559
  palmar digital branches, 484, 578
  recurrent branch, 559, 561, 563, 566, 567
meningeal, recurrent, 304
mental, 629, 631t, 828, 829
musculocutaneous, 345, 480, 502, 506, 507t, 508, 510, 521, 525, 540, 600
mylohyoid, 681, 763, 778, 779, 828, 829
nasal, external, 631t
nasociliary, 652–654, 656, 825
nasopalatine, 683, 692, 702, 826, 827
obturator, 118, 172, 173, 202, 205, 212, 250, 345, 356, 358t, 359, 372, 382, 394, 399
occipital, 333, 785
  greater, 330, 331, 333, 784
  lesser, 754
oculomotor, 640, 641, 643–645, 652, 654, 656, 734, 812–814, 815t, 821, 822, 822t, 823, 841, 841t, 842, 844
olfactory, 640, 692, 812–814, 815t, 818, 841
ophthalmic, 640, 644, 824t, 825
optic, 640, 641, 652, 653, 655–657, 660, 719, 721, 727, 728, 732–734, 738, 739, 812–814, 815t, 819, 820, 841, 842
palatine
  greater, 671, 683, 692, 702, 826, 827
  lesser, 671, 683, 692, 702, 826, 827
pectoral
  lateral, 500, 503, 506, 507t, 508, 509
  medial, 500, 503, 506, 507t, 508, 509
perineal, 202, 231, 265, 269
petrosal
  deep, 701, 831
  greater, 701, 831
  lesser, 834, 835
pharyngeal, 692, 826, 827
phrenic, 67, 72, 80, 755, 762, 772, 773, 807
  left, 25, 42, 48, 73, 81
  right, 25, 42, 48, 73
plantar, 451
  lateral, 345, 356, 359, 438, 443, 446, 456, 458
  medial, 345, 356, 359, 438, 443, 446, 456, 458
pterygopalatine, 700–702
pudendal, 206, 207, 207t, 212, 214, 218, 222, 230, 231, 246, 250, 265, 269, 270, 274, 392t, 399
radial, 345, 481, 502, 506, 507t, 509, 510, 521, 527, 528, 540, 549, 579, 600
  deep branch, 481, 540, 555–557, 577
  dorsal digital branch, 569, 578
  superficial branch, 481, 484, 485t, 540, 555–557, 559, 578, 582, 584, 602

Nerve—*continued*
  rectal
    inferior, 202, 278
    superior, 214
  saphenous, 345, 359, 373, 382,
      438, 457
  scapular, dorsal, 506, 507t, 529
  sciatic, 172, 173, 206, 207, 207t,
      212, 216, 218, 222, 230,
      250, 268, 275, 345, 356,
      358t, 390, 391, 392t, 399,
      470
  scrotal, posterior, 231, 261
  spinal, 123, 169, 334, 336,
      338–340, 343, 344, 352, 481
  spinal accessory, 333, 334, 511,
      529, 642, 662, 663, 667,
      720, 755, 762, 763, 766,
      785, 807, 812–814, 815t,
      838, 841, 841t, 843
  splanchnic, 17, 85, 123, 125
    greater, 73, 80–83, 85, 176–178,
      179t, 183
    least, 176–178, 179t
    lesser, 82, 176–178, 179t, 183
    lumbar, 176–178, 179t, 214,
      230, 231, 246
    pelvic, 176–178, 179t, 206, 207,
      207t, 210, 214, 230, 231,
      246, 249
    sacral, 176–178, 179t, 231
  subclavian, 506, 507t
  subcostal, 85, 100, 101, 163,
      170–173, 359, 496
  suboccipital, 330, 331, 784
  subscapular
    lower, 506, 507t, 508–511
    upper, 503, 506, 507t, 509–511
  supraclavicular, 3, 484, 485t, 494,
      746, 754
  supraorbital, 629, 630, 631t, 651,
      825
  suprascapular, 481, 509, 510, 528,
      529, 537
  supratrochlear, 629, 630, 631t, 651,
      825
  sural, 359, 403, 430, 457
  sural cutaneous
    lateral, 359
    medial, 359, 434
  temporal, 629
    deep, 668
  tentorial, 638
  thoracic, 17, 112
    lateral, 508
    long, 7, 100, 496, 502, 503, 506,
      507t, 508, 509, 511
    posterior ramus, 18
  thoracoabdominal, 100–102, 496
  thoracodorsal, 502, 506, 507t,
      508–510
  tibial, 345, 356, 358t, 359, 402,
      403, 434–438, 443, 451,
      457, 472
    anterior recurrent, 425
    posterior, 269
  trigeminal, 631, 631t, 640–643,
      812–814, 815t, 824, 841,
      842, 844
    cutaneous branches, 630
    groove for, 615
    mandibular division, 824t,
      828–829
    maxillary division, 824t,
      826–827

  motor root, 645, 646, 734
  ophthalmic division, 824t, 825
  sensory root, 644–646, 734
  spinal tract, 734
  trochlear, 640–645, 652, 656,
      812–814, 815t, 821, 822,
      822t, 823, 841
  tympanic, 710, 834–835
  ulnar, 345, 476, 477, 480, 484,
      485t, 502, 506, 507t, 508,
      521, 525, 527, 540, 542,
      543, 549, 555, 556, 558,
      559, 566, 571, 579, 600,
      602, 604, 605
    communicating branch, 567
    deep branch, 480, 567, 570, 571,
      591
    dorsal branch, 484, 559, 578,
      582, 587
    dorsal cutaneous branch, 566
    dorsal digital branch, 578
    palmar branch, 579
    palmar digital branch, 578
    superficial branch, 484, 567, 571
  ulnar collateral, 525
  vagus, 181, 640–642, 662, 663,
      667, 720, 766, 771, 772,
      785, 807, 812–814, 815t,
      836–837, 841, 843
    in abdomen, 181
    auricular branch, 703
    inferior cardiac branch, 772
    left, 25, 42, 48, 49, 65, 67–69,
      81, 84, 85, 773, 836
    right, 25, 42, 48, 67, 68, 72, 80,
      84, 85, 773, 836
  vestibular, 709, 715, 734, 735,
      832–833
  vestibulocochlear, 640–642, 709,
      715, 734, 735, 738, 739,
      812–814, 815t, 832–833,
      841, 843
  zygomatic, 630, 631t, 700, 701,
      826, 827
  zygomaticofacial, 630
Nerve blocks, during pregnancy, 247
Nerve point of neck, 754
Nipple, 5–7, 100, 496, 497
Node
  atrioventricular, 64
  lymph. *See* Lymph nodes
  sinoatrial, 64
  superficial parotid, 762
Nose
  bones, 690
  cartilage, 690
  lateral wall, 623
  surface anatomy, 690
Nostril, 690
Notch
  acetabular, 396
  cardiac, 26, 32, 34, 35, 96
  cardial, 129
  clavicular, 12
  costal, 12
  fibular, 652
  interarytenoid, 790
  intertragic, 703
  jugular, 10, 12, 499
  mandibular, 612, 664
  mastoid, 615, 625
  notch, 625
  pterygoid, 624
  radial, 544, 548
  sacrococcygeal, 313

  sciatic
    greater, 197, 312, 381, 397
    lesser, 197, 202, 312, 381, 397
  supraorbital, 650
  suprascapular, 518, 532
  suprasternal, 2, 495
  tentorial, 643
  trochlear, 544, 546, 547
  ulnar, 589
  vertebral, 289, 302
Nuchal region, 333
  superior, 350
Nucleus
  amygdaloid, 726, 727, 729, 741
  caudate, 727, 729–734, 740–742
  cingulate, 742
  cochlear, 735
  cranial nerve, 816–817
  dentate, 740
  geniculate
    lateral, 741, 820
    medial, 741
  habenular, 731
  lentiform, 726, 727, 730–734, 740,
      741
  red, 732, 733, 738, 739, 741
  reticular, 741
  thalamic
    anterior, 741
    lateral, 741
    medial, 741
  vestibular, 735
Nucleus pulposus, 306–308

Occipital bone, 350, 608, 609, 613,
      617, 619, 664, 738, 739
  basilar part, 617, 618, 795
  lateral part, 618
  squamous part, 614, 617, 618
Olecranon, 519, 521, 524, 526, 527,
      542–544, 546–549, 574,
      600
Olive, 639, 734
Omentum
  greater, 119–121, 124, 136, 137
  lesser, 119–121, 123–126, 147, 148
Opening
  aortic, 172, 173
  coronary sinus, 56, 64
  esophageal, 125, 172
  saphenous, 103, 107, 112, 368,
      370, 371
Ora serrata, 660
Orbicular zone, 395
Orbit
  arteries, 657, 657t
  lateral aspect, 654–655
  muscles, 658–659, 658t, 659t, 821
  nerves, 656, 821
  veins, 656
Orifice
  of appendix, 139
  atrioventricular
    left, 58, 59
    right, 56
  cardial, 129
  ileocecal, 139
  maxillary, 695, 696
  pyloric, 129
  ureteric, 234
  urethral, 271–273
    external, 216, 253, 255
    internal, 216
  vaginal, 255, 271–273
Oropharynx, 128, 721, 790, 810

Os trigonum, 467
Ossicles, 704, 707
Otolith, 715
Ovary, 208, 232, 234, 240, 280–283
  fetal, 114
  left, 122

Pain, referred, 180
Palate, 28, 682–684, 808
  hard, 623, 682, 684t, 697, 719,
      721, 743
  soft, 682, 684t, 713, 721, 743, 790,
      792, 794, 810
Palatine bone, 617, 623, 664, 682,
      691, 695, 700, 702
  horizontal plate, 615, 682
  orbital process, 650
  pyramidal process, 682
Palm
  compartments, 562
  deep dissection, 570–571
  fascia, 560, 562
  muscular layers, 564
  spaces, 562
  superficial dissection, 566–567
  synovial sheaths, 568
Pancreas, 96, 97, 120–122, 125–128,
      131, 135, 145, 152, 154,
      155, 160, 162, 188
  blood supply, 135
  body, 125, 133, 134, 156, 187
  dorsal, 157
  head, 127, 133, 134, 153, 156, 187,
      189
  lymphatic drainage, 184
  neck, 127, 133, 156
  relationships, 134
  tail, 125, 133, 134, 156, 162, 164,
      187, 189
    artery to, 135
  ultrasound, 190
  uncinate process, 187, 189
  ventral, 157
Papilla
  inferior lacrimal, 651
  lingual, 676
  major duodenal, 133, 156
  minor duodenal, 133, 156
  renal, 166, 167
Paracolic gutter, 122
Parietal bone, 609, 611, 613, 614,
      617, 619, 634, 636
Parotid bed, 666
Parotid region, 662–663
Pars tensa, 706
Patella, 354, 355, 374, 375, 380, 406,
      407, 410, 411, 420–422
  bipartite, 467
  radiograph, 418
Pecten, anal, 211
Pectoral girdle, 530
Pectoral region
  female, 4
  male, 2–3, 494, 495
  superficial dissection, 3, 4
  surface anatomy, 2
Pedicle, 289, 296, 301–303, 310, 334,
      337
Peduncle
  cerebellar, 734, 735, 737–739, 816
  cerebral, 732, 733, 742
Pelvic brim, 200
Pelvic girdle, 197
  female, 195, 198t–199t
  male, 194, 198t–199t

Pelvis
  anatomical position, 197
  angiography, 277
  bifid, 168
  bones, 196, 311
  divisions, 196
  female, 205, 208, 232–251
    arteries, 241–243, 243t
    autonomic nerves, 248–249
    hysterosalpingogram, 284
    innervation, 246–249
    laparoscopic view, 233
    lymphatic drainage, 244–245,
      245t
    magnetic resonance imaging,
      279–282
    organs, 232–239
    subperitoneal region, 250–251
    supporting and
      compressor/sphincteric
      muscles, 260
    transverse section, 249
    ultrasound, 282–283
    veins, 242
    vessels, 240–243
  floor, 203–205, 203t
  greater, 128
  ligaments, 200, 201, 314, 315
  male, 204, 209, 216–231
    arteries, 224, 225, 225t, 226
    innervation, 230–231
    lymphatic drainage, 228–229,
      229t
    magnetic resonance imaging,
      276–279
    organs, 216–223
    posterior view, 218–219
    supporting and
      compressor/sphincteric
      muscles, 260
    transrectal ultrasound, 223
    transverse sections, 222
    veins, 224, 227
    vessels, 224–227
  posterior, neurovascular structures,
    212
  radiograph, 311
  renal, 143, 165, 166, 187
  viscera, 246, 247, 251
  walls, 203t, 204–205
Penis, 264
  body, 252, 264, 266, 268
  bulb of, 209, 216, 217, 262,
    266–268, 276, 277, 279
  corona, 252, 264
  cross sections, 267
  crura, 262, 266, 267, 276, 277
  distal, urethral aspect, 268
  dorsal artery, 116, 254, 264, 267
  dorsal nerve, 116, 202, 231, 254,
    264, 265, 267
  dorsal vein, 116, 216, 224, 254,
    264, 267, 268
  fascia, 258, 265
  fundiform ligament, 107
  glans, 116, 216, 217, 252, 264,
    266–268
  layers, 265
  nerves, 265
  prepuce, 264, 265
  root, 252, 264, 266, 268, 276, 277
  septum, 267
  subcutaneous tissue, 258
  surface anatomy, 264
  suspensory ligament, 112, 116, 264

Perforated area
  anterior, 734
  posterior, 734
Pericardium, 48–51, 53, 67
  fibrous, 25, 29, 51, 65, 66
  magnetic resonance imaging,
    88–89, 91
  posterior relationships, 65
  relationship to sternum, 48
  serous, 29, 50, 51
    parietal layer, 25, 51, 65
    visceral layer, 25, 50
  subdivisions, 29
Pericranium, 634, 636, 743
Perilymph
  cochlear, 738, 739
  vestibular, 738, 739
Perineum, 196
  compartments, 254–255, 258, 259
  female, 269–275
    compartments, 259
    fascia, 259
    innervation, 270
    lymphatic drainage, 244–245,
      245t
    magnetic resonance imaging,
      279–282
    surface anatomy, 253
  male
    compartments, 258
    dissection, 261–263
    fascia, 258
    innervation, 230–231
    lymphatic drainage, 228–229,
      229t
    magnetic resonance imaging,
      276–279
    surface anatomy, 252
  muscles, 256t–257t, 257
Peripheral nerves, 345
Peristaltic wave, 132
Peritoneum, 129, 152, 153, 157, 212,
    218, 219
  female pelvis, 208
  male pelvis, 209
  parietal, 105, 118, 120, 121, 124,
    136, 164
  of posterior abdominal cavity, 144
  visceral, 120, 121, 124, 164
Perpendicular plate of ethmoid bone,
    610, 690
Pes hippocampi, 741
Phalanx, 431, 476–479, 574, 598
  distal, 427, 444, 466, 552, 574,
    586, 588, 589, 595, 599
  middle, 427, 444, 466, 552, 588,
    589, 595, 599
  proximal, 427, 444, 466, 552, 569,
    574, 586, 588, 589, 595,
    599
Pharyngeal constrictor
  inferior, 770, 786–788, 788t, 789,
    806, 807
  middle, 786–788, 788t, 789
  superior, 712, 713, 786–788, 788t,
    789, 791, 792, 795, 797
Pharyngotympanic tube, 28, 615,
    681, 695, 704, 705,
    710–713, 720, 785, 790,
    794
Pharynx, 28, 128, 738, 739, 742, 743,
    790–791, 806, 808
  cavity, 678
  external, 786–787, 789
  internal, 790–791

  muscles, 681, 788, 788t, 797
Pinching movements, 596, 597
Pinna, 738, 739
Pisiform, 552, 558, 559, 566, 571,
    587–589, 591–594, 599,
    604
Placenta, 238, 239
Plane
  interspinous, 128
  orbitomeatal, 612, 613
  transpyloric, 128
Plate
  cribriform, 618, 619, 743, 808
  horizontal, 615, 617, 682
  perpendicular, of ethmoid bone,
    610, 690
  pterygoid
    lateral, 617, 624, 702, 712, 720
    medial, 617, 624, 702
  tarsal
    inferior, 629, 630
    superior, 629, 630
  tympanic, 615
Plateau, tibial, 411
Pleura, 129
  cervical, 66–69
  costal, 73
  diaphragmatic, 73
  mediastinal, 73
  parietal, 20, 28, 72, 78, 83, 123,
    334
    cervical, 773
    costal part, 80, 81
    extent of, 30–31
    mediastinal part, 25, 80, 81
    sternal reflection, 72
    surface markings, 31t, 45
  visceral, 28, 31t
Plexus
  abdominopelvic, 176–178, 179t
  aortic, 84, 85, 230
  arterial, pial, 342
  brachial, 22, 82, 503, 756, 757,
    776, 807
    branches, 507t
    illustration, 506
    inferior trunk, 72
    lateral cord, 508, 510
    medial cord, 508, 510
    posterior cord, 509, 510
  cardiac, 68, 84
  carotid
    external, 717
    internal, 701, 717
  celiac, 176, 177, 181
  cervical, 762, 807
  choroid, 639, 727, 729, 731–733,
    740
  coccygeal, 206, 207, 207t
  esophageal, 42, 65, 80, 85
  hypogastric
    inferior, 176, 177, 214, 230, 231,
      246, 249
    superior, 145, 214, 215, 230,
      231, 246
  intermesenteric, 176, 177
  lumbar, 172
    nerves, 173
  lymphatic
    deep, 43
    of palm, 489
    subareolar, 9
    subpleural, 43
  mesenteric
    inferior, 176, 177

    superior, 176, 177
  ovarian, 246
  para-aortic, 214, 246
  pelvic, 214, 246
  periarterial, sympathetic, 805
  pharyngeal, 787
  phrenic, inferior, 163
  prostatic, 230, 231
  pulmonary, 42, 67
    anterior, 49, 68
    left, 84
    right, 84
  renal, 176, 177
  sacral, 205, 206, 207t, 214, 246
  subtrapezial, 514
  suprarenal, 176, 177
  tympanic, 834–835
  ureterovaginal, 249
  uterine, 246
  uterovaginal, 246
  venous
    basilar, 639
    pampiniform, 113, 116, 216,
      264
    pial, 342
    prostatic, 222, 224, 279
    pterygoid, 639
    rectal, 211, 224
    uterine, 242
    vaginal, 242
    vertebral, 309, 333, 339, 342,
      639, 785, 807
    vesical, 224, 242
  vesical, 230, 231
Plica semilunaris, 651
Pole
  frontal, 728, 742
  occipital, 728, 742
  temporal, 639, 742
Pons, 639, 722, 723, 734, 738–740,
    742, 743, 808
Popliteal region, 354, 405
Porta hepatis, 124, 147, 154, 155
Portacaval system, 161
Portal confluence, 187, 189
Portal triad, 123–125, 134, 147,
    149–153, 162
Pouch
  rectouterine, 120, 208, 232, 233,
    238, 250
  rectovesical, 121, 209, 215–217,
    219, 279
  superficial perineal, 258, 259
  vesicouterine, 208, 232, 279
Precuneus, 728
Pregnancy, pelvic visceral innervation
    during, 247
Process
  accessory, 300, 303
  acromion, 532, 535
  alveolar
    of mandible, 611, 613, 664
    of maxilla, 611, 613, 617, 721
  articular, 289
    inferior, 296, 297, 300, 302, 303,
      310
    superior, 15
  axillary, of breast, 4
  caudate, 147, 148
  ciliary, 660
  clinoid
    anterior, 618, 619, 624, 702
    posterior, 615, 618, 619, 624,
      643, 702
  condylar, of mandible, 612

Process—*continued*
  coracoid, 27, 498, 508, 511, 518, 522, 523, 525, 530–532, 535, 536, 598
  coronoid, 544, 546, 548, 549, 552, 613, 667, 720
  digital, of fat, 269, 271, 274
  frontal
    of maxilla, 611, 613, 650, 690, 721
    of zygomatic bone, 611, 613
  jugular, 617
  lateral, 433, 444, 450, 690
  mamillary, 300, 303
  mastoid, 350, 352, 609, 612, 614–617, 711–713, 720, 750, 785
  medial, 433, 444, 450, 456
  palatine, 615, 650, 682
  pterygoid, 624, 699, 701
  spinous, 11, 14, 88–89, 123, 187, 286, 288, 289, 295–297, 300–303, 310, 311, 330, 331, 350, 351, 750, 751, 810
  styloid, 552, 574, 585, 587, 589–592, 612, 614–617, 625, 663, 681, 712, 713, 720, 785, 797
  superior articular, 197, 296, 300, 302, 303, 310, 338
  supracondylar, 541
  transverse, 14–18, 187, 288–290, 295–297, 300–303, 310–313, 324, 339, 350, 351, 751, 807
    atlas, 750
    lumbar, 171, 200
    vertebral, 132
  uncal, 296
  uncinate, 127, 133, 134, 187, 189, 295, 296
  vaginal, 624
  xiphoid, 2, 10, 12, 29, 48, 98, 128, 187, 300, 499
  zygomatic, 611, 613, 617, 625, 664
Prominence, laryngeal, 749
Prominens, vertebral, 512
Promontory, 708, 710
  sacral, 196, 197, 199, 313
Protrusion, synovial, 395
Protuberance
  external occipital, 295, 328, 330, 331, 350, 613–615, 617, 743, 750, 785, 808
  internal occipital, 618, 619, 621, 743, 808
  mental, 610, 612, 664
Pterion, 612, 635
Pubic bone, 234, 280, 281
Pubis, 196, 197, 202, 222, 250, 312, 397
  anterior aspect, 197
  body, 197, 311, 312, 380
  pecten, 197–199, 312, 380
  ramus, 380
    inferior, 197, 199, 397
    superior, 106, 197, 198, 311, 312, 380, 396
Pulp, tooth, 687
Pulse, carotid, 768
Pulvinar, 730, 732, 733, 735
Punctum, inferior lacrimal, 651
Pupil, 650, 651, 660
Putamen, 732, 733, 740, 741

Pyelogram, 165
Pylorus, of stomach, 96, 125, 128, 129, 132, 134, 156, 189
Pyramid, 639, 708, 734, 738–740
  renal, 166

Radiations, optic, 726, 728, 729, 732–734
Radiograph
  ankle, 453, 454
  biliary passages, 158
  chest, 27
  colon, 138
  cranium, 608, 609, 620–621, 697, 698
  duodenum, 132
  elbow joint, 544, 547
  esophagus, 132
  foot, 453
  forearm, 545
  glenohumeral (shoulder) joint, 536
  hand, 586, 589
  hip joint, 398
  hyoid bone, 750
  knee, 418, 420
  pelvis, 311
  pregnant uterus, 239
  stomach, 132
  teeth, 685
  uterus and uterine tube, 284
  vertebrae
    cervical, 292, 296, 297, 750
    lumbar, 293, 302, 310
    thoracic, 310
Radius, 476–479, 518, 519, 523, 545, 548, 552, 557, 574, 586, 590, 591, 593, 594, 598, 602
  distal end, 592, 598
  dorsal tubercle, 574, 581, 586
  dysplasia, 131
  head, 518, 519, 544, 546, 547, 549, 552, 574
  neck, 544, 546, 547
  proximal, 598
  styloid process, 552, 574, 585, 589–592
  ulnar notch, 589
Ramus
  anterior, 17, 20, 333, 336, 338, 339, 345, 351, 352, 511, 642, 757, 773, 785
    anterior abdominal branches, 103
    sacral, 202, 205, 210, 212, 249
  ischiopubic, 197–199, 263, 267, 273, 311, 312, 380
  of ischium, 197, 199, 312, 397
  of mandible, 350, 608, 610–613, 664
  posterior, 17, 20, 83, 304, 327, 330, 331, 334, 336, 338, 339, 345, 352, 514, 642
  pubic, 380
    inferior, 197, 199, 397
    superior, 106, 197, 198, 311, 312, 380, 396
Ramus communicans, 17, 20, 80, 81, 83, 334, 339
  gray, 173, 230
  white, 230
Raphe
  perineal, 252
  pharyngeal, 333, 785
  pterygomandibular, 797

scrotal, 252
Recess
  anterior, of ischioanal fossa, 118
  apical, 808
  articular, superior, 312, 313
  costodiaphragmatic, 27, 28, 73, 78, 90, 118, 119, 123–125, 163, 164
  costomediastinal, 29, 73
  epitympanic, 708
  hepatorenal, 123, 147, 152
  ileocecal
    inferior, 139
    superior, 139
  pharyngeal, 713, 720, 790
  piriform, 790, 807
  sacciform, 548, 591
  spheno-ethmoidal, 694, 696
  splenic, 164
  subphrenic, 147
  superior, 148
  suprapineal, 741
Rectum, 97, 120–122, 128, 138, 160, 205, 209, 212, 216, 222, 233, 250, 254, 275–281
  ampulla, 208, 232
  autonomic stimulation effects, 230t
  innervation, 214
  in situ, 215
  vasculature, 213
Referred pain, 180
Reflex
  calcaneal (Achilles), 357
  quadriceps, 357
Renal column, 166
Renal corpuscle, 167
Renal medulla, 166, 167
Respiration, muscles of, 24, 24t
Respiratory system, 28
Rete testis, 117
Retina, 660
Retinaculum, 398
  extensor, 368, 458, 576, 577, 581, 582, 587
    inferior, 422, 424, 426, 430, 431
    superior, 422, 425
  fibular
    inferior, 425, 430
    superior, 430, 434
  flexor, 434, 436–438, 493, 554, 564, 567, 568, 570, 571, 591–593, 604, 605
  patellar, 410
    lateral, 375, 406
    medial, 375, 406
Retroinguinal passage, 372, 373
Rib, 123, 290
  anomalies, 16
  atypical, 13
  bicipital, 16
  bifid, 16
  cervical, 16
  costovertebral articulations, 14
  eighth, 10, 11, 13, 18, 26, 511
  eleventh, 10, 11, 13, 164, 165
  facets, 13, 14
  fifth, 10, 11
  first, 10, 11, 13, 23, 24, 26, 27, 39, 66–69, 75, 508, 530, 536, 773
  floating, 11
  fourth, 10, 11, 22, 26, 511
  head, 13–15, 88–89
  neck, 13
  ninth, 10, 11, 19, 164

second, 10, 11, 13, 23, 24, 511
  seventh, 10, 11, 14, 18, 124, 301
  shaft, 13
  sixth, 10, 11, 13, 14, 26
  tenth, 10, 11, 26, 124, 163, 164
  third, 10, 11
  tubercle, 13, 14
  twelfth, 10, 11, 13, 164, 165, 169–172, 174, 310
  typical, 13
Ridge
  supraepicondylar, 547
    lateral, 519, 544, 552, 574
    medial, 518, 544, 552
  transverse, 12
Rima glottidis, 799, 804, 806
Ring
  femoral, 371, 372
  fibrous, 59
  inguinal
    deep, 108, 109, 111, 112, 118, 233
    superficial, 102, 106, 107, 110, 116, 264, 372, 373
  tendinous, common, 656
  tracheal, 749, 807
  umbilical, 105

Sac
  dural, 83, 300, 334, 336–337
  endolymphatic, 714
  greater, 120, 122, 123
  lacrimal, 651
  pericardial, 51, 73, 80, 81, 119
Saccule, 714, 715, 807
Sacrum, 165, 194–198, 202, 208–210, 232, 278–282, 312, 313, 316
  ala, 196–198, 310, 311, 313, 317
  body, 197, 198
  cornu, 194, 195
  overview, 286, 288
  promontory, 196, 197, 199
Scalp, 634, 636
Scaphoid, 552, 559, 574, 585, 586, 588, 589, 591–594, 599
Scapula, 10, 11, 97, 476–479, 503, 518, 519, 537, 598
  anastomoses, 487
  coracoid process, 498, 518
  inferior angle, 11, 511, 518, 522, 523, 535
  lateral border, 535, 536
  medial border, 512, 522
  movements, 515
  spine, 11, 518, 519, 527, 529, 532, 536
  superior angle, 511, 518, 523, 529, 536
  superior border, 536
  vertebral border, 536
Scapular region
  dorsal, 528
  surface anatomy, 526
Sclera, 661
Scrotum, 113, 117, 216, 252, 264
  fascia, 258
  lymphatic drainage, 117
Seminal vesicle, 118, 278
Seminiferous tubule, 117
Septum
  interatrial, 58, 61
  intermuscular
    anterior, 369, 472
    anteromedial, 470

fascial, 457
lateral, 409, 470, 493, 521, 543, 600
medial, 493, 521, 525, 540, 543, 600
posterior, 369, 437, 470, 472
posteromedial, 470
transverse, 369, 436–438
interventricular, 57, 58
inferior, 3-D volume reconstruction and CT angiogram, 92–93
magnetic resonance imaging, 88–89
membranous part, 59, 61
muscular part, 59, 64
membranous, 63
nasal, 690–693, 697, 719–721, 738, 739, 743, 790, 808
orbital, 630
inferior, 629, 630
superior, 629, 630
rectovesical, 216, 263
prostatic, 220
Septum pellucidum, 723, 727–733, 740, 743
Sesamoid, 443, 445, 447, 463, 589, 606
anomalous, 467
lateral, 439
medial, 439, 452
Sheath
arachnoid, 655
axillary, 502, 503
carotid, 678, 747, 769
digital, fibrous, 443, 446, 561, 566–569, 571
dural, 655
femoral, 112, 371, 373
hypogastric, 218, 251
pial, 655
rectus
anterior, 102–104, 107, 496, 497
layers, 105
posterior, 101, 103, 112, 118
synovial, 561, 568
tendon, intertubercular, 532
Shoulder region, 476, 477
Sialogram, 680
Sinus
aortic, 55, 59
cavernous, 639, 644, 740
confluence of, 724
coronal, 50
coronary, 47, 53
opening, 56, 64
valve of, 56
frontal, 620, 638, 695–698, 743
intercavernous, 639
lactiferous, 4, 5
maxillary, 620, 621, 691, 695–698, 700, 719, 720, 738, 739
occipital, 639
pericardial
oblique, 29, 60
anterior wall, 50
posterior wall, 51
transverse, 29, 49–51, 60
petrosal
groove, 618
inferior, 615, 639
superior, 615, 639
renal, 166, 171
sagittal
inferior, 636, 638, 639

superior, 618, 636–639, 724, 738–740, 743
sigmoid, 615, 619, 639, 713, 767
sphenoidal, 621, 624, 695–698, 702, 713, 721
sphenoparietal, 639
straight, 638, 639, 724, 732, 733, 738–740, 742
tonsil, 792, 793
transverse, 619, 639, 742
groove, 618, 619
right, 639
venous, scleral, 660
Sinus venarum, 56
Sinusoids, 151
Siphon, carotid, 740
Skin, 105, 743
Skull base, 350, 785
Small intestine, 96, 97, 128, 162, 187–189, 352
interior, 136
lymphatic drainage, 184
Smooth muscle, 256t, 257, 274
Somatic nervous system, 343
Space
infracolic, 122
intercostal
contents, 20
eighth, 10
inferior, 18, 19
ninth, 11
vertebral ends, 17, 18
intervertebral disc, 302
lateral pharyngeal, 713, 720
midpalmar, 562, 606
palmar, 606
perivertebral, 218
quadrangular, 510, 527, 528, 537
retromammary, 5
retropharyngeal, 350, 678, 807, 808
retropubic, 208, 209, 216, 218–220, 232
subaponeurotic areolar, 606
subarachnoid, 286, 337, 352, 655, 724, 738, 739, 806, 810
subhepatic, 121, 147
suprasternal, 808
thenar, 562
triangular, 528
Speech area, 722
Spermatic cord, 102, 106, 107, 109, 113, 216, 222, 268
coverings, 103, 112, 113
dissection, 116
internal spermatic fascia covering, 108
Sphenoid bone, 609, 611, 613, 614, 617, 619, 624, 650, 664, 691, 695, 701, 702, 721
body, 618, 701
greater wing, 613, 618, 624, 650, 701, 702, 721
lesser wing, 618, 620, 624, 650, 701, 702
spine, 615, 624
Sphincter
anal
external, 209–213, 216, 256t, 257, 261–263, 273
internal, 209–211, 216, 262, 263
pyloric, 129
urethral
external, 202, 209, 210, 216, 220, 254, 256t, 257, 260

internal, 209, 210, 216, 260, 282
urethrovaginal, 254, 256t, 257, 260, 273
Spinal cord, 83, 123, 187, 286, 300, 334–342, 350, 352, 639, 721, 742, 806–808, 810
blood supply, 341–342
cervical, 334, 338, 340
developmental changes, 344
lumbar, 334, 340
magnetic resonance imaging, 88–89
rootlets, 334, 335, 337, 339, 340
sacral, 340
termination, 337
thoracic, 340
Spine
ethmoidal, 619, 624
iliac
anterior inferior, 196–198, 200, 312, 380, 396, 397
anterior superior, 96, 98, 100–103, 106, 109, 110, 128, 194–198, 200, 311, 312, 354, 372, 373, 380, 382, 396, 397, 496, 497
posterior inferior, 197, 311, 312, 320, 381, 390, 391, 397
posterior superior, 194, 195, 197, 201, 312, 381, 390, 397, 512
ischial, 196, 197, 199, 202, 311, 312, 315, 381, 390, 397
nasal
anterior, 610, 612, 690
posterior, 615
scapular, 11, 518, 519, 527, 529, 532, 536
Spiral organ (of Corti), 715, 833
Spleen, 96, 97, 119, 124, 127, 128, 130, 133, 135, 160, 162–164, 187–189, 352
blood supply, 135
lymphatic drainage, 184
surface anatomy, 131
Spondylolisthesis, 319
Spondylolysis, 319
Spur, bony, 318
Stapes, 704, 706, 707, 710
Sternum, 12, 23, 29, 72, 174
3-D volume reconstruction and CT angiogram, 92–93
anatomy, 10
anomalies, 16
body, 10, 12, 21, 48, 300, 497–499
magnetic resonance imaging, 88–89
manubrium, 24, 498, 810
ossification, 16
Stomach, 82, 96, 119, 121, 123–128, 132, 135, 148, 154, 157, 160–162, 164, 187–189, 352
air-fluid level, 186
anterior view, 129–130
body, 129
greater curvature, 124, 125, 129, 132
lesser curvature, 124, 129
lymphatic drainage, 184
muscular layers, 129
pylorus of, 96, 125, 128, 129, 132, 134, 156, 189
radiograph, 132
Stria medullaris thalami, 728

Subcallosal region, 728, 729
Subcutaneous triangular area, 449
Subdeltoid region, 528
Suboccipital region, 330–333
Substantia nigra, 738–741
Sulcus
calcarine, 723, 728, 729, 742
callosal, 728
carotid, 624
central, 722, 725
cingulate, 728, 742
collateral, 728
coronary, 46
frontal, superior, 742
hippocampal, 728, 729
hypothalamic, 728
interatrial, 50
intraparietal, 725
lateral, 722, 725
marginal, 728
parieto-occipital, 723, 725, 728
postcentral, 725
precentral, 725
prechiasmatic, 624
temporal, superior, 742
terminal, 49, 676, 790
Sulcus limitans, 735
Suprascapular region, 529
Sustentaculum tali, 433, 438, 444, 445, 447, 448, 450, 452, 453, 456, 458, 464, 465
Sutural bone, 613, 614
Suture
coronal, 609, 613, 614
frontal, 608–610
frontonasal, 690
infraorbital, 650
intermaxillary, 608, 610
internasal, 608, 610
lambdoid, 609, 613, 614
median palatine, 682
occipitomastoid, 614
palatine, 617
parietomastoid, 614
sagittal, 609, 614, 615
Swallowing, 808
Symphysis
mandibular, 608–610
pubic, 98, 106, 120, 194, 196–200, 202, 208, 210, 217, 222, 232, 250, 263, 267, 272, 273, 275, 278, 279, 311, 354, 380
Synchondrosis, sternocostal, 10
Syndesmosis, tibiofibular, 442
Synostosis, 318
Systole, 62

T tube, 158
Taenia coli, 136, 137, 139, 140, 144
Talus, 427, 430, 431, 442, 450, 453–457, 459, 461, 466, 472
head, 444, 448, 452, 454, 455, 459
medial tubercle, 433, 438, 452
neck, 448, 452, 455, 459
Tapetum, 729
Tarsal bones, 459
Tarsal tunnel, 453
Teeth
canine, 685, 688, 689t
incisor, 685, 687, 688, 689t
innervation, 687
magnetic resonance imaging, 806
mandibular, 686, 688

Teeth—*continued*
  maxillary, 686, 688
  molar, 685, 687, 688, 689t, 719
  permanent, 685–686
  primary, 688, 689t
  secondary, 689t
Tegmen tympani, 712, 713
Telencephalon, 722, 723, 725–733
Temporal bone, 133, 608, 609, 611, 613, 614, 617, 619, 625, 702
  mastoid part, 613
  petrous part, 618, 620, 621, 625, 714
  squamous part, 613, 618, 625, 664, 721
  tympanic part, 613, 625, 664
  zygomatic process, 613, 664
Tendinous cords, 57–59, 63
Tendon
  abductor pollicis longus, 558, 559, 591
  Achilles, 453
  biceps brachii, 522, 523, 539, 540, 546, 549, 557
  biceps femoris, 409, 428
  calcaneal, 428, 430, 433–439, 450–452, 454, 458, 472
  central, 24, 29, 73, 174
  common extensor, 518, 542, 549, 552, 574
  common flexor, 518, 549, 552
  conjoint, 103, 107–109, 111, 112
  digastric, 787
  extensor digitorum longus, 422
  extensor hallucis longus, 422
  fibularis brevis, 431
  fibularis longus, 431
  flexor carpi radialis, 558, 592
  flexor carpi ulnaris, 558
  flexor digitorum longus, 445
  flexor digitorum profundus, 557, 569
  flexor digitorum superficialis, 559, 569
  flexor hallucis brevis, 447
  flexor hallucis longus, 445, 446, 451
  flexor pollicis longus, 559, 570
  long head of biceps brachii, 531, 532, 534, 535, 537
  obturator internus, 389, 395
  palmaris longus, 558, 559, 561, 563, 566
  pectoralis minor, 522
  peroneus longus, 464
  popliteus, 409
  quadriceps, 376, 420, 421
  rotator cuff, 534
  sartorius, 406
  subscapularis, 532–534
  supraspinatus, 517, 531, 532, 534
  synovial covering, 569
  tensor tympani, 708
  terminal, 583
  tibialis anterior, 422, 424
  tibialis posterior, 429
  triceps, 524, 526–528, 542
Tenia coli, 122
Tentorium cerebelli, 638, 639, 740, 743
Terminale, filum, 334, 336, 337
Terminalis
  crista, 56
  lamina, 728

stria, 729, 731, 741
sulcus, 49, 676, 790
Testis, 116, 209, 210, 216, 217, 264
  blood supply, 117
  coverings, 112, 113
  fetal, 114
  lymphatic drainage, 117
  rete, 117
Thalamus, 728, 730–733, 735, 740–742
Thigh, 354
  anteromedial aspect, 382
  arteries, 393t
  bones, 380, 381
  lateral aspect, 383
  magnetic resonance imaging, 470–471
  muscles
    anterior, 375, 376, 377t
    medial, 375, 376, 378t, 379
    posterior, 384, 385, 387t, 388, 389
  posterior aspect, 384, 385, 387t, 388, 389
  surface anatomy, 374
  transverse sections, 470–471
Thoracic cage, 128
Thoracic wall
  anterior, internal aspect, 23
  external aspect, 22
  muscles, 21, 21t
Thorax
  3-D volume reconstruction and CT angiogram, 92–93
  autonomic innervation, 84–85
  bony, 10–11
  contents, 25
  lymphatic drainage, 86–87
  magnetic resonance imaging, 88–91
  viscera, 96, 97
3-D volume reconstruction
  heart, 46, 47
  thorax, 41, 92–93
Thumb, movements, 596, 597
Thymus, 88–89, 749, 759, 808
Thyroid disease, 773
Tibia, 354, 355, 380, 381, 410, 419, 420, 422, 423, 425, 429, 433, 442, 448, 450, 453–455, 472–473
Tibiofibular syndesmosis, 442
Tissue
  areolar, 108
    loose, 634, 636
  glandular, 5
  subcutaneous, 3–5, 370, 494, 743
    cervical, 747
    fatty layer, 102, 105, 106, 110, 258, 259
    membranous layer, 102, 105, 106, 110, 111, 258, 259, 261
Tongue, 28, 128, 676–677, 677t, 678–680, 719, 721, 738, 739, 743, 782, 790, 808, 810, 829
Tonsil
  cerebellar, 736, 740, 808, 810
  cerebral, 742
  lingual, 676
  palatine, 712, 716, 792, 793
  pharyngeal, 716, 720, 743, 794, 808, 810
Trabecula, septomarginal, 57, 64

Trabeculae, 398
Trabeculae carneae, 57–59
Trachea, 25, 28, 29, 38–40, 43, 48, 66–69, 71, 72, 74, 75, 82, 84, 128, 300, 716, 750, 770, 773, 808, 810
  arterial supply, 75
  autonomic innervation, 84
  bifurcation, 69
  general anatomy, 39–40
  lymphatic drainage, 805
  magnetic resonance imaging, 88–90
  relationship to great vessels, 66
Tracheobronchial tree, 39–40
Tracheostomy, 749
Tract
  corticospinal, 740
  iliotibial, 368, 369, 372, 373, 380, 383–385, 399, 406, 409, 419, 422, 425, 428, 470
  olfactory, 639, 726, 728, 818
  optic, 639, 721, 727, 732–734, 740, 741, 819, 820
  upper respiratory, 694
  urinary, autonomic stimulation effects, 230t
Tragus, 703
Trapezium, 552, 570, 571, 574, 586, 589, 591, 593, 594, 599, 604, 605
  tubercle, 588, 591, 593
Trapezoid, 552, 574, 586, 588, 589, 593, 594, 599, 604, 605
Triangle
  anal, 255, 273
  of auscultation, 512, 514
  carotid, 752, 752t, 762, 763, 766
  clavipectoral, 3, 490, 491, 494, 495
  cystohepatic, 154
  femoral, 372, 373
  lumbar, 514
  muscular, 752, 752t
  occipital, 752, 752t
  omoclavicular, 752, 752t, 757
  submandibular, 752, 752t
  submental, 752, 752t, 760
  suboccipital, 784
  urogenital, 255, 273
  vertebrocostal, 174
Triangular interval, 510, 528
Trigone
  bladder, 217, 221, 234
  collateral, 727
  habenular, 730, 735
  hypoglossal, 735
  vagal, 735
Triquetrum, 552, 574, 587–589, 591–594, 599
Trochanter
  greater, 311, 354, 380, 381, 390, 391, 394, 395, 398, 399
  lesser, 311, 354, 380, 381, 390, 391, 394, 398
Trochlea, 41, 518, 544, 546, 549, 552, 598, 651
  fibular, 431
Trunk
  anterolateral aspect, 497
  brachiocephalic, 29, 46–49, 68, 70, 74, 80, 82, 90, 486, 772, 773, 808
  celiac, 75, 85, 120, 123, 127, 130, 131, 133–135, 154, 163, 174, 175, 184, 185, 190

cervicodorsal, 486, 529, 772
costocervical, 74, 75, 764, 765, 765t
lumbosacral, 172, 173, 202, 206, 207, 212, 230, 231
lymphatic
  bronchomediastinal, 9, 43, 76, 716
  intestinal, 182, 184
  jugular, 9, 76, 716, 805
  lumbar, 182, 184
  subclavian, 9, 76, 716
  pulmonary, 26, 41, 42, 46, 49–52, 57–59, 61, 65, 68, 84
  3-D volume reconstruction and CT angiogram, 92–93
  magnetic resonance imaging, 88–89
subclavian, 43
superficial dissection, 496
sympathetic, 17, 20, 72, 73, 80–85, 163, 172, 183, 212, 230, 231, 249, 334, 339, 720, 772, 773, 776, 786, 805, 807
  left, 123
  lumbar, 214, 246
  thyrocervical, 70, 74, 486, 504, 505t, 529, 764, 765, 765t, 773
  vagal, 181, 836
    anterior, 85
    posterior, 85, 163
Tube, left uterine, 122
Tubercle, 301
  adductor, 373, 380, 381, 385, 433
  anterior, 296, 297, 350, 444, 465, 730, 742, 807
  articular, 617, 625, 675
  of auricle, 703
  carotid, 750, 773, 775
  corniculate, 804
  cuneate, 734, 735
  cuneiform, 466, 804
  dorsal, 574, 581, 586
  gracile, 734, 735
  greater, 503, 517–519, 522, 532, 536, 537
  infraglenoid, 536
  jugular, 335, 615, 619
  lateral, 431, 455, 457
  lesser, 518, 537
  medial, 433, 438, 452, 455, 457
  mental, 610, 613, 664
  pharyngeal, 617, 721
  posterior, 296, 297, 330, 331, 350, 807, 810
  postglenoid, 675
  pubic, 106, 108–111, 194–200, 311, 372, 373, 380, 397
  of rib, 13, 14
  of scaphoid, 559, 588, 591
  of trapezium, 588, 593
Tuberculum cinereum, 732, 733
Tuberculum sellae, 619, 624
Tuberosity
  biceps brachii, 544
  calcaneal, 427, 443–445, 447, 457, 464
  cuboid, 444
  deltoid, 518, 519
  gluteal, 381
  iliac, 197, 312

ischial, 194, 195, 197, 201, 202, 250, 261–263, 268, 272, 273, 311, 312, 354, 368, 380, 381, 390, 391, 396, 397
  maxillary, 702
  navicular, 439, 452
  pronator, 552, 574
  radial, 544, 546, 547, 552
  sacral, 312, 313, 316
  subtendinous bursa, 544
  tibial, 406, 420–422, 425
  ulnar, 518, 544, 552
Tubule
  convoluted
    distal, 167
    proximal, 167
  seminiferous, 117
Tunica albuginea, 117
Tunica vaginalis, 112, 113, 116, 117

Ulna, 478, 479, 518, 519, 523, 544–548, 552, 557, 574, 590, 591, 593, 594, 598, 602
  distal, 598
  head, 552, 574, 580, 589, 590
  proximal, 598
  styloid process, 552, 574, 587, 589–592
  subcutaneous part, 587
Ultrasound
  abdomen, 190–191
  glenohumeral (shoulder) joint, 537
  hepatic veins, 149
  internal carotid artery, 809
  pelvis
    female, 282–283
    male, 223
Umbilical cord, 239
Umbilicus, 98, 100, 106, 118, 161, 219, 238, 496, 497
Uncus, 728, 729, 738, 739
Upper limb
  arteries and arterial anastomoses, 486, 487
  bones, 476–479, 598–599
  cutaneous nerves, 484, 485t
  deep fascia, 492, 493
  dermatomes, 483
  epiphyseal sites, 598–599
  joints, 476, 477
  lymphatic drainage, 489
  motor innervation, 480, 481
  myotatic (deep tendon) reflexes, 482
  myotomes, 482
  proximal
    arteries, 504, 505t
    bones, 518–519
  regions, 476, 477
  veins
    deep, 488
    superficial, 489–491
Ureter, 97, 118, 145, 152, 153, 162–166, 202, 212, 215–220, 226, 233, 240
  anomalies, 168
  bifid, 168
  intramural part, 217
  left, 133, 165
  magnetic resonance imaging, 186–187
  pelvic part, 217
  relationship to uterine artery, 240

retrocaval, 168
right, 122, 133, 143
Urethra, 120, 165, 208, 217, 219, 222, 232, 250, 254, 255, 268, 275–278, 280–282
  compressor, 202
  intermediate, 209, 216, 217, 220, 268
  intramural, 217
  muscles compressing, 260
  prostatic, 209, 216, 217, 221, 263, 268
  spongy, 209, 216, 217, 267, 268
Urinary bladder, 96, 97, 118, 120–122, 128, 136, 165, 205, 208–210, 215, 276–283, 311, 470
  female, 232, 233, 250
  male, 216–222
  trigone, 217, 221, 234
Urogenital system, male, 266
Uterine tube, 208, 232–234, 284
Uterus, 120, 122, 208, 232, 280–283
  adnexa, 237
  bicornate, 284
  blood supply, 235
  body, 279
  cervix, 237, 279
  fundus, 234, 237, 279, 282
  pregnant, 238, 239
  radiograph, 284
Utricle, 714, 715
  prostatic, 220, 221
Uvula, 221, 790

Vagina, 120, 205, 208, 232, 250, 254, 275, 279–282
  muscles compressing, 260
  posterior fornix, 208, 232
  vestibule, 269, 273, 280, 281
  wall, 272, 273
Valve
  aortic, 29, 55, 59, 60, 63, 88–89
  atrioventricular, 63
  during cardiac cycle, 62
  coronary sinus, 56
  heart
    auscultation, 44
    surface markings, 44
  mitral, 58, 59, 61, 63
    3-D volume reconstruction and CT angiogram, 92–93
  pulmonary, 57, 60, 61
  semilunar, 63
  tricuspid, 57, 61, 63
Vasa recta, 140, 141
Vasa recta duodeni, 135
Vein
  acetabular, 401
  anal, inferior, 269
  angular, 633, 633t, 656
  appendicular, 160
  auricular, posterior, 331, 662, 716, 748
  axillary, 22, 488, 489, 501, 503, 508
  azygos, 29, 73, 75, 76, 80, 82, 83, 119, 123, 161, 175, 186, 227, 339
    3-D volume reconstruction and CT angiogram, 92–93
    arch, 47, 49, 68, 69, 74, 80
    magnetic resonance imaging, 88–90
    overview, 78–79

basilic, 488–491, 501, 502, 509, 521, 525, 538, 539, 587, 600, 602
basivertebral, 309, 342
brachial, 488, 489, 501, 502, 539
  deep, 488, 521, 600
brachiocephalic, 23, 748
  left, 29, 46, 48, 66, 67, 76, 78, 80, 81, 91, 488, 716, 749, 773, 808
  right, 46, 48, 49, 66, 67, 72, 76, 78, 80, 88–90, 488, 773
cardiac, 53
  anterior, 46, 49, 53
  great, 46, 47, 49, 50, 53, 58
  middle, 47, 50, 53
  small, 46, 47, 50, 53
  smallest, 53
central, 151
cephalic, 3, 4, 488–491, 494, 500–502, 508, 521, 538, 584, 600, 602
cerebral
  anterior, 649
  deep middle, 649
  great, 638, 639, 649, 724, 732, 733, 740, 743
  internal, 727, 741
  superior, 638, 743
cervical
  deep, 330, 331, 784
  transverse, 763
ciliary
  anterior, 661
  long posterior, 661
  short posterior, 661
circumflex femoral
  lateral, 363
  medial, 363, 373
circumflex fibular, 363
circumflex humeral
  anterior, 488
  posterior, 488
circumflex iliac
  deep, 108, 109, 111, 118, 224, 242, 363
  superficial, 364, 370
circumflex scapular, 488
colic, 161
  left, 160
  middle, 122, 126, 127, 160
  right, 127, 134, 160, 188
collateral, of elbow, 488
communicating
  anterior, 649
  posterior, 649
cremasteric, 108
cubital, median, 489–491, 538
cystic, 154, 160
  anterior, 154
  posterior, 154
digital
  dorsal, 364, 490, 582
  palmar, 488, 490
  plantar, 363
diploic, 634
dorsal
  of penis, 116, 216, 224, 254, 264, 267, 268
  superficial, 272, 490, 491
emissary, 712
  condylar, 785
  mastoid, 785
epigastric, 161, 227

inferior, 108, 109, 111, 118, 218, 219, 224, 242, 363
  superficial, 102, 364, 370
esophageal, 161, 227
facial, 627, 633, 633t, 639, 656, 662, 666, 716, 721, 748, 762, 807
  common, 748, 762
  deep, 633, 633t
femoral, 109, 118, 222, 250, 275, 363, 364, 370–373, 382, 399, 470
fibular, 363, 365
gastric
  left, 126, 127, 129, 134, 154, 155, 160, 161, 227
  right, 127, 129, 154, 155, 160
  short, 129, 131, 160
gastro-omental
  left, 126, 127, 129, 160
  right, 126, 127, 129, 130, 160
genicular
  descending, 363
  lateral inferior, 363
  lateral superior, 363
  medial inferior, 363, 435
  medial superior, 363
gluteal
  inferior, 224, 242, 363
  superior, 224, 242, 351, 363
gonadal, 175
hemiazygos, 78, 79, 81, 83, 175, 186, 339, 352
  accessory, 78, 79, 81
  magnetic resonance imaging, 88–89
hepatic, 146, 149, 150, 163, 175
  intermediate, 186
  left, 186
  middle, 188, 189
  right, 187
ileal, 160
ileocolic, 127, 134, 160
iliac
  common, 79, 145, 163, 175, 216, 224, 242, 363
  external, 109, 111, 163, 175, 202, 213, 215, 216, 218, 224, 225, 225t, 226, 242, 363
  internal, 175, 216, 224, 226, 242, 351, 363
iliolumbar, 79
infraorbital, 656
intercostal
  anterior, 22, 23
  left superior, 67, 76, 78, 79, 81
  posterior, 17, 79–83, 175, 339
  right posterior, 78
  superior, 72
internal, thoracic, 23
interosseous, anterior, 488
intervertebral, 342, 740
jejunal, 160
jugular, 713
  anterior, 716, 748, 763
  external, 488, 501, 662, 716, 748, 754, 806, 807
  internal, 333, 350, 488, 501, 662, 663, 667, 681, 710–713, 716, 720, 721, 738, 739, 748, 762, 763, 767, 771–773, 785, 806, 807
  confluence, 88–89

Vein—*continued*
   inferior bulb, 767
      left, 9, 43, 48, 76, 88–89, 716,
         767
      right, 26, 43, 48, 76
      superior bulb, 767
   lumbar, 79, 175
   marginal, 53
   maxillary, 639, 748
   median, of forearm, 490, 491, 538
   meningeal, middle, 637
   mesenteric
      inferior, 122, 127, 133, 134, 160,
         161, 163, 174, 186, 215,
         227
      superior, 122, 126, 127, 133,
         134, 145, 156, 160–162,
         187–189, 227
   oblique, 47, 50, 53, 79
   obturator, 118, 224, 242, 250, 363,
         399
   occipital, 331, 784
   ophthalmic
      inferior, 639, 656
      superior, 639, 656
   ovarian, 233
   palatine
      ascending, 712
      external, 796
   pancreatic, 160
   pancreaticoduodenal, 160
      posterior superior, 154
   paraumbilical, 118, 161, 227
   perforating, 363, 365, 538, 539,
         584
   phrenic, inferior, 175
   plantar, 365
   popliteal, 363, 365, 402, 419, 420,
         435, 437
   portal, 160, 188, 189, 227
      hepatic, 122–124, 126, 127, 133,
         134, 147, 149–155, 160,
         161, 187
   pudendal
      external, 269, 364, 370
      inferior, 213
      internal, 213, 222, 224, 242,
         250, 274, 363
   pulmonary, 34, 35, 81
      imaging of, 41, 92–93
      inferior, 80
      left, 29, 33, 46, 47, 50, 51, 64,
         65, 88–89
      left inferior, 58, 68, 92–93
      left superior, 41, 58, 60, 68,
         92–93
      right, 29, 33, 46, 47, 50–52, 58,
         60, 65, 88–89
      right inferior, 58, 68, 92–93
      right superior, 41, 58, 68, 92–93
   radial, 488
   rectal
      inferior, 161
      middle, 213, 224, 242
      portal and systemic, 227
      superior, 160, 161, 213

recurrent
   radial, 488
   ulnar, 488
renal, 162, 164, 166
   left, 78, 79, 127, 175, 186, 188,
         189
   right, 153, 175, 187
retinal, central, 660, 661
retromandibular, 350, 633, 633t,
         662, 716, 720, 721, 748,
         762
retroperitoneal, 161, 227
sacral
   lateral, 224, 242
   median, 175
saphenous, 382
   great, 102, 103, 112, 275,
         363–367, 370, 372, 382,
         438, 457, 470, 472
   small, 364, 430, 457, 472
scapular, dorsal, 488, 501
sigmoid, 160
spinal
   anterior, 342
   posterior, 342
splenic, 122, 125, 127, 134, 160,
         161, 164, 187–189, 227
subclavian, 22, 80, 488, 501, 511,
         748, 757, 762, 772, 773
   left, 43, 48, 76, 81, 716, 767,
         773
   right, 26, 43, 48, 76, 716, 767
subcostal, 79
subscapular, 488
supraorbital, 633, 633t, 639, 656
suprarenal, 175
suprascapular, 488, 501, 748
supratrochlear, 633, 633t
temporal, superficial, 633, 633t,
         662, 716, 721, 748
testicular, 113, 127, 145, 152, 153,
         162, 163, 215, 226
thalamostriate, 730
of thigh
   deep, 363, 373
   lateral cutaneous, 364
   medial cutaneous, 364
thoracic
   internal, 22, 66, 72, 80, 81,
         88–89, 773
   lateral, 488
   superior, 488
thoraco-acromial, 488, 500
thoracodorsal, 488
thymic, 66
thyroid
   inferior, 66, 749, 768, 773
   middle, 768, 807
   superior, 762, 768, 807
tibial
   anterior, 363, 437, 472
   posterior, 363, 365, 451, 472
ulnar, 488
uterine, 242
varicose, 365
ventricular, left posterior, 47, 53

vertebral, 772, 773, 807
   anterior, 773
vesical, 224, 242
   inferior, 224
vorticose, 656, 660, 661
Velum, medullary
   inferior, 735
   superior, 742
Vena cava
   inferior, 46, 47, 50, 51, 56, 58, 65,
         73, 76, 78–80, 82, 119,
         122–124, 133, 146–150,
         152–154, 157, 160–163,
         165, 174, 175, 186, 188,
         189, 215, 227, 351, 363
      computed tomography, 6
      magnetic resonance imaging,
         90, 91
      radiograph, 27
      tributaries, 175
      valve of, 56
   superior, 41, 46, 47, 49–52, 56–58,
         60, 64, 65, 67, 72, 76,
         78–80, 488, 716
      3-D volume reconstruction and
         CT angiogram, 92–93
      magnetic resonance imaging,
         88–91
      radiograph, 27
Venae cordis minimae, 53
Ventricle
   of brain, 724
   fourth, 723, 724, 738–740, 742, 743
   of larynx, 801
   lateral, 724, 727, 729–733,
         738–742
   left, 27, 29, 46, 47, 49, 50, 53,
         58–60, 84
      3-D volume reconstruction and
         CT angiogram, 92–93
      computed tomography, 6
      interior, 58, 59
      magnetic resonance imaging,
         90, 91
      wall, 64
   radiograph, 27
   right, 29, 46, 47, 49, 50, 53, 59, 60,
         84
      3-D volume reconstruction and
         CT angiogram, 92–93
      interior, 57
      magnetic resonance imaging,
         90, 91
      wall, 64
   third, 723, 724, 728, 730–733, 735,
         740, 741
Venule, inferior temporal retinal, 661
Vermis
   inferior, 738–740
   superior, 736, 738–740
Vertebrae
   3-D volume reconstruction and
         CT angiogram, 92–93
   anomalies, 318
   cervical, 16, 290, 291. *See also*
         Atlas; Axis

CT scan, 296, 350
   features, 751
   lower, 338
   magnetic resonance imaging, 352
   movements, 292
   overview, 286, 288, 294, 294t
   radiograph, 292, 296, 297, 750
   typical, 294, 294t
homologous parts, 290
levels, 133
lumbar, 145, 171, 290, 291, 351
   CT scan, 351
   magnetic resonance imaging,
         343
   movements, 293
   overview, 286, 288, 302–303,
         302t
   radiograph, 293, 302, 310
lumbosacral, transitional, 318
movements, 291
sacral, 290, 351
spondylolisthesis, 319
spondylolysis, 319
thoracic, 10, 11, 290, 291
   magnetic resonance imaging,
         300, 352
   overview, 286, 288, 300–301,
         300t
   radiograph, 310
   typical, 289
Vertebral column
   curvatures, 287
   imaging of, 350–352
   lumbar region, 308, 337
   overview, 286, 288
Vestibule, 234, 714
   aortic, 59
   bulb of, 272, 274
   nasal, 694
   vaginal, 269, 273, 280, 281
Viscera
   abdominal, 96, 97, 162, 163
   pelvic, 246, 247, 251
   peritoneal, 120, 121, 124, 164
   pleural, 28, 31t
   thoracic, 96, 97
Visual pathway, 820
Vocalis, 802, 802t
Vomer, 610, 611, 613, 615, 617, 690,
         691, 702, 720

White matter, 732, 733, 738–740,
         742
Window
   oval, 714
   round, 710, 714
Wrist, 476, 477
   anterior aspect, 558, 559
   coronal section, 590
   imaging of, 589
   lateral aspect, 584–586
   medial aspect, 587
   surface anatomy, 560

Zygomatic bone, 608, 609, 611, 613,
         617, 650, 651, 664, 699